SO-EHX-204

S A U N D E R S

PHARMACEUTICAL WORD BOOK

2000

ELLEN DRAKE, CMT
RANDY DRAKE, BS

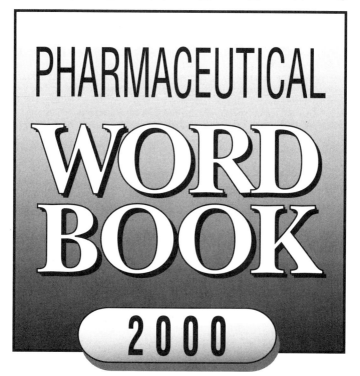

S A U N D E R S

PHARMACEUTICAL
WORD
BOOK

2000

W.B. SAUNDERS COMPANY
A Harcourt Health Sciences Company
Philadelphia London Toronto Montreal Sydney Tokyo

W.B. SAUNDERS COMPANY

A Harcourt Health Sciences Company

The Curtis Center
Independence Square West
Philadelphia, Pennsylvania 19106

www.wbsaunders.com

NOTICE

We have carefully checked the generic and trade names, approved indications and uses, and dosages of pharmaceuticals appearing in this book. Medicine is an ever-changing field, however, and the information listed here may have changed since its publication. While we have made every attempt to include as much necessary information as possible, we have by no means tried to provide *prescribing information* as defined by the FDA. The given uses and actions for a particular drug are not all-inclusive, and the indications, contraindications, and side effects are not listed. Physicians should consult the package insert or some other acceptable source for prescribing information.

Herbal and natural remedies are also listed in this book. The indications and uses listed are the historical or traditional uses of the remedy. In most cases, the efficacy of a remedy for a particular indication has been neither proven nor disproven by modern scientific methods. Some of the plants used in herbal remedies are poisonous and may cause illness or death if not properly prepared and used. Therefore, both the authors and publisher disclaim responsibility for the use or misuse of any information contained herein.

SAUNDERS PHARMACEUTICAL WORD BOOK 2000   ISBN 0–7216–8944–2

ISSN 1072–7779

Printed in the United States of America.

Last digit is the print number: 9   8   7   6   5   4   3   2   1

To the Lord Jesus

How lovely on the mountains
Are the feet of him who brings good news,
Who announces peace
And brings good news of happiness,
Who announces salvation,
And says to Zion, "Your God reigns!"

— Isaiah 52:7

Contents

Preface

We are happy to announce the publication of a brand-new companion to this book, the *Saunders Pharmaceutical Xref Book*. The *Xref Book* is the result of readers' suggestions and requests we've received over the past seven years.

Since our first edition in 1993, we have used feedback from our readers to expand and change our concept of the ultimate pharmaceutical reference book. We added dosage information, herbal and natural medicines, street drug slang, therapeutic serum level information, and a quick reference to the most-prescribed drugs to subsequent editions in direct response to users' requests. But with all these changes, our core concept has not changed: to provide the most complete and up-to-date listing of pharmaceuticals in a format allied health professionals find quick and intuitive. (That includes proper capitalization and sound-alikes, which were unheard-of in 1993!) Our concept was then and is now to provide this information in one main alphabetical listing. We could not see the logic of requiring the reader to search through multiple lists of generic drugs, brand name drugs, chemotherapy protocols, and more, as do some other references. We also thought it unethical to keep long-discontinued drugs listed, just to increase the page count and book price.

Two suggestions we received almost from the beginning, however, were the inclusion of a cross-reference between generic drugs and the brands that contain them, and a listing of drugs by indication (also known as the drug's "designated use," "approved use," or "therapeutic action"). As we pondered these suggestions, we recognized two problems: first and most importantly, these two lists could easily double the size of the book (increasing its price, of course); and second, the idea of separate lists went against our core concept.

Our new companion book solves those problems. It contains both of the cross-references mentioned above, plus a comprehensive listing of over 3000 hazardous materials and their potential adverse effects. The Investigational Codes appendix and Street Drug Slang appendix have been moved from this book to the *Xref Book*, allowing more extensive updating without increasing the page count. We urge you to take a moment to study the contents of our companion book; it will be well worth your time!

We welcome your comments regarding additions, inconsistencies, or inaccuracies in either book. Please send them to us via e-mail at the address below, or via regular mail to W.B. Saunders Company, The Curtis Center, Independence Square West, Philadelphia, PA 19106-3399.

Authors' e-mail address:
PharmaceuticalWordBook@Saunders.net

ELLEN DRAKE, CMT
RANDY DRAKE, BS
Orlando, Florida

Notes on Using the Text

The purpose of the *Saunders Pharmaceutical Word Book* is to provide the medical transcriptionist (as well as medical record administrators and technicians, coders, nurses, ward clerks, court reporters, legal secretaries, medical assistants, allied health students, physicians, and even pharmacists) a quick, easy-to-use reference that gives not only the correct spellings and capitalizations of drugs, but the designated uses of those drugs, the cross-referencing of brand names to generics, and the usual methods of administration (e.g., capsule, IV, cream). The indication of the preferred nonproprietary (generic) names and the agencies adopting these names (e.g., USAN, USP) should be particularly useful to those writing for publication. The reader will also find various trademarked or proprietary names (e.g., Spansule, Dosepak) that are not drugs but are closely associated with the packaging or administration of drugs.

There are four different ways to refer to drugs. One of these ways is not the name of the drug itself but the class to which it belongs—aminoglycosides, for example. Inexperienced transcriptionists sometimes confuse these classes with the names of drugs. We have included some 200 drug classes in the main list, with a brief description of the therapeutic use and/or method of action common to drugs in the class. Beyond a class description, each drug has three names. The first is the *chemical name*, which describes its chemical composition and how the molecules are arranged. It is often long and complex, sometimes containing numbers, Greek letters, italicized letters, and hyphens between elements. This name is rarely used in dictation except in research hospitals and sometimes in the laboratory section when the blood or urine is examined for traces of the drug. The second name for a drug is the *nonproprietary* or *generic name*. This is a name chosen by the discovering manufacturer or agency and submitted to a nomenclature committee (the United States Adopted Names Council, for example). The name is simpler than the chemical name but often reflects the chemical entity. It is arrived at by using guidelines provided by the nomenclature committee—beta-blockers must end in "olol," for example—and must be unique. There is increasing emphasis on the adoption of the same nonproprietary name by various nomenclature committees worldwide (see the list on page xiii). The third name for a drug is the *trade* or *brand name*. There may be several trade names for the same generic drug, each marketed by a different company. These are the ones that are highly advertised, and sometimes have unusual capitalization. An interesting article on the naming of drugs is "Pharmaceutical Nomenclature: The Lawless Language" in *Perspectives on the Medical Transcription Profession*.[1] *Understanding Pharmacology*[2] also discusses the naming of drugs.

We have included many foreign names of drugs for our Canadian friends, and also because we have so many visitors to the United States from other countries (and they get sick, too). The international and British spellings of generic drugs are cross-referenced to the American spellings, and vice versa. Occasionally there will be three different spellings—one American, one international, and another British—which are all cross-referenced to each other. Other special features that may be useful, especially for students, are the commonly used prescribing abbreviations and the sound-alike lists that are found in the appendices. Another appendix gives the investigational codes (assigned to drugs before they are named), cross-referenced to their subsequent generic names. The Most Prescribed Drugs and Therapeutic Drug Levels appendices will be useful as well.

This information was compiled using a variety of sources including direct communication with over 500 drug companies. The orphan entries are taken directly from the latest list issued by the FDA. When sources differed, we ranked our sources as to reliability and went with what we thought was the most reliable source. We recognize that there may be several published ways in which to type a single drug, but we have chosen to use only one of those ways. In the instance of internal capitalization (e.g., pHisoHex), it should be recognized that in most instances it is acceptable to type such words with initial capitalization only (Phisohex).

How the Book Is Arranged

While other pharmaceutical references have separate listings for brand names and generics, or put entries into separate sections by body system or therapeutic use, we have chosen to list all entries in one comprehensive alphabetical listing. Therefore, it is not necessary to know if the term sought is a brand name, a generic, a drug class, a chemotherapy protocol, approved or investigational, or slang; what it's used for; or which body system it affects. If it's given to a patient, it's in "the list." In addition to strict pharmaceuticals, we have included other "consumable" products, such as *in vitro* testing kits, radiographic contrast and other imaging agents, wound dressings, etc.

All entries are in alphabetical order by word. Initial numbers, chemical prefixes (*N*-, *p*-, L-, D-, etc.), and punctuation (prime, ampersands, etc.) are ignored. For example, L-dopa would be alphabetized under "dopa," but levodopa under "levo."

We have indicated brand names with initial capital letters unless an unusual combination of capitals and lowercase has been designated by the manufacturer (e.g., pHisoHex, ALternaGEL). Generic names are rendered in lowercase. Where the same name can be either generic or brand, both have been included.

The general format of a *generic* entry is:

entry council(s) *designated use* [other references] dosages 🔊 sound-alike(s)

| #1 | | #2 | | #3 | | #4 | | #5 | | #6 |

1. The name of the drug (in bold).
2. The various agencies that have approved the name, shown in small caps, which may be any or all of the following (listed according to appearance in the book):

   USAN   United States Adopted Name Council
   USP   United States Pharmacopeial Convention
   NF   National Formulary
   FDA   U.S. Food and Drug Administration
   INN   International Nonproprietary Name (a project of the World Health Organization)
   BAN   British Approved Name
   JAN   Japanese Accepted Name
   DCF   Dénomination Commune Française (French)

3. The indications, sometimes referred to as the drug's "designated use," "approved use," or "therapeutic action." This is provided only for official FDA-approved names or other names for the same substance (e.g., the British name of an official U.S. generic). This entry is always in italic.
4. The entry in brackets is one of four cross-references:

   see: refers the reader to the "official" name(s).
   now: for an older generic name no longer used, refers reader to the current official name(s).
   also: a substance that has two or more different names, each officially recognized by one of the above groups, will cross-reference the other name(s).
   q.v.   Latin for quod vide; which see. Used exclusively for abbreviations, it invites the reader to turn to the reference in parentheses.

   If there is more than one cross reference, alternate names will follow the order of the above agency list; i.e., U.S. names, then international names, then British, Japanese, and French names. The first cross-reference will always be to the approved U.S. name, unless the entry itself is the U.S. name.

5. Dosage information, including the delivery form(s), is given for medications that may be dispensed generically. No dosage information appears for drugs dispensed only under the brand name, or for those containing multiple ingredients. Some drugs may be available in more than one strength, indicated by a comma in the dosage field:

   erythromycin stearate USP, BAN *macrolide antibiotic* 250, 500 mg oral

   A semicolon in the dosage field separates different delivery forms, such as:

   nitroglycerin USP *coronary vasodilator; antianginal; antihypertensive* [also: glyceryl trinitrate] 2.5, 6.5, 9 mg oral; 5 mg/mL injection; 16–187.5 mg transdermal; 2% topical

   (Note that the oral and transdermal forms come in multiple strengths.)

6. Sound-alike drugs follow the "ear" icon.

The general format for a *brand name* entry is:

Entry ⒸⒶⓃ form(s) ℞/OTC *designated use* [generics] dosages ⑨ sound-alike(s)

#1	#2	#3	#4	#5	#6	#7	#8

1. The drug name (in bold), which almost always starts with a capital letter.
2. If a brand is not marketed in the U.S., an icon designates the country where it is available. Canadian brands are designated by ⒸⒶⓃ.
3. The form of administration; e.g., tablets, capsules, syrup. (Sometimes these words are slurred by the dictator, causing confusion regarding the name.)
4. The ℞ or OTC status. A few drugs may be either ℞ or OTC depending on strength or various state laws.[3]
5. The designated use in italics as for generics. These are more complete or less complete as supplied by the individual drug companies.
6. The brackets that follow contain the generic names of the active ingredients to which the reader may refer for further information.
7. Dosage information follows the generics. For multi-ingredient drugs, a bullet separates the dosages of each ingredient, listed in the same order as the generics. For example,

   > **Ser-Ap-Es** tablets ℞ *antihypertensive; vasodilator; diuretic* [hydrochlorothiazide; reserpine; hydralazine HCl] 15•0.1•25 mg

   shows a three-ingredient product containing 15 mg hydrochlorothiazide, 0.1 mg reserpine, and 25 mg hydralazine HCl.

   Some drugs may have more than one strength, indicated by a comma in the dosage field:

   > **Norpace** capsules ℞ *antiarrhythmic* [disopyramide phosphate] 100, 150 mg

   A semicolon in the dosage field separates either different products listed together, such as:

   > **Pred Mild; Pred Forte** eye drop suspension ℞ *topical ophthalmic corticosteroidal anti-inflammatory* [prednisolone acetate] 0.12%; 1%

   Or different delivery forms:

   > **Phenergan** tablets, suppositories, injection ℞ *antihistamine; sedative; antiemetic; motion sickness relief* [promethazine HCl] 12.5, 25, 50 mg; 12.5, 25, 50 mg; 25, 50 mg/mL

   (Note that all three forms of Phenergan come in multiple strengths.)

   Liquid delivery forms show the strength per usual dose where appropriate. Thus injectables and drops are usually shown per milliliter (mL), with oral liquids and syrups shown per 5 mL or 15 mL.

   The ⚌ symbol indicates that dosage information has not been supplied by the manufacturer for one or more ingredients.

   The ± symbol is used when a value *cannot* be given because the generic entry refers to multiple ingredients.
8. Sound-alike drugs follow the "ear" icon.

Experimental, Investigational, and Orphan Drugs

Before a drug can be advertised or sold in the United States, it must first be approved for marketing by the U.S. Food and Drug Administration. With a few exceptions, FDA approval is contingent solely upon the manufacturer demonstrating that the proposed drug is both safe and effective.

To provide such proof, the manufacturer undertakes a series of tests. Preclinical (before human) research is done through computer simulation, then *in vitro* (L. "in glass," meaning laboratory) tests, then in animals. In most cases neither the public nor the general medical community hears about "experimental drugs" in this stage of testing. Neither are they listed in this reference.

If safety and efficacy are successfully demonstrated during the preclinical stage, an Investigational New Drug (IND) application is filed with the FDA. There are three phases of clinical trials, designated Phase I, Phase II, and Phase III. After each phase, the FDA will review the findings and approve or deny further testing.

Phase I trials involve 20 to 100 patients, primarily to establish safety. Phase II trials may involve several hundred patients for up to two years. The goal in this phase is to determine the drug's effectiveness for the proposed indication. Phase III trials, which routinely last up to four years and involve several thousand patients, determine the optimum effective, but safe, dosage. The manufacturer will then file a New Drug Application (NDA) with the FDA, requesting final marketing approval. Only 20% of drugs entering Phase I trials will ultimately be approved for marketing, at an average cost of $359 million and 8½ years in testing.[4]

An orphan drug is a drug or biological product for the diagnosis, treatment, or prevention of a rare disease or condition. A rare disease is one that affects less than 200,000 persons or for which there is no reasonable expectation that the cost of development and testing will be recovered through U.S. sales of the product. Federal subsidies are provided to the manufacturer or sponsor for the development of orphan drugs. Applications for orphan status are made through the FDA, and may be made during drug development or after marketing approval.

A Brief Note on the Transcription of Drugs

Many references are available describing several acceptable ways to transcribe drug information when dictated. We offer the following only as brief guidelines.

Although some institutions favor capitalizing every drug, others promote not capitalizing any drug, and yet others put drugs in all capital letters, the generally accepted style today for the transcription of medical reports for hospital and doctors' office charts (see the American Medical Association *Manual of Style*[5] for publications) is to capitalize the initial letter of brand name drugs and lowercase generic name drugs. The institution may also designate that brand name drugs with unusual capitalization may be typed with initial capital letter only, or typed using the manufacturer's scheme.

In general, commas are omitted between the drug name, the dosage, and the instructions for purposes of simplification. Items in a series may be separated by either commas (if no internal commas are used) or semicolons. A simple series might be typed thus:

> Procardia, nitroglycerin sublingual, and Tolinase

or

> Procardia 10 mg three times a day, nitroglycerin 1/150 p.r.n., and Tolinase 100 mg twice a day.

or

> Procardia 10 mg t.i.d., nitroglycerin 1/150 p.r.n., and Tolinase 100 mg b.i.d.

A more complex or lengthy list of medications, or a list with internal commas, may require the use of semicolons to separate the items in a series. For example,

> Procardia 10 mg, one t.i.d.; nitroglycerin 1/150 p.r.n., to take one with onset of pain, a second in five minutes, and a third five minutes later, if no relief to go immediately to the ER; Tolinase 100 mg, one b.i.d.; and Coumadin 2.5 mg on Mondays, Wednesdays, and Fridays, and 5 mg on Tuesdays, Thursdays, and Saturdays...

Note that the "one" following Procardia 10 mg and Tolinase 100 mg is not necessary, but many doctors dictate something like this; when they do, it is acceptable to place a comma after the dosage. In addition, when two numbers are adjacent to each other, write out one number and use a numeral for the other.

The typing of chemicals with superscripts or subscripts, italics, small capitals, and Greek letters often presents a problem to the medical transcriptionist. In general, Greek letters are written out (alpha-, beta-, gamma-, etc.). Italics and small capitals are written as standard letters followed by a hyphen (dl-alpha-tocopherol, L-dopa).

When typing nonproprietary (generic) isotope names, element symbols should be included with the name. It may appear to be redundant, but it is the correct form. Therefore, we would type sodium pertechnetate Tc 99m, iodohippurate sodium I 131, or sodium iodide I 125. Occasionally the physician may simply dictate isotopes such as Tc 99m, iodine 131 or I 131, or sodium iodide I 125, and unless he is indicating a trademarked name, it should be typed with a space, no hyphen, and no superscript. This reference indicates proper capitalization, spacing, and hyphenation of isotope entries.

Other combinations of letters and numbers are usually written without spaces or hyphens (OKT1, OKT3, T101, SC1), but this is a complex subject and is dealt with extensively in the AMA *Manual of Style*.

---

[1] Dirckx, John, M.D.: "Pharmaceutical Nomenclature: The Lawless Language," *Perspectives on the Medical Transcription Profession*, Vol. 1, No. 4. Modesto: Health Professions Institute, 1991, p. 9.

[2] Turley, Susan M., CMT: *Understanding Pharmacology*. Englewood Cliffs: Regents/Prentice Hall, 1991.

[3] Some states are moving toward the creation of a third class of drugs between ℞ and oTc. These medications, while not being readily available on the shelf, could be dispensed by a licensed pharmacist without a doctor's prescription.

[4] *FDA Consumer*, January, 1995. www.fda.gov/fdac/special/newdrug/ndd_toc.html

[5] American Medical Association: *Manual of Style*, 9th ed. Baltimore: Williams & Wilkins, 1997.

A (vitamin A) [q.v.]

A and D ointment OTC *moisturizer; emollient* [fish liver oil (vitamins A and D); cholecalciferol; lanolin] ≥

A and D Medicated ointment OTC *topical diaper rash treatment* [zinc oxide; vitamins A and D] ≥

A + D (ara-C, daunorubicin) *chemotherapy protocol*

A-200 shampoo concentrate (discontinued 1995) OTC *pediculicide for lice* [pyrethrins; piperonyl butoxide] 0.33%•4%

AA (ara-C, Adriamycin) *chemotherapy protocol*

AA-HC Otic ear drops ℞ *topical corticosteroidal anti-inflammatory; antibacterial; antifungal* [hydrocortisone; acetic acid] 1%•2%

abacavir succinate USAN *antiviral nucleoside reverse transcriptase inhibitor for HIV*

abacavir sulfate USAN *antiviral nucleoside reverse transcriptase inhibitor for HIV*

abafilcon A USAN *hydrophilic contact lens material*

abamectin USAN, INN *antiparasitic*

abanoquil INN, BAN

abarelix USAN *investigational (Phase III) LHRH antagonist for medical castration (androgen ablation), prostate cancer, uterine fibroids, endometriosis, and precocious puberty*

Abbokinase powder for IV or intracoronary artery infusion ℞ *thrombolytic enzymes for pulmonary embolism or coronary artery thrombosis* [urokinase] 250 000 IU/vial

Abbokinase Open-Cath powder for catheter clearance ℞ *thrombolytic enzymes* [urokinase] 5000 IU/mL

Abbo-Pac (trademarked packaging form) *unit dose package*

Abbott HIVAB HIV-1 EIA test kit (name changed to HIVAB HIV-1 EIA in 1995)

Abbott HIVAG-1 test kit (name changed to HIVAG-1 in 1995)

Abbott HTLV I EIA test kit (name changed to Human T-Lymphotropic Virus Type I EIA in 1995)

Abbott HTLV III Confirmatory EIA test kit for professional use (discontinued 1995) *in vitro diagnostic aid for HTLV III antibody* [enzyme immunoassay (EIA)]

Abbott TestPack Plus hCG-Urine Plus test kit for professional use *in vitro diagnostic aid for urine pregnancy test* [monoclonal antibody-based enzyme immunoassay]

Abbott TestPack Strep A kit (name changed to Test Pack in 1995)

ABC (Adriamycin, BCNU, cyclophosphamide) *chemotherapy protocol*

ABC to Z tablets OTC *vitamin/mineral/iron supplement* [multiple vitamins & minerals; ferrous fumarate; folic acid; biotin] ±•18 mg•0.4 mg•30 μg

abciximab USAN, INN *antithrombotic monoclonal antibody; antiplatelet agent for acute arterial occlusive disorders*

ABCM (Adriamycin, bleomycin, cyclophosphamide, mitomycin) *chemotherapy protocol*

ABD (Adriamycin, bleomycin, DTIC) *chemotherapy protocol*

ABDIC (Adriamycin, bleomycin, DIC, [CCNU, prednisone]) *chemotherapy protocol*

ABDV (Adriamycin, bleomycin, DTIC, vinblastine) *chemotherapy protocol*

ABE (antitoxin botulism equine) [see: botulism equine antitoxin, trivalent]

abecarnil INN *investigational anxiolytic*

Abelcet suspension for IV infusion ℞ *systemic polyene antifungal for aspergillosis and other resistant fungal infections (orphan)* [amphotericin B lipid complex (ABLC)] 100 mg/20 mL

Abelmoschus moschatus *medicinal herb* [see: ambrette]

Abenol Ⓒ (U.S. product: Tylenol) suppositories OTC *analgesic; antipyretic* [acetaminophen] 120, 325, 650 mg

Abitrexate IV or IM injection ℞ *antimetabolite antineoplastic for leukemia; systemic antipsoriatic; antirheumatic* [methotrexate sodium]

ABLC [see: TLC ABLC]

ABLC (amphotericin B lipid complex) [q.v.]

ablukast USAN, INN *antiasthmatic; leukotriene antagonist*

ablukast sodium USAN *antiasthmatic; leukotriene antagonist*

Abolic *a veterinary steroid abused as a street drug*

abortifacients *a class of agents that stimulate uterine contractions sufficient to produce uterine evacuation*

ABP (Adriamycin, bleomycin, prednisone) *chemotherapy protocol*

ABPP (aminobromophenylpyrimidinone) [see: bropirimine]

Abrus precatorius **medicinal herb** [see: precatory bean]

ABS-205 *investigational (Phase I) treatment for age-related cognitive decline and neurodegeneration*

absinthe; absinthites; absinthium *medicinal herb* [see: wormwood]

absorbable cellulose cotton [see: cellulose, oxidized]

absorbable collagen sponge [see: collagen sponge, absorbable]

absorbable dusting powder [see: dusting powder, absorbable]

absorbable gelatin film [see: gelatin film, absorbable]

absorbable gelatin powder [see: gelatin powder, absorbable]

absorbable gelatin sponge [see: gelatin sponge, absorbable]

absorbable surgical suture [see: suture, absorbable surgical]

Absorbase OTC *ointment base* [water-in-oil emulsion of cholesterolized petrolatum and purified water]

absorbent gauze [see: gauze, absorbent]

Absorbine Antifungal cream, powder (discontinued 1998) OTC *topical antifungal* [tolnaftate] 1%

Absorbine Antifungal Foot aerosol powder OTC *topical antifungal* [miconazole nitrate; alcohol 10%] 2%

Absorbine Arthritis Strength Liquid with Capsaicin OTC *topical analgesic; counterirritant* [menthol; capsaicin] 4%•0.025%

Absorbine Athlete's Foot cream OTC *topical antifungal* [tolnaftate] 1%

Absorbine Athlete's Foot Care liquid (name changed to Absorbine Footcare in 1998)

Absorbine Footcare spray liquid OTC *topical antifungal* [tolnaftate] 1%

Absorbine Jock Itch powder (discontinued 1998) OTC *topical antifungal* [tolnaftate] 1%

Absorbine Jr. liniment OTC *topical analgesic; counterirritant* [menthol] 1.27%, 4%

Absorbine Jr. Antifungal spray liquid (discontinued 1998) OTC *topical antifungal* [tolnaftate] 1%

Absorbine Jr. Extra Strength liquid OTC *topical analgesic; counterirritant* [menthol] 4%

Absorbine Power gel (discontinued 1998) OTC *topical analgesic; counterirritant* [menthol] 4%

ABT-719 *investigational quinolizidine antibiotic*

abunidazole INN

ABV (actimomycin D, bleomycin, vincristine) *chemotherapy protocol*

ABV (Adriamycin, bleomycin, vinblastine) *chemotherapy protocol*

ABVD (Adriamycin, bleomycin, vinblastine, dacarbazine) *chemotherapy protocol*

ABVD/MOPP (alternating cycles of ABVD and MOPP) *chemotherapy protocol*

ABX-CBL *investigational (Phase II) monoclonal antibody for graft vs. host disease that reverses unwanted immune response without general immune system suppression*

AC (Adriamycin, carmustine) *chemotherapy protocol*

AC (Adriamycin, CCNU) *chemotherapy protocol*

AC (Adriamycin, cisplatin) *chemotherapy protocol*

AC; A-C (Adriamycin, cyclophosphamide) *chemotherapy protocol*

acacia NF, JAN *suspending agent; emollient; demulcent*

acacia *(Acacia senegal; A. verek)* gum *medicinal herb for colds, cough, periodontal disease, and wound healing*

acadesine USAN, INN, BAN *platelet aggregation inhibitor*

A-Caine Rectal ointment (discontinued 1995) OTC *topical anesthetic; vasoconstrictor; astringent* [diperodon HCl; pyrilamine maleate; phenylephrine HCl; bismuth subcarbonate; zinc oxide] 0.25%•0.1%•0.25%•0.2%•5%

acamprosate 6473 INN

acamylophenine [see: camylofin]

Acanthopanax senticosus medicinal herb [see: Siberian ginseng]

acaprazine INN

acarbose USAN, INN, BAN *α-glucosidase inhibitor for type 2 diabetes mellitus*

ACAT (acylCoA transferase) inhibitor *investigational agent to lower serum cholesterol levels*

Accolate film-coated tablets ℞ *leukotriene receptor antagonist (LTRA) for prevention and chronic treatment of asthma* [zafirlukast] 20 mg

Accu-Chek Advantage reagent strips for home use OTC *in vitro diagnostic aid for blood glucose*

Accu-Pak (trademarked packaging form) *unit dose blister pack*

Accupep HPF powder OTC *enteral nutritional therapy for GI impairment*

Accupril film-coated tablets ℞ *antihypertensive; angiotensin-converting enzyme (ACE) inhibitor* [quinapril HCl] 5, 10, 20, 40 mg

Accurbron syrup ℞ *antiasthmatic; bronchodilator* [theophylline; alcohol 7.5%] 150 mg/15 mL ② Accutane

Accuretic ⒶⓃ film-coated tablets ℞ *antihypertensive; angiotensin-converting enzyme (ACE) inhibitor; diuretic* [quinapril HCl; hydrochlorothiazide] 10•12.5, 20•12.5 mg

Accusens T multi-sample kit (discontinued 1995) *in vitro diagnostic aid for taste dysfunction*

AccuSite injectable gel ℞ *investigational (NDA filed) treatment for genital warts; development discontinued in 1997* [fluorouracil; epinephrine]

Accutane capsules ℞ *internal keratolytic for severe recalcitrant cystic acne* [isotretinoin] 10, 20, 40 mg ② Accurbron

Accuzyme ointment ℞ *topical enzyme for wound debridement; vulnerary* [papain; urea] 11 000 IU/g•10%

ACD solution (acid citrate dextrose; anticoagulant citrate dextrose) [see: anticoagulant citrate dextrose solution]

ACD whole blood [see: blood, whole]

ACe (Adriamycin, cyclophosphamide) *chemotherapy protocol*

ACE (Adriamycin, cyclophosphamide, etoposide) *chemotherapy protocol* [also: CAE]

ACE inhibitors (angiotensin-converting enzyme inhibitors) [q.v.]

acebrochol INN, DCF

aceburic acid INN, DCF

acebutolol USAN, INN, BAN *antihypertensive; antiarrhythmic; antiadrenergic (β-receptor)* [also: acebutolol HCl]

acebutolol HCl JAN *antihypertensive; antiarrhythmic; antiadrenergic (β-receptor)* [also: acebutolol] 200, 400 mg oral

acecainide INN *antiarrhythmic* [also: acecainide HCl]

acecainide HCl USAN *antiarrhythmic* [also: acecainide]

acecarbromal INN *CNS depressant; sedative; hypnotic*

aceclidine USAN, INN *cholinergic*

aceclofenac INN, BAN

acedapsone USAN, INN, BAN *antimalarial; antibacterial; leprostatic*

acediasulfone sodium INN, DCF

acedoben INN
acefluranol INN, BAN
acefurtiamine INN
acefylline clofibrol INN
acefylline piperazine INN, DCF [also: acepifylline]
aceglaton JAN [also: aceglatone]
aceglatone INN [also: aceglaton]
aceglutamide INN *antiulcerative* [also: aceglutamide aluminum]
aceglutamide aluminum USAN, JAN *antiulcerative* [also: aceglutamide]
ACEIs (angiotensin-converting enzyme inhibitors) [q.v.]
Acel-Imune IM injection ℞ *immunization against diphtheria, tetanus and pertussis* [diphtheria & tetanus toxoids & acellular pertussis (DTaP) vaccine] 7.5 LfU•5 LfU•300 HAU per 0.5 mL
Acel-P ⓐ suspension for IM injection ℞ *active immunization against pertussis* [pertussis vaccine, acellular adsorbed] 300 HAU/0.5 mL
acemannan USAN, INN *investigational (Phase I) antiviral and immunomodulator for AIDS*
acemetacin INN, BAN, JAN
acemethadone [see: methadyl acetate]
aceneuramic acid INN
acenocoumarin [see: acenocoumarol]
acenocoumarol NF, INN [also: nicoumalone]
aceperone INN
Acephen suppositories OTC *analgesic; antipyretic* [acetaminophen] 120, 325, 650 mg
acephenazine dimaleate [see: acetophenazine maleate]
acepifylline BAN [also: acefylline piperazine]
acepromazine INN, BAN *veterinary sedative* [also: acepromazine maleate]
acepromazine maleate USAN *veterinary sedative* [also: acepromazine]
aceprometazine INN, DCF
acequinoline INN, DCF
acerola *(Malpighia glabra; M. punicifolia)* fruit *natural dietary source of vitamin C*

acesulfame INN, BAN
Aceta tablets, elixir OTC *analgesic; antipyretic* [acetaminophen] 325, 500 mg; 120 mg/5 mL
Aceta with Codeine tablets ℞ *narcotic analgesic* [codeine phosphate; acetaminophen] 30•300 mg
Aceta-Gesic tablets OTC *antihistamine; analgesic* [phenyltoloxamine citrate; acetaminophen] 30•325 mg
p-**acetamidobenzoic acid** [see: acedoben]
6-acetamidohexanoic acid [see: acexamic acid]
4-acetamidophenyl acetate [see: diacetamate]
acetaminocaproic acid [see: acexamic acid]
acetaminophen USP *analgesic; antipyretic* [also: paracetamol] 80, 325, 500, 650 mg, 100 mg/mL, 120, 160 mg/5 mL, 500/15 mL oral; 120, 300, 325, 650 mg suppository
acetaminophen & butalbital & caffeine *analgesic; sedative* 325•50•40 mg oral
acetaminophen & hydrocodone bitartrate *analgesic; antitussive* 650•10, 750•7.5 mg oral
acetaminophen & codeine *narcotic analgesic* 300•15, 300•30, 300•60 mg oral; 30•12 mg/5 mL oral
acetaminophenol [see: acetaminophen]
acetaminosalol INN, DCF
acetanilid (or acetanilide) NF
acetannin [see: acetyltannic acid]
acetarsol INN, BAN, DCF [also: acetarsone]
acetarsone NF [also: acetarsol]
acetarsone salt of arecoline [see: drocarbil]
Acetasol ear drops ℞ *antibacterial; antifungal* [acetic acid] 2%
Acetasol HC ear drops ℞ *topical corticosteroidal anti-inflammatory; antibacterial; antifungal* [hydrocortisone; acetic acid] 1%•2%
acetazolamide USP, INN, BAN, JAN *carbonic anhydrase inhibitor; diuretic; anticonvulsant; antiglaucoma; treat-*

ment for acute mountain sickness 125, 250 mg oral; 500 mg injection

acetazolamide sodium USP, JAN *carbonic anhydrase inhibitor; diuretic; anticonvulsant; antiglaucoma; treatment for acute mountain sickness*

acetcarbromal [see: acecarbromal]

acet-dia-mer-sulfonamide (sulfacetamide, sulfadiazine & sulfamerazine) [q.v.]

acetergamine INN

Acetest reagent tablets for professional use *in vitro diagnostic aid for acetone (ketones) in the urine or blood*

acetiamine INN

acetic acid NF, JAN *acidifying agent* 0.25%

acetic acid, aluminum salt [see: aluminum acetate]

acetic acid, calcium salt [see: calcium acetate]

acetic acid, diluted NF *bladder irrigant*

acetic acid, ethyl ester [see: ethyl acetate]

acetic acid, glacial USP, INN *acidifying agent*

acetic acid, potassium salt [see: potassium acetate]

acetic acid, sodium salt trihydrate [see: sodium acetate]

acetic acid, zinc salt dihydrate [see: zinc acetate]

acetic acid 5-nitrofurfurylidenehydrazide [see: nihydrazone]

aceticyl [see: aspirin]

acetilum acidulatum [see: aspirin]

acetiromate INN

acetohexamide USAN, USP, INN, BAN, JAN *sulfonylurea antidiabetic* 250, 500 mg oral

acetohydroxamic acid (AHA) USAN, USP, INN *urease enzyme inhibitor for chronic urea-splitting urinary infections*

acetol [see: aspirin]

acetomenaphthone BAN

acetomeroctol

acetone NF *solvent; antiseptic*

acetophen [see: aspirin]

acetophenazine INN *antipsychotic* [also: acetophenazine maleate]

acetophenazine maleate USAN, USP *antipsychotic* [also: acetophenazine]

p-**acetophenetidide** *(withdrawn from market)* [see: phenacetin]

acetophenetidin *(withdrawn from market)* [now: phenacetin]

acetorphine INN, BAN *enkephalinase inhibitor for acute diarrhea; investigational for opioid withdrawal and GERD*

acetosal [see: aspirin]

acetosalic acid [see: aspirin]

acetosalin [see: aspirin]

acetosulfone sodium USAN *antibacterial; leprostatic* [also: sulfadiasulfone sodium]

acetoxyphenylmercury [see: phenylmercuric acetate]

acetoxythymoxamine [see: moxisylyte]

acetphenarsine [see: acetarsone]

acetphenetidin *(withdrawn from market)* [now: phenacetin]

acetphenolisatin [see: oxyphenisatin acetate]

acetrizoate sodium USP [also: sodium acetrizoate]

acetrizoic acid USP

acetryptine INN

acetsalicylamide [see: salacetamide]

acet-theocin sodium [see: theophylline sodium acetate]

aceturate USAN, INN *combining name for radicals or groups*

acetyl adalin [see: acetylcarbromal]

acetyl sulfisoxazole [see: sulfisoxazole acetyl]

l-**acetyl-α-methadol (LAAM)** [see: levomethadyl acetate]

p-**acetylaminobenzaldehyde thiosemicarbazone** [see: thioacetazone; thiacetazone]

acetylaminobenzene [see: acetanilid]

N-acetyl-*p*-aminophenol (APAP; NAPA) [see: acetaminophen]

acetylaniline [see: acetanilid]

acetylated polyvinyl alcohol *viscosity-increasing agent*

acetyl-bromo-diethylacetylcarbamide [see: acecarbromal]

acetylcarbromal [see: acecarbromal]

acetylcholine chloride USP, INN, BAN, JAN *cardiac depressant; cholinergic; miotic; peripheral vasodilator*

acetylcholinesterase (AChE) inhibitors *a class of drugs that alter acetylcholine neurotransmitters, used as a cognition adjuvant in Alzheimer's dementia* [also called: cholinesterase inhibitors]

acetylcysteine (N-acetylcysteine) USAN, USP, INN, BAN *mucolytic inhaler; treatment for severe acetaminophen overdose (orphan); investigational immunomodulator for AIDS* [also: N-acetyl-L-cysteine]

acetylcysteine sodium *mucolytic inhaler 10%, 20% inhalation*

acetyldigitoxin (α-acetyldigitoxin) NF, INN

acetyldihydrocodeinone [see: thebacon]

N-acetyl-DL-leucine [see: acetylleucine]

acetylin [see: aspirin]

acetylkitasamycin JAN *antibacterial* [also: kitasamycin; kitasamycin tartrate]

N-acetyl-L-cysteine JAN *mucolytic inhaler* [also: acetylcysteine]

N-acetyl-L-cysteine salicylate [see: salnacedin]

acetylleucine (N-acetyl-DL-leucine) INN

acetylmethadol INN, DCF *narcotic analgesic* [also: methadyl acetate]

acetyloleandomycin [see: troleandomycin]

2-acetyloxybenzoic acid [see: aspirin]

acetylpheneturide JAN [also: pheneturide]

acetylphenylisatin [see: oxyphenisatin acetate]

N-acetyl-procainamide (NAPA) *investigational (orphan) preventative for ventricular arrhythmias in procainamide-induced lupus*

acetylpropylorvinol [see: acetorphine]

acetylresorcinol [see: resorcinol monoacetate]

acetylsal [see: aspirin]

N-acetylsalicylamide [see: salacetamide]

acetylsalicylate aluminum [see: aspirin aluminum]

acetylsalicylic acid (ASA) [now: aspirin]

acetylsalicylic acid, phenacetin & caffeine [see: APC]

acetylspiramycin JAN *macrolide antibiotic* [also: spiramycin]

acetylsulfamethoxazole JAN *broad-spectrum sulfonamide bacteriostatic* [also: sulfamethoxazole; sulphamethoxazole; sulfamethoxazole sodium]

N^1-acetylsulfanilamide [see: sulfacetamide]

acetyltannic acid USP

acetyltannin [see: acetyltannic acid]

acevaltrate INN

acexamic acid INN, DCF

ACFUCY (actinomycin D, fluorouracil, cyclophosphamide) *chemotherapy protocol*

AChE (acetylcholinesterase) inhibitors [q.v.]

Aches-N-Pain tablets (discontinued 1996) OTC *nonsteroidal anti-inflammatory drug (NSAID); antiarthritic; analgesic* [ibuprofen] 200 mg

Achillea millefolium *medicinal herb* [see: yarrow]

Achromycin eye drop suspension, ophthalmic ointment (discontinued 1995) ℞ *topical ophthalmic antibiotic* [tetracycline HCl] 10 mg/mL; 10 mg/g ⓢ actinomycin; Aureomycin

Achromycin topical ointment (discontinued 1995) OTC *broad-spectrum antibacterial* [tetracycline HCl] 3%

Achromycin V capsules, oral suspension ℞ *broad-spectrum antibiotic* [tetracycline HCl] 250, 500 mg; 125 mg/5 mL

aciclovir INN, JAN *antiviral* [also: acyclovir]

acid acriflavine [see: acriflavine HCl]

acid alpha-glucosidase, human [see: human acid alpha-glucosidase]

acid citrate dextrose (ACD) [see: anticoagulant citrate dextrose solution]

acid histamine phosphate [see: histamine phosphate]

Acid Mantle OTC *cream base*

acid trypaflavine [see: acriflavine HCl]

acidogen [see: glutamic acid HCl]

acidol HCl [see: betaine HCl]

acidophilus (*Lactobacillus acidophilus*) *natural bacteria for replenishment of normal flora in the gastrointestinal tract and vagina; not generally regarded as safe and effective as an antidiarrheal*

acidulated phosphate fluoride (sodium fluoride & hydrofluoric acid) *dental caries prophylactic*

acidum acetylsalicylicum [see: aspirin]

Acid-X tablets OTC *analgesic; antipyretic; antacid* [acetaminophen; calcium carbonate] 500•250 mg

acifran USAN, INN *antihyperlipoproteinemic*

aciglumin [see: glutamic acid HCl]

Aci-jel vaginal jelly OTC *acidity modifier* [acetic acid; oxyquinolone sulfate] 0.921%•0.025%

acinitrazole BAN *veterinary antibacterial* [also: nithiamide; aminitrozole]

Aciphex ℞ *investigational (NDA filed) proton pump inhibitor for gastroesophageal reflux disease and ulcers* [rabeprazole sodium]

acipimox INN, BAN

acistrate INN *combining name for radicals or groups*

acitemate INN

acitretin USAN, INN, BAN *systemic antipsoriatic; retinoic acid analog*

acivicin USAN, INN *antineoplastic*

ackee (*Blighia sapida*) *medicinal herb for colds, fever, edema, and epilepsy; not generally regarded as safe and effective as seeds and unripened fruit are highly toxic*

aclacinomycin A [now: aclarubicin]

aclantate INN

aclarubicin USAN, INN, BAN *antibiotic antineoplastic* [also: aclarubicin HCl]

aclarubicin HCl JAN *antibiotic antineoplastic* [also: aclarubicin]

aclatonium napadisilate INN, BAN, JAN

Aclophen long-acting tablets ℞ *decongestant; antihistamine; analgesic* [phenylephrine HCl; chlorpheniramine maleate; acetaminophen] 40•8•500 mg

Aclovate ointment, cream ℞ *topical corticosteroidal anti-inflammatory* [alclometasone dipropionate] 0.05%

ACM (Adriamycin, cyclophosphamide, methotrexate) *chemotherapy protocol*

A.C.N. tablets OTC *vitamin supplement* [vitamins A, B₃, and C] 25 000 IU•25 mg•250 mg

Acne Lotion 10 OTC *antibacterial and exfoliant for acne* [colloidal sulfur] 10%

Acne-5 lotion, mask OTC *topical keratolytic for acne* [benzoyl peroxide] 5%

Acne-10 lotion OTC *topical keratolytic for acne* [benzoyl peroxide] 10%

Acno lotion OTC *topical acne treatment* [sulfur] 3%

Acno Cleanser liquid OTC *topical cleanser for acne* [isopropyl alcohol] 60%

Acnomel cream OTC *topical acne treatment* [sulfur; resorcinol; alcohol] 8%•2%•11%

Acnotex lotion OTC *topical acne treatment* [sulfur; resorcinol; isopropyl alcohol] 8%•2%•20%

acodazole INN *antineoplastic* [also: acodazole HCl]

acodazole HCl USAN *antineoplastic* [also: acodazole]

aconiazide INN *investigational (orphan) for tuberculosis*

aconite (*Aconitum napellus*) *plant and root medicinal herb for fever, hypertension, and neuralgia; not generally regarded as safe and effective as it is highly toxic*

aconitine USP

ACOP (Adriamycin, cyclophosphamide, Oncovin, prednisone) *chemotherapy protocol*

ACOPP; A-COPP (Adriamycin, cyclophosphamide, Oncovin, procarbazine, prednisone) *chemotherapy protocol*

acortan [see: corticotropin]

Acorus calamus medicinal herb [see: calamus]

acoxatrine INN

9-acridinamine monohydrochloride [see: aminacrine HCl]

acridinyl anisidide [see: amsacrine]

acridinylamine methanesulfon anisidide (AMSA) [see: amsacrine]

acridorex INN

acrids a class of agents that have a pungent taste or cause heat and irritation when applied to the skin

acriflavine NF

acriflavine HCl NF [also: acriflavinium chloride]

acriflavinium chloride INN [also: acriflavine HCl]

acrihellin INN

acrinol JAN [also: ethacridine lactate; ethacridine]

acrisorcin USAN, USP, INN antifungal

acrivastine USAN, INN, BAN antihistamine

acrocinonide INN, DCF

acronine USAN, INN antineoplastic

acrosoxacin BAN antibacterial [also: rosoxacin]

AcryDerm Strands wound dressing high-exudate absorbent dressing for cavitated wounds

ACT oral rinse OTC topical dental caries preventative [sodium fluoride; alcohol 7%] 0.05%

Actaea alba; A. pachypoda; A. rubra medicinal herb [see: white cohosh]

Actaea racemosa medicinal herb [see: black cohosh]

actagardin INN

Actagen tablets, syrup OTC decongestant; antihistamine [pseudoephedrine HCl; triprolidine HCl] 60•2.5 mg; 30•1.25 mg/5 mL

Actagen-C Cough syrup ℞ narcotic antitussive; decongestant; antihistamine [codeine phosphate; pseudoephedrine HCl; triprolidine HCl] 10•30•2 mg/5 mL

Actamin; Actamin Extra tablets OTC analgesic; antipyretic [acetaminophen]

actaplanin USAN, INN, BAN veterinary growth stimulant

actarit INN

ACTH powder for IM or subcu injection ℞ corticosteroid; anti-inflammatory [corticotropin] 40 U/vial

ACTH (adrenocorticotropic hormone) [see: corticotropin]

ACTH-80 subcu or IM injection ℞ corticosteroid; anti-inflammatory [corticotropin repository] 80 U/mL

Acthar powder for IM or subcu injection ℞ corticosteroid; anti-inflammatory [corticotropin] 25, 40 U/vial

Acthar Gel [see: H.P. Acthar Gel]

ActHIB powder for injection ℞ pediatric vaccine for meningitis caused by Haemophilus influenzae type b (HIB) virus [Hemophilus b conjugate vaccine; tetanus toxoid] 10•24 μg/0.5 mL

ActHIB/acellular DTP (formula changed and released as ActHIB/Tripedia in 1996)

ActHIB/DTacP (pre-marketing name; released as ActHIB/Tripedia in 1996)

ActHIB/DTP (pre-marketing name; released as ActHIB/Tripedia in 1996)

ActHIB/Tripedia IM injection ℞ pediatric vaccine for children younger than 5 months old [Hemophilus b conjugate vaccine; diphtheria & tetanus toxoids & acellular pertussis (DTaP) vaccine] 10 μg•6.7 LfU•5 LfU•46.8 μg per 0.5 mL

Acthrel IV infusion ℞ diagnostic aid for adrenocorticotropic hormone (ACTH)-dependent Cushing syndrome (orphan) [corticorelin ovine triflutate] 100 μg

ActiBath effervescent tablets OTC moisturizer; emollient [colloidal oatmeal] 20%

Acticin cream ℞ pediculicide for lice; scabicide [permethrin] 5%

Acticort 100 lotion ℞ topical corticosteroidal anti-inflammatory [hydrocortisone] 1%

Actidil syrup (discontinued 1996) OTC antihistamine [triprolidine HCl; alcohol 4%] 1.25 mg/5 mL ② Actifed

Actidose with Sorbitol oral suspension OTC *adsorbent antidote for poisoning; reduces intestinal transit time* [activated charcoal; sorbitol] 25•⅖ g/120 mL; 50•⅖ g/240 mL

Actidose-Aqua oral suspension OTC *adsorbent antidote for poisoning* [activated charcoal] 25 g/120 mL, 50 g/240 mL

Actifed syrup (discontinued 1995) OTC *decongestant; antihistamine* [pseudoephedrine HCl; triprolidine HCl] 30•1.25 mg/5 mL ☑ Actidil

Actifed tablets OTC *decongestant; antihistamine* [pseudoephedrine HCl; triprolidine HCl] 60•2.5 mg ☑ Actidil

Actifed Allergy daytime caplets + nighttime caplets OTC *decongestant; (antihistamine/sleep aid added at night)* [pseudoephedrine HCl; (diphenhydramine HCl added at night)] 30 mg; 30•25 mg ☑ Actidil

Actifed Plus caplets, tablets OTC *decongestant; antihistamine; analgesic* [pseudoephedrine HCl; triprolidine HCl; acetaminophen] 30•1.25•500 mg ☑ Actidil

Actifed Sinus daytime caplets + nighttime caplets OTC *decongestant; analgesic; (antihistamine/sleep aid added at night)* [pseudoephedrine HCl; acetaminophen; (diphenhydramine HCl added at night)] 30•325 mg; 30•500•25 mg ☑ Actidil

Actifed with Codeine Cough syrup (discontinued 1997) R *narcotic antitussive; decongestant; antihistamine* [codeine phosphate; pseudoephedrine HCl; triprolidine HCl; alcohol 4.3%] 10•30•1.25 mg/5 mL ☑ Actidil

Actigall capsules R *gallstone dissolving agent; also for primary biliary cirrhosis (orphan)* [ursodiol] 300 mg

Actimmune subcu injection R *immunoregulator for chronic granulomatous disease (orphan); investigational (orphan) for renal cell carcinoma and severe congenital osteopetrosis* [interferon gamma-1b] 100 μg (3 million U)

Actinex cream R *antineoplastic for actinic keratoses (AK)* [masoprocol] 10%

actinium *element (Ac)*

actinomycin C BAN *antibiotic antineoplastic* [also: cactinomycin] ☑ Achromycin; Aureomycin

actinomycin D JAN *antibiotic antineoplastic* [also: dactinomycin] ☑ Achromycin; Aureomycin

actinoquinol INN *ultraviolet screen* [also: actinoquinol sodium]

actinoquinol sodium USAN *ultraviolet screen* [also: actinoquinol]

actinospectocin [see: spectinomycin]

Actiq "lollipops" R *oral transmucosal narcotic analgesic for breakthrough pain in cancer patients* [fentanyl citrate] 200, 400, 600, 800, 1200, 1600 μg

Actisite periodontal fiber R *oral antibiotic for periodontitis* [tetracycline] 12.7 mg/23 cm

actisomide USAN, INN *antiarrhythmic*

Activase powder for IV infusion R *tissue plasminogen activator (tPA) thrombolytic for acute myocardial infarction, acute ischemic stroke, or pulmonary embolism* [alteplase] 50, 100 mg/vial (29, 58 million IU/vial)

activated attapulgite [see: attapulgite, activated]

activated carbon

activated charcoal [see: charcoal, activated]

activated 7-dehydrocholesterol [see: cholecalciferol]

activated ergosterol [see: ergocalciferol]

activated prothrombin complex BAN

Activelle R *investigational (NDA filed) hormone replacement therapy for postmenopausal vasomotor symptoms* [norethindrone acetate; estradiol]

actodigin USAN, INN *cardiotonic*

Actonel film-coated tablets R *bisphosphonate bone resorption inhibitor for Paget's disease* [risedronate sodium] 30 mg

Actos tablets R *thiazolidinedione antidiabetic; increases cellular response to insulin without increasing insulin secretion* [pioglitazone HCl] 15, 30, 45 mg

Act-O-Vial (trademarked packaging form) *vial system*

Actron tablets OTC *nonsteroidal anti-inflammatory drug (NSAID); analgesic; antiarthritic* [ketoprofen] 12.5 mg

ACU-dyne ointment, perineal wash concentrate, prep solution, skin cleanser, prep swabs, swabsticks OTC *broad-spectrum antimicrobial* [povidone-iodine]

ACU-dyne Douche concentrate OTC *antiseptic/germicidal; vaginal cleanser and deodorizer* [povidone-iodine]

Acular; Acular PF eye drops ℞ *topical ophthalmic nonsteroidal anti-inflammatory drug (NSAID) for allergic conjunctivitis or cataract extraction* [ketorolac tromethamine] 0.5%

Acupaque (name changed to Visipaque upon release in 1996)

AcuTect ℞ *radiopharmaceutical diagnostic aid for acute venous thrombosis* [technetium Tc 99m apcitide]

Acutrim 16 Hour; Acutrim Late Day; Acutrim II precision-release tablets OTC *diet aid* [phenylpropanolamine HCl] 75 mg

AcuTrim Diet chewing gum OTC *diet aid* [phenylpropanolamine HCl] 75 mg

acycloguanosine [see: acyclovir]

acyclovir USAN, USP, BAN *antiviral* [also: aciclovir] 200, 400, 800 mg oral

acyclovir CD *investigational (Phase I) controlled-delivery antiviral*

acyclovir redox [see: redox-acyclovir]

acyclovir sodium USAN *antiviral* 200 mg oral; 50 mg/mL injection

acylCoA transferase (ACAT) inhibitor *investigational agent to lower serum cholesterol levels*

acylpyrin [see: aspirin]

AD-32 *investigational (NDA filed) novel anthracycline for treatment of bladder cancer*

AD-439 *investigational (Phase II) antiviral for HIV and AIDS*

AD-519 *investigational (Phase II) antiviral for HIV and AIDS*

ad5CMV-p53 [see: adenoviral p53 gene]

AD7C *investigational urinary test for Alzheimer's disease*

ADA (adenosine deaminase) [see: pegademase bovine; pegademase]

adafenoxate INN

Adagen IM injection ℞ *adenosine deaminase (ADA) enzyme replacement for severe combined immunodeficiency disease (orphan)* [pegademase bovine] 250 U/mL

Adalat capsules ℞ *antianginal; antihypertensive; calcium channel blocker* [nifedipine] 10, 20 mg

Adalat CC; Adalat Oros sustained-release tablets ℞ *antianginal; antihypertensive; calcium channel blocker* [nifedipine] 30, 60, 90 mg

adamantanamine [see: amantadine]

adamantanamine HCl [see: amantadine HCl]

adamexine INN

adapalene USAN, INN, BAN *synthetic retinoid analog for topical treatment of acne*

Adapettes solution OTC *rewetting solution for hard contact lenses*

Adapettes Especially for Sensitive Eyes solution OTC *rewetting solution for soft contact lenses*

Adapin capsules (discontinued 1996) ℞ *tricyclic antidepressant; anxiolytic* [doxepin HCl] 10, 25, 50, 75, 100, 150 mg ⊡ Atabrine; Ativan; Betapen

adaprolol maleate USAN *ophthalmic antihypertensive (β-blocker)*

Adapt solution (discontinued 1995) OTC *wetting/rewetting solution for hard contact lenses*

adatanserin INN *anxiolytic; antidepressant* [also: adatanserin HCl]

adatanserin HCl USAN *anxiolytic; antidepressant* [also: adatanserin]

AdatoSil 5000 intraocular injection ℞ *retinal tamponade for retinal detachment* [polydimethylsiloxane] 10, 15 mL

Adavite tablets OTC *vitamin supplement* [multiple vitamins; folic acid; biotin] ≛•400•35 μg

Adavite-M tablets OTC *vitamin/mineral/iron supplement* [multiple vitamins & minerals; iron; folic acid; biotin] ± • 27 mg • 0.4 mg • 30 μg

ADBC (Adriamycin, DTIC, bleomycin, CCNU) *chemotherapy protocol*

ADC with Fluoride drops ℞ *pediatric vitamin supplement and dental caries preventative* [vitamins A, C, and D; fluoride] 1500 IU • 35 mg • 400 IU • 0.5 mg per mL

Adcon-L gel ℞ *investigational (NDA filed) postsurgical wound dressing to inhibit the formation of scars and adhesions following lumbar discectomy surgery* [carbohydrate polymer gel]

Adcon-P Adhesion Control Barrier ℞ *investigational postsurgical wound dressing to inhibit the formation of scars and adhesions in the peritoneal cavity*

Adderall tablets ℞ *CNS stimulant for attention deficit hyperactivity disorder (ADHD), narcolepsy, and obesity* [amphetamines (amphetamine aspartate; amphetamine sulfate; dextroamphetamine sulfate; dextroamphetamine saccharate)] 5, 10, 20, 30 mg (1.25 • 1.25 • 1.25 • 1.25, 2.5 • 2.5 • 2.5 • 2.5, 5 • 5 • 5 • 5, 7.5 • 7.5 • 7.5 • 7.5 mg)

adder's mouth *medicinal herb* [see: chickweed]

adder's tongue (Erythronium americanum) *bulb and leaves medicinal herb used as an emetic, antiscrofulous agent, and emollient*

ADD-Vantage (trademarked delivery system) *intravenous drug admixture system*

ADE (ara-C, daunorubicin, etoposide) *chemotherapy protocol*

Adeflor M tablets ℞ *pediatric vitamin deficiency and dental caries prevention* [multiple vitamins; fluoride; calcium; iron] ± • 1 • 250 • 30 mg

adefovir dipivoxil *investigational (Phase III) oral reverse transcriptase inhibitor for HIV and AIDS; investigational (Phase III) treatment for chronic hepatitis B virus (HBV) infection*

ADEKs chewable tablets OTC *vitamin/ mineral supplement* [multiple vita-

mins & minerals; folic acid; biotin] ± • 200 • 50 μg

ADEKs pediatric drops OTC *vitamin/ mineral supplement* [multiple vitamins & minerals; biotin] ± • 15 μg

adelmidrol INN

ademetionine INN

adenine USP, JAN *amino acid*

adenine arabinoside (ara-A) [see: vidarabine]

adeno-associated viral-based vector cystic fibrosis gene therapy *investigational (orphan) for cystic fibrosis*

Adenocard IV injection ℞ *antiarrhythmic* [adenosine] 3 mg/mL

Adenoscan IV infusion ℞ *cardiac diagnostic aid; cardiac stressor; adjunct to thallium 201 myocardial perfusion scintigraphy* [adenosine] 3 mg/mL

adenosine USAN, BAN *antiarrhythmic for paroxysmal supraventricular tachycardia; diagnostic aid; orphan status withdrawn 1996*

adenosine deaminase (ADA) [see: pegademase bovine; pegademase]

adenosine monophosphate (AMP) [see: adenosine phosphate]

adenosine phosphate USAN, INN, BAN *nutrient; treatment for varicose veins and herpes infections* 25 mg/mL IM injection

adenosine triphosphate (ATP) disodium JAN

adenoviral p53 gene *investigational (Phase II) gene therapy for cancer* [also: p53 adenoviral gene]

5'-adenylic acid [see: adenosine phosphate]

adepsine oil [see: mineral oil]

adhesive bandage [see: bandage, adhesive]

adhesive tape [see: tape, adhesive]

adibendan INN

A-DIC (Adriamycin, dacarbazine) *chemotherapy protocol*

adicillin INN, BAN

adimolol INN

adinazolam USAN, INN, BAN *antidepressant; sedative*

adinazolam mesylate USAN *antidepressant*

Adipex-P tablets ℞ *anorexiant; CNS stimulant* [phentermine HCl] 37.5 mg

adiphenine INN *smooth muscle relaxant* [also: adiphenine HCl]

adiphenine HCl USAN *smooth muscle relaxant* [also: adiphenine]

adipiodone INN, JAN *parenteral radiopaque contrast medium* [also: iodipamide]

adipiodone meglumine JAN *parenteral radiopaque contrast medium (49.42% iodine)* [also: iodipamide meglumine]

Adipost slow-release capsules ℞ *anorexiant; CNS stimulant* [phendimetrazine tartrate] 105 mg

aditeren INN

aditoprim INN

AdjuVax-100a ℞ *investigational (Phase I/II) liposomal cancer vaccine synergist*

Adlone injection ℞ *corticosteroid; anti-inflammatory* [methylprednisolone acetate] 40, 80 mg/mL

adnephrine [see: epinephrine]

ADOAP (Adriamycin, Oncovin, ara-C, prednisone) *chemotherapy protocol*

Adolph's Salt Substitute OTC *salt substitute* [potassium chloride] 64 mEq/5 g; 35 mEq/5 g

Adolph's Seasoned Salt Substitute (discontinued 1997) OTC *salt substitute* [potassium chloride] 35 mEq/5 g

ADOP (Adriamycin, Oncovin, prednisone) *chemotherapy protocol*

adosopine INN

adozelesin USAN, INN *antineoplastic*

Adprin-B coated tablets OTC *analgesic; antipyretic; anti-inflammatory; antirheumatic* [aspirin (buffered with calcium carbonate, magnesium oxide, and magnesium carbonate)] 325, 500 mg

ADR (Adriamycin) [see: Adriamycin; doxorubicin HCl]

adrafinil INN

adrenal [see: epinephrine]

adrenal cortical steroids *a class of steroid hormones that stimulate the adrenal cortex*

Adrenalin Chloride eye drops ℞ *topical antiglaucoma agent* [epinephrine HCl]

Adrenalin Chloride nose drops ℞ *nasal decongestant* [epinephrine HCl] 0.1%

Adrenalin Chloride solution for inhalation ℞ *sympathomimetic bronchodilator* [epinephrine HCl] 1:100, 1:1000

Adrenalin Chloride subcu, IV, IM or intracardiac injection ℞ *sympathomimetic bronchodilator for bronchial asthma, bronchospasm, and COPD; vasopressor for shock* [epinephrine HCl] 1:1000 (1 mg/mL)

adrenaline BAN *vasoconstrictor; sympathomimetic bronchodilator; topical antiglaucoma agent; vasopressor for shock* [also: epinephrine] ☐ adrenalone

adrenaline bitartrate [see: epinephrine bitartrate]

adrenaline HCl [see: epinephrine HCl]

adrenalone USAN, INN *ophthalmic adrenergic* ☐ adrenaline

adrenamine [see: epinephrine]

adrenergic agonists *a class of bronchodilators that relax the bronchial muscles, reducing bronchospasm; a class of cardiac agents that increase myocardial contractility, causing a vasopressor effect to counteract shock (inadequate tissue perfusion)* [also called: sympathomimetics]

adrenine [see: epinephrine]

adrenochromazone [see: carbazochrome salicylate]

adrenochrome [see: carbazochrome salicylate]

adrenochrome guanylhydrazone mesilate JAN

adrenochrome monoaminoguanidine sodium methylsulfonate [see: adrenochrome guanylhydrazone mesilate]

adrenochrome monosemicarbazone sodium salicylate [see: carbazochrome salicylate]

adrenocorticotrophin [see: corticotropin]

adrenocorticotropic hormone (ACTH) [see: corticotropin]

adrenone [see: adrenalone]

Adria + BCNU (Adriamycin, BCNU) *chemotherapy protocol*

Adria-L-PAM (Adriamycin, L-phenylalanine mustard) *chemotherapy protocol*

Adriamycin PFS (preservative-free solution) IV injection ℞ *anthracycline antibiotic antineoplastic* [doxorubicin HCl] 2 mg/mL

Adriamycin RDF (rapid dissolution formula) powder for IV injection ℞ *anthracycline antibiotic antineoplastic* [doxorubicin HCl] 10, 20, 50, 150 mg/vial

Adria-Oncoline Chemo-Pin (trademarked delivery system)

Adrucil IV injection ℞ *antimetabolite antineoplastic for colorectal (orphan), breast, stomach, and pancreatic cancers; investigational (orphan) adjuvant to esophageal cancer* [fluorouracil] 50 mg/mL

ADS (azodisal sodium) [now: olsalazine sodium]

adsorbed diphtheria toxoid [see: diphtheria toxoid, adsorbed]

Adsorbocarpine eye drops ℞ *topical antiglaucoma agent; direct-acting miotic* [pilocarpine HCl] 1%, 2%, 4%

Adsorbonac eye drops OTC *corneal edema-reducing agent* [sodium chloride (hypertonic saline solution)] 2%, 5%

Adsorbotear eye drops (discontinued 1998) OTC *ocular moisturizer/lubricant* [hydroxyethylcellulose] 0.4%

ADT (trademarked dosage form) *alternate-day therapy*

Advair Diskus (powder for inhalation) ℞ *investigational (NDA filed) bronchodilator and corticosteroidal anti-inflammatory combination for asthma* [salmeterol xinafoate; fluticasone propionate]

Advance test stick for home use OTC *in vitro diagnostic aid for urine pregnancy test*

Advanced Care Cholesterol Test kit for home use OTC *in vitro diagnostic aid for cholesterol in the blood*

"Advanced Formula" products [see under product name]

Advantage 24 vaginal gel OTC *spermicidal contraceptive (for use with a diaphragm)* [nonoxynol 9] 3.5%

Advera liquid OTC *enteral nutritional therapy for HIV and AIDS patients* [lactose-free formula] 240 mL

Advil tablets, caplets, Liqui-Gels (soft liquid-filled gelatin capsules) OTC *nonsteroidal anti-inflammatory drug (NSAID); antiarthritic; analgesic* [ibuprofen] 200 mg ② Avail

Advil, Children's oral suspension OTC *nonsteroidal anti-inflammatory drug (NSAID); analgesic* [ibuprofen] 100 mg/5 mL

Advil, Junior Strength coated tablets OTC *nonsteroidal anti-inflammatory drug (NSAID); analgesic* [ibuprofen] 100 mg

Advil Cold & Sinus caplets OTC *decongestant; analgesic* [pseudoephedrine HCl; ibuprofen] 30•200 mg

Advil Pediatric Drops oral suspension OTC *nonsteroidal anti-inflammatory drug (NSAID); analgesic* [ibuprofen] 100 mg/2.5 mL

AE-941 *investigational (Phase III) angiogenesis inhibitor for osteoarthritis, rheumatoid arthritis, and various cancers*

AEDs (anti-epileptic drugs) [see: anticonvulsants]

A-E-R pads OTC *astringent* [hamamelis water] 50%

Aeroaid spray OTC *antiseptic; antibacterial; antifungal* [thimerosal; alcohol 72%] 1:1000

AeroBid; AeroBid-M oral inhalation aerosol ℞ *corticosteroidal anti-inflammatory for chronic asthma* [flunisolide] 250 μg/dose

AeroCaine aerosol solution OTC *topical local anesthetic* [benzocaine; benzethonium chloride] 13.6%•0.5%

AeroChamber (trademarked form) *aerosol holding chamber*

Aerodine aerosol OTC *broad-spectrum antimicrobial* [povidone-iodine]

Aerofreeze spray OTC *topical vapo-coolant anesthetic* [trichloromonofluoromethane; dichlorodifluoromethane] ≗ • ≗

Aerolate Sr.; Aerolate Jr.; Aerolate III timed-action capsules ℞ *antiasthmatic; bronchodilator* [theophylline] 260 mg; 130 mg; 65 mg

Aeropin ℞ *investigational (orphan) for cystic fibrosis* [heparin, 2-0-desulfated]

Aeroseb-Dex aerosol spray ℞ *topical corticosteroidal anti-inflammatory* [dexamethasone] 0.01%

Aeroseb-HC aerosol spray (discontinued 1997) ℞ *topical corticosteroidal anti-inflammatory; antiseborrheic* [hydrocortisone] 0.5%

aerosol OT [see: docusate sodium]

aerosolized pooled immune globulin [see: globulin, aerosolized pooled immune]

Aerosporin powder for IV, IM or intrathecal injection (discontinued 1996) ℞ *bactericidal antibiotic* [polymyxin B sulfate] 500 000 U

AeroTherm aerosol solution OTC *topical local anesthetic* [benzocaine; benzethonium chloride] 13.6%•0.5%

Aerotrol (trademarked form) *inhalation aerosol*

AeroZoin spray OTC *skin protectant* [benzoin; isopropyl alcohol 44.8%] 30%

AERx ℞ *investigational (Phase II) system that delivers morphine directly to the lungs* [morphine sulfate]

Aesculus hippocastanum; A. californica; A. glabra medicinal herb [see: horse chestnut]

Aethusa cynapium medicinal herb [see: dog poison]

aethylis chloridum [see: ethyl chloride]

afalanine INN

afloqualone INN, JAN

AFM (Adriamycin, fluorouracil, methotrexate [with leucovorin rescue]) *chemotherapy protocol*

afovirsen INN *antisense antiviral*

afovirsen sodium USAN *antisense antiviral; investigational for genital warts*

African ginger *medicinal herb* [see: ginger]

African pepper; African red pepper *medicinal herb* [see: cayenne]

Afrin extended-release tablets OTC *nasal decongestant* [pseudoephedrine sulfate] 120 mg ⊘ aspirin

Afrin nasal spray, nose drops OTC *nasal decongestant* [oxymetazoline HCl] 0.05% ⊘ aspirin

Afrin Children's Nose Drops OTC *nasal decongestant* [oxymetazoline HCl] 0.025% ⊘ aspirin

Afrin Moisturizing Saline Mist solution OTC *nasal moisturizer* [sodium chloride (saline solution)] 0.64% ⊘ aspirin

Afrin Saline Mist solution (name changed to Afrin Moisturizing Saline Mist in 1996)

Afrin Sinus nasal spray OTC *nasal decongestant* [oxymetazoline HCl] 0.05% ⊘ aspirin

Aftate for Athlete's Foot spray powder, spray liquid OTC *topical antifungal* [tolnaftate] 1%

Aftate for Jock Itch spray powder OTC *topical antifungal* [tolnaftate] 1%

afurolol INN

A/G Pro tablets OTC *dietary supplement* [protein hydrolysate; multiple vitamins & minerals; multiple amino acids] 542• ± mg

AG-3340 *investigational (Phase II/III) matrix metalloprotease inhibitor for lung and prostate cancer; investigational (Phase II) for age-related macular degeneration*

aganodine INN

agar NF, JAN *suspending agent*

agar-agar [see: agar]

Agathosma betulina medicinal herb [see: buchu]

agave (Agave americana) plant *medicinal herb used as an antiseptic, diuretic, and laxative and for jaundice and liver disease, pulmonary tuberculosis, and syphilis; also used to combat* *putrefactive bacteria in the stomach and intestines*

age cross-link breakers *a class of investigational antiaging compounds that break age-mediated bonds between proteins*

Agenerase capsules, oral solution ℞ *antiviral protease inhibitor for HIV* [amprenavir] 50, 150 mg; 15 mg/mL

Aggrastat IV infusion ℞ *GP IIb/IIIa platelet aggregation inhibitor for acute coronary syndrome, unstable angina, myocardial infarction, and cardiac surgery* [tirofiban HCl] 50, 250 μg/mL

aggregated albumin [see: albumin, aggregated]

aggregated radio-iodinated I 131 serum albumin [see: albumin, aggregated iodinated I 131 serum]

Aggrenox extended-release tablets ℞ *investigational (NDA filed) platelet aggregation inhibitor for stroke* [dipyridamole; aspirin] 200•25 mg

aglepristone INN

agofollin [see: estradiol]

Agoral emulsion OTC *laxative* [mineral oil; phenolphthalein] 4.2•0.2 g/15 mL ☒ Argyrol

Agoral Plain emulsion (discontinued 1997) OTC *emollient laxative* [mineral oil] 1.4 g/5 mL

agrimony *(Agrimonia eupatoria)* plant *medicinal herb for diarrhea, gastroenteritis, jaundice, kidney stones, liver disorders, mucous membrane inflammation with discharge; also used topically as an astringent and antiseptic*

agrimony, hemp *medicinal herb* [see: hemp agrimony]

Agropyron repens medicinal herb [see: couch grass]

Agrylin capsules ℞ *thrombolytic and antiplatelet agent for essential thrombocytopenia (orphan); investigational (orphan) for thrombocytosis and polycythemia vera* [anagrelide HCl] 0.5, 1 mg

ague tree *medicinal herb* [see: sassafras]

agurin [see: theobromine sodium acetate]

AHA (acetohydroxamic acid) [q.v.]

AHA (alpha hydroxy acids) [see: glycolic acid]

AH-chew chewable tablets ℞ *decongestant; antihistamine; anticholinergic* [phenylephrine HCl; chlorpheniramine maleate; methscopolamine nitrate] 10•2•1.25 mg

AH-chew D chewable tablets ℞ *decongestant* [phenylephrine HCl] 10 mg

AHF (antihemophilic factor) [q.v.]

AHG (antihemophilic globulin) [see: antihemophilic factor]

A-Hydrocort IV or IM injection ℞ *corticosteroid; anti-inflammatory* [hydrocortisone sodium succinate] 100, 250, 500, 1000 mg/vial

AIDS vaccine (several different compounds are included in this general category; e.g., gp120, rgp160, rgp160 MN, rp24) *investigational (Phase I–III) antiviral for HIV and AIDS treatment and prophylaxis* [also: gp120; rgp160; rp24]

AIDSVax ℞ *investigational (Phase III) bivalent HIV vaccine*

AIIRAs (angiotensin II receptor antagonists) [q.v.]

air, compressed [see: air, medical]

air, medical USP *medicinal gas*

Airet solution for inhalation ℞ *sympathomimetic bronchodilator* [albuterol sulfate] 0.083%

Airomir ⒶⓃ (U.S. product: Proventil HFA) CFC-free inhalation aerosol *sympathomimetic bronchodilator* [salbutamol sulfate] 100 μg/dose

AI-RSA *investigational (orphan) for autoimmune uveitis*

ajmaline JAN

Akarpine eye drops ℞ *topical antiglaucoma agent; direct-acting miotic* [pilocarpine HCl] 1%, 2%, 4%

AKBeta eye drops ℞ *topical antiglaucoma agent (β-blocker)* [levobunolol HCl] 0.25%, 0.5%

AK-Chlor eye drops, ophthalmic ointment ℞ *topical ophthalmic antibiotic* [chloramphenicol] 5 mg/mL; 10 mg/g

AK-Con eye drops ℞ *topical ophthalmic decongestant and vasoconstrictor* [naphazoline HCl] 0.1%

AK-Con-A eye drops (discontinued 1995) ℞ *topical ophthalmic decongestant and antihistamine* [naphazoline HCl; pheniramine maleate] 0.025%•0.3%

AK-Dex eye drops ℞ *topical ophthalmic corticosteroidal anti-inflammatory* [dexamethasone sodium phosphate] 0.1%

AK-Dex ophthalmic ointment ℞ *topical ophthalmic corticosteroidal anti-inflammatory* [dexamethasone sodium phosphate] 0.05%

AK-Dilate eye drops ℞ *topical ophthalmic decongestant and vasoconstrictor; mydriatic* [phenylephrine HCl] 2.5%, 10%

AK-Fluor antecubital venous injection ℞ *ophthalmic diagnostic agent* [fluorescein] 10%, 25%

AK-Homatropine eye drops (discontinued 1998) ℞ *mydriatic; cycloplegic* [homatropine hydrobromide] 5%

Akineton IV or IM injection ℞ *anticholinergic; antiparkinsonian* [biperiden lactate] 5 mg/mL

Akineton tablets ℞ *anticholinergic; antiparkinsonian* [biperiden HCl] 2 mg

aklomide USAN, INN, BAN *coccidiostat for poultry*

AK-Mycin ophthalmic ointment (discontinued 1995) ℞ *topical ophthalmic antibiotic* [erythromycin] 5 mg/g ⊡ Akne-Mycin

AK-NaCl eye drops, ophthalmic ointment OTC *corneal edema-reducing agent* [sodium chloride (hypertonic saline solution)] 5%

AK-Nefrin eye drops OTC *topical ophthalmic decongestant* [phenylephrine HCl] 0.12%

Akne-mycin ointment, topical solution ℞ *topical antibiotic for acne* [erythromycin] 2% ⊡ Ak-Mycin

AK-Neo-Dex eye drops ℞ *topical ophthalmic corticosteroidal anti-inflammatory; antibiotic* [dexamethasone sodium phosphate; neomycin sulfate] 0.1%•0.35%

Akoline C.B. capsules, caplets (discontinued 1995) OTC *dietary lipotropic with vitamin supplementation* [choline; inositol; methionine; multiple B vitamins; vitamin C; lemon bioflavonoids] 111•111•28• ≐ •100•100 mg

Akoline CB with Zinc caplets OTC *dietary lipotropic with vitamin and zinc supplementation* [choline; inositol; methionine; multiple B vitamins; vitamin C; bioflavonoid; zinc amino acid chelate]

AK-Pentolate eye drops ℞ *mydriatic; cycloplegic* [cyclopentolate HCl] 1%

AK-Poly-Bac ophthalmic ointment ℞ *topical ophthalmic antibiotic* [polymyxin B sulfate; bacitracin zinc] 10 000•500 U/g

AK-Pred eye drops ℞ *topical ophthalmic corticosteroidal anti-inflammatory* [prednisolone sodium phosphate] 0.125%, 1%

AKPro eye drops ℞ *topical antiglaucoma agent* [dipivefrin HCl] 0.1%

AK-Rinse ophthalmic solution OTC *extraocular irrigating solution* [sterile isotonic solution]

AK-Spore eye drops ℞ *topical ophthalmic antibiotic* [polymyxin B sulfate; neomycin sulfate; gramicidin] 10 000 U•1.75 mg•0.025 mg per mL

AK-Spore ophthalmic ointment ℞ *topical ophthalmic antibiotic* [polymyxin B sulfate; neomycin sulfate; bacitracin zinc] 10 000 U•3.5 mg•400 U per g

AK-Spore H.C. ear drops, otic suspension ℞ *topical corticosteroidal anti-inflammatory; antibiotic* [hydrocortisone; neomycin sulfate; polymyxin B sulfate] 1%•5 mg•10 000 U per mL

AK-Spore H.C. eye drop suspension ℞ *topical ophthalmic corticosteroidal anti-inflammatory; antibiotic* [hydrocortisone; neomycin sulfate; polymyxin B sulfate] 1%•0.35%•10 000 U per mL

AK-Spore H.C. ophthalmic ointment ℞ *topical ophthalmic corticosteroidal*

anti-inflammatory; antibiotic [hydrocortisone; neomycin sulfate; bacitracin zinc; polymyxin B sulfate] 1%•0.35%•400 U/g•10 000 U/g

AK-Sulf eye drops, ophthalmic ointment ℞ *topical ophthalmic antibiotic* [sulfacetamide sodium] 10%

AK-Taine eye drops (discontinued 1995) ℞ *topical ophthalmic anesthetic* [proparacaine HCl] 0.5%

AKTob eye drops ℞ *topical ophthalmic antibiotic* [tobramycin] 0.3%

AK-Tracin ophthalmic ointment ℞ *ophthalmic antibiotic* [bacitracin] 500 U/g

AK-Trol eye drop suspension, ophthalmic ointment ℞ *topical ophthalmic corticosteroidal anti-inflammatory; antibiotic* [dexamethasone; neomycin sulfate; polymyxin B sulfate] 0.1%•0.35%•10 000 U/mL; 0.1%•0.35%•10 000 U/g

Akwa Tears eye drops OTC *ophthalmic moisturizer/lubricant* [polyvinyl alcohol] 1.4%

Akwa Tears ophthalmic ointment OTC *ocular moisturizer/lubricant* [white petrolatum; mineral oil]

AL-721 *investigational (Phase I/II) antiviral for HIV and AIDS*

ALA (alpha lipoic acid) *natural antioxidant* [q.v.]

ALA; 5-ALA HCl [see: aminolevulinic acid HCl]

ALA Photodynamic Therapy ℞ *investigational (Phase III) treatment for psoriasis and actinic keratoses*

alacepril INN, JAN

Ala-Cort cream, lotion ℞ *topical corticosteroidal anti-inflammatory* [hydrocortisone] 1%

alafosfalin INN, BAN

Alamag oral suspension OTC *antacid* [aluminum hydroxide; magnesium hydroxide] 225•200 mg/5 mL ② Alma-Mag

Alamag Plus oral suspension OTC *antacid; antiflatulent* [aluminum hydroxide; magnesium hydroxide; simethicone] 225•200•25 mg/5 mL

alamecin USAN *antibacterial*

alanine (L-alanine) USAN, USP, INN *nonessential amino acid; symbols: Ala, A*

alanine nitrogen mustard [see: melphalan]

alanosine INN

alaproclate USAN, INN *antidepressant*

Ala-Quin cream ℞ *topical corticosteroidal anti-inflammatory; antifungal; antibacterial* [hydrocortisone; clioquinol] 0.5%•3%

Ala-Scalp lotion ℞ *topical corticosteroidal anti-inflammatory* [hydrocortisone] 2%

AlaSTAT lab test for professional use ℞ *test for allergic reaction to latex*

Alasulf vaginal cream ℞ *broad-spectrum antibiotic; antiseptic; vulnerary* [sulfanilamide; aminacrine HCl; allantoin] 15%•0.2%•2%

alatrofloxacin mesylate USAN *broad-spectrum fluoroquinolone antibiotic*

alazanine triclofenate INN

Albalon eye drops ℞ *topical ophthalmic decongestant and vasoconstrictor and lubricant* [naphazoline HCl; polyvinyl alcohol] 0.1%•1.4%

Albamycin capsules ℞ *bacteriostatic antibiotic* [novobiocin sodium] 250 mg

Albay subcu or IM injection ℞ *venom sensitivity testing (subcu); venom desensitization therapy (IM)* [extracts of honeybee, yellow jacket, yellow hornet, white-faced hornet, mixed vespid, and wasp venom]

albendazole USAN, INN, BAN *anthelmintic for neurocysticercosis and hydatid cyst disease (orphan); investigational (Phase III) for AIDS-related microsporidiosis*

albendazole oxide INN, BAN

Albenza Tiltab (film-coated tablets) ℞ *anthelmintic for neurocysticercosis (tapeworm) and cestode-induced hydatid cyst disease (orphan)* [albendazole]

Albright solution (sodium citrate and citric acid) *urine alkalizer; compounding agent*

albucid [see: sulfacetamide]

albumin, aggregated USAN *lung imaging aid (with technetium Tc 99m)*

albumin, aggregated iodinated I 131 serum USAN, USP *radioactive agent*

albumin, chromated Cr 51 serum USAN *radioactive agent*

albumin, human USP *blood volume supporter* 5%, 25% injection

albumin, human (sonicated with chlorofluorocarbons) *ultrasound contrast medium for cardiac imaging; investigational (Phase III) diagnostic aid for infertility due to obstructed fallopian tubes*

albumin, iodinated (^{125}I) human serum INN *radioactive agent; blood volume test* [also: albumin, iodinated I 125 serum]

albumin, iodinated (^{131}I) human serum INN, JAN *radioactive agent; intrathecal imaging agent; blood volume test* [also: albumin, iodinated I 131 serum]

albumin, iodinated I 125 USP *radioactive agent; blood volume test*

albumin, iodinated I 125 serum USAN, USP *radioactive agent; blood volume test* [also: iodinated (^{125}I) human serum albumin]

albumin, iodinated I 131 USP *radioactive agent; intrathecal imaging agent; blood volume test*

albumin, iodinated I 131 serum USAN, USP *radioactive agent; intrathecal imaging agent; blood volume test* [also: iodinated (^{131}I) human serum albumin]

albumin, normal human serum [now: albumin, human]

Albuminar-5; Albuminar-25 IV infusion ℞ *blood volume expander for shock, burns, and hypoproteinemia* [human albumin] 5%; 25%

Albunex injection ℞ *ultrasound heart imaging agent; investigational (Phase III) diagnostic aid for infertility due to obstructed fallopian tubes* [human albumin, sonicated] 5%

Albustix reagent strips for professional use *in vitro diagnostic aid for albumin (protein) in the urine*

Albutein 5%; Albutein 25% IV infusion ℞ *blood volume expander for shock, burns, and hypoproteinemia* [human albumin] 5%; 25%

albuterol USAN, USP *sympathomimetic bronchodilator* [also: salbutamol] 90 μg inhalation

albuterol sulfate USAN, USP *sympathomimetic bronchodilator* [also: salbutamol sulfate] 2, 4 mg oral; 2 mg/5 mL oral; 0.083%, 0.5% inhalation

albutoin USAN, INN *anticonvulsant*

Alcaine Drop-Tainers (eye drops) ℞ *topical ophthalmic anesthetic* [proparacaine HCl] 0.5%

alcanna *medicinal herb* [see: henna (Alkanna)]

Alcare foam OTC *topical antiseptic* [ethyl alcohol] 62%

Alchemilla xanthochlora; A. vulgaris *medicinal herb* [see: lady's mantle]

alclofenac USAN, INN, BAN, JAN *anti-inflammatory*

alclometasone INN, BAN *topical corticosteroidal anti-inflammatory* [also: alclometasone dipropionate]

alclometasone dipropionate USAN, USP, JAN *topical corticosteroidal anti-inflammatory* [also: alclometasone]

alcloxa USAN, INN *astringent; keratolytic* [also: aluminum chlorohydroxy allantoinate]

Alco-Gel OTC *topical antiseptic for instant sanitation of hands* [ethyl alcohol] 60% ⌧ aloe gel

alcohol USP *topical anti-infective/antiseptic; astringent; solvent; a widely abused "legal street drug" used to produce euphoria* [also: ethanol]

alcohol, dehydrated USP *antidote* [also: ethanol, dehydrated]

alcohol, diluted NF *solvent*

alcohol, rubbing USP, INN *rubefacient*

5% Alcohol and 5% Dextrose in Water; 10% Alcohol and 5% Dextrose in Water IV infusion ℞ *for*

caloric replacement and rehydration
[dextrose; alcohol] 5%•5%; 10%•5%

Alcon Saline Especially for Sensitive Eyes solution OTC *rinsing/storage solution for soft contact lenses* [sodium chloride (preserved saline solution)]

Alconefrin nose drops, nasal spray OTC *nasal decongestant* [phenylephrine HCl] 0.25%, 0.5%

Alconefrin 12 nose drops OTC *nasal decongestant* [phenylephrine HCl] 0.16%

alcuronium chloride USAN, INN, BAN, JAN *skeletal muscle relaxant*

Aldactazide tablets R̸ *antihypertensive; diuretic* [spironolactone; hydrochlorothiazide] 25•25, 50•50 mg ⧈ Aldactone

Aldactone tablets R̸ *antihypertensive; potassium-sparing diuretic* [spironolactone] 25, 50, 100 mg ⧈ Aldactazide

Aldara cream R̸ *immunomodulator for external genital and perianal warts* [imiquimod] 5% in 250 mg single-use packets

alder, spotted *medicinal herb* [see: witch hazel]

alder, striped *medicinal herb* [see: winterberry; witch hazel]

alder buckthorn; European black alder *medicinal herb* [see: buckthorn]

alderlin [see: pronethalol]

aldesleukin USAN, INN, BAN *immunostimulant; biological response modifier; antineoplastic for metastatic melanoma and renal cell carcinoma (orphan); investigational (Phase II, orphan) for immunodeficiency diseases; investigational (Phase III, orphan) for acute myelogenous leukemia (AML)*

aldesulfone sodium INN, DCF *antibacterial; leprostatic* [also: sulfoxone sodium]

aldioxa USAN, INN, JAN *astringent; keratolytic*

Aldoclor-150; Aldoclor-250 film-coated tablets R̸ *antihypertensive* [chlorothiazide; methyldopa] 150•250 mg; 250•250 mg

aldocorten [see: aldosterone]

Aldomet film-coated tablets, oral suspension R̸ *antihypertensive* [methyldopa] 125, 250, 500 mg; 250 mg/5 mL

Aldomet; Aldomet Ester HCl IV injection R̸ *antihypertensive* [methyldopate HCl] 50 mg/mL

Aldoril 15; Aldoril 25; Aldoril D30; Aldoril D50 film-coated tablets R̸ *antihypertensive; diuretic* [hydrochlorothiazide; methyldopa] 15•250 mg; 25•250 mg; 30•500 mg; 50•500 mg ⧈ Elavil; Eldepryl; Enovil; Equanil; Mellaril

aldosterone INN, BAN, DCF

Alec R̸ *investigational (orphan) for neonatal respiratory distress syndrome* [colfosceril palmitate; phosphatidylglycerol]

alendronate sodium USAN *bisphosphonate bone resorption inhibitor for postmenopausal and corticosteroid-induced osteoporosis and Paget's disease*

alendronic acid INN, BAN

Alenic Alka chewable tablets OTC *antacid* [aluminum hydroxide; magnesium trisilicate] 80•20 mg

Alenic Alka liquid OTC *antacid* [aluminum hydroxide; magnesium carbonate] 31.7•137.3 mg/5 mL

Alenic Alka, Extra Strength chewable tablets OTC *antacid* [aluminum hydroxide; magnesium carbonate] 160•105 mg

alentemol INN *antipsychotic; dopamine agonist* [also: alentemol hydrobromide]

alentemol hydrobromide USAN *antipsychotic; dopamine agonist* [also: alentemol]

alepride INN

Alersule sustained-release capsules (discontinued 1995) R̸ *decongestant; antihistamine* [phenylephrine HCl; chlorpheniramine maleate] 20•8 mg

Alertec ⒸⒶⓃ (U.S. product: Provigil) R̸ *analeptic for excessive daytime sleepiness of narcolepsy* [modafinil]

Alesse tablets (21 or 28 per pack) R̸ *monophasic oral contraceptive* [levonorgestrel; ethinyl estradiol] 100•20 μg

alestramustine INN

aletamine HCl USAN *antidepressant* [also: alfetamine]

Aletris farinosa *medicinal herb* [see: star grass]

Aleurites moluccana; A. cordata medicinal herb [see: tung seed]

Aleve tablets, gelcaps OTC *nonsteroidal anti-inflammatory drug (NSAID); antiarthritic; analgesic* [naproxen (from naproxen sodium)] 200 (220) mg

alexidine USAN, INN *antibacterial*

alexitol sodium INN, BAN

alexomycin USAN *veterinary growth promoter for poultry and swine*

alfacalcidol INN, BAN, JAN

alfadex INN

alfadolone INN, DCF [also: alphadolone]

alfalfa *(Medicago sativa)* leaves and flowers *medicinal herb for anemia, appetite stimulation, arthritis, atherosclerosis, blood cleansing, diabetes, hemorrhages, kidney cleansing, lowering cholesterol levels, nausea, pituitary disorders, and peptic ulcers*

alfaprostol USAN, INN, BAN *veterinary prostaglandin*

alfaxalone INN, JAN, DCF [also: alphaxalone]

Alfenta IV or IM injection ℞ *narcotic analgesic; anesthetic* [alfentanil HCl] 500 μg/mL

alfentanil INN, BAN *narcotic analgesic* [also: alfentanil HCl]

alfentanil HCl USAN *narcotic analgesic* [also: alfentanil]

Alferon LDO (low dose oral) ℞ *investigational (Phase I/II) cytokine for AIDS and ARC* [interferon alfa-n3]

Alferon N ℞ *investigational (Phase III) injectable cytokine for HIV, AIDS, ARC, and hepatitis C; investigational (Phase II) gel for intravaginal warts* [interferon alfa-n3]

alfetamine INN *antidepressant* [also: aletamine HCl]

alfetamine HCl [see: aletamine HCl]

alfuzosin INN, BAN *antihypertensive (α-blocker)* [also: alfuzosin HCl]

alfuzosin HCl USAN *antihypertensive (α-blocker)* [also: alfuzosin]

algeldrate USAN, INN *antacid*

Algenic Alka liquid OTC *antacid* [aluminum hydroxide; magnesium carbonate; EDTA]

Algenic Alka Improved chewable tablets OTC *antacid* [aluminum hydroxide; sodium bicarbonate; magnesium trisilicate]

algestone INN *anti-inflammatory* [also: algestone acetonide]

algestone acetonide USAN, BAN *anti-inflammatory* [also: algestone]

algestone acetophenide USAN *progestin*

algin [see: sodium alginate]

alginic acid NF, BAN *tablet binder and emulsifying agent*

alginic acid, sodium salt [see: sodium alginate]

alglucerase USAN, INN, BAN *glucocerebrosidase enzyme replacement for Gaucher's disease type I (orphan); investigational (orphan) for types II and III*

alibendol INN, DCF

aliconazole INN

alidine dihydrochloride [see: anileridine]

alidine phosphate [see: anileridine]

alifedrine INN

aliflurane USAN, INN *inhalation anesthetic*

alimadol INN

alimemazine INN *phenothiazine antihistamine; antipruritic* [also: trimeprazine tartrate; trimeprazine; alimemazine tartrate]

alimemazine tartrate JAN *phenothiazine antihistamine; antipruritic* [also: trimeprazine tartrate; alimemazine; trimeprazine]

Alimentum ready-to-use liquid OTC *hypoallergenic infant food* [casein protein formula]

Aliminase ℞ *investigational (Phase III) immunostimulant for ulcerative colitis*

alinidine INN, BAN

alipamide USAN, INN, BAN *diuretic; antihypertensive*

aliphatic alcohol compound *investigational (Phase III) topical antiviral treatment for herpes simplex*

alisactide [see: alsactide]

alisobumal [see: butalbital]

alitame USAN *sweetener*

alitretinoin USAN *topical treatment for cutaneous lesions of AIDS-related Kaposi sarcoma (orphan); investigational (Phase III, orphan) for acute promyelocytic leukemia*

alizapride INN

Alkaban-AQ IV injection (discontinued 1995) ℞ *antineoplastic* [vinblastine sulfate] 1 mg/mL

Alka-Mints chewable tablets OTC *antacid* [calcium carbonate] 850 mg

Alkanna tinctoria *medicinal herb* [see: henna]

Alka-Seltzer effervescent tablets OTC *antacid; analgesic* [sodium bicarbonate; citric acid; aspirin; phenylalanine] 1700•1000•325•9 mg

Alka-Seltzer, Extra Strength effervescent tablets OTC *antacid; analgesic* [sodium bicarbonate; citric acid; aspirin] 1985•1000•500 mg

Alka-Seltzer, Gold effervescent tablets OTC *antacid* [sodium bicarbonate; citric acid; potassium bicarbonate] 958•832•312 mg

Alka-Seltzer, Original effervescent tablets OTC *antacid; analgesic* [sodium bicarbonate; citric acid; aspirin] 1916•1000•325 mg

Alka-Seltzer Plus Allergy Liqui-Gels; Alka-Seltzer Plus Cold Liqui-Gels (capsules) OTC *decongestant; antihistamine; analgesic* [pseudoephedrine HCl; chlorpheniramine maleate; acetaminophen] 30•2•250 mg

Alka-Seltzer Plus Cold & Cough tablets OTC *antitussive; decongestant; antihistamine; analgesic; antipyretic* [dextromethorphan hydrobromide; phenylpropanolamine bitartrate; chlorpheniramine maleate; aspirin] 10•20•2•325 mg

Alka-Seltzer Plus Cold & Cough Liqui-Gels (capsules) OTC *antitussive; decongestant; antihistamine; analgesic* [dextromethorphan hydrobromide; pseudoephedrine HCl;

chlorpheniramine maleate; acetaminophen] 10•30•2•250 mg

Alka-Seltzer Plus Cold Medicine; Alka-Seltzer Plus Cold Tablets for oral solution OTC *decongestant; antihistamine; analgesic; antipyretic* [phenylpropanolamine bitartrate; brompheniramine maleate; aspirin] 20•2•325 mg; 24.08•2•325 mg

Alka-Seltzer Plus Cold & Sinus capsules OTC *decongestant; analgesic* [pseudoephedrine HCl; acetaminophen] 30•325 mg

Alka-Seltzer Plus Cold & Sinus effervescent tablets OTC *decongestant; analgesic; antipyretic* [phenylpropanolamine bitartrate; aspirin] 20•325 mg

Alka-Seltzer Plus Flu & Body Aches Non-Drowsy Liqui-Gels (capsules) OTC *antitussive; decongestant; analgesic* [dextromethorphan hydrobromide; pseudoephedrine HCl; acetaminophen] 10•30•250 mg

Alka-Seltzer Plus Night-Time Cold tablets OTC *antitussive; decongestant; antihistamine; analgesic; antipyretic* [dextromethorphan hydrobromide; phenylpropanolamine bitartrate; doxylamine succinate; aspirin] 10•20•6.25•500 mg

Alka-Seltzer Plus Night-Time Cold Liqui-Gels (capsules) OTC *antitussive; decongestant; antihistamine; analgesic* [dextromethorphan hydrobromide; pseudoephedrine HCl; doxylamine succinate; acetaminophen] 10•30•6.25•250 mg

Alka-Seltzer Plus Sinus tablets OTC *decongestant; analgesic; antipyretic* [phenylpropanolamine bitartrate; aspirin] 20•325 mg

Alka-Seltzer Plus Sinus Allergy tablets (discontinued 1995) OTC *decongestant; antihistamine; analgesic; antipyretic* [phenylpropanolamine bitartrate; brompheniramine maleate; aspirin] 24.08•2•500 mg

Alka-Seltzer with Aspirin effervescent tablets OTC *antacid; analgesic* [sodium bicarbonate; citric acid;

aspirin] 1900•1000•325, 1900•
1000•500 mg

alkavervir (Veratrum viride alka-loids)

Alkeran tablets, powder for IV infu-sion ℞ *nitrogen mustard-type alkylat-ing antineoplastic for multiple myeloma (orphan) and ovarian cancer; investiga-tional (orphan) for metastatic mela-noma* [melphalan] 2 mg; 50 mg

Alkets chewable tablets OTC *antacid* [calcium carbonate] 500, 750 mg

alkyl aryl sulfonate *surfactant/wet-ting agent*

alkylamines *a class of antihistamines*

alkylbenzyldimethylammonium chloride [see: benzalkonium chloride]

alkyldimethylbenzylammonium chloride [see: benzalkonium chloride]

alkylpolyaminoethylglycine JAN

alkylpolyaminoethylglycine HCl JAN

allantoin USAN, BAN *topical vulnerary*

Allbee C-800 film-coated tablets OTC *vitamin supplement* [multiple B vita-mins; vitamins C and E] ±•800•45 mg

Allbee C-800 plus Iron film-coated tablets OTC *vitamin/iron supplement* [ferrous fumarate; multiple B vita-mins; vitamins C and E; folic acid] 27 mg• ±•800 mg•45 IU•0.4 mg

Allbee with C caplets OTC *vitamin supplement* [multiple B vitamins; vitamin C] ±•300 mg

Allbee-T tablets OTC *vitamin supple-ment* [multiple B vitamins; vitamin C] ±•500 mg

Allegra capsules ℞ *nonsedating antihis-tamine* [fexofenadine HCl] 60 mg

Allegra-D capsules ℞ *decongestant; nonsedating antihistamine* [pseudo-ephedrine HCl; fexofenadine HCl] 120•60 mg

allegron [see: nortriptyline]

Allelix ℞ *investigational (Phase III) agent to increase bone mineral content and density in postmenopausal osteo-porosis* [parathyroid hormone (1-84), recombinant human]

Allent sustained-release capsules ℞ *decongestant; antihistamine* [pseudo-ephedrine HCl; brompheniramine maleate] 120•12 mg

Aller-Chlor tablets, syrup OTC *antihis-tamine* [chlorpheniramine maleate] 4 mg; 2 mg/5 mL

Allercon tablets OTC *decongestant; antihistamine* [pseudoephedrine HCl; triprolidine HCl] 60•2.5 mg

Allercreme Skin lotion OTC *moistur-izer; emollient*

Allercreme Ultra Emollient cream OTC *moisturizer; emollient*

Allerest eye drops OTC *topical ophthal-mic decongestant and vasoconstrictor* [naphazoline HCl] 0.012%

Allerest tablets OTC *decongestant; anti-histamine* [pseudoephedrine HCl; chlorpheniramine maleate] 30•2 mg

Allerest, Children's chewable tablets OTC *pediatric decongestant and antihis-tamine* [phenylpropanolamine HCl; chlorpheniramine maleate] 9.4•1 mg

Allerest 12 Hour nasal spray OTC *nasal decongestant* [oxymetazoline HCl] 0.05%

Allerest 12 Hour sustained-release caplets OTC *decongestant; antihistamine* [phenylpropanolamine HCl; chlor-pheniramine maleate] 75•12 mg

Allerest Headache; Allerest Sinus Pain Formula tablets OTC *deconges-tant; antihistamine; analgesic* [pseudo-ephedrine HCl; chlorpheniramine maleate; acetaminophen] 30•2•325 mg; 30•2•500 mg

Allerest No Drowsiness tablets OTC *decongestant; analgesic* [pseudoephed-rine HCl; acetaminophen] 30•325 mg

Allerfrim tablets, syrup OTC *decongestant; antihistamine* [pseudoephedrine HCl; triprolidine HCl] 60•2.5 mg; 30•1.25 mg/5 mL

Allerfrin with Codeine syrup ℞ *nar-cotic antitussive; decongestant; antihis-tamine* [codeine phosphate; pseudo-ephedrine HCl; triprolidine HCl] 10•30•1.25 mg/5 mL

Allergan Enzymatic tablets OTC *enzymatic cleaner for soft contact lenses* [papain] ② allergen; Auralgan

Allergan Hydrocare [see: Hydrocare]

Allergen Ear Drops ℞ *topical local anesthetic; analgesic* [benzocaine; antipyrine] 1.4% • 5.4%

allergenic extracts *a class of agents derived from various biological sources containing antigens that possess immunologic activity*

allergenic extracts (aqueous, glycerinated, or alum-precipitated) *over 900 allergens available for diagnosis of and desensitization to specific allergies*

Allergy tablets OTC *antihistamine* [chlorpheniramine maleate] 4 mg

Allergy Cold tablets (discontinued 1995) OTC *decongestant; antihistamine* [pseudoephedrine HCl; triprolidine HCl] 60 • 2.5 mg

Allergy Drops eye drops OTC *topical ophthalmic decongestant and vasoconstrictor* [naphazoline HCl] 0.012%; 0.03%

Allergy Relief Medicine tablets (discontinued 1995) OTC *decongestant; antihistamine* [phenylpropanolamine HCl; chlorpheniramine maleate] 25 • 4 mg

AlleRid capsules OTC *decongestant* [pseudoephedrine HCl]

AllerMax caplets OTC *antihistamine* [diphenhydramine HCl] 50 mg

AllerMax liquid (name changed to AllerMax Allergy & Cough Formula in 1997)

AllerMax Allergy & Cough Formula liquid OTC *antihistamine* [diphenhydramine HCl] 6.25 mg/5 mL

Allermed capsules OTC *nasal decongestant* [pseudoephedrine HCl] 60 mg

Allerphed syrup OTC *decongestant; antihistamine* [pseudoephedrine HCl; triprolidine HCl] 30 • 1.25 mg/5 mL

alletorphine BAN, INN

all-heal *medicinal herb* [see: mistletoe; valerian]

Allium cepa medicinal herb [see: onion]

Allium porrum medicinal herb [see: leek]

Allium sativum medicinal herb [see: garlic]

All-Nite Cold Formula liquid OTC *antitussive; decongestant; antihistamine; analgesic* [dextromethorphan hydrobromide; pseudoephedrine HCl; doxylamine succinate; acetaminophen; alcohol 25%] 5 • 10 • 1.25 • 167 mg/5 mL

allobarbital USAN, INN *hypnotic*

allobarbitone [see: allobarbital]

alloclamide INN, DCF

allocupreide sodium INN, DCF

AlloDerm *investigational acellular connective tissue skin graft for third-degree burns and plastic surgery* [processed human donor skin]

allomethadione INN, DCF [also: aloxidone]

allopurinol USAN, USP, INN, BAN, JAN *xanthine oxidase inhibitor for gout and hyperuricemia* 100, 300 mg oral

allopurinol riboside *orphan status withdrawn 1996*

allopurinol sodium *antineoplastic for leukemia, lymphoma, and solid tumor malignancies (orphan)*

Allovectin-7 ℞ *investigational (Phase II) treatment for head and neck cancer*

Allpyral subcu or IM injection ℞ *allergenic sensitivity testing (subcu); allergenic desensitization therapy (IM)* [allergenic extracts, alum-precipitated]

allspice (Eugenia pimenta; Pimenta dioica; P. officinalis) *unripe fruit and leaves medicinal herb for diarrhea and gas; also used as a purgative and tonic*

all-trans-retinoic acid [see: tretinoin]

allyl isothiocyanate USAN, USP

allylamines *a class of antifungals*

allylbarbituric acid [now: butalbital]

allylestrenol INN, JAN [also: allyloestrenol]

allyl-isobutylbarbituric acid [see: butalbital]

allylisopropylmalonylurea [see: aprobarbital]

4-allyl-2-methoxyphenol [see: eugenol]

N-allylnoretorphine [see: alletorphine]

N-allylnoroxymorphone HCl [see: naloxone HCl]

allyloestrenol BAN [also: allylestrenol]

allylprodine INN, BAN, DCF

5-allyl-5-*sec*-butylbarbituric acid [see: talbutal]

allylthiourea INN

allypropymal [see: aprobarbital]

Almacone chewable tablets, liquid OTC *antacid; antiflatulent* [aluminum hydroxide; magnesium hydroxide; simethicone] 200•200•20 mg; 200•200•20 mg/5 mL

Almacone II liquid OTC *antacid; antiflatulent* [aluminum hydroxide; magnesium hydroxide; simethicone] 400•400•40 mg/5 mL

almadrate sulfate USAN, INN *antacid*

almagate USAN, INN *antacid*

almagodrate INN

almasilate INN, BAN

Almebex Plus B₁₂ liquid OTC *vitamin supplement* [multiple B vitamins] ±

almecillin INN

almestrone INN

alminoprofen INN, JAN

almitrine INN, BAN

almokalant INN *investigational antiarrhythmic*

almond (*Prunus amygdalus*) kernels *medicinal herb used as a demulcent, emollient, and pectoral*

almond oil NF *emollient and perfume; oleaginous vehicle*

Almora tablets OTC *magnesium supplement* [magnesium gluconate] 500 mg

almotriptan USAN, INN *investigational 5-HT₁D agonist for migraine*

almotriptan malate USAN *5-HT₁D agonist for migraine*

almoxatone INN

alnespirone INN

alniditan dihydrochloride USAN *serotonin 5-HT₁D agonist for migraine*

Alnus glutinosa *medicinal herb* [see: black alder]

Alodopa-15; Alodopa-25 tablets ℞ *antihypertensive; diuretic* [hydrochlorothiazide; methyldopa]

aloe USP ② Alco-Gel

aloe (*Aloe vera* and over 500 other species) leaves and juice *medicinal herb for burns, hemorrhoids, insect bites, and scalds; also used as a deodorant and to aid digestion and limit scarring; not generally regarded as safe and effective as a cathartic*

Aloe Grande lotion OTC *moisturizer; emollient; skin protectant* [vitamins A and E; aloe] 3333.3•50• ± U/g

Aloe Vesta Perineal solution OTC *emollient/protectant* [propylene glycol; aloe vera gel]

alofilcon A USAN *hydrophilic contact lens material*

aloin BAN

ALOMAD (Adriamycin, Leukeran, Oncovin, methotrexate, actinomycin D, dacarbazine) *chemotherapy protocol* ② Alomide

Alomide Drop-Tainers (eye drops) ℞ *topical antiallergic for vernal keratoconjunctivitis (orphan)* [lodoxamide tromethamine] 0.1% ② ALOMAD

alonacic INN

alonimid USAN, INN *sedative; hypnotic*

Alophen Pills tablets (discontinued 1998) OTC *stimulant laxative* [phenolphthalein] 60 mg

Alophen Pills No. 973 tablets (name changed to Alophen Pills in 1995)

Alor 5/500 tablets ℞ *narcotic analgesic* [hydrocodone bitartrate; aspirin] 5•500 mg

Alora transdermal patch ℞ *estrogen replacement therapy for postmenopausal disorders* [estradiol] 50, 75, 100 μg/day

aloracetam INN

alosetron INN, BAN *antiemetic* [also: alosetron HCl]

alosetron HCl USAN *antiemetic; investigational (Phase II) for irritable bowel syndrome* [also: alosetron]

alovudine USAN, INN *antiviral*

aloxidone BAN [also: allomethadione]

aloxiprin INN, BAN, DCF

aloxistatin INN

***Aloysiatriphylla* spp.** *medicinal herb* [see: lemon verbena] alozafone INN

alpertine USAN, INN *antipsychotic*

alpha amylase (α-amylase) USAN *anti-inflammatory*

alpha hydroxy acids (AHA) [see: glycolic acid]

alpha interferon-2A [see: interferon alfa-2A]

alpha interferon-2B [see: interferon alfa-2B]

alpha interferon-N1 [see: interferon alfa-N1]

alpha interferon-N3 [see: interferon alfa-N3]

Alpha Keri Moisturizing Soap bar OTC *therapeutic skin cleanser*

Alpha Keri Spray; Alpha Keri Therapeutic Bath Oil OTC *bath emollient*

alpha lipoic acid (ALA) *natural antioxidant that is both fat- and water-soluble and readily crosses cell membranes; used in the treatment of AIDS, diabetes, liver ailments, oxidative stress injuries, and various cancers*

d-**alpha tocopherol** [see: vitamin E]

dl-**alpha tocopherol** [see: vitamin E]

d-**alpha tocopheryl acetate** [see: vitamin E]

dl-**alpha tocopheryl acetate** [see: vitamin E]

d-**alpha tocopheryl acid succinate** [see: vitamin E]

dl-**alpha tocopheryl acid succinate** [see: vitamin E]

alpha$_1$ PI (alpha$_1$-proteinase inhibitor) [q.v.]

alpha$_1$-antitrypsin (AAT), recombinant *investigational (orphan) for alpha$_1$-antitrypsin deficiency in the ZZ phenotype population*

alpha$_1$-antitrypsin, transgenic human *investigational (Phase II, orphan) for cystic fibrosis*

alpha$_1$-proteinase inhibitor (alpha$_1$ PI) *chronic replacement therapy for hereditary alpha$_1$ PI deficiency, which leads to progressive panacinar emphysema (orphan); investigational (Phase II) antiviral for HIV*

l-**alpha-acetyl-methadol (LAAM)** *orphan status withdrawn 1996*

alphacemethadone [see: alphacetyl-methadol]

alphacetylmethadol BAN, INN, DCF

alpha-chymotrypsin [see: chymotrypsin]

alpha-cypermethrin BAN

alpha-D-galactosidase *digestive enzyme*

alphadolone BAN [also: alfadolone]

alpha-estradiol [see: estradiol]

alpha-estradiol benzoate [see: estradiol benzoate]

alpha-ethyltryptamine (alpha-EtT) *a hallucinogenic street drug chemically related to MDMA* [see also: MDMA; alpha-methyltryptamine]

alphafilcon A USAN *hydrophilic contact lens material*

alpha-galactosidase A *investigational (orphan) enzyme replacement therapy for Fabry's disease*

alpha-galactosidase A & ceramide trihexosidase (CTH) *investigational (orphan) for Fabry's disease*

Alphagan eye drops ℞ *selective α$_2$ agonist for open-angle glaucoma and ocular hypertension* [brimonidine tartrate] 0.2%

alpha-glucosidase, human acid [see: human acid alpha-glucosidase]

1-alpha-hydroxy vitamin D$_2$ *investigational osteoporosis treatment*

alpha-hypophamine [see: oxytocin]

alpha-L-iduronidase, recombinant *investigational (orphan) enzyme for mucopolysaccharidosis I (MPS-I)*

alpha-melanocyte stimulating hormone *investigational (orphan) agent for the prevention and treatment of acute renal failure due to ischemia*

alphameprodine INN, BAN, DCF

alphamethadol INN, BAN, DCF

alpha-methyldopa [now: methyldopa]

alpha-methyltryptamine (alpha-MeT) *a hallucinogenic street drug chemically related to MDMA* [see also: MDMA; alpha-ethyltryptamine]

Alphanate powder for IV injection ℞ *antihemophilic; investigational (orphan)* *for von Willebrand's disease* [antihemophilic factor VIII:C, solvent/detergent treated] ₂

AlphaNine IV injection (discontinued 1997; replaced by AlphaNine SD) ℞ *antihemophilic for factor IX deficiency (hemophilia B; Christmas disease) (orphan)* [coagulation factor IX, human]

AlphaNine SD IV injection ℞ *antihemophilic for factor IX deficiency (hemophilia B; Christmas disease) (orphan)* [coagulation factors II, VII, IX, and X, solvent/detergent treated]

alpha-phenoxyethyl penicillin, potassium [see: phenethicillin potassium]

alphaprodine INN, BAN [also: alphaprodine HCl]

alphaprodine HCl USP [also: alphaprodine]

alphasone acetophenide [now: algestone acetonide]

Alphatrex cream, ointment, lotion ℞ *topical corticosteroidal anti-inflammatory* [betamethasone dipropionate] 0.05%

alphaxalone BAN [also: alfaxalone]

Alphosyl lotion OTC *topical antipsoriatic; antiseborrheic; vulnerary* [coal tar extract; allantoin]

alpidem USAN, INN, BAN *anxiolytic*

Alpinia officinarum; A. galanga medicinal herb [see: galangal]

Alpinia oxyphylla; A. fructus medicinal herb [see: bitter cardamom]

Alpinia speciosa medicinal herb for edema, fungal infections, hypertension, and thrombosis

alpiropride INN

alprafenone INN

alprazolam USAN, USP, INN, BAN, JAN *benzodiazepine anxiolytic; sedative; treatment of panic disorders and agoraphobia* 0.25, 0.5, 1, 2 mg, 0.5 mg/5 mL, 1 mg/mL oral

alprenolol INN, BAN *antiadrenergic (β-receptor)* [also: alprenolol HCl]

alprenolol HCl USAN, JAN *antiadrenergic (β-receptor)* [also: alprenolol]

alprenoxime HCl USAN *antiglaucoma agent*

alprostadil USAN, USP, INN, BAN, JAN *vasodilator for erectile dysfunction; platelet aggregation inhibitor; investigational (orphan) for peripheral arterial occlusive disease*

alprostadil, liposomal *investigational (Phase III) for erectile dysfunction; investigational (orphan) for acute respiratory distress and ischemic ulcerations due to peripheral artery disease*

alprostadil alfadex BAN

Alprox-TD cream ℞ *investigational (Phase III) topical therapy for erectile dysfunction* [alprostadil]

Alramucil effervescent powder OTC *bulk laxative* [psyllium hydrophilic mucilloid] 3.6 g/packet

Alredase ℞ *investigational (NDA filed) aldose reductase inhibitor for diabetic neuropathy* [tolrestat]

alrestatin INN *aldose reductase enzyme inhibitor* [also: alrestatin sodium]

alrestatin sodium USAN *aldose reductase enzyme inhibitor* [also: alrestatin]

Alrex eye drop suspension ℞ *corticosteroidal anti-inflammatory* [loteprednol etabonate] 0.2%

alsactide INN

alseroxylon JAN *antihypertensive; rauwolfia derivative*

ALT (autolymphocyte therapy) [q.v.]

Altace capsules ℞ *antihypertensive; angiotensin-converting enzyme (ACE) inhibitor* [ramipril] 1.25, 2.5, 5, 10 mg

altanserin INN *serotonin antagonist* [also: altanserin tartrate]

altanserin tartrate USAN *serotonin antagonist* [also: altanserin]

altapizone INN

alteconazole INN

alteplase USAN, INN, BAN, JAN *tissue plasminogen activator (tPA) for acute myocardial infarction, acute ischemic stroke, or pulmonary embolism*

alteratives *a class of agents that produce gradual beneficial changes in the body, usually by improving nutrition, without having any marked specific effect*

ALternaGEL liquid OTC *antacid* [aluminum hydroxide gel] 600 mg/5 mL

Althaea officinalis *medicinal herb* [see: marsh mallow]

althiazide USAN *antihypertensive* [also: altizide]

altizide INN, DCF *antihypertensive* [also: althiazide]

altoqualine INN

Altracin *investigational (orphan) for pseudomembranous enterocolitis* [bacitracin]

altrenogest USAN, INN, BAN *veterinary progestin*

altretamine USAN, INN, BAN *antineoplastic for advanced ovarian adenocarcinoma (orphan)*

Altropane ℞ *investigational (Phase II) radioimaging agent for Parkinson's disease*

altumomab USAN, INN *radiodiagnostic monoclonal antibody for colorectal carcinoma; anticarcinoembryonic antigen (anti-CEA)* [also: indium In 111 altumomab pentetate]

altumomab pentetate USAN *monoclonal antibody conjugate* [also: indium In 111 altumomab pentetate]

Alu-Cap capsules OTC *antacid* [aluminum hydroxide gel] 400 mg

Aludrox oral suspension OTC *antacid; antiflatulent* [aluminum hydroxide; magnesium hydroxide; simethicone] 307•103•2̲ mg/5 mL

alukalin [see: kaolin]

alum, ammonium USP *topical astringent*

alum, potassium USP *topical astringent* [also: aluminum potassium sulfate]

alum root *(Geranium maculatum) medicinal herb used as an astringent, hemostatic, and antiseptic*

Alumadrine tablets ℞ *decongestant; antihistamine; analgesic* [phenylpropanolamine HCl; chlorpheniramine maleate; acetaminophen] 25•4•500 mg

alumina & magnesia USP *antacid*

aluminopara-aminosalicylate calcium (alumino *p*-aminosalicylate calcium) JAN

aluminosilicic acid, magnesium salt hydrate [see: silodrate]

aluminum *element (Al)*

aluminum, micronized *astringent*

aluminum acetate USP *topical astringent; Burow solution*

aluminum aminoacetate [see: dihydroxyaluminum aminoacetate]

aluminum ammonium sulfate dodecahydrate [see: alum, ammonium]

aluminum bismuth oxide [see: bismuth aluminate]

aluminum carbonate, basic USAN, USP *antacid*

aluminum chlorhydroxide [now: aluminum chlorohydrate]

aluminum chlorhydroxide alcohol soluble complex [now: aluminum chlorohydrex]

aluminum chloride USP *topical astringent for hyperhidrosis*

aluminum chloride, basic [see: aluminum sesquichlorohydrate]

aluminum chloride hexahydrate [see: aluminum chloride]

aluminum chloride hydroxide hydrate [see: aluminum chlorohydrate]

aluminum chlorohydrate USAN *anhidrotic*

aluminum chlorohydrex USAN *topical astringent*

aluminum chlorohydrol propylene glycol complex [now: aluminum chlorohydrex]

aluminum chlorohydroxy allantoinate JAN *astringent; keratolytic* [also: alcloxa]

aluminum clofibrate INN, BAN, JAN

aluminum dihydroxyaminoacetate [see: dihydroxyaluminum aminoacetate]

aluminum flufenamate JAN

aluminum glycinate, basic [see: dihydroxyaluminum aminoacetate]

aluminum hydroxide gel USP *antacid* 320, 450, 600 mg/5 mL oral

aluminum hydroxide gel, dried USP, JAN *antacid*

aluminum hydroxide glycine [see: dihydroxyaluminum aminoacetate] aluminum hydroxide hydrate [see: algeldrate]

aluminum hydroxychloride [now: aluminum chlorohydrate]

aluminum magnesium carbonate hydroxide dihydrate [see: almagate]

aluminum magnesium hydroxide carbonate hydrate [see: hydrotalcite]

aluminum magnesium hydroxide oxide sulfate [see: almadrate sulfate]

aluminum magnesium hydroxide oxide sulfate hydrate [see: almadrate sulfate]

aluminum magnesium hydroxide sulfate [see: magaldrate]

aluminum magnesium hydroxide sulfate hydrate [see: magaldrate]

aluminum monostearate NF, JAN

aluminum oxide

Aluminum Paste ointment OTC occlusive skin protectant [metallic aluminum] 10%

aluminum phosphate gel USP antacid (disapproved for use as an antacid in 1989)

aluminum potassium sulfate JAN topical astringent [also: alum, potassium]

aluminum potassium sulfate dodecahydrate [see: alum, potassium]

aluminum sesquichlorohydrate USAN anhidrotic

aluminum silicate, natural JAN

aluminum silicate, synthetic JAN

aluminum sodium carbonate hydroxide [see: dihydroxyaluminum sodium carbonate]

aluminum subacetate USP topical astringent

aluminum sulfate USP anhidrotic

aluminum sulfate hydrate [see: aluminum sulfate]

aluminum zirconium glycine tetrachloro hydrate complex [see: aluminum zirconium tetrachlorohydrex gly]

aluminum zirconium glycine trichloro hydrate complex [see: aluminum zirconium trichlorohydrex gly]

aluminum zirconium octachlorohydrate USP anhidrotic

aluminum zirconium octachlorohydrex gly USP anhidrotic

aluminum zirconium pentachlorohydrate USP anhidrotic

aluminum zirconium pentachlorohydrex gly USP anhidrotic

aluminum zirconium tetrachlorohydrate USP anhidrotic

aluminum zirconium tetrachlorohydrex gly USAN, USP anhidrotic

aluminum zirconium trichlorohydrate USP anhidrotic

aluminum zirconium trichlorohydrex gly USAN, USP anhidrotic

Alupent tablets (discontinued 1999) R sympathomimetic bronchodilator [metaproterenol sulfate] 10, 20 mg

Alupent syrup, inhalation aerosol powder, solution for inhalation R sympathomimetic bronchodilator [metaproterenol sulfate] 10 mg/5 mL; 0.65 mg/dose; 0.4%, 0.6%, 5%

Alurate elixir R sedative; hypnotic [aprobarbital] 40 mg/5 mL

alusulf INN

Alu-Tab film-coated tablets OTC antacid [aluminum hydroxide gel] 500 mg

ALVAC-120TMG investigational (Phase I) vaccine for HIV

ALVAC-HIV 1 R investigational (Phase I) vaccine for HIV [AIDS vaccine gp160 MN]

alverine INN, BAN anticholinergic [also: alverine citrate]

alverine citrate USAN, NF anticholinergic [also: alverine]

alvircept sudotox USAN, INN antiviral; investigational (Phase II) for AIDS

amabevan [see: carbarsone]

amacetam HCl [now: pramiracetam HCl]

amacetam sulfate [now: pramiracetam sulfate]

Amacodone tablets (discontinued 1995) R narcotic analgesic [hydrocodone bitartrate; acetaminophen] 5•500 mg

amadinone INN progestin [also: amadinone acetate]

amadinone acetate USAN *progestin* [also: amadinone]

amafolone INN, BAN

amalgucin

Amanita muscaria **mushrooms** *a species that produces muscarine and ibotenic acid, a psychotropic substance ingested as a street drug*

amanozine INN

amantadine INN, BAN *antiviral for influenza A virus; dopaminergic antiparkinsonian* [also: amantadine HCl]

amantadine HCl USAN, USP, JAN *antiviral for influenza A virus; dopaminergic antiparkinsonian* [also: amantadine] 100 mg oral; 50 mg/5 mL oral

amantanium bromide INN

amantocillin INN

Amaphen capsules ℞ *analgesic; sedative* [acetaminophen; caffeine; butalbital] 325•40•50 mg

Amaphen with Codeine #3 capsules (discontinued 1995) ℞ *narcotic analgesic; sedative* [codeine phosphate; acetaminophen; caffeine; butalbital] 30•325•40•50 mg

amara; amargo *medicinal herb* [see: quassia]

amaranth (*Amaranthus* spp.) leaves and flowers *medicinal herb for diarrhea, dysentery, excessive menstruation, and nosebleeds*

amaranth (FD&C Red No. 2) USP

amargo; amara *medicinal herb* [see: quassia]

amarsan [see: acetarsone]

Amaryl tablets ℞ *once-daily sulfonylurea antidiabetic* [glimepiride] 1, 2, 4 mg

Amatine (name changed to ProAmatine upon release in 1996)

ambamustine INN

ambasilide INN *investigational antiarrhythmic*

ambazone INN, BAN, DCF

ambenonium chloride USP, INN, BAN, JAN *anticholinesterase muscle stimulant*

ambenoxan INN, BAN

Ambenyl Cough syrup ℞ *narcotic antitussive; antihistamine* [codeine phosphate; bromodiphenhydramine HCl; alcohol 5%] 10•12.5 mg/5 mL
② Aventyl

Ambenyl-D liquid OTC *antitussive; decongestant; expectorant* [dextromethorphan hydrobromide; pseudoephedrine HCl; guaifenesin; alcohol 9.5%] 10•30•100 mg/5 mL

amber; amber touch-and-heal *medicinal herb* [see: St. John's wort]

Ambi 10 bar OTC *therapeutic skin cleanser*

Ambi 10 cream OTC *topical keratolytic for acne* [benzoyl peroxide] 10%

Ambi Skin Tone cream OTC *hyperpigmentation bleaching agent; sunscreen* [hydroquinone; padimate O]

ambicromil INN, BAN *prophylactic antiallergic* [also: probicromil calcium]

ambicromil calcium [see: probicromil calcium]

Ambien film-coated tablets ℞ *imidazopyridine sedative/hypnotic* [zolpidem tartrate] 5, 10 mg

AmBisome powder for IV infusion ℞ *systemic polyene antifungal for cryptococcal meningitis, visceral leishmaniasis, and histoplasmosis (orphan)* [amphotericin B lipid complex (ABLC)] 50 mg/vial

ambomycin USAN, INN *antineoplastic*

ambrette (*Abelmoschus moschatus*) seeds and oil *medicinal herb for gastric cancer, gonorrhea, hysteria, and respiratory disorders; also used as a fragrance in cosmetics and a flavoring in alcoholic beverages, bitters, and coffees; not generally regarded as safe and effective for medicinal uses*

ambroxol INN [also: ambroxol HCl]

ambroxol HCl JAN [also: ambroxol]

ambruticin USAN, INN *antifungal*

ambucaine INN, DCF

ambucetamide INN, BAN

ambuphylline USAN *diuretic; smooth muscle relaxant* [also: bufylline]

ambuside USAN, INN, BAN *diuretic*

ambuterol [see: mabuterol]

ambutonium bromide BAN

ambutoxate [see: ambucaine]

amcinafal USAN, INN *anti-inflammatory*

amcinafide USAN, INN *anti-inflammatory*

amcinonide USAN, USP, INN, BAN, JAN *topical corticosteroidal anti-inflammatory*

Amcort IM injection ℞ *corticosteroid; anti-inflammatory* [triamcinolone diacetate] 40 mg/mL

amdinocillin USAN, USP *aminopenicillin antibiotic* [also: mecillinam]

amdinocillin pivoxil USAN *antibacterial* [also: pivmecillinam; pivmecillinam HCl]

ameban [see: carbarsone]

amebarsone [see: carbarsone]

amebicides *a class of drugs that kill amoebae*

amebucort INN

amechol [see: methacholine chloride]

amedalin INN *antidepressant* [also: amedalin HCl]

amedalin HCl USAN *antidepressant* [also: amedalin]

Amelorad *investigational agent to reduce chemotherapy side effects (clinical trials discontinued 1998)* [EF-27 (code name—generic name not yet assigned)]

ameltolide USAN, INN, BAN *anticonvulsant*

Amen tablets ℞ *progestin for secondary amenorrhea, abnormal uterine bleeding, and endometrial hyperplasia* [medroxyprogesterone acetate] 10 mg

amenozine [see: amanozine]

Amerge film-coated tablets ℞ *vascular serotonin 5-HT$_1$ receptor agonist for migraine headache* [naratriptan HCl] 1, 2.5 mg

Americaine ointment, anorectal ointment, aerosol spray OTC *topical local anesthetic* [benzocaine] 20%

Americaine Anesthetic Lubricant gel ℞ *anesthetic lubricant for upper GI procedures* [benzocaine] 20%

Americaine First Aid ointment OTC *topical local anesthetic* [benzocaine] 20%

Americaine Otic ear drops ℞ *topical local anesthetic* [benzocaine] 20%

American angelica *medicinal herb* [see: angelica]

American aspen *medicinal herb* [see: poplar]

American centaury (Sabatia angularis) *plant medicinal herb used as a bitter tonic, emmenagogue, febrifuge, and vermifuge*

American elder *medicinal herb* [see: elderberry]

American elm *medicinal herb* [see: slippery elm]

American foxglove *medicinal herb* [see: feverweed]

American ginseng (Panax quinquefolia) *medicinal herb* [see: ginseng]

American hellebore (Veratrum viride) [see: hellebore]

American ivy (Parthenocissus quinquefolia) *bark and twigs medicinal herb used as an alterative, astringent, and expectorant*

American nightshade *medicinal herb* [see: pokeweed]

American pepper; American red pepper *medicinal herb* [see: cayenne]

American saffron *medicinal herb* [see: safflower]

American valerian *medicinal herb* [see: lady's slipper]

American vegetable tallow tree; American vegetable wax *medicinal herb* [see: bayberry]

American woodbine *medicinal herb* [see: American ivy]

americium *element (Am)*

amesergide USAN, INN *serotonin antagonist; investigational antidepressant*

ametantrone INN *antineoplastic* [also: ametantrone acetate]

ametantrone acetate USAN *antineoplastic* [also: ametantrone]

ametazole BAN [also: betazole HCl; betazole]

A-Methapred powder for injection ℞ *corticosteroid; anti-inflammatory; immunosuppressant* [methylprednisolone sodium succinate] 40, 125, 500, 1000 mg/vial

amethocaine BAN *topical anesthetic* [also: tetracaine]

amethocaine HCl BAN *local anesthetic* [also: tetracaine HCl]

amethopterin [now: methotrexate]

amezepine INN

amezinium metilsulfate INN, JAN

amfebutamone INN *aminoketone antidepressant; non-nicotine aid to smoking cessation* [also: bupropion HCl; bupropion]

amfebutamone HCl [see: bupropion HCl]

amfecloral INN, BAN *anorectic* [also: amphecloral]

amfenac INN, BAN *anti-inflammatory* [also: amfenac sodium]

amfenac sodium USAN, JAN *anti-inflammatory* [also: amfenac]

amfepentorex INN, DCF

amfepramone INN, DCF *anorexiant* [also: diethylpropion HCl; diethylpropion]

amfepramone HCl *anorexiant* [see: diethylpropion HCl]

amfetamine INN *CNS stimulant* [also: amphetamine sulfate; amphetamine]

amfetaminil INN

amfilcon A USAN *hydrophilic contact lens material*

amflutizole USAN, INN *gout suppressant*

amfodyne [see: imidecyl iodine]

amfomycin INN, DCF *antibacterial* [also: amphomycin]

amfonelic acid USAN, INN, BAN *CNS stimulant*

Amgenal Cough syrup ℞ *narcotic antitussive; antihistamine* [codeine phosphate; bromodiphenhydramine HCl] 10•12.5 mg/5 mL

amibiarson [see: carbarsone]

Amicar tablets, syrup, IV infusion ℞ *systemic hemostatic to control excessive bleeding* [aminocaproic acid] 500 mg; 250 mg/mL; 250 mg/mL ⃞ Amikin

amicarbalide INN, BAN

amicibone INN

amicloral USAN *veterinary food additive*

amicycline USAN, INN *antibacterial*

amidantel INN, BAN

amidapsone USAN, INN *antiviral for poultry*

Amidate IV injection ℞ *rapid-acting nonbarbiturate general anesthetic* [etomidate] 2 mg/mL

amidefrine mesilate INN *adrenergic* [also: amidephrine mesylate; amidephrine]

amidephrine BAN *adrenergic* [also: amidephrine mesylate; amidefrine mesilate]

amidephrine mesylate USAN *adrenergic* [also: amidefrine mesilate; amidephrine]

amidofebrin [see: aminopyrine]

amidol [see: dimepheptanol]

amidone HCl [see: methadone HCl]

amidopyrazoline [see: aminopyrine]

amidopyrine [now: aminopyrine]

amidotrizoate sodium [see: diatrizoate sodium]

amidotrizoic acid JAN *radiopaque contrast medium* [also: diatrizoic acid]

Ami-Drix sustained-release tablets (discontinued 1995) ℞ *decongestant; antihistamine* [pseudoephedrine sulfate; dexbrompheniramine maleate] 120•6 mg

amiflamine INN

amifloverine INN, DCF

amifloxacin USAN, INN, BAN *broad-spectrum fluoroquinolone antibiotic*

amifloxacin mesylate USAN *antibacterial*

amifostine USAN, INN, BAN *chemoprotective agent for cisplatin and paclitaxel chemotherapy (orphan); radioprotective agent; investigational (orphan) for cyclophosphamide rescue*

Amigesic film-coated tablets, film-coated caplets, capsules ℞ *analgesic; antipyretic; anti-inflammatory; antirheumatic* [salsalate] 500 mg; 750 mg; 500 mg

amikacin USP, INN, BAN *aminoglycoside antibiotic*

amikacin sulfate USAN, USP, JAN *aminoglycoside antibiotic* 50, 250 mg/mL injection

amikhelline INN

Amikin IV or IM injection, pediatric injection ℞ *aminoglycoside antibiotic* [amikacin sulfate] 250 mg/mL; 50 mg/mL ⑨ Amicar

amilomer INN

amiloride INN, BAN *antihypertensive; potassium-sparing diuretic* [also: amiloride HCl]

amiloride HCl USAN, USP *antihypertensive; potassium-sparing diuretic; investigational (orphan) inhalant for cystic fibrosis* [also: amiloride]

aminacrine BAN *topical anti-infective/antiseptic* [also: aminacrine HCl; aminoacridine]

aminacrine HCl USAN *vaginal antibacterial/antiseptic* [also: aminoacridine; aminacrine]

Amin-Aid Instant Drink powder (discontinued 1997) OTC *enteral nutritional therapy for acute or chronic renal failure* [essential amino acids]

aminarsone [see: carbarsone]

amindocate INN

amine resin [see: polyamine-methylene resin]

amineptine INN

Aminess 5.2% IV infusion ℞ *nutritional therapy for renal failure* [multiple essential amino acids]

aminicotin [see: niacinamide]

aminitrozole INN *veterinary antibacterial* [also: nithiamide; acinitrazole]

2-amino-2-deoxyglucose [see: glucosamine]

aminoacetic acid JAN *nonessential amino acid; urologic irrigant; symbols:* Gly, G [also: glycine]

aminoacridine INN *topical anti-infective/antiseptic* [also: aminacrine HCl; aminacrine]

aminoacridine HCl [see: aminacrine HCl]

9-aminoacridine monohydrochloride [see: aminacrine HCl]

p-aminobenzenearsonic acid [see: arsanilic acid]

p-aminobenzenesulfonamide [see: sulfanilamide]

p-aminobenzene-sulfonylacetylimide [see: sulfacetamide]

aminobenzoate potassium USP *analgesic; "possibly effective" for scleroderma and other skin diseases, and Peyronie's disease*

aminobenzoate sodium USP *analgesic*

p-aminobenzoic acid [see: aminobenzoic acid]

aminobenzoic acid (4-aminobenzoic acid) USP *ultraviolet screen*

aminobenzylpenicillin [see: ampicillin]

γ-amino-β-hydroxybutyric acid JAN

aminobromophenylpyrimidinone (ABPP) [see: bropirimine]

γ-aminobutyric acid JAN

9-aminocamptothecin (9-AC) *investigational (Phase I/II) anticancer agent*

aminocaproic acid USAN, USP, INN, BAN *systemic hemostatic; investigational (orphan) topical treatment for traumatic hyphema of the eye* [also: ε-aminocaproic acid] 250 mg/mL injection

ε-aminocaproic acid JAN *systemic hemostatic* [also: aminocaproic acid]

aminocardol [see: aminophylline]

Amino-Cerv pH 5.5 vaginal cream ℞ *emollient; antifungal; anti-inflammatory* [urea; sodium propionate; methionine; cystine; inositol] 8.34%•0.5%•0.83%•0.35%•0.83%

aminodeoxykanamycin [see: bekanamycin]

2-aminoethanethiol [see: cysteamine]

2-aminoethanethiol HCl [see: cysteamine HCl]

2-aminoethanol [see: monoethanolamine]

aminoethyl nitrate (2-aminoethyl nitrate) INN, DCF

amino-ethyl-propanol [see: ambuphylline]

aminoethylsulfonic acid JAN [also: taurine]

aminoform [see: methenamine]

aminoglutethimide USP, INN, BAN *adrenal steroid inhibitor; antisteroidal antineoplastic*

aminoglycosides *a class of bactericidal antibiotics effective against gram-negative organisms*

aminoguanidine monohydrochloride [see: pimagedine HCl]

6-aminohexanoic acid [see: aminocaproic acid]

aminohippurate sodium USP *diagnostic aid for renal function* [also: *p*-aminohippurate sodium] 20% injection

p-**aminohippurate sodium** JAN *renal function test* [also: aminohippurate sodium]

aminohippuric acid (*p*-aminohippuric acid) USP

aminohydroxypropylidene diphosphonate (APD) [see: pamidronate disodium]

aminoisobutanol [see: ambuphylline]

aminoisometradine [see: methionine]

aminoketones *a class of oral antidepressants*

5-aminolevulinic acid HCl (5-ALA HCl) USAN *investigational (Phase III) photosensitizer for photodynamic therapy of precancerous actinic keratoses of the skin*

aminometradine INN, BAN

Amino-Min-D capsules OTC *dietary supplement* [calcium carbonate; multiple minerals; vitamin D] 250 mg• ± •100 IU

aminonat [see: protein hydrolysate]

Amino-Opti-C sustained-release tablets OTC *dietary supplement* [vitamin C; lemon & rose hips bioflavonoids; rutin; hesperidin] 1000• 250• ± • ± mg

Amino-Opti-E capsules OTC *dietary supplement* [vitamin E] 165 mg

aminopenicillins *a subclass of penicillins (q.v.)*

aminopentamide sulfate [see: dimevamide]

aminophenazone INN [also: aminopyrine]

aminophenazone cyclamate INN

p-**aminophenylarsonic acid** [see: arsanilic acid]

aminophylline USP, INN, BAN, JAN *smooth muscle relaxant; bronchodilator* 100, 200 mg oral; 105 mg/5 mL oral; 250 mg/10 mL injection; 250, 500 suppositories

aminopromazine INN, DCF [also: proquamezine]

aminopterin sodium INN, BAN, DCF *investigational (Phase II) antifolate for breast and ovarian cancer*

4-aminopyridine [see: fampridine]

aminopyrine NF, JAN [also: aminophenazone]

aminoquin naphthoate [see: pamaquine naphthoate]

aminoquinol INN

aminoquinoline [see: aminoquinol]

4-aminoquinoline [see: chloroquine phosphate]

8-aminoquinoline [see: primaquine phosphate]

aminoquinuride INN

aminorex USAN, INN, BAN *anorectic*

aminosalicylate calcium USP [also: calcium para-aminosalicylate]

aminosalicylate potassium USP

aminosalicylate sodium (*p*-aminosalicylate sodium) USP *bacteriostatic; tuberculosis retreatment agent; investigational (orphan) for Crohn's disease*

aminosalicylic acid (4-aminosalicylic acid) USP *antibacterial; tuberculostatic (orphan); investigational (orphan) for ulcerative colitis*

5-aminosalicylic acid (5-ASA) [see: mesalamine]

aminosalyle sodium [see: aminosalicylate sodium]

aminosidine *investigational (orphan) for tuberculosis, Mycobacterium avium complex, and visceral leishmaniasis*

aminosidine sulfate [see: paromomycin sulfate]

21-aminosteroids *a class of potent antioxidants that can protect against oxygen radical–mediated lipid peroxidation and progressive neuronal degeneration following brain or spinal trauma, subarachnoid hemorrhage, or stroke* [also called: lazaroids]

aminosuccinic acid [see: aspartic acid]

Aminosyn 3.5% (5%, 7%, 8.5%, 10%); Aminosyn (pH6) 10%; Aminosyn II 3.5% (5%, 7%, 8.5%, 10%, 15%); Aminosyn-PF 7% (10%) IV infusion ℞ *total parenteral nutrition (except 3.5%); peripheral parenteral nutrition (all)* [multiple essential and nonessential amino acids]

Aminosyn 3.5% M; Aminosyn II 3.5% M IV infusion ℞ *peripheral parenteral nutrition* [multiple essential and nonessential amino acids; electrolytes]

Aminosyn 7% (8.5%) with Electrolytes; Aminosyn II 7% (8.5%, 10%) with Electrolytes IV infusion ℞ *total parenteral nutrition; peripheral parenteral nutrition* [multiple essential and nonessential amino acids; electrolytes]

Aminosyn II 3.5% in 5% (25%) Dextrose; Aminosyn II 4.25% in 10% (20%, 25%) Dextrose; Aminosyn II 5% in 25% Dextrose IV infusion ℞ *total parenteral nutrition (except 3.5% in 5%); peripheral parenteral nutrition (not 20% and 25%)* [multiple essential and nonessential amino acids; dextrose]

Aminosyn II 3.5% M in 5% Dextrose; Aminosyn II 4.25% M in 10% Dextrose IV infusion ℞ *total parenteral nutrition (4.25% in 10% only); peripheral parenteral nutrition (both)* [multiple essential and nonessential amino acids; electrolytes; dextrose]

Aminosyn-HBC 7% IV infusion ℞ *nutritional therapy for high metabolic stress* [multiple branched-chain essential and nonessential amino acids; electrolytes]

Aminosyn-RF 5.2% IV infusion ℞ *nutritional therapy for renal failure* [multiple essential amino acids]

aminothiazole INN

aminotrate phosphate [see: trolnitrate phosphate]

aminoxaphen [see: aminorex]

aminoxytriphene INN

aminoxytropine tropate HCl [see: atropine oxide HCl]

Amio-Aqueous ℞ *antiarrhythmic for acute ventricular tachycardia and fibrillation (orphan)* [amiodarone HCl]

amiodarone USAN, INN, BAN *ventricular antiarrhythmic*

amiodarone HCl *ventricular antiarrhythmic for acute ventricular tachycardia and fibrillation (orphan)* 200 mg oral

Amipaque powder for injection (discontinued 1999) ℞ *radiopaque contrast medium* [metrizamide (48.25% iodine)] 13.5%, 18.75%

amiperone INN

amiphenazole INN, BAN

amipizone INN

amipramidine [see: amiloride HCl]

amiprilose INN *anti-inflammatory* [also: amiprilose HCl]

amiprilose HCl USAN *investigational (Phase III) anti-inflammatory for rheumatoid arthritis* [also: amiprilose]

amiquinsin INN *antihypertensive* [also: amiquinsin HCl]

amiquinsin HCl USAN *antihypertensive* [also: amiquinsin]

amisometradine NF, INN, BAN

amisulpride INN

amiterol INN

Ami-Tex LA long-acting tablets ℞ *decongestant; expectorant* [phenylpropanolamine HCl; guaifenesin] 75•400 mg

amithiozone [see: thioacetazone; thiacetazone]

amitivir INN *investigational influenza vaccine*

Amitone chewable tablets OTC *antacid* [calcium carbonate] 350 mg

amitraz USAN, INN, BAN *scabicide*

amitriptyline (AMT) INN, BAN *tricyclic antidepressant* [also: amitriptyline HCl] ② nortriptyline

amitriptyline HCl USP, JAN *tricyclic antidepressant* [also: amitriptyline] 10, 25, 50, 75, 100, 150 mg oral

amitriptylinoxide INN

amixetrine INN, DCF
AmLactin cream, lotion OTC *moisturizer; emollient* [ammonium lactate] 12%
amlexanox USAN, INN, JAN *antiallergic; anti-inflammatory; aphthous ulcer treatment*
amlintide USAN *antidiabetic for type 1 diabetes mellitus*
amlodipine INN, BAN *antianginal; antihypertensive; calcium channel blocker* [also: amlodipine besylate]
amlodipine besylate USAN *antianginal; antihypertensive; calcium channel blocker* [also: amlodipine]
amlodipine maleate USAN *antianginal; antihypertensive*
ammi *(Ammi majus; A. visnaga)* dried ripe fruits *medicinal herb for angina, bronchial asthma, diabetes, diuresis, kidney and bladder stones, psoriasis, respiratory diseases, and vitiligo*
ammoidin [see: methoxsalen]
[^{13}N]ammonia [see: ammonia N 13]
ammonia [see: ammonia spirit, aromatic]
ammonia N 13 USAN, USP *radioactive diagnostic aid for cardiac and liver imaging*
ammonia solution, strong NF *solvent; source of ammonia* [also: ammonia water]
ammonia spirit, aromatic USP *respiratory stimulant*
ammonia water JAN *solvent; source of ammonia* [also: ammonia solution, strong]
ammoniated mercury [see: mercury, ammoniated]
ammonio methacrylate copolymer NF *coating agent*
ammonium alum [see: alum, ammonium]
ammonium benzoate USP
ammonium biphosphate *urinary acidifier*
ammonium carbonate NF *source of ammonia*

ammonium chloride USP, JAN *urinary acidifier; diuretic; expectorant* 486, 500 mg oral; 5 mEq/mL (26.75%) injection
ammonium 2-hydroxypropanoate [see: ammonium lactate]
ammonium ichthosulfonate [see: ichthammol]
ammonium lactate (lactic acid neutralized with ammonium hydroxide) USAN *antipruritic; emollient for xerosis*
ammonium mandelate USP
ammonium molybdate USP *dietary molybdenum supplement* 25 μg/mL injection
ammonium molybdate tetrahydrate [see: ammonium molybdate]
ammonium phosphate NF *pharmaceutic aid*
ammonium salicylate NF
ammonium tetrathiomolybdate *investigational (orphan) for Wilson's disease*
ammonium valerate NF
ammophyllin [see: aminophylline]
Amnaranthus spp. *medicinal herb* [see: amaranth]
AMO Endosol; AMO Endosol Extra ophthalmic solution ℞ *intraocular irrigating solution* [sodium chloride (balanced saline solution)]
AMO Vitrax intraocular injection ℞ *viscoelastic agent for ophthalmic surgery* [hyaluronate sodium] 30 mg/mL
amobarbital USP, INN, JAN *sedative; hypnotic; anticonvulsant; also abused as a street drug* [also: amylobarbitone]
amobarbital sodium USP, JAN *hypnotic; sedative; anticonvulsant; also abused as a street drug*
amocaine chloride [see: amolanone HCl]
amocarzine INN
amodiaquine USP, INN, BAN *antiprotozoal*
amodiaquine HCl USP *antimalarial*
Amodopa tablets (discontinued 1998) ℞ *antihypertensive* [methyldopa] 125, 250, 500 mg
amogastrin INN, JAN

amolanone INN
amolanone HCl [see: amolanone]
amonafide INN *investigational antineo-plastic*
Amoni-Opti-E capsules OTC *vitamin supplement* [vitamin E]
amoproxan INN, DCF
amopyroquine INN
amorolfine USAN, INN, BAN *antimycotic*
Amorphophallus konjac medicinal herb [see: glucomannan]
Amosan powder OTC *oral antibacterial* [sodium peroxyborate monohydrate]
amoscanate INN
amosulalol INN [also: amosulalol HCl]
amosulalol HCl JAN [also: amosulalol]
amotriphene [see: aminoxytriphene]
amoxapine USAN, USP, INN, BAN, JAN *tricyclic antidepressant* 25, 50, 100, 150 mg oral ② amoxicillin; Amoxil
amoxecaine INN
amoxicillin USAN, USP, JAN *aminopenicillin antibiotic* [also: amoxicilline; amoxycillin] 125, 250, 500 mg oral; 125, 250 mg/5 mL oral ② amoxapine
amoxicillin sodium USAN *aminopenicillin antibiotic*
amoxicilline INN *aminopenicillin antibiotic* [also: amoxicillin; amoxycillin]
Amoxil capsules, tablets, chewable tablets, powder for oral suspension, pediatric drops ℞ *aminopenicillin antibiotic* [amoxicillin] 250, 500 mg; 500, 875 mg; 125, 250 mg; 125, 250 mg/5 mL; 50 mg/mL ② amoxapine
amoxycillin BAN *aminopenicillin antibiotic* [also: amoxicillin; amoxicilline]
amoxydramine camsilate INN [also: amoxydramine camsylate]
amoxydramine camsylate DCF [also: amoxydramine camsilate]
AMP; A₅MP (adenosine monophosphate) [see: adenosine phosphate]
amperozide INN, BAN *investigational antipsychotic for schizophrenia*
amphecloral USAN *anorectic* [also: amfecloral]
amphenidone INN
amphetamine BAN *CNS stimulant; widely abused as a street drug, which*
causes strong psychic dependence [also: amphetamine sulfate; amfetamine]
***d*-amphetamine** [see: dextroamphetamine]
(+)-amphetamine [see: dextroamphetamine]
***l*-amphetamine** [see: levamphetamine]
(−)-amphetamine [see: levamphetamine]
amphetamine aspartate *CNS stimulant*
amphetamine complex (resin complex of amphetamine & dextroamphetamine) [q.v.]
amphetamine phosphate, dextro [see: dextroamphetamine phosphate]
amphetamine succinate, levo [see: levamphetamine succinate]
amphetamine sulfate USP *CNS stimulant; widely abused as a street drug, which causes strong psychic dependence* [also: amfetamine; amphetamine] 5, 10 mg oral
amphetamine sulfate, dextro [see: dextroamphetamine sulfate]
amphetamines *a class of CNS stimulants that includes amphetamine, dextroamphetamine, levamphetamine, methamphetamine, and their salts*
amphocortrin [see: amphomycin]
Amphojel tablets, oral suspension OTC *antacid* [aluminum hydroxide gel] 300, 600 mg; 320 mg/5 mL ② Amphocil
amphomycin USAN, BAN *antibacterial* [also: amfomycin]
amphotalide INN, DCF
Amphotec powder for IV infusion ℞ *systemic polyene antifungal for invasive aspergillosis* [amphotericin B cholesteryl sulfate] 50, 100 mg
amphotericin B USP, INN, BAN, JAN *polyene antifungal*
amphotericin B cholesteryl sulfate *systemic polyene antifungal for invasive aspergillosis*
amphotericin B deoxycholate *systemic polyene antifungal* 50 mg injection
amphotericin B lipid complex (ABLC) *systemic polyene antifungal*

for meningitis, leishmaniasis, histoplasmosis, and other invasive infections (orphan)

ampicillin USAN, USP, INN, BAN, JAN *aminopenicillin antibiotic* 250, 500 mg oral; 125, 250 mg/5 mL oral

ampicillin sodium USAN, USP, JAN *aminopenicillin antibiotic* 125, 250, 500 mg, 1, 2, 10 g injection

ampiroxicam INN, BAN

Amplicor Chlamydia test kit for professional use *in vitro diagnostic aid for Chlamydia trachomatis* [DNA amplification test]

Amplicor HIV-1 Monitor test kit for professional use *in vitro diagnostic aid for HIV-1 in blood* [polymerase chain reaction (PCR) test]

Amplicor MTB test kit for professional use *in vitro diagnostic aid for Mycobacterium tuberculosis* [polymerase chain reaction (PCR) test]

Ampligen ℞ *investigational (Phase III, orphan) RNA synthesis inhibitor and immunomodulator for AIDS, renal cell carcinoma, metastatic melanoma, and chronic fatigue syndrome* [poly I: poly C12U]

amprenavir USAN *antiviral protease inhibitor for HIV*

amprocidum [see: amprolium]

amprolium USP, INN, BAN *coccidiostat for poultry*

amprotropine phosphate

ampyrimine INN

ampyzine INN *CNS stimulant* [also: ampyzine sulfate]

ampyzine sulfate USAN *CNS stimulant* [also: ampyzine]

amquinate USAN, INN *antimalarial*

amrinone USAN, INN, BAN *cardiotonic*

amrinone lactate *vasodilator for congestive heart failure*

amrubicin INN

AMSA; m-AMSA (acridinylamine methanesulfon anisidide) [see: amsacrine]

amsacrine USAN, INN, BAN *investigational (NDA filed) antineoplastic for*

acute adult leukemias (AML, APL, and ALL) and lymphomas

Amsidyl ℞ *investigational (NDA filed) antineoplastic for acute adult leukemias (AML, APL, and ALL) and lymphomas* [amsacrine]

amsonate INN, BAN *combining name for radicals or groups*

AMT (amitriptyline HCl) [q.v.]

amtolmetin guacil INN

Amvisc; Amvisc Plus intraocular injection ℞ *viscoelastic agent for ophthalmic surgery* [hyaluronate sodium] 12 mg/mL; 16 mg/mL

amyl alcohol, tertiary [see: amylene hydrate]

amyl nitrite USP, JAN *vasodilator; antianginal; also abused as a euphoric street drug and sexual stimulant* 0.3 mL inhalant

amylase *digestive enzyme* [100 IU/mg in pancrelipase; 25 IU/mg in pancreatin]

amylase [see: alpha amylase]

amylene hydrate NF *solvent*

amylin [see: amlintide]

amylmetacresol INN, BAN

amylobarbitone BAN *sedative; hypnotic; anticonvulsant* [also: amobarbital]

amylocaine BAN

amylopectin sulfate, sodium salt [see: sodium amylosulfate]

amylosulfate sodium [see: sodium amylosulfate]

Amytal Sodium powder for injection ℞ *sedative; hypnotic; anxiolytic; anticonvulsant; also abused as a street drug* [amobarbital sodium]

anabolic steroids *a class of hormones derived from or closely related to testosterone that increase anabolic (tissue-building) and decrease catabolic (tissue-depleting) processes*

Anacin caplets, tablets OTC *analgesic; antipyretic; anti-inflammatory* [aspirin; caffeine] 400•32 mg; 400•32, 500•32 mg ⊘ Unisom; Unasyn

Anacin, Aspirin Free tablets, caplets, gelcaps OTC *analgesic; antipyretic* [acetaminophen] 500 mg ⊘ Unisom; Unasyn

Anacin P.M., Aspirin Free film-coated caplets OTC *antihistaminic sleep aid; analgesic* [diphenhydramine HCl; acetaminophen] 25•500 mg ② Unisom; Unasyn

Anadrol-50 tablets ℞ *anabolic steroid for anemias; also abused as a street drug* [oxymetholone] 50 mg

anafebrina [see: aminopyrine]

Anafranil capsules ℞ *tricyclic antidepressant for obsessive-compulsive disorders* [clomipramine HCl] 25, 50, 75 mg ② enalapril

anagestone INN *progestin* [also: anagestone acetate]

anagestone acetate USAN *progestin* [also: anagestone]

anagrelide INN *antithrombotic/antiplatelet drug for essential thrombocythemia (orphan); investigational (orphan) for thrombocytosis and polycythemia vera* [also: anagrelide HCl]

anagrelide HCl USAN *antithrombotic/ antiplatelet drug for essential thrombocythemia (orphan); investigational (orphan) for thrombocytosis and polycythemia vera* [also: anagrelide]

Ana-Guard subcu or IM injection ℞ *sympathomimetic bronchodilator for emergency treatment of anaphylaxis; vasopressor for shock* [epinephrine] 1:1000

anakinra USAN, INN *nonsteroidal anti-inflammatory for inflammatory bowel disease; investigational (orphan) for juvenile rheumatoid arthritis and graft vs. host disease*

Ana-Kit ℞ *emergency treatment of anaphylaxis* [epinephrine; chlorpheniramine maleate; alcohol; tourniquet] 1:100 000•2 mg

analeptics *a class of central nervous system stimulants used to maintain or improve alertness*

Analgesia Creme OTC *topical analgesic* [trolamine salicylate] 10%

Analgesic Balm OTC *topical analgesic; counterirritant* [methyl salicylate; menthol]

analgesics *a class of drugs that relieve pain or reduce sensitivity to pain without causing loss of consciousness*

analgesine [see: antipyrine]

Analpram-HC anorectal cream ℞ *topical corticosteroidal anti-inflammatory; local anesthetic* [hydrocortisone acetate; pramoxine] 1%•1%, 2.5%•1% ② Analbalm

Anamine syrup ℞ *decongestant; antihistamine* [pseudoephedrine HCl; chlorpheniramine maleate] 30•2 mg/5 mL

Anamine T.D. sustained-release capsules ℞ *decongestant; antihistamine* [pseudoephedrine HCl; chlorpheniramine maleate] 120•8 mg

Anamirta cocculus; A. paniculata medicinal herb [see: levant berry]

ananain *investigational (orphan) proteolytic enzymes for debridement of severe burns*

Ananas comosus medicinal herb [see: pineapple]

Anandron ⓐ (U.S. product: Nilandron) tablets (also available in Europe and Latin America) ℞ *antiandrogen antineoplastic adjunct to surgical or chemical castration for metastatic prostate cancer* [nilutamide] 50, 100 mg

Anaphalis margaritacea; Gnaphalium polycephalum; G. uliginosum medicinal herb [see: everlasting]

anaphrodisiacs *a class of agents that reduce sexual desire or potency*

Anaplex liquid ℞ *decongestant; antihistamine* [pseudoephedrine HCl; chlorpheniramine maleate] 30•2 mg/5 mL

Anaplex HD syrup ℞ *narcotic antitussive; decongestant; antihistamine* [hydrocodone bitartrate; phenylephrine HCl; chlorpheniramine maleate] 1.7•5•2 mg/5 mL

Anaplex SR sustained-release capsules (discontinued 1995) ℞ *decongestant; antihistamine* [pseudoephedrine HCl; chlorpheniramine maleate] 120•8 mg

Anaprox; Anaprox DS film-coated tablets ℞ *nonsteroidal anti-inflammatory drug (NSAID); antiarthritic; anal-*

gesic [naproxen (from naproxen sodium)] 250 (275) mg; 500 (550) mg

anarel [see: guanadrel sulfate]

anaritide INN, BAN *antihypertensive; diuretic* [also: anaritide acetate]

anaritide acetate USAN *antihypertensive; diuretic; investigational (orphan) for acute renal failure and renal transplants; clinical trials discontinued 1997; orphan status withdrawn 1998*

Anaspaz tablets ℞ *GI antispasmodic; anticholinergic* [hyoscyamine sulfate] 0.125 mg

anastrozole USAN, INN, BAN *hormone antagonist antineoplastic/aromatase inhibitor for advanced breast cancer*

Anatrast rectal paste ℞ *radiopaque contrast medium for defecography* [barium sulfate] 100%

Anatrofin *brand name for stenbolone acetate, an anabolic steroid abused as a street drug*

Anatuss film-coated tablets ℞ *antitussive; decongestant; expectorant; analgesic* [dextromethorphan hydrobromide; phenylpropanolamine HCl; guaifenesin; acetaminophen] 15•25•100•325 mg

Anatuss syrup OTC *antitussive; decongestant; expectorant* [dextromethorphan hydrobromide; phenylpropanolamine HCl; guaifenesin] 15•25•100 mg/5 mL

Anatuss DM tablets, syrup OTC *antitussive; decongestant; expectorant* [dextromethorphan hydrobromide; pseudoephedrine HCl; guaifenesin] 20•60•400 mg; 10•30•100 mg/5 mL

Anatuss LA long-acting tablets ℞ *decongestant; expectorant* [pseudoephedrine HCl; guaifenesin] 120•400 mg

Anavar *brand name for oxandrolone, an anabolic steroid abused as a street drug*

anaxirone INN

anayodin [see: chiniofon]

anazocine INN

anazolene sodium USAN, INN *blood volume and cardiac output test* [also: sodium anoxynaphthonate]

Anbesol liquid, gel OTC *topical oral anesthetic; antipruritic/counterirritant; antiseptic* [benzocaine; phenol; alcohol 70%] 6.3%•0.5%

Anbesol, Baby gel OTC *topical oral anesthetic* [benzocaine] 7.5%

Anbesol, Maximum Strength liquid, gel OTC *mucous membrane anesthetic* [benzocaine; alcohol 60%] 20%

ancarolol INN

Ancef powder or frozen premix for IV or IM injection ℞ *cephalosporin antibiotic* [cefazolin sodium] 0.5, 1, 5, 10 g

ancestim USAN *investigational (NDA filed) hematopoietic growth factor; investigational (orphan) adjunct to myelosuppressive and myeloablative therapy*

Ancet liquid OTC *soap-free therapeutic skin cleanser*

anchusa *medicinal herb* [see: henna (Alkanna)]

ancitabine INN [also: ancitabine HCl]

ancitabine HCl JAN [also: ancitabine]

Ancobon capsules ℞ *antifungal* [flucytosine] 250, 500 mg ② Oncovin

ancrod USAN, INN, BAN *anticoagulant enzyme derived from the venom of the Malayan pit viper; investigational (orphan) antithrombotic for heparin-induced thrombocytopenia or thrombosis*

andolast INN

andrachne *(Andrachne aspera; A. cordifolia; A. phyllanthoides)* root *medicinal herb for eye inflammation; not generally regarded as safe and effective*

Andro 100; Andro 200 [see: depAndro 100; depAndro 200]

Andro L.A. 200 IM injection ℞ *androgen replacement for delayed puberty or breast cancer* [testosterone enanthate] 200 mg/mL

Androcur *orphan status withdrawn 1996* [cyproterone acetate]

Androderm transdermal patch (for nonscrotal area) ℞ *hormone replacement therapy for hypogonadism* [testosterone] 2.5, 5 mg/day

Andro/Fem IM injection (discontinued 1995) ℞ *estrogen/androgen for*

menopausal vasomotor symptoms [estradiol cypionate; testosterone cypionate] 2•50 mg/mL

Androgel *investigational (orphan) for AIDS-wasting syndrome; investigational (NDA filed) for testosterone deficiency in men* [testosterone]

Androgel-DHT ℞ *investigational (Phase III) transdermal testosterone replacement in elderly men; investigational (orphan) for AIDS-wasting syndrome* [dihydrotestosterone]

androgens *a class of sex hormones responsible for the development of the male sex organs and secondary sex characteristics*

Androgyn [see: depAndrogyn]

Android-10; Android-25 tablets ℞ *androgen for male hypogonadism, cryptorchidism, impotence, and female breast cancer* [methyltestosterone] 10 mg; 25 mg

Androlone-D 200 IM injection ℞ *anabolic steroid for anemia of renal insufficiency* [nandrolone decanoate] 200 mg/mL

Andropogon citratus medicinal herb [see: lemongrass]

Andropository-200 IM injection ℞ *androgen replacement for delayed puberty or breast cancer* [testosterone enanthate] 200 mg/mL

androstanazole [now: stanozolol]

androstane [see: androstanolone; stanolone]

androstanolone INN *investigational (orphan) for AIDS-wasting syndrome* [also: stanolone]

androtest P [see: testosterone propionate]

Androtest-SL sublingual tablets ℞ *investigational (NDA filed) treatment for hypogonadism; investigational (orphan) for delay of growth and puberty in boys* [testosterone]

Androvite tablets OTC *vitamin/mineral/ iron supplement* [multiple vitamins & minerals; iron; folic acid; biotin] ±• 3•0.06• ≟ mg

anecortave acetate USAN *angiostatic steroid for neovascularization of the eye*

Anectine IV or IM injection, Flo-Pack (powder for injection) ℞ *muscle relaxant; anesthesia adjunct* [succinylcholine chloride] 20 mg/mL; 500, 1000 mg

Anemone patens medicinal herb [see: pasque flower]

Anergan 25 injection (discontinued 1995) ℞ *antihistamine; motion sickness; sleep aid; antiemetic; sedative* [promethazine HCl] 25 mg/mL

Anergan 50 IM injection ℞ *antihistamine; sedative; antiemetic; motion sickness relief* [promethazine HCl] 50 mg/mL

anertan [see: testosterone propionate]

AnervaX *investigational (Phase II) therapeutic peptide vaccine for rheumatoid arthritis*

Anestacon jelly ℞ *mucous membrane anesthetic* [lidocaine HCl] 2%

anesthesin [see: benzocaine]

anesthetics *a class of agents that abolish the sensation of pain*

anesthrone [see: benzocaine]

anethaine [see: tetracaine HCl]

anethole NF *flavoring agent*

anetholtrithion JAN

Anethum foeniculum medicinal herb [see: fennel]

Anethum graveolens medicinal herb [see: dill]

aneurine HCl [see: thiamine HCl]

Anexsia 5/500; Anexsia 7.5/650; Anexsia 10/660 tablets ℞ *narcotic analgesic* [hydrocodone bitartrate; acetaminophen] 5•500 mg; 7.5•650 mg; 10•660 mg

angelica (*Angelica atropurpurea*) root *medicinal herb for appetite stimulation, bronchial disorders, colds, colic, cough, exhaustion, gas, heartburn, and rheumatism; also used as a tonic*

Angelica levisticum medicinal herb [see: lovage]

Angelica polymorpha; A. sinensis; A. dahurica medicinal herb [see: dong quai]

Angio-Conray injection (discontinued 1999) ℞ *radiopaque contrast medium for angiography* [iothalamate sodium (59.9% iodine)] 800 mg/mL (480 mg/mL)

AngioMark injection ℞ *investigational (Phase II) MRI contrast medium for multiple cardiovascular indications* [MS-325 (code name—generic name not yet assigned)]

angiotensin II INN

angiotensin II receptor antagonists (AIIRAs) *a class of antihypertensives that reduce the vasoconstricting effects of angiotensin II by blocking the angiotensin II receptor sites in the vascular smooth muscles* [compare to: angiotensin-converting enzyme inhibitors]

angiotensin amide USAN, NF, BAN *vasoconstrictor* [also: angiotensinamide]

angiotensinamide INN *vasoconstrictor* [also: angiotensin amide]

angiotensin-converting enzyme inhibitors (ACEIs) *a class of antihypertensives that reduce the vasoconstricting effects of angiotensin II by blocking the enzyme (kininase II) that converts angiotensin I to angiotensin II* [compare to: angiotensin II receptor antagonists]

Angiovist 282 injection (discontinued 1999) ℞ *radiopaque contrast medium* [diatrizoate meglumine] 60%

Angiovist 292; Angiovist 370 injection (discontinued 1999) ℞ *radiopaque contrast medium* [diatrizoate meglumine; diatrizoate sodium (48.7% total iodine)] 52%•8% (29.3%); 66%•10% (37%)

anhidrotics *a class of agents that reduce or suppress perspiration* [also called: anidrotics; antihydrotics]

anhydrohydroxyprogesterone [now: ethisterone]

anhydrous lanolin [see: lanolin, anhydrous]

anidoxime USAN, INN, BAN *analgesic*

anidrotics *a class of agents that reduce or suppress perspiration* [also called: anhidrotics; antihydrotics]

anilamate INN

anileridine USP, INN, BAN *narcotic analgesic*

anileridine HCl USP *narcotic analgesic*

anilopam INN *analgesic* [also: anilopam HCl]

anilopam HCl USAN *analgesic* [also: anilopam]

Animal Shapes chewable tablets OTC *vitamin supplement* [multiple vitamins; folic acid] ±•0.3 mg

Animal Shapes + Iron chewable tablets OTC *vitamin/iron supplement* [multiple vitamins; iron; folic acid] ±•15•0.3 mg

anion exchange resin [see: polyamine-methylene resin]

anipamil INN

aniracetam USAN, INN *mental performance enhancer*

anirolac USAN, INN *anti-inflammatory; analgesic*

anisacril INN

anisatil USAN *combining name for radicals or groups*

anise (Pimpinella anisum) oil and seeds *medicinal herb for colic, convulsions, cough, gas, intestinal cleansing, iron-deficiency anemia, mucous discharge, promoting expectoration, and psoriasis; also used as an antibacterial, antimicrobial, and antiseptic*

anise oil NF

anise root; sweet anise *medicinal herb* [see: sweet cicely]

anisindione NF, INN, BAN *indandione-derivative anticoagulant*

anisopirol INN

anisopyradamine [see: pyrilamine maleate]

anisotropine methylbromide USAN, JAN *anticholinergic; peptic ulcer adjunct* [also: octatropine methylbromide] 50 mg oral

anisoylated plasminogen streptokinase activator complex (APSAC) [see: anistreplase]

anistreplase USAN, INN, BAN *fibrinolytic; thrombolytic enzyme for acute myocardial infarction*

Anisum officinarum; A. vulgare medicinal herb [see: anise]

anitrazafen USAN, INN *topical anti-inflammatory*

anodynes *a class of agents that lessen or relieve pain*

anodynine [see: antipyrine]

anodynon [see: ethyl chloride]

Anodynos tablets (discontinued 1995) OTC *analgesic; antipyretic; anti-inflammatory* [aspirin; salicylamide; caffeine] 420.6•34.4•34.4 mg

Anogesic ℞ *investigational (Phase III) topical treatment for hemorrhoids and anal fissures* [nitroglycerin]

Anoquan capsules ℞ *analgesic; sedative* [acetaminophen; caffeine; butalbital] 325•40•50 mg

anorectics *a class of central nervous system stimulants that suppress the appetite* [also called: anorexiants; anorexigenics]

Anorex capsules (discontinued 1996) ℞ *anorexiant; CNS stimulant* [phendimetrazine tartrate] 35 mg

anorexiants *a class of central nervous system stimulants that suppress the appetite* [also called: anorectics; anorexigenics]

anorexigenics *a class of central nervous system stimulants that suppress the appetite* [also called: anorexiants; anorectics]

anovlar [see: norethindrone & ethinyl estradiol]

anoxomer USAN *antioxidant; food additive*

anoxynaphthonate sodium [see: anazolene sodium]

anpirtoline INN

Ansaid tablets ℞ *nonsteroidal anti-inflammatory drug (NSAID); antiarthritic* [flurbiprofen] 50, 100 mg

ansamycin [see: rifabutin]

ansoxetine INN

Answer; Answer 2; Answer Plus 2 test kit for home use (discontinued 1995) OTC *in vitro diagnostic aid for urine pregnancy test*

Answer Ovulation test kit for home use OTC *in vitro diagnostic aid to predict ovulation time*

Answer Plus; Answer Quick & Simple test kit for home use OTC *in vitro diagnostic aid for urine pregnancy test*

Antabuse tablets ℞ *deterrent to alcohol consumption* [disulfiram] 250, 500 mg

Antacid chewable tablets OTC *antacid* [calcium carbonate] 500, 750 mg

Antacid oral suspension OTC *antacid* [aluminum hydroxide; magnesium hydroxide] 225•200 mg/5 mL

antacids *a class of drugs that neutralize gastric acid*

antafenite INN

antastan [see: antazoline HCl]

antazoline INN, BAN [also: antazoline HCl]

antazoline HCl USP [also: antazoline]

antazoline phosphate USP *antihistamine*

antazoline phosphate & naphazoline HCl *topical ocular antihistamine and decongestant* 0.5%•0.05%

Antazoline-V eye drops (discontinued 1995) ℞ *topical ophthalmic decongestant and antihistamine* [naphazoline HCl; antazoline phosphate] 0.05%•0.5%

antazonite INN

Antegren ℞ *investigational humanized monoclonal antibody for treatment of multiple sclerosis*

antelmycin INN *anthelmintic* [also: anthelmycin]

anterior pituitary

anthelmintics *a class of drugs effective against parasitic infections* [also called: vermicides; vermifuges]

anthelmycin USAN *anthelmintic* [also: antelmycin]

Anthemis nobilis medicinal herb [see: chamomile]

anthiolimine INN

Anthoxanthum odoratum medicinal herb [see: sweet vernal grass]

anthracyclines *a class of antibiotic antineoplastics*

Anthra-Derm ointment ℞ *topical antipsoriatic* [anthralin] 0.1%, 0.25%, 0.5%, 1%

anthralin USP *topical antipsoriatic* [also: dithranol]

anthramycin USAN *antineoplastic* [also: antramycin]

anthraquinone of cascara [see: cascara sagrada]

Anthriscus cerefolium *medicinal herb* [see: chervil]

anti pan T lymphocyte MAb *orphan status withdrawn 1996* [also: anti-T lymphocyte immunotoxin XMMLY-H65-RTA]

anti-A blood grouping serum USP *in vitro blood testing*

antiadrenergics *a class of cardiovascular drugs that block the passage of impulses through the sympathetic nervous system* [also called: sympatholytics]

antiandrogens *a class of hormonal antineoplastics*

antib [see: thioacetazone; thiacetazone]

anti-B blood grouping serum USP *in vitro blood testing*

anti-B4-blocked ricin [see: ricin (blocked) ...]

antibason [see: methylthiouracil]

AntibiOtic ear drops, otic suspension R *topical corticosteroidal anti-inflammatory; antibiotic* [hydrocortisone; neomycin sulfate; polymyxin B sulfate] 1%•5 mg•10 000 U per mL

Antibiotic Ear Solution R *topical corticosteroidal anti-inflammatory; antibiotic* [hydrocortisone; neomycin sulfate; polymyxin B sulfate] 1%•5 mg•10 000 U per mL

Antibiotic Ear Suspension R *topical corticosteroidal anti-inflammatory; antibiotic* [hydrocortisone; neomycin sulfate; polymyxin B sulfate] 1%•5 mg•10 000 U per mL

antibiotics *a class of agents that destroy or arrest the growth of micro-organisms*

antibromics *a class of agents that mask undesirable or offensive odors* [also called: deodorants]

anti-C blood grouping serum [see: blood grouping serum, anti-C]

anti-c blood grouping serum [see: blood grouping serum, anti-c]

anti-CD3 [see: muromonab-CD3]

anti-CD11a monoclonal antibodies [see: HU-1124]

anticholinergics *a class of agents that block parasympathetic nerve impulses, producing antiemetic, antinausea, and antispasmodic effects; also used to dry mucosal secretions*

anticoagulant citrate dextrose (ACD) solution USP *anticoagulant for storage of whole blood and during cardiac surgery*

anticoagulant citrate phosphate dextrose adenine solution USP *anticoagulant for storage of whole blood*

anticoagulant citrate phosphate dextrose solution USP *anticoagulant for storage of whole blood*

anticoagulant heparin solution USP *anticoagulant for storage of whole blood*

anticoagulant sodium citrate solution USP *anticoagulant for plasma and for blood for fractionation*

anticoagulants *a class of therapeutic agents that inhibit or inactivate blood clotting factors*

anticonvulsants *a class of drugs that prevent seizures by suppressing abnormal neuronal discharges in the central nervous system* [also called: anti-epileptic drugs (AEDs)]

anti-D antibodies [see: $Rh_0(D)$ immune globulin]

antidopaminergics *a class of antiemetic drugs*

antidotes *a class of drugs that counteract the effects of toxic doses of other drugs or toxic substances*

anti-E blood grouping serum [see: blood grouping serum, anti-E]

anti-e blood grouping serum [see: blood grouping serum, anti-e]

antiemetics *a class of agents that prevent or alleviate nausea and vomiting* [also called: antinauseants]

antiendotoxin MAb E5 [now: edobacomab]

antienite INN

antiepilepsirine [now: ilepcimide]

anti-epileptic drugs (AEDs) *a class of drugs that prevent seizures by suppressing abnormal neuronal discharges in the central nervous system* [also called: anticonvulsants]

antiestrogen [see: tamoxifen citrate]

antiestrogens *a class of hormonal antineoplastics*

antifebriles *a class of agents that relieve or reduce fever* [also called: antipyretics; antithermics; febricides; febrifuges]

antifebrin [see: acetanilide]

antifolic acid [see: methotrexate]

antiformin, dental JAN [also: sodium hypochlorite, diluted]

antihemophilic factor (AHF) USP *antihemophilic; systemic hemostatic; investigational (orphan) for von Willebrand's disease*

Antihemophilic Factor (Porcine) Hyate:C powder for IV injection ℞ *antihemophilic to correct coagulation deficiency* [antihemophilic factor VIII:C] 400–700 porcine units/vial

antihemophilic factor, human [now: antihemophilic factor]

antihemophilic factor, recombinant (rFVIII) *antihemophilic for treatment of hemophilia A and presurgical prophylaxis for hemophiliacs (orphan)*

antihemophilic factor A [see: antihemophilic factor]

antihemophilic factor B [see: factor IX complex]

antihemophilic globulin (AHG) [see: antihemophilic factor]

antihemophilic human plasma [now: plasma, antihemophilic human]

antihemophilic plasma, human [now: plasma, antihemophilic human]

antiheparin [see: protamine sulfate]

Antihist-1 tablets OTC *antihistamine* [clemastine fumarate] 1.34 mg

antihistamines *a class of drugs that counteract the effect of histamine*

Antihist-D tablets OTC *decongestant; antihistamine* [phenylpropanolamine HCl (extended release); clemastine fumarate (immediate release)] 75 • 1.34 mg

anti-HIV T-cell *investigational (Phase I/II) gene therapy for HIV*

anti-human thymocyte immunoglobulin, rabbit *investigational (Phase III) immunosuppressant for kidney transplants*

antihydrotics *a class of agents that reduce or suppress perspiration* [also called: anhidrotics; anidrotics]

antihyperlipidemic agents *a class of drugs that lower serum lipid levels* [also called: antilipemics]

anti-inhibitor coagulant complex *antihemophilic*

antilipemics *a class of drugs that lower serum lipid levels* [also called: antihyperlipidemics]

Antilirium IV or IM injection ℞ *cholinergic to reverse anticholinergic overdose; investigational (orphan) for Friedreich's and other inherited ataxias* [physostigmine salicylate] 1 mg/mL

antilithics *a class of agents that prevent the formation of stone or calculus* [see also: litholytics]

antilymphocyte immunoglobulin BAN

antimelanoma antibody XMMME-001-DTPA 111 indium *orphan status withdrawn 1996*

antimelanoma antibody XMMME-001-RTA *orphan status withdrawn 1996*

Antiminth oral suspension OTC *anthelmintic for ascariasis (roundworm) and enterobiasis (pinworm)* [pyrantel pamoate] 50 mg/mL

antimony *element (Sb)*

antimony potassium tartrate USP *antischistosomal*

antimony sodium tartrate USP, JAN *antischistosomal*

antimony sodium thioglycollate USP

antimony sulfide [see: antimony trisulfide colloid]

antimony trisulfide colloid USAN *pharmaceutic aid*

antimonyl potassium tartrate [see: antimony potassium tartrate]

antimuscarinics *a class of anticholinergic agents*

anti-MY9-blocked ricin [see: ricin (blocked) ...]

antinauseants *a class of agents that prevent or alleviate nausea and vomiting* [also called: antiemetics]

antineoplastics *a class of chemotherapeutic agents capable of selective action on neoplastic (abnormally proliferating) tissues*

antineoplastons *a class of naturally occurring peptides that suppress cancer oncogenes and stimulate the body's cancer suppressor genes*

Antiox capsules OTC *vitamin supplement* [vitamins C and E; beta carotene] 120 mg•100 IU•25 mg

anti-pellagra vitamin [see: niacin]

antiperiodics *a class of agents that prevent periodic or intermittent recurrence of symptoms, as in malaria*

anti-pernicious anemia principle [see: cyanocobalamin]

antiphlogistics *a class of agents that reduce inflammation and fever*

antipyretics *a class of agents that relieve or reduce fever* [also called: antifebriles; antithermics; febricides; febrifuges]

antipyrine USP, JAN *analgesic; orphan status withdrawn 1996* [also: phenazone]

N-antipyrinylnicotinamide [see: nifenazone]

antirabies serum (ARS) USP *passive immunizing agent*

anti-Rh antibodies [see: $Rh_0(D)$ immune globulin]

anti-Rh typing serums [now: blood grouping serums]

antiscorbutic vitamin [see: ascorbic acid]

antiscorbutics *a class of agents that are sources of vitamin C and are effective in the prevention or relief of scurvy*

antiscrofulous herbs *a class of agents that counteract scrofuloderma (tuberculous cervical lymphadenitis)*

antisense drugs *a class of antiviral drugs that interfere with the replication of viral protein*

antiseptics *a class of agents that inhibit the growth and development of microorganisms, usually on a body surface, without necessarily killing them* [see also: disinfectants; germicides]

Antispas IM injection ℞ *GI antispasmodic* [dicyclomine HCl] 10 mg/mL

Antispasmodic elixir ℞ *GI antispasmodic; anticholinergic; sedative* [atropine sulfate; scopolamine hydrobromide; hyoscyamine sulfate; phenobarbital] 0.0194•0.0065•0.1037•16.2 mg/5 mL

antispasmodics *a class of agents that relieve spasms or cramps, usually of gastrointestinal tract or blood vessels*

antisterility vitamin [see: vitamin E]

anti-T lymphocyte immunotoxin XMMLY-H65-RTA *orphan status withdrawn 1996* [also: anti pan T lymphocyte monoclonal antibody]

anti-tac, humanized; SMART anti-tac [now: dacliximab]

anti-TAP-72 immunotoxin *orphan status withdrawn 1996*

antithermics *a class of agents that relieve or reduce fever* [also called: antifebriles; antipyretics; febricides; febrifuges]

antithrombin III (AT-III) INN, BAN *for thrombosis and pulmonary emboli of congenital AT-III deficiency (orphan); investigational (Phase II) for coronary artery bypass grafts*

antithrombin III, human [see: antithrombin III]

antithrombin III, recombinant human (rhATIII) [see: antithrombin III]

antithrombin III concentrate IV [see: antithrombin III]

antithymocyte globulin [see: lymphocyte immune globulin, antithymocyte]

antithymocyte serum [see: lymphocyte immune globulin, antithymocyte]

anti-TNF (tumor necrosis factor) MAb [now: nerelimomab]

antitoxin botulism equine (ABE) [see: botulism equine antitoxin, trivalent]

antitoxins *a class of drugs used for passive immunization that consist of antibodies which combine with toxins to neutralize them*

α₁-antitrypsin [see: alpha₁-antitrypsin]

antituberculous agents *a class of antibiotics, divided into primary and retreatment agents*

Anti-Tuss syrup OTC *expectorant* [guaifenesin; alcohol 3.5%] 100 mg/5 mL

antitussives *a class of drugs that prevent or relieve cough*

antivenin (Crotalidae) polyvalent USP *passive immunizing agent for pit viper (rattlesnake, copperhead, and cottonmouth moccasin) bites*

antivenin (Crotalidae) polyvalent (ovine) Fab *investigational (orphan) treatment of Crotalidae snake bites*

antivenin (Crotalidae) purified (avian) *investigational (orphan) treatment of Crotalidae snake bites*

antivenin (*Latrodectus mactans*) USP *passive immunizing agent for black widow spider bites* 6000 U/vial

antivenin (Micrurus fulvius) USP *passive immunizing agent for coral snake bites*

antivenins *a class of drugs used for passive immunization against venomous bites and stings*

Antivert; Antivert/25; Antivert/50 tablets ℞ *anticholinergic; antihistamine; antivertigo agent; motion sickness preventative* [meclizine HCl] 12.5 mg; 25 mg; 50 mg

Antivert/25 chewable tablets (discontinued 1995) ℞ *anticholinergic; antihistamine; antivertigo agent; motion sickness preventative* [meclizine HCl] 25 mg

antivirals *a class of drugs effective against viral infections*

antixerophthalmic vitamin [see: vitamin A]

Antizol injection ℞ *alcohol dehydrogenase inhibitor for methanol or ethylene glycol poisoning (orphan)* [fomepizole] 1 g/mL

antler (deer and elk) *natural remedy for aging, energy, hormone balancing, impotence, infertility, and longevity*

antrafenine INN

antramycin INN *antineoplastic* [also: anthramycin]

Antril ℞ *nonsteroidal anti-inflammatory drug (NSAID) for inflammatory bowel disease; investigational (orphan) for juvenile rheumatoid arthritis and graft vs. host disease* [anakinra]

Antrizine tablets ℞ *anticholinergic; antihistamine; antivertigo agent; motion sickness preventative* [meclizine HCl] 12.5, 25, 50 mg

Antrocol capsules, tablets (discontinued 1995) ℞ *GI anticholinergic; sedative* [atropine sulfate; phenobarbital] 0.195•16 mg

Antrocol elixir ℞ *GI anticholinergic; sedative* [atropine sulfate; phenobarbital] 0.195•16 mg/5 mL

Antrypol (available only from the Centers for Disease Control) ℞ *antiparasitic for African trypanosomiasis and onchocerciasis* [suramin sodium]

antrypol [see: suramin sodium]

Anturane tablets, capsules ℞ *uricosuric for gout* [sulfinpyrazone] 100 mg; 200 mg ② Artane

Anucort HC rectal suppositories ℞ *corticosteroidal anti-inflammatory* [hydrocortisone acetate] 25 mg

Anumed rectal suppositories OTC *temporary relief of hemorrhoidal symptoms* [bismuth subgallate; bismuth resorcin compound; benzyl benzoate; zinc oxide; peruvian balsam] 2.25%•1.75%•1.2%•11%•1.8%

Anumed HC rectal suppositories ℞ *corticosteroidal anti-inflammatory* [hydrocortisone acetate] 10 mg

Anuprep HC rectal suppositories (discontinued 1995) ℞ *corticosteroidal anti-inflammatory; antipruritic* [hydrocortisone acetate] 25 mg

Anuprep Hemorrhoidal rectal suppositories (discontinued 1995) OTC *temporary relief of hemorrhoidal symptoms* [bismuth subgallate; bismuth resorcin compound; benzyl benzoate; peruvian balsam; zinc oxide] 2.25%• 1.75%•1.2%•1.8%•11%

Anusol anorectal ointment OTC *topical local anesthetic; astringent* [pramoxine HCl; zinc oxide] 1%•12.5% ② Aplisol

Anusol rectal suppositories OTC *emollient* [topical starch] 51%

Anusol-HC anorectal cream ℞ *topical corticosteroidal anti-inflammatory* [hydrocortisone] 2.5%

Anusol-HC rectal suppositories ℞ *corticosteroidal anti-inflammatory* [hydrocortisone acetate] 25 mg

Anusol-HC 1 ointment ℞ *topical corticosteroidal anti-inflammatory* [hydrocortisone acetate] 1%

Anxanil film-coated tablets (discontinued 1998) ℞ *anxiolytic; minor tranquilizer* [hydroxyzine HCl] 25 mg

Anzemet tablets, IV injection ℞ *antiemetic for nausea following chemotherapy, radiation therapy, or operations; selective serotonin 5-HT₃ receptor antagonist* [dolasetron mesylate] 50, 100 mg; 20 mg/mL

AOD-9604 *investigational (Phase II) antiobesity drug*

AOPA (ara-C, Oncovin, prednisone, asparaginase) *chemotherapy protocol*

AOPE (Adriamycin, Oncovin, prednisone, etoposide) *chemotherapy protocol*

Aosept solution + Aodisc (tablet) OTC *two-step chemical disinfecting system for soft contact lenses* [hydrogen peroxide based] 3%

AP (Adriamycin, Platinol) *chemotherapy protocol*

Apacet chewable tablets, drops OTC *analgesic; antipyretic* [acetaminophen] 80 mg; 100 mg/mL

apafant USAN, INN *platelet activating factor antagonist for allergies, asthma, and acute pancreatitis*

apalcillin sodium USAN, INN *antibacterial*

Apanol ℞ *investigational phospholipase A2 inhibitor* [IPL-576 (code name— generic name not yet assigned)]

APAP (N-acetyl-p-aminophenol) [see: acetaminophen]

Apatate chewable tablets, liquid OTC *vitamin supplement* [vitamins B₁, B₆, and B₁₂] 15•0.5•0.025 mg; 15•0.5•0.025 mg/5 mL

Apatate with Fluoride liquid ℞ *pediatric vitamin supplement and dental caries preventative* [vitamins B₁, B₆, and B₁₂; fluoride] 15•0.5•0.025•0.5 mg/5 mL

apaxifylline USAN, INN *selective adenosine A₁ antagonist for cognitive deficits*

apazone USAN *anti-inflammatory* [also: azapropazone]

APC (AMSA, prednisone, chlorambucil) *chemotherapy protocol*

APC (aspirin, phenacetin & caffeine) [q.v.]

APC-366 *investigational (Phase II) tryptase inhibitor for asthma*

apcitide [see: technetium Tc 99m apcitide]

APD (aminohydroxypropylidene diphosphonate) [see: pamidronate disodium]

APE (Adriamycin, Platinol, etoposide) *chemotherapy protocol*

APE (ara-C, Platinol, etoposide) *chemotherapy protocol*

aperients *a class of agents that have a mild purgative or laxative effect* [see also: aperitives]

aperitives *a class of agents that stimulate the appetite or have a mild purgative or laxative effect* [see also: aperients]

Apetil liquid OTC *vitamin/mineral supplement* [multiple B vitamins; multiple minerals] ± • ±

aphrodisiacs *a class of agents that arouse or increase sexual desire or potency*

Aphrodyne tablets ℞ *no FDA-approved uses; sympatholytic; mydriatic; aphrodisiac* [yohimbine HCl] 5.4 mg

Aphthasol oral paste ℞ *anti-inflammatory for aphthous ulcers* [amlexanox] 5%

apicillin [see: ampicillin]

apicycline INN

apiquel fumarate [see: aminorex]

Apium graveolens medicinal herb [see: celery]

A.P.L. powder for IM injection ℞ *hormone for prepubertal cryptorchidism and hypogonadism; ovulation stimulant* [chorionic gonadotropin] 500, 1000, 2000 U/mL

APL 400-020 investigational (orphan) for cutaneous T-cell lymphoma

Apligraf ℞ *living skin construct for diabetic foot ulcers and pressure sores* [graftskin]

Aplisol intradermal injection ℞ *tuberculosis skin test* [tuberculin purified protein derivative] 5 U/0.1 mL ⑨ Anusol; Apresoline

Aplitest single-use intradermal puncture test device ℞ *tuberculosis skin test* [tuberculin purified protein derivative] 5 U

aplonidine HCl [see: apraclonidine HCl]

APO (Adriamycin, prednisone, Oncovin) chemotherapy protocol

Apo-Acyclovir ⒸⒶⓃ (U.S. product: Zovirax) tablets ℞ *antiviral for herpes infections* [acyclovir] 200, 400, 800 mg

Apo-Cefaclor ⒸⒶⓃ (U.S. product: Ceclor) capsules, oral suspension ℞ *cephalosporin antibiotic* [cefaclor] 250, 500 mg; 125, 250, 375 mg/5 mL

Apo-Cromolyn ⒸⒶⓃ (U.S. product: Intal) Sterules (solution for nebulization) ℞ *anti-inflammatory/mast cell stabilizer for the prophylaxis of asthma and bronchospasm* [cromolyn sodium (sodium cromoglycate)] 1% (20 mg/2 mL dose)

Apo-Cromolyn ⒸⒶⓃ (U.S. product: NasalCrom) nasal spray ℞ *anti-inflammatory/mast cell stabilizer for the prophylaxis of allergic rhinitis* [cromolyn sodium (sodium cromoglycate)] 2% (5.2 mg/dose)

Apocynum androsaemifolium medicinal herb [see: dogbane]

apodol [see: anileridine HCl]

Apo-Domperidone ⒸⒶⓃ film-coated tablets ℞ *antiemetic for diabetic gastroparesis and chronic gastritis* [domperidone maleate] 10 mg

Apo-Etodolac ⒸⒶⓃ (U.S. product: Lodine) capsules ℞ *nonsteroidal anti-inflammatory drug (NSAID); analgesic; antiarthritic* [etodolac] 200, 300 mg

Apo-Fluphenazine ⒸⒶⓃ (U.S. product: Prolixin) tablets ℞ *conventional (typical) antipsychotic* [fluphenazine HCl] 1, 2, 5 mg

Apo-Gemfibrozil ⒸⒶⓃ (U.S. product: Lopid) capsules, tablets ℞ *antihyperlipidemic for hypertriglyceridemia and coronary heart disease* [gemfibrozil] 300 mg; 600 mg

Apo-Ipravent ⒸⒶⓃ (U.S. product: Atrovent) solution for inhalation ℞ *anticholinergic bronchodilator for bronchospasm; antisecretory for rhinorrhea* [ipratropium bromide] 250 µg/mL

Apo-Ketoconazole ⒸⒶⓃ (U.S. product: Nizoral) tablets ℞ *systemic antifungal* [ketoconazole] 200 mg

Apokinon injection ℞ *investigational (orphan) treatment for late-stage Parkinson's disease* [apomorphine HCl]

Apo-Loxapine ⒸⒶⓃ (U.S. product: Loxitane) film-coated tablets ℞ *conventional (typical) antipsychotic for schizophrenia* [loxapine succinate] 5, 10, 25, 50 mg

Apo-Moclobemide ⒸⒶⓃ film-coated tablets ℞ *antidepressant; MAO inhibitor* [moclobemide] 100, 150 mg

apomorphine BAN *emetic* [also: apomorphine HCl]

apomorphine HCl USP *emetic; investigational (orphan) for late-stage Parkinson's disease* [also: apomorphine]

Apo-Oflox ⒸⒶⓃ (U.S. product: Floxin) film-coated tablets ℞ *broad-spectrum fluoroquinolone antibiotic* [ofloxacin] 200, 300, 400 mg

Apo-Perphenazine ⒸⒶⓃ (U.S. product: Trilafon) film-coated tablets ℞ *conventional (typical) antipsychotic; antiemetic* [perphenazine] 4, 8, 16 mg

Apo-Terazosin ⒸⒶⓃ (U.S. product: Hytrin) tablets ℞ *antihypertensive (α-blocker); treatment for benign prostatic hyperplasia (BPH)* [terazosin HCl] 1, 2, 5, 10 mg

Apo-Thioridazine ⒸⒶⓃ (U.S. product: Mellaril) film-coated tablets ℞ *conventional (typical) antipsychotic* [thioridazine HCl] 10, 25 mg

Apo-Ticlopidine ⒸⒶⓃ (U.S. product: Ticlid) film-coated tablets ℞ *platelet aggregation inhibitor for stroke* [ticlopidine HCl] 250 mg

Apo-Trifluoperazine ⒸⒶⓃ (U.S. product: Stelazine) film-coated tablets ℞ *conventional (typical) antipsychotic; anxiolytic* [trifluoperazine HCl] 1, 2, 5, 10, 20 mg

apovincamine INN

Appedrine tablets OTC *nonprescription diet aid; vitamin/mineral supplement* [phenylpropanolamine HCl; multiple vitamins & minerals; folic acid] 25•⚕•0.4 mg ② aprindine; ephedrine

appetizers *a class of agents that stimulate the appetite* [see also: aperitives]

APPG (aqueous penicillin G procaine) [see: penicillin G procaine]

apple *(Pyrus malus)* fruit *medicinal herb for constipation and diarrhea, dysentery, fever, heart ailments, scurvy, and warts*

apple, ground *medicinal herb* [see: chamomile]

apple, hog; Indian apple; May apple *medicinal herb* [see: mandrake]

Appli-Kit (trademarked form) *ointment and adhesive dosage covers*

Appli-Ruler (trademarked name) OTC *dose-determining pads*

Appli-Tape (trademarked name) OTC *dosage covers*

apraclonidine INN, BAN *topical adrenergic for glaucoma* [also: apraclonidine HCl]

apraclonidine HCl USAN *topical adrenergic for glaucoma* [also: apraclonidine]

apramycin USAN, INN, BAN *antibacterial*

Aprazone capsules ℞ *uricosuric for gout* [sulfinpyrazone]

Apresazide 25/25; Apresazide 50/50; Apresazide 100/50 capsules ℞ *antihypertensive; vasodilator; diuretic* [hydralazine HCl; hydrochlorothiazide] 25•25 mg; 50•50 mg; 100•50 mg

Apresoline tablets ℞ *antihypertensive; vasodilator* [hydralazine HCl] 10, 25, 50, 100 mg

apricot *(Prunus armeniaca)* fruit, seeds, and kernel oil *medicinal herb for asthma, constipation, cough, eye inflammation, hemorrhage, infertility, spasm, and vaginal infections; not generally regarded as safe and effective as apricot kernel ingestion causes cyanide poisoning*

apricot kernel water JAN

aprikalim INN *investigational antianginal*

aprindine USAN, INN, BAN *antiarrhythmic* ② Appedrine; ephedrine

aprindine HCl USAN, JAN *antiarrhythmic*

aprobarbital NF, INN, DCF *sedative*

Aprodine tablets, syrup OTC *decongestant; antihistamine* [pseudoephedrine HCl; triprolidine HCl] 60•2.5 mg; 30•1.25 mg/5 mL

Aprodine with Codeine syrup ℞ *narcotic antitussive; decongestant; antihistamine* [codeine phosphate; pseudoephedrine HCl; triprolidine HCl] 10•30•1.25 mg/5 mL

aprofene INN

aprosulate sodium INN

aprotinin USAN, INN, BAN, JAN *systemic hemostatic to reduce blood loss in coronary surgery (orphan); protease inhibitor*

Aprozide 25/25; Aprozide 50/50; Aprozide 100/50 capsules ℞ *antihypertensive; vasodilator; diuretic* [hydrochlorothiazide; hydralazine HCl]

A.P.S. (aspirin, phenacetin & salicylamide) [q.v.]

APSAC (anisoylated plasminogen streptokinase activator complex) [see: anistreplase]

aptazapine INN *antidepressant* [also: aptazapine maleate]

aptazapine maleate USAN *antidepressant* [also: aptazapine]

aptiganel HCl USAN *investigational (Phase III) NMDA ion channel blocker for stroke and traumatic brain injury*

aptocaine INN, BAN, DCF

apyron [see: magnesium salicylate]

Aqua-Ban enteric-coated tablets OTC *diuretic* [ammonium chloride; caffeine] 325•100 mg

Aqua-Ban, Maximum Strength tablets OTC *diuretic* [pamabrom] 50 mg

Aqua-Ban Plus enteric-coated tablets OTC *diuretic; iron supplement* [ammonium chloride; caffeine; ferrous sulfate] 650•200•6 mg

Aquabase OTC *ointment base*

Aquacare cream, lotion OTC *moisturizer; emollient; keratolytic* [urea] 10%

Aquachloral Supprettes (suppositories) ℞ *sedative; hypnotic* [chloral hydrate] 324, 648 mg

aquaday [see: menadione]

aquakay [see: menadione]

AquaMEPHYTON IM or subcu injection ℞ *coagulant; correct anticoagulant-induced prothrombin deficiency; vitamin K supplement* [phytonadione] 2, 10 mg/mL

Aquanil lotion OTC *moisturizer; emollient*

Aquanil Cleanser lotion OTC *soap-free therapeutic skin cleanser*

Aquaphilic OTC *ointment base*

Aquaphilic with Carbamide OTC *ointment base* [urea] 10%, 20%

Aquaphor OTC *ointment base*

Aquaphyllin syrup ℞ *antiasthmatic; bronchodilator* [theophylline] 80 mg/15 mL

AquaSite eye drops OTC *ophthalmic moisturizer/lubricant* [polyethylene glycol 400] 0.2%

Aquasol A capsules, IM injection ℞ *vitamin deficiency therapy* [vitamin A] 25 000, 50 000 IU; 50 000 IU/mL

Aquasol A drops OTC *vitamin supplement* [vitamin A] 5000 IU/0.1 mL

Aquasol E capsules, drops OTC *vitamin supplement* [vitamin E] 73.5 mg, 400 IU; 50 mg/mL

AquaTar gel OTC *topical antipsoriatic; antiseborrheic* [coal tar extract] 2.5%

Aquatensen tablets ℞ *diuretic; antihypertensive* [methyclothiazide] 5 mg

Aquavit-E drops ℞ *vitamin supplement* [vitamin E] 15 IU/0.3 mL

aqueous penicillin G procaine (APPG) [see: penicillin G procaine]

Aquest IM injection (discontinued 1998) ℞ *estrogen replacement therapy for postmenopausal disorders; palliative therapy for inoperable prostatic and breast cancer* [estrone] 2 mg/mL

Aquilegia vulgaris medicinal herb [see: columbine]

aquinone [see: menadione]

AR-177 *investigational (Phase I) antiviral/oligonucleotide/integrase inhibitor for HIV*

ara-A (adenine arabinoside) [see: vidarabine]

ara-AC (azacytosine arabinoside) [see: fazarabine]

arabinofuranosylcytosine [see: cytarabine]

arabinoluranosylcytosine HCl [see: cytarabine HCl]

arabinosyl cytosine [see: cytarabine]

ara-C (cytosine arabinoside) [see: cytarabine] ☒ ERYC

ara-C + 6-TG (ara-C, thioguanine) *chemotherapy protocol*

ara-C + ADR (ara-C, Adriamycin) *chemotherapy protocol*

ara-C + DNR + PRED + MP (ara-C, daunorubicin, prednisolone, mercaptopurine) *chemotherapy protocol*

arachis oil [see: peanut oil]

ara-C-HU (ara-C, hydroxyurea) *chemotherapy protocol*

ara-cytidine [see: cytarabine]

Aralen HCl IM injection ℞ *antimalarial; amebicide* [chloroquine HCl] 50 mg/mL ☒ Arlidin

Aralen Phosphate film-coated tablets ℞ *antimalarial; amebicide* [chloroquine phosphate] 500 mg

Aralen Phosphate injection (discontinued 1996) ℞ *antimalarial; amebicide* [chloroquine phosphate] 5 mg

**Aralen Phosphate with Primaquine
Phosphate** tablets (discontinued
1996) ℞ *malaria prophylaxis* [chloro-
quine phosphate; primaquine phos-
phate] 500•79 mg
Aralia racemosa medicinal herb [see:
spikenard]
Aralia spp. medicinal herb [see: ginseng]
Aramine IV, subcu or IM injection ℞
*vasopressor for acute hypotensive
shock, anaphylaxis, or traumatic shock*
[metaraminol bitartrate] 10 mg/mL
aranidipine INN
aranotin USAN, INN *antiviral*
araprofen INN
Arava film-coated tablets ℞ *anti-
inflammatory for rheumatoid arthritis*
[leflunomide] 10, 20, 30 mg
arbaprostil USAN, INN *gastric antisecretory*
arbekacin INN
arberry *medicinal herb* [see: uva ursi]
arbutamine INN, BAN *cardiac stressor
for diagnosis of coronary artery disease*
[also: arbutamine HCl]
arbutamine HCl USAN *cardiac stressor
for diagnosis of coronary artery disease*
[also: arbutamine]
Arbutus uva ursi medicinal herb [see:
uva ursi]
Arcet tablets (discontinued 1995) ℞
sedative; analgesic; antipyretic [butal-
bital; acetaminophen; caffeine] 50•
325•40 mg
archangel *medicinal herb* [see: angelica]
arcitumomab USAN *imaging agent for
detection of recurrent or metastatic thyroid cancers* (orphan)
arclofenin USAN, INN *hepatic function
test*
Arcobee with C caplets OTC *vitamin
supplement* [multiple B vitamins;
vitamin C] ±•300 mg
Arco-Lase chewable tablets OTC *digestive enzymes* [amylase; protease;
lipase; cellulase] 30•6•25•2 mg
Arco-Lase Plus tablets ℞ *digestive
enzymes; GI antispasmodic; sedative*
[amylase; protease; lipase; cellulase;
hyoscyamine sulfate; atropine sul-

fate; phenobarbital] 30•6•25•2•
0.1•0.02•7.5 mg
Arcotinic tablets (discontinued 1995)
OTC *hematinic* [ferrous fumarate &
ferrous sulfate; liver, desiccated;
ascorbic acid] 102.5•200•250 mg
*Arctium lappa; A. majus; A. minus
medicinal herb* [see: burdock]
Arctostaphylos uva ursi medicinal herb
[see: uva ursi]
ardacin INN
ardeparin sodium USAN, INN *low molecular weight heparin-type anticoagulant and antithrombotic for the prevention of deep vein thrombosis (DVT)
following knee replacement surgery*
Arduan powder for IV injection ℞
*nondepolarizing neuromuscular blocker;
adjunct to anesthesia* [pipecuronium
bromide] 10 mg/vial
arecoline acetarsone salt [see: dro-
carbil]
arecoline hydrobromide NF
Aredia powder for IV infusion ℞ *bisphosphonate bone resorption inhibitor
for Paget's disease, hypercalcemia of
malignancy, breast cancer, and multiple
myeloma* [pamidronate disodium] 30,
60, 90 mg
arfalasin INN
arfendazam INN
Arfonad IV infusion (discontinued
1995) ℞ *antihypertensive for hypertensive emergency* [trimethaphan camsy-
late] 50 mg/mL
argatroban USAN, INN, JAN *investigational (NDA filed) thrombin inhibitor
for heparin-induced thrombocytopenia
(HIT) and thrombosis (NDA disapproved in 1998); investigational (Phase
II) for myocardial infarction*
Argesic cream OTC *topical analgesic;
counterirritant* [methyl salicylate; tro-
lamine]
Argesic-SA tablets ℞ *analgesic; anti-
inflammatory* [salsalate] 500 mg
argimesna INN
arginine (L-arginine) USP, INN *nonessential amino acid; ammonia detoxi-*

cant; *diagnostic aid for pituitary function; symbols: Arg, R*
arginine butanoate [see: arginine butyrate]
arginine butyrate (L-arginine butyrate) USAN *investigational (orphan) for beta-hemoglobinopathies, beta-thalassemia, and sickle cell disease*
arginine glutamate (L-arginine L-glutamate) USAN, BAN, JAN *ammonia detoxicant*
arginine HCl USAN, USP, JAN *ammonia detoxicant; pituitary (growth hormone) function diagnostic aid*
L-arginine monohydrochloride [see: arginine HCl]
8-L-arginine vasopressin [see: vasopressin]
8-arginineoxytocin [see: argiprestocin]
8-L-argininevasopressin tannate [see: argipressin tannate]
argipressin INN, BAN *antidiuretic* [also: argipressin tannate]
argipressin tannate USAN *antidiuretic* [also: argipressin]
argiprestocin INN
argon *element (Ar)*
argyn [see: silver protein, mild]
Argyrol S.S. 20% eye drops (discontinued 1995) ℞ *ophthalmic mucus staining and coagulating agent; topical antiseptic* [silver protein, mild] 20%
Aricept tablets ℞ *reversible acetylcholinesterase (AChE) inhibitor; cognition adjuvant for Alzheimer's dementia* [donepezil HCl] 5, 10 mg ⊡ Erycette
arildone USAN, INN *antiviral*
Arimidex film-coated tablets ℞ *hormonal antineoplastic/aromatase inhibitor for advanced breast cancer* [anastrozole] 1 mg
aripiprazole USAN *antischizophrenic*
Aristocort ointment, cream ℞ *topical corticosteroidal anti-inflammatory* [triamcinolone acetonide] 0.1%, 0.5%; 0.025%, 0.1%, 0.5%
Aristocort tablets ℞ *corticosteroid; anti-inflammatory* [triamcinolone] 1, 2, 4, 8 mg

Aristocort A ointment, cream ℞ *topical corticosteroidal anti-inflammatory* [triamcinolone acetonide in a water-washable base] 0.1%; 0.025%, 0.1%, 0.5%
Aristocort Forte IM injection ℞ *corticosteroid; anti-inflammatory* [triamcinolone diacetate] 40 mg/mL
Aristocort Intralesional injection ℞ *corticosteroid; anti-inflammatory* [triamcinolone diacetate] 25 mg/mL
Aristolochia clematitis medicinal herb [see: birthwort]
Aristospan Intra-articular injection ℞ *corticosteroid; anti-inflammatory* [triamcinolone hexacetonide] 20 mg/mL
Aristospan Intralesional injection ℞ *corticosteroid; anti-inflammatory* [triamcinolone hexacetonide] 5 mg/mL
Arkin Z (commercially available in Japan) ℞ *investigational treatment for congestive heart failure (clinical trials discontinued 1996)* [vesnarinone]
A.R.M. (Allergy Relief Medicine) caplets OTC *decongestant; antihistamine* [phenylpropanolamine HCl; chlorpheniramine maleate] 25•4 mg
Arm-A-Med (trademarked packaging form) *single-dose plastic vial*
Arm-A-Vial (trademarked packaging form) *single-dose plastic vial*
Armoracia rusticana; A. lapathiofolia medicinal herb [see: horseradish]
Armour Thyroid tablets ℞ *thyroid replacement therapy for hypothyroidism or thyroid cancer* [thyroid, desiccated] 15, 30, 60, 90, 120, 180, 240, 300 mg
arnica (*Arnica montana; A. cordifolia; A. fulgens*) flowers *medicinal herb used as a topical counterirritant and vulnerary for acne, bruises, rashes, and other dermal lesions; not generally regarded as safe and effective taken internally as it is highly toxic*
arnolol INN
arofylline USAN *phosphodiesterase IV inhibitor for asthma*
aromatase inhibitors *a class of hormonal antineoplastics*
aromatic ammonia spirit [see: ammonia spirit, aromatic]

aromatic cascara fluidextract [see: cascara fluidextract, aromatic]

aromatic cascara sagrada [see: cascara fluidextract, aromatic]

aromatic elixir NF *flavored and sweetened vehicle*

aromatics *a class of agents that have an agreeable odor and stimulating qualities; also, substances with a specific molecular structure in organic chemistry*

aronixil INN

arotinolol INN [also: arotinolol HCl]

arotinolol HCl JAN [also: arotinolol]

arprinocid USAN, INN, BAN *coccidiostat*

arpromidine INN

Arrestin IM injection ℞ *anticholinergic; antiemetic* [trimethobenzamide HCl] 100 mg/mL

arrow wood; Indian arrow wood; Indian arrow *medicinal herb* [see: wahoo]

ARS (antirabies serum) [q.v.]

arsambide [see: carbarsone]

arsanilic acid INN, BAN *investigational (Phase I/II) immunomodulator for AIDS; orphan status withdrawn 1996*

arseclor [see: dichlorophenarsine HCl]

arsenic *element (As)*

arsenic acid, sodium salt [see: sodium arsenate]

arsenic trioxide JAN *investigational (orphan) antineoplastic for renal cell carcinoma*

arsenobenzene [see: arsphenamine]

arsenobenzol [see: arsphenamine]

arsenphenolamine [see: arsphenamine]

Arsobal (available only from the Centers for Disease Control) ℞ *investigational anti-infective for trypanosomiasis* [melarsoprol]

arsphenamine USP

arsthinenol DCF [also: arsthinol]

arsthinol INN [also: arsthinenol]

Artane tablets, elixir, Sequels (sustained-release capsules) ℞ *anticholinergic; antiparkinsonian* [trihexyphenidyl HCl] 2, 5 mg; 2 mg/5 mL; 5 mg ② Anturane

arteflene USAN, INN *antimalarial*

artegraft USAN *arterial prosthetic aid*

artemether INN

Artemisia absinthium *medicinal herb* [see: wormwood]

Artemisia dracunculus *medicinal herb* [see: tarragon]

Artemisia vulgaris *medicinal herb* [see: mugwort]

artemisinin INN

arterenol [see: norepinephrine bitartrate]

artesunate INN

Artha-G tablets OTC *analgesic; anti-inflammatory* [salsalate] 750 mg

ArthriCare, Double Ice gel OTC *topical analgesic; counterirritant* [menthol; camphor] 4%•3.1%

ArthriCare, Odor Free rub OTC *topical analgesic; counterirritant* [menthol; methyl nicotinate; capsaicin] 1.25%•0.25%•0.025%

ArthriCare Triple Medicated gel OTC *topical analgesic; counterirritant* [methyl salicylate; menthol; methyl nicotinate] 30%•1.5%•0.7%

Arthriten tablets OTC *analgesic; antipyretic* [acetaminophen; magnesium salicylate; caffeine (buffered with magnesium carbonate, magnesium oxide, and calcium carbonate)] 250•250•32.5 mg

"Arthritis Formula"; "Arthritis Strength" products [see under product name]

Arthritis Foundation Ibuprofen tablets (discontinued 1997) OTC *nonsteroidal anti-inflammatory drug (NSAID); antiarthritic; analgesic* [ibuprofen] 200 mg

Arthritis Foundation Nighttime caplets (discontinued 1997) OTC *antihistaminic sleep aid; analgesic* [diphenhydramine HCl; acetaminophen] 25•500 mg

Arthritis Foundation Pain Reliever tablets OTC *analgesic; antipyretic; anti-inflammatory; antirheumatic* [aspirin] 500 mg

Arthritis Foundation Pain Reliever, Aspirin Free caplets (discontinued

1997) OTC *analgesic; antipyretic* [acetaminophen] 500 mg

Arthritis Hot Creme OTC *topical analgesic; counterirritant* [methyl salicylate; menthol] 15%•10%

Arthritis Pain Formula caplets OTC *analgesic; antipyretic; anti-inflammatory; antirheumatic* [aspirin (buffered with magnesium hydroxide and aluminum hydroxide)] 500 mg

Arthritis Pain Formula Aspirin-Free tablets (discontinued 1997) OTC *analgesic; antipyretic* [acetaminophen] 500 mg

Arthropan IM injection ℞ *analgesic; antipyretic; anti-inflammatory; antirheumatic* [choline salicylate] 870 mg/5 mL

Arthrotec tablets ℞ *antiarthritic NSAID with a coating to protect gastric mucosa* [diclofenac sodium (enteric-coated core); misoprostol (coating)] 50•0.2, 75•0.2 mg

articaine INN *amide local anesthetic for dentistry* [also: carticaine]

artichoke *(Cynara scolymus)* flower heads *medicinal herb for albuminuria, bile stimulation, diabetes, diuresis, dyspepsia, jaundice, liver diseases, and postoperative anemia*

Articulose L.A. IM injection ℞ *corticosteroid; anti-inflammatory* [triamcinolone diacetate] 40 mg/mL

Articulose-50 IM injection (discontinued 1998) ℞ *corticosteroid; anti-inflammatory* [prednisolone acetate] 50 mg/mL

Artificial Tears eye drops OTC *ocular moisturizer/lubricant*

Artificial Tears ophthalmic ointment OTC *ocular moisturizer/lubricant* [white petrolatum; mineral oil; lanolin]

Artificial Tears Plus eye drops OTC *ophthalmic moisturizer/lubricant* [polyvinyl alcohol] 1.4%

artilide INN *antiarrhythmic* [also: artilide fumarate]

artilide fumarate USAN *antiarrhythmic* [also: artilide]

Arvin (available in Canada as Viprinex) ℞ *anticoagulant; orphan status withdrawn 1997* [ancrod]

arzoxifene HCl USAN *selective estrogen receptor modulator (SERM) for breast cancer, uterine fibroids, endometriosis, and dysfunctional uterine bleeding*

AS-013 [see: prostaglandin E_1 enol ester]

⁷⁴As [see: sodium arsenate As 74]

A.S.A. Enseals (enteric-release tablets), suppositories OTC *analgesic; antipyretic; anti-inflammatory* [aspirin]

5-ASA (5-aminosalicylic acid) [see: mesalamine]

ASA (acetylsalicylic acid) [see: aspirin]

Asacol delayed-release tablets ℞ *treatment of active ulcerative colitis, proctosigmoiditis and proctitis* [mesalamine] 400 mg

asafetida; asafoetida *(Ferula assafoetida; F. foetida; F. rubricaulis)* gum resin from dried roots and rhizomes *medicinal herb for abdominal tumors, amenorrhea, asthma, colic, convulsions, corns and calluses, edema; also used as an expectorant; not generally regarded as safe and effective in children as it may induce methemoglobinemia*

asafoetida *medicinal herb* [see: asafetida]

Asarum canadense *medicinal herb* [see: wild ginger]

Asbron-G Inlay-Tabs (tablets), elixir (discontinued 1996) ℞ *antiasthmatic; bronchodilator; expectorant* [theophylline; guaifenesin] 150•100 mg; 150•100 mg/15 mL

Asclepias geminata *medicinal herb* [see: gymnema]

Asclepias syriaca *medicinal herb* [see: milkweed]

Asclepias tuberosa *medicinal herb* [see: pleurisy root]

ascorbic acid (L-ascorbic acid) USP, INN, BAN, JAN *vitamin C; antiscorbutic; urinary acidifier* 25, 50, 100, 250, 500, 1000, 1500 oral; 500 mg/5 mL oral; 250, 500 mg/mL injection

L-ascorbic acid, monosodium salt [see: sodium ascorbate]

L-ascorbic acid 6-palmitate [see: ascorbyl palmitate]

Ascorbicap timed-release capsules OTC *vitamin supplement* [ascorbic acid] 500 mg

ascorbyl palmitate NF *antioxidant*

Ascriptin; Ascriptin A/D coated tablets OTC *analgesic; antipyretic; anti-inflammatory; antirheumatic* [aspirin (buffered with magnesium hydroxide, aluminum hydroxide, and calcium carbonate)] 325, 500 mg; 325 mg

Asendin tablets ℞ *tricyclic antidepressant* [amoxapine] 25, 50, 100, 150 mg

aseptichrome [see: merbromin]

ash, bitter *medicinal herb* [see: quassia; wahoo]

ash, mountain; American mountain ash; European mountain ash *medicinal herb* [see: mountain ash]

ash, poison *medicinal herb* [see: fringe tree]

ASHAP; A-SHAP (Adriamycin, Solu-Medrol, high-dose ara-C, Platinol) *chemotherapy protocol*

Asimina triloba medicinal herb [see: pawpaw]

Asmalix elixir ℞ *antiasthmatic; bronchodilator* [theophylline] 80 mg/15 mL

asobamast INN, BAN

asocainol INN

Aspalathus linearis; A. contaminata; Borbonia pinifolia medicinal herb [see: red bush tea]

asparaginase (L-asparaginase) USAN, JAN *antineoplastic for acute lymphocytic leukemia* [also: colaspase]

asparagine (L-asparagine) *nonessential amino acid; symbols: Asn, N*

L-asparagine amidohydrolase [see: asparaginase]

asparagus (Asparagus officinalis) roots, seeds *medicinal herb for acne, constipation, contraception, edema, neuritis, parasites, rheumatism, stimulating hair growth, and toothache*

aspartame USAN, NF, INN, BAN *sweetener*

L-aspartate potassium JAN

aspartic acid (L-aspartic acid) USAN, INN *nonessential amino acid; symbols: Asp, D*

L-aspartic acid insulin [see: insulin aspart]

aspartocin USAN, INN *antibacterial*

A-Spas S/L sublingual tablets ℞ *GI antispasmodic; anticholinergic* [hyoscyamine sulfate] 0.125 mg

aspen, European *medicinal herb* [see: black poplar]

aspen poplar; American aspen; quaking aspen *medicinal herb* [see: poplar]

Aspercreme cream OTC *topical analgesic* [trolamine salicylate] 10%

Aspercreme Rub lotion OTC *topical analgesic* [trolamine salicylate] 10%

Aspergillus oryase proteinase [see: asperkinase]

Aspergum chewing gum tablets OTC *analgesic; antipyretic; anti-inflammatory; antirheumatic* [aspirin] 227.5 mg

asperkinase

asperlin USAN *antibacterial; antineoplastic*

Asperula odorata medicinal herb [see: sweet woodruff]

aspidium (Dryopteris filix-mas) plant *medicinal herb for bloody nose, menorrhagia, worm infections including tapeworm and ringworm, and wound healing; not generally regarded as safe and effective for internal use as it is highly toxic*

aspidosperma USP

aspirin USP, BAN, JAN *analgesic; antipyretic; anti-inflammatory; antirheumatic* 325, 500, 650, 975 mg oral; 120, 200, 300, 600 mg suppositories ② Afrin

aspirin, buffered USP *analgesic; antipyretic; anti-inflammatory; antirheumatic* 325 mg oral

aspirin aluminum NF, JAN

aspirin & butalbital & caffeine *analgesic; sedative* 325•50•40 mg oral

aspirin DL-lysine JAN

Aspirin with Codeine No. 2, No. 3, and No. 4 tablets ℞ *narcotic analgesic* [codeine phosphate; aspirin] 15•325 mg; 30•325 mg; 60•325 mg

Aspirin-Free Pain Relief tablets, caplets OTC *analgesic; antipyretic* [acetaminophen] 325, 500 mg; 500 mg

Aspirol (trademarked delivery form) *crushable ampule for inhalation*

aspogen [see: dihydroxyaluminum aminoacetate]

aspoxicillin INN, JAN

Asprimox; Asprimox Extra Protection for Arthritis Pain tablets, caplets OTC *analgesic; antipyretic; antiinflammatory; antirheumatic* [aspirin (buffered with aluminum hydroxide, magnesium hydroxide, and calcium carbonate)] 325 mg

aspro [see: aspirin]

astatine *element (At)*

Astelin nasal spray ℞ *antihistamine* [azelastine HCl] 137 µg/spray

astemizole USAN, INN, BAN *antiallergic; second-generation piperidine antihistamine*

AsthmaHaler inhalation aerosol OTC *sympathomimetic bronchodilator* [epinephrine bitartrate] 0.35 mg/dose

AsthmaNefrin solution for inhalation OTC *sympathomimetic bronchodilator* [racepinephrine HCl] 2.25%

astifilcon A USAN *hydrophilic contact lens material*

Astracaine; Astracaine Forte ⓒᴬ intraoral injection ℞ *local anesthetic for dentistry* [articaine HCl; epinephrine] 4%•1:200 000; 4%•1:100 000

astragalus (Astragalus membranaceus) root *medicinal herb for cancer, chronic fatigue, and Epstein-Barr syndrome; also used to strengthen the immune system, especially after chemotherapy and HIV treatments*

Astramorph PF (preservative free) IV, subcu or IM injection ℞ *narcotic analgesic* [morphine sulfate] 0.5, 1 mg/mL

astringents *a class of agents that contract tissue, reducing secretions or discharges* [see also: hemostatics; styptics]

Astroglide vaginal gel OTC *lubricant* [glycerin; propylene glycol]

astromicin INN *antibacterial* [also: astromicin sulfate]

astromicin sulfate USAN, JAN *antibacterial* [also: astromicin]

AT·III (antithrombin III) [q.v.]

Atacand tablets ℞ *antihypertensive; angiotensin II receptor antagonist* [candesartan cilexetil] 4, 8, 16, 32 mg

atamestane INN *investigational aromatase inhibitor for cancer*

ataprost INN

Atarax tablets, syrup ℞ *anxiolytic; minor tranquilizer; antihistamine for allergic pruritus* [hydroxyzine HCl] 10, 25, 50 mg; 10 mg/5 mL ⊡ Marax

Atarax 100 tablets ℞ *anxiolytic; minor tranquilizer; antihistamine for allergic pruritus* [hydroxyzine HCl] 100 mg ⊡ Marax

atarvet [see: acepromazine]

atenolol USAN, INN, BAN, JAN *antihypertensive; antiadrenergic (β-receptor)* 25, 50, 100 mg oral ⊡ timolol

atevirdine INN *antiviral* [also: atevirdine mesylate]

atevirdine mesylate USAN *antiviral; investigational (Phase I) for HIV and AIDS* [also: atevirdine]

Atgam IV infusion ℞ *immunizing agent for allograft rejection* [lymphocyte immune globulin, antithymocyte (equine)] 50 mg/mL

athyromazole [see: carbimazole]

atipamezole USAN, INN, BAN *α_2-receptor antagonist*

atiprimod dihydrochloride USAN *immunomodulator; anti-inflammatory; antiarthritic*

atiprimod dimaleate USAN *immunomodulator; anti-inflammatory; antiarthritic*

atiprosin INN *antihypertensive* [also: atiprosin maleate]

atiprosin maleate USAN *antihypertensive* [also: atiprosin]

Ativan IV or IM injection ℞ *benzodiazepine anxiolytic; anticonvulsive* [lorazepam] 2, 4 mg/mL ⊡ Adapin; Avitene

Ativan tablets ℞ *benzodiazepine anxiolytic* [lorazepam] 0.5, 1, 2 mg ⊡ Adapin; Avitene

atlafilcon A USAN *hydrophilic contact lens material*

ATM·027 *investigational (Phase I) monoclonal antibody for multiple sclerosis*

ATnativ powder for IV infusion (discontinued 1999) ℞ *for thrombosis and pulmonary emboli of congenital AT-III deficiency (orphan)* [antithrombin III] 500 IU

atolide USAN, INN *anticonvulsant*

Atolone tablets ℞ *corticosteroid; antiinflammatory* [triamcinolone] 4 mg

atorvastatin calcium USAN *HMG-CoA reductase inhibitor for hypercholesterolemia, dysbetalipoproteinemia, and hypertriglyceridemia*

atosiban USAN, INN *oxytocin antagonist*

atovaquone USAN, INN, BAN *antipneumocystic for Pneumocystis carinii pneumonia (orphan); antimalarial; investigational (orphan) antiprotozoal for Toxoplasma gondii encephalitis*

ATP (adenosine triphosphate) [see: adenosine triphosphate disodium]

ATPase (adenosine triphosphatase) inhibitors *a class of gastric antisecretory agents that inhibit the ATPase "proton pump" within the gastric parietal cell* [also called: proton pump inhibitors; substituted benzimidazoles]

atracurium besilate INN *skeletal muscle relaxant; nondepolarizing neuromuscular blocker; adjunct to anesthesia* [also: atracurium besylate]

atracurium besylate USAN, BAN *skeletal muscle relaxant; nondepolarizing neuromuscular blocker; adjunct to anesthesia* [also: atracurium besilate]

Atragen ℞ *investigational (NDA filed, orphan) antineoplastic for acute promyelocytic leukemia; investigational (orphan) for other leukemias and ophthalmic squamous metaplasia* [tretinoin]

atreleuton USAN *5-lipoxygenase inhibitor for asthma*

Atretol tablets ℞ *anticonvulsant; analgesic for trigeminal neuralgia; antipsychotic* [carbamazepine] 200 mg

Atridox gel ℞ *subgingival antibiotic for periodontal disease* [doxycycline hyclate] 10%

Atrigel (trademarked delivery system) *sustained-release delivery*

atrimustine INN

atrinositol INN

Atrisorb FreeFlow GTR Barrier ℞ *guided tissue regeneration (GTR) therapy for severe periodontal disease*

Atrohist Pediatric oral suspension ℞ *pediatric decongestant and antihistamine* [phenylephrine tannate; chlorpheniramine tannate; pyrilamine tannate] 5•2•12.5 mg/5 mL

Atrohist Pediatric sustained-release capsules ℞ *pediatric decongestant and antihistamine* [pseudoephedrine HCl; chlorpheniramine maleate] 60•4 mg

Atrohist Plus sustained-release tablets ℞ *decongestant; antihistamine; anticholinergic* [phenylpropanolamine HCl; phenylephrine HCl; chlorpheniramine maleate; hyoscyamine sulfate; atropine sulfate; scopolamine hydrobromide] 50•25•8•0.19• 0.04•0.01 mg

Atrohist Sprinkle sustained-release capsules (name changed to Atrohist Pediatric in 1995)

atromepine INN, DCF

Atromid-S capsules ℞ *cholesterol-lowering antihyperlipidemic; also for primary dysbetalipoproteinemia* [clofibrate] 500 mg (1 g available in Canada)

Atropa belladonna *medicinal herb* [see: belladonna]

AtroPen auto-injector (automatic IM injection device) ℞ *antidote for organophosphorous or carbamate insecticides* [atropine sulfate] ²⁄

atropine USP, BAN *anticholinergic*

Atropine Care eye drops ℞ *mydriatic; cycloplegic* [atropine sulfate] 1%

atropine methonitrate INN, BAN *anticholinergic* [also: methylatropine nitrate]

atropine methylnitrate [see: methylatropine nitrate]

atropine oxide INN *anticholinergic* [also: atropine oxide HCl]

atropine oxide HCl USAN *anticholinergic* [also: atropine oxide]

atropine propionate [see: prampine]

atropine sulfate USP, JAN GI *antispasmodic; bronchodilator; cycloplegic; mydriatic* [also: atropine sulphate] 0.4, 0.6 mg oral; 1%, 2% eye drops; 0.05, 0.1, 0.3, 0.4, 0.5, 0.8, 1 mg/mL injection

atropine sulphate BAN GI *antispasmodic; bronchodilator; cycloplegic; mydriatic* [also: atropine sulfate]

Atropine-1 eye drops ℞ *mydriatic; cycloplegic* [atropine sulfate] 1%

Atropisol Dropperettes (eye drops) ℞ *cycloplegic; mydriatic* [atropine sulfate] 1%

Atrosept sugar-coated tablets ℞ *urinary antibiotic; analgesic; antispasmodic; acidifier* [methenamine; phenyl salicylate; atropine sulfate; methylene blue; hyoscyamine sulfate; benzoic acid] 40.8•18.1•0.03•5.4•0.03•4.5 mg

Atrovent nasal spray, solution for inhalation, inhalation aerosol ℞ *anticholinergic bronchodilator for bronchospasm; antisecretory for rhinorrhea* [ipratropium bromide] 0.03%, 0.06%; 0.02%; 18 μg/dose ② Trovan

A/T/S topical solution, gel ℞ *topical antibiotic for acne* [erythromycin] 2%

Attain liquid OTC *enteral nutritional therapy* [lactose-free formula]

attapulgite, activated USP *suspending agent; GI adsorbent*

Attenuvax powder for subcu injection ℞ *measles vaccine* [measles virus vaccine, live attenuated] 0.5 mL

Atuss DM syrup ℞ *antitussive; decongestant; antihistamine* [dextromethorphan hydrobromide; phenylephrine HCl; chlorpheniramine maleate] 15•5•2 mg/5 mL

Atuss EX syrup ℞ *narcotic antitussive; expectorant* [hydrocodone bitartrate; guaifenesin] 5•100 mg/5 mL

Atuss G syrup ℞ *narcotic antitussive; decongestant; expectorant* [hydrocodone bitartrate; phenylephrine HCl; guaifenesin] 2•10•100 mg/5 mL

Atuss HD liquid ℞ *narcotic antitussive; decongestant; antihistamine* [hydrocodone bitartrate; phenylephrine HCl; chlorpheniramine maleate] 2.5•5•2 mg/5 mL

"atypical" antipsychotics [see: novel antipsychotics]

[198]Au [see: gold Au 198]

augmented betamethasone dipropionate *topical corticosteroid*

Augmentin film-coated tablets, chewable tablets, powder for oral suspension ℞ *aminopenicillin antibiotic* [amoxicillin; clavulanate potassium] 250•125, 500•125, 875•125 mg; 125•31.25, 200•28.5, 250•62.5, 400•57 mg; 125•31.25, 200•28.5, 250•62.5, 400•57 mg/5 mL

Augmentin IV injection ℞ *aminopenicillin antibiotic* [amoxicillin sodium; clavulanate potassium]

Auralgan Otic ear drops ℞ *topical local anesthetic; analgesic* [benzocaine; antipyrine] 1.4%•5.4% ② Allergan; allergen

auranofin USAN, INN, BAN, JAN *antirheumatic (29% gold)*

Aureomycin ointment (discontinued 1996) OTC *topical antibiotic* [chlortetracycline HCl] 3% ② Achromycin; actinomycin

Aureomycin ophthalmic ointment (discontinued 1995) ℞ *topical ophthalmic antibiotic* [chlortetracycline HCl] 10 mg/g

aureoquin [now: quinetolate]

Auriculin *investigational (orphan) for acute renal failure and renal transplants; clinical trials discontinued 1997; orphan status withdrawn 1998* [anaritide acetate]

Auro Ear Drops OTC *agent to emulsify and disperse ear wax* [carbamide peroxide] 6.5%

Auro-Dri ear drops OTC *antibacterial; antifungal* [boric acid] 2.75%

Aurolate IM injection ℞ *antirheumatic* [gold sodium thiomalate] 50 mg/mL
aurolin [see: gold sodium thiosulfate]
auropin [see: gold sodium thiosulfate]
aurosan [see: gold sodium thiosulfate]
aurothioglucose USP *antirheumatic (50% gold)*
aurothioglycanide INN, DCF
aurothiomalate disodium [see: gold sodium thiomalate]
aurothiomalate sodium [see: gold sodium thiomalate]
Auroto Otic ear drops ℞ *topical local anesthetic; analgesic* [antipyrine; benzocaine] 1.4%•5.4%
Australian tea tree *medicinal herb* [see: tea tree oil]
Autohaler (delivery form) *breath-activated metered-dose inhaler*
auto-injector (delivery device) *automatic IM injection device*
autolymphocyte therapy (ALT) *investigational (orphan) for metastatic renal cell carcinoma (clinical trials discontinued 1998)*
Autoplex T IV injection or drip ℞ *antihemophilic to correct factor VIII deficiency and coagulation deficiency* [anti-inhibitor coagulant complex, heat treated] (each bottle is labeled with dosage)
autoprothrombin I [see: factor VII]
autoprothrombin II [see: factor IX]
autumn crocus *(Colchicum autumnale; C. speciosum; C. vernum)* plant and corm *medicinal herb for edema, gonorrhea, gout, prostate enlargement, and rheumatism; not generally regarded as safe and effective as it is highly toxic because of its colchicine content*
AV (Adriamycin, vincristine) *chemotherapy protocol*
Avail tablets OTC *vitamin/mineral/iron supplement* [multiple vitamins & minerals; iron; folic acid] ≟•18•0.4 mg ⅀ Advil
Avakine (name changed to Remicade upon release in 1998)

Avalide tablets ℞ *antihypertensive; angiotensin II receptor antagonist; diuretic* [irbesartan; hydrochlorothiazide] 150•12.5, 300•12.5 mg
Avandia film-coated tablets ℞ *thiazolidinedione antidiabetic; increases cellular response to insulin without increasing insulin secretion* [rosiglitazone maleate] 2, 4, 8 mg
Avapro tablets ℞ *antihypertensive; angiotensin II receptor antagonist* [irbesartan] 75, 150, 300 mg
avasimbe USAN *acylCoA transferase (ACAT) inhibitor for hyperlipidemia and atherosclerosis*
AVC vaginal cream, vaginal suppositories ℞ *broad-spectrum antibiotic* [sulfanilamide] 15%; 1.05 g
Aveeno lotion OTC *moisturizer; emollient* [colloidal oatmeal] 1%
Aveeno Anti-Itch cream, lotion OTC *topical poison ivy treatment* [calamine; pramoxine HCl; camphor] 3%•1%•0.3%
Aveeno Cleansing bar OTC *soap-free therapeutic skin cleanser* [colloidal oatmeal] 51%
Aveeno Cleansing for Acne-Prone Skin bar OTC *medicated cleanser for acne* [salicylic acid; colloidal oatmeal]
Aveeno Moisturizing cream OTC *moisturizer; emollient* [colloidal oatmeal] 1%
Aveeno Oilated Bath packets OTC *bath emollient* [colloidal oatmeal; mineral oil] 43%•≟
Aveeno Regular Bath packets OTC *bath emollient* [colloidal oatmeal] 100%
Aveeno Shave gel OTC *moisturizer; emollient* [oatmeal flour] ≟
Aveeno Shower & Bath oil OTC *bath emollient* [colloidal oatmeal] 5%
Avena sativa *medicinal herb* [see: oats]
Aventyl HCl Pulvules (capsules), oral solution ℞ *tricyclic antidepressant* [nortriptyline HCl] 10, 25 mg; 10 mg/5 mL ⅀ Ambenyl; Bentyl
avertin [see: tribromoethanol]
avicatonin INN

Avicidin ℞ *investigational (Phase II) antineoplastic for prostate, colon, and lung cancers*

Avicine ℞ *investigational (Phase III) theraccine for pancreatic cancer; investigational (Phase II) for prostate and advanced colorectal cancers*

avilamycin USAN, INN, BAN *antibacterial*

avinar [see: uredepa]

Avita cream, gel ℞ *topical keratolytic for acne* [tretinoin] 0.025% ☑ Evista

Avitene Hemostat fiber (discontinued 1996) ℞ *topical hemostatic aid for surgery* [microfibrillar collagen hemostat] ☑ Ativan

Avitene Hemostat nonwoven web ℞ *topical hemostatic aid for surgery* [microfibrillar collagen hemostat] ☑ Ativan

avitriptan fumarate USAN *serotonin 5-HT$_1$ agonist for migraine*

avizafone INN, BAN

avobenzone USAN, INN *sunscreen*

avocado *(Persea americana; P. gratissima)* fruit and seed *medicinal herb for diarrhea, dysentery, inducing menstruation, lowering total cholesterol and improving overall lipid profile, promoting hair growth, and stimulating wound healing; also used as an aphrodisiac*

Avonex powder for IM injection ℞ *immunomodulator for relapsing remitting multiple sclerosis (orphan); investigational (orphan) for non-A, non-B hepatitis and brain tumors* [interferon beta-1a] 33 μg (6.6 million IU)/vial

avoparcin USAN, INN, BAN *glycopeptide antibiotic*

AVP (actinomycin D, vincristine, Platinol) *chemotherapy protocol*

avridine USAN, INN *antiviral*

Award *hydrophilic contact lens material* [hilafilcon A]

axamozide INN

axerophthol [see: vitamin A]

axetil USAN, INN *combining name for radicals or groups*

Axid Pulvules (capsules) ℞ *histamine H$_2$ antagonist for treatment of gastric and duodenal ulcers* [nizatidine] 150, 300 mg ☑ Biaxin

Axid AR ("acid reducer") tablets OTC *histamine H$_2$ antagonist for heartburn* [nizatidine] 75 mg

Axocet capsules ℞ *analgesic; antipyretic; sedative* [acetaminophen; butalbital] 650•50 mg

Axokine ℞ *investigational agent for the treatment of obesity associated with type 2 diabetes*

Axotal tablets (discontinued 1997) ℞ *analgesic; sedative* [aspirin; butalbital] 650•50 mg

Aygestin tablets ℞ *progestin for amenorrhea, abnormal uterine bleeding, or endometriosis* [norethindrone acetate] 5 mg

Ayr Saline nasal mist, nose drops, nasal gel OTC *nasal moisturizer* [sodium chloride (saline solution)] 0.65%

5-AZA (5-azacitidine) [see: azacitidine]

azabon USAN, INN *CNS stimulant*

azabuperone INN

azacitidine (5-AZA; 5-AZC) USAN, INN *antineoplastic*

azaclorzine INN *coronary vasodilator* [also: azaclorzine HCl]

azaclorzine HCl USAN *coronary vasodilator* [also: azaclorzine]

azaconazole USAN, INN *antifungal*

azacosterol INN *avian chemosterilant* [also: azacosterol HCl]

azacosterol HCl USAN *avian chemosterilant* [also: azacosterol]

AZA-CR [see: azacitidine]

Azactam powder for IV or IM injection ℞ *monobactam bactericidal antibiotic* [aztreonam] 0.5, 1, 2 g

azacyclonol INN, BAN [also: azacyclonol HCl]

azacyclonol HCl NF [also: azacyclonol]

5-azacytosine arabinoside (ara-AC) [see: fazarabine]

5-aza-2′-deoxycytidine *investigational (orphan) for acute leukemia*

Azadirachta indica *medicinal herb* [see: neem tree]

azaftozine INN

azalanstat dihydrochloride USAN *hypolipidemic*

azalomycin INN, BAN

azaloxan INN *antidepressant* [also: azaloxan fumarate]

azaloxan fumarate USAN *antidepressant* [also: azaloxan]

azamethiphos BAN

azamethonium bromide INN, BAN

azamulin INN

azanator INN *bronchodilator* [also: azanator maleate]

azanator maleate USAN *bronchodilator* [also: azanator]

azanidazole USAN, INN, BAN *antiprotozoal*

azaperone USAN, INN, BAN *antipsychotic*

azapetine BAN

azapetine phosphate [see: azapetine]

azaprocin INN

azapropazone INN, BAN, DCF *antiinflammatory* [also: apazone]

azaquinzole INN

azaribine USAN, INN, BAN *antipsoriatic*

azarole USAN *immunoregulator*

azaserine USAN, INN *antifungal*

azasetron INN

azaspirium chloride INN

azaspirones *a class of anxiolytics*

azastene

azatadine INN, BAN *piperidine antihistamine* [also: azatadine maleate]

azatadine maleate USAN, USP *piperidine antihistamine* [also: azatadine]

azatepa INN *antineoplastic* [also: azetepa]

azathioprine USAN, USP, INN, BAN, JAN *immunosuppressant*

azathioprine sodium USP *immunosuppressant* 100 mg injection

5-AZC (5-azacitidine) [see: azacitidine]

Azdone tablets ℞ *narcotic analgesic* [hydrocodone bitartrate; aspirin] 5•500 mg

azdU (azidouridine) [q.v.]

azelaic acid USAN, INN *topical antimicrobial and keratolytic for acne*

azelastine INN, BAN *phthalazinone antihistamine; antiallergic; antiasthmatic* [also: azelastine HCl]

azelastine HCl USAN, JAN *phthalazinone antihistamine; antiallergic; antiasthmatic* [also: azelastine]

Azelex cream ℞ *antimicrobial and keratolytic for inflammatory acne vulgaris* [azelaic acid] 20%

azelnidipine INN

azepexole INN, BAN

azephine [see: azapetine phosphate]

azepinamide [see: glypinamide]

azepindole USAN, INN *antidepressant*

azetepa USAN, BAN *antineoplastic* [also: azatepa]

azetirelin INN

azidamfenicol INN, BAN, DCF

azidoamphenicol [see: azidamfenicol]

azidocillin INN, BAN

azidothymidine (AZT) [now: zidovudine]

azidouridine (azdU) *investigational (Phase I) antiviral for HIV and AIDS*

azimexon INN

azimilide dihydrochloride USAN *investigational (NDA filed) antiarrhythmic and antifibrillatory*

azintamide INN

azinthiamide [see: azintamide]

azipramine INN *antidepressant* [also: azipramine HCl]

azipramine HCl USAN *antidepressant* [also: azipramine]

aziridinyl benzoquinone [see: diaziquone]

azithromycin USAN, USP, INN, BAN *macrolide antibiotic*

azlocillin USAN, INN, BAN *penicillin antibiotic*

azlocillin sodium USP *penicillin antibiotic*

Azmacort oral inhalation aerosol ℞ *corticosteroidal anti-inflammatory for chronic asthma* [triamcinolone acetonide] 100 μg/dose

Azo Gantanol film-coated tablets (discontinued 1995) ℞ *urinary anti-infective; urinary analgesic* [sulfamethoxazole; phenazopyridine HCl] 500•100 mg

Azo Gantrisin film-coated tablets (discontinued 1995) ℞ *urinary anti-infective; urinary analgesic* [sulfisoxazole; phenazopyridine HCl] 500•50 mg

Azo Test Strips reagent strips for home use *in vitro diagnostic aid for urinary tract infections*

azoconazole [now: azaconazole]

azodisal sodium (ADS) [now: olsalazine sodium]

"azoles" *a class of fungicides that include all with generic names ending in "azole," such clotrimazole, fluconazole, etc.*

azolimine USAN, INN *diuretic* ⊡ Azulfidine

Azopt eye drop suspension ℞ *carbonic anhydrase inhibitor for glaucoma* [brinzolamide] 1%

azosemide USAN, INN, JAN *diuretic*

Azo-Standard tablets OTC *urinary analgesic* [phenazopyridine HCl] 95 mg

Azostix reagent strips for professional use *in vitro diagnostic aid to estimate the amount of BUN in whole blood*

Azo-Sulfisoxazole tablets ℞ *urinary anti-infective; urinary analgesic* [sulfisoxazole; phenazopyridine HCl] 500•50 mg

azotomycin USAN, INN *antibiotic antineoplastic*

azovan blue BAN *blood volume test* [also: Evans blue]

azovan sodium [see: Evans blue]

AZT (azidothymidine) [now: zidovudine]

Aztec ℞ *investigational (Phase III) controlled-release formulation for early HIV and AIDS* [zidovudine]

AZT-P-ddI *investigational (Phase I) antiviral for AIDS*

aztreonam USAN, USP, INN, BAN, JAN *monobactam bactericidal antibiotic*

azulene sulfonate sodium JAN [also: sodium gualenate]

Azulfidine oral suspension (discontinued 1995) ℞ *broad-spectrum bacteriostatic; antirheumatic; anti-inflammatory for ulcerative colitis* [sulfasalazine] 250 mg/5 mL ⊡ azolimine

Azulfidine tablets ℞ *broad-spectrum bacteriostatic; antirheumatic; anti-inflammatory for ulcerative colitis* [sulfasalazine] 500 mg ⊡ Silvadene

Azulfidine EN-tabs enteric-coated tablets ℞ *broad-spectrum bacteriostatic; antirheumatic; anti-inflammatory for ulcerative colitis* [sulfasalazine] 500 mg

azumolene INN *skeletal muscle relaxant* [also: azumolene sodium]

azumolene sodium USAN *skeletal muscle relaxant* [also: azumolene]

azure A carbacrylic resin [see: azuresin]

azuresin NF, BAN

B

B Complex + C timed-release tablets OTC *vitamin supplement* [multiple B vitamins; vitamin C] ≛•500 mg

B Complex with C and B-12 injection ℞ *parenteral vitamin supplement* [multiple vitamins] ≛

B Complex-50 sustained-release tablets OTC *vitamin supplement* [multiple B vitamins; folic acid; biotin] ≛•400•50 μg

B Complex-150 sustained-release tablets OTC *vitamin supplement* [multiple B vitamins; folic acid; biotin] ≛•400•150 μg

B & O Suprettes No. 15A; B & O Suprettes No. 16A suppositories ℞ *narcotic analgesic* [belladonna extract; opium] 16.2•30 mg; 16.2•60 mg

B vitamins [see: vitamin B]

B₁ (vitamin B₁) [see: thiamine HCl]

B₂ (vitamin B₂) [see: riboflavin]

B₃ (vitamin B₃) [see: niacin; niacinamide]

B₅ (vitamin B₅) [see: calcium pantothenate]

B$_6$ (vitamin B$_6$) [see: pyridoxine HCl]

B$_8$ (vitamin B$_8$) [see: adenosine phosphate]

B$_{12}$ (vitamin B$_{12}$) [see: cyanocobalamin]

B$_{12a}$ (vitamin B$_{12a}$) [see: hydroxocobalamin]

B$_{12b}$ (vitamin B$_{12b}$) [see: hydroxocobalamin]

B-50 tablets OTC *vitamin supplement* [multiple B vitamins; folic acid; biotin] ≠•100•50 μg

B-50 timed-release tablets (discontinued 1995) OTC *vitamin supplement* [multiple B vitamins; folic acid; biotin] ≠•100•50 μg

B-100 tablets, timed-release tablets OTC *vitamin supplement* [multiple B vitamins; folic acid; biotin] ≠•100• 100 μg; ≠•400•50 μg

B2036-PEG *investigational (orphan) growth hormone antagonist for acromegaly*

B$_c$ (vitamin B$_c$) [see: folic acid]

B$_t$ (vitamin B$_t$) [see: carnitine]

Babee Teething lotion OTC *topical oral anesthetic; antiseptic* [benzocaine; cetalkonium chloride] 2.5%•0.02%

Baby Vitamin drops OTC *vitamin supplement* [multiple vitamins] ≠

Baby Vitamin with Iron drops OTC *vitamin/iron supplement* [multiple vitamins; iron] ≠•10 mg/mL

Babylax [see: Fleet Babylax]

BAC (BCNU, ara-C, cyclophosphamide) *chemotherapy protocol*

BAC (benzalkonium chloride) [q.v.]

bacampicillin INN, BAN *aminopenicillin antibiotic* [also: bacampicillin HCl]

bacampicillin HCl USAN, USP, JAN *aminopenicillin antibiotic* [also: bacampicillin]

bachelor's buttons *medicinal herb* [see: cornflower; feverfew; tansy; buttercup]

BACI ℞ *investigational anti-infective for AIDS-related cryptosporidiosis* [*Cryptosporidium parvum* bovine colostrum IgG concentrate]

Bacid capsules OTC *dietary supplement; fever blister treatment; not generally*

regarded as safe and effective as an antidiarrheal [*Lactobacillus acidophilus*] 500 million cultures ② Banacid

Baciguent ointment OTC *topical antibiotic* [bacitracin] 500 U/g

Baci-IM powder for IM injection ℞ *bactericidal antibiotic* [bacitracin] 50 000 U

bacillus Calmette-Guérin (BCG) vaccine [see: BCG vaccine]

bacitracin USP, INN, BAN, JAN *bactericidal antibiotic; investigational (orphan) for pseudomembranous enterocolitis* 500 U/g topical; 50 000 U/vial injection ② Bacitrin; Bactrim

bacitracin zinc USP, BAN *bactericidal antibiotic*

bacitracins zinc complex [see: bacitracin zinc]

Backache Maximum Strength Relief film-coated caplets OTC *analgesic; antirheumatic* [magnesium salicylate] 467 mg

Back-Pack (trademarked packaging form) *unit-of-use package*

baclofen (L-baclofen) USAN, USP, INN, BAN, JAN *skeletal muscle relaxant for intractable spasticity due to spinal cord injury or disease (orphan); investigational (orphan) for trigeminal neuralgia* 10, 20 mg oral

bacmecillinam INN

Bacmin tablets ℞ *vitamin/mineral/iron supplement* [multiple vitamins & minerals; iron; folic acid; biotin] ≠• 27•0.8•0.15 mg

BACOD (bleomycin, Adriamycin, CCNU, Oncovin, dexamethasone) *chemotherapy protocol*

BACON (bleomycin, Adriamycin, CCNU, Oncovin, nitrogen mustard) *chemotherapy protocol*

BACOP (bleomycin, Adriamycin, cyclophosphamide, Oncovin, prednisone) *chemotherapy protocol*

BACT (BCNU, ara-C, cyclophosphamide, thioguanine) *chemotherapy protocol*

bactericidal and permeability-increasing (BPI) protein, recombi-

nant *investigational (Phase III, orphan) treatment for gram-negative sepsis, hemorrhagic shock, and meningococcemia*

bactericidal/permeability-increasing protein [see: rBPI-21]

bacteriostatic sodium chloride [see: sodium chloride]

Bacteriostatic Sodium Chloride Injection ℞ *IV diluent* [sodium chloride (normal saline solution)] 0.9% (normal)

Bacti-Cleanse liquid OTC *soap-free therapeutic skin cleanser* [benzalkonium chloride] ≟

Bacticort eye drop suspension (discontinued 1995) ℞ *topical ophthalmic corticosteroidal anti-inflammatory; antibiotic* [hydrocortisone; neomycin sulfate; polymyxin B sulfate] 1%•0.35%•10 000 U/mL

Bactigen B Streptococcus-CS slide test for professional use *in vitro diagnostic aid for Group B streptococcal antigens in vaginal and cervical swabs*

Bactigen Meningitis Panel slide test for professional use *in vitro diagnostic aid for H influenzae, N meningitidis, and S pneumoniae in various fluids* [latex agglutination test]

Bactigen N meningitidis slide test for professional use ℞ *in vitro diagnostic aid for Neisseria meningitidis* [latex agglutination test]

Bactigen S Pneumonia test kit for professional use (discontinued 1996) *in vitro diagnostic aid for Streptococcus pneumoniae antigens in various fluids*

Bactigen Salmonella-Shigella slide test for professional use *in vitro diagnostic aid for salmonella and shigella* [latex agglutination test]

Bactigen Strep B slide test for professional use (discontinued 1996) *in vitro diagnostic aid for Group B streptococcal antigens in various fluids*

Bactine Antiseptic Anesthetic aerosol (discontinued 1995) OTC *topical local anesthetic; antiseptic* [lidocaine HCl; benzalkonium chloride] 2.5%•0.13%

Bactine Antiseptic Anesthetic liquid, spray OTC *topical local anesthetic; antiseptic* [lidocaine HCl; benzalkonium chloride] 2.5%•0.13%

Bactine First Aid Antibiotic ointment OTC *topical antibiotic* [polymyxin B sulfate; neomycin sulfate; bacitracin]

Bactine First Aid Antibiotic Plus Anesthetic ointment OTC *topical antibiotic; topical local anesthetic* [polymyxin B sulfate; neomycin sulfate; bacitracin; diperodon HCl] 5000 U•3.5 mg•400 U•10 mg per g

Bactine Hydrocortisone; Maximum Strength Bactine cream OTC *topical corticosteroidal anti-inflammatory* [hydrocortisone] 0.5%; 1%

Bactocill capsules (discontinued 1998) ℞ *penicillinase-resistant penicillin antibiotic* [oxacillin sodium] 250, 500 mg Ⓓ Pathocil

Bactocill powder for IV or IM injection ℞ *penicillinase-resistant penicillin antibiotic* [oxacillin sodium] 0.5, 1, 2, 4, 10 g Ⓓ Pathocil

BactoShield aerosol foam, solution OTC *broad-spectrum antimicrobial; germicidal* [chlorhexidine gluconate; alcohol 4%] 4%

BactoShield 2 solution OTC *broad-spectrum antimicrobial; germicidal* [chlorhexidine gluconate; alcohol 4%] 2%

Bactrim; Bactrim DS tablets ℞ *anti-infective; antibacterial* [trimethoprim; sulfamethoxazole] 80•400 mg; 160•800 mg Ⓓ bacitracin

Bactrim IV infusion ℞ *anti-infective; antibacterial* [trimethoprim; sulfamethoxazole] 80•400 mg/5 mL

Bactrim Pediatric oral suspension ℞ *anti-infective; antibacterial* [trimethoprim; sulfamethoxazole] 40•200 mg/5 mL

Bactroban cream ℞ *topical antibiotic* [mupirocin calcium] 2%

Bactroban ointment ℞ *topical antibiotic for impetigo* [mupirocin] 2%

Bactroban Nasal ointment in single-use tubes ℞ *antibiotic for iatrogenic*

*methicillin-resistant Staphylococcus
aureus (MRSA) infections* [mupirocin
calcium] 2%

bakeprofen INN

baker's yeast *natural source of protein
and B-complex vitamins*

BAL (British antilewisite) [now:
dimercaprol]

BAL in Oil *deep IM injection* ℞ *antidote for arsenic, gold, and mercury poisoning; lead poisoning adjunct* [dimer-
caprol in peanut oil] 100 mg/mL

balafilcon A USAN *hydrophilic contact
lens material*

balipramine BAN [also: depramine]

balm *medicinal herb* [see: lemon balm]

balm, eye; eye root *medicinal herb*
[see: goldenseal]

balm, mountain *medicinal herb* [see:
yerba santa]

balm, squaw; squaw mint *medicinal
herb* [see: pennyroyal]

**balm of Gilead (Populus balsam-
ifera; P. candicans)** *buds medicinal
herb used as an antiscorbutic, balsamic,
diuretic, stimulant, and vulnerary*

Balmex *ointment* OTC *astringent; moisturizer; emollient* [zinc oxide] 11.3%

Balmex Baby *powder* OTC *topical diaper rash treatment* [zinc oxide; peruvian balsam; corn starch]

Balmex Emollient *lotion* OTC *moisturizer; emollient*

balmony *medicinal herb* [see: turtle-
bloom]

Balneol Perianal Cleansing *lotion*
OTC *emollient/protectant* [mineral oil;
lanolin]

Balnetar *bath oil* OTC *antipsoriatic;
antiseborrheic; antipruritic; emollient*
[coal tar] 2.5%

balsalazide INN, BAN *investigational
(NDA filed) gastrointestinal anti-
inflammatory for ulcerative colitis* [also:
balsalazide disodium]

balsalazide disodium USAN *investigational (Phase III) gastrointestinal anti-
inflammatory for acute ulcerative colitis*
[also: balsalazide]

balsalazide sodium [see: balsalazide
disodium]

balsalazine [see: balsalazide disodium;
balsalazide]

balsam apple; balsam pear *medicinal
herb* [see: bitter melon]

balsam Peru [see: peruvian balsam;
balsam tree]

balsam poplar *medicinal herb* [see:
balm of Gilead]

balsam tree *medicinal herb* [see: Peruvian balsam]

balsamics; balsams *a class of agents
that soothe or heal; balms; also, certain
resinous substances of vegetable origin*

*Balsamodendron myrrha medicinal
herb* [see: myrrh]

balsan [see: peruvian balsam]

bamaluzole INN

bambermycin INN, BAN *antibacterial
antibiotic* [also: bambermycins]

bambermycins USAN *antibacterial antibiotic* [also: bambermycin]

bambuterol INN, BAN

bamethan INN, BAN *vasodilator* [also:
bamethan sulfate]

bamethan sulfate USAN, JAN *vasodilator* [also: bamethan]

bamifylline INN, BAN *bronchodilator*
[also: bamifylline HCl]

bamifylline HCl USAN *bronchodilator*
[also: bamifylline]

bamipine INN, BAN, DCF

bamnidazole USAN, INN *antiprotozoal
(Trichomonas)*

**BAMON (bleomycin, Adriamycin,
methotrexate, Oncovin, nitrogen
mustard)** *chemotherapy protocol*

Banadyne-3 *solution* OTC *topical oral
anesthetic; analgesic; counterirritant;
antiseptic* [lidocaine; menthol; alcohol 45%] 4%•1%

Banalg *lotion* OTC *topical analgesic;
counterirritant* [methyl salicylate;
camphor; menthol] 4.9%•2%•1%

Banalg Hospital Strength *lotion* OTC
topical analgesic; counterirritant [methyl
salicylate; menthol] 14%•3%

Bancap HC capsules ℞ *narcotic analgesic* [hydrocodone bitartrate; acetaminophen] 5•500 mg

bandage, adhesive USP *surgical aid*

bandage, gauze USP *surgical aid*

Banex liquid ℞ *decongestant; expectorant* [phenylpropanolamine HCl; phenylephrine HCl; guaifenesin]

Banflex IV or IM injection ℞ *skeletal muscle relaxant* [orphenadrine citrate] 30 mg/mL

banocide [see: diethylcarbamazine citrate]

Banophen caplets, capsules OTC *antihistamine* [diphenhydramine HCl] 25 mg

Banophen elixir OTC *antihistamine* [diphenhydramine HCl] 12.5 mg/5 mL

Banophen Decongestant capsules OTC *decongestant; antihistamine* [pseudoephedrine HCl; diphenhydramine HCl] 60•25 mg ☑ Barophen

BanSmoke gum (discontinued 1995) OTC *smoking deterrent* [benzocaine] 6 mg

Banthīne tablets ℞ *anticholinergic; peptic ulcer treatment adjunct* [methantheline bromide] 50 mg ☑ Brethine; Vantin

Bantron tablets (discontinued 1999) OTC *smoking deterrent* [lobeline sulfate alkaloids; tribasic calcium phosphate; magnesium carbonate] 2•130•130 mg ☑ Vantin

Baptisia tinctoria medicinal herb [see: wild indigo]

baquiloprim INN, BAN

Barbados aloe *medicinal herb* [see: aloe]

barbenyl [see: phenobarbital]

barberry (*Berberis vulgaris*) bark *medicinal herb for bacteria-associated diarrhea, blood cleansing, cough, fever, indigestion, jaundice, liver disorders, sciatica, and sore throat*

barberry, California *medicinal herb* [see: Oregon grape]

barbexaclone INN

Barbidonna elixir (discontinued 1995) ℞ *GI antispasmodic; anticholinergic; sedative* [atropine sulfate; scopolamine hydrobromide; hyoscy-amine hydrobromide; phenobarbital] 0.034•0.01•0.174•21.6 mg/5 mL

Barbidonna; Barbidonna No. 2 tablets ℞ *GI antispasmodic; anticholinergic; sedative* [atropine sulfate; scopolamine hydrobromide; hyoscyamine hydrobromide; phenobarbital] 0.025•0.0074•0.1286•16 mg; 0.025•0.0074•0.1286•32 mg

barbiphenyl [see: phenobarbital]

barbital NF, INN, JAN [also: barbitone]

barbital, soluble [now: barbital sodium]

barbital sodium NF, INN [also: barbitone sodium]

barbitone BAN [also: barbital]

barbitone sodium BAN [also: barbital sodium]

barbiturates *a class of sedative/hypnotics that produce a wide range of mood alteration; also widely abused as addictive street drugs*

Barc liquid OTC *pediculicide for lice* [pyrethrins; piperonyl butoxide; petroleum distillate] 0.18%•2.2%•5.52%

bardana *medicinal herb* [see: burdock]

Baricon powder for oral suspension ℞ *radiopaque contrast medium for gastrointestinal imaging* [barium sulfate] 98%

Baridium tablets ℞ *urinary analgesic* [phenazopyridine HCl] 100 mg

barium *element (Ba)*

barium hydroxide lime USP *carbon dioxide absorbent*

barium sulfate USP, JAN *oral/rectal radiopaque contrast medium for gastrointestinal imaging*

barley (*Hordeum vulgare*) juice powder *medicinal herb for anemia, arthritis, blood cleansing, boils, bronchitis, cancer, metal poisoning, poor circulation, and reducing total and LDL cholesterol and increasing HDL cholesterol*

barmastine USAN, INN *antihistamine*

BarnesHind Saline for Sensitive Eyes solution OTC *rinsing/storage solution for soft contact lenses* [sodium chloride (preserved saline solution)]

barnidipine INN

Barobag rectal suspension ℞ *radiopaque contrast medium for gastrointestinal imaging* [barium sulfate] 97%

Baro-cat oral suspension ℞ *radiopaque contrast medium for gastrointestinal imaging* [barium sulfate] 1.5%

Baroflave powder for oral suspension (discontinued 1999) ℞ *radiopaque contrast medium for gastrointestinal imaging* [barium sulfate]

Barophen elixir (discontinued 1995) ℞ *GI antispasmodic; anticholinergic; sedative* [atropine sulfate; scopolamine hydrobromide; hyoscyamine sulfate; phenobarbital] 0.0194•0.0065•0.1037•16.2 mg/5 mL ▣ Banophen

Baros effervescent granules ℞ *adjunct to gastrointestinal imaging* [sodium bicarbonate; tartaric acid; simethicone] 460•420• ² mg/g

Barosma betulina; B. cenulata; B. serratifolia medicinal herb [see: buchu]

barosmin [see: diosmin]

Barosperse powder for oral suspension ℞ *radiopaque contrast medium for gastrointestinal imaging* [barium sulfate] 95%

Barosperse, Liquid oral/rectal suspension ℞ *radiopaque contrast medium for gastrointestinal imaging* [barium sulfate] 60%

barucainide INN

BAS (benzyl analogue of serotonin) [see: benanserin HCl]

Basaljel tablets, capsules, suspension OTC *antacid* [aluminum carbonate gel, basic] 500 mg; 500 mg; 400 mg/5 mL

basic aluminum acetate [see: aluminum subacetate]

basic aluminum aminoacetate [see: dihydroxyaluminum aminoacetate]

basic aluminum carbonate [see: aluminum carbonate, basic]

basic aluminum chloride [see: aluminum sesquichlorohydrate]

basic aluminum glycinate [see: dihydroxyaluminum aminoacetate]

basic bismuth carbonate [see: bismuth subcarbonate]

basic bismuth gallate [see: bismuth subgallate]

basic bismuth nitrate [see: bismuth subnitrate]

basic bismuth potassium bismuthotartrate [see: bismuth potassium tartrate]

basic bismuth salicylate [see: bismuth subsalicylate]

basic fibroblast growth factor (bFGF) [see: ersofermin]

basic fuchsin [see: fuchsin, basic]

basic zinc acetate [see: zinc acetate, basic]

basifungin USAN, INN *antifungal*

basil (Ocimum basilicum) leaves *medicinal herb for colds, headache, indigestion, insect and snake bites, and whooping cough*

basiliximab *immunosuppressant; IL-2 receptor antagonist for the prevention of acute rejection of renal transplants (orphan)*

basswood; bast tree *medicinal herb* [see: linden tree]

bastard hemp *medicinal herb* [see: hemp nettle]

bastard saffron *medicinal herb* [see: safflower]

batanopride INN *antiemetic* [also: batanopride HCl]

batanopride HCl USAN *antiemetic* [also: batanopride]

batebulast INN

batelapine INN *antipsychotic* [also: batelapine HCl]

batelapine maleate USAN *antipsychotic* [also: batelapine]

batilol INN

batimastat USAN, INN *investigational (Phase III) antineoplastic; matrix metalloproteinase (MMP) inhibitor*

batoprazine INN

batroxobin INN, JAN

batyl alcohol [see: batilol]

batylol [see: batilol]

BAVIP (bleomycin, Adriamycin, vinblastine, imidazole carboxamide, prednisone) *chemotherapy protocol*

baxitozine INN

bay; bay laurel; bay tree; Indian bay; sweet bay *medicinal herb* [see: laurel]

bay, holly; red bay; white bay *medicinal herb* [see: magnolia]

bayberry (Myrica cerifera) bark, berries, root bark *medicinal herb for cholera, diarrhea, dysentery, glands, goiter, indigestion, jaundice, excessive menstruation, scrofuloderma, and uterine hemorrhage; not generally regarded as safe and effective because of its high tannin content*

Baycol tablets ℞ *HMG-CoA reductase inhibitor for hypercholesterolemia, mixed hyperlipidemia, hypertriglyceridemia, and elevated apolipoprotein B* [cerivastatin sodium] 0.2, 0.3, 0.4 mg

Bayer Arthritis Regimen delayed-release enteric-coated tablets OTC *analgesic; antipyretic; anti-inflammatory; antirheumatic* [aspirin] 500 mg

Bayer Aspirin, Genuine; Maximum Bayer Aspirin film-coated tablets, film-coated caplets OTC *analgesic; antipyretic; anti-inflammatory; antirheumatic* [aspirin] 325 mg; 500 mg

Bayer Aspirin Regimen delayed-release enteric-coated tablets and caplets OTC *analgesic; antipyretic; anti-inflammatory; antirheumatic* [aspirin] 81, 325 mg

Bayer Buffered Aspirin tablets OTC *analgesic; antipyretic; anti-inflammatory; antirheumatic* [aspirin, buffered] 325 mg

Bayer Children's Aspirin chewable tablets OTC *analgesic; antipyretic; anti-inflammatory; antirheumatic* [aspirin] 81 mg

Bayer Enteric 500 delayed-release enteric-coated caplets (name changed to Bayer Arthritis Regimen in 1995)

Bayer Enteric Coated delayed-release enteric-coated caplets (name changed to Bayer Aspirin Regimen in 1995)

Bayer Low Adult Strength delayed-release enteric-coated tablets (name changed to Bayer Aspirin Regimen in 1995)

Bayer Plus caplets OTC *analgesic; antipyretic; anti-inflammatory; antirheumatic* [aspirin (buffered with calcium carbonate, magnesium carbonate and magnesium oxide)] 500 mg

Bayer Select Allergy Sinus, Aspirin-Free caplets OTC *decongestant; antihistamine; analgesic* [pseudoephedrine HCl; chlorpheniramine maleate; acetaminophen] 30•2•500 mg

Bayer Select Backache caplets OTC *analgesic; antipyretic; anti-inflammatory; antirheumatic* [magnesium salicylate] 580 mg

Bayer Select Chest Cold caplets OTC *antitussive; analgesic* [dextromethorphan hydrobromide; acetaminophen] 15•500 mg

Bayer Select Flu Relief caplets OTC *antitussive; decongestant; antihistamine; analgesic* [dextromethorphan hydrobromide; pseudoephedrine HCl; chlorpheniramine maleate; acetaminophen] 15•30•2•500 mg

Bayer Select Head & Chest Cold, Aspirin-Free caplets OTC *antitussive; decongestant; expectorant; analgesic* [dextromethorphan hydrobromide; pseudoephedrine HCl; guaifenesin; acetaminophen] 10•30•100•325 mg

Bayer Select Head Cold; Bayer Select Sinus Pain Relief caplets OTC *decongestant; analgesic; antipyretic* [pseudoephedrine HCl; acetaminophen] 30•500 mg

Bayer Select Headache caplets OTC *analgesic; antipyretic* [acetaminophen; caffeine] 500•65 mg

Bayer Select Menstrual caplets OTC *analgesic; antipyretic; diuretic* [acetaminophen; pamabrom] 500•25 mg

Bayer Select Night Time Cold caplets OTC *antitussive; decongestant; antihistamine; analgesic* [dextromethorphan hydrobromide; pseudoephedrine HCl; triprolidine HCl; acetaminophen] 15•30•1.25•500 mg

Bayer Select Night Time Pain Relief caplets OTC *antihistaminic sleep aid; analgesic* [diphenhydramine HCl; acetaminophen] 25•500 mg

Bayer Select Pain Relief Formula caplets OTC *nonsteroidal anti-inflammatory drug (NSAID); analgesic* [ibuprofen] 200 mg

Bayer Timed Release, 8-Hour caplets OTC *analgesic; antipyretic; anti-inflammatory; antirheumatic* [aspirin] 650 mg

Baylocaine 2% Viscous; Baylocaine 4% solution ℞ *topical anesthetic for mouth and pharynx* [lidocaine HCl]

Baypress ℞ *investigational (NDA filed) antihypertensive; calcium channel blocker* [nitrendipine]

bazinaprine INN

BB-2893 *investigational disease-modifying oral anti-inflammatory (discontinued 1997)*

BBVP-M (BCNU, bleomycin, VePesid, prednisone, methotrexate) *chemotherapy protocol*

BC tablets, powder OTC *analgesic; antipyretic; anti-inflammatory* [aspirin; salicylamide; caffeine] 325•95•16 mg; 650•145•32 mg/packet

B$_c$ (vitamin B$_c$) [see: folic acid]

BC Arthritis Strength powder OTC *analgesic; antipyretic; anti-inflammatory* [aspirin; salicylamide; caffeine] 742•222•36 mg

BC Cold Powder Non-Drowsy Formula packets (name changed to BC Cold-Sinus Powder in 1995)

BC Cold-Sinus Powder packets OTC *decongestant; analgesic; antipyretic* [phenylpropanolamine HCl; aspirin] 25•650 mg

BC Cold-Sinus-Allergy Powder packets OTC *decongestant; antihistamine; analgesic; antipyretic* [phenylpropanolamine HCl; chlorpheniramine maleate; aspirin] 25•4•650 mg

BC Multi Symptom Cold Powder packets (name changed to BC Cold-Sinus-Allergy Powder in 1995)

B-C with Folic Acid tablets ℞ *vitamin supplement* [multiple B vitamins; vitamin C; folic acid] ≐•500•0.5 mg

B-C with Folic Acid Plus tablets ℞ *vitamin/mineral/iron supplement* [multiple vitamins & minerals; ferrous fumarate; folic acid; biotin] ≐•27•0.8•0.15 mg

BCAA (branched-chain amino acids) [see: isoleucine; leucine; valine]

BCAP (BCNU, cyclophosphamide, Adriamycin, prednisone) *chemotherapy protocol*

BCAVe; B-CAVe (bleomycin, CCNU, Adriamycin, Velban) *chemotherapy protocol*

B-C-Bid caplets OTC *vitamin supplement* [multiple B vitamins; vitamin C] ≐•300 mg

BCD (bleomycin, cyclophosphamide, dactinomycin) *chemotherapy protocol*

BCG vaccine (bacillus Calmette-Guérin) USP *active bacterin for tuberculosis; antineoplastic for urinary bladder cancer*

B-CHOP (bleomycin, Cytoxin, hydroxydaunomycin, Oncovin, prednisone) *chemotherapy protocol*

BCMF (bleomycin, cyclophosphamide, methotrexate, fluorouracil) *chemotherapy protocol*

BCNU (bis-chloroethyl-nitrosourea) [see: carmustine]

B-Complex elixir OTC *vitamin supplement* [multiple B vitamins] ≐

B-Complex and B-12 tablets OTC *vitamin supplement* [multiple B vitamins; protease] ≐•10 mg

B-Complex with B-12 tablets OTC *vitamin supplement* [multiple B vitamins] ≐

B-Complex/Vitamin C caplets OTC *vitamin supplement* [multiple B vitamins; vitamin C] ≐•300 mg

BCOP (BCNU, cyclophosphamide, Oncovin, prednisone) *chemotherapy protocol*

BCP (BCNU, cyclophosphamide, prednisone) *chemotherapy protocol*

BC-Vite tablets OTC *vitamin supplement* [multiple B vitamins; vitamin C]

BCVP (BCNU, cyclophosphamide, vincristine, prednisone) *chemotherapy protocol*

BCVPP (BCNU, cyclophosphamide, vinblastine, procarbazine, prednisone) *chemotherapy protocol*

BCX-1470 *investigational (Phase I) agent for use in patients receiving heparin during cardiopulmonary bypass surgery*

BCX-34 *investigational (Phase III) agent for psoriasis, cutaneous T-cell lymphoma, and HIV (clinical trials discontinued 1997)* [now: peldesine]

B-D glucose chewable tablets OTC *glucose elevating agent* [glucose] 5 g

BDNF (brain-derived neurotrophic factor) [q.v.]

B-DOPA (bleomycin, DTIC, Oncovin, prednisone, Adriamycin) *chemotherapy protocol*

BEAC (BCNU, etoposide, ara-C, cyclophosphamide) *chemotherapy protocol*

BEAM (BCNU, etoposide, ara-C, melphalan) *chemotherapy protocol*

bean herb *medicinal herb* [see: summer savory]

bean trefoil *medicinal herb* [see: buckbean]

Beano liquid, tablets OTC *digestive aid* [alpha-D-galactosidase enzyme]

bearberry *medicinal herb* [see: uva ursi]

beard, old man's *medicinal herb* [see: fringe tree; woodbine]

Bear-E-Bag Pediatric rectal suspension R *radiopaque contrast medium for gastrointestinal imaging* [barium sulfate] 95%

Bear-E-Yum CT oral suspension R *radiopaque contrast medium for gastrointestinal imaging* [barium sulfate] 1.5%

Bear-E-Yum GI oral/rectal suspension R *radiopaque contrast medium for gastrointestinal imaging* [barium sulfate] 60%

bear's grape *medicinal herb* [see: uva ursi]

bear's weed *medicinal herb* [see: yerba santa]

bearsfoot *medicinal herb* [see: hellebore]

Beaumont root *medicinal herb* [see: Culver's root]

beaver tree *medicinal herb* [see: magnolia]

BEC-2 *investigational (Phase III) anti-idiotype monoclonal antibody for small cell lung cancer*

becanthone HCl USAN *antischistosomal* [also: becantone]

becantone INN *antischistosomal* [also: becanthone HCl]

becantone HCl [see: becanthone HCl]

becaplermin USAN *recombinant platelet-derived growth factor B for chronic diabetic foot ulcers*

Because vaginal foam OTC *spermicidal contraceptive* [nonoxynol 9] 8%

beciparcil INN

beclamide INN, BAN, DCF

becliconazole INN

beclobrate INN, BAN

Becloforte Inhaler ⓒ (U.S. product: Beclovent) oral inhalation aerosol R *corticosteroidal anti-inflammatory for chronic asthma* [beclomethasone dipropionate] 250 μg/dose

beclometasone INN *corticosteroidal inhalant for asthma; intranasal steroid* [also: beclomethasone dipropionate; beclomethasone; beclometasone dipropionate]

beclometasone dipropionate JAN *corticosteroidal inhalant for asthma; intranasal steroid* [also: beclomethasone dipropionate; beclomethasone; beclometasone]

beclomethasone BAN *corticosteroidal anti-inflammatory for chronic asthma* [also: beclomethasone dipropionate; beclometasone; beclometasone dipropionate]

beclomethasone dipropionate USAN, USP *corticosteroidal anti-inflammatory for chronic asthma and rhinitis; investigational (orphan) oral treatment for intestinal graft vs. host disease* [also: beclometasone; beclomethasone; beclometasone dipropionate]

beclotiamine INN

Beclovent oral inhalation aerosol ℞ *corticosteroidal anti-inflammatory for chronic asthma* [beclomethasone dipropionate] 42 μg/dose

Beclovent Inhaler ⓒⒶⓃ oral inhalation aerosol ℞ *corticosteroidal anti-inflammatory for chronic asthma* [beclomethasone dipropionate] 50 μg/dose

Becomject-100 injection (discontinued 1996) ℞ *parenteral vitamin therapy* [multiple B vitamins] ±

Beconase nasal inhalation aerosol ℞ *corticosteroidal anti-inflammatory for seasonal or perennial rhinitis* [beclomethasone dipropionate] 42 μg/dose

Beconase AQ nasal spray ℞ *corticosteroidal anti-inflammatory for seasonal or perennial rhinitis* [beclomethasone dipropionate] 0.042%

bectumomab USAN *monoclonal antibody; investigational (Phase III, orphan) diagnostic aid for non-Hodgkin's lymphoma and AIDS-related lymphoma* [also: technetium Tc 99m bectumomab]

bedstraw (Galium aparine; G. verum) plant *medicinal herb used as an antispasmodic, aperient, diaphoretic, diuretic, and vulnerary*

bee balm *medicinal herb* [see: lemon balm]

bee pollen *natural remedy for anemia, bodily weakness, cerebral hemorrhage, colitis, constipation, enteritis, and weight loss; also used as an anti-aging agent and prenatal nutritional supplement; not generally regarded as safe and effective because of widespread allergic reactions*

bee venom (derived from Apis mellifera) *natural remedy for arthritis and multiple sclerosis, and for hyposensitization of persons highly sensitive to bee stings*

beechwood creosote [see: creosote carbonate]

beef tallow JAN

Beelith tablets OTC *dietary supplement* [vitamin B$_6$; magnesium oxide] 20•362 mg

Beepen-VK tablets, powder for oral solution ℞ *natural penicillin antibiotic* [penicillin V potassium] 250, 500 mg; 125, 250 mg/5 mL

bee's nest plant *medicinal herb* [see: carrot]

beeswax, white JAN [also: wax, white]

beeswax, yellow JAN [also: wax, yellow]

Bee-T-Vites film-coated tablets (discontinued 1995) OTC *vitamin supplement* [multiple B vitamins; vitamin C] ±•300 mg

Bee-Zee tablets OTC *vitamin/zinc supplement* [multiple vitamins; zinc] ±•22.5 mg

befiperide INN

befloxatone INN

befunolol INN [also: befunolol HCl]

befunolol HCl JAN [also: befunolol]

befuraline INN

behepan [see: cyanocobalamin]

bekanamycin INN *antibiotic* [also: bekanamycin sulfate]

bekanamycin sulfate JAN *antibiotic* [also: bekanamycin]

belarizine INN

belfosdil USAN, INN *antihypertensive; calcium channel blocker*

Belganyl (available only from the Centers for Disease Control) ℞ *antiparasitic for African trypanosomiasis and onchocerciasis* [suramin sodium]

Belix elixir (discontinued 1997) OTC *antihistamine* [diphenhydramine HCl] 12.5 mg/5 mL

Bellacane elixir ℞ *GI antispasmodic; anticholinergic; sedative* [atropine sulfate; scopolamine hydrobromide; hyoscyamine sulfate; phenobarbital] 0.0194•0.0065•0.1037•16.2 mg/5 mL

Bellacane tablets ℞ *GI antispasmodic; anticholinergic; sedative* [hyoscyamine sulfate; phenobarbital] 0.125•15 mg

Bellacane SR sustained-release tablets ℞ *GI anticholinergic; sedative; analgesic* [belladonna alkaloids; phenobarbital; ergotamine tartrate] 0.2•40•0.6 mg

belladonna (Atropa belladonna) leaves, tops, and berries *medicinal* *herb used as an antispasmodic, calmative, diaphoretic, diuretic, and narcotic*

belladonna extract USP *GI/GU anticholinergic/antispasmodic; antiparkinsonian* 27–33 mg/100 mL oral

Bellafoline tablets (discontinued 1998) ℞ *GI anticholinergic; antispasmodic; antiparkinsonian agent* [belladonna extract] 0.25 mg

Bell/ans tablets OTC *antacid* [sodium bicarbonate] 520 mg

Bellatal tablets ℞ *long-acting barbiturate sedative, hypnotic, and anticonvulsant* [phenobarbital] 16.2 mg

Bellergal-S tablets ℞ *GI anticholinergic; sedative; analgesic* [belladonna extract; phenobarbital; ergotamine tartrate] 0.2•40•0.6 mg

Bellis perennis medicinal herb [see: wild daisy]

bells, May *medicinal herb* [see: lily of the valley]

beloxamide USAN, INN *antihyperlipoproteinemic*

beloxepin USAN *norepinephrine uptake inhibitor for depression*

Bel-Phen-Ergot SR sustained-release tablets ℞ *GI anticholinergic; sedative; analgesic* [belladonna alkaloids; phenobarbital; ergotamine tartrate] 0.2•40•0.6 mg

bemarinone INN *cardiotonic; positive inotropic; vasodilator* [also: bemarinone HCl]

bemarinone HCl USAN *cardiotonic; positive inotropic; vasodilator* [also: bemarinone]

bemegride USP, INN, BAN, JAN

bemesetron USAN, INN *antiemetic*

bemetizide INN, BAN

Beminal 500 tablets OTC *vitamin supplement* [multiple B vitamins; vitamin C] ±•500 mg ⊘ Benemid

bemitradine USAN, INN *antihypertensive; diuretic*

bemoradan USAN, INN *cardiotonic*

BEMP (bleomycin, Eldisine, mitomycin, Platinol) *chemotherapy protocol*

benactyzine INN, BAN

benactyzine HCl *mild antidepressant; anticholinergic*

Bena-D 10; Bena-D 50 injection (discontinued 1996) ℞ *antihistamine; motion sickness preventative; sleep aid; antiparkinsonian* [diphenhydramine HCl] 10 mg/mL; 50 mg/mL

Benadryl elixir (name changed to Benadryl Allergy in 1995)

Benadryl injection ℞ *antihistamine; motion sickness preventative; sleep aid; antiparkinsonian* [diphenhydramine HCl] 50 mg/mL ⊘ Bentyl; Benylin; Caladryl

Benadryl Kapseals (capsules), tablets (name changed to Benadryl Allergy in 1997)

Benadryl; Benadryl 2% cream, spray OTC *topical antihistamine* [diphenhydramine HCl] 1%; 2% ⊘ Bentyl; Benylin; Caladryl

Benadryl 25 capsules (name changed to Benadryl Allergy Kapseals in 1997)

Benadryl 25 tablets (name changed to Benadryl Allergy Ultratabs in 1997)

Benadryl Allergy Kapseals (sealed capsules), Ultratabs (tablets), chewable tablets OTC *antihistamine* [diphenhydramine HCl] 25 mg; 25 mg; 12.5 mg ⊘ Bentyl; Benylin; Caladryl

Benadryl Allergy liquid ℞ *antihistamine* [diphenhydramine HCl] 6.25 mg/5 mL ⊘ Bentyl; Benylin; Caladryl

Benadryl Allergy Decongestant liquid OTC *pediatric decongestant and antihistamine* [pseudoephedrine HCl; diphenhydramine HCl] 30•12.5 mg/5 mL ⊘ Bentyl; Benylin; Caladryl

Benadryl Allergy/Sinus Headache caplets OTC *decongestant; antihistamine; analgesic* [pseudoephedrine HCl; diphenhydramine HCl; acetaminophen] 30•12.5•500 mg ⊘ Bentyl; Benylin; Caladryl

Benadryl Cold Nighttime Formula liquid (discontinued 1995) OTC *decongestant; antihistamine; analgesic* [pseudoephedrine HCl; diphenhydramine HCl; acetaminophen; alco-

hol 10%] 10•8.3•167 mg/5 mL ⊠
Bentyl; Benylin; Caladryl

Benadryl Cold/Flu tablets (discontinued 1996) OTC *decongestant; antihistamine; analgesic* [pseudoephedrine HCl; diphenhydramine HCl; acetaminophen] 30•12.5•500 mg ⊠ Bentyl; Benylin; Caladryl

Benadryl Decongestant elixir (name changed to Benadryl Allergy Decongestant in 1995)

Benadryl Decongestant Allergy film-coated tablets OTC *decongestant; antihistamine* [pseudoephedrine HCl; diphenhydramine HCl] 60•25 mg ⊠ Bentyl; Benylin; Caladryl

Benadryl Dye-Free Allergy Liqui Gels (soft capsules), liquid OTC *antihistamine* [diphenhydramine HCl] 25 mg; 6.25 mg/5 mL ⊠ Bentyl; Benylin; Caladryl

Benadryl Itch Relief spray, cream, stick OTC *topical antihistamine; astringent* [diphenhydramine HCl; zinc acetate] 2%•0.1% ⊠ Bentyl; Benylin; Caladryl

Benadryl Itch Relief, Children's spray, cream OTC *topical antihistamine; astringent* [diphenhydramine HCl; zinc acetate] 1%•0.1% ⊠ Bentyl; Benylin; Caladryl

Benadryl Itch Stopping Gel; Benadryl Itch Stopping Gel Children's Formula OTC *topical antihistamine; astringent* [diphenhydramine HCl; zinc acetate] 2%•1%; 1%•1% ⊠ Bentyl; Benylin; Caladryl

Benadryl Junior ⒸⒶⓃ chewable tablets OTC *antihistamine* [diphenhydramine HCl] 12.5 mg

benafentrine INN

Benahist 10; Benahist 50 injection (discontinued 1996) ℞ *antihistamine; motion sickness preventative; sleep aid; antiparkinsonian* [diphenhydramine HCl] 10 mg/mL; 50 mg/mL

Ben-Allergin-50 injection (discontinued 1997) ℞ *antihistamine; motion sickness preventative; sleep aid; anti-*

parkinsonian [diphenhydramine HCl] 50 mg/mL

benanserin HCl

benapen [see: benethamine penicillin]

benaprizine INN *anticholinergic* [also: benapryzine HCl; benapryzine]

benapryzine BAN *anticholinergic* [also: benapryzine HCl; benaprizine]

benapryzine HCl USAN *anticholinergic* [also: benaprizine; benapryzine]

benaxibine INN

benazepril INN, BAN *antihypertensive; angiotensin-converting enzyme (ACE) inhibitor* [also: benazepril HCl]

benazepril HCl USAN *antihypertensive; angiotensin-converting enzyme (ACE) inhibitor* [also: benazepril]

benazeprilat USAN, INN *angiotensin-converting enzyme inhibitor*

bencianol INN

bencisteine INN, DCF

benclonidine INN

bencyclane INN [also: bencyclane fumarate]

bencyclane fumarate JAN [also: bencyclane]

bendacalol mesylate USAN *antihypertensive*

bendamustine INN

bendazac USAN, INN, BAN, JAN *antiinflammatory*

bendazol INN, DCF

benderizine INN

bendrofluazide BAN *diuretic; antihypertensive* [also: bendroflumethiazide]

bendroflumethiazide USP, INN *diuretic; antihypertensive* [also: bendrofluazide]

BeneFin ℞ *investigational (Phase III) angiogenesis inhibitor for the treatment of solid tumors* [squalamine (shark cartilage powder)]

Benefix powder for IV injection ℞ *antihemophilic for factor IX deficiency (hemophilia B; Christmas disease) (orphan)* [coagulation factor IX, recombinant] 250, 500, 1000 IU

Benemid ⒸⒶⓃ tablets (discontinued in U.S. 1996) ℞ *uricosuric for gout* [probenecid] 500 mg ⊠ Beminal

benethamine penicillin INN, BAN

benexate INN
benexate HCl JAN
benfluorex INN, DCF
benfosformin INN, DCF
benfotiamine INN, JAN, DCF
benfurodil hemisuccinate INN, DCF
bengal gelatin [see: agar]
Ben-Gay, Arthritis Formula cream OTC *topical analgesic; counterirritant* [methyl salicylate; menthol] 30%•8%
Ben-Gay Extra Strength cream (name changed to Arthritis Formula Ben-Gay in 1999)
Ben-Gay Original ointment OTC *topical analgesic; counterirritant* [methyl salicylate; menthol] 18.3%•16%
Ben-Gay Regular Strength cream OTC *topical analgesic; counterirritant* [methyl salicylate; menthol] 15%•10%
Ben-Gay SPA cream OTC *topical analgesic; counterirritant* [menthol] 10%
Ben-Gay Ultra Strength cream OTC *topical analgesic; counterirritant* [methyl salicylate; menthol; camphor] 30%•10%•4%
Ben-Gay Vanishing Scent gel OTC *topical analgesic; counterirritant* [menthol; camphor] 3%• 2
benhepazone INN
benidipine INN
benmoxin INN, DCF
Benoject-10; Benoject-50 injection (discontinued 1996) ℞ *antihistamine; motion sickness preventative; sleep aid; antiparkinsonian* [diphenhydramine HCl] 10 mg/mL; 50 mg/mL
benolizime INN
Benoquin cream ℞ *depigmenting agent for vitiligo* [monobenzone] 20%
benorilate INN, DCF [also: benorylate]
benorterone USAN, INN *antiandrogen*
benorylate BAN [also: benorilate]
benoxafos INN
benoxaprofen USAN, INN, BAN *antiinflammatory; analgesic*
benoxinate HCl USP *topical ophthalmic anesthetic* [also: oxybuprocaine; oxybuprocaine HCl]

Benoxyl #5 lotion, mask OTC *topical keratolytic for acne* [benzoyl peroxide] 5% ② PanOxyl
Benoxyl 10 lotion OTC *topical keratolytic for acne* [benzoyl peroxide] 10%
benpenolisin INN
benperidol USAN, INN, BAN *antipsychotic*
benproperine INN [also: benproperine phosphate]
benproperine phosphate JAN [also: benproperine]
benrixate INN, DCF
Bensal HP ointment ℞ *topical antifungal; keratolytic* [benzoic acid; salicylic acid] 6%•3%
bensalan USAN, INN *disinfectant*
benserazide USAN, INN, BAN *decarboxylase inhibitor; antiparkinsonian adjunct* [also: benserazide HCl]
benserazide HCl JAN *decarboxylase inhibitor; antiparkinsonian adjunct* [also: benserazide]
bensuldazic acid INN, BAN
Bensulfoid cream OTC *topical acne treatment* [colloidal sulfur; resorcinol; alcohol] 8%•2%•12%
bensylyte HCl [see: phenoxybenzamine HCl]
bentazepam USAN, INN *sedative*
bentemazole INN
bentiamine INN
bentipimine INN
bentiromide USAN, INN, BAN, JAN *diagnostic aid for pancreas function*
bentonite NF, JAN *suspending agent*
bentoquatam USAN *topical skin protectant for allergic contact dermatitis*
Bentyl capsules, tablets, IM injection, syrup ℞ *GI antispasmodic* [dicyclomine HCl] 10 mg; 20 mg; 10 mg/mL; 10 mg/5 mL ② Aventyl; Benadryl; Bontril
benurestat USAN, INN *urease enzyme inhibitor*
Benuryl ⒸⒶⓃ tablets ℞ *uricosuric for gout* [probenecid] 500 mg
Benylin Adult oral liquid OTC *antitussive* [dextromethorphan hydrobromide; alcohol 5%] 15 mg/5 mL ② Benadryl

Benylin Cough syrup (name changed to Benylin Adult in 1995)

Benylin Decongestant liquid (discontinued 1995) OTC *decongestant; antihistamine* [pseudoephedrine HCl; diphenhydramine HCl; alcohol 5%] 30 • 12.5 mg/5 mL ☑ Benadryl

Benylin DM syrup OTC *antitussive* [dextromethorphan hydrobromide] 10 mg/5 mL ☑ Benadryl

Benylin DM 12-Hour; Benylin DM for Children 12-Hour ⊛ controlled-release syrup OTC *antitussive* [dextromethorphan polistirex] 30 mg/5 mL; 15 mg/5 mL ☑ Benadryl

Benylin DM-D; Children's Benylin DM-D ⊛ syrup OTC *antitussive; decongestant* [dextromethorphan hydrobromide; pseudoephedrine HCl] 15 • 30 mg/5 mL; 7.5 • 15 mg/5 mL ☑ Benadryl

Benylin DM-D-E ⊛ syrup OTC *antitussive; decongestant; expectorant* [dextromethorphan hydrobromide; pseudoephedrine HCl; guaifenesin; alcohol 5%] 15 • 30 • 100, 15 • 30 • 200 mg/5 mL ☑ Benadryl

Benylin DM-E ⊛ syrup OTC *antitussive; expectorant* [dextromethorphan hydrobromide; guaifenesin; alcohol 5%] 15 • 100 mg/5 mL ☑ Benadryl

Benylin Expectorant liquid OTC *antitussive; expectorant* [dextromethorphan hydrobromide; guaifenesin] 5 • 100 mg/5 mL ☑ Benadryl

Benylin Multi-Symptom liquid OTC *antitussive; decongestant; expectorant* [dextromethorphan hydrobromide; pseudoephedrine HCl; guaifenesin] 5 • 15 • 100 mg/5 mL ☑ Benadryl

Benylin Pediatric oral liquid OTC *antitussive* [dextromethorphan hydrobromide] 7.5 mg/5 mL ☑ Benadryl

Benz 42 *hydrophilic contact lens material* [hefilcon A]

Benza solution OTC *topical antiseptic* [benzalkonium chloride] 1:750

Benzac AC 2½; Benzac W 2½; Benzac 5; Benzac AC 5; Benzac W 5; Benzac 10; Benzac AC 10;

Benzac W 10 gel ℞ *topical keratolytic for acne* [benzoyl peroxide] 2.5%; 2.5%; 5%; 5%; 5%; 10%; 10%; 10%

Benzac AC Wash 2½; Benzac AC Wash 5; Benzac W Wash 5; Benzac AC Wash 10; Benzac W Wash 10 liquid ℞ *topical keratolytic for acne* [benzoyl peroxide] 2.5%; 5%; 5%; 10%; 10%

5 Benzagel; 10 Benzagel gel ℞ *topical keratolytic for acne* [benzoyl peroxide] 5%; 10%

benzaldehyde NF *flavoring agent*

benzalkonium chloride (BAC) NF, INN, BAN, JAN *preservative; bacteriostatic antiseptic; surfactant/wetting agent* 17% topical

Benzamycin gel ℞ *topical antibiotic and keratolytic for acne* [erythromycin; benzoyl peroxide] 30 • 50 mg/mL

benzaprinoxide INN

benzarone INN, DCF

Benzashave shaving cream ℞ *topical keratolytic for acne* [benzoyl peroxide] 5%, 10%

benzathine benzylpenicillin INN *natural penicillin antibiotic* [also: penicillin G benzathine; benzathine penicillin; benzylpenicillin benzathine]

benzathine penicillin BAN *natural penicillin antibiotic* [also: penicillin G benzathine; benzathine benzylpenicillin; benzylpenicillin benzathine]

benzathine penicillin G [see: penicillin G benzathine]

benzatropine INN *antiparkinsonian; anticholinergic* [also: benztropine mesylate; benztropine]

benzazoline HCl [see: tolazoline HCl]

benzbromaron JAN *uricosuric* [also: benzbromarone]

benzbromarone USAN, INN, BAN *uricosuric* [also: benzbromaron]

benzchinamide [see: benzquinamide]

benzchlorpropamide [see: beclamide]

Benzedrex inhaler ℞ *nasal decongestant* [propylhexedrine] 250 mg

benzene ethanol [see: phenylethyl alcohol]

benzene hexachloride, gamma
[now: lindane]
benzeneacetic acid, sodium salt
[see: sodium phenylacetate]
benzenebutanoic acid, sodium salt
[see: sodium phenylbutyrate]
1,3-benzenediol [see: resorcinol]
benzenemethanol [see: benzyl alcohol]
benzestrofol [see: estradiol benzoate]
benzestrol USP, INN, BAN
benzethacil [see: penicillin G benza-
thine]
benzethidine INN, BAN, DCF
benzethonium chloride USP, INN, BAN,
JAN *topical anti-infective; preservative*
benzetimide INN *anticholinergic* [also:
benzetimide HCl]
benzetimide HCl USAN *anticholinergic*
[also: benzetimide]
benzfetamine INN *anorexiant; CNS
stimulant* [also: benzphetamine HCl;
benzphetamine]
benzhexol BAN *anticholinergic; antiparkinsonian* [also: trihexyphenidyl HCl;
trihexyphenidyl]
N-benzhydryl-N-methylpiperazine
[see: cyclizine HCl]
benzilone bromide [see: benzilonium
bromide]
benzilonium bromide USAN, INN,
BAN *anticholinergic*
2-benzimidazolepropionic acid [see:
procodazole]
benzimidazoles, substituted *a class of
gastric antisecretory agents that inhibit
the ATPase "proton pump" within the
cell* [also called: proton pump inhibitors; ATPase inhibitors]
benzin, petroleum JAN
benzindamine HCl [see: benzydamine HCl]
benzindopyrine INN *antipsychotic*
[also: benzindopyrine HCl]
benzindopyrine HCl USAN *antipsychotic* [also: benzindopyrine]
benzinoform [see: carbon tetrachloride]
benziodarone INN, BAN, DCF
benzisoxazoles *a class of novel (atypical) antipsychotic agents*
benzmalecene INN

benzmethoxazone [see: chlorthenox-
azine]
benznidazole INN
benzoaric acid [see: ellagic acid]
benzoate & phenylacetate [see:
sodium benzoate & sodium phenyl-
acetate]
benzobarbital INN
benzocaine USP, INN, BAN *topical anesthetic; nonprescription diet aid* [also:
ethyl aminobenzoate] 5% topical
benzoclidine INN
Benzocol cream (discontinued 1995)
OTC *topical local anesthetic* [benzo-
caine] 5%
benzoctamine INN, BAN *sedative; muscle relaxant* [also: benzoctamine HCl]
benzoctamine HCl USAN, INN *sedative;
muscle relaxant* [also: benzoctamine]
Benzodent ointment OTC *topical oral
anesthetic* [benzocaine] 20%
benzodepa USAN, INN *antineoplastic*
benzodiazepine HCl [see: medazepam HCl]
benzodiazepines *a class of nonbarbiturate sedative/hypnotics and anticonvulsants*
benzododecinium chloride INN
benzogynestryl [see: estradiol benzoate]
benzoic acid USP, JAN *antifungal; urinary acidifier*
benzoic acid, phenylmethyl ester
[see: benzyl benzoate]
benzoic acid, potassium salt [see:
potassium benzoate]
benzoic acid, sodium salt [see:
sodium benzoate]
benzoin USP, JAN *topical protectant*
Benzoin Compound tincture OTC
skin protectant [benzoin; aloe; alcohol
74–80%]
benzol [see: benzene ...]
benzonatate USP, INN, BAN *antitussive*
100 mg oral
benzophenone
benzopyrrolate [see: benzopyrronium]
benzopyrronium bromide INN
**benzoquinone amidoinohydrazone
thiosemicarbazone hydrate** [see:
ambazone]

benzoquinonium chloride

benzorphanol [see: levophenacylmorphan]

benzosulfinide [see: saccharin]

benzosulphinide sodium [see: saccharin sodium]

benzothiazepines *a class of calcium channel blockers*

benzothiozon [see: thioacetazone; thiacetazone]

benzotript INN

Benzox-10 gel ℞ *topical keratolytic for acne* [benzoyl peroxide] 10%

benzoxiquine USAN, INN *antiseptic/disinfectant*

benzoxonium chloride INN

benzoyl p-aminosalicylate (B-PAS) [see: benzoylpas calcium]

benzoyl peroxide USAN, USP *keratolytic* 5%, 10% topical

m-benzoylhydratropic acid [see: ketoprofen]

benzoylmethylecgonine [see: cocaine]

benzoylpas calcium USAN, USP *antibacterial; tuberculostatic* [also: calcium benzamidosalicylate]

benzoylsulfanilamide [see: sulfabenzamide]

benzoylthiamindisulfide [see: bisbentiamine]

benzoylthiaminmonophosphate [see: benfotiamine]

benzphetamine BAN *anorexiant; CNS stimulant* [also: benzphetamine HCl; benzfetamine]

benzphetamine chloride [see: benzphetamine HCl]

benzphetamine HCl NF *anorexiant; CNS stimulant* [also: benzfetamine; benzphetamine]

benzpiperylon [see: benzpiperylone]

benzpiperylone INN

benzpyrinium bromide NF, INN

benzquercin INN

benzquinamide USAN, INN, BAN *postanesthesia antinauseant and antiemetic*

benzthiazide USP, INN, BAN *diuretic; antihypertensive*

benztropine BAN *anticholinergic; antiparkinsonian* [also: benztropine mesylate; benzatropine]

benztropine mesylate USP *anticholinergic; antiparkinsonian* [also: benzatropine; benztropine] 0.5, 1, 2 mg oral

benztropine methanesulfonate [see: benztropine mesylate]

benzydamine INN, BAN *analgesic; antipyretic; anti-inflammatory* [also: benzydamine HCl]

benzydamine HCl USAN, JAN *analgesic; antipyretic; anti-inflammatory; investigational (orphan) radioprotectant for oral mucosa* [also: benzydamine]

benzydroflumethiazide [see: bendroflumethiazide]

benzyl alcohol NF, INN, JAN *antimicrobial agent; antiseptic; local anesthetic*

benzyl analogue of serotonin (BAS) [see: benanserin HCl]

benzyl antiserotonin [see: benanserin HCl]

benzyl benzoate USP, JAN

benzyl carbinol [see: phenylethyl alcohol]

S-benzyl thiobenzoate [see: tibenzate]

benzylamide [see: beclamide]

benzylamines *a class of antifungals structurally related to the allylamines*

N-benzylanilinoacetamidoxime [see: cetoxime]

2-benzylbenzimidazole [see: bendazol]

benzyldimethyltetradecylammonium chloride [see: miristalkonium chloride]

benzyldodecyldimethylammonium chloride [see: benzododecinium chloride]

benzylhexadecyldimethylammonium [see: cetalkonium]

benzylhexadecyldimethylammonium chloride [see: cetalkonium chloride]

benzylhydrochlorothiazide JAN

p-benzyloxyphenol [see: monobenzone]

benzylpenicillin INN, BAN *natural penicillin antibiotic; investigational* *(orphan) for penicillin hypersensitivity assessment*

benzylpenicillin benzathine JAN *natural penicillin antibiotic* [also: penicillin G benzathine; benzathine benzylpenicillin; benzathine penicillin]

benzylpenicillin potassium BAN, JAN *natural penicillin antibiotic* [also: penicillin G potassium]

benzylpenicillin procaine *natural penicillin antibiotic* [see: penicillin G procaine]

benzylpenicillin sodium BAN *natural penicillin antibiotic* [also: penicillin G sodium]

benzylpenicilloic acid [see: benzylpenicillin]

benzylpenicilloyl polylysine USP *diagnostic aid for penicillin sensitivity*

benzylpenilloic acid [see: benzylpenicillin]

benzylsulfamide INN, DCF

benzylsulfanilamide [see: benzylsulfamide]

BEP (bleomycin, etoposide, Platinol) *chemotherapy protocol*

bepafant INN

bepanthen [see: panthenol]

beperidium iodide INN

bephene oxinaphthoate [see: bephenium hydroxynaphthoate]

bephenium embonate [see: bephenium hydroxynaphthoate]

bephenium hydroxynaphthoate USP, INN, BAN

bepiastine INN, DCF

bepridil INN, BAN *vasodilator; antianginal; calcium channel blocker* [also: bepridil HCl]

bepridil HCl USAN *vasodilator; antianginal; calcium channel blocker* [also: bepridil]

beractant USAN *pulmonary surfactant for neonatal respiratory distress syndrome or respiratory failure (orphan)*

beraprost USAN, INN *platelet aggregation inhibitor*

beraprost sodium USAN *platelet aggregation inhibitor*

berberine chloride JAN

berberine sulfate JAN

berberine tannate JAN

Berberis vulgaris medicinal herb [see: barberry]

berculon A [see: thioacetazone; thiacetazone]

berefrine USAN, INN *mydriatic*

bergamot, scarlet *medicinal herb* [see: Oswego tea]

bergamot, wild *medicinal herb* [see: wild bergamot]

bergamot oil (*Citrus aurantium; C. bergamia*) *fruit peel medicinal herb used in conjunction with long-wave UV light therapy for psoriasis and vitiligo; not generally regarded as safe and effective because of its photosensitizing properties*

bergenin JAN

Berinert-P ℞ *investigational (orphan) for acute angioedema* [C1-esterase-inhibitor, human]

berkelium *element (Bk)*

berlafenone INN

bermastine [see: barmastine]

bermoprofen INN

Berocca tablets ℞ *vitamin supplement* [multiple B vitamins; vitamin C; folic acid] ±•500•0.5 mg

Berocca Parenteral Nutrition injection (discontinued 1997) ℞ *parenteral vitamin supplement* [multiple vitamins; folic acid; biotin] ±•400•60 μg/mL

Berocca Plus tablets ℞ *vitamin/mineral/iron supplement* [multiple vitamins & minerals; ferrous fumarate; folic acid; biotin] ±•27•0.8•0.15 mg

Berotec ℞ *investigational (NDA filed) bronchodilator; antiasthmatic* [fenoterol hydrobromide]

Berplex Plus tablets ℞ *vitamin/mineral/iron supplement* [multiple vitamins & minerals; ferrous fumarate; folic acid; biotin] ±•27•0.8•0.15 mg

bertosamil INN

beryllium *element (Be)*

berythromycin USAN, INN *antiamebic; antibacterial*

besigomsin INN

besilate INN *combining name for radicals or groups* [also: besylate]

besipirdine INN *cognition enhancer for Alzheimer's disease* [also: besipiridine HCl]

besipirdine HCl USAN *cognition enhancer for Alzheimer's disease* [also: besipiridine]

besulpamide INN

besunide INN

besylate USAN *combining name for radicals or groups* [also: besilate]

beta alethine *investigational (orphan) for multiple myeloma and metastatic melanoma*

beta blockers (β-blockers) *a class of cardiac agents characterized by their antihypertensive, antiarrhythmic, and antianginal actions; a class of topical antiglaucoma agents* [also called: beta-adrenergic antagonists]

beta carotene USAN, USP *vitamin A precursor* [also: betacarotene] 15 mg (25 000 IU) oral

beta cyclodextrin (β-cyclodextrin) *(previously used NF name)* [now: betadex]

Beta-2 solution for inhalation (discontinued 1999) ℞ *sympathomimetic bronchodilator* [isoetharine HCl] 1%

betacarotene INN *vitamin A precursor* [also: beta carotene]

betacetylmethadol INN, BAN

Betachron E-R extended-release capsules ℞ *antianginal; antihypertensive; antiarrhythmic; β-blocker; migraine preventative* [propranolol HCl] 60, 80, 120, 160 mg

betadex USAN, INN *sequestering agent* [previous NF name: beta cyclodextrin]

beta-D-galactosidase *digestive enzyme* [see: tilactase]

Betadine aerosol, gauze pads, lubricating gel, cream, mouthwash, ointment, perineal wash, skin cleanser, foam, solution, swab, swabsticks, surgical scrub OTC *broad-spectrum antimicrobial* [povidone-iodine] 5%; 10%; 5%; 5%; 0.5%; 10%; 10%; 7.5%; 7.5%; 10%; 10%; 10%; 7.5%

Betadine shampoo OTC *broad-spectrum antimicrobial for dandruff* [povidone-iodine] 7.5%

Betadine 5% Sterile Ophthalmic Prep solution ℞ *broad-spectrum antimicrobial for eye surgery* [povidone-iodine] 5%

Betadine First Aid Antibiotics + Moisturizer ointment OTC *topical antibiotic* [polymyxin B sulfate; bacitracin zinc] 10 000•500 IU/g

Betadine Medicated vaginal suppositories, vaginal gel OTC *antiseptic/germicidal; vaginal cleanser and deodorant* [povidone-iodine] 10%

Betadine Medicated Douche; Betadine Medicated Disposable Douche; Betadine Premixed Medicated Disposable Douche solution OTC *antiseptic/germicidal; vaginal cleanser and deodorant* [povidone-iodine] 10%

Betadine Plus First Aid Antibiotics and Pain Reliever ointment OTC *topical antibiotic and anesthetic* [polymyxin B sulfate; bacitracin zinc; pramoxine HCl] 10 000 IU•500 IU•10 mg per g

beta-estradiol [see: estradiol]

beta-estradiol benzoate [see: estradiol benzoate]

betaeucaine HCl [now: eucaine HCl]

Betafectin ℞ *investigational (Phase III) immunotherapeutic to prevent postsurgical infections in non-colorectal GI surgery patients (clinical trials discontinued 1999)* [PGG glucan]

Betagan Liquifilm eye drops ℞ *topical antiglaucoma agent (β-blocker)* [levobunolol HCl] 0.25%, 0.5% ☑ Betagen

Betagen ointment, solution, surgical scrub OTC *broad-spectrum antimicrobial* [povidone-iodine] 1%; 10%; 7.5% ☑ Betagan

beta-glucocerebrosidase [see: alglucerase]

betahistine INN, BAN *vasodilator* [also: betahistine HCl; betahistine mesilate]

betahistine HCl USAN *vasodilator* [also: betahistine; betahistine mesilate]

betahistine mesilate JAN *vasodilator* [also: betahistine HCl; betahistine]

beta-hypophamine [see: vasopressin]

betaine HCl USP *electrolyte replenisher for homocystinuria (orphan)*

beta-lactams *a class of antibiotics*

beta-lactone [see: propiolactone]

betameprodine INN, BAN, DCF

betamethadol INN, BAN, DCF

betamethasone USAN, USP, INN, BAN, JAN *corticosteroid; anti-inflammatory*

betamethasone acetate USP, JAN *corticosteroid; anti-inflammatory*

betamethasone acibutate INN, BAN *corticosteroid; anti-inflammatory*

betamethasone benzoate USAN, USP, BAN *topical corticosteroidal anti-inflammatory*

betamethasone dipropionate USAN, USP, BAN, JAN *topical corticosteroidal anti-inflammatory* 0.05% topical

betamethasone dipropionate, augmented *topical corticosteroidal anti-inflammatory*

betamethasone sodium phosphate USP, BAN, JAN *corticosteroid; anti-inflammatory* 4 mg/mL injection

betamethasone valerate USAN, USP, BAN, JAN *topical corticosteroidal anti-inflammatory; investigational (NDA filed) mousse for scalp psoriasis* 0.1% topical

betamicin INN *antibacterial* [also: betamicin sulfate]

betamicin sulfate USAN *antibacterial* [also: betamicin]

betamipron INN

betanaphthol NF

betanidine INN *antihypertensive* [also: bethanidine sulfate; bethanidine; betanidine sulfate]

betanidine sulfate JAN *antihypertensive* [also: bethanidine sulfate; betanidine; bethanidine]

Betapace tablets R̥ *antiarrhythmic (β-blocker) for life-threatening ventricular arrhythmias (orphan)* [sotalol HCl] 80, 120, 160, 240 mg

Betapen-VK film-coated tablets, powder for oral solution (discontinued 1998) R̥ *natural penicillin antibiotic* [penicillin V potassium] 250, 500 mg; 125, 250 mg/5 mL ② Adapin; Phenaphen

betaprodine INN, BAN, DCF

beta-propiolactone [see: propiolactone]

beta-pyridylcarbinol [see: nicotinyl alcohol]

BetaRx *investigational (orphan) antidiabetic for type 1 patients on immunosuppression* [porcine islet preparation, encapsulated]

Betasept liquid OTC *broad-spectrum antimicrobial; germicidal* [chlorhexidine gluconate; alcohol 4%] 4%

Betaseron powder for subcu injection R̥ *immunomodulator for relapsing-remitting multiple sclerosis (orphan); investigational (Phase II/III) cytokine for AIDS* [interferon beta-1b] 0.3 mg (9.6 mIU)/vial

Betathine *investigational (orphan) for multiple myeloma and metastatic melanoma* [beta alethine]

Beta-Tim ⓒⒶⓃ (U.S. product: Timoptic) eye drops R̥ *topical antiglaucoma agent (β-blocker)* [timolol maleate] 0.25%, 0.5%

Betatrex cream, ointment, lotion R̥ *topical corticosteroidal anti-inflammatory* [betamethasone valerate] 0.1%

Beta-Val cream, lotion R̥ *topical corticosteroidal anti-inflammatory* [betamethasone valerate] 0.1%

betaxolol INN, BAN *antianginal; antihypertensive; topical antiglaucoma agent (β-blocker)* [also: betaxolol HCl]

betaxolol HCl USAN, USP *antianginal; antihypertensive; topical antiglaucoma agent (β-blocker)* [also: betaxolol]

betazole INN [also: betazole HCl; ametazole]

betazole HCl USP [also: betazole; ametazole]

betazolium chloride [see: betazole HCl]

betel nut (Areca catechu) leaves and quids (a mixture of tobacco, powdered or sliced areca nut, and slaked lime wrapped in a *Piper betel* leaf)

*medicinal herb used as a digestive aid
and mild stimulant; not generally
regarded as safe and effective as it
causes leukoplakia and oral cancer*

beth root *medicinal herb* [see: birthroot]

bethanechol chloride USP, BAN, JAN
*cholinergic urinary stimulant for post-
surgical and postpartum urinary retention* 5, 10, 25, 50 mg oral

bethanidine BAN *antihypertensive* [also:
bethanidine sulfate; betanidine;
betanidine sulfate]

bethanidine sulfate USAN *antihypertensive; orphan status withdrawn 1996*
[also: betanidine; bethanidine;
betanidine sulfate]

betiatide USAN, INN, BAN *pharmaceutic
aid*

Betimol eye drops ℞ *topical antiglaucoma agent (β-blocker)* [timolol hemi-
hydrate] 0.25%, 0.5%

Betonica officinalis medicinal herb
[now: *Stachys officinalis*] [see: betony]

betony (Stachys officinalis) plant
*medicinal herb for anxiety, delirium,
diarrhea, fever, jaundice, liver and
spleen sclerosis, migraine headache,
mouth or throat irritation, nervousness,
palpitations, and toothache; also used
as a purgative and emetic agent*

Betoptic; Betoptic S Drop-Tainer (eye
drops) ℞ *topical antiglaucoma agent
(β-blocker)* [betaxolol HCl] 0.5%
(5.6 mg/mL); 0.25% (2.8 mg/mL)

betoxycaine INN

betoxycaine HCl [see: betoxycaine]

betula oil [see: methyl salicylate]

Betula spp. medicinal herb [see: birch]

Betuline lotion OTC *topical analgesic;
counterirritant* [methyl salicylate;
camphor; menthol; peppermint oil]

bevantolol INN, BAN *antianginal; antihypertensive; antiarrhythmic* [also:
bevantolol HCl]

bevantolol HCl USAN *antianginal;
antihypertensive; antiarrhythmic* [also:
bevantolol]

bevonium methylsulphate BAN
[also: bevonium metilsulfate]

bevonium metilsulfate INN [also:
bevonium methylsulphate]

bexarotene USAN *investigational synthetic retinoid analog antineoplastic for
cutaneous T-cell lymphoma; antidiabetic*

Bexxar ℞ *investigational (Phase III)
treatment for low-grade non-Hodgkin's
lymphoma* [iodine I 131 tositumomab]

bezafibrate USAN, INN, BAN, JAN *antihyperlipidemic*

bezitramide INN, BAN, DCF

bezomil INN *combining name for radicals or groups*

**bFGF (basic fibroblast growth fac-
tor)** [see: ersofermin]

B.F.I. Antiseptic powder OTC *topical
antiseptic* [bismuth-formic-iodide] 16%

BHA (butylated hydroxyanisole)
[q.v.]

BHAPs (bisheteroarylpiperazines)
a class of antiviral drugs

**BHD (BCNU, hydroxyurea, dacar-
bazine)** *chemotherapy protocol*

**BHDV; BHD-V (BCNU, hydroxy-
urea, dacarbazine, vincristine)**
chemotherapy protocol

BHT (butylated hydroxytoluene)
[q.v.]

bialamicol INN, BAN *antiamebic* [also:
bialamicol HCl]

bialamicol HCl USAN *antiamebic* [also:
bialamicol]

biallylamicol [see: bialamicol]

biantrazole [now: losoxantrone HCl]

biapenem USAN, INN *antibacterial*

Biavax II powder for subcu injection
℞ *mumps and rubella vaccine* [mumps
and rubella virus vaccine, live]
1000•20 000 U/0.5 mL

Biaxin Filmtabs (film-coated tablets),
granules for oral suspension ℞ *macrolide antibiotic* [clarithromycin] 250,
500 mg; 125, 250 mg/5 mL ☒ Axid

bibapcitide USAN *glycoprotein (GP)
IIb/IIIa receptor antagonist; investigational (Phase III) diagnostic imaging
aid for deep vein thrombosis*

bibenzonium bromide INN, BAN

bibrocathin [see: bibrocathol]

bibrocathol INN, DCF

bicalutamide USAN, INN, BAN *antiandrogen antineoplastic for prostatic cancer*

Bichloracetic Acid liquid ℞ *cauterant; keratolytic* [dichloroacetic acid] 10 mL ② dichloroacetic acid

bicifadine INN *analgesic* [also: bicifadine HCl]

bicifadine HCl USAN *analgesic* [also: bicifadine]

Bicillin C-R; Bicillin C-R 900/300 IM injection, Tubex (cartridge-needle unit) ℞ *natural penicillin antibiotic* [penicillin G benzathine; penicillin G procaine] 150•150, 300•300, 600•600, 1200•1200 thousand U; 900•300 thousand U ② V-Cillin; Wycillin

Bicillin L-A IM injection, Tubex (cartridge-needle units) ℞ *natural penicillin antibiotic* [penicillin G benzathine] 300, 600, 1200, 2400 thousand U

biciromab USAN, INN, BAN *antifibrin monoclonal antibody*

Bicitra oral solution ℞ *urinary alkalinizing agent* [sodium citrate; citric acid] 500•334 mg/5 mL

biclodil INN *antihypertensive; vasodilator* [also: biclodil HCl]

biclodil HCl USAN *antihypertensive; vasodilator* [also: biclodil]

biclofibrate INN, DCF

biclotymol INN, DCF

BiCNU powder for IV injection ℞ *nitrosourea-type alkylating antineoplastic* [carmustine] 100 mg

bicozamycin INN

Bicozene cream OTC *topical local anesthetic; antifungal* [benzocaine; resorcinol] 6%•1.67%

bicyclomycin [see: bicozamycin]

bidCAP (trademarked dosage form) *twice-daily capsule*

bidimazium iodide INN, BAN

bidisomide USAN, INN *antiarrhythmic*

Biebrich scarlet red [see: scarlet red]

Biebrich scarlet-picroaniline blue

bietamiverine INN

bietamiverine HCl [see: bietamiverine]

bietaserpine INN, DCF

bifemelane INN [also: bifemelane HCl]

bifemelane HCl JAN [also: bifemelane]

bifepramide INN

bifeprofen INN

bifluranol INN, BAN

bifonazole USAN, INN, BAN, JAN *antifungal*

Bignonia sempervirens medicinal herb [see: gelsemium]

bilberry (*Myrtilli fructus; Vaccinium myrtillus*) fruit *medicinal herb for cold hands and feet, diarrhea, edema, increasing microvascular blood flow, mild gastroenteritis, mucous membrane inflammation, night blindness, and varicose veins*

bile acid sequestrants *a class of antihyperlipidemic agents*

bile acids, oxidized [see: dehydrocholic acid]

bile salts BAN *digestive enzymes; laxative*

Bilezyme tablets (discontinued 1995) ℞ *digestive enzymes; choleretic* [amylase; protease; dehydrocholic acid; desoxycholic acid] 30•6•200•50 mg

Bili-Labstix reagent strips *in vitro diagnostic aid for multiple urine products*

Bilivist capsules (discontinued 1999) ℞ *radiopaque contrast medium for cholecystography* [ipodate sodium (61.4% iodine)] 500 mg (307 mg)

Bilopaque capsules ℞ *radiopaque contrast medium for cholecystography* [tyropanoate sodium (57.4% iodine)] 750 mg (430.5 mg)

Biltricide film-coated tablets ℞ *anthelmintic for schistosomiasis (flukes)* [praziquantel] 600 mg

bimakalim INN

bimazol [see: carbimazole]

bimethadol [see: dimepheptanol]

bimethoxycaine lactate

bimoclomol *investigational (Phase II) agent for microalbuminuria and diabetic neuropathy*

bindarit USAN, INN *antirheumatic; investigational (orphan) for lupus nephritis*

bindazac [see: bendazac]

binedaline INN

binfloxacin USAN, INN *veterinary antibacterial*

binifibrate INN

biniramycin USAN, INN *antibacterial antibiotic*

binizolast INN

binodaline [see: binedaline]

binospirone INN *anxiolytic* [also: binospirone mesylate]

binospirone mesylate USAN *anxiolytic* [also: binospirone]

Bio-Acerola C Complex wafers OTC *dietary supplement* [vitamin C; citrus bioflavonoids; rutin] 500•10•5 mg

bioallethrin BAN

Biocef capsules, powder for oral suspension ℞ *cephalosporin antibiotic* [cephalexin] 500 mg; 250 mg/5 mL

Bioclate powder for IV injection ℞ *antihemophilic to correct coagulation deficiency* [antihemophilic factor VIII, recombinant] 250, 500, 1000 IU

BioCox intradermal injection ℞ *diagnostic aid for coccidioidomycosis* [coccidioidin] 1:100, 1:10

Biocult-GC culture paddles for professional use *in vitro diagnostic aid for Neisseria gonorrhoeae*

Bioday with Iron tablets OTC *vitamin/iron supplement* [multiple vitamins; iron; folic acid]

Biodel Implant/BCNU (name changed to Gliadel upon marketing release in 1998)

Biodine Topical solution OTC *broad-spectrum antimicrobial* [povidone-iodine] 1%

Bioferon (working name during investigational testing; name changed to Avonex upon product launch in 1996)

bioflavonoids *vitamin P*

biogastrone [see: carbenoxolone]

Biohist-LA timed-release tablets ℞ *decongestant; antihistamine* [pseudoephedrine HCl; carbinoxamine maleate] 120•8 mg

biological indicator for dry-heat sterilization USP *sterilization indicator*

biological indicator for ethylene oxide sterilization USP *sterilization indicator*

biological indicator for steam sterilization USP *sterilization indicator*

Biomox capsules, powder for oral suspension (discontinued 1998) ℞ *aminopenicillin antibiotic* [amoxicillin] 250, 500 mg; 250 mg/5 mL

Bion Tears eye drops OTC *ophthalmic moisturizer/lubricant* [hydroxypropyl methylcellulose] 0.3%

bioral [see: carbenoxolone]

Bio-Rescue ℞ *investigational (orphan) for acute iron poisoning* [dextran; deferoxamine]

bioresmethrin INN

bios I [see: inositol]

bios II [see: biotin]

Biosynject ℞ *investigational (orphan) for newborn hemolytic disease and ABO blood incompatibility of organ or bone marrow transplants* [trisaccharides A and B]

biosynthetic human parathyroid hormone (1-34) [see: teriparatide]

Bio-Tab film-coated tablets ℞ *tetracycline antibiotic* [doxycycline hyclate] 100 mg

Biotab tablets OTC *decongestant; antihistamine; analgesic* [phenylpropanolamine HCl; phenyltoloxamine citrate; acetaminophen]

Biotel diabetes test kit (discontinued 1995) *in vitro diagnostic aid for urine glucose*

Biotel kidney reagent strips *in vitro diagnostic aid for urine hemoglobin, RBCs, and albumin (predictor of kidney diseases)*

Biotel u.t.i. test kit for home use (discontinued 1995) *in vitro diagnostic aid for urine nitrite (predictor of urinary tract infections)*

biotexin [see: novobiocin]

biotin USP, INN, JAN *B complex vitamin; vitamin H*

Biotin Forte tablets OTC *vitamin supplement* [multiple B vitamins; vitamin C; folic acid; biotin] $\pm \bullet 200 \bullet$ 0.8•3 mg, $\pm \bullet 100 \bullet 0.8 \bullet 5$ mg

BioTropin *orphan status withdrawn 1997* [somatropin]

BIP (bleomycin, ifosfamide [with mesna rescue], Platinol) *chemotherapy protocol*

bipenamol INN *antidepressant* [also: bipenamol HCl]

bipenamol HCl USAN *antidepressant* [also: bipenamol]

biperiden USP, INN, BAN, JAN *anticholinergic; antiparkinsonian*

biperiden HCl USP, BAN, JAN *anticholinergic; antiparkinsonian*

biperiden lactate USP, BAN, JAN *anticholinergic; antiparkinsonian*

biphasic insulin [see: insulin, biphasic]

biphenamine HCl USAN *topical anesthetic; antibacterial; antifungal* [also: xenysalate]

biprofenide [see: bifepramide]

birch (Betula spp.) bark and leaves *medicinal herb for bladder problems, blood cleansing, and eczema*

birch oil, sweet [see: methyl salicylate]

bird lime *medicinal herb* [see: mistletoe]

bird pepper *medicinal herb* [see: cayenne]

bird's nest root *medicinal herb* [see: carrot]

biricodar dicitrate USAN *investigational (Phase II) multi–drug-resistance inhibitor for prostate and ovarian cancers*

biriperone INN

birthroot (Trillium erectum; T. grandiflorum; T. pendulum) plant *medicinal herb for insect and snake bites, stimulating menses and diaphoresis, and stopping bleeding after childbirth; also used as an antiseptic and astringent*

birthwort (Aristolochia clematitis) root and flowering plant *medicinal herb used as a diaphoretic, emmenagogue, febrifuge, oxytocic, and stimulant*

bisacodyl USP, INN, BAN, JAN *stimulant laxative* 5 mg oral; 10 mg suppositories

bisacodyl tannex USAN *stimulant laxative*

bisantrene INN *antineoplastic* [also: bisantrene HCl]

bisantrene HCl USAN *antineoplastic* [also: bisantrene]

bisaramil INN

bisatin [see: oxyphenisatin acetate]

bisbendazole INN

bisbentiamine INN, JAN

bisbutiamine [see: bisbutitiamine]

bisbutitiamine JAN

bis-chloroethyl-nitrosourea (BCNU) [see: carmustine]

Bisco-Lax suppositories OTC *stimulant laxative* [bisacodyl] 10 mg

bisdequalinium diacetate JAN

bisfenazone INN, DCF

bisfentidine INN

bisheteroarylpiperazines (BHAPs) *a class of antiviral drugs*

bishop's wort *medicinal herb* [see: nutmeg; betony]

bishydroxycoumarin [now: dicumarol]

bisibutiamine JAN [also: sulbutiamine]

Bismatrol chewable tablets, liquid OTC *antidiarrheal; antinauseant* [bismuth subsalicylate] 262 mg; 524 mg/5 mL

bismucatebrol [see: bibrocathol]

bismuth *element (Bi)*

bismuth, milk of USP *antacid; astringent*

bismuth aluminate USAN

bismuth betanaphthol USP

bismuth carbonate USAN

bismuth carbonate, basic [see: bismuth subcarbonate]

bismuth citrate USP

bismuth cream [see: bismuth, milk of]

bismuth gallate, basic [see: bismuth subgallate]

bismuth glycollylarsanilate BAN [also: glycobiarsol]

bismuth hydroxide [see: bismuth, milk of]

bismuth hydroxide nitrate oxide [see: bismuth subnitrate]

bismuth magma [now: bismuth, milk of]

bismuth magnesium aluminosilicate JAN

bismuth oxycarbonate [see: bismuth subcarbonate]

bismuth potassium tartrate NF
bismuth sodium triglycollamate USP
bismuth subcarbonate USAN, JAN *antacid; GI adsorbent*
bismuth subgallate USAN, USP *antacid; GI adsorbent*
bismuth subnitrate USP, JAN *skin protectant*
bismuth subsalicylate (BSS) USAN, JAN *antiperistaltic; antacid; GI adsorbent*
bisnafide dimesylate USAN *antineoplastic; DNA and RNA synthesis inhibitor*
bisobrin INN *fibrinolytic* [also: bisobrin lactate]
bisobrin lactate USAN *fibrinolytic* [also: bisobrin]
bisoprolol USAN, INN, BAN *antihypertensive (β-blocker)*
bisoprolol fumarate USAN, JAN *antihypertensive (β-blocker)*
bisorcic INN
bisoxatin INN, BAN *laxative* [also: bisoxatin acetate]
bisoxatin acetate USAN *laxative* [also: bisoxatin]
Bispan ℞ *investigational agent for rheumatoid arthritis* [IPL-423 (code name —generic name not yet assigned)]
bispecific antibody 520C9x22 *investigational (orphan) for ovarian cancer*
bisphosphonates *a class of calcium-regulating agents that inhibit normal and abnormal bone resorption*
bispyrithione magsulfex USAN *antibacterial; antidandruff; antifungal*
bistort (Polygonum bistorta) *root medicinal herb for bleeding, cholera, cuts, diarrhea, dysentery, gum disease (mouthwash), and hemorrhoids*
bis-tropamide [now: tropicamide]
bithionol NF, INN, BAN, JAN *investigational anti-infective for paragonimiasis and fascioliasis*
bithionolate sodium USAN *topical anti-infective* [also: sodium bitionolate]
bithionoloxide INN
Bitin (available only from the Centers for Disease Control) ℞ *investigational anti-infective for paragonimiasis and fascioliasis* [bithionol]

bitipazone INN
bitolterol INN, BAN *sympathomimetic bronchodilator* [also: bitolterol mesylate; bitolterol mesilate]
bitolterol mesilate JAN *sympathomimetic bronchodilator* [also: bitolterol mesylate; bitolterol]
bitolterol mesylate USAN *sympathomimetic bronchodilator* [also: bitolterol; bitolterol mesilate]
bitoscanate INN
bitter ash *medicinal herb* [see: quassia; wahoo]
bitter ash; bitter quassia; bitter wood *medicinal herb* [see: quassia]
bitter buttons *medicinal herb* [see: tansy]
bitter cardamom (Alpinia fructus; A. oxyphylla) *medicinal herb for dementia, excessive water loss, and gastric lesions*
bitter cucumber *medicinal herb* [see: bitter melon]
bitter dogbane *medicinal herb* [see: dogbane]
bitter grass *medicinal herb* [see: star grass]
bitter herb *medicinal herb* [see: centaury]
bitter melon (Momordica charantia) *fruit, leaves, seeds, oil medicinal herb used as an antimicrobial and hypoglycemic; also used to reduce fertility in both males and females, and can act as an abortifacient*
bitter quassia; bitter ash; bitter wood *medicinal herb* [see: quassia tree]
bitter tonics; bitters *a class of agents that have a bitter taste, used as tonics, alteratives, or appetizers*
bitter wintergreen *medicinal herb* [see: pipsissewa]
bitter wood; bitter ash; bitter quassia *medicinal herb* [see: quassia tree]
bitterroot; bitterwort *medicinal herb* [see: dogbane; gentian]
bitters; bitter tonics *a class of agents that have a bitter taste, used as tonics, alteratives, or appetizers*
bittersweet herb; bittersweet twigs *medicinal herb* [see: bittersweet nightshade]

bittersweet nightshade (*Solanum dulcamara*) *medicinal herb for topical application on abrasions and felons; not generally regarded as safe and effective for internal use as it is highly toxic*

bitterweed *medicinal herb* [see: fleabane; horseweed]

bitterwort; bitterroot *medicinal herb* [see: gentian]

bivalirudin USAN *anticoagulant; antithrombotic for DVT and unstable angina, and to prevent reocclusion in MI and angioplasty*

bizelesin USAN, INN *antineoplastic*

B-Ject-100 injection ℞ *parenteral vitamin therapy* [multiple B vitamins] ≛

black alder (*Alnus glutinosa*) bark and leaves *medicinal herb used as an astringent, demulcent, emetic, hemostatic, and tonic*

black alder dogwood *medicinal herb* [see: buckthorn; cascara sagrada]

black birch *medicinal herb* [see: birch]

black cherry; poison black cherry *medicinal herb* [see: belladonna]

black choke *medicinal herb* [see: wild black cherry]

black cohosh (*Cimicifuga racemosa*) root and rhizome *medicinal herb for asthma, bronchitis, dysmenorrhea, dyspepsia, epilepsy, hypertension, hormone imbalance, lung disorders, menopause, rheumatism, snake bite, sore throat, St. Vitus dance, and tuberculosis*

black currant (*Ribes nigrum*) *medicinal herb* [see: currant]

black dogwood *medicinal herb* [see: buckthorn; cascara sagrada]

black elder *medicinal herb* [see: elderberry]

black false hellebore (*Veratrum niger*) [see: hellebore]

black ginger *medicinal herb* [see: ginger]

black hellebore (*Helleborus niger*) [see: hellebore]

black mulberry (*Morus nigra*) *medicinal herb* [see: mulberry]

black oak (*Quercus tinctoria*) *medicinal herb* [see: white oak]

black poplar (*Populus nigra; P. tremula*) buds *medicinal herb used as a diaphoretic, diuretic, expectorant, and vulnerary*

black root *medicinal herb* [see: Culver's root]

black sanicle *medicinal herb* [see: sanicle]

black snakeroot *medicinal herb* [see: black cohosh; sanicle]

black walnut (*Juglans nigra*) hulls and leaves *medicinal herb for parasites, ringworm, skin rashes, and stopping lactation; also used as an external antiseptic*

black widow spider antivenin [see: antivenin (Latrodectus mactans)]

black willow (*Salix nigra*) *medicinal herb* [see: willow]

blackberry (*Rubus fructicosus; R. villosus*) berries, leaves, and root bark *medicinal herb for bleeding, cholera, diarrhea in children, dysentery, sinus drainage, and vomiting*

Black-Draught syrup OTC *stimulant laxative* [casanthranol; senna extract] 90•≛ mg/15 mL

Black-Draught tablets, granules OTC *stimulant laxative* [senna concentrate] 600 mg; 1.65 g per ½ tsp.

blackwort *medicinal herb* [see: comfrey]

bladder fucus; bladderwrack *medicinal herb* [see: kelp (*Fucus*)]

bladderpod *medicinal herb* [see: lobelia]

Blairex Lens Lubricant solution OTC *rewetting solution for soft contact lenses*

Blairex Sterile Saline aerosol solution OTC *rinsing/storage solution for soft contact lenses* [sodium chloride (saline solution)]

blastomycin NF

blazing star *medicinal herb* [see: star grass]

blazing star (*Liatris scariosa; L. spicata; L. squarrosa*) root *medicinal herb used as a diuretic*

BlemErase lotion OTC *topical keratolytic for acne* [benzoyl peroxide] 10%

Blenoxane powder for IM, IV, subcu, or intrapleural injection ℞ *antibiotic* *antineoplastic for lymphomas, testicular and squamous cell carcinomas and malignant pleural effusion (orphan)* [bleomycin sulfate] 15 U

BLEO-COMF (bleomycin, cyclophosphamide, Oncovin, methotrexate, fluorouracil) *chemotherapy protocol*

bleomycin (BLM) INN, BAN *glycopeptide antibiotic antineoplastic* [also: bleomycin sulfate; bleomycin HCl] ② Cleocin

bleomycin HCl JAN *glycopeptide antibiotic antineoplastic* [also: bleomycin sulfate; bleomycin]

bleomycin sulfate USAN, USP, JAN *glycopeptide antibiotic antineoplastic for multiple carcinomas and malignant pleural effusion (orphan)* [also: bleomycin; bleomycin HCl]

Bleph-10 eye drops, ophthalmic ointment Ŗ *topical ophthalmic antibiotic* [sulfacetamide sodium] 10%

Blephamide eye drop suspension, ophthalmic ointment Ŗ *topical ophthalmic corticosteroidal anti-inflammatory; antibiotic* [prednisolone acetate; sulfacetamide sodium] 0.2%•10%

blessed cardus; holy thistle *medicinal herb* [see: blessed thistle]

blessed thistle (Cnicus benedictus) plant *medicinal herb for blood cleansing, digestive disorders, headache, hormonal imbalance, lactation disorders, liver and gallbladder ailments, menstrual disorders, poor circulation, and strengthening heart and lungs*

Blighia sapida medicinal herb [see: ackee]

blind nettle (Lamium album) plant and flowers *medicinal herb used as an antispasmodic, astringent, expectorant, and styptic*

Blinx ophthalmic solution OTC *extraocular irrigating solution* [sterile isotonic solution]

BlisterGard liquid OTC *skin protectant*

Blistex ointment OTC *topical antipruritic/counterirritant; mild local anesthetic; vulnerary* [camphor; phenol; allantoin] 0.5%•0.5%•1%

Blistik lip balm OTC *antipruritic/counterirritant; mild local anesthetic; skin protectant; sunscreen (SPF 10)* [camphor; phenol; allantoin; dimethicone; padimate O; oxybenzone] 0.5%•0.5%•1%•2%•6.6%•2.5%

Blis-To-Sol liquid OTC *topical antifungal; keratolytic* [tolnaftate] 1%

Blis-To-Sol powder OTC *topical antifungal* [zinc undecylenate] 12%

BLM (bleomycin) [q.v.]

Blocadren tablets Ŗ *antihypertensive; antianginal; migraine preventative; β-blocker* [timolol maleate] 5, 10, 20 mg

blocked ricin conjugated murine MAb [see: ricin (blocked) conjugated murine MAb]

blood, whole USP *blood replenisher*

blood, whole human [now: blood, whole]

blood cells, human red [now: blood cells, red]

blood cells, red USP *blood replenisher*

blood group specific substances A, B & AB USP *blood neutralizer*

blood grouping serum, anti-A [see: anti-A blood grouping serum]

blood grouping serum, anti-B [see: anti-B blood grouping serum]

blood grouping serum, anti-C USP *for in vitro blood testing*

blood grouping serum, anti-c USP *for in vitro blood testing*

blood grouping serum, anti-D USP *for in vitro blood testing*

blood grouping serum, anti-E USP *for in vitro blood testing*

blood grouping serum, anti-e USP *for in vitro blood testing*

blood mononuclear cells, allogenic peripheral *investigational (orphan) treatment for pancreatic cancer*

blood staunch *medicinal herb* [see: fleabane; horseweed]

blood volume expanders *a class of therapeutic blood modifiers used to increase the volume of circulating blood* [also called: plasma expanders]

bloodroot (Sanguinaria canadensis) root and rhizome *medicinal herb for*

*diuresis, fever, inducing emesis, nasal
polyps, rheumatism, sedation, skin
cancer, stimulating menstrual flow, and
warts; also used in toothpaste and
mouthwash; not generally regarded as
safe and effective for internal use*

BLP-25 *investigational liposomal formulation of MUC-1, an investigational
cancer vaccine*

Bluboro powder packets OTC *astringent
wet dressing (modified Burow solution)*
[aluminum sulfate; calcium acetate]

**blue cohosh (Caulophyllum thalic-
troides)** root *medicinal herb for
cramps, epilepsy, induction of labor,
menstrual flow stimulant, nerves, and
chronic uterine problems*

blue curls *medicinal herb* [see: wound-
wort]

blue flag (Iris versicolor) root *medicinal herb used as a cathartic, diuretic,
laxative, sialagogue, and vermifuge*

Blue Gel OTC *pediculicide for lice* [pyre-
thrins; piperonyl butoxide; petro-
leum distillate] 0.3%•3%•1.2%

Blue Gel Muscular Pain Reliever
gel OTC *topical analgesic; counterirritant* [menthol] 2

blue ginseng *medicinal herb* [see: blue
cohosh]

blue gum tree *medicinal herb* [see:
eucalyptus]

blue mountain tea *medicinal herb*
[see: goldenrod]

blue pimpernel; blue skullcap
medicinal herb [see: skullcap]

blue vervain (Verbena hastata) plant
*medicinal herb for asthma, bladder and
bowel disorders, bronchitis, colds, convulsions, cough, fever, insomnia, pulmonary tuberculosis, stomach upset,
and worms*

blueberry *medicinal herb* [see: bilberry;
blue cohosh]

bluebonnet; bluebottle *medicinal herb*
[see: cornflower]

**blue-green algae (Chloroplast mem-
brane sulfolipids)** *nutritional supplement for boosting the immune system*

bluensomycin INN *antibiotic*

**B-MOPP (bleomycin, nitrogen
mustard, Oncovin, procarbazine,
prednisone)** *chemotherapy protocol*

**BMP (BCNU, methotrexate, pro-
carbazine)** *chemotherapy protocol*

BMS-234475 *investigational (Phase III)
protease inhibitor for HIV*

BNP-7787 *investigational (Phase I)
chemotherapy protective agent*

**BOAP (bleomycin, Oncovin, Adri-
amycin, prednisone)** *chemotherapy
protocol*

Bo-Cal tablets OTC *dietary supplement*
[calcium; vitamin D; magnesium]
250 mg•100 IU•125 mg

boforsin [see: colforsin]

bofumustine INN

bogbean; bog myrtle *medicinal herb*
[see: buckbean]

Boil-Ease ointment OTC *topical local
anesthetic* [benzocaine] 20%

bolandiol INN *anabolic* [also: bolandiol
dipropionate]

bolandiol dipropionate USAN, JAN
anabolic [also: bolandiol]

bolasterone USAN, INN *anabolic steroid; also abused as a street drug*

bolazine INN

**BOLD (bleomycin, Oncovin,
lomustine, dacarbazine)** *chemotherapy protocol*

Boldea fragrans *medicinal herb* [see:
boldo]

boldenone INN, BAN *veterinary anabolic steroid; also abused as a street
drug* [also: boldenone undecylenate]

boldenone undecylenate USAN *veterinary anabolic steroid; also abused as a
street drug* [also: boldenone]

boldo (Peumus boldus) plant and
leaves *medicinal herb for bile stimulation, colds, constipation, digestive disorders, earache, edema, gallstones,
gonorrhea, gout, liver disease, rheumatism, syphilis, and worms*

Boldu boldus *medicinal herb* [see: boldo]

bolenol USAN, INN *anabolic*

bolmantalate USAN, INN, BAN *anabolic*

bolus alba [see: kaolin]

Bombay aloe *medicinal herb* [see: aloe]

bometolol INN
BOMP (bleomycin, Oncovin, Matulane, prednisone) *chemotherapy protocol*
BOMP (bleomycin, Oncovin, mitomycin, Platinol) *chemotherapy protocol*
Bonamil Infant Formula with Iron powder, oral liquid OTC *total or supplementary infant feeding* 453 g; 384, 946 mL
Bondronat ℞ *bone resorption inhibitor for postmenopausal osteoporosis, metastatic bone disease, hypercalcemia of malignancy, and Paget's disease* [ibandronate sodium]
bone ash [see: calcium phosphate, tribasic]
Bone Meal tablets OTC *dietary supplement* [calcium; phosphorus] 236•118 mg
bone powder, purified [see: calcium phosphate, tribasic]
Bonefos ℞ *investigational (orphan) for increased bone resorption due to malignancy* [disodium clodronate tetrahydrate]
boneset (*Eupatorium perfoliatum*) plant *medicinal herb for chills, colds, constipation, dengue fever, edema, fever, flu, pneumonia, and rheumatism*
Bonine chewable tablets OTC *anticholinergic; antihistamine; antivertigo agent; motion sickness preventative* [meclizine HCl] 25 mg
Bontril slow-release capsules ℞ *anorexiant; CNS stimulant* [phendimetrazine tartrate] 105 mg ② Bentyl; Vontrol
Bontril PDM tablets ℞ *anorexiant; CNS stimulant* [phendimetrazine tartrate] 35 mg
Bonviva ℞ *bone resorption inhibitor for postmenopausal osteoporosis, metastatic bone disease, hypercalcemia of malignancy, and Paget's disease* [ibandronate sodium]
bookoo *medicinal herb* [see: buchu]
Boost liquid, pudding OTC *enteral nutritional therapy* [milk-based formula] 237 mL

BOP (BCNU, Oncovin, prednisone) *chemotherapy protocol*
BOPAM (bleomycin, Oncovin, prednisone, Adriamycin, mechlorethamine, methotrexate) *chemotherapy protocol*
bopindolol INN
BOPP (BCNU, Oncovin, procarbazine, prednisone) *chemotherapy protocol*
boracic acid [see: boric acid]
borage (*Borago officinalis*) leaves *medicinal herb for bronchitis, colds, eye inflammation, hay fever, strengthening of heart, lactation stimulation, rashes, rheumatism, ringworm; not generally regarded as safe and effective*
borax [see: sodium borate]
Borbonia pinifolia *medicinal herb* [see: red bush tea]
boric acid NF, JAN *acidifying agent; ophthalmic emollient; antiseptic; astringent* 10% topical
2-bornanone [see: camphor]
bornaprine INN, BAN
bornaprolol INN
bornelone USAN, INN *ultraviolet screen*
bornyl acetate USAN
borocaptate sodium B 10 USAN *antineoplastic; radioactive agent* [also: sodium borocaptate (^{10}B)]
Borocell ℞ *investigational (orphan) for boron neutron capture therapy (BNCT) for glioblastoma multiforme* [sodium monomercaptoundecahydro-closo-dodecaborate]
Borofair Otic ear drops ℞ *antibacterial; antifungal; astringent* [acetic acid; aluminum acetate] 2%• ②
Borofax Skin Protectant ointment OTC *astringent* [zinc oxide] 15%
boroglycerin NF
boron *element (B); trace mineral for enhancing mental acuity and improving alertness; not generally regarded as safe and effective as it is highly toxic if taken internally or absorbed through broken skin*
Boropak powder packets OTC *astringent wet dressing (modified Burrow*

solution) [aluminum sulfate; calcium acetate]

bosentan USAN, INN *investigational endothelin receptor antagonist for vasospastic diseases*

Boston Advance Cleaner; Boston Cleaner solution OTC *cleaning solution for rigid gas permeable contact lenses*

Boston Advance Comfort Formula solution OTC *disinfecting/wetting/soaking solution for rigid gas permeable contact lenses*

Boston Advance Conditioning Solution (name changed to Boston Advance Comfort Formula in 1995)

Boston Advance Rewetting Drops (name changed to Boston Rewetting Drops in 1995)

Boston Conditioning Solution OTC *disinfecting/wetting/soaking solution for rigid gas permeable contact lenses*

Boston Rewetting Drops OTC *rewetting solution for rigid gas permeable contact lenses*

Boswellia serrata medicinal herb [see: frankincense]

botiacrine INN

Botox powder for extraocular muscle injection ℞ *blepharospasm and strabismus of dystonia (orphan); investigational (orphan) for pediatric cerebral palsy and cervical dystonia* [botulinum toxin, type A] 100 U

BottomBetter ointment OTC *topical diaper rash treatment*

botulinum toxin, type A *blepharospasm and strabismus of dystonia (orphan); investigational (orphan) for pediatric cerebral palsy and cervical dystonia*

botulinum toxin, type B *investigational (Phase III, orphan) for cervical dystonia*

botulinum toxin, type F *investigational (orphan) for spasmodic torticollis (cervical dystonia) and essential blepharospasm*

botulinum toxoid, pentavalent (ABCDE) *investigational vaccine (available only from the Centers for Disease Control and Prevention)*

botulism antitoxin USP *passive immunizing agent*

botulism equine antitoxin, trivalent *passive immunizing agent*

botulism immune globulin *investigational (orphan) for infant botulism*

Bounty Bears chewable tablets OTC *vitamin supplement* [multiple vitamins; folic acid] ± •0.3 mg

Bounty Bears Plus Iron chewable tablets OTC *vitamin/iron supplement* [multiple vitamins; iron; folic acid] ± •15•0.3 mg

bourbonal [see: ethyl vanillin]

bovactant BAN

bovine colostrum [see: *Cryptosporidium parvum* bovine colostrum IgG concentrate]

bovine fibrin BAN

bovine immunoglobulin concentrate [see: *Cryptosporidium parvum* bovine colostrum IgG concentrate]

bovine myelin *investigational (Phase III) oral treatment for multiple sclerosis*

bovine superoxide dismutase (bSOD) [see: orgotein]

bovine whey protein concentrate [see: *Cryptosporidium parvum* bovine colostrum IgG concentrate]

bower, virgin's medicinal herb [see: woodbine]

Bowman's root medicinal herb [see: Culver's root]

box, mountain medicinal herb [see: uva ursi]

boxberry medicinal herb [see: wintergreen]

boxidine USAN, INN *antihyperlipoproteinemic*

Boyol salve OTC *topical anti-infective; anesthetic* [ichthammol; benzocaine] 10%• ± 🔲 boil

B-PAS (benzoyl para-aminosalicylate) [see: benzoylpas calcium]

BPD-MA (benzoporphyrin derivative) [see: verteporfin]

BPI (bactericidal and permeability-increasing) protein [q.v.]

BPI-21 *investigational agent for multiple drug-resistant bacteria, alone or in combination with antibiotics*

B-Plex tablets R *vitamin supplement* [multiple B vitamins; vitamin C; folic acid] ± • 500 • 0.5 mg

brain-derived neurotrophic factor (BDNF) *investigational (Phase III) treatment for brain and nerve degenerative diseases; clinical trials for ALS discontinued 1997*

brallobarbital INN

bramble *medicinal herb* [see: blackberry]

BranchAmin 4% IV infusion R *nutritional therapy for high metabolic stress* [multiple branched-chain essential amino acids]

branched-chain amino acids (BCAA) *investigational (orphan) for amyotrophic lateral sclerosis* [see: isoleucine; leucine; valine]

brandy mint *medicinal herb* [see: peppermint]

Brasivol cream OTC *abrasive cleanser for acne* [aluminum oxide]

brasofensine *investigational dopamine reuptake inhibitor for Parkinson's disease*

Brassica alba *medicinal herb* [see: mustard]

Bravavir R *investigational (NDA filed) antiviral for varicella zoster and herpes zoster in AIDS; orphan status withdrawn 1997* [sorivudine]

brazergoline INN

Breathe Free nasal spray OTC *nasal moisturizer* [sodium chloride (saline solution)] 0.65%

Breezee Mist Aerosol powder OTC *topical antifungal; analgesic; anhidrotic* [undecylenic acid; menthol; aluminum chlorohydrate]

Breezee Mist Antifungal powder OTC *topical antifungal* [miconazole nitrate (note: one of two different products with the same name)] 2%

Breezee Mist Antifungal powder OTC *topical antifungal* [tolnaftate (note: one of two different products with the same name)] 1%

Breezee Mist Foot Powder OTC *topical anhidrotic* [talc; aluminum chlorohydrate]

brefonalol INN

bremazocine INN

Breonesin capsules OTC *expectorant* [guaifenesin] 200 mg

brequinar INN *antineoplastic* [also: brequinar sodium]

brequinar sodium USAN *antineoplastic* [also: brequinar]

bretazenil USAN, INN *anxiolytic*

Brethaire oral inhalation aerosol R *sympathomimetic bronchodilator* [terbutaline sulfate] 0.2 mg/dose

Brethine tablets, IV or subcu injection R *sympathomimetic bronchodilator* [terbutaline sulfate] 2.5, 5 mg; 1 mg/mL ② Banthine

bretylium tosilate INN *antiadrenergic; antiarrhythmic* [also: bretylium tosylate]

bretylium tosylate USAN, BAN *antiadrenergic; antiarrhythmic* [also: bretylium tosilate] 500, 1000 mg/vial injection

Bretylol IV or IM injection (discontinued 1997) R *antiarrhythmic* [bretylium tosylate] 50 mg/mL ② Brevital

BrevaRex R *investigational (Phase II, orphan) therapeutic vaccine for solid tumors* [monoclonal antibody B43.13]

Brevibloc IV infusion R *antiarrhythmic; β-blocker for supraventricular tachycardia* [esmolol HCl] 10, 250 mg/mL

Brevicon tablets R *monophasic oral contraceptive* [norethindrone; ethinyl estradiol] 0.5 mg • 35 μg

Brevital Sodium powder for IV injection R *barbiturate general anesthetic* [methohexital sodium] 0.5, 2.5, 5 g ② Bretylol

Brevoxyl gel R *keratolytic for acne* [benzoyl peroxide] 4%

brewer's yeast *natural source of protein and B-complex vitamins*

Brexidol R *investigational analgesic, anti-inflammatory, and antirheumatic* [piroxicam betadex]

Brexin-L.A. sustained-release capsules ℞ *decongestant; antihistamine* [pseudoephedrine HCl; chlorpheniramine maleate] 120•8 mg

Bricanyl tablets, IV or subcu injection ℞ *sympathomimetic bronchodilator* [terbutaline sulfate] 2.5, 5 mg; 1 mg/mL

Brietal Sodium ⓐ (U.S. product: Brevital Sodium) powder for IV injection ℞ *barbiturate general anesthetic* [methohexital sodium] 10 mg/mL

brifentanil INN *narcotic analgesic* [also: brifentanil HCl]

brifentanil HCl USAN *narcotic analgesic* [also: brifentanil]

Brigham tea; Brigham Young weed *medicinal herb* [see: ephedra]

Brik-Paks (trademarked delivery form) *ready-to-use liquid containers*

brimonidine INN *ophthalmic α₂-adrenergic agonist for open-angle glaucoma and ocular hypertension* [also: brimonidine tartrate]

brimonidine tartrate USAN *ophthalmic α₂-adrenergic agonist for open-angle glaucoma and ocular hypertension* [also: brimonidine]

brinaldix [see: clopamide]

brinase INN [also: brinolase]

brinazarone INN

brindoxime INN

brinolase USAN *fibrinolytic enzyme* [also: brinase]

brinzolamide USAN, INN *carbonic anhydrase inhibitor for glaucoma*

Bristoject (trademarked delivery form) *prefilled disposable syringe*

British antilewisite (BAL) [now: dimercaprol]

British tobacco *medicinal herb* [see: coltsfoot]

brivudine INN

brobactam INN

brobenzoxaldine [see: broxaldine]

broclepride INN

brocresine USAN, INN, BAN *histidine decarboxylase inhibitor*

brocrinat USAN, INN *diuretic*

brodimoprim INN

brofaromine INN *investigational reversible/selective MAO inhibitor*

Brofed elixir ℞ *decongestant; antihistamine* [pseudoephedrine HCl; brompheniramine maleate] 30•4 mg/5 mL

brofezil INN, BAN

brofoxine USAN, INN *antipsychotic*

brolaconazole INN

brolamfetamine INN

Brolene eye drops *investigational (orphan) for Acanthamoeba keratitis* [propamidine isethionate] 0.1%

bromacrylide INN

bromadel [see: carbromal]

Bromadine-DM syrup ℞ *antitussive; decongestant; antihistamine* [dextromethorphan hydrobromide; pseudoephedrine HCl; brompheniramine maleate] 10•30•2 mg/5 mL

Bromadine-DX syrup ℞ *antitussive; decongestant; antihistamine* [dextromethorphan hydrobromide; pseudoephedrine HCl; brompheniramine maleate] 10•30•2 mg/5 mL

bromadoline INN *analgesic* [also: bromadoline maleate]

bromadoline maleate USAN *analgesic* [also: bromadoline]

Bromaline elixir OTC *decongestant; antihistamine* [phenylpropanolamine HCl; brompheniramine maleate] 12.5•2 mg/5 mL

Bromaline Plus captabs (discontinued 1995) OTC *decongestant; antihistamine; analgesic* [phenylpropanolamine HCl; brompheniramine maleate; acetaminophen] 12.5•2•500 mg

bromamid INN

Bromanate elixir OTC *decongestant; antihistamine* [phenylpropanolamine HCl; brompheniramine maleate] 12.5•2 mg/5 mL

Bromanate DC Cough syrup ℞ *narcotic antitussive; decongestant; antihistamine* [codeine phosphate; phenylpropanolamine HCl; brompheniramine maleate; alcohol] 10•12.5•2 mg/5 mL

Bromanyl syrup ℞ *narcotic antitussive; antihistamine* [codeine phosphate;

bromodiphenhydramine HCl] 10•
12.5 mg/5 mL

bromanylpromide [see: bromamid]

Bromarest DX Cough syrup ℞ *antitussive; decongestant; antihistamine* [dextromethorphan hydrobromide; pseudoephedrine HCl; brompheniramine maleate; alcohol 0.95%] 10•30•2 mg/5 mL

Bromatane DX Cough syrup ℞ *antitussive; decongestant; antihistamine* [dextromethorphan hydrobromide; pseudoephedrine HCl; brompheniramine maleate] 10•30•2 mg/5 mL

Bromatapp elixir (name changed to Cold & Allergy in 1995)

Bromatapp extended-release tablets OTC *decongestant; antihistamine* [phenylpropanolamine HCl; brompheniramine maleate] 75•12 mg

bromauric acid NF

bromazepam USAN, INN, BAN, JAN *benzodiazepine anxiolytic; minor tranquilizer*

bromazine INN, DCF *antihistamine* [also: bromodiphenhydramine HCl; bromodiphenhydramine]

bromazine HCl [see: bromodiphenhydramine HCl]

brombenzonium [see: bromhexine HCl]

bromchlorenone USAN, INN *topical anti-infective*

bromebric acid INN, BAN

bromelain JAN *anti-inflammatory; proteolytic enzymes* [also: bromelains]

bromelains USAN, INN, BAN *anti-inflammatory; proteolytic enzymes* [also: bromelain]

bromelin [see: bromelains]

bromerguride INN

brometenamine INN, DCF

bromethol [see: tribromoethanol]

Bromfed syrup OTC *decongestant; antihistamine* [pseudoephedrine HCl; brompheniramine maleate] 30•2 mg/5 mL ⓓ Bromphen

Bromfed tablets, timed-release capsules ℞ *decongestant; antihistamine* [pseudoephedrine HCl; brompheniramine maleate] 60•4 mg; 120•12 mg

Bromfed-DM Cough syrup ℞ *antitussive; decongestant; antihistamine* [dextromethorphan hydrobromide; pseudoephedrine HCl; brompheniramine maleate] 10•30•2 mg/5 mL

Bromfed-PD timed-release capsules ℞ *pediatric decongestant and antihistamine* [pseudoephedrine HCl; brompheniramine maleate] 60•6 mg

bromfenac INN *long-acting nonsteroidal anti-inflammatory drug (NSAID); analgesic; antipyretic* [also: bromfenac sodium]

bromfenac sodium USAN *long-acting nonsteroidal anti-inflammatory drug (NSAID); analgesic; antipyretic* [also: bromfenac]

Bromfenex extended-release capsules ℞ *decongestant; antihistamine* [pseudoephedrine HCl; brompheniramine maleate] 120•12 mg

Bromfenex PD extended-release capsules ℞ *pediatric decongestant and antihistamine* [pseudoephedrine HCl; brompheniramine maleate] 60•6 mg

bromhexine INN, BAN *expectorant; mucolytic; investigational (orphan) for keratoconjunctivitis sicca of Sjögren syndrome* [also: bromhexine HCl]

bromhexine HCl USAN, JAN *expectorant; mucolytic* [also: bromhexine]

bromindione USAN, INN, BAN *anticoagulant*

bromine *element (Br)*

bromisoval INN [also: bromisovalum; bromvalerylurea; bromovaluree]

bromisovalum NF [also: bromisoval; bromvalerylurea; bromovaluree]

2-bromo-α-ergocryptine [see: bromocriptine]

bromocamphor [see: camphor, monobromated]

bromociclen INN [also: bromocyclen]

bromocriptine USAN, INN, BAN *dopamine agonist; prolactin enzyme inhibitor; antiparkinsonian*

bromocriptine mesilate JAN *dopamine agonist; prolactin enzyme inhibitor; antiparkinsonian* [also: bromocriptine mesylate]

bromocriptine mesylate USAN, USP *dopamine agonist; prolactin enzyme inhibitor; antiparkinsonian; investigational (NDA filed) agent for diabetic control of hypoglycemia; investigational (Phase II/III) treatment for obesity* [also: bromocriptine mesilate]

bromocyclen BAN [also: bromociclen]

bromodeoxyuridine [now: broxuridine]

bromodiethylacetylurea [see: carbromal]

bromodiphenhydramine BAN *antihistamine* [also: bromodiphenhydramine HCl; bromazine]

bromodiphenhydramine HCl USP *antihistamine* [also: bromazine; bromodiphenhydramine]

bromofenofos INN

bromoform USP

bromofos INN

1-bromoheptadecafluorooctane [see: perflubron]

bromoisovaleryl urea (BVU) [see: bromisovalum]

Bromophen T.D. sustained-release tablets ℞ *decongestant; antihistamine* [phenylpropanolamine HCl; phenylephrine HCl; brompheniramine maleate] 15•15•12 mg ② Bromphen

bromophenol blue

bromophin [see: apomorphine HCl]

bromophos [see: bromofos]

bromopride INN, DCF

Bromo-Seltzer effervescent granules OTC *antacid; analgesic; antipyretic* [sodium bicarbonate; citric acid; acetaminophen] 2781•2224•325 mg/dose

bromotheophyllinate aminoisobutanol [see: pamabrom]

bromotheophyllinate pyranisamine [see: pyrabrom]

bromotheophyllinate pyrilamine [see: pyrabrom]

8-bromotheophylline [see: pamabrom]

Bromotuss with Codeine syrup ℞ *narcotic antitussive; antihistamine* [codeine phosphate; bromodiphenhydramine HCl] 10•12.5 mg/5 mL

bromovaluree DCF [also: bromisovalum; bromisoval; bromvalerylurea]

11-bromovincamine [see: brovincamine]

bromovinyl arabinosyluracil (BV-araU) [see: sorivudine]

bromoxanide USAN, INN *anthelmintic*

bromperidol USAN, INN, BAN, JAN *antipsychotic*

bromperidol decanoate USAN, BAN *antipsychotic*

Bromphen elixir (discontinued 1997) OTC *antihistamine* [brompheniramine maleate] 2 mg/5 mL ② Bromfed; Bromophen

Bromphen sustained-release tablets, elixir (discontinued 1995) OTC *decongestant; antihistamine* [phenylpropanolamine HCl; brompheniramine maleate] 75•12 mg; 12.5•2 mg/5 mL ② Bromfed; Bromophen

Bromphen DC with Codeine Cough syrup ℞ *narcotic antitussive; decongestant; antihistamine* [codeine phosphate; phenylpropanolamine HCl; brompheniramine maleate] 10•12.5•2 mg/5 mL

Bromphen DX Cough syrup ℞ *antitussive; decongestant; antihistamine* [dextromethorphan hydrobromide; pseudoephedrine HCl; brompheniramine maleate; alcohol 0.95%] 10•30•2 mg/5 mL

brompheniramine INN, BAN *alkylamine antihistamine* [also: brompheniramine maleate]

Brompheniramine Cough syrup OTC *antitussive; decongestant; antihistamine* [dextromethorphan hydrobromide; pseudoephedrine HCl; brompheniramine maleate; alcohol 0.95%] 10•30•2 mg/5 mL

Brompheniramine DC Cough syrup ℞ *narcotic antitussive; decongestant; antihistamine* [codeine phosphate; phenylpropanolamine HCl; brompheniramine maleate; alcohol 1.15%] 10•12.5•2 mg/5 mL

brompheniramine maleate USP *alkylamine antihistamine* [also: brompheniramine] 10 mg/mL injection

Brompton's Cocktail; Brompton's Mixture (refers to any oral narcotic/ alcoholic solution containing morphine and either cocaine or a phenothiazine derivative) *prophylaxis for chronic, severe pain*

bromvalerylurea JAN [also: bromisovalum; bromisoval; bromovaluree]

Bronalide Ⓒᴬᴺ (U.S. product: AeroBid) oral inhalation aerosol ℞ *corticosteroid for bronchial asthma* [flunisolide] 250 μg/dose

Bronchial capsules ℞ *antiasthmatic; bronchodilator; expectorant* [theophylline; guaifenesin] 150•90 mg

Broncho Saline solution OTC *diluent for inhalation bronchodilators; solution for tracheal lavage* [sodium chloride (saline solution)] 0.9%

Broncholate softgels, syrup ℞ *decongestant; expectorant* [ephedrine HCl; guaifenesin] 12.5•200 mg; 6.25•100 mg/5 mL ② Brondelate

Brondelate elixir ℞ *antiasthmatic; bronchodilator; expectorant* [theophylline; guaifenesin] 192•150 mg/15 mL ② Broncholate

Bronitin Mist inhalation aerosol (discontinued 1999) OTC *sympathomimetic bronchodilator* [epinephrine bitartrate] 0.3 mg/dose

Bronkaid tablets (discontinued 1995) OTC *antiasthmatic; bronchodilator; decongestant; expectorant* [theophylline; ephedrine sulfate; guaifenesin] 100•24•100 mg

Bronkaid Dual Action caplets OTC *decongestant; expectorant* [ephedrine sulfate; guaifenesin] 25•400 mg

Bronkaid Mist inhalation aerosol (discontinued 1999) OTC *sympathomimetic bronchodilator* [epinephrine nitrate & epinephrine HCl] 0.5%

Bronkephrine subcu or IM injection (discontinued 1996) ℞ *sympathomimetic bronchodilator* [ethylnorepinephrine HCl] 2 mg/mL

Bronkodyl capsules ℞ *antiasthmatic; bronchodilator* [theophylline] 100, 200 mg

Bronkolixir elixir (discontinued 1995) OTC *antiasthmatic; bronchodilator; decongestant; expectorant; sedative* [theophylline; ephedrine sulfate; guaifenesin; phenobarbital] 3•2.4•10•0.8 mg/mL

Bronkometer inhalation aerosol (discontinued 1999) ℞ *sympathomimetic bronchodilator* [isoetharine mesylate] 0.61% (340 μg/dose)

Bronkosol solution for inhalation (discontinued 1999) ℞ *sympathomimetic bronchodilator* [isoetharine HCl] 1%

Bronkotabs tablets (discontinued 1995) OTC *antiasthmatic; bronchodilator; decongestant; expectorant; sedative* [theophylline; ephedrine sulfate; guaifenesin; phenobarbital] 100•24•100•8 mg

Bronkotuss Expectorant liquid ℞ *decongestant; antihistamine; expectorant* [ephedrine sulfate; chlorpheniramine maleate; guaifenesin; hydriodic acid; alcohol 5%] 8.2•4•100•1.67 mg/5 mL

bronopol INN, BAN, JAN

Brontex tablets, liquid ℞ *narcotic antitussive; expectorant* [codeine phosphate; guaifenesin] 10•300 mg; 2.5•75 mg/5 mL

brook bean *medicinal herb* [see: buckbean]

brooklime (Veronica beccabunga) plant *medicinal herb used as a diuretic, emmenagogue, and febrifuge*

broom (Cytisus scoparius) plant and bloom *medicinal herb for inducing bowel evacuation, diuresis, and emesis; also used as a homeopathic remedy for arrhythmias, diphtheria, and head and throat congestion*

broom, butcher's *medicinal herb* [see: butcher's broom]

broom, dyer's; green broom *medicinal herb* [see: dyer's broom]

broparestrol INN, DCF

broperamole USAN, INN *anti-inflammatory*

bropirimine USAN, INN *antineoplastic; antiviral*

broquinaldol INN

brosotamide INN, DCF

brosuximide INN

Brotane DX Cough syrup ℞ *antihistamine; antitussive* [pseudoephedrine HCl; brompheniramine maleate; dextromethorphan hydrobromide]

brotianide INN, BAN

brotizolam USAN, INN, BAN, JAN *hypnotic*

brovanexine INN

brovavir [see: sorivudine]

brovincamine INN [also: brovincamine fumarate]

brovincamine fumarate JAN [also: brovinacamine]

brown algae *medicinal herb* [see: kelp (*Laminaria*)]

brownwort *medicinal herb* [see: woundwort]

broxaldine INN, DCF

broxaterol INN

Broxine ℞ *investigational (NDA filed, orphan) radiosensitizer for breast and brain tumors* [broxuridine]

broxitalamic acid INN

broxuridine INN *investigational (NDA filed, orphan) radiosensitizer for breast and brain tumors*

broxyquinoline INN, DCF

brucine sulfate NF

bruisewort *medicinal herb* [see: comfrey; soapwort]

bryony (*Bryonia alba; B. dioica*) root *medicinal herb used as a pectoral and purgative; not generally regarded as safe and effective as root is poisonous in high doses (ingestion of as few as 40 berries can be fatal in adults, 15 in children)*

B-Salt Forte ophthalmic solution ℞ *intraocular irrigating solution* [sodium chloride (balanced saline solution)]

bSOD (bovine superoxide dismutase) [see: orgotein]

BSS (bismuth subsalicylate) [q.v.]

BSS; BSS Plus ophthalmic solution ℞ *intraocular irrigating solution* [sodium chloride (balanced saline solution)]

BTA Rapid Urine Test test kit for professional use ℞ *in vitro diagnostic aid for bladder tumor analytes in the urine*

BTA Stat Test test kit for home use ℞ *in vitro diagnostic aid for bladder tumor analytes in the urine* [rapid immunoassay (RIA)]

BTI-322 *investigational (Phase II) monoclonal antibody for graft vs. host disease*

bucainide INN *antiarrhythmic* [also: bucainide maleate]

bucainide maleate USAN *antiarrhythmic* [also: bucainide]

Bucast ℞ *investigational (Phase II) antiviral glucosidase inhibitor for HIV* [celgosivir HCl]

bucco *medicinal herb* [see: buchu]

Bucet capsules ℞ *sedative; analgesic* [butalbital; acetaminophen] 50•650 mg

bucetin INN, BAN, JAN

buchu (*Agathosma betulina; Barosma betulina; B. cenulata; B. serratifolia*) leaves *medicinal herb for edema, gas, gout, inflammation, kidney and urinary tract infections, and prostatitis; also used as a douche for leukorrhea and vaginal yeast infections*

buciclovir INN

bucillamine INN, JAN

bucindolol INN, BAN *antihypertensive* [also: bucindolol HCl]

bucindolol HCl USAN *antihypertensive* [also: bucindolol]

buckbean (*Menyanthes trifoliata*) leaves *medicinal herb used as a tonic, cathartic, diuretic, anthelmintic, and emetic*

buckeye; California buckeye; Ohio buckeye *medicinal herb* [see: horse chestnut]

buckhorn brake (*Osmunda cinnamomea; O. regalis*) root *medicinal herb used as a demulcent and tonic*

buckthorn (*Rhamnus cathartica; R. frangula*) bark and berries *medicinal* *herb for bleeding, bowel disorders, chronic constipation, fever, gallstones, lead poisoning, and liver disorders* [also see: cascara sagrada]

bucku *medicinal herb* [see: buchu]

bucladesine INN [also: bucladesine sodium]

bucladesine sodium JAN [also: bucladesine]

buclizine INN, BAN *antinauseant; antiemetic; anticholinergic; motion sickness relief* [also: buclizine HCl]

buclizine HCl USAN *antinauseant; antiemetic; anticholinergic; motion sickness relief* [also: buclizine]

buclosamide INN, BAN, DCF

bucloxic acid INN, DCF

bucolome INN, JAN

bucricaine INN

bucrilate INN *tissue adhesive* [also: bucrylate]

bucromarone USAN, INN *antiarrhythmic*

bucrylate USAN *tissue adhesive* [also: bucrilate]

bucumolol INN [also: bucumolol HCl]

bucumolol HCl JAN [also: bucumolol]

budesonide USAN, INN, BAN, JAN *corticosteroidal anti-inflammatory for chronic asthma, rhinitis, and inflammatory bowel disease*

budipine INN

budotitane INN

budralazine INN, JAN

bufenadine [see: bufenadrine]

bufenadrine INN

bufeniode INN, DCF

bufetolol INN [also: bufetolol HCl]

bufetolol HCl JAN [also: bufetolol]

bufexamac INN, BAN, JAN, DCF

bufezolac INN

buffered aspirin [see: aspirin, buffered]

Bufferin coated tablets, coated caplets OTC *analgesic; antipyretic; anti-inflammatory; antirheumatic* [aspirin (buffered with calcium carbonate, magnesium oxide, and magnesium carbonate)] 325, 500 mg

Bufferin AF Nite Time tablets OTC *antihistaminic sleep aid; analgesic* [diphenhydramine HCl; acetaminophen] 30•500 mg

Buffets II tablets OTC *analgesic; antipyretic; anti-inflammatory; antacid* [acetaminophen; aspirin; caffeine; aluminum hydroxide] 162•227•32.4•50 mg

Buffex tablets OTC *analgesic; antipyretic; anti-inflammatory; antirheumatic* [aspirin (buffered with aluminum glycinate and magnesium carbonate)] 325 mg

bufilcon A USAN *hydrophilic contact lens material*

buflomedil INN, BAN, DCF

bufogenin INN

buformin USAN, INN *antidiabetic*

Buf-Puf Acne Cleansing bar (discontinued 1997) OTC *medicated cleanser for acne* [salicylic acid; vitamin E] 2%•²⁄

Buf-Puf Medicated pads OTC *medicated cleansing pad for acne* [salicylic acid; alcohol]

bufrolin INN, BAN

bufuralol INN, BAN

bufylline BAN *diuretic; smooth muscle relaxant* [also: ambuphylline]

bugbane *medicinal herb* [see: hellebore; black cohosh]

bugleweed (*Lycopus virginicus*) plant *medicinal herb for cough, excessive menses, nervous indigestion, and other nervous disorders*

bugloss *medicinal herb* [see: borage]

Bugs Bunny Complete chewable tablets OTC *vitamin/mineral/calcium/iron supplement* [multiple vitamins & minerals; calcium; iron; folic acid; biotin] ≛•100•18•0.4•0.04 mg

Bugs Bunny Plus Iron chewable tablets OTC *vitamin/iron supplement* [multiple vitamins; iron; folic acid] ≛•15•0.3 mg

Bugs Bunny with Extra C Children's chewable tablets OTC *vitamin supplement* [multiple vitamins; folic acid] ≛•0.3 mg

bugwort *medicinal herb* [see: black cohosh]

buku *medicinal herb* [see: buchu]
bull's foot *medicinal herb* [see: coltsfoot]
bumadizone INN, DCF
bumecaine INN
bumepidil INN
bumetanide USAN, USP, INN, BAN, JAN
  loop diuretic 0.25 mg/mL injection
bumetrizole USAN, INN *ultraviolet screen*
Bumex tablets, IV or IM injection ℞
  loop diuretic [bumetanide] 0.5, 1, 2
  mg; 0.25 mg/mL
Buminate 5%; Buminate 25% IV
  infusion ℞ *blood volume expander for
  shock, burns, and hypoproteinemia*
  [human albumin] 5%; 25%
bunaftine INN
bunamidine INN, BAN *anthelmintic*
  [also: bunamidine HCl]
bunamidine HCl USAN *anthelmintic*
  [also: bunamidine]
bunamiodyl INN [also: buniodyl]
bunamiodyl sodium [see:
  bunamiodyl; buniodyl]
bunaprolast USAN, INN *antiasthmatic;
  5-lipoxygenase inhibitor*
bunapsilate INN *combining name for
  radicals or groups*
bunazosin INN [also: bunazosin HCl]
bunazosin HCl JAN [also: bunazosin]
bundlin [now: sedecamycin]
buniodyl BAN [also: bunamiodyl]
bunitrolol INN [also: bunitrolol HCl]
bunitrolol HCl JAN [also: bunitrolol]
bunolol INN *antiadrenergic (β-receptor)*
  [also: bunolol HCl]
bunolol HCl USAN *antiadrenergic (β-
  receptor)* [also: bunolol]
Bupap tablets ℞ *analgesic; antipyretic;
  sedative* [acetaminophen; butalbital]
  650•50 mg
buparvaquone INN, BAN
buphenine INN, BAN *peripheral vasodilator* [also: nylidrin HCl]
Buphenyl tablets, powder for oral
  solution ℞ *antihyperammonemic for
  urea cycle disorders (orphan); investigational (orphan) for various sickling
  disorders* [sodium phenylbutyrate]
  500 mg; 3 g/tsp, 8.6 g/tbsp
bupicomide USAN, INN *antihypertensive*

bupivacaine INN, BAN *injectable local
  anesthetic* [also: bupivacaine HCl]
bupivacaine HCl USAN, USP, JAN
  injectable local anesthetic [also: bupi-
  vacaine] 0.25%, 0.5%, 0.75%
bupranol [see: bupranolol]
bupranolol INN, DCF [also: bupranolol HCl]
bupranolol HCl JAN [also: bupranolol]
Buprenex IV or IM injection ℞ *narcotic agonist-antagonist analgesic*
  [buprenorphine HCl] 0.324 mg/mL
buprenorphine INN, BAN *narcotic agonist-antagonist analgesic* [also: buprenorphine HCl]
buprenorphine HCl USAN, JAN *narcotic agonist-antagonist analgesic;
  investigational (orphan) for opiate
  addictions* [also: buprenorphine]
**buprenorphine HCl & naloxone
  HCl** *investigational (orphan) for opiate
  addictions*
bupropion BAN *aminoketone antidepressant; non-nicotine aid to smoking
  cessation* [also: bupropion HCl; amfe-
  butamone]
bupropion HCl USAN *aminoketone
  antidepressant; non-nicotine aid to
  smoking cessation* [also: amfebutamone; bupropion]
buquineran INN, BAN
buquinolate USAN, INN *coccidiostat
  for poultry*
buquiterine INN
buramate USAN, INN *anticonvulsant;
  antipsychotic*
**burdock (Arctium lappa; A. majus;
  A. minus)** *root medicinal herb for
  arthritis, blood cleansing, dandruff,
  eczema, edema, fever, gout, kidney
  and lung disorders, rheumatism, skin
  diseases, and tumors; also used as an
  antimicrobial and diaphoretic*
burefrine [now: berefrine]
**burnet (Pimpinella magna; P. saxi-
  frage)** *root medicinal herb used as an
  antispasmodic, astringent, carminative,
  diaphoretic, diuretic, stimulant, and
  stomachic*

burning bush *medicinal herb* [see: fraxinella; wahoo]

burodiline INN

Buro-Sol solution OTC *astringent wet dressing (Burow solution)* [aluminum sulfate] 0.23%

Burow solution [see: aluminum acetate]

burr seed; turkey burr seed; clotbur; hareburr; hurr-burr; thorny burr *medicinal herb* [see: burdock]

burrage *medicinal herb* [see: borage]

buserelin INN, BAN *hormonal antineoplastic; gonad-stimulating principle; luteinizing hormone-releasing hormone analog* [also: buserelin acetate]

buserelin acetate USAN, JAN *hormonal antineoplastic; gonad-stimulating principle; luteinizing hormone-releasing hormone analog* [also: buserelin]

BuSpar tablets ℞ *azaspirone anxiolytic* [buspirone HCl] 5, 10, 15 mg

BuSpar transdermal patch ℞ *investigational (Phase III) delivery form for anxiety and ADHD* [buspirone HCl]

buspirone INN, BAN *azaspirone anxiolytic; minor tranquilizer* [also: buspirone HCl]

buspirone HCl USAN *azaspirone anxiolytic; minor tranquilizer; investigational (Phase III) transdermal delivery form for anxiety and ADHD* [also: buspirone]

busulfan USP, INN, JAN *alkylating antineoplastic for chronic myelogenous leukemia (CML); pretreatment for bone marrow transplants (orphan)* [also: busulphan]

Busulfex IV infusion ℞ *alkylating antineoplastic for chronic myelogenous leukemia (CML); pretreatment for bone marrow and stem cell transplants (orphan)* [busulfan] 6 mg/mL

busulphan BAN *alkylating antineoplastic* [also: busulfan]

butabarbital USP *sedative; hypnotic* [also: secbutobarbitone] ☒ butalbital

butabarbital sodium USP *sedative; hypnotic* [also: secbutabarbital sodium] 15, 30 mg oral; 30 mg/5 mL oral

butacaine INN, BAN [also: butacaine sulfate]

butacaine sulfate USP [also: butacaine]

butacetin USAN *analgesic; antidepressant*

butacetoluide [see: butanilicaine]

butaclamol INN *antipsychotic* [also: butaclamol HCl]

butaclamol HCl USAN *antipsychotic* [also: butaclamol]

butadiazamide INN

butafosfan INN, BAN

butalamine INN, BAN

butalbital USAN, USP, INN *sedative* ☒ butabarbital; Butibel

butalbital & acetaminophen & caffeine *analgesic; sedative* 50•325•40 mg oral

butalbital & aspirin & caffeine *analgesic; sedative* 50•325•40 mg oral

Butalbital Compound tablets, capsules ℞ *analgesic; sedative* [aspirin; caffeine; butalbital] 325•40•50 mg

butalgin [see: methadone HCl]

butallylonal NF

butamben USAN, USP *topical anesthetic*

butamben picrate USAN *topical local anesthetic* 1% topical

butamirate INN *antitussive* [also: butamirate citrate; butamyrate]

butamirate citrate USAN *antitussive* [also: butamirate; butamyrate]

butamisole INN *veterinary anthelmintic* [also: butamisole HCl]

butamisole HCl USAN *veterinary anthelmintic* [also: butamisole]

butamiverine [see: butaverine]

butamoxane INN

butamyrate BAN *antitussive* [also: butamirate citrate; butamirate]

butane (n-butane) NF *aerosol propellant*

butanilicaine INN, BAN

butanixin INN

butanserin INN

butantrone INN

butaperazine USAN, INN *antipsychotic*

butaperazine maleate USAN *antipsychotic*

butaprost USAN, INN, BAN *bronchodilator*

butaverine INN, DCF

butaxamine INN *antidiabetic; antihyperlipoproteinemic* [also: butoxamine HCl; butoxamine]

butcher's broom (*Ruscus aculeatus*) rhizomes *medicinal herb for atherosclerosis, circulatory disorders, hemorrhoids, thrombosis, varicose veins, and venous insufficiency; not generally regarded as safe and effective*

butedronate tetrasodium USAN *bone imaging aid*

butedronic acid INN

butelline [see: butacaine sulfate]

butenafine INN *antifungal*

butenafine HCl USAN *topical benzylamine antifungal*

butenemal [see: vinbarbital]

buteprate INN *former combining name for radicals or groups (name rescinded by USAN)* [now: probutate]

buterizine USAN, INN *peripheral vasodilator*

Butesin Picrate ointment OTC *topical local anesthetic* [butamben picrate] 1%

butetamate INN [also: butethamate]

butethal NF [also: butobarbitone]

butethamate BAN [also: butetamate]

butethamine HCl NF

butethanol [see: tetracaine]

buthalital sodium INN [also: buthalitone sodium]

buthalitone sodium BAN [also: buthalital sodium]

buthiazide USAN *diuretic; antihypertensive* [also: butizide]

Butibel tablets, elixir ℞ *GI anticholinergic; sedative* [belladonna extract; butabarbital sodium] 15•15 mg; 15•15 mg/5 mL ⑨ butalbital

butibufen INN

butidrine INN, DCF

butikacin USAN, INN, BAN *antibacterial*

butilfenin USAN, INN *hepatic function test*

butinazocine INN

butinoline INN

butirosin INN *antibacterial antibiotic* [also: butirosin sulfate; butirosin sulphate]

butirosin sulfate USAN *antibacterial antibiotic* [also: butirosin; butirosin sulphate]

butirosin sulphate BAN *antibacterial antibiotic* [also: butirosin sulfate; butirosin]

Butisol Sodium tablets, elixir ℞ *sedative; hypnotic* [butabarbital sodium] 15, 30, 50, 100 mg; 30 mg/5 mL ⑨ Butazolidin

butixirate USAN, INN *analgesic; antirheumatic*

butixocort INN

butizide INN *diuretic; antihypertensive* [also: buthiazide]

butobarbitone BAN [also: butethal]

butobendine INN

butoconazole INN, BAN *antifungal* [also: butoconazole nitrate]

butoconazole nitrate USAN, USP *antifungal* [also: butoconazole]

butocrolol INN

butoctamide INN [also: butoctamide semisuccinate]

butoctamide semisuccinate JAN [also: butoctamide]

butofilolol INN

butonate USAN, INN *anthelmintic*

butopamine USAN, INN *cardiotonic*

butopiprine INN, DCF

butoprozine INN *antiarrhythmic; antianginal* [also: butoprozine HCl]

butoprozine HCl USAN *antiarrhythmic; antianginal* [also: butoprozine]

butopyrammonium iodide INN

butopyronoxyl USP

butorphanol USAN, INN, BAN *analgesic; antitussive*

butorphanol tartrate USAN, USP, BAN, JAN *narcotic agonist-antagonist analgesic; antitussive* 1, 2 mg injection

butoxamine BAN *antidiabetic; antihyperlipoproteinemic* [also: butoxamine HCl; butaxamine]

butoxamine HCl USAN *antidiabetic; antihyperlipoproteinemic* [also: butaxamine; butoxamine]

2-butoxyethyl nicotinate [see: nicoboxil]

butoxylate INN

butoxyphenylacethydroxamic acid [see: bufexamac]

butriptyline INN, BAN *antidepressant* [also: butriptyline HCl]

butriptyline HCl USAN *antidepressant* [also: butriptyline]

butropium bromide INN, JAN

butterbur *(Petasites hybridus)* leaves and root *medicinal herb used as an analgesic for migraines and as an antispasmodic for asthma, cough, and gastrointestinal and urinary tract disorders; not generally regarded as safe and effective due to organ damage and carcinogenic properties*

buttercup *(Ranunculus acris; R. bulbosus; R. sceratus)* plant *medicinal herb used as an acrid, anodyne, antispasmodic, diaphoretic, and rubefacient*

butterfly weed *medicinal herb* [see: pleurisy root]

butternut *(Juglans cinerea)* bark, leaves, flowers *medicinal herb used as an anthelmintic, antiseptic, cathartic, cholagogue, and nervine*

butterweed *medicinal herb* [see: fleabane; horseweed]

butydrine [see: butidrine]

butyl alcohol NF *solvent*

butyl aminobenzoate (butyl *p*-aminobenzoate) [now: butamben]

butyl *p*-aminobenzoate picrate [see: butamben picrate]

butyl chloride NF

butyl 2-cyanoacrylate [see: enbucrilate]

butyl DNJ (deoxynojirimycin) [see: deoxynojirimycin]

butyl *p*-hydroxybenzoate [see: butylparaben]

butyl methoxydibenzoylmethane [see: avobenzone]

butyl nitrite; isobutyl nitrite *amyl nitrite substitutes, sold as euphoric street drugs, which produce a quick but short-lived "rush"* [see also: amyl nitrite; volatile nitrites]

butyl parahydroxybenzoate JAN *antifungal agent* [also: butylparaben]

***p*-butylaminobenzoyldiethylaminoethyl HCl** JAN

butylated hydroxyanisole (BHA) NF, BAN *antioxidant*

butylated hydroxytoluene (BHT) NF, BAN *antioxidant*

α-butylbenzyl alcohol [see: fenipentol]

1-butylbiguanide [see: buformin]

N-butyl-deoxynojirimycin [see: deoxynojirimycin]

1,5-(butylimino)-1,5-dideoxy-D-glucitol *investigational (orphan) for Fabry's disease and Gaucher's disease*

butylmesityl oxide [see: butopyronoxyl]

butylparaben NF *antifungal agent* [also: butyl parahydroxybenzoate]

butylphenamide

butylphenylsalicylamide [see: butylphenamide]

butylscopolamine bromide JAN

butynamine INN

butyrate propionate [see: probutate; buteprate]

butyrophenones *a class of dopamine receptor antagonists with conventional (typical) antipsychotic activity* [also called: phenylbutylpiperadines]

butyrylcholesterinase *investigational (orphan) for reduction and clearance of serum cocaine levels and postsurgical apnea*

butyrylperazine [see: butaperazine]

O-butyrylthiamine disulfide [see: bisbutitiamine]

butyvinyl [see: vinylbital]

buzepide metiodide INN, DCF

BVAP (BCNU, vincristine, Adriamycin, prednisone) *chemotherapy protocol*

BV-araU (bromovinyl arabinosyluracil) [see: sorivudine]

BVCPP (BCNU, vinblastine, cyclophosphamide, procarbazine, prednisone) *chemotherapy protocol*

BVDS (bleomycin, Velban, doxorubicin, streptozocin) *chemotherapy protocol*

BVPP (BCNU, vincristine, procarbazine, prednisone) *chemotherapy protocol*

BVU (bromoisovaleryl urea) [see: bromisovalum]

BW 12C *orphan status discontinued 1996*

Byclomine capsules, tablets ℞ *GI antispasmodic* [dicyclomine HCl] 10 mg; 20 mg ⊡ Hycomine

Bydramine Cough syrup (discontinued 1997) OTC *antihistamine; antitussive* [diphenhydramine HCl; alcohol 5%] 12.5 mg/5 mL ⊡ Hydramine

C (vitamin C) [see: ascorbic acid]

C & E softgels OTC *vitamin supplement* [vitamins C and E] 500•400 mg

C Factors "1000" Plus tablets OTC *dietary supplement* [vitamin C; citrus & rose hips bioflavonoids; rutin; hesperidin complex] 1000•250•50•25 mg

C Speridin sustained-release tablets OTC *dietary supplement* [ascorbic acid; hesperidin; lemon bioflavonoids] 500•100•100

C vitamin [see: ascorbic acid]

¹⁴C urea *diagnostic aid for H. pylori in the stomach* [also: carbon C 14 urea]

C1-esterase-inhibitor, human *investigational (orphan) for acute angioedema*

C-225 *investigational (Phase III) monoclonal antibody antineoplastic for advanced squamous head and neck cancers; investigational (Phase II) for metastatic renal cell carcinoma*

C242-DM1 *investigational colon cancer therapy*

CA (cyclophosphamide, Adriamycin) *chemotherapy protocol*

cA2 MAb (chimeric A2 MAb) [see: infliximab]

⁴⁵Ca [see: calcium chloride Ca 45]

⁴⁷Ca [see: calcium chloride Ca 47]

cabastine INN

cabbage, cow *medicinal herb* [see: masterwort; white pond lily]

cabbage, meadow; swamp cabbage *medicinal herb* [see: skunk cabbage]

cabbage, water *medicinal herb* [see: white pond lily]

cabergoline USAN, INN *dopamine agonist for hyperprolactinemia; investigational treatment for Parkinson's disease and gynecologic disorders*

cabis bromatum [see: bibrocathol]

CABOP; CA-BOP (Cytoxin, Adriamycin, bleomycin, Oncovin, prednisone) *chemotherapy protocol*

CABS (CCNU, Adriamycin bleomycin, streptozocin) *chemotherapy protocol*

cabufocon A USAN *hydrophobic contact lens material*

cabufocon B USAN *hydrophobic contact lens material*

CAC (cisplatin, ara-C, caffeine) *chemotherapy protocol*

cacao butter JAN

Cachexon ℞ *investigational (orphan) for AIDS-related cachexia* [L-glutathione, reduced]

cactinomycin USAN, INN *antibiotic antineoplastic* [also: actinomycin C]

CAD (cyclophosphamide, Adriamycin, dacarbazine) *chemotherapy protocol*

CAD (cytarabine [and] daunorubicin) *chemotherapy protocol*

cade oil [see: juniper tar]

cadexomer INN

cadexomer iodine USAN, INN, BAN *antiseptic; antiulcerative*

cadmium *element (Cd)*

cadralazine INN, BAN, JAN

CAE (cyclophosphamide, Adriamycin, etoposide) *chemotherapy protocol* also: ACE

CAF (cyclophosphamide, Adria-mycin, fluorouracil) *chemotherapy protocol*

cafaminol INN

Cafatine suppositories ℞ *migraine-specific vasoconstrictor* [ergotamine tartrate; caffeine] 2•200 mg

Cafatine-PB tablets ℞ *migraine treatment; vasoconstrictor; anticholinergic; sedative* [ergotamine tartrate; caffeine; pentobarbital sodium; belladonna extract] 1•100•30•0.125 mg

cafedrine INN, BAN

Cafergot tablets, suppositories ℞ *migraine treatment; vasoconstrictor* [ergotamine tartrate; caffeine] 1•100 mg; 2•100 mg

Cafetrate suppositories ℞ *migraine-specific vasoconstrictor* [ergotamine tartrate; caffeine] 2•100 mg

Caffedrine tablets OTC *CNS stimulant; analeptic* [caffeine] 200 mg

caffeic acid phenethyl ester (CAPE) *antimicrobial substance found in bee propolis*

caffeine USP, BAN, JAN *methylxanthine analeptic; CNS stimulant; diuretic; investigational (orphan) for apnea of prematurity*

caffeine, citrated NF

caffeine monohydrate [see: caffeine, citrated]

caffeine nut *medicinal herb* [see: kola nut]

caffeine & sodium benzoate *analeptic for respiratory depression due to an overdose of CNS depressants* 250 mg/mL injection

CAFP (cyclophosphamide, Adria-mycin, fluorouracil, prednisone) *chemotherapy protocol*

CAFTH (cyclophosphamide, Adria-mycin, fluorouracil, tamoxifen, Halotestin) *chemotherapy protocol*

CAFVP (cyclophosphamide, Adria-mycin, fluorouracil, vincristine, prednisone) *chemotherapy protocol*

Cal Carb-HD powder OTC *calcium supplement* [calcium carbonate] 2.5 g/packet

Caladryl cream OTC *topical antihistamine; astringent; antipruritic/anesthetic* [diphenhydramine HCl; calamine] 1%•8% ⧉ Benadryl

Caladryl lotion OTC *topical poison ivy treatment* [calamine; pramoxine HCl; alcohol 2.2%] 8%•1%

Caladryl Clear lotion OTC *topical poison ivy treatment* [pramoxine HCl; zinc acetate; alcohol 2%] 1%•0.1%

Caladryl for Kids cream OTC *topical poison ivy treatment* [calamine; pramoxine HCl] 8%•1%

Cala-gen lotion OTC *topical antihistamine; antipruritic/anesthetic* [diphenhydramine HCl; alcohol 2%] 1%

Calamatum spray OTC *topical poison ivy treatment* [calamine; zinc oxide; menthol; camphor; benzocaine]

calamine USP, JAN *topical protectant; astringent*

calamint (Calamintha officinalis) *medicinal herb* [see: summer savory]

Calamintha hortensis *medicinal herb* [see: summer savory]

Calamintha montana *medicinal herb* [see: winter savory]

Calamox ointment OTC *topical poison ivy treatment* [calamine] 17 g/100 g ⧉ Camalox

calamus (Acorus calamus) *rhizome medicinal herb for anxiety, bad breath from smoking, colic, digestive disorders, fever, gas, irritated throat, and promoting wound healing; not generally regarded as safe and effective and is prohibited in the U.S. as a food additive or supplement*

Calamycin lotion OTC *topical antihistamine; astringent; anesthetic* [pyrilamine maleate; zinc oxide; calamine; benzocaine; chloroxylenol; alcohol 2%]

Calan film-coated tablets ℞ *antianginal; antiarrhythmic; antihypertensive; calcium channel blocker* [verapamil HCl] 40, 80, 120 mg ⧉ kaolin; Kaon

Calan SR film-coated sustained-release tablets ℞ *antihypertensive; antianginal; antiarrhythmic; calcium*

channel blocker [verapamil HCl] 120, 180, 240 mg ⑫ kaolin; Kaon

calanolide A *investigational (Phase I) non-nucleoside reverse transcriptase inhibitor (NNRTI) for HIV and AIDS*

Calcet tablets OTC *dietary supplement* [calcium; vitamin D] 152.8 mg•100 IU

Calcet Plus tablets OTC *vitamin/calcium/iron supplement* [multiple vitamins; calcium; iron; folic acid] ±• 152.8•18•0.8 mg

Calcibind powder for oral solution ℞ *antiurolithic to prevent stone formation in absorptive calciuria type I* [cellulose sodium phosphate] 300 g bulk pack

CalciCaps tablets OTC *dietary supplement* [dibasic calcium phosphate; calcium gluconate; calcium carbonate; vitamin D] 125 mg (Ca)•60 mg (P)•67 IU

CalciCaps with Iron tablets OTC *dietary supplement* [dibasic calcium phosphate; calcium gluconate; calcium carbonate; vitamin D; ferrous gluconate] 125 mg (Ca)•60 mg (P)•67 IU•7 mg

Calci-Chew chewable tablets OTC *calcium supplement* [calcium carbonate] 1.25 g

Calciday-667 tablets OTC *calcium supplement* [calcium carbonate] 667 mg

calcidiol [see: calcifediol]

Calcidrine syrup ℞ *narcotic antitussive; expectorant* [codeine phosphate; calcium iodide; alcohol 6%] 8.4• 152 mg/5 mL

calcifediol USAN, USP, INN *vitamin D; calcium regulator for hypocalcemia and hypoparathyroidism*

calciferol [now: ergocalciferol]

Calciferol tablets, IM injection ℞ *vitamin deficiency therapy* [ergocalciferol (vitamin D₂)] 50 000 IU; 500 000 IU/mL

Calciferol Drops OTC *vitamin supplement* [ergocalciferol (vitamin D₂)] 8000 IU/mL

Calcijex injection ℞ *vitamin D therapy for hypocalcemia and hypoparathyroidism* [calcitriol] 1, 2 μg/mL

Calcimar subcu or IM injection ℞ *calcium regulator for hypercalcemia, Paget's disease, and postmenopausal osteoporosis* [calcitonin (salmon)] 200 IU/mL

Calci-Mix capsules OTC *calcium supplement* [calcium carbonate] 1250 mg

Calciparine IV or deep subcu injection (discontinued 1995) ℞ *anticoagulant* [heparin calcium] 5000 U/dose

calcipotriene USAN *topical antipsoriatic* [also: calcipotriol]

calcipotriol INN, BAN *topical antipsoriatic* [also: calcipotriene]

calcitonin (human) USAN, INN, BAN, JAN *calcium regulator for symptomatic Paget's disease (osteitis deformans) (orphan)* ⑫ calcitriol

calcitonin (salmon) USAN, INN, BAN *calcium regulator for hypercalcemia, postmenopausal osteoporosis, and Paget's disease; orphan status withdrawn 1996*

calcitonin salmon (synthesis) JAN *synthetic analog of calcitonin (salmon); calcium regulator* [also: salcatonin]

calcitonin salmon, recombinant *investigational (Phase III) calcium regulator for hypercalcemia, postmenopausal osteoporosis, and Paget's disease*

calcitriol USAN, INN, BAN, JAN *vitamin D; calcium regulator for hypocalcemia and hypoparathyroidism* ⑫ calcitonin

calcium *element (Ca)*

calcium, oyster shell [see: calcium carbonate]

Calcium 600 tablets OTC *dietary supplement* [calcium carbonate] 600 mg

Calcium 600 + D tablets OTC *dietary supplement* [calcium; vitamin D] 600 mg•125 IU

Calcium 600 with Vitamin D tablets OTC *dietary supplement* [calcium; vitamin D] 600 mg•100 IU

calcium acetate USP, JAN *buffering agent for hyperphosphatemia of end-stage renal disease (orphan)*

calcium alginate fiber *topical local hemostatic*

calcium aminacyl B-PAS (benzoyl para-aminosalicylate) [see: benzoylpas calcium]

calcium 4-aminosalicylate trihydrate [see: aminosalicylate calcium]

calcium amphomycin [see: amphomycin]

calcium antagonists *a class of coronary vasodilators that inhibit cardiac muscle contraction and slow cardiac electrical conduction velocity* [also called: calcium channel blockers; slow channel blockers]

calcium ascorbate USP *vitamin C; antiscorbutic* 500 mg oral; 1652 mg/ ½ tsp. oral

calcium benzamidosalicylate INN, BAN *antibacterial; tuberculostatic* [also: benzoylpas calcium]

calcium benzoyl *p*-aminosalicylate (B-PAS) [see: benzoylpas calcium]

calcium benzoylpas [see: benzoylpas calcium]

calcium bis-dioctyl sulfosuccinate [see: docusate calcium]

calcium bromide JAN

calcium carbimide INN [also: cyanamide]

calcium carbonate USP *antacid; calcium replenisher; investigational (orphan) for hyperphosphatemia of end-stage renal disease* [also: precipitated calcium carbonate] 500, 600, 650, 1250 mg oral; 1250 mg/5 mL oral

calcium carbonate, precipitated [now: calcium carbonate]

calcium carbophil *bulk laxative*

calcium caseinate *dietary supplement; infant formula modifier*

calcium channel blockers *a class of coronary vasodilators that inhibit cardiac muscle contraction and slow cardiac electrical conduction velocity* [also called: calcium antagonists; slow channel blockers]

calcium chloride USP, JAN *calcium replenisher*

calcium chloride Ca 45 USAN *radioactive agent*

calcium chloride Ca 47 USAN *radioactive agent*

calcium chloride dihydrate [see: calcium chloride]

calcium citrate USP *calcium supplement*

calcium citrate tetrahydrate [see: calcium citrate]

calcium clofibrate INN

calcium cyanamide [see: calcium carbimide]

calcium D-glucarate tetrahydrate [see: calcium saccharate]

calcium D-gluconate lactobionate monohydrate [see: calcium glubionate]

calcium dioctyl sulfosuccinate [see: docusate calcium]

calcium disodium edathamil [see: edetate calcium disodium]

calcium disodium edetate JAN *heavy metal chelating agent* [also: edetate calcium disodium; sodium calcium edetate; sodium calciumedetate]

Calcium Disodium Versenate IM, IV, or subcu injection ℞ *lead chelation therapy; antidote to lead poisoning and lead encephalopathy* [edetate calcium disodium] 200 mg/mL

calcium dobesilate INN

calcium doxybensylate [see: calcium dobesilate]

calcium edetate sodium [see: edetate calcium disodium]

calcium EDTA (ethylene diamine tetraacetic acid) [see: edetate calcium disodium]

calcium folinate INN, BAN, JAN *antianemic; folate replenisher; antidote to folic acid antagonist* [also: leucovorin calcium]

calcium glubionate USAN, INN *calcium replenisher*

calcium gluceptate USP *calcium replenisher* [also: calcium glucoheptonate] 1100 mg/5 mL injection

calcium glucoheptonate INN, DCF *calcium replenisher* [also: calcium gluceptate]

calcium gluconate (calcium D-gluconate) USP *calcium replenisher; investigational (orphan) for hydrofluoric acid burns* 500, 650, 975, 1000 mg oral; 10% injection

calcium glycerinophosphate [see: calcium glycerophosphate]

calcium glycerophosphate NF, JAN

calcium hopantenate JAN

calcium hydroxide USP *astringent*

calcium hydroxide phosphate [see: calcium phosphate, tribasic]

calcium hypophosphite NF

calcium iodide *expectorant*

calcium iododocosanoate [see: iodobehenate calcium]

calcium lactate USP, JAN *calcium replenisher* 325, 650 mg oral

calcium lactate hydrate [see: calcium lactate]

calcium lactate pentahydrate [see: calcium lactate]

calcium lactobionate USP *calcium supplement*

calcium lactobionate dihydrate [see: calcium lactobionate]

calcium lactophosphate NF

calcium L-aspartate JAN

calcium levofolinate [see: levoleucovorin calcium]

calcium levulate [see: calcium levulinate]

calcium levulinate USP *calcium replenisher*

calcium levulinate dihydrate [see: calcium levulinate]

calcium mandelate USP

calcium oxide [see: lime]

calcium pantothenate (calcium D-pantothenate) USP, INN, JAN *vitamin B_5; enzyme cofactor* [also: pantothenic acid] 25, 100, 218, 250, 500, 545 mg oral

calcium pantothenate, racemic (calcium DL-pantothenate) USP *vitamin; enzyme cofactor*

calcium para-aminosalicylate JAN [also: aminosalicylate calcium]

calcium phosphate, dibasic USP, JAN *calcium replenisher; tablet base*

calcium phosphate, monocalcium [see: calcium phosphate, dibasic]

calcium phosphate, tribasic NF *calcium replenisher* [also: durapatite; hydroxyapatite]

calcium polycarbophil USAN, USP *bulk laxative*

calcium polystyrene sulfonate JAN *ion exchange resin for hyperkalemia*

calcium polysulfide & calcium thiosulfate [see: lime, sulfurated]

calcium saccharate USP, INN *stabilizer*

calcium silicate NF *tablet excipient*

calcium sodium ferriclate INN *hematinic* [also: ferriclate calcium sodium]

calcium stearate NF, JAN *tablet and capsule lubricant*

calcium sulfate NF *tablet and capsule diluent*

calcium tetracemine disodium [see: edetate calcium disodium]

calcium trisodium pentetate INN, BAN *plutonium chelating agent* [also: pentetate calcium trisodium]

calcium 10-undecenoate [see: calcium undecylenate]

calcium undecylenate USAN *antifungal*

calciumedetate sodium [see: edetate calcium disodium]

CaldeCort aerosol spray (discontinued 1997) OTC *topical corticosteroidal anti-inflammatory* [hydrocortisone] 0.5%

CaldeCort Anti-Itch; CaldeCort Light with Aloe cream (discontinued 1997) OTC *topical corticosteroidal anti-inflammatory* [hydrocortisone acetate] 0.5%

Calderol capsules ℞ *vitamin D therapy for hypocalcemia or hypoparathyroidism* [calcifediol] 20, 50 μg

Caldesene ointment OTC *moisturizer; emollient; astringent; antiseptic* [cod liver oil (vitamins A and D); zinc oxide; lanolin]

Caldesene powder OTC *topical antifungal* [calcium undecylenate] 10%

caldiamide INN *pharmaceutic aid* [also: caldiamide sodium]

caldiamide sodium USAN, BAN *pharmaceutic aid* [also: caldiamide]

Calel D tablets OTC *dietary supplement* [calcium carbonate; cholecalciferol] 500 mg•200 IU

Calendula officinalis medicinal herb [see: marigold]

CALF (cyclophosphamide, Adriamycin, leucovorin [rescue], fluorouracil) *chemotherapy protocol*

calfactant USAN *surface-active extract of saline lavage of calf lungs, used for prevention of respiratory distress syndrome (RDS) in premature infants*

CALF-E (cyclophosphamide, Adriamycin, leucovorin [rescue], fluorouracil, ethinyl estradiol) *chemotherapy protocol*

Calglycine chewable tablets (discontinued 1998) OTC *antacid* [calcium carbonate; glycine] 420•150 mg

Calgonate wash ℞ *investigational (orphan) emergency treatment for hydrofluoric acid burns* [calcium gluconate]

Cal-Guard softgels OTC *calcium supplement* [calcium carbonate] 50 mg

California barberry *medicinal herb* [see: Oregon grape]

California buckthorn *medicinal herb* [see: buckthorn; cascara sagrada]

California false hellebore (Veratrum californicum) [see: hellebore]

californium *element (Cf)*

calioben [see: calcium iodobehenate]

Calluna vulgaris medicinal herb [see: heather]

calmatives *a class of soothing agents that reduce excitement, nervousness, distress, or irritation* [also called: sedatives]

Calmol 4 rectal suppositories OTC *emollient; astringent* [cocoa butter; zinc oxide] 80%•10%

Calm-X tablets OTC *anticholinergic; antiemetic; antivertigo agent; motion sickness preventative* [dimenhydrinate] 50 mg

Calmylin ⒸⒶⓃ oral solution OTC *antitussive; decongestant; expectorant* [dextromethorphan hydrobromide; pseudoephedrine HCl; guaifenesin] 3•6•20 mg/mL

Calmylin #1 ⒸⒶⓃ syrup OTC *antihistamine* [dextromethorphan hydrobromide] 3 mg/mL

Calmylin #2 ⒸⒶⓃ oral solution OTC *antitussive; decongestant* [dextromethorphan hydrobromide; pseudoephedrine HCl] 3•6 mg/mL

Calmylin #4 ⒸⒶⓃ oral solution OTC *antitussive; antihistamine; expectorant* [dextromethorphan hydrobromide; diphenhydramine HCl; ammonium chloride] 2.5•3•25 mg/mL

Calmylin Codeine ⒸⒶⓃ oral solution ℞ *narcotic antitussive; decongestant; expectorant* [codeine phosphate; pseudoephedrine HCl; guaifenesin] 0.66•6•20 mg/mL

Calmylin Cough & Cold ⒸⒶⓃ oral solution OTC *antitussive; decongestant; expectorant; analgesic* [dextromethorphan hydrobromide; pseudoephedrine HCl; guaifenesin; acetaminophen] 1•2•6.67•21.67 mg/mL

Calmylin Expectorant ⒸⒶⓃ syrup OTC *expectorant* [guaifenesin] 20 mg/mL

Calmylin Pediatric ⒸⒶⓃ syrup OTC *pediatric antitussive and decongestant* [dextromethorphan hydrobromide; pseudoephedrine HCl] 1.5•3 mg/mL

calomel NF

Calphosan IV injection ℞ *calcium replacement* [calcium glycerophosphate; calcium lactate] 50•50 mg/10 mL (0.08 mEq/mL)

Calphron tablets OTC *buffering agent for hyperphosphatemia in end-stage renal failure (orphan)* [calcium acetate] 667 mg

Cal-Plus tablets OTC *calcium supplement* [calcium carbonate] 1.5 g

calteridol INN *pharmaceutic aid* [also: calteridol calcium]

calteridol calcium USAN, BAN *pharmaceutic aid* [also: calteridol]

Caltha palustris medicinal herb [see: cowslip]

Caltrate 600 film-coated tablets OTC *calcium supplement* [calcium carbonate] 1.5 g

Caltrate 600 + D tablets OTC *dietary supplement* [calcium carbonate; vitamin D] 600 mg•200 IU

Caltrate 600 + Iron/Vitamin D film-coated tablets OTC *dietary supplement* [calcium carbonate; ferrous fumarate; vitamin D] 600 mg•18 mg•125 IU

Caltrate Jr. chewable tablets OTC *calcium supplement* [calcium carbonate] 750 mg

Caltrate Plus tablets OTC *dietary supplement* [calcium carbonate; vitamin D; multiple minerals] 600 mg•200 IU• ±

Caltro tablets OTC *dietary supplement* [calcium; vitamin D] 250 mg•125 IU

calumba; calumba root; calumbo *medicinal herb* [see: colombo]

calusterone USAN, INN *antineoplastic*

Calypte test kit for professional use ℞ *urine test for HIV-1 antibodies*

CAM (cyclophosphamide, Adriamycin, methotrexate) *chemotherapy protocol*

Cama Arthritis Pain Reliever tablets OTC *analgesic; antipyretic; anti-inflammatory; antirheumatic* [aspirin (buffered with magnesium oxide and aluminum hydroxide)] 500 mg

Cam-Ap-Es tablets (discontinued 1995) ℞ *antihypertensive; vasodilator; diuretic* [hydrochlorothiazide; reserpine; hydralazine HCl] 15•0.1•25 mg

camazepam INN

CAMB (Cytoxin, Adriamycin, methotrexate, bleomycin) *chemotherapy protocol*

cambendazole USAN, INN, BAN *anthelmintic*

CAMELEON (cytosine arabinoside, methotrexate, Leukovorin, Oncovin) *chemotherapy protocol*

camellia oil JAN

Camellia sinensis *medicinal herb* [see: green tea]

CAMEO (cyclophosphamide, Adriamycin, methotrexate, etoposide, Oncovin) *chemotherapy protocol*

Cameo Oil OTC *bath emollient*

CAMF (cyclophosphamide, Adriamycin, methotrexate, folinic acid) *chemotherapy protocol*

camiglibose USAN, INN *antidiabetic*

camiverine INN

camomile *medicinal herb* [see: chamomile]

camonagrel INN

camostat INN [also: camostat mesilate]

camostat mesilate JAN [also: camostat]

CAMP (cyclophosphamide, Adriamycin, methotrexate, procarbazine HCl) *chemotherapy protocol*

Campath 1H ℞ *investigational immunosuppressant for non-Hodgkin's lymphoma, rheumatoid arthritis; investigational (orphan) for chronic lymphocytic leukemia (CLL)*

camphetamide [see: camphotamide]

Campho-Phenique liquid, gel OTC *mild anesthetic; anti-infective; counterirritant* [camphor; phenol; eucalyptus oil] 10.8%•4.7%• ²⁄

Campho-Phenique Antibiotic Plus Pain Reliever ointment OTC *topical antibiotic; local anesthetic* [polymyxin B sulfate; neomycin sulfate; bacitracin zinc; lidocaine] 5000 U•3.5 mg•500 U•40 mg per g

camphor (*d*-camphor; *dl*-camphor) USP, JAN *topical antipruritic; mild local anesthetic; counterirritant* [also: trans-π-oxocamphor]

camphor, monobromated USP

camphorated opium tincture [now: paregoric]

camphorated parachlorophenol [see: parachlorophenol, camphorated]

camphoric acid USP

camphotamide INN, DCF

Camptosar IV infusion ℞ *topoisomerase I inhibitor; antineoplastic for metastatic cervical, colon, and rectal cancers* [irinotecan HCl]

camptothecin-11 (CPT-11) [see: irinotecan]

camsilate INN *combining name for radicals or groups* [also: camsylate]

camsylate USAN, BAN *combining name for radicals or groups* [also: camsilate] camylofin INN, DCF

Canada fleabane *medicinal herb* [see: fleabane; horseweed]

Canada pitch tree *medicinal herb* [see: hemlock]

Canada root *medicinal herb* [see: pleurisy root]

Canada tea *medicinal herb* [see: wintergreen]

canaigre *(Rumex hymenosepalus)* *medicinal herb for a variety of disease states and used as a purported substitute for ginseng; not generally regarded as safe and effective because of high tannin content and possible mutagenic effect when used internally*

canbisol INN

candesartan USAN, INN *antihypertensive; angiotensin II receptor antagonist*

candesartan cilexetil USAN *antihypertensive; angiotensin II receptor antagonist*

candicidin USAN, USP, INN, BAN *polyene antifungal*

Candida albicans skin test antigen *diagnostic aid for diminished cellular immunity; test for HIV patients to assess TB antigen response*

CandidaSure *reagent slides for professional use* in vitro *diagnostic aid for Candida albicans in the vagina*

Candin *intradermal injection* ℞ *diagnostic aid for diminished cellular immunity; test for HIV patients to assess TB antigen response* [Candida albicans skin test antigen] 0.1 mL

candleberry; candleberry myrtle *medicinal herb* [see: bayberry; tung seed]

candocuronium iodide INN

candoxatril USAN, INN, BAN *antihypertensive*

candoxatrilat USAN, INN, BAN *antihypertensive*

cankerroot *medicinal herb* [see: gold thread]

cannabinol INN, BAN *antiemetic; antinauseant; a nonpsychoactive derivative of the Cannabis sativa plant*

Cannabis sativa (marijuana; marihuana; hashish) *euphoric/hallucinogenic street drug made from the resin or dried leaves and flowering tops of the cannabis plant; medicinal herb for asthma, analgesia, leprosy, and loss of appetite*

canrenoate potassium USAN *aldosterone antagonist* [also: canrenoic acid; potassium canrenoate]

canrenoic acid INN, BAN *aldosterone antagonist* [also: canrenoate potassium; potassium canrenoate]

canrenone USAN, INN *aldosterone antagonist*

cantharides JAN

cantharidin *topical keratolytic*

Cantil *tablets* ℞ *treatment for peptic ulcer* [mepenzolate bromide] 25 mg

CAO (cyclophosphamide, Adriamycin, Oncovin) *chemotherapy protocol*

CAP (cellulose acetate phthalate) [q.v.]

CAP (cyclophosphamide, Adriamycin, prednisone) *chemotherapy protocol*

CAP; CAP-I (cyclophosphamide, Adriamycin, Platinol) *chemotherapy protocol*

CAP-II (cyclophosphamide, Adriamycin, high-dose Platinol) *chemotherapy protocol*

Capastat Sulfate *powder for IM injection* ℞ *tuberculostatic* [capreomycin sulfate] 1 g/10 mL ② Cepastat

CAP-BOP (cyclophosphamide, Adriamycin, procarbazine, bleomycin, Oncovin, prednisone) *chemotherapy protocol*

CAPE (caffeic acid phenethyl ester) *antimicrobial substance found in bee propolis*

Cape aloe *medicinal herb* [see: aloe]

cape gum *medicinal herb* [see: acacia]

capecitabine USAN, INN *antineoplastic (5-FU prodrug) for metastatic breast cancer; investigational (NDA filed) for colorectal cancer*

capers *(Capparis spinosa)* *flower buds and leaves medicinal herb for skin dis-*

orders and reducing the effects of enlarged capillaries

Capital with Codeine oral suspension ℞ *narcotic analgesic* [codeine phosphate; acetaminophen] 12•120 mg/ 5 mL

Capitrol shampoo ℞ *antiseborrheic; antibacterial; antifungal* [chloroxine] 2% ② captopril

caplet (dosage form) *capsule-shaped tablet*

capmul 8210 [see: monoctanoin]

capobenate sodium USAN *antiarrhythmic*

capobenic acid USAN, INN *antiarrhythmic*

Capoten tablets ℞ *antihypertensive; angiotensin-converting enzyme (ACE) inhibitor* [captopril] 12.5, 25, 50, 100 mg

Capozide 25/15; Capozide 25/25; Capozide 50/15; Capozide 50/25 tablets ℞ *antihypertensive; angiotensin-converting enzyme (ACE) inhibitor; diuretic* [captopril; hydrochlorothiazide] 25•15 mg; 25•25 mg; 50• 15 mg; 50•25 mg

Capparis spinosa medicinal herb [see: capers]

CAPPr (cyclophosphamide, Adriamycin, Platinol, prednisone) *chemotherapy protocol*

capreomycin INN, BAN *bactericidal antibiotic; tuberculostatic* [also: capreomycin sulfate]

capreomycin sulfate USAN, USP, JAN *bactericidal antibiotic; tuberculostatic* [also: capreomycin]

Caprogel ℞ *investigational (orphan) topical treatment for traumatic hyphema of the eye* [aminocaproic acid]

capromab INN *monoclonal antibody for diagnosis of prostate cancer* [also: capromab pendetide]

capromab pendetide USAN *monoclonal antibody for diagnosis of prostate cancer* [also: capromab]

caproxamine INN, BAN

capsaicin *topical analgesic; counterirritant*

Capsella bursa-pastoris medicinal herb [see: shepherd's purse]

Capsicum frutescens; C. annuum medicinal herb [see: cayenne]

capsicum oleoresin *topical analgesic; counterirritant*

Capsin lotion OTC *topical analgesic* [capsaicin] 0.025%, 0.075%

Capsulets (trademarked form) *sustained-release caplet*

captab (dosage form) *capsule-shaped tablet*

captamine INN *depigmentor* [also: captamine HCl]

captamine HCl USAN *depigmentor* [also: captamine]

captodiame INN, BAN

captodiame HCl [see: captodiame]

captodiamine HCl [see: captodiame]

captopril USAN, USP, INN, BAN, JAN *antihypertensive; angiotensin-converting enzyme (ACE) inhibitor* 12.5, 25, 50, 100 mg oral ② Capitrol

Captrix cream OTC *topical analgesic* [capsaicin]

capuride USAN, INN *hypnotic*

Capzasin-P cream OTC *topical analgesic* [capsaicin] 0.025%

caracemide USAN, INN *antineoplastic*

Carafate tablets, oral suspension ℞ *treatment for duodenal ulcer* [sucralfate] 1 g; 1 g/10 mL

caramel NF *coloring agent*

caramiphen INN, BAN *antitussive*

caramiphen edisylate *antitussive*

caramiphen HCl [see: caramiphen]

caraway (Carum carvi) NF seeds *medicinal herb for acid indigestion, appetite stimulation, colic, gas, gastrointestinal spasms, and uterine cramps*

caraway oil NF

carazolol INN, BAN

carbacephems *a class of bactericidal antibiotics similar to second-generation cephalosporins (q.v.)*

carbachol USP, INN, BAN, JAN *ophthalmic cholinergic; miotic for surgery; antiglaucoma agent* [also: carbacholine chloride]

carbacholine chloride DCF *ophthalmic cholinergic; miotic for surgery; antiglaucoma agent* [also: carbachol]

carbacrylamine resins
carbadipimidine HCl [see: carpipramine dihydrochloride]
carbadox USAN, INN, BAN *antibacterial*
carbaldrate INN
carbamate choline chloride [see:
carbachol]
carbamazepine USAN, USP, INN, BAN,
JAN *anticonvulsant; analgesic for
trigeminal neuralgia* 100, 200 mg oral
carbamide [see: urea]
carbamide peroxide USP *topical dental
anti-infective; cerumenolytic to emulsify and disperse ear wax*
N-carbamoylarsanilic acid [see: car-
barsone]
carbamoylcholine chloride [see: car-
bachol]
O-carbamoylsalicylic acid lactam
[see: carsalam]
carbamylcholine chloride [see: car-
bachol]
carbamylglutamic acid *investigational
(orphan) treatment for N-acetylgluta-
mate synthetase deficiency*
carbamylmethylcholine chloride
[see: bethanechol chloride]
carbantel INN *anthelmintic* [also: carbantel lauryl sulfate]
carbantel lauryl sulfate USAN *anthelmintic* [also: carbantel]
carbaril INN [also: carbaryl]
carbarsone USP, INN
carbaryl BAN [also: carbaril]
carbasalate calcium INN *analgesic*
[also: carbaspirin calcium]
carbaspirin calcium USAN *analgesic*
[also: carbasalate calcium]
Carbastat solution ℞ *direct-acting
miotic for ophthalmic surgery* [carba-
chol] 0.01%
Carbatrol extended-release capsules ℞
*anticonvulsant; analgesic for trigeminal
neuralgia; antipsychotic* [carbamaze-
pine] 200, 300 mg
carbazeran USAN, INN *cardiotonic*
carbazochrome INN, JAN
carbazochrome salicylate INN
carbazochrome sodium sulfonate
INN

carbazocine INN
carbenicillin INN, BAN *extended-spectrum penicillin antibiotic* [also: carbenicillin disodium; carbenicillin sodium]
carbenicillin disodium USAN, USP
extended-spectrum penicillin antibiotic
[also: carbenicillin; carbenicillin
sodium]
carbenicillin indanyl sodium USAN,
USP *extended-spectrum penicillin antibiotic* [also: carindacillin]
carbenicillin phenyl sodium USAN
antibacterial [also: carfecillin]
carbenicillin potassium USAN *antibacterial*
carbenicillin sodium JAN *antibacterial*
[also: carbenicillin disodium; car-
benicillin]
carbenoxolone INN, BAN *corticosteroid; anti-inflammatory* [also: carbenoxolone sodium]
carbenoxolone sodium USAN *corticosteroid; anti-inflammatory* [also: car-
benoxolone]
carbenzide INN
carbesilate INN *combining name for
radicals or groups*
carbetapentane citrate NF *antitussive*
[also: pentoxyverine]
carbetapentane tannate *antitussive*
carbetimer USAN, INN *antineoplastic*
carbetocin INN, BAN
Carbex tablets ℞ *dopaminergic antiparkinsonian (orphan)* [selegiline
HCl] 5 mg
carbidopa USAN, USP, INN, JAN
*decarboxylase inhibitor; antiparkinso-
nian adjunct*
carbidopa & levodopa *antiparkinsonian*
10•100, 25•100, 25•250 mg oral
carbifene INN *analgesic* [also: carbiphene HCl; carbiphene]
carbimazole INN, BAN
carbinoxamine INN, BAN *antihistamine*
[also: carbinoxamine maleate]
Carbinoxamine Compound syrup,
pediatric drops ℞ *antitussive; decongestant; antihistamine* [dextromethor-
phan hydrobromide; pseudoephed-

rine HCl; carbinoxamine maleate]
15•60•4 mg/5 mL; 4•25•2 mg/mL

carbinoxamine maleate USP *antihistamine* [also: carbinoxamine]

carbinoxamine maleate & pseudoephedrine HCl *antihistamine; decongestant* 4•60 mg/5 mL oral; 2•25 mg/mL oral

carbiphene BAN *analgesic* [also: carbiphene HCl; carbifene]

carbiphene HCl USAN *analgesic* [also: carbifene; carbiphene]

Carbiset tablets ℞ *decongestant; antihistamine* [pseudoephedrine HCl; carbinoxamine maleate] 60•4 mg

Carbiset-TR timed-release tablets ℞ *decongestant; antihistamine* [pseudoephedrine HCl; carbinoxamine maleate] 120•8 mg

Carbocaine injection ℞ *injectable local anesthetic* [mepivacaine HCl] 1%, 1.5%, 2%, 3%

Carbocaine with Neo-Cobefrin injection ℞ *injectable local anesthetic* [mepivacaine HCl; levonordefrin] 2%•1:20 000

carbocisteine INN, BAN *mucolytic* [also: carbocysteine]

carbocloral USAN, INN, BAN *hypnotic*

carbocromen INN *coronary vasodilator* [also: chromonar HCl]

carbocysteine USAN *mucolytic* [also: carbocisteine]

Carbodec tablets, syrup ℞ *decongestant; antihistamine* [pseudoephedrine HCl; carbinoxamine maleate] 60•4 mg; 60•4 mg/5 mL

Carbodec DM syrup, pediatric drops ℞ *antitussive; decongestant; antihistamine* [dextromethorphan hydrobromide; pseudoephedrine HCl; carbinoxamine maleate] 15•60•4 mg/5 mL; 4•25•2 mg/mL

Carbodec TR timed-release tablets ℞ *decongestant; antihistamine* [pseudoephedrine HCl; carbinoxamine maleate] 120•8 mg

carbodimid calcium [see: calcium carbimide]

carbofenotion INN [also: carbophenothion]

carbohydrate polymer gel *investigational (NDA filed) postsurgical dressing to inhibit scar formation*

carbol-fuchsin solution (or paint) USP *antifungal*

carbolic acid [see: phenol]

carbolin [see: carbachol]

Carbolith ⓒ (U.S. product: Eskalith) capsules ℞ *antipsychotic for manic episodes* [lithium carbonate] 150, 300, 600 mg

carbolonium bromide BAN [also: hexcarbacholine bromide]

carbomer INN, BAN *emulsifying and suspending agent* [also: carbomer 910]

carbomer 1342 NF *emulsifying and suspending agent*

carbomer 910 USAN, NF *emulsifying and suspending agent* [also: carbomer]

carbomer 934 USAN, NF *emulsifying and suspending agent*

carbomer 934P USAN, NF *emulsifying and suspending agent*

carbomer 940 USAN, NF *emulsifying and suspending agent*

carbomer 941 USAN, NF *emulsifying and suspending agent*

carbomycin INN

carbon *element* (C)

carbon, activated

carbon C 14 urea *diagnostic aid for H. pylori in the stomach* [also: ^{14}C urea]

carbon dioxide (CO_2) USP *respiratory stimulant*

carbon tetrachloride NF *solvent*

carbonic acid, calcium salt [see: calcium carbonate]

carbonic acid, dilithium salt [see: lithium carbonate]

carbonic acid, dipotassium salt [see: potassium carbonate]

carbonic acid, disodium salt [see: sodium carbonate]

carbonic acid, magnesium salt [see: magnesium carbonate]

carbonic acid, monoammonium salt [see: ammonium carbonate]

carbonic acid, monopotassium salt [see: potassium bicarbonate]

carbonic acid, monosodium salt [see: sodium bicarbonate]

carbonic anhydrase inhibitors *a class of diuretic agents that reduce the rate of aqueous humor formation, resulting in decreased intraocular pressure; available in both systemic (tablets) and topical (eye drops) forms*

carbonis detergens, liquor (LCD) [see: coal tar]

carbonyl iron *hematinic (100% elemental iron as microparticles)*

carbophenothion BAN [also: carbofenotion]

carboplatin USAN, INN, BAN *alkylating antineoplastic for ovarian and other cancers*

carboprost USAN, INN, BAN *oxytocic*

carboprost methyl USAN *oxytocic*

carboprost trometanol BAN *oxytocic; prostaglandin-type abortifacient* [also: carboprost tromethamine]

carboprost tromethamine USAN, USP *oxytocic; prostaglandin-type abortifacient* [also: carboprost trometanol]

Carboptic Drop-Tainers (eye drops) ℞ *topical antiglaucoma agent; direct-acting miotic* [carbachol] 3%

carboquone INN

carbose D [see: carboxymethylcellulose sodium]

carbovir *investigational (orphan) for AIDS and symptomatic HIV*

carboxyimamidate [see: carbetimer]

carboxymethylcellulose calcium NF *tablet disintegrant*

carboxymethylcellulose sodium USP *bulk laxative; suspending and viscosity-increasing agent; ophthalmic moisturizer; tablet excipient* [also: carmellose; carmellose sodium]

carboxymethylcellulose sodium 12 NF *suspending and viscosity-increasing agent*

carbromal NF, INN

carbubarb INN

carbubarbital [see: carbubarb]

carburazepam INN

carbutamide INN, BAN

carbuterol INN, BAN *bronchodilator* [also: carbuterol HCl]

carbuterol HCl USAN *bronchodilator* [also: carbuterol]

carcainium chloride INN

carcinoembryonic antigen (CEA)

cardamom seed NF

cardamom [see: bitter cardamom]

Cardec-DM syrup, pediatric syrup, pediatric drops ℞ *antitussive; decongestant; antihistamine* [dextromethorphan hydrobromide; pseudoephedrine HCl; carbinoxamine maleate] 15•60•4 mg/5 mL; 15•60•4 mg/5 mL; 4•25•2 mg/mL

Cardec-S syrup ℞ *decongestant; antihistamine* [pseudoephedrine HCl; carbinoxamine maleate] 60•4 mg/5 mL

Cardene capsules ℞ *antianginal; antihypertensive; calcium channel blocker* [nicardipine HCl] 20, 30 mg ② Cardizem

Cardene I.V. injection ℞ *antihypertensive; calcium channel blocker* [nicardipine HCl] 2.5 mg/mL

Cardene SR sustained-release capsules ℞ *antihypertensive; calcium channel blocker* [nicardipine HCl] 30, 45, 60 mg

cardiac glycosides *a class of cardiovascular drugs that increase the force of cardiac contractions* [also called: digitalis glycosides]

Cardiac T test ℞ *in vitro diagnostic aid for troponin T (indicator of cardiac damage) in whole blood*

cardiacs *a class of agents that stimulate or otherwise affect the heart (a term used in folk medicine)*

cardiamid [see: nikethamide]

Cardilate oral or sublingual tablets (discontinued 1995) ℞ *antianginal* [erythrityl tetranitrate] 10 mg

cardin *medicinal herb* [see: blessed thistle]

Cardio-Green (CG) powder for IV injection ℞ *in vivo diagnostic aid for cardiac output, hepatic function, or ophthalmic angiography* [indocyanine green] 25, 50 mg

Cardiolite injection ℞ *myocardial perfusion agent for cardiac SPECT imaging* [technetium Tc 99m sestamibi] 5 mL

Cardi-Omega 3 capsules OTC *dietary supplement* [omega-3 fatty acids; multiple vitamins & minerals] 1000• ± mg

cardioplegic solution (calcium chloride, magnesium chloride, potassium chloride, sodium chloride) [q.v.]

cardioprotective agents *a class of potent intracellular chelating agents which protect the heart from the effects of doxorubicin*

Cardioquin tablets ℞ *antiarrhythmic* [quinidine polygalacturonate] 275 mg

Cardizem IV injection, Lyo-Ject (prefilled syringe) ℞ *calcium channel blocker for atrial fibrillation or paroxysmal supraventricular tachycardia (PSVT)* [diltiazem HCl] 5 mg/mL ⊉ Cardene

Cardizem tablets ℞ *antianginal; antihypertensive; antiarrhythmic; calcium channel blocker* [diltiazem HCl] 30, 60, 90, 120 mg

Cardizem SR; Cardizem CD sustained-release capsules ℞ *antihypertensive; antianginal; antiarrhythmic; calcium channel blocker* [diltiazem HCl] 60, 90, 120 mg; 120, 180, 240, 300 mg

cardophyllin [see: aminophylline]

Cardura tablets ℞ *antihypertensive (α-blocker); treatment for benign prostatic hyperplasia* [doxazosin mesylate] 1, 2, 4, 8 mg

carebastine INN

carena [see: aminophylline]

carfecillin INN, BAN *antibacterial* [also: carbenicillin phenyl sodium]

carfenazine INN *antipsychotic* [also: carphenazine maleate; carphenazine]

carfentanil INN *narcotic analgesic* [also: carfentanil citrate]

carfentanil citrate USAN *narcotic analgesic* [also: carfentanil]

carfimate INN

Carfin tablets ℞ *anticoagulant* [warfarin sodium]

cargentos [see: silver protein]

cargutocin INN

Carica papaya *medicinal herb* [see: papaya]

Cariel ℞ *investigational (Phase III) wound healing treatment*

carindacillin INN, BAN *extended-spectrum penicillin antibiotic* [also: carbenicillin indanyl sodium]

carisoprodol USP, INN, BAN *skeletal muscle relaxant* 350 mg oral

carline thistle (Carlina acaulis) root *medicinal herb used as a carminative, diaphoretic, digestive, diuretic, febrifuge, and, in large doses, an emetic and purgative*

carmantadine USAN, INN *antiparkinsonian*

carmellose INN *suspending agent; tablet excipient* [also: carboxymethylcellulose sodium; carmellose sodium]

carmellose sodium BAN *suspending agent; tablet excipient* [also: carboxymethylcellulose sodium; carmellose]

carmetizide INN

carminatives *a class of agents that relieve flatulence*

carminomycin HCl [now: carubicin HCl]

carmofur INN

Carmol 10 lotion OTC *moisturizer; emollient; keratolytic* [urea] 10%

Carmol 20 cream OTC *moisturizer; emollient; keratolytic* [urea] 20%

Carmol HC cream ℞ *topical corticosteroidal anti-inflammatory; moisturizer; emollient* [hydrocortisone acetate; urea] 1%•10%

carmoxirole INN

carmustine USAN, INN, BAN *nitrosourea-type alkylating antineoplastic; polymer implant for recurrent malignant glioma (orphan)*

Carnation Follow-Up; Carnation GoodStart liquid, powder OTC *total or supplementary infant feeding*

carnauba wax [see: wax, carnauba]

carnidazole USAN, INN, BAN *antiprotozoal*

carnitine INN *vitamin B_t*

L-carnitine [see: levocarnitine]

Carnitor tablets, oral solution, IV injection or infusion ℞ *dietary amino acid for primary and secondary genetic carnitine deficiency (orphan); investigational (orphan) for end-stage renal disease and pediatric cardiomyopathy* [levocarnitine] 330 mg; 100 mg/mL; 500 mg/2.5 mL, 1 g/5 mL

carocainide INN

β-carotene [see: beta carotene]

caroverine INN

caroxazone USAN, INN *antidepressant*

carpenter's herb *medicinal herb* [see: woundwort]

carpenter's square *medicinal herb* [see: figwort]

carperidine INN, BAN

carperone INN

carphenazine BAN *antipsychotic* [also: carphenazine maleate; carfenazine]

carphenazine maleate USAN, USP *antipsychotic* [also: carfenazine; carphenazine]

carpindolol INN

carpipramine INN

carpipramine dihydrochloride [see: carpipramine]

carpolene [now: carbomer 934P]

carprazidil INN

carprofen USAN, INN, BAN *nonsteroidal anti-inflammatory drug (NSAID); analgesic; antipyretic*

carpronium chloride INN

Carpuject (trademarked delivery system) *prefilled cartridge-needle unit*

Carpuject Smartpak (trademarked delivery system) *prefilled cartridge-needle unit package*

carrageenan NF *suspending and viscosity-increasing agent*

Carrisyn ℞ *investigational (Phase I) antiviral and immunomodulator for AIDS* [acemannan]

carrot (Daucus carota) oil from the dried seed and root *medicinal herb for edema, gas, and worms; also used as a nutritional and vitamin supplement and stimulant; may possibly protect the heart and liver*

carsalam INN, BAN

carsatrin INN *cardiotonic* [also: carsatrin succinate]

carsatrin succinate USAN *cardiotonic* [also: carsatrin]

cartazolate USAN, INN *antidepressant*

carteolol INN, BAN *antiadrenergic; topical antiglaucoma agent (β-blocker)* [also: carteolol HCl]

carteolol HCl USAN *antiadrenergic; topical antiglaucoma agent (β-blocker)* [also: carteolol]

Carthamus tinctorius *medicinal herb* [see: safflower]

carticaine BAN *amide local anesthetic for dentistry* [also: articaine]

Carticel ℞ *investigational process to grow autologous cartilage cells to correct cartilage damage due to acute or chronic trauma* [chondrocytes, cultured autologous]

Cartrix (delivery system) *prefilled syringes*

Cartrol Filmtabs (film-coated tablets) OTC *antihypertensive; β-blocker* [carteolol HCl] 2.5, 5 mg

carubicin INN *antineoplastic* [also: carubicin HCl]

carubicin HCl USAN *antineoplastic* [also: carubicin]

Carum carvi NF *medicinal herb* [see: caraway]

carumonam INN, BAN *antibacterial* [also: carumonam sodium]

carumonam sodium USAN *antibacterial* [also: carumonam]

carvedilol USAN, INN, BAN, JAN *antianginal; antihypertensive; α- and β-blocker for congestive heart failure*

carvotroline HCl USAN *antipsychotic*

Caryophyllus aromaticus *medicinal herb* [see: cloves]

carzelesin USAN *antineoplastic*

carzenide INN

casanthranol USAN, USP *stimulant laxative*

cascara fluidextract, aromatic USP *laxative*

cascara sagrada USP *stimulant laxative* 325 mg oral

cascara sagrada *(Frangula purshi-ana; Rhamnus purshiana)* bark *medicinal herb for constipation, cough, and gallbladder, intestinal, and liver disorders; chronic use can cause hypokalemia and melanosis coli* [also see: buckthorn]

cascara sagrada fluid extract *investigational (orphan) for oral drug overdose*

cascarin [see: casanthranol]

Casec powder OTC *protein supplement* [calcium caseinate]

Casodex film-coated tablets ℞ *antiandrogen antineoplastic for prostatic cancer* [bicalutamide] 50 mg

caspofungin acetate USAN *antifungal*

Cassia acutifolia; C. angustifolia; C. senna medicinal herb [see: senna]

cassia oil [see: cinnamon oil]

CAST (Color Allergy Screening Test) reagent sticks for professional use *in vitro diagnostic aid for immunoglobulin E in serum*

Castaderm liquid OTC *topical antifungal; astringent; antiseptic* [resorcinol; boric acid; acetone; basic fuchsin; phenol; alcohol 9%]

Castel Minus; Castel Plus liquid OTC *topical antifungal* [resorcinol; acetone; basic fuchsin; alcohol 11.5%]

Castellani Paint solution (name changed to Castellani Paint Modified in 1996)

Castellani Paint Modified solution ℞ *topical antifungal; antibacterial; keratolytic* [basic fuchsin; phenol; resorcinol]

Castellani's paint [see: carbol-fuchsin solution]

Castile soap

castor oil USP *stimulant laxative*

CAT (cytarabine, Adriamycin, thioguanine) *chemotherapy protocol*

Cataflam tablets ℞ *nonsteroidal anti-inflammatory drug (NSAID); antiarthritic; analgesic for primary dysmenorrhea* [diclofenac potassium] 50 mg

catalase *catalytic neutralizing agent and rinse for contact lenses*

Catapres tablets ℞ *antihypertensive* [clonidine HCl] 0.1, 0.2, 0.3 mg ② Catarase; Combipres; Ser-Ap-Es

Catapres-TTS-1; Catapres-TTS-2; Catapres-TTS-3 7-day transdermal patch ℞ *antihypertensive* [clonidine HCl] 0.1 mg/day (2.5 mg); 0.2 mg/day (5 mg); 0.3 mg/day (7.5 mg)

Catarase 1:5000 ophthalmic solution (discontinued 1999) ℞ *enzymatic zonulolytic for intracapsular lens extraction* [chymotrypsin] 300 U ② Catapres

Catatrol ℞ *investigational (NDA filed) bicyclic antidepressant* [viloxazine]

catchfly *medicinal herb* [see: dogbane]

catchweed *medicinal herb* [see: bedstraw]

catechol-O-methyltransferase (COMT) [see: COMT inhibitors]

catgut suture [see: absorbable surgical suture]

Catha edulis the plant from which cathinone, a naturally occurring stimulant, is derived [see also: cathinone; methcathinone]

Catharanthus roseus medicinal herb [see: periwinkle]

cathartics *a class of agents that cause vigorous evacuation of the bowels by increasing bulk, stimulating peristaltic action, etc.* [also called: purgatives]

cathine INN

cathinone INN *an extract of the Catha edulis plant, a naturally occurring stimulant* [see also: Catha edulis; methcathinone]

cathomycin sodium [see: novobiocin sodium]

catkins willow *medicinal herb* [see: willow]

catmint *medicinal herb* [see: catnip]

catnip *(Nepeta cataria)* plant *medicinal herb for colds, colic, convulsions, diarrhea, digestion, fever, flu, gas, hives, nervous conditions, and stimulating delayed menses*

Catrix Correction cream OTC *moisturizer; emollient*

catrup *medicinal herb* [see: catnip]

cat's claw *(Uncaria guianensis; U. tomentosa)* inner bark *medicinal herb for cancer,* Candida *infections, chronic fatigue, contraception, Crohn's disease, diverticulitis, hypertension, irritable bowel, lupus, parasites, PMS, ulcers, and viral infections; also used as immune booster*

catswort *medicinal herb* [see: catnip]

Caucasian walnut *medicinal herb* [see: English walnut]

Caulophyllum thalictroides *medicinal herb* [see: blue cohosh]

caustics *a class of escharotic or corrosive agents that destroy living tissue* [also called: cauterants]

cauterants *a class of escharotic or corrosive agents that destroy living tissue* [also called: caustics]

CAV (cyclophosphamide, Adriamycin, vinblastine) *chemotherapy protocol*

CAV (cyclophosphamide, Adriamycin, vincristine) *chemotherapy protocol* [also: VAC]

CAVe; CA-Ve (CCNU, Adriamycin, vinblastine) *chemotherapy protocol*

CAVE (cyclophosphamide, Adriamycin, vincristine, etoposide) *chemotherapy protocol*

Caverject powder for intracavernosal injection, PenInject single-use autoinjector ℞ *vasodilator for erectile dysfunction* [alprostadil] 5, 10, 20 μg/mL

CAVP16 (cyclophosphamide, Adriamycin, VP-16) *chemotherapy protocol*

cayenne *(Capsicum annuum; C. frutescens)* fruit *medicinal herb for arthritis, bleeding, cold feet, diabetes, high blood pressure, kidney disorders, rheumatism, poor circulation, strokes, topical neuritis syndromes, tumors, and ulcers*

C-B Time; C-B Time 500 timed-release tablets (discontinued 1995) OTC *vitamin supplement* [multiple B vitamins; vitamin C] ± •200 mg; ± •500 mg

CBV (cyclophosphamide, BCNU, VePesid) *chemotherapy protocol*

CBV (cyclophosphamide, BCNU, VP-16-213) *chemotherapy protocol*

CC (carboplatin, cyclophosphamide) *chemotherapy protocol*

CC-Galactosidase ℞ *investigational (orphan) enzyme replacement therapy for Fabry's disease* [alpha-galactosidase A]

CCM (cyclophosphamide, CCNU, methotrexate) *chemotherapy protocol*

CCNU (chloroethyl-cyclohexyl-nitrosourea) [see: lomustine]

C-Crystals crystals OTC *vitamin supplement* [vitamin C]

CCV-AV (CCNU, cyclophosphamide, vincristine [alternates with] Adriamycin, vincristine) *chemotherapy protocol*

CCVPP (CCNU, cyclophosphamide, Velban, procarbazine, prednisone) *chemotherapy protocol*

CD (cytarabine, daunorubicin) *chemotherapy protocol*

CD4, human truncated 369 AA polypeptide *orphan status withdrawn 1996*

CD4, recombinant soluble human (rCD4) *investigational (Phase II, orphan) antiviral for AIDS*

CD4 immunoadhesin [see: CD4 immunoglobulin G, recombinant human]

CD4 immunoglobulin G, recombinant human *investigational (Phase I) antiviral for maternal/fetal transfer of HIV; investigational (orphan) for AIDS*

CD4-IgG [see: CD4 immunoglobulin G, recombinant human]

CD4-PE40 [see: alvircept sudotox]

CD5-T lymphocyte immunotoxin *orphan status withdrawn 1997*

CD19 [see: anti-B4-blocked ricin]

CD20 *investigational for low-grade non-Hodgkin's lymphoma*

CD-33 [see: ricin (blocked) conjugated murine MCA myeloid cells]

CD-40 ligand *investigational (Phase I) cytokine for rheumatoid arthritis, AIDS, and hyperimmunoglobulin M (HIM) syndrome*

CD-45 monoclonal antibodies
orphan status withdrawn 1996

CD-45RB monoclonal antibodies
investigational antirejection antibody

CdA (2-chloro-2'-deoxyadenosine)
[see: cladribine]

CDC (carboplatin, doxorubicin, cyclophosphamide) *chemotherapy protocol*

CDDP; C-DDP (cis-diamminedi-chloroplatinum) [see: cisplatin]

CDDP/VP (CDDP, VePesid) *chemotherapy protocol*

CDE (cyclophosphamide, doxorubicin, etoposide) *chemotherapy protocol*

CDP571 *investigational (orphan) for Crohn's disease*

CDP-cholin [see: citicoline]

CEA (carcinoembryonic antigen)

CEA-Cide ℞ *investigational (orphan) antineoplastic for pancreatic and small cell lung cancer* [monoclonal antibody to CEA, humanized]

CEAker *orphan status withdrawn 1997* [indium In 111 murine anti-CEA MAb, type ZCE 025]

Ceanothus americanus medicinal herb [see: New Jersey tea]

CEA-Scan powder for injection ℞ *imaging agent for detection of recurrent or metastatic colorectal cancer* [arcitumomab] 1.25 mg

CEB (carboplatin, etoposide, bleomycin) *chemotherapy protocol*

Cebid Timecelles (sustained-release capsules) OTC *vitamin supplement* [ascorbic acid] 500 mg

CECA (cisplatin, etoposide, cyclophosphamide, Adriamycin) *chemotherapy protocol*

Ceclor Pulvules (capsules), powder for oral suspension ℞ *cephalosporin antibiotic* [cefaclor] 250, 500 mg; 125, 187, 250, 375 mg/5 mL

Ceclor CD extended-release tablets ℞ *cephalosporin antibiotic* [cefaclor] 375, 500 mg

Ceclor SR (pre-marketing name; released as Ceclor CD in 1996)

Cecon solution OTC *vitamin supplement* [vitamin C] 100 mg/mL

Cedax capsules, oral suspension ℞ *cephalosporin antibiotic* [ceftibuten] 400 mg; 90, 180 mg/mL

cedefingol USAN *antipsoriatic; antineoplastic adjunct*

cedelizumab USAN *monoclonal antibody; prophylaxis of rejection of solid organ allograft; immunomodulator for autoimmune diseases*

CeeNu capsules, dose pack ℞ *nitrosourea-type alkylating antineoplastic for brain tumors and Hodgkin's disease* [lomustine] 10, 40, 100 mg; 2 × 100 mg + 2 × 40 mg + 2 × 10 mg

CEF (cyclophosphamide, epirubicin, fluorouracil) *chemotherapy protocol*

cefacetrile INN *antibacterial* [also: cephacetrile sodium]

cefacetrile sodium [see: cephacetrile sodium]

cefaclor USAN, USP, INN, BAN, JAN *second-generation cephalosporin antibiotic* 250, 500 mg oral; 125, 187, 250, 375 mg/5 mL oral

cefadroxil USAN, USP, INN, BAN *first-generation cephalosporin antibiotic* 500, 1000 mg oral

Cefadyl powder for IV or IM injection ℞ *cephalosporin antibiotic* [cephapirin sodium] 1 g ◙ Cefzil

cefalexin INN, JAN *first-generation cephalosporin antibiotic* [also: cephalexin]

cefaloglycin INN *antibacterial* [also: cephaloglycin]

cefalonium INN [also: cephalonium]

cefaloram INN [also: cephaloram]

cefaloridine INN *antibacterial* [also: cephaloridine]

cefalotin INN *first-generation cephalosporin antibiotic* [also: cephalothin sodium; cephalothin]

cefalotin sodium [see: cephalothin sodium]

cefamandole USAN, INN *second-generation cephalosporin antibiotic* [also: cephamandole]

cefamandole nafate USAN, USP *second-generation cephalosporin antibiotic* [also: cephamandole nafate]

cefamandole sodium USP *second-generation cephalosporin antibiotic*

Cefanex capsules (discontinued 1995) ℞ *cephalosporin antibiotic* [cephalexin] 250, 500 mg

cefaparole USAN, INN *antibacterial*

cefapirin INN, BAN *first-generation cephalosporin antibiotic* [also: cephapirin sodium]

cefapirin sodium [see: cephapirin sodium]

cefatrizine USAN, INN, BAN *antibacterial*

cefazaflur INN *antibacterial* [also: cefazaflur sodium]

cefazaflur sodium USAN *antibacterial* [also: cefazaflur]

cefazedone INN, BAN

cefazolin USP, INN *first-generation cephalosporin antibiotic* [also: cephazolin] ☑ cephalothin; Zefazone

cefazolin sodium USAN, USP *first-generation cephalosporin antibiotic* [also: cephazolin sodium] 0.25, 0.5, 1, 5, 10, 20 g injection ☑ cephalothin; Zefazone

cefbuperazone USAN, INN *antibacterial*

cefcanel INN

cefcanel daloxate INN

cefdinir USAN, INN *third-generation cephalosporin antibiotic*

cefedrolor INN

cefempidone INN, BAN

cefepime USAN, INN *third-generation cephalosporin antibiotic*

cefepime HCl USAN *third-generation cephalosporin antibiotic*

cefetamet USAN, INN *veterinary antibacterial*

cefetecol USAN, INN, BAN *antibacterial*

cefetrizole INN

cefivitril INN

cefixime USAN, USP, INN, BAN *third-generation cephalosporin antibiotic*

Cefizox powder or frozen premix for IV or IM injection ℞ *cephalosporin antibiotic* [ceftizoxime sodium] 0.5, 1, 2, 10 g

cefmenoxime INN *antibacterial* [also: cefmenoxime HCl]

cefmenoxime HCl USAN, USP *antibacterial* [also: cefmenoxime]

cefmepidium chloride INN

cefmetazole USAN, INN *second-generation cephalosporin antibiotic*

cefmetazole sodium USAN, USP, JAN *second-generation cephalosporin antibiotic*

cefminox INN

Cefobid powder or frozen premix for IV or IM injection ℞ *cephalosporin antibiotic* [cefoperazone sodium] 1, 2, 10 g

cefodizime INN *investigational cephalosporin antibiotic*

Cefol Filmtabs (film-coated tablets) ℞ *vitamin supplement* [multiple vitamins; folic acid] ≛ •0.5 mg

cefonicid INN, BAN *second-generation cephalosporin antibiotic* [also: cefonicid monosodium]

cefonicid monosodium USAN *second-generation cephalosporin antibiotic* [also: cefonicid]

cefonicid sodium USAN, USP *second-generation cephalosporin antibiotic*

cefoperazone INN, BAN *third-generation cephalosporin antibiotic* [also: cefoperazone sodium]

cefoperazone sodium USAN, USP *third-generation cephalosporin antibiotic* [also: cefoperazone]

ceforanide USAN, USP, INN, BAN *bactericidal antibiotic*

Cefotan powder or frozen premix for IV or IM injection ℞ *cephamycin antibiotic* [cefotetan disodium] 1, 2, 10 g

cefotaxime INN, BAN *third-generation cephalosporin antibiotic* [also: cefotaxime sodium] ☑ cefoxitin

cefotaxime sodium USAN, USP *third-generation cephalosporin antibiotic* [also: cefotaxime]

cefotetan USAN, INN, BAN *cephamycin antibiotic*

cefotetan disodium USAN, USP *cephamycin antibiotic*

cefotiam INN, BAN *antibacterial* [also: cefotiam HCl]

cefotiam HCl USAN *antibacterial* [also: cefotiam]

cefoxazole INN [also: cephoxazole]

cefoxitin USAN, INN, BAN *cephamycin antibiotic* ⚕ cefotaxime

cefoxitin sodium USAN, USP, BAN *cephamycin antibiotic*

cefpimizole USAN, INN *antibacterial*

cefpimizole sodium USAN, JAN *antibacterial*

cefpiramide USAN, USP, INN *antibacterial*

cefpiramide sodium USAN, JAN *antibacterial*

cefpirome INN, BAN *antibacterial* [also: cefpirome sulfate]

cefpirome sulfate USAN, JAN *antibacterial* [also: cefpirome]

cefpodoxime INN, BAN *broad-spectrum third-generation cephalosporin antibiotic* [also: cefpodoxime proxetil]

cefpodoxime proxetil USAN, JAN *broad-spectrum third-generation cephalosporin antibiotic* [also: cefpodoxime]

cefprozil USAN, INN *second-generation cephalosporin antibiotic*

cefprozil monohydrate

cefquinome INN, BAN *veterinary antibacterial*

cefquinome sulfate USAN *veterinary antibacterial*

cefradine INN *first-generation cephalosporin antibiotic* [also: cephradine]

cefrotil INN

cefroxadine USAN, INN *antibacterial*

cefsulodin INN, BAN *antibacterial* [also: cefsulodin sodium]

cefsulodin sodium USAN *antibacterial* [also: cefsulodin]

cefsumide INN

ceftazidime USAN, USP, INN, BAN, JAN *third-generation cephalosporin antibiotic*

cefteram INN

ceftezole INN

ceftibuten USAN, INN, BAN *third-generation cephalosporin antibiotic*

Ceftin film-coated tablets, oral suspension ℞ *cephalosporin antibiotic* [cefuroxime axetil] 125, 250, 500 mg; 125, 250 mg/5 mL

ceftiofur INN, BAN *veterinary antibacterial* [also: ceftiofur HCl]

ceftiofur HCl USAN *veterinary antibacterial* [also: ceftiofur]

ceftiofur sodium USAN *veterinary antibacterial*

ceftiolene INN

ceftioxide INN

ceftizoxime INN, BAN *third-generation cephalosporin antibiotic* [also: ceftizoxime sodium] ⚕ cefuroxime

ceftizoxime sodium USAN, USP *third-generation cephalosporin antibiotic* [also: ceftizoxime]

ceftriaxone INN, BAN *third-generation cephalosporin antibiotic* [also: ceftriaxone sodium]

ceftriaxone sodium USAN, USP *third-generation cephalosporin antibiotic* [also: ceftriaxone]

cefuracetime INN, BAN

cefuroxime USAN, INN, BAN *second-generation cephalosporin antibiotic* ⚕ ceftizoxime

cefuroxime axetil USAN, USP, BAN *second-generation cephalosporin antibiotic*

cefuroxime pivoxetil USAN *second-generation cephalosporin antibiotic*

cefuroxime sodium USP, BAN *second-generation cephalosporin antibiotic* 0.75, 1.5, 7.5 g injection

cefuzonam INN

Cefzil film-coated tablets, powder for oral suspension ℞ *cephalosporin antibiotic* [cefprozil] 250, 500 mg; 125, 250 mg/5 mL ⚕ Cefadyl; Kefzol

Cefzon (foreign name for U.S. product Omnicef)

celandine (Chelidonium majus) root and plant *medicinal herb used as an analgesic, antispasmodic, caustic, diaphoretic, diuretic, narcotic, and purgative*

Celebra (name changed to Celebrex upon release in 1999)

Celebrex capsules ℞ *COX-2 inhibitor anti-inflammatory and analgesic for osteoarthritis and rheumatoid arthritis* [celecoxib] 100, 200 mg ⚕ Cerebyx

celecoxib USAN *COX-2 inhibitor anti-inflammatory and analgesic for osteoarthritis and rheumatoid arthritis*

celery (Apium graveolens) root, stem, and seeds *medicinal herb for aiding digestion, arthritis, cancer, diuresis, gas, headache, hysteria, inducing menstruation, lumbago, nervousness, rheumatism, and terminating lactation*

Celestone tablets, syrup *corticosteroid; anti-inflammatory* [betamethasone] 0.6 mg; 0.6 mg/5 mL

Celestone Phosphate IV, IM injection ℞ *corticosteroid; anti-inflammatory* [betamethasone sodium phosphate] 4 mg/mL

Celestone Soluspan intrabursal, intra-articular, intralesional injection ℞ *corticosteroid; anti-inflammatory* [betamethasone sodium phosphate; betamethasone acetate] 3•3 mg/mL

Celexa film-coated tablets ℞ *selective serotonin reuptake inhibitor (SSRI) for depression; investigational for Alzheimer's disease* [citalopram hydrobromide] 20, 40 mg

celgosivir HCl USAN *antiviral; α-glucosidase I inhibitor for HIV*

celiprolol INN, BAN *antiadrenergic (β-receptor)* [also: celiprolol HCl]

celiprolol HCl USAN *antiadrenergic (β-receptor)* [also: celiprolol]

cellacefate INN *tablet-coating agent* [also: cellulose acetate phthalate; cellacephate]

cellacephate BAN *tablet-coating agent* [also: cellulose acetate phthalate; cellacefate]

CellCept capsules, tablets ℞ *immunosuppressant for allogenic kidney and heart transplants* [mycophenolate mofetil] 250 mg; 500 mg

CellCept powder for IV infusion ℞ *immunosuppressant for allogenic kidney and heart transplants* [mycophenolate mofetil HCl] 500 mg

Cellufresh eye drops (discontinued 1998) OTC *ophthalmic moisturizer/lubricant* [carboxymethylcellulose] 0.5%

cellulase USAN *digestive enzyme*

cellulolytic enzyme [see: cellulase]

cellulose, absorbable [see: cellulose, oxidized]

cellulose, ethyl ester [see: ethylcellulose]

cellulose, hydroxypropyl methyl ether [see: hydroxypropyl methylcellulose]

cellulose, microcrystalline NF *tablet and capsule diluent* [also: dispersible cellulose]

cellulose, oxidized USP *topical local hemostatic*

cellulose, oxidized regenerated USP *local hemostatic*

cellulose, sodium carboxymethyl [see: carboxymethylcellulose sodium]

cellulose acetate NF *tablet-coating agent; insoluble polymer membrane*

cellulose acetate butyrate [see: cabufocon A; cabufocon B]

cellulose acetate dibutyrate [see: porofocon A; porofocon B]

cellulose acetate phthalate (CAP) NF *tablet-coating agent* [also: cellacefate; cellacephate]

cellulose carboxymethyl ether, sodium salt [see: carboxymethylcellulose sodium]

cellulose diacetate [see: cellulose acetate]

cellulose dihydrogen phosphate, disodium salt [see: cellulose sodium phosphate]

cellulose disodium phosphate [see: cellulose sodium phosphate]

cellulose ethyl ether [see: ethylcellulose]

cellulose gum, modified [now: croscarmellose sodium]

cellulose methyl ether [see: methylcellulose]

cellulose nitrate [see: pyroxylin]

cellulose sodium phosphate (CSP) USAN, USP *antiurolithic to prevent stone formation in absorptive hypercalciuria Type I*

cellulosic acid [see: cellulose, oxidized]

Celluvisc solution OTC *ophthalmic moisturizer/lubricant* [carboxymethyl-cellulose] 1%

celmoleukin INN *immunostimulant*

Celontin Kapseals (capsules) ℞ *anticonvulsant* [methsuximide] 150, 300 mg

celucloral INN, BAN

Cel-U-Jec IV, IM injection ℞ *corticosteroid; anti-inflammatory* [betamethasone sodium phosphate] 4 mg/mL

CEM (cytosine arabinoside, etoposide, methotrexate) *chemotherapy protocol*

Cenafed syrup OTC *nasal decongestant* [pseudoephedrine HCl] 30 mg/5 mL

Cenafed Plus tablets OTC *decongestant; antihistamine* [pseudoephedrine HCl; triprolidine HCl] 60•2.5 mg

Cena-K liquid ℞ *potassium supplement* [potassium chloride] 20, 40 mEq/15 mL

Cenestin film-coated tablets ℞ *estrogen replacement therapy for postmenopausal disorders* [conjugated estrogens, synthetic] 0.625, 0.9 mg

Cenolate IV, IM, or subcu injection ℞ *antiscorbutic* [sodium ascorbate] 562.5 mg/mL

Centara ℞ *investigational treatment for arthritis and multiple sclerosis; transplant rejection preventative* [priliximab]

Centaurea cyanus *medicinal herb* [see: cornflower]

centaury (Erythraea centaurium) plant *medicinal herb for aiding digestion, blood cleansing, fever, and promoting menstruation*

Centella asiatica *medicinal herb* [see: gotu kola]

Center-Al subcu or IM injection ℞ *allergenic sensitivity testing (subcu); allergenic desensitization therapy (IM)* [allergenic extracts, alum-precipitated]

CentoRx (name changed to ReoPro upon its release in 1995)

Centoxin ℞ *investigational (orphan) for gram-negative bacteremia in endotoxin shock* [nebacumab]

Centrafree tablets OTC *antianemic* [ferrous fumarate; multiple vitamins]

Centrax capsules, tablets (discontinued 1995) ℞ *anxiolytic; sedative* [prazepam] 5, 10, 20 mg; 10 mg

centrazene [see: simtrazene]

centrophenoxine [see: meclofenoxate]

Centrovite Advanced Formula tablets (name changed to Cerovite Advanced Formula in 1995)

Centrovite Jr. tablets (name changed to Cerovite Jr. in 1995)

Centrum tablets OTC *antianemic* [ferrous fumarate; multiple vitamins]

Centrum, Advanced Formula liquid OTC *vitamin/mineral/iron supplement* [multiple vitamins & minerals; ferrous fumarate; biotin; alcohol 6.7%] ±•9•0.3 mg/15 mL

Centrum, Advanced Formula tablets OTC *vitamin/mineral/iron supplement* [multiple vitamins & minerals; ferrous fumarate; folic acid; biotin] ±•18 mg•0.4 mg•30 µg

Centrum Jr. + Extra C; Centrum Jr. + Extra Calcium chewable tablets OTC *vitamin/mineral/calcium/iron supplement* [multiple vitamins & minerals; calcium; iron; folic acid; biotin] ±•108•18•0.4•0.045 mg; ±•160•18•0.4•0.045 mg

Centrum Jr. with Iron tablets OTC *vitamin/mineral/iron supplement* [multiple vitamins & minerals; iron; folic acid; biotin] ±•18 mg•0.4 mg•45 µg

Centrum Silver tablets OTC *geriatric vitamin/mineral supplement* [multiple vitamins & minerals; folic acid; biotin] ±•400•30 µg

Centurion A-Z tablets (name changed to Multi-Vitamin Mineral with Beta-Carotene in 1995)

Ceo-Two suppository OTC *laxative* [sodium bicarbonate; potassium bitartrate]

CEP (CCNU, etoposide, prednimustine) *chemotherapy protocol*

Cēpacol mouthwash/gargle OTC *oral antiseptic* [cetylpyridinium chloride] 0.05%

Cēpacol, Children's oral liquid OTC *pediatric decongestant and analgesic*

[pseudoephedrine HCl; acetamino-phen] 15•160 mg/5 mL

Cēpacol Anesthetic troches OTC *topical oral anesthetic; antiseptic* [benzocaine; cetylpyridinium chloride] 10 mg•0.07%

Cēpacol Maximum Strength lozenges OTC *topical oral anesthetic* [benzocaine] 10 mg

Cēpacol Throat lozenges OTC *oral antiseptic* [cetylpyridinium chloride] 0.07%

Cēpastat Sore Throat lozenges OTC *topical antipruritic/counterirritant; mild local anesthetic* [phenol] 14.5, 29 mg ▣ Capastat

cephacetrile sodium USAN, USP *antibacterial* [also: cefacetrile]

cephalexin USAN, USP, BAN *first-generation cephalosporin antibiotic* [also: cefalexin] 250, 500, 1000 mg oral; 125, 250 mg/5 mL oral ▣ cefazolin; cephalothin

cephalexin HCl USAN, USP *first-generation cephalosporin antibiotic*

cephaloglycin USAN, USP, BAN *antibacterial* [also: cefaloglycin]

cephalonium BAN [also: cefalonium]

cephaloram BAN [also: cefaloram]

cephaloridine USAN, USP, BAN *antibacterial* [also: cefaloridine]

cephalosporin N [see: adicillin]

cephalosporins *a class of bactericidal antibiotics, divided into first-, second-, and third-generation cephalosporins; higher generations have increasing efficacy against gram-negative and decreasing efficacy against gram-positive bacteria*

cephalothin BAN *first-generation cephalosporin antibiotic* [also: cephalothin sodium; cefalotin] ▣ cefazolin

cephalothin sodium USAN, USP *first-generation cephalosporin antibiotic* [also: cefalotin; cephalothin]

cephamandole BAN *second-generation cephalosporin antibiotic* [also: cefamandole]

cephamandole nafate BAN *second-generation cephalosporin antibiotic* [also: cefamandole nafate]

cephamycins *a class of bactericidal antibiotics similar to second-generation cephalosporins (q.v.)*

cephapirin sodium USAN, USP *first-generation cephalosporin antibiotic* [also: cefapirin] ▣ cephradine

cephazolin BAN *first-generation cephalosporin antibiotic* [also: cefazolin]

cephazolin sodium BAN *first-generation cephalosporin antibiotic* [also: cefazolin sodium]

cephoxazole BAN [also: cefoxazole]

cephradine USAN, USP, BAN *first-generation cephalosporin antibiotic* [also: cefradine] 250, 500 mg oral; 125, 250 mg/5 mL oral ▣ cephapirin

Cephulac syrup ℞ *prevent and treat portal-systemic encephalopathy* [lactulose] 10 g/15 mL

Ceprate SC ℞ *investigational (Phase III) stem cell concentration/purification system for multiple myeloma and bone marrow transplants for breast cancer* [monoclonal antibodies]

Ceptaz powder for IV or IM injection ℞ *cephalosporin antibiotic* [ceftazidime pentahydrate] 1, 2, 10 g

ceramide trihexosidase (CTH) & alpha-galactosidase A *investigational (orphan) for Fabry's disease*

CerAxon ℞ *investigational (Phase III) brain tissue protector for cerebral infarction following ischemic stroke* [citicoline sodium]

Cerebyx IV or IM injection ℞ *hydantoin anticonvulsant for grand mal status epilepticus (orphan)* [fosphenytoin sodium (phenytoin sodium equivalent)] 75 (50) mg/mL ▣ Celebrex

CereCRIB ℞ *investigational (Phase II) cellular pain control implant*

Ceredase IV infusion ℞ *glucocerebrosidase enzyme replacement in Gaucher's disease type I (orphan); investigational (orphan) for types II and III* [alglucerase] 10, 80 U/mL

cerelose [see: glucose]

Ceresine ℞ *investigational pyruvate dehydrogenase stimulator for acute head trauma*

Cerespan timed-release capsules (discontinued 1996) ℞ *peripheral vasodilator; smooth muscle relaxant for cerebral, myocardial, and peripheral ischemias* [papaverine HCl] 150 mg

Cerestat ℞ *investigational (Phase III) treatment for traumatic brain injury (clinical trials discontinued 1997); investigational (Phase III) treatment for stroke* [aptiganel HCl]

Cerezyme powder for IV infusion ℞ *enzyme replacement therapy for types I, II, and III Gaucher's disease (orphan)* [imiglucerase] 40 U/mL

cerium *element (Ce)*

cerium oxalate USP

cerivastatin sodium USAN *HMG-CoA reductase inhibitor for hyperlipidemia*

Cernevit-12 powder for IV injection ℞ *parenteral vitamin therapy* [multiple vitamins; folic acid; biotin] ≚•_?_•_?_

ceronapril USAN, INN *antihypertensive*

Cerose-DM liquid OTC *antitussive; decongestant; antihistamine* [dextromethorphan hydrobromide; phenylephrine HCl; chlorpheniramine maleate; alcohol 2.4%] 15•10•4 mg/5 mL

Cerovite; Cerovite Advanced Formula tablets OTC *vitamin/mineral/iron supplement* [multiple vitamins & minerals; ferrous fumarate; folic acid; biotin] ≚•18 mg•0.4 mg•30 μg

Cerovite Jr. tablets OTC *vitamin/mineral/iron supplement* [multiple vitamins & minerals; ferrous fumarate; folic acid; biotin] ≚•18 mg•0.4 mg•45 μg

Cerovite Senior tablets OTC *geriatric vitamin/mineral supplement* [multiple vitamins & minerals; folic acid; biotin] ≚•200•30 μg

Certagen film-coated tablets OTC *vitamin/mineral/iron supplement* [multiple vitamins & minerals; ferrous fumarate; folic acid; biotin] ≚•18 mg•0.4 mg•30 μg

Certagen liquid OTC *vitamin/mineral/iron supplement* [multiple vitamins & minerals; iron; biotin; alcohol 6.6%] ≚•9•0.3 mg

Certagen Senior tablets OTC *geriatric vitamin/mineral supplement* [multiple vitamins & minerals; folic acid; biotin] ≚•200•30 μg

CertaVite tablets OTC *vitamin/mineral/iron supplement* [multiple vitamins & minerals; ferrous fumarate; folic acid; biotin] ≚•18 mg•0.4 mg•30 μg

Certa-Vite Golden tablets OTC *geriatric vitamin/mineral supplement* [multiple vitamins & minerals; biotin] ≚•30 μg

Certiva IM injection ℞ *active immunizing agent for diphtheria, tetanus, and pertussis* [diphtheria & tetanus toxoids & acellular pertussis (DTaP) vaccine] 15 Lf•6 Lf•40 μg per 0.5 mL

Cerubidine powder for IV injection ℞ *antibiotic antineoplastic for multiple nonlymphocytic leukemias* [daunorubicin HCl] 20 mg

ceruletide USAN, INN, BAN *gastric secretory stimulant*

ceruletide diethylamine USAN *gastric secretory stimulant*

Cerumenex ear drops ℞ *cerumenolytic to emulsify and disperse ear wax* [trolamine polypeptide oleate-condensate] 10%

Cervidil vaginal insert ℞ *prostaglandin for cervical ripening at term* [dinoprostone] 10 mg

cesium *element (Cs)*

cesium (^{131}Cs) chloride INN *radioactive agent* [also: cesium chloride Cs 131]

cesium chloride Cs 131 USAN *radioactive agent* [also: cesium (^{131}Cs) chloride]

Ceta liquid OTC *soap-free therapeutic skin cleanser*

Ceta Plus capsules ℞ *narcotic analgesic* [hydrocodone bitartrate; acetaminophen] 5•500 mg

cetaben INN *antihyperlipoproteinemic* [also: cetaben sodium]

cetaben sodium USAN *antihyperlipoproteinemic* [also: cetaben]

Cetacaine gel, liquid, ointment, aerosol ℞ *topical local anesthetic; antiseptic* [benzocaine; tetracaine HCl; butamben] 14%•2%•2%

Cetacort lotion ℞ *topical corticosteroidal anti-inflammatory* [hydrocortisone] 0.25%, 0.5%

cetalkonium *antiseptic*

cetalkonium chloride USAN, INN, BAN *topical anti-infective*

Cetamide ophthalmic ointment ℞ *topical ophthalmic antibiotic* [sulfacetamide sodium] 10%

cetamolol INN *antiadrenergic (β-receptor)* [also: cetamolol HCl]

cetamolol HCl USAN *antiadrenergic (β-receptor)* [also: cetamolol]

Cetaphil cream, lotion, cleansing bar, cleansing solution OTC *soap-free therapeutic skin cleanser*

Cetapred ophthalmic ointment ℞ *topical ophthalmic corticosteroidal anti-inflammatory; antibiotic* [prednisolone acetate; sulfacetamide sodium] 0.25%•10%

cethexonium chloride INN

cetiedil INN *peripheral vasodilator* [also: cetiedil citrate]

cetiedil citrate USAN *peripheral vasodilator* [also: cetiedil]

cetirizine INN, BAN *second-generation piperazine antihistamine* [also: cetirizine HCl]

cetirizine HCl USAN *second-generation piperazine antihistamine* [also: cetirizine]

cetobemidone [see: ketobemidone]

cetocycline INN *antibacterial* [also: cetocycline HCl]

cetocycline HCl USAN *antibacterial* [also: cetocycline]

cetofenicol INN *antibacterial* [also: cetophenicol]

cetohexazine INN

cetomacrogol 1000 INN, BAN

cetophenicol USAN *antibacterial* [also: cetofenicol]

cetophenylbutazone [see: kebuzone]

cetostearyl alcohol NF *emulsifying agent*

cetotetrine HCl [now: cetocycline HCl]

cetotiamine INN

cetoxime INN, BAN

cetoxime HCl [see: cetoxime]

Cetraria islandica *medicinal herb* [see: Iceland moss]

cetraxate INN *GI antiulcerative* [also: cetraxate HCl]

cetraxate HCl USAN *GI antiulcerative* [also: cetraxate]

cetrimide INN, BAN *topical antiseptic*

cetrimonium bromide INN *topical antiseptic* [also: cetrimonium chloride]

cetrimonium chloride BAN *topical antiseptic* [also: cetrimonium bromide]

cetyl alcohol NF *emulsifying and stiffening agent*

cetyl esters wax NF *stiffening agent*

cetyldimethylbenzyl ammonium chloride [see: cetalkonium chloride]

cetylpyridinium chloride USP, INN, BAN *topical antiseptic; preservative*

cetyltrimethyl ammonium bromide

CEV (cyclophosphamide, etoposide, vincristine) *chemotherapy protocol*

Cevalin IV, IM, or subcu injection ℞ *antiscorbutic* [ascorbic acid] 500 mg/mL

Cevi-Bid timed-release capsules OTC *vitamin supplement* [ascorbic acid] 500 mg

Cevi-Fer timed-release capsules ℞ *hematinic* [ferrous fumarate; ascorbic acid; folic acid] 20•300•1 mg

cevimeline HCl USAN *muscarinic receptor agonist for Alzheimer's disease*

Ce-Vi-Sol drops OTC *vitamin supplement* [ascorbic acid; alcohol 5%] 35 mg/0.6 mL

cevitamic acid [see: ascorbic acid]

cevitan [see: ascorbic acid]

ceylon gelatin [see: agar]

Cezin capsules OTC *vitamin/mineral supplement* [multiple vitamins & minerals]

Cezin-S capsules ℞ *geriatric vitamin/ mineral supplement* [multiple vitamins & minerals; folic acid] ±•0.5 mg

CF (carboplatin, fluorouracil) *chemotherapy protocol*

CF (cisplatin, fluorouracil) *chemotherapy protocol*

CFL (cisplatin, fluorouracil, leucovorin [rescue]) *chemotherapy protocol*

CFM (cyclophosphamide, fluorouracil, mitoxantrone) *chemotherapy protocol* [also: CNF; FNC]

CFP (cyclophosphamide, fluoro-uracil, prednisone) *chemotherapy protocol*

CFPT (cyclophosphamide, fluoro-uracil, prednisone, tamoxifen) *chemotherapy protocol*

CFTR (cystic fibrosis transmembrane conductance regulator) [q.v.]

CG (Cardio-Green) [q.v.]

CG (chorionic gonadotropin) [see: gonadotropin, chorionic]

CGF (Control Gel Formula) dressing [see: DuoDERM CGF]

CGP-64128A *investigational (Phase I) antisense anticancer compound*

CGP-69846A *investigational (Phase II) anticancer agent for solid tumors*

CH1VPP; Ch1VPP (chlorambucil, vinblastine, procarbazine, prednisone) *chemotherapy protocol*

CHAD (cyclophosphamide, hexamethylmelamine, Adriamycin, DDP) *chemotherapy protocol*

chalk, precipitated [see: calcium carbonate, precipitated]

Chamaelirium luteum medicinal herb [see: false unicorn]

CHAMOCA (Cytoxan, hydroxyurea, actinomycin D, methotrexate, Oncovin, calcium folinate, Adriamycin) *chemotherapy protocol*

chamomile *(Anthemis nobilis; Matricaria chamomilla)* flowers *medicinal herb for appetite stimulation, bronchitis, excessive menstruation with cramps, fever, gastrointestinal cramps, hysteria, inflammation, insomnia, nervousness, rheumatic disorders, and parasites*

CHAP (cyclophosphamide, Hexalen, Adriamycin, Platinol) *chemotherapy protocol*

CHAP (cyclophosphamide, hexamethylmelamine, Adriamycin, Platinol) *chemotherapy protocol*

Chap Stick Medicated Lip Balm stick, jar, squeezable tube OTC *topical analgesic; counterirritant; moisturizer; protectant; emollient* [camphor; menthol; phenol] 1%•0.6%•0.5%

chaparral *(Larrea divaricata; L. glutinosa; L. tridentata)* leaves and stems *medicinal herb for arthritis, blood cleansing, bronchitis, cancer, chickenpox, colds, leukemia, rheumatic pain, stomach pain, and tumors; not generally regarded as safe and effective because of liver toxicity and stimulation of some tumors*

CharcoAid oral suspension OTC *adsorbent antidote for poisoning* [activated charcoal] 15 g/120 mL, 30 g/150 mL

CharcoAid 2000 oral liquid, granules OTC *adsorbent antidote for poisoning* [activated charcoal] 15 g/120 mL, 50 g/240 mL; 15 g

charcoal *gastric adsorbent/detoxicant; antiflatulent* 260 mg oral

charcoal, activated USP *general purpose antidote/adsorbent* 15, 30, 40, 120, 240 g, 208 mg/mL oral

Charcoal Plus enteric-coated tablets OTC *adsorbent; detoxicant* [activated charcoal] 250 mg

CharcoCaps capsules OTC *adsorbent; detoxicant; antiflatulent* [charcoal] 260 mg

Chardonna-2 tablets ℞ *GI anticholinergic; sedative* [belladonna extract; phenobarbital] 15•15 mg

chaste tree *(Vitex agnus-castus)* dried ripe fruit *medicinal herb for acne, balancing progesterone and estrogen production, increasing lactation, ovarian insufficiency, premenstrual breast pain, regulating menstrual cycle, and uterine bleeding*

chaulmosulfone INN

checkerberry *medicinal herb* [see: squaw vine; wintergreen]

cheese plant; cheeseflower *medicinal herb* [see: mallow]

cheese rennet *medicinal herb* [see: bedstraw]

chelafrin [see: epinephrine]

Chelated Magnesium tablets OTC *magnesium supplement* [magnesium amino acid chelate] 500 mg

Chelated Manganese tablets OTC *manganese supplement* [manganese] 20, 50 mg

chelating agents *a class of agents that prevent bodily absorption of and cause the excretion of substances such as heavy metals*

chelen [see: ethyl chloride]

Chelidonium majus *medicinal herb* [see: celandine]

Chelone glabra *medicinal herb* [see: turtlebloom]

Chemet capsules ℞ *heavy metal chelating agent for lead poisoning (orphan); investigational (orphan) for cystine kidney stones and mercury poisoning* [succimer] 100 mg

Chemo-Pin (trademarked form) *chemical-dispensing pin*

Chemstrip 2 GP; Chemstrip 2 LN; Chemstrip 4 the OB; Chemstrip 6; Chemstrip 7; Chemstrip 8; Chemstrip 9; Chemstrip 10 with SG; Chemstrip uGK reagent strips *in vitro diagnostic aid for multiple urine products*

Chemstrip bG reagent strips for home use OTC *in vitro diagnostic aid for blood glucose*

Chemstrip K reagent strips for professional use *in vitro diagnostic aid for acetone (ketones) in the urine*

Chemstrip Micral reagent strips for professional use *in vitro diagnostic aid for albumin (protein) in the urine*

Chemstrip uG reagent strips for home use OTC *in vitro diagnostic aid for urine glucose*

chenic acid [now: chenodiol]

Chenix tablets ℞ *anticholelithogenic for radiolucent gallstones (orphan)* [chenodiol] 250 mg

chenodeoxycholic acid INN, BAN *anticholelithogenic* [also: chenodiol]

chenodiol USAN *anticholelithogenic for radiolucent gallstones (orphan)* [also: chenodeoxycholic acid]

Cheracol Cough syrup ℞ *narcotic antitussive; expectorant* [codeine phosphate; guaifenesin; alcohol 1.75%] 10•100 mg/5 mL

Cheracol D Cough liquid OTC *antitussive; expectorant* [dextromethorphan hydrobromide; guaifenesin; alcohol 4.75%] 10•100 mg/5 mL

Cheracol Nasal spray OTC *nasal decongestant* [oxymetazoline HCl] 0.05%

Cheracol Plus liquid OTC *antitussive; decongestant; antihistamine* [dextromethorphan hydrobromide; phenylpropanolamine HCl; chlorpheniramine maleate; alcohol 8%] 6.7•8.3•1.3 mg/5 mL

Cheracol Sinus sustained-action tablets (discontinued 1995) OTC *decongestant; antihistamine* [pseudoephedrine sulfate; dexbrompheniramine maleate] 120•6 mg

Cheracol Sore Throat spray OTC *topical antipruritic/counterirritant; mild local anesthetic* [phenol] 1.4%

cherry, black; choke cherry; rum cherry *medicinal herb* [see: wild black cherry]

cherry, black; poison black cherry *medicinal herb* [see: belladonna]

cherry birch *medicinal herb* [see: birch]

cherry juice NF

chervil (*Anthriscus cerefolium*) *flowering plant medicinal herb used as a digestive, diuretic, expectorant, and stimulant*

chervil, sweet *medicinal herb* [see: sweet cicely]

chestnut *medicinal herb* [see: horse chestnut]

Chewable C chewable tablets OTC *vitamin supplement* [sodium ascorbate & ascorbic acid] 100, 250, 300, 500 mg

Chewable Multivitamins with Fluoride tablets ℞ *pediatric vitamin supplement and dental caries preventative* [multiple vitamins; fluoride; folic acid] ±•1•0.3 mg

Chewable Triple Vitamins with Fluoride tablets ℞ *pediatric vitamin supplement and dental caries preventative* [vitamins A, C, and D; fluoride] 2500 IU•60 mg•400 IU•1 mg

Chew-Vites chewable tablets OTC *vitamin supplement* [multiple vitamins; folic acid]

ChexUP; Chex-Up; CHEX-UP (cyclophosphamide, hexamethylmelamine, fluorouracil, Platinol) *chemotherapy protocol*

CHF (cyclophosphamide, hexamethylmelamine, fluorouracil) *chemotherapy protocol*

Chibroxin Ocumeter (eye drops) ℞ *topical ophthalmic antibiotic* [norfloxacin] 3 mg/mL

chicken's toes *medicinal herb* [see: coral root]

chickweed *(Stellaria media)* plant *medicinal herb for appetite suppression, bleeding, blood cleansing, convulsions, obesity, skin rashes, and ulcers; also used as a homeopathic remedy for psoriasis and rheumatic pain*

chicory *(Chicorium intybus)* plant and root *medicinal herb for blood cleansing, cardiac disease, jaundice, liver disorders, promoting expectoration, and removal of calcium deposits*

Chiggerex ointment OTC *topical local anesthetic; analgesic; counterirritant* [benzocaine; camphor; menthol] ≟

Chigger-Tox liquid OTC *topical local anesthetic* [benzocaine] ≟

Chikusetsu ginseng *(Panax pseudoginseng)* *medicinal herb* [see: ginseng]

Children's Formula Cough syrup OTC *pediatric antitussive and expectorant* [dextromethorphan hydrobromide; guaifenesin] 5•50 mg/5 mL

chili pepper; chilies *medicinal herb* [see: cayenne]

chillifolinum [see: quillifoline]

Chimaphila umbellata *medicinal herb* [see: pipsissewa]

chimeric (murine variable, human constant) MAb (C2B8) to CD20 [now: rituximab]

chimeric A2 (human-murine) IgG monoclonal anti-TNF antibody (cA2) [see: infliximab]

chimeric M-T412 (human-murine) IgG monoclonal anti-CD4 *orphan* status withdrawn 1997 [now: priliximab]

ChimeriVax ℞ *investigational chimeric flavivirus vaccine*

chinchona *medicinal herb* [see: quinine]

Chinese cucumber *(Trichosanthes kirilowii)* gourd and root *medicinal herb for abscesses, amenorrhea, cough, diabetes, edema, fever, inducing abortion, invasive moles, jaundice, polyuria, and tumors*

Chinese gelatin [see: agar]

Chinese isinglass [see: chiniofon]

Chinese rhubarb *medicinal herb* [see: rhubarb]

chinethazone [see: quinethazone]

chiniofon NF, INN

Chionanthus virginica *medicinal herb* [see: fringe tree]

Chirocaine ℞ *investigational (NDA filed) long-acting local anesthetic* [levobupivacaine]

chitosamine [see: glucosamine]

chitosan *natural cellulose-like biopolymer extracted from marine animal exoskeletons and used as a treatment for hypercholesterolemia, hyperlipidemia, and obesity; also used topically as an antimicrobial and vulnerary*

chittem bark *medicinal herb* [see: buckthorn; cascara sagrada]

CHL + PRED (chlorambucil, prednisone) *chemotherapy protocol*

Chlamydiazyme reagent kit for professional use *in vitro diagnostic aid for Chlamydia trachomatis* [solid phase enzyme immunoassay]

Chlo-Amine chewable tablets OTC *antihistamine* [chlorpheniramine maleate] 2 mg

chlophedianol BAN *antitussive* [also: chlophedianol HCl; clofedanol]

chlophedianol HCl USAN *antitussive* [also: clofedanol; chlophedianol]

chlophenadione [see: clorindione]

chloquinate [see: cloquinate]

Chlor-100 injection (discontinued 1997) ℞ *antihistamine; anaphylaxis* [chlorpheniramine maleate] 100 mg/mL

chloracyzine INN
Chlorafed liquid OTC *decongestant; antihistamine* [pseudoephedrine HCl; chlorpheniramine maleate] 30•2 mg/5 mL
Chlorafed; Chlorafed HS Timecelles (sustained-release capsules) ℞ *decongestant; antihistamine* [pseudoephedrine HCl; chlorpheniramine maleate] 120•8 mg; 60•4 mg
chloral betaine USAN, NF, BAN *sedative* [also: cloral betaine]
chloral hydrate USP, BAN *hypnotic; sedative; also abused as a street drug* 500 mg oral; 250, 500 mg/5 mL oral
chloral hydrate betaine [see: chloral betaine]
chloralformamide USP
chloralodol INN [also: chlorhexadol]
chloralose (α-chloralose) INN
chloralurethane [see: carbocloral]
chlorambucil USP, INN, BAN *nitrogen mustard-type alkylating antineoplastic for multiple leukemias and lymphomas*
chloramidobenzol [see: clofenamide]
chloramine [now: chloramine-T]
chloramine-T NF [also: tosylchloramide sodium]
chloramiphene [see: clomiphene citrate]
chloramphenicol USP, INN, BAN, JAN *bacteriostatic antibiotic; antirickettsial* 250 mg oral; 5 mg/mL eye drops; 10 mg/g topical
chloramphenicol palmitate USP, JAN *antibacterial; antirickettsial* 150 mg/5 mL oral
chloramphenicol pantothenate complex USAN *antibacterial; antirickettsial* [also: cloramfenicol pantotenate complex]
chloramphenicol sodium succinate USP, JAN *antibacterial; antirickettsial* 100 mg/mL injection
chloranautine [see: dimenhydrinate]
chlorarsen [see: dichlorophenarsine HCl]
Chloraseptic mouthwash/gargle OTC *topical antipruritic/counterirritant; mild local anesthetic* [phenol] 1.4%

Chloraseptic, Children's lozenges OTC *topical oral anesthetic* [benzocaine] 5 mg
Chloraseptic, Children's throat spray OTC *topical antipruritic/counterirritant; mild local anesthetic* [phenol] 0.5%
Chloraseptic Sore Throat lozenges OTC *topical oral anesthetic; analgesic; counterirritant* [benzocaine; menthol] 6•10 mg
Chlorate tablets (discontinued 1997) OTC *antihistamine* [chlorpheniramine maleate] 4 mg
chlorazanil INN
chlorazanil HCl [see: chlorazanil]
chlorazodin INN [also: chloroazodin]
chlorazone [see: chloramine-T]
chlorbenzoxamine INN
chlorbenzoxamine HCl [see: chlorbenzoxamine]
chlorbetamide INN, BAN
chlorbutanol [see: chlorobutanol]
chlorbutin [see: chlorambucil]
chlorbutol BAN *antimicrobial agent* [also: chlorobutanol]
chlorcinnazine [see: clocinizine]
chlorcyclizine INN, BAN *topical antihistamine* [also: chlorcyclizine HCl]
chlorcyclizine HCl USP *topical antihistamine* [also: chlorcyclizine]
chlordantoin USAN, BAN *antifungal* [also: clodantoin]
chlordiazepoxide USP, INN, BAN, JAN *benzodiazepine anxiolytic; minor tranquilizer; alcohol withdrawal therapy*
chlordiazepoxide HCl USAN, USP, BAN, JAN *benzodiazepine anxiolytic; sedative; sometimes abused as a street drug* 5, 10, 25 mg oral
chlordiazepoxide HCl & clidinium bromide *anxiolytic; GI anticholinergic* 5•2.5 mg
chlordimorine INN
Chlordrine S.R. sustained-release capsules ℞ *decongestant; antihistamine* [pseudoephedrine HCl; chlorpheniramine maleate] 120•8 mg
Chloresium ointment, solution OTC *vulnerary and deodorant for wounds,*

burns, and ulcers [chlorophyllin copper complex] 0.5%; 0.2%

Chloresium tablets OTC *systemic deodorant for ostomy, breath, and body odors* [chlorophyllin copper complex] 14 mg

chlorethate [see: clorethate]

chlorethyl [see: ethyl chloride]

chlorfenisate [see: clofibrate]

chlorfenvinphos BAN [also: clofenvinfos]

Chlorgest-HD liquid (discontinued 1997) ℞ *narcotic antitussive; decongestant; antihistamine* [hydrocodone bitartrate; phenylephrine HCl; chlorpheniramine maleate] 1.67•5•4 mg/5 mL

chlorguanide HCl [see: chloroguanide HCl]

chlorhexadol BAN [also: chloralodol]

chlorhexidine INN, BAN *antimicrobial* [also: chlorhexidine gluconate]

chlorhexidine gluconate USAN *antimicrobial; investigational (orphan) for oral mucositis in bone marrow transplant patients* [also: chlorhexidine]

chlorhexidine HCl USAN, BAN *topical anti-infective*

chlorhexidine phosphanilate USAN *antibacterial*

chlorimiphenin [see: imiclopazine]

chlorimpiphenine [see: imiclopazine]

chlorinated & iodized peanut oil [see: chloriodized oil]

chlorindanol USAN *spermaticide* [also: clorindanol]

chlorine *element (Cl)*

chloriodized oil USP

chlorisondamine chloride INN, BAN

chlorisondamone chloride [see: chlorisondamine chloride]

chlormadinone INN, BAN *progestin* [also: chlormadinone acetate]

chlormadinone acetate USAN, NF *progestin* [also: chlormadinone]

chlormerodrin NF, INN, BAN

chlormerodrin (^{197}Hg) INN *renal function test; radioactive agent* [also: chlormerodrin Hg 197]

chlormerodrin Hg 197 USAN, USP *renal function test; radioactive agent* [also: chlormerodrin (^{197}Hg)]

chlormerodrin Hg 203 USAN, USP *renal function test; radioactive agent*

chlormeroprin [see: chlormerodrin]

chlormethazanone [see: chlormezanone]

chlormethiazole BAN [also: clomethiazole]

chlormethine INN *nitrogen mustard-type alkylating antineoplastic* [also: mechlorethamine HCl; mustine; nitrogen mustard N-oxide HCl]

chlormethylencycline [see: clomocycline]

chlormezanone INN, BAN *mild anxiolytic*

chlormidazole INN, BAN

chlornaphazine INN

chloroacetic acid [see: monochloroacetic, dichloroacetic, or trichloroacetic acid]

chloroazodin USP [also: chlorazodin]

5-chlorobenzoxazolinone [see: chlorzoxazone]

chlorobutanol NF, INN *antimicrobial agent; preservative* [also: chlorbutol]

chlorochine [see: chloroquine]

chlorocresol USAN, NF, INN *antiseptic; disinfectant*

2-chloro-2'-deoxyadenosine (CdA) [now: cladribine]

chlorodeoxylincomycin [see: clindamycin]

chloroethane [see: ethyl chloride]

chloroform NF *solvent*

chloroguanide HCl USP *antimalarial; dihydrofolate reductase inhibitor* [also: proguanil]

chloroguanide triazine pamoate [see: cycloguanil pamoate]

chloro-iodohydroxyquinoline [see: clioquinol]

chlorolincomycin [see: clindamycin]

chloromethapyrilene citrate [see: chlorothen citrate]

Chloromycetin Kapseals (capsules) (discontinued 1996) ℞ *broad-spectrum bacteriostatic antibiotic* [chloramphenicol] 250 mg

Chloromycetin powder for eye drops, ophthalmic ointment ℞ *topical ophthalmic antibiotic* [chloramphenicol] 25 mg/15 mL; 10 mg/g

Chloromycetin Hydrocortisone powder for eye drops ℞ *topical ophthalmic corticosteroidal anti-inflammatory; broad-spectrum antibiotic* [hydrocortisone acetate; chloramphenicol] 0.5%•0.25%

Chloromycetin Otic ear drops ℞ *broad-spectrum antibiotic* [chloramphenicol] 0.5%

Chloromycetin Sodium Succinate powder for IV injection ℞ *broad-spectrum bacteriostatic antibiotic* [chloramphenicol sodium succinate] 100 mg/mL

p-chlorophenol [see: parachlorophenol]

chlorophenothane NF [also: clofenotane; dicophane]

chlorophenoxamide [see: clefamide]

chlorophenylmercury [see: phenylmercuric chloride]

chlorophyll, water soluble [see: chlorophyllin]

chlorophyllin *vulnerary; oral deodorant for ostomy, breath, and body odors; topical deodorant for wounds and ulcers* 20 mg oral

chlorophyllin copper complex USAN *oral deodorant for ostomy, breath, and body odors; topical deodorant for wounds and ulcers*

chloroprednisone INN

chloroprednisone acetate [see: chloroprednisone]

chloroprocaine INN *local anesthetic* [also: chloroprocaine HCl]

chloroprocaine HCl USP *injectable local anesthetic* [also: chloroprocaine]

Chloroptic eye drops ℞ *topical ophthalmic antibiotic* [chloramphenicol] 5 mg/mL

Chloroptic S.O.P. ophthalmic ointment ℞ *topical ophthalmic antibiotic* [chloramphenicol] 10 mg/g

chloropyramine INN [also: halopyramine]

chloropyrilene INN, BAN [also: chlorothen citrate]

chloroquine USP, INN, BAN *amebicide; antimalarial*

chloroquine diphosphate [see: chloroquine phosphate]

chloroquine HCl USP *amebicide; antimalarial* [also: chloroquine]

chloroquine phosphate USP, BAN *amebicide; antimalarial; lupus erythematosus suppressant* 250 mg oral

chloroserpidine INN

Chloroserpine tablets (discontinued 1995) ℞ *antihypertensive* [chlorothiazide; reserpine] 250•0.125 mg

N-chlorosuccinimide [see: succinchlorimide]

chlorothen citrate NF [also: chloropyrilene]

chlorothenium citrate [see: chlorothen citrate]

chlorothenylpyramine [see: chlorothen]

chlorothiazide USP, INN, BAN *diuretic; antihypertensive* 250, 500 mg oral

chlorothiazide sodium USAN, USP *diuretic; antihypertensive*

chlorothymol NF

chlorotrianisene USP, INN, BAN *estrogen for hormone replacement therapy or inoperable prostatic cancer*

chloroxine USAN *antiseborrheic*

chloroxylenol USP, INN, BAN *bacteriostatic*

chlorozone [see: chloramine-T]

chlorpenthixol [see: clopenthixol]

Chlorphed-LA nasal spray OTC *nasal decongestant* [oxymetazoline HCl] 0.05%

Chlorphedrine SR sustained-release capsules ℞ *decongestant; antihistamine* [pseudoephedrine HCl; chlorpheniramine maleate] 120•8 mg

chlorphenamine INN *antihistamine* [also: chlorpheniramine maleate; chlorpheniramine]

chlorphenamine maleate [see: chlorpheniramine maleate]

chlorphenecyclane [see: clofenciclan]

chlorphenesin INN, BAN *skeletal muscle relaxant* [also: chlorphenesin carbamate]

chlorphenesin carbamate USAN, JAN *skeletal muscle relaxant* [also: chlorphenesin]

chlorphenindione [see: clorindione]

chlorpheniramine BAN *alkylamine antihistamine* [also: chlorpheniramine maleate; chlorphenamine] ☒ chlorphentermine

chlorpheniramine maleate USP *alkylamine antihistamine* [also: chlorphenamine; chlorpheniramine] 4 mg oral; 10 mg/mL injection

chlorpheniramine polistirex USAN *alkylamine antihistamine*

chlorpheniramine tannate, pyrilamine tannate, and phenylephrine tannate *alkylamine antihistamine; decongestant* 8•25•25 mg oral

chlorphenoctium amsonate INN, BAN

chlorphenotane [see: chlorophenothane]

chlorphenoxamine INN, BAN [also: chlorphenoxamine HCl]

chlorphenoxamine HCl USP [also: chlorphenoxamine]

chlorphentermine INN, BAN *anorectic* [also: chlorphentermine HCl] ☒ chlorpheniramine

chlorphentermine HCl USAN *anorectic* [also: chlorphentermine]

chlorphenylindandione [see: clorindione]

chlorphthalidone [see: chlorthalidone]

Chlor-Pro injection (discontinued 1997) ℞ *antihistamine* [chlorpheniramine maleate] 10, 100 mg/mL

chlorprocaine chloride [see: chloroprocaine HCl]

chlorproethazine INN [also: chlorproethazine HCl]

chlorproethazine HCl [also: chlorproethazine]

chlorproguanil INN, BAN

chlorproguanil HCl [see: chlorproguanil]

chlorpromazine USP, INN, BAN *phenothiazine antipsychotic; antiemetic; intractable hiccough relief*

chlorpromazine HCl USP, BAN, JAN *phenothiazine antipsychotic; antiemetic; intractable hiccough relief* 10, 25, 50, 100, 200 mg oral; 30, 100 mg/mL oral; 25 mg/mL injection

chlorpromazine hibenzate JAN *phenothiazine antipsychotic; antiemetic*

chlorpromazine phenolphthalinate JAN *phenothiazine antipsychotic; antiemetic*

chlorpromazine tannate USP, INN, BAN *phenothiazine antipsychotic; antiemetic*

chlorpropamide USP, INN, BAN, JAN *sulfonylurea antidiabetic* 100, 250 mg oral

chlorprophenpyridamine maleate [see: chlorpheniramine maleate]

chlorprothixene USAN, USP, INN, BAN *thioxanthene antipsychotic*

chlorprothixene HCl *thioxanthene antipsychotic*

chlorprothixene lactate *thioxanthene antipsychotic*

chlorpyrifos BAN

chlorquinaldol INN, BAN

Chlor-Rest tablets OTC *decongestant; antihistamine* [phenylpropanolamine HCl; chlorpheniramine maleate] 18.7•2 mg

Chlorspan-12 timed-release capsules (discontinued 1997) ℞ *antihistamine* [chlorpheniramine maleate] 12 mg

Chlortab-4 tablets (discontinued 1996) ℞ *antihistamine* [chlorpheniramine maleate] 4 mg

Chlortab-8 timed-release tablets (discontinued 1996) ℞ *antihistamine* [chlorpheniramine maleate] 8 mg

chlortalidone INN *antihypertensive; diuretic* [also: chlorthalidone]

chlortetracycline INN, BAN *antibacterial antibiotic; antiprotozoal* [also: chlortetracycline bisulfate]

chlortetracycline bisulfate USP *antibacterial; antiprotozoal* [also: chlortetracycline]

chlortetracycline calcium

chlortetracycline HCl USP, BAN *antibacterial antibiotic; antiprotozoal*

chlorthalidone USAN, USP, BAN *antihypertensive; diuretic* [also: chlortalidone] 25, 50, 100 mg oral

chlorthenoxazin BAN [also: chlorthenoxazine]

chlorthenoxazine INN [also: chlorthenoxazin]

chlorthiazide [see: chlorothiazide]

chlortrianisestrol [see: chlorotrianisene]

Chlor-Trimeton IV injection (discontinued 1997) ℞ *antihistamine for anaphylaxis* [chlorpheniramine maleate] 10 mg/mL

Chlor-Trimeton syrup (name changed to Chlor-Trimeton Allergy in 1997)

Chlor-Trimeton 4 Hour Relief tablets OTC *decongestant; antihistamine* [pseudoephedrine sulfate; chlorpheniramine maleate] 60•4 mg

Chlor-Trimeton 12 Hour Relief sustained-release tablets OTC *decongestant; antihistamine* [pseudoephedrine sulfate; chlorpheniramine maleate] 120•8 mg

Chlor-Trimeton Allergy 4 Hour syrup OTC *antihistamine* [chlorpheniramine maleate] 2 mg/5 mL

Chlor-Trimeton Allergy 4 Hour tablets OTC *antihistamine* [chlorpheniramine maleate] 4 mg

Chlor-Trimeton Allergy 8 Hour; Chlor-Trimeton Allergy 12 Hour timed-release tablets OTC *antihistamine* [chlorpheniramine maleate] 8 mg; 12 mg

Chlor-Trimeton Allergy-Sinus caplets OTC *decongestant; antihistamine; analgesic* [phenylpropanolamine HCl; chlorpheniramine maleate; acetaminophen] 12.5•2•500 mg

chlorzoxazone USP, INN, BAN, JAN *skeletal muscle relaxant* 250, 500 mg oral

chlosudimeprimylum [see: clopamide]

ChlVPP (chlorambucil, vinblastine, procarbazine, prednisone) *chemotherapy protocol*

ChlVPP/EVA (chlorambucil, vinblastine, procarbazine, prednisone, etoposide, vincristine, Adriamycin) *chemotherapy protocol*

CHO (cyclophosphamide, hydroxydaunomycin, Oncovin) *chemotherapy protocol*

CHO cells, recombinant [see: CD4, human truncated]

CHOB (cyclophosphamide, hydroxydaunomycin, Oncovin, bleomycin) *chemotherapy protocol*

CHOD (cyclophosphamide, hydroxydaunomycin, Oncovin, dexamethasone) *chemotherapy protocol*

choice dielytra *medicinal herb* [see: turkey corn]

Choice dm oral liquid OTC *enteral nutritional therapy for abnormal glucose tolerance* [lactose-free formula] 240 mL

choke cherry; black choke *medicinal herb* [see: wild black cherry]

Cholac syrup ℞ *prevent and treat portal-systemic encephalopathy* [lactulose] 10 g/15 mL

cholagogues *a class of agents that stimulate the flow of bile into the duodenum*

cholalic acid [see: dehydrocholic acid]

Cholan-HMB tablets (discontinued 1998) OTC *laxative; hydrocholeretic* [dehydrocholic acid] 250 mg

Cholebrine tablets (discontinued 1999) ℞ *radiopaque contrast medium for cholecystography* [iocetamic acid (62% iodine)] 750 mg

cholecalciferol USP, BAN, JAN *vitamin D_3; antirachitic* [also: colecalciferol] 1000 IU oral

Choledyl tablets, pediatric syrup, elixir (discontinued 1996) ℞ *antiasthmatic; bronchodilator* [oxtriphylline] 100, 200 mg; 50 mg/5 mL; 100 mg/5 mL

Choledyl SA sustained-action tablets ℞ *antiasthmatic; bronchodilator* [oxtriphylline] 400, 600 mg

cholera vaccine USP *active bacterin for cholera (Vibrio cholerae)* 16 U/mL injection

CholestaGel ℞ *investigational (Phase III) bile acid sequestrant used in combination with lovastatin to lower cholesterol levels* [colesevelam HCl]

cholesterin [see: cholesterol]

cholesterol NF *emulsifying agent*

cholestrin [see: cholesterol]

cholestyramine BAN *bile salts ion-exchange resin; antihyperlipoproteinemic* [also: cholestyramine resin; colestyramine]

cholestyramine resin USP *bile salts ion-exchange resin; antihyperlipidemic* [also: colestyramine; cholestyramine] 4 g powder for oral solution

cholic acid [see: dehydrocholic acid]

Cholidase tablets OTC *dietary lipotropic with vitamin supplementation* [choline; inositol; vitamins B$_6$, B$_{12}$, and E] 185•150•2.5•0.005•7.5 mg

choline *dietary lipotropic supplement* 250, 300, 500, 650 mg oral

choline alfoscerate INN

choline bitartrate NF 250 mg oral

choline bromide hexamethylenedicarbamate [see: hexacarbacholine bromide]

choline chloride INN *investigational (orphan) for choline deficiency of long-term parenteral nutrition*

choline chloride acetate [see: acetylcholine chloride]

choline chloride carbamate [see: carbachol]

choline chloride succinate [see: succinylcholine chloride]

choline dihydrogen citrate NF 650 mg oral

choline gluconate INN

choline glycerophosphate [see: choline alfoscerate]

choline magnesium trisalicylate (choline salicylate + magnesium salicylate) *nonsteroidal anti-inflammatory drug (NSAID)* [q.v.] 500, 750, 1000 mg (293•362, 440•544, 587•725 mg) oral

choline perchlorate, nitrate ester [see: nitricholine perchlorate]

choline salicylate USAN, INN, BAN *analgesic; antipyretic; anti-inflammatory; antirheumatic*

choline theophyllinate INN, BAN *bronchodilator* [also: oxtriphylline]

cholinergic agonists *a class of agents that produce effects similar to those of the parasympathetic nervous system* [also called: parasympathomimetics]

cholinesterase inhibitors *a class of drugs which increase acetylcholine neurotransmitters, used as a cognition adjuvant in Alzheimer's dementia* [also called: acetylcholinesterase (AChE) inhibitors]

Cholinoid capsules OTC *dietary lipotropic with vitamin supplementation* [choline; inositol; multiple B vitamins; vitamin C; lemon bioflavonoids] 111•111•≛•100•100 mg

Cholografin Meglumine injection ℞ *radiopaque contrast medium for cholecystography and cholangiography* [iodipamide meglumine (49.2% iodine)] 520 mg/mL (257 mg/mL)

Choloxin tablets (discontinued 1999) ℞ *antihyperlipidemic for hypercholesterolemia* [dextrothyroxine sodium] 2, 4 mg

chondodendron tomentosum [see: tubocurarine chloride]

chondrocyte-alginate *investigational (orphan) gel suspension for vesicoureteral reflux in children*

chondroitin 4-sulfate [see: danaparoid sodium]

chondroitin 6-sulfate [see: danaparoid sodium]

chondroitin sulfate *natural remedy for arthritis, blood clots, and extravasation from needle sticks after certain chemotherapy treatments*

chondroitin sulfate sodium JAN

chondroitin sulfuric acid *natural remedy* [see: chondroitin sulfate]

chondroitinase *investigational (orphan) for vitrectomy*

Chondrus crispus *medicinal herb* [see: Irish moss]

chonsurid *natural remedy* [see: chondroitin sulfate]

Chooz chewable tablets OTC *antacid* [calcium carbonate] 500 mg

CHOP (cyclophosphamide, hydroxydaunomycin, Oncovin, prednisone) *chemotherapy protocol*

CHOP-BLEO (cyclophosphamide, hydroxydaunomycin, Oncovin, prednisone, bleomycin) *chemotherapy protocol*

CHOPE (cyclophosphamide, hydroxydaunomycin, Oncovin, prednisone, etoposide) *chemotherapy protocol*

CHOR (cyclophosphamide, hydroxydaunomycin, Oncovin, radiation therapy) *chemotherapy protocol*

Chorex-5; Chorex-10 powder for IM injection ℞ *hormone for prepubertal cryptorchidism and hypogonadism; ovulation stimulant* [chorionic gonadotropin] 500 U/mL; 1000 U/mL

Chorigon powder for injection (discontinued 1995) ℞ *hormone for prepubertal cryptorchidism and hypogonadism; ovulation stimulant* [chorionic gonadotropin] 1000 U/mL

chorionic gonadotrophin [see: gonadotropin, chorionic]

chorionic gonadotropin (CG) [see: gonadotropin, chorionic]

Choron-10 powder for IM injection ℞ *hormone for prepubertal cryptorchidism and hypogonadism; ovulation stimulant* [chorionic gonadotropin] 1000 U/mL

CHP (chlorhexidine phosphanilate) [q.v.]

Christmas factor [see: factor IX complex]

Chromagen capsules ℞ *hematinic* [ferrous fumarate; cyanocobalamin; ascorbic acid; intrinsic factor concentrate] 66 mg•10 μg•250 mg•100 mg

Chromagen FA; Chromagen Forte capsules OTC *vitamin/iron supplement* [vitamins B₁₂ & C; iron; folic acid] 0.01•250•66•1 mg; 0.01•60•151•1 mg

Chroma-Pak IV injection ℞ *intravenous nutritional therapy* [chromic chloride hexahydrate] 20.5, 102.5 μg/mL

chromargyre [see: merbromin]

chromated albumin [see: albumin, chromated Cr 51 serum]

Chromelin Complexion Blender OTC *skin darkening agent for vitiligo and hypopigmented areas* [dihydroxyacetone] 5%

chromic acid, disodium salt [see: sodium chromate Cr 51]

chromic chloride USP *dietary chromium supplement* 4, 20 μg/mL injection

chromic chloride Cr 51 USAN *radioactive agent*

chromic chloride hexahydrate [see: chromic chloride]

chromic phosphate Cr 51 USAN *radioactive agent*

chromic phosphate P 32 USAN, USP *antineoplastic; radioactive agent*

chromium *element (Cr); trace mineral important in glucose metabolism*

Chromium Chloride IV injection ℞ *intravenous nutritional therapy* [chromic chloride hexahydrate] 4 μg/mL

chromium chloride [see: chromic chloride Cr 51]

chromium chloride hexahydrate [see: chromic chloride]

chromium picolinate *trace mineral important in glucose metabolism*

chromium polynicotinate *trace mineral important in glucose metabolism*

chromocarb INN

chromonar HCl USAN *coronary vasodilator* [also: carbocromen]

Chronosule (trademarked dosage form) *sustained-action capsule*

Chronotab (trademarked dosage form) *sustained-action tablet*

Chronovera ⓐ (U.S. product: Verelan PM) delayed-onset, extended-release tablets ℞ *antihypertensive; calcium channel blocker* [verapamil HCl] 180, 240 mg

Chronulac syrup ℞ *laxative* [lactulose] 10 g/15 mL

Chrysanthemum parthenium *medicinal herb* [see: feverfew]

Chrysanthemum vulgare *medicinal herb* [see: tansy]

chrysazin *(withdrawn from market by FDA)* [see: danthron]

CHVP (cyclophosphamide, hydroxydaunomycin, VM-26, prednisone) *chemotherapy protocol*

Chymex solution ℞ *diagnostic aid for pancreatic function* [bentiromide] 500 mg/7.5 mL

Chymodiactin powder for intradiscal injection ℞ *proteolytic enzyme for herniated nucleus pulposus* [chymopapain] 4 nKat

chymopapain USAN, INN, BAN *proteolytic enzyme for herniated lumbar discs*

chymotrypsin USP, INN, BAN *proteolytic enzyme; zonulolytic for intracapsular lens extraction*

C.I. acid orange 24 monosodium salt (color index) [see: resorcin brown]

C.I. basic violet 3 (color index) [see: gentian violet]

C.I. basic violet 14 monohydrochloride (color index) [see: fuchsin, basic]

C.I. direct blue 53 tetrasodium salt (color index) [see: Evans blue]

C.I. mordant yellow 5, disodium salt (color index) [see: olsalazine sodium]

CI-1012 *investigational (Phase I) antiviral for HIV*

CI-1020 *investigational (Phase I) antiviral for HIV*

ciadox INN

ciamexon INN, BAN

cianergoline INN

cianidanol INN

cianidol [see: cianidanol]

cianopramine INN

ciapilome INN

Ciba Vision Cleaner for Sensitive Eyes solution OTC *surfactant cleaning solution for soft contact lenses*

Ciba Vision Saline aerosol solution OTC *rinsing/storage solution for soft contact lenses* [sodium chloride (saline solution)]

Cibacalcin subcu or IM injection ℞ *calcium regulator for Paget's disease (osteitis deformans) (orphan)* [calcitonin (human)] 0.5 mg/vial

cibenzoline INN, BAN *antiarrhythmic* [also: cifenline]

cibenzoline succinate JAN *antiarrhythmic* [also: cifenline succinate]

cicaprost INN *prostacyclin analog*

cicarperone INN

cicely, sweet *medicinal herb* [see: sweet cicely]

Cichorium intybus *medicinal herb* [see: chicory]

ciclacillin INN, BAN *antibacterial* [also: cyclacillin]

ciclactate INN

ciclafrine INN *antihypotensive* [also: ciclafrine HCl]

ciclafrine HCl USAN *antihypotensive* [also: ciclafrine]

ciclazindol USAN, INN, BAN *antidepressant*

cicletanine USAN, INN, BAN *antihypertensive*

ciclindole INN *antidepressant* [also: cyclindole]

cicliomenol INN

ciclobendazole INN, BAN *anthelmintic* [also: cyclobendazole]

ciclofenazine INN *antipsychotic* [also: cyclophenazine HCl]

ciclofenazine HCl [see: cyclophenazine HCl]

cicloheximide INN *antipsoriatic* [also: cycloheximide]

ciclonicate INN

ciclonium bromide INN

ciclopirox USAN, INN, BAN *antifungal*

ciclopirox olamine USAN, USP, JAN *antifungal*

ciclopramine INN

cicloprofen USAN, INN, BAN *anti-inflammatory*

cicloprolol INN *antiadrenergic (β-receptor)* [also: cicloprolol HCl; cycloprolol]

cicloprolol HCl USAN *antiadrenergic (β-receptor)* [also: cicloprolol; cycloprolol]

ciclosidomine INN, BAN

ciclosporin INN *immunosuppressive*
[also: cyclosporine; cyclosporin]
ciclotate INN *combining name for radicals or groups*
ciclotizolam INN, BAN
ciclotropium bromide INN
cicloxilic acid INN
cicloxolone INN, BAN
cicortonide INN
cicrotoic acid INN
cideferron INN
Cidex; Cidex-7; Cidex Plus 28 solution OTC *broad-spectrum antimicrobial* [glutaral] 2%; 2%; 3.2%
cidofovir USAN, INN *antiviral for AIDS-related cytomegalovirus retinitis*
cidoxepin INN *antidepressant* [also: cidoxepin HCl]
cidoxepin HCl USAN *antidepressant* [also: cidoxepin]
cifenline USAN *antiarrhythmic* [also: cibenzoline]
cifenline succinate USAN *antiarrhythmic* [also: cibenzoline succinate]
cifostodine INN
ciglitazone USAN, INN *antidiabetic*
cignolin [see: anthralin]
ciheptolane INN
ciladopa INN, BAN *antiparkinsonian; dopaminergic agent* [also: ciladopa HCl]
ciladopa HCl USAN *antiparkinsonian; dopaminergic agent* [also: ciladopa]
cilansetron INN *investigational treatment for irritable bowel syndrome*
cilastatin INN, BAN *enzyme inhibitor* [also: cilastatin sodium]
cilastatin sodium USAN, JAN *enzyme inhibitor* [also: cilastatin]
cilazapril USAN, INN, BAN, JAN *antihypertensive; ACE inhibitor*
cilazaprilat INN, BAN
cilexetil USAN *combining name for radicals or groups*
ciliary neurotrophic factor *investigational (orphan) for amyotrophic lateral sclerosis*
ciliary neurotrophic factor, recombinant human *orphan status withdrawn 1997*

cilmostim USAN *hematopoietic; macrophage colony-stimulating factor*
cilobamine INN *antidepressant* [also: cilobamine mesylate]
cilobamine mesylate USAN *antidepressant* [also: cilobamine]
cilofungin USAN, INN *antifungal*
ciloprost [see: iloprost]
cilostamide INN
cilostazol USAN, INN *vasodilator; antithrombotic; phosphodiesterase (PDE) III platelet aggregation inhibitor for intermittent claudication*
Ciloxan Drop-Tainers (eye drops), ointment R *topical ophthalmic antibiotic* [ciprofloxacin HCl] 3.5 mg/mL; 0.3%
ciltoprazine INN
cilutazoline INN
cimaterol USAN, INN *repartitioning agent*
cimemoxin INN
cimepanol INN
cimetidine USAN, USP, INN, BAN, JAN *histamine H₂ antagonist for gastric ulcers* 200, 300, 400, 800 mg oral ② dimethicone
cimetidine HCl USAN *histamine H₂ antagonist for gastric ulcers* 300 mg/5 mL oral; 300 mg/2 mL injection
cimetropium bromide INN
Cimicifuga racemosa medicinal herb [see: black cohosh]
cimoxatone INN
cinalukast USAN, INN *antiasthmatic*
cinametic acid INN
cinamolol INN
cinanserin INN *serotonin inhibitor* [also: cinanserin HCl]
cinanserin HCl USAN *serotonin inhibitor* [also: cinanserin]
cinaproxen INN
cincaine chloride [see: dibucaine HCl]
cinchocaine INN, BAN *local anesthetic* [also: dibucaine]
cinchocaine HCl BAN *local anesthetic* [also: dibucaine HCl]
Cinchona succirubra; C. ledgeriana; C. calisaya medicinal herb [see: quinine]
cinchonidine sulfate NF
cinchonine sulfate NF
cinchophen NF, INN, BAN

cinecromen INN
cinepaxadil INN
cinepazet INN, BAN *antianginal* [also: cinepazet maleate]
cinepazet maleate USAN *antianginal* [also: cinepazet]
cinepazic acid INN
cinepazide INN, BAN
cinfenine INN
cinfenoac INN, BAN
cinflumide USAN, INN *muscle relaxant*
cingestol USAN, INN *progestin*
cinitapride INN
cinmetacin INN
cinnamaldehyde NF
cinnamaverine INN
cinnamedrine USAN, INN *smooth muscle relaxant*
cinnamedrine HCl *smooth muscle relaxant*
cinnamic aldehyde [now: cinnamaldehyde]
cinnamon NF
cinnamon oil NF
cinnamon (*Cinnamonum zeylanicum*) bark and oil *medicinal herb for diarrhea, dysmenorrhea, gastrointestinal upset, microbial and fungal infections, and gas pain; also used as an aromatic, astringent, and stimulant*
cinnamon wood *medicinal herb* [see: sassafras]
cinnarizine USAN, INN, BAN *antihistamine*
cinnarizine clofibrate INN
cinnofuradione INN
cinnofuron [see: cinnofuradione]
cinnopentazone INN *anti-inflammatory* [also: cintazone]
cinnopropazone [see: apazone]
Cinobac capsules ℞ *urinary antibacterial* [cinoxacin] 250, 500 mg
cinoctramide INN
cinodine HCl USAN *veterinary antibacterial*
cinolazepam INN
cinoquidox INN
cinoxacin USAN, USP, INN, BAN *urinary antibacterial*

cinoxate USAN, USP, INN *ultraviolet screen*
cinoxolone INN, BAN
cinoxopazide INN
cinperene USAN, INN *antipsychotic*
cinprazole INN
cinpropazide INN
cinquefoil (*Potentilla anserina; P. canadensis; P. reptans*) plant *medicinal herb used as an antispasmodic and astringent*
cinromide USAN, INN *anticonvulsant*
cintazone USAN *anti-inflammatory* [also: cinnopentazone]
cintramide INN *antipsychotic* [also: cintriamide]
cintriamide USAN *antipsychotic* [also: cintramide]
cinuperone INN
cioteronel USAN, INN *antiandrogen*
cipamfylline USAN *antiviral agent; tumor necrosis factor alpha inhibitor*
cipionate INN *combining name for radicals or groups* [also: cypionate]
ciprafamide INN
Cipralan ℞ *investigational antiarrhythmic* [cifenline succinate]
Cipramil (name changed to Celexa upon marketing release in 1998)
ciprazafone INN
ciprefadol INN *analgesic* [also: ciprefadol succinate]
ciprefadol succinate USAN *analgesic* [also: ciprefadol]
Cipro film-coated tablets, Cystitis Pack (6 tablets), oral suspension, IV infusion ℞ *broad-spectrum fluoroquinolone antibiotic* [ciprofloxacin] 100, 250, 500, 750 mg; 100 mg; 250, 500 mg/5 mL; 200, 400 mg ② Septa; Septra
Cipro HC Otic ear drop suspension ℞ *topical broad-spectrum fluoroquinolone antibiotic; corticosteroidal anti-inflammatory* [ciprofloxacin; hydrocortisone] 0.2%•1% (2•10 mg/mL)
ciprocinonide USAN, INN *adrenocortical steroid*
ciprofibrate USAN, INN, BAN *antihyperlipoproteinemic*

ciprofloxacin USAN, INN, BAN *broad-spectrum bactericidal antibiotic*
ciprofloxacin HCl USAN, USP, JAN *broad-spectrum bactericidal antibiotic*
cipropride INN
ciproquazone INN
ciproquinate INN *coccidiostat for poultry* [also: cyproquinate]
ciprostene INN *platelet antiaggregatory agent* [also: ciprostene calcium]
ciprostene calcium USAN *platelet antiaggregatory agent* [also: ciprostene]
ciproximide INN *antipsychotic; antidepressant* [also: cyproximide]
ciramadol USAN, INN *analgesic*
ciramadol HCl USAN *analgesic*
cirazoline INN
Circavite-T tablets OTC *vitamin/mineral/iron supplement* [multiple vitamins & minerals; iron] ± • 12 mg
cirolemycin USAN, INN *antineoplastic; antibacterial*
cisapride USAN, INN, BAN, JAN *peristaltic stimulant; treatment for nocturnal heartburn due to gastroesophageal reflux disease*
cisatracurium besylate USAN *nondepolarizing neuromuscular blocker*
CISCA; CisCA (cisplatin, cyclophosphamide, Adriamycin) *chemotherapy protocol*
CISCA_{II}/VB_{IV} (cisplatin, cyclophosphamide, Adriamycin, vinblastine, bleomycin) *chemotherapy protocol*
cisclomiphene [now: enclomiphene]
cisconazole USAN, INN *antifungal*
cis-DDP (diamminedichloroplatinum) [see: cisplatin]
cis-diamminedichloroplatinum (DDP) [see: cisplatin]
cismadinone INN
cisplatin USAN, USP, INN, BAN *alkylating antineoplastic for testicular, ovarian, and bladder cancer*
cisplatin & epinephrine *investigational (Phase II) injectable gel for inoperable primary liver cancer*
cis-platinum [now: cisplatin]
cis-platinum II [now: cisplatin]

9-cis-retinoic acid [see: alitretinoin]
13-cis-retinoic acid [see: isotretinoin]
cistinexine INN
citalopram INN, BAN *selective serotonin reuptake inhibitor (SSRI) for depression*
citalopram hydrobromide *selective serotonin reuptake inhibitor (SSRI) for depression; investigational for Alzheimer's disease*
Citanest Forte injection ℞ *injectable local anesthetic for dental procedures* [prilocaine HCl; epinephrine] 4% • 1:200 000
Citanest Plain injection ℞ *injectable local anesthetic for dental procedures* [prilocaine HCl] 4%
citatepine INN
citenamide USAN, INN *anticonvulsant*
citenazone INN
citicoline INN, JAN *investigational (Phase III) oral treatment for ischemic stroke and head trauma* [also: citicoline sodium]
citicoline & dizocilpine maleate *investigational (Phase III) neuroprotective treatment for stroke*
citicoline sodium USAN *investigational (Phase III) oral treatment for ischemic stroke and head trauma* [also: citicoline]
citiolone INN, DCF
Citra pH oral solution OTC *antacid* [sodium citrate] 450 mg/5 mL
Citracal tablets OTC *calcium supplement* [calcium citrate] 900 mg ⍰ Citrucel
Citracal Caplets + D OTC *dietary supplement* [calcium citrate; vitamin D] 315 mg•200 IU ⍰ Citrucel
Citracal Liquitab effervescent tablets OTC *calcium supplement* [calcium citrate] 23.76 mg ⍰ Citrucel
Citralax effervescent granules OTC *laxative* [magnesium citrate; magnesium sulfate]
citrate dextrose [see: ACD solution]
citrate of magnesia [see: magnesium citrate]
citrate phosphate dextrose [see: anticoagulant citrate phosphate dextrose solution]

citrate phosphate dextrose adenine [see: anticoagulant citrate phosphate dextrose adenine solution]

citrated caffeine [see: caffeine, citrated]

citric acid USP *pH adjusting agent*

citric acid, glucono-delta-lactone & magnesium carbonate *irrigant for renal and bladder apatite or struvite calculi (orphan)*

citric acid, magnesium oxide & sodium carbonate [see: Suby solution G]

citrin [see: bioflavonoids]

Citrocarbonate effervescent granules OTC *antacid* [sodium bicarbonate; sodium citrate] 780•1820 mg/dose

Citro-Flav 200 capsules OTC *dietary supplement* [citrus bioflavonoids complex] 200 mg

Citrolith tablets ℞ *urinary alkalinizing agent* [potassium citrate; sodium citrate] 50•950 mg

citronella (Cymbopogon nardus; C. winterianus) oil *medicinal herb for gastrointestinal spasms, promoting diuresis, and worms; also used as an antibacterial; not generally regarded as safe and effective for internal use as it is highly toxic*

Citrotein powder, liquid OTC *enteral nutritional therapy* [lactose-free formula]

citrovorum factor [see: leucovorin calcium]

Citrucel powder OTC *bulk laxative* [methylcellulose] 2 g/tbsp. ⊠ Citracal

Citrucel Sugar Free powder OTC *bulk laxative* [methylcellulose; phenylalanine] 2 g•52 mg per tbsp. ⊠ Citracal

Citrus bergamia; C. aurantium medicinal herb [see: bergamot oil]

citrus bioflavonoids [see: bioflavonoids]

Citrus limon medicinal herb [see: lemon]

Citrus paradisi medicinal herb [see: grapefruit]

Citrus-flav C 500 tablets OTC *dietary supplement* [vitamin C; citrus & acerola bioflavonoids; hesperidin; rutin] 200•250•40•10 mg

CIVPP (chlorambucil, vinblastine, procarbazine, prednisone) *chemotherapy protocol*

cladribine *antimetabolite antineoplastic for hairy-cell leukemia (orphan); investigational (orphan) for chronic lymphocytic leukemia, multiple sclerosis, and non-Hodgkin's lymphoma*

Claforan powder or frozen premix for IV or IM injection ℞ *cephalosporin antibiotic* [cefotaxime sodium] 0.5, 1, 2, 10 g

clamidoxic acid INN, BAN

clamoxyquin BAN *antiamebic* [also: clamoxyquin HCl; clamoxyquine]

clamoxyquin HCl USAN *antiamebic* [also: clamoxyquine; clamoxyquin]

clamoxyquine INN *antiamebic* [also: clamoxyquin HCl; clamoxyquin]

clanfenur INN

clanobutin INN

clantifen INN

clara cell 10kDa protein *investigational (orphan) prevention of bronchopulmonary dysplasia in neonates with respiratory distress syndrome* ⊠ Clearasil

claretin-12 [see: cyanocobalamin] ⊠ Claritin; Clarityne

clarithromycin USAN, INN, BAN, JAN *macrolide antibiotic*

Claritin tablets, RediTabs (rapidly disintegrating tablets), syrup ℞ *nonsedating antihistamine; treatment for chronic urticaria* [loratadine] 10 mg; 10 mg; 1 mg/mL ⊠ claretin; Clarityne

Claritin-D; Claritin-D 12 Hour; Claritin-D 24 Hour extended-release film-coated tablets ℞ *decongestant; nonsedating antihistamine* [pseudoephedrine sulfate; loratadine] 120•5 mg; 120•5 mg; 240•10 mg

Clarityne (Mexican name for U.S. product Claritin) ⊠ claretin; Claritin

Claviceps purpurea medicinal herb [see: ergot]

clavulanate potassium USAN, USP *β-lactamase inhibitor; penicillin synergist*

clavulanic acid INN, BAN *β-lactamase inhibitor; penicillin synergist*

claw, scaly dragon's; turkey claw *medicinal herb* [see: coral root]

clay, kaolin *natural material* [see: kaolin]

clazolam USAN, INN *minor tranquilizer*

clazolimine USAN, INN *diuretic*

clazuril USAN, INN, BAN *coccidiostat for pigeons*

Clean-N-Soak solution OTC *cleaning/ soaking solution for hard contact lenses*

Clear By Design gel OTC *topical keratolytic for acne* [benzoyl peroxide] 2.5%

Clear Eyes eye drops OTC *topical ophthalmic decongestant and vasoconstrictor* [naphazoline HCl] 0.012%

Clear Eyes ACR eye drops OTC *topical ophthalmic decongestant and astringent* [naphazoline HCl; zinc sulfate] 0.012%•0.25%

Clear Total Lice Elimination System kit (shampoo + egg remover enzymes + nit comb) OTC *pediculicide for lice* [pyrethrins; piperonyl butoxide] 0.3%•3%

Clear Tussin 30 liquid OTC *antitussive; expectorant* [dextromethorphan hydrobromide; guaifenesin] 15•100 mg/5 mL

Clearasil cream, lotion OTC *topical keratolytic for acne* [benzoyl peroxide] 10% ☑ clara cell

Clearasil Acne-Fighting Pads OTC *topical keratolytic for acne* [salicylic acid; alcohol ≟%] 2%

Clearasil Adult Care cream OTC *topical acne treatment* [sulfur; resorcinol; alcohol 10%]

Clearasil Antibacterial Soap bar OTC *medicated cleanser for acne* [triclosan]

Clearasil Clearstick liquid OTC *topical keratolytic for acne* [salicylic acid; alcohol 39%] 1.25%, 2%

Clearasil Daily Face Wash liquid OTC *medicated cleanser for acne* [triclosan] 0.3%

Clearasil Double Clear; Clearasil Double Textured medicated pads OTC *topical keratolytic for acne* [salicylic acid; alcohol 40%] 1.25%, 2%; 2%

Clearasil Medicated Deep Cleanser liquid OTC *topical keratolytic cleanser for acne* [salicylic acid; alcohol 42%] 0.5%

Clearblue test kit for home use (discontinued 1995) OTC *in vitro diagnostic aid for urine pregnancy test*

Clearblue Easy test stick for home use OTC *in vitro diagnostic aid for urine pregnancy test*

Clearly Cala-gel OTC *topical antihistamine* [diphenhydramine HCl] ≟

Clearplan Easy test kit for home use OTC *in vitro diagnostic aid to predict ovulation time*

Clearview Chlamydia test for professional use *in vitro diagnostic aid for Chlamydia trachomatis* [color-label immunoassay]

Clearview hCG test kit for professional use (discontinued 1996) *in vitro diagnostic aid for urine pregnancy test*

cleavers; cleaverwort *medicinal herb* [see: bedstraw]

clebopride USAN, INN *antiemetic*

clefamide INN, BAN

clemastine USAN, BAN *ethanolamine antihistamine*

clemastine fumarate USAN, USP, BAN *ethanolamine antihistamine* 1.34, 2.68 mg oral; 0.5 mg/5 mL

Clematis cirrhosa; C. virginiana *medicinal herb* [see: woodbine]

clemeprol INN, BAN

clemizole INN, BAN

clemizole penicillin INN, BAN

clenbuterol INN, BAN

clenoliximab *investigational (Phase I/II) anti-CD4 antibody for the treatment of rheumatoid arthritis*

clenpirin INN [also: clenpyrin]

clenpyrin BAN [also: clenpirin]

Clens solution (discontinued 1995) OTC *cleaning solution for hard contact lenses*

clentiazem INN *calcium channel antagonist* [also: clentiazem maleate]

clentiazem maleate USAN *calcium channel antagonist* [also: clentiazem]

Cleocin capsules ℞ *lincosamide antibiotic; investigational (orphan) for AIDS-related Pneumocystis carinii* *pneumonia* [clindamycin HCl] 75, 150, 300 mg ⧉ bleomycin; Lincocin

Cleocin vaginal cream ℞ *lincosamide antibiotic for bacterial vaginosis* [clindamycin phosphate] 2%

Cleocin Pediatric granules for oral solution ℞ *lincosamide antibiotic* [clindamycin palmitate HCl] 75 mg/5 mL

Cleocin Phosphate IV infusion, IM injection ℞ *lincosamide antibiotic; investigational (orphan) for AIDS-related Pneumocystis carinii pneumonia* [clindamycin phosphate] 150 mg/mL

Cleocin T gel, topical solution, lotion, pads ℞ *topical antibiotic for acne* [clindamycin phosphate] 10 mg/mL

Clerz 2 solution OTC *rewetting solution for hard or soft contact lenses*

cletoquine INN, BAN

Clexane (European name for U.S. product Lovenox)

clibucaine INN

clidafidine INN

clidanac INN

clidinium bromide USAN, USP, INN, BAN *GI anticholinergic; peptic ulcer adjunct*

clidinium bromide & chlordiazepoxide HCl *GI anticholinergic; anxiolytic* 2.5•5 mg

Climara transdermal patch ℞ *estrogen replacement therapy for postmenopausal disorders* [estradiol] 25, 50, 75, 100 µg/day

climazolam INN

climbazole INN, BAN

climiqualine INN

clinafloxacin HCl USAN *quinolone antibacterial*

Clinda-Derm topical solution ℞ *topical antibiotic for acne* [clindamycin phosphate] 10 mg/mL

clindamycin USAN, INN, BAN *lincosamide antibiotic; investigational (orphan) for AIDS-related Pneumocystis carinii pneumonia*

clindamycin HCl USP, BAN *lincosamide antibiotic* 75, 150 mg oral

clindamycin HCl & primaquine phosphate *investigational (orphan)*

for AIDS-associated Pneumocystis carinii pneumonia

clindamycin palmitate HCl USAN, USP *lincosamide antibiotic*

clindamycin phosphate USAN, USP *lincosamide antibiotic* 10 mg/mL topical; 150 mg/mL injection

Clindets pledgets ℞ *topical antibiotic for acne* [clindamycin] 1% (10 mg/mL)

Clindex capsules (discontinued 1998) ℞ *GI anticholinergic; anxiolytic* [clidinium bromide; chlordiazepoxide HCl] 2.5•5 mg

Clinipak (trademarked packaging form) *unit dose package*

Clinistix reagent strips for home use OTC *in vitro diagnostic aid for urine glucose*

Clinitest reagent tablets for home use OTC *in vitro diagnostic aid for urine glucose*

clinocaine HCl [see: procaine HCl]

clinofibrate INN

clinolamide INN

Clinoril tablets ℞ *nonsteroidal anti-inflammatory drug (NSAID); antiarthritic; analgesic* [sulindac] 150, 200 mg

Clinoxide capsules (discontinued 1995) ℞ *GI anticholinergic; anxiolytic* [clidinium bromide; chlordiazepoxide HCl] 2.5•5 mg ⧉ clioxanide; Clipoxide

clioquinol USP, INN, BAN *topical antibacterial; antifungal*

clioxanide USAN, INN, BAN *anthelmintic* ⧉ Clinoxide

clipoxamine [see: cliropamine]

Clipoxide capsules (discontinued 1995) ℞ *GI anticholinergic; anxiolytic* [clidinium bromide; chlordiazepoxide HCl] 2.5•5 mg ⧉ Clinoxide

cliprofen USAN, INN *anti-inflammatory*

cliropamine INN

clobamine mesylate [now: cilobamine mesylate]

clobazam USAN, INN, BAN *minor benzodiazepine tranquilizer; anxiolytic*

clobedolum [see: clonitazene]

clobenoside INN

clobenzepam INN

clobenzorex INN

clobenztropine INN

clobetasol INN, BAN *topical corticosteroidal anti-inflammatory* [also: clobetasol propionate]

clobetasol propionate USAN *topical corticosteroidal anti-inflammatory* [also: clobetasol] 0.05% topical

clobetasone INN, BAN *topical corticosteroidal anti-inflammatory* [also: clobetasone butyrate]

clobetasone butyrate USAN *topical corticosteroidal anti-inflammatory* [also: clobetasone]

clobutinol INN

clobuzarit INN, BAN

clocanfamide INN

clocapramine INN

clociguanil INN, BAN

clocinizine INN

clocortolone INN *topical corticosteroid* [also: clocortolone acetate]

clocortolone acetate USAN *topical corticosteroid* [also: clocortolone]

clocortolone pivalate USAN, USP *topical corticosteroid*

clocoumarol INN

Clocream cream OTC *moisturizer; emollient* [cod liver oil (vitamins A and E); cholecalciferol; vitamin A palmitate]

clodacaine INN

clodanolene USAN, INN *skeletal muscle relaxant*

clodantoin INN *antifungal* [also: chlordantoin]

clodazon INN *antidepressant* [also: clodazon HCl]

clodazon HCl USAN *antidepressant* [also: clodazon]

Cloderm cream ℞ *topical corticosteroidal anti-inflammatory* [clocortolone pivalate] 0.1%

clodoxopone INN

clodronate disodium *bisphosphonate bone resorption inhibitor for hypercalcemia of malignancy* [also: disodium clodronate]

clodronic acid USAN, INN, BAN *calcium regulator*

clofazimine USAN, INN, BAN *bactericidal; tuberculostatic; leprostatic (orphan)*

clofedanol INN *antitussive* [also: chlophedianol HCl; chlophedianol]

clofedanol HCl [see: chlophedianol HCl]

clofenamic acid INN

clofenamide INN

clofenciclan INN

clofenetamine INN

clofenetamine HCl [see: clofenetamine]

clofenotane INN [also: chlorophenothane; dicophane]

clofenoxyde INN

clofenpyride [see: nicofibrate]

clofenvinfos INN [also: chlorfenvinphos]

clofeverine INN

clofexamide INN

clofezone INN

clofibrate USAN, USP, INN, BAN *antihyperlipidemic*

clofibric acid INN

clofibride INN

clofilium phosphate USAN, INN *antiarrhythmic*

clofinol [see: nicofibrate]

cloflucarban USAN *disinfectant* [also: halocarban]

clofluperol INN, BAN *antipsychotic* [also: seperidol HCl]

clofluperol HCl [see: seperidol HCl]

clofoctol INN

cloforex INN

clofurac INN

clogestone INN, BAN *progestin* [also: clogestone acetate]

clogestone acetate USAN *progestin* [also: clogestone]

cloguanamil INN, BAN [also: cloguanamile]

cloguanamile BAN [also: cloguanamil]

clomacran INN, BAN *antipsychotic* [also: clomacran phosphate]

clomacran phosphate USAN *antipsychotic* [also: clomacran]

clomegestone INN *progestin* [also: clomegestone acetate]

clomegestone acetate USAN *progestin* [also: clomegestone]

clometacin INN

clometerone INN *antiestrogen* [also: clometherone]

clometherone USAN *antiestrogen* [also: clometerone]

clomethiazole INN [also: chlormethiazole]

clometocillin INN

Clomid tablets ℞ *ovulation stimulant* [clomiphene citrate] 50 mg

clomide [see: aklomide]

clomifene INN *gonad-stimulating principle; ovulation stimulant* [also: clomiphene citrate; clomiphene]

clomifenoxide INN

clominorex USAN, INN *anorectic*

clomiphene BAN *gonad-stimulating principle; ovulation stimulant* [also: clomiphene citrate; clomifene] ② clonidine

clomiphene citrate USAN, USP *gonad-stimulating principle; ovulation stimulant* [also: clomifene; clomiphene] 50 mg oral

clomipramine INN, BAN *tricyclic antidepressant for obsessive-compulsive disorders* [also: clomipramine HCl]

clomipramine HCl USAN *tricyclic antidepressant for obsessive-compulsive disorders* [also: clomipramine] 25, 50, 75 mg oral

clomocycline INN, BAN

clomoxir INN

Clomycin ointment OTC *topical antibiotic; anesthetic* [polymyxin B sulfate; bacitracin; neomycin sulfate; lidocaine] 5000 U•500 U•3.5 mg•40 mg per g

clonazepam USAN, USP, INN, BAN *anticonvulsant; investigational (orphan) for hyperexplexia (startle disease)* 0.5, 1, 2 mg oral

clonazoline INN

clonidine USAN, INN, BAN *centrally acting antiadrenergic antihypertensive; adjunct to epidural opioid analgesics for severe cancer pain (orphan)* ② clomiphene; Klonopin; quinidine

clonidine HCl USAN, USP, BAN *centrally acting antiadrenergic antihypertensive; adjunct to epidural opioid analgesics for severe cancer pain (orphan)* 0.1, 0.2, 0.3 mg oral

clonitazene INN, BAN

clonitrate USAN, INN *coronary vasodilator*

clonixeril USAN, INN *analgesic*

clonixin USAN, INN *analgesic*

clopamide USAN, INN, BAN *antihypertensive; diuretic*

clopenthixol USAN, INN, BAN *antipsychotic*

cloperastine INN

cloperidone INN *sedative* [also: cloperidone HCl]

cloperidone HCl USAN *sedative* [also: cloperidone]

clophenoxate [see: meclofenoxate]

clopidogrel INN, BAN *platelet aggregation inhibitor for stroke, myocardial infarction, and peripheral artery disease*

clopidogrel bisulfate USAN *platelet aggregation inhibitor for stroke, myocardial infarction, and peripheral artery disease*

clopidol USAN, INN, BAN *coccidiostat for poultry*

clopimozide USAN, INN *antipsychotic*

clopipazan INN *antipsychotic* [also: clopipazan mesylate]

clopipazan mesylate USAN *antipsychotic* [also: clopipazan]

clopirac USAN, INN, BAN *anti-inflammatory*

cloponone INN, BAN

clopoxide [see: chlordiazepoxide]

clopoxide chloride [see: chlordiazepoxide HCl]

Clopra tablets ℞ *antidopaminergic; antiemetic for chemotherapy; peristaltic* [metoclopramide HCl] 10 mg

cloprednol USAN, INN, BAN *corticosteroid; anti-inflammatory*

cloprostenol INN, BAN *prostaglandin* [also: cloprostenol sodium]

cloprostenol sodium USAN *prostaglandin* [also: cloprostenol]

cloprothiazole INN

cloquinate INN, BAN

cloquinozine INN

cloracetadol INN

cloral betaine INN *sedative* [also: chloral betaine]

cloramfenicol pantotenate complex INN *antibacterial; antirickettsial* [also: chloramphenicol pantothenate complex]

cloranolol INN

clorarsen [see: dichlorophenarsine HCl]

clorazepate dipotassium USAN, USP *benzodiazepine anxiolytic; minor tranquilizer; anticonvulsant adjunct; alcohol withdrawal aid* [also: dipotassium clorazepate] 3.75, 7.5, 15 mg oral

clorazepate monopotassium USAN *minor tranquilizer*

clorazepic acid BAN

cloretate INN *sedative; hypnotic* [also: clorethate]

clorethate USAN *sedative; hypnotic* [also: cloretate]

clorexolone USAN, INN, BAN *diuretic*

clorgiline INN [also: clorgyline]

clorgyline BAN [also: clorgiline]

cloricromen INN

cloridarol INN

clorindanic acid INN

clorindanol INN *spermaticide* [also: chlorindanol]

clorindione INN, BAN

clormecaine INN

clorofene INN *disinfectant* [also: clorophene]

cloroperone INN *antipsychotic* [also: cloroperone HCl]

cloroperone HCl USAN *antipsychotic* [also: cloroperone]

clorophene USAN *disinfectant* [also: clorofene]

cloroqualone INN

clorotepine INN

Clorpactin WCS-90 powder for solution OTC *topical antimicrobial* [oxychlorosene sodium] 2 g

clorprenaline INN, BAN *adrenergic; bronchodilator* [also: clorprenaline HCl]

clorprenaline HCl USAN *adrenergic; bronchodilator* [also: clorprenaline]

clorquinaldol [see: chlorquinaldol]

clorsulon USAN, INN *antiparasitic; fasciolicide*

clortermine INN *anorectic* [also: clortermine HCl]

clortermine HCl USAN *anorectic* [also: clortermine]

closantel USAN, INN, BAN *anthelmintic*

closilate INN *combining name for radicals or groups* [also: closylate]

closiramine INN *antihistamine* [also: closiramine aceturate]

closiramine aceturate USAN *antihistamine* [also: closiramine]

clostebol INN [also: clostebol acetate]

clostebol acetate BAN [also: clostebol]

clostridial collagenase *investigational (Phase II, orphan) for advanced Dupuytren's disease*

Clostridium botulinum toxin [see: botulinum toxin]

closylate USAN, BAN *combining name for radicals or groups* [also: closilate]

clotbur *medicinal herb* [see: burdock]

clothiapine USAN, BAN *antipsychotic* [also: clotiapine]

clothixamide maleate USAN *antipsychotic* [also: clotixamide]

clotiapine INN *antipsychotic* [also: clothiapine]

clotiazepam INN

cloticasone INN, BAN *anti-inflammatory* [also: cloticasone propionate]

cloticasone propionate USAN *anti-inflammatory* [also: cloticasone]

clotioxone INN

clotixamide INN *antipsychotic* [also: clothixamide maleate]

clotixamide maleate [see: clothixamide maleate]

clotrimazole (CLT) USAN, USP, INN, BAN, JAN *broad-spectrum antifungal* 1% topical; 100 mg vaginal ② co-trimoxazole

clotrimidazole *investigational (orphan) for sickle cell disease*

cloudberry *medicinal herb* [see: blackberry]

clove oil NF

clover, king's; sweet clover *medicinal herb* [see: melilot]

clover, marsh *medicinal herb* [see: buckbean]

clover, purple; wild clover *medicinal herb* [see: red clover]

clover, winter *medicinal herb* [see: squaw vine]

cloves (*Caryophyllus aromaticus; Eugenia caryophyllata; Syzygium aromaticum*) seed and oil *medicinal herb for bad breath, bronchial secretions, dizziness, earache, fever, nausea, platelet aggregation inhibition, poor circulation, and thrombosis; also used topically as an analgesic and antiseptic*

clovoxamine INN

cloxacepride INN

cloxacillin INN, BAN *penicillinase-resistant penicillin antibiotic* [also: cloxacillin benzathine]

cloxacillin benzathine USP *penicillinase-resistant penicillin antibiotic* [also: cloxacillin]

cloxacillin sodium USAN, USP *penicillinase-resistant penicillin antibiotic* 250, 500 mg oral; 125 mg/5 mL oral

Cloxapen capsules R *penicillinase-resistant penicillin antibiotic* [cloxacillin sodium] 250, 500 mg

cloxazolam INN

cloxestradiol INN

cloxifenol [see: triclosan]

cloximate INN

cloxiquine INN *antibacterial* [also: cloxyquin]

cloxotestosterone INN

cloxphendyl [see: cloxypendyl]

cloxypendyl INN

cloxyquin USAN *antibacterial* [also: cloxiquine]

clozapine USAN, INN, BAN *dibenzodiazepine antipsychotic for severe schizophrenia; sedative* 25, 100 mg oral

Clozaril tablets R *novel (atypical) antipsychotic for severe schizophrenia* [clozapine] 25, 100 mg

CLT (clotrimazole) [q.v.]

club, shepherd's *medicinal herb* [see: mullein]

club moss (*Lycopodium clavatum*) spores *medicinal herb used as a hemostatic and vulnerary*

cluster, wax *medicinal herb* [see: wintergreen]

Clysodrast powder for oral solution R *pre-procedure bowel evacuant* [bisacodyl tannex] 2.5 g/packet

C-Max gradual-release tablets OTC *vitamin/mineral supplement* [multiple minerals; vitamin C] ± •1 g

CMC (carboxymethylcellulose) gum [see: carboxymethylcellulose sodium]

CMC (cyclophosphamide, methotrexate, CCNU) *chemotherapy protocol*

CMC-VAP (cyclophosphamide, methotrexate, CCNU, vincristine, Adriamycin, procarbazine) *chemotherapy protocol*

CMF (cyclophosphamide, methotrexate, fluorouracil) *chemotherapy protocol*

CMF/AV (cyclophosphamide, methotrexate, fluorouracil, Adriamycin, Oncovin) *chemotherapy protocol*

CMFAVP (cyclophosphamide, methotrexate, fluorouracil, Adriamycin, vincristine, prednisone) *chemotherapy protocol*

CMFP; CMF-P (cyclophosphamide, methotrexate, fluorouracil, prednisone) *chemotherapy protocol*

CMFPT (cyclophosphamide, methotrexate, fluorouracil, prednisone, tamoxifen) *chemotherapy protocol*

CMFPTH (cyclophosphamide, methotrexate, fluorouracil, prednisone, tamoxifen, Halotestin) *chemotherapy protocol*

CMFT (cyclophosphamide, methotrexate, fluorouracil, tamoxifen) *chemotherapy protocol*

CMFVAT (cyclophosphamide, methotrexate, fluorouracil, vincristine, Adriamycin, testosterone) *chemotherapy protocol*

CMFVP (cyclophosphamide, methotrexate, fluorouracil, vincris-

tine, prednisone) *chemotherapy protocol* [two dosing protocols: Cooper's protocol and SWOG protocol]

CMH (cyclophosphamide, *m*-AMSA, hydroxyurea) *chemotherapy protocol*

C-MOPP (cyclophosphamide, mechlorethamine, Oncovin, procarbazine, prednisone) *chemotherapy protocol*

CMV (cisplatin, methotrexate, vinblastine) *chemotherapy protocol*

CMV-IGIV (cytomegalovirus immune globulin intravenous) [see: globulin, immune]

CN2 HCl [see: mechlorethamine HCl]

CNF (cyclophosphamide, Novantrone, fluorouracil) *chemotherapy protocol* [also: CFM; FNC]

Cnicus benedictus medicinal herb [see: blessed thistle]

CNOP (cyclophosphamide, Novantrone, Oncovin, prednisone) *chemotherapy protocol*

CNS-5161 *investigational (Phase I) for neuropathic pain and migraine*

Co I (coenzyme I) [see: nadide]

Co Tinic IM injection ℞ antianemic [ferrous gluconate; multiple B vitamins; procaine]

CO$_2$ (carbon dioxide) [q.v.]

^{57}Co [see: cobaltous chloride Co 57]

^{57}Co [see: cyanocobalamin Co 57]

^{58}Co [see: cyanocobalamin (^{58}Co)]

^{60}Co [see: cobaltous chloride Co 60]

^{60}Co [see: cyanocobalamin Co 60]

coachweed medicinal herb [see: bedstraw]

coagulants *a class of agents that promote or accelerate clotting of the blood*

coagulation factor VIIa [see: factor VIIa, recombinant]

coagulation factor IX (human) [see: factor IX complex]

coakum medicinal herb [see: pokeweed]

coal tar USP *topical antieczematic; antiseborrheic*

co-amoxiclav (amoxicillin & potassium clavulanate) [q.v.]

COAP (cyclophosphamide, Oncovin, ara-C, prednisone) *chemotherapy protocol*

Co-Apap tablets OTC *antitussive; decongestant; antihistamine; analgesic* [dextromethorphan hydrobromide; pseudoephedrine HCl; chlorpheniramine maleate; acetaminophen] 15•30•2•325 mg

COAP-BLEO (cyclophosphamide, Oncovin, ara-C, prednisone, bleomycin) *chemotherapy protocol*

COB (cisplatin, Oncovin, bleomycin) *chemotherapy protocol*

cobalamin concentrate USP *vitamin B$_{12}$; hematopoietic*

cobalt *element (Co)*

cobalt-labeled vitamin B$_{12}$ [see: cyanocobalamin Co 57 & Co 60]

cobaltous chloride Co 57 USAN *radioactive agent*

cobaltous chloride Co 60 USAN *radioactive agent*

cobamamide INN

cocaine USP, BAN *topical anesthetic for mucous membranes; widely abused as a street drug, derived from coca leaves* 4%, 10% topical

cocaine, crack *street drug made by converting cocaine HCl into a form that can be smoked, which causes a faster, more intense effect*

cocaine HCl USP *topical anesthetic for mucous membranes; widely abused as a street drug, derived from coca leaves* 135 mg oral; 4%, 10% topical

Cocaine Viscous topical solution ℞ *topical mucosal anesthesia* [cocaine] 4%, 10%

cocarboxylase INN [also: co-carboxylase]

co-carboxylase BAN [also: cocarboxylase]

cocashweed medicinal herb [see: life root]

coccidioidin USP *dermal coccidioidomycosis test*

cocculin [see: picrotoxin]

Cocculus lacunosus; C. suberosus medicinal herb [see: levant berry]

Cocculus palmatus medicinal herb [see: colombo]

Cochlearia armoracia medicinal herb [see: horseradish]

cocklebur medicinal herb [see: agrimony; burdock]

cockspur pepper medicinal herb [see: cayenne]

cockspur rye medicinal herb [see: ergot]

cocoa NF

cocoa (*Theobromo cacao*) bean medicinal herb used as a cardiac stimulant, diuretic, and vasodilator

cocoa butter NF suppository base; emollient/protectant

cocowort medicinal herb [see: shepherd's purse]

cod liver oil USP, BAN vitamins A and D source; emollient/protectant

cod liver oil, nondestearinated NF

codactide INN, BAN

Codamine syrup, pediatric syrup ℞ narcotic antitussive; decongestant [hydrocodone bitartrate; phenylpropanolamine HCl] 5•25 mg/5 mL; 2.5•12.5 mg/5 mL

CODE (cisplatin, Oncovin, doxorubicin, etoposide) chemotherapy protocol

Codegest Expectorant liquid ℞ narcotic antitussive; decongestant; expectorant [codeine phosphate; phenylpropanolamine HCl; guaifenesin] 10•12.5•100 mg/5 mL ② Codehist

Codehist DH elixir ℞ narcotic antitussive; decongestant; antihistamine [codeine phosphate; pseudoephedrine HCl; chlorpheniramine maleate; alcohol 5.7%] 10•30•2 mg/5 mL ② Codegest

codehydrogenase I [see: nadide]

codeine USP, BAN narcotic analgesic used as an antitussive; sometimes abused as a street drug ② Kaodene

codeine & acetaminophen narcotic analgesic 15•300, 30•300, 60•300 mg oral; 12•30 mg/5 mL oral

codeine phosphate USP, BAN narcotic analgesic used as an antitussive 15 mg/5 mL oral; 30, 60 mg injection

codeine phosphate & guaifenesin antitussive; narcotic analgesic; expectorant 10•300 mg oral; 10•100 mg/5 mL oral

codeine polistirex USAN narcotic analgesic used as an antitussive

codeine sulfate USP narcotic analgesic used as an antitussive 15, 30, 60 mg oral

codelcortone [see: prednisolone]

co-dergocrine mesylate BAN cognition adjuvant [also: ergoloid mesylates]

Codiclear DH syrup ℞ narcotic antitussive; expectorant [hydrocodone bitartrate; guaifenesin] 5•100 mg/5 mL

Codimal capsules, film-coated tablets OTC decongestant; antihistamine; analgesic [pseudoephedrine HCl; chlorpheniramine maleate; acetaminophen] 30•2•325 mg

Codimal DH syrup ℞ narcotic antitussive; decongestant; antihistamine [hydrocodone bitartrate; phenylephrine HCl; pyrilamine maleate] 1.66•5•8.33 mg/5 mL

Codimal DM syrup OTC antitussive; decongestant; antihistamine [dextromethorphan hydrobromide; phenylephrine HCl; pyrilamine maleate] 10•5•8.33 mg/5 mL

Codimal PH syrup OTC narcotic antitussive; decongestant; antihistamine [codeine phosphate; phenylephrine HCl; pyrilamine maleate] 10•5•8.33 mg/5 mL

Codimal-L.A.; Codimal-L.A. Half extended-release capsules ℞ decongestant; antihistamine [pseudoephedrine HCl; chlorpheniramine maleate] 120•8 mg; 60•4 mg

codorphone [now: conorphone HCl]

codoxime USAN, INN antitussive

coenzyme Q10 natural enzyme used as a cardiac protectant, free radical scavenger, membrane stabilizer; investigational (Phase I) immune stimulant for AIDS

COF/COM (cyclophosphamide, Oncovin, fluorouracil + cyclophosphamide, Oncovin, methotrexate) chemotherapy protocol

coffeine [see: caffeine]
cofisatin INN
cofisatine [see: cofisatin]
cogazocine INN
Cogentin tablets, IV or IM injection ℞ *anticholinergic; antiparkinsonian* [benztropine mesylate] 0.5, 1, 2 mg; 1 mg/mL
Co-Gesic tablets ℞ *narcotic analgesic* [hydrocodone bitartrate; acetaminophen] 5•500 mg
Cognex capsules ℞ *cognition adjuvant for Alzheimer's dementia; reversible cholinesterase inhibitor* [tacrine HCl] 10, 20, 30, 40 mg
Co-Hist tablets OTC *decongestant; antihistamine; analgesic* [pseudoephedrine HCl; chlorpheniramine maleate; acetaminophen] 30•2•325 mg
cohosh *medicinal herb* [see: black cohosh; blue cohosh; white cohosh]
Cola acuminata medicinal herb [see: kola nut]
Colabid tablets ℞ *uricosuric for gout* [probenecid; colchicine]
Colace capsules, syrup, drops OTC *stool softener* [docusate sodium] 50, 100 mg; 60 mg/15 mL; 150 mg/15 mL
colaspase BAN *antineoplastic for acute lymphocytic leukemia (ALL)* [also: asparaginase]
Co-Lav powder for oral solution ℞ *pre-procedure bowel evacuant* [polyethylene glycol-electrolyte solution; electrolytes] 60 g/L
Colax tablets OTC *stimulant laxative; stool softener* [phenolphthalein; docusate sodium] 65•100 mg
Colazide (commercially available in Europe) ℞ *investigational (NDA filed) gastrointestinal anti-inflammatory for acute ulcerative colitis* [balsalazide disodium]
ColBenemid tablets (discontinued 1997) ℞ *treatment for frequent, recurrent attacks of gouty arthritis* [probenecid; colchicine] 500•0.5 mg
colchamine [see: demecolcine]

colchicine USP, JAN *gout suppressant; orphan status withdrawn 1997* 0.5, 0.6 mg oral; 1 mg injection
colchicine & probenecid *treatment for frequent, recurrent attacks of gouty arthritis*
Colchicum autumnale; C. speciosum; C. vernum medicinal herb [see: autumn crocus]
Cold & Allergy elixir OTC *decongestant; antihistamine* [phenylpropanolamine HCl; brompheniramine maleate] 12.5•2 mg/5 mL
cold cream USP
Cold Relief tablets OTC *antitussive; decongestant; antihistamine; analgesic* [dextromethorphan hydrobromide; phenylpropanolamine HCl; chlorpheniramine maleate; acetaminophen] 10•12.5•2•325 mg
Cold Symptoms Relief tablets OTC *antitussive; decongestant; antihistamine; analgesic* [dextromethorphan hydrobromide; pseudoephedrine HCl; chlorpheniramine maleate; acetaminophen] 10•30•2•325 mg
Cold-Gest sustained-release capsules OTC *decongestant; antihistamine* [phenylpropanolamine HCl; chlorpheniramine maleate] 75•8 mg
Coldloc liquid ℞ *decongestant; expectorant* [phenylpropanolamine HCl; phenylephrine HCl; guaifenesin] 20•5•100 mg/5 mL
Coldloc-LA sustained-release caplets ℞ *decongestant; expectorant* [phenylpropanolamine HCl; guaifenesin] 75•600 mg
Coldrine tablets OTC *decongestant; analgesic* [pseudoephedrine HCl; acetaminophen] 30•325 mg
colecalciferol INN *vitamin D_3; antirachitic* [also: cholecalciferol]
colesevelam HCl USAN *bile acid sequestrant for hypercholesterolemia*
Colestid tablets, granules ℞ *cholesterol-lowering antihyperlipidemic* [colestipol HCl] 1 g; 5 g/dose ⨂
colistin

colestipol INN, BAN *antihyperlipidemic; bile acid sequestrant* [also: colestipol HCl] ⑨ colistin

colestipol HCl USAN, USP *antihyperlipidemic; bile acid sequestrant* [also: colestipol]

colestolone USAN, INN *hypolipidemic*

colestyramine INN *bile salts ion-exchange resin; antihyperlipoproteinemic* [also: cholestyramine resin; cholestyramine]

colestyramine resin [see: cholestyramine resin]

colextran INN

Colfed-A sustained-release capsules ℞ *decongestant; antihistamine* [pseudoephedrine HCl; chlorpheniramine maleate] 120•8 mg

colfenamate INN

colforsin USAN, INN *antiglaucoma agent*

colfosceril palmitate USAN, INN, BAN *pulmonary surfactant for hyaline membrane disease and neonatal respiratory distress syndrome (orphan); investigational (orphan) for adult respiratory distress syndrome (ARDS)*

colfosceril palmitate & phosphatidylglycerol *investigational (orphan) for neonatal respiratory distress syndrome*

colic root *medicinal herb* [see: blazing star; star grass; wild yam]

colimecycline INN

colistimethate sodium USAN, USP, INN *bactericidal antibiotic* [also: colistin sulphomethate]

colistin INN, BAN *bactericidal antibiotic* [also: colistin sulfate] ⑨ Colestid; colestipol

colistin methanesulfonate [see: colistimethate sodium]

colistin sulfate USP *bactericidal antibiotic* [also: colistin]

colistin sulphomethate BAN *bactericidal antibiotic* [also: colistimethate sodium]

collagen *ophthalmic implant to block puncta and retain moisture; urethral injection for stress urinary incontinence*

collagen, purified type II *investigational (Phase III, orphan) oral treatment for juvenile rheumatoid arthritis*

collagen sponge, absorbable *topical local hemostat for surgery*

collagenase *topical proteolytic enzymes for necrotic tissue debridement; investigational (orphan) for Peyronie's disease*

collagenase, clostridial [see: clostridial collagenase]

collard *medicinal herb* [see: skunk cabbage]

Collastin Oil Free Moisturizer lotion (discontinued 1998) OTC *moisturizer; emollient* [collagen] ②

Collinsonia canadensis medicinal herb [see: stone root]

collodion USP *topical protectant*

colloidal aluminum hydroxide [see: aluminum hydroxide gel]

colloidal oatmeal *demulcent*

colloidal silicon dioxide [see: silicon dioxide, colloidal]

Colloral *investigational (Phase III, orphan) oral treatment for juvenile rheumatoid arthritis* [collagen, purified type II]

Collyrium for Fresh Eyes ophthalmic solution OTC *extraocular irrigating solution* [sterile isotonic solution]

Collyrium Fresh eye drops OTC *topical ophthalmic decongestant and vasoconstrictor* [tetrahydrozoline HCl] 0.05%

ColoCare test kit for home use OTC *in vitro diagnostic aid for fecal occult blood*

colombo (Cocculus palmatus) root *medicinal herb used as an antiemetic and febrifuge*

Colomed enema ℞ *investigational (orphan) for left-sided ulcerative colitis and chronic radiation proctitis* [short chain fatty acids]

colony-stimulating factors *a class of glycoproteins that stimulate the production of granulocytes and macrophages*

Color Allergy Screening Test (CAST) reagent assay tubes ℞ *in vitro diagnostic aid for immunoglobulin E in serum*

Color Ovulation Test kit for home use OTC *in vitro diagnostic aid to predict ovulation time*

ColoScreen slide test for professional use *in vitro diagnostic aid for fecal occult blood*

Colovage powder for oral solution ℞ *pre-procedure bowel evacuant* [polyethylene glycol-electrolyte solution]

Col-Probenecid tablets (discontinued 1998) ℞ *treatment for frequent, recurrent attacks of gouty arthritis* [probenecid; colchicine] 500•0.5 mg

colterol INN *bronchodilator* [also: colterol mesylate]

colterol mesylate USAN *bronchodilator* [also: colterol]

colt's tail *medicinal herb* [see: fleabane; horseweed]

coltsfoot *(Tussilago farfara)* buds, flowers, and leaves *medicinal herb for asthma, bronchitis, dry cough, hay fever, lung disorders, excess mucus, and throat irritation*

columbine *(Aquilegia vulgaris)* plant *medicinal herb used as an astringent, diaphoretic, and diuretic*

Coly-Mycin M powder for IV or IM injection ℞ *bactericidal antibiotic* [colistimethate sodium] 150 mg

Coly-Mycin S powder for oral suspension (discontinued 1996) ℞ *bactericidal antibiotic* [colistin sulfate] 25 mg/5 mL

Coly-Mycin S Otic suspension ℞ *topical corticosteroidal anti-inflammatory; antibiotic* [hydrocortisone acetate; neomycin sulfate; colistin sulfate] 1%•4.71 mg•3 mg per mL

Colyte powder for oral solution ℞ *pre-procedure bowel evacuant* [polyethylene glycol-electrolyte solution]

COM (cyclophosphamide, Oncovin, MeCCNU) *chemotherapy protocol*

COM (cyclophosphamide, Oncovin, methotrexate) *chemotherapy protocol*

COMA-A (cyclophosphamide, Oncovin, methotrexate/citrovorum factor, Adriamycin, ara-C) *chemotherapy protocol*

COMB (cyclophosphamide, Oncovin, MeCCNU, bleomycin) *chemotherapy protocol*

COMB (Cytoxin, Oncovin, methotrexate, bleomycin) *chemotherapy protocol*

Combidex ℞ *investigational (Phase III) MRI diagnostic aid for lymph node metastases* [ferumoxtran-10]

CombiPatch transdermal patch ℞ *estrogen/progesterone for hormone replacement therapy* [estradiol; norethindrone acetate] 0.05•0.14, 0.05•0.25 mg/day

Combipres 0.1; Combipres 0.2; Combipres 0.3 tablets ℞ *antihypertensive; diuretic* [clonidine HCl; chlorthalidone] 0.1•15 mg; 0.2•15 mg; 0.3•15 mg ⊉ Catapres

Combistix reagent strips *in vitro diagnostic aid for multiple urine products*

Combivent oral inhalation aerosol ℞ *anticholinergic bronchodilator for chronic bronchospasm with COPD* [ipratropium bromide; albuterol sulfate] 18•103 μg/spray

Combivir film-coated tablets ℞ *nucleoside reverse transcriptase inhibitor combination for HIV* [lamivudine; zidovudine] 150•300 mg

COMe (Cytoxin, Oncovin, methotrexate) *chemotherapy protocol*

COMF (cyclophosphamide, Oncovin, methotrexate, fluorouracil) *chemotherapy protocol*

Comfort eye drops OTC *topical ophthalmic decongestant and vasoconstrictor* [naphazoline HCl] 0.03%

Comfort Tears eye drops OTC *ocular moisturizer/lubricant* [hydroxyethylcellulose] ≟

ComfortCare GP Wetting & Soaking solution OTC *disinfecting/wetting/soaking solution for rigid gas permeable contact lenses*

Comfortine ointment OTC *moisturizer; emollient; astringent; antiseptic* [vitamins A and D; lanolin; zinc oxide]

comfrey *(Symphytum officinale; S. tuberosum)* leaves and roots *medici-*

nal herb for anemia, arthritis, blood cleansing, boils and sores, bruises, burns, edema, emphysema, fractures, gastric ulcers, hemorrhoids, and sprains; not generally regarded as safe and effective as it may be carcinogenic and hepatotoxic

comfrey, spotted medicinal herb [see: lungwort]

Comhist tablets ℞ decongestant; antihistamine [phenylephrine HCl; chlorpheniramine maleate; phenyltoloxamine citrate] 10•2•25 mg

Comhist LA long-acting capsules ℞ decongestant; antihistamine [phenylephrine HCl; chlorpheniramine maleate; phenyltoloxamine citrate] 20•4•50 mg

COMLA (cyclophosphamide, Oncovin, methotrexate, leucovorin [rescue], ara-C) chemotherapy protocol

Commiphora abssynica; C. molmol; C. myrrha medicinal herb [see: myrrh]

Commiphora mukul medicinal herb [see: guggul]

common bugloss medicinal herb [see: borage]

common elder medicinal herb [see: elderberry]

common flax medicinal herb [see: flaxseed]

comosain investigational (orphan) proteolytic enzymes for debridement of severe burns

COMP (CCNU, Oncovin, methotrexate, procarbazine) chemotherapy protocol

COMP (cyclophosphamide, Oncovin, methotrexate, prednisone) chemotherapy protocol

Compazine suppositories ℞ conventional (typical) antipsychotic; antiemetic [prochlorperazine] 2.5, 5, 25 mg

Compazine syrup, IV or IM injection ℞ conventional (typical) antipsychotic; antiemetic [prochlorperazine edisylate] 5 mg/5 mL; 5 mg/mL

Compazine tablets, Spansules (sustained-release capsules) ℞ conven-

tional (typical) antipsychotic; antiemetic [prochlorperazine maleate] 5, 10 mg; 10, 15 mg

Compete tablets OTC vitamin/iron supplement [multiple vitamins; ferrous gluconate; folic acid] ±•27•0.4 mg

Compleat Modified Formula closed system containers OTC enteral nutritional therapy [lactose-free formula]

Compleat Modified Formula ready-to-use liquid OTC enteral nutritional therapy [lactose-free formula]

Compleat Regular Formula ready-to-use liquid OTC enteral nutritional therapy [milk-based formula]

complement receptor type I, soluble recombinant human investigational (orphan) for adult respiratory distress syndrome

Complete solution OTC rewetting solution for soft contact lenses

Complete All-in-One solution OTC cleaning/disinfecting/rinsing/storage solution for soft contact lenses

Complete Multi-Purpose solution (name changed to Complete All-In-One in 1995)

Complete Weekly Enzymatic Cleaner effervescent tablets OTC enzymatic cleaner for soft contact lenses [subtilisin A]

Complex 15 Face cream OTC moisturizer; emollient

Complex 15 Hand & Body cream, lotion OTC moisturizer; emollient

Comply liquid OTC enteral nutritional therapy [lactose-free formula]

compound 42 [see: warfarin]

compound CB3025 [see: melphalan]

compound E [see: cortisone acetate]

compound F [see: hydrocortisone]

compound orange spirit [see: orange spirit, compound]

compound Q [see: trichosanthin]

compound S [see: zidovudine]

compound solution of sodium chloride INN fluid and electrolyte replenisher [also: Ringer's injection]

compound solution of sodium lactate INN electrolyte and fluid replen-

isher; systemic alkalizer [also: Ringer's injection, lactated]

Compound W liquid, gel OTC *topical keratolytic* [salicylic acid in collodion] 17%

Compoz gel caps OTC *antihistaminic sleep aid* [diphenhydramine HCl] 25 mg

Compoz Nighttime Sleep Aid tablets OTC *antihistaminic sleep aid* [diphenhydramine HCl] 50 mg

compressible sugar [see: sugar, compressible]

Computer Eye Drops OTC *ophthalmic moisturizer and emollient* [glycerin] 1%

COMT inhibitors (catechol-O-methyltransferase) *a class of antiparkinson agents that stabilize serum levodopa levels by inhibiting an enzyme that breaks down the levodopa before it reaches the brain*

Comtan (commercially available in Europe) ℞ *investigational (NDA filed) COMT inhibitor for Parkinson's disease* [entacapone]

Comtrex caplets, tablets (name changed to Comtrex Multi-Symptom Cold & Flu Relief in 1995)

Comtrex liquid OTC *antitussive; decongestant; antihistamine; analgesic* [dextromethorphan hydrobromide; pseudoephedrine HCl; chlorpheniramine maleate; acetaminophen] 3.3•10•0.67•108.3 mg/5 mL

Comtrex, Cough Formula liquid OTC *antitussive; decongestant; expectorant; analgesic* [dextromethorphan hydrobromide; pseudoephedrine HCl; guaifenesin; acetaminophen; alcohol 20%] 7.5•15•50•125 mg/5 mL

Comtrex, Day & Night daytime caplets + nighttime tablets (discontinued 1995) OTC *antitussive; decongestant; analgesic; (antihistamine added nighttime)* [dextromethorphan hydrobromide; pseudoephedrine HCl; acetaminophen; (chlorpheniramine maleate added nighttime)] 15•30•500 mg daytime; 15•30•500•2 mg nighttime

Comtrex Allergy-Sinus caplets, tablets OTC *decongestant; antihistamine; analgesic* [pseudoephedrine HCl; chlorpheniramine maleate; acetaminophen] 30•2•500 mg

Comtrex Hot Flu Relief powder (discontinued 1995) OTC *antitussive; decongestant; antihistamine; analgesic* [dextromethorphan hydrobromide; pseudoephedrine HCl; chlorpheniramine maleate; acetaminophen] 20•60•4•500 mg/packet

Comtrex Liqui-Gels (liquid-filled capsules) OTC *antitussive; decongestant; antihistamine; analgesic* [dextromethorphan hydrobromide; phenylpropanolamine HCl; chlorpheniramine maleate; acetaminophen] 10•12.5•2•325, 15•12.5•2•500 mg

Comtrex Multi-Symptom, Day & Night daytime caplets + nighttime tablets (discontinued 1995) OTC *antitussive; decongestant; analgesic; (antihistamine added nighttime)* [dextromethorphan hydrobromide; pseudoephedrine HCl; acetaminophen; (chlorpheniramine maleate added nighttime)] 10•30•325 mg daytime; 10•30•325•2 mg nighttime

Comtrex Multi-Symptom Cold & Flu Relief tablets, caplets OTC *antitussive; decongestant; antihistamine; analgesic* [dextromethorphan hydrobromide; pseudoephedrine HCl; chlorpheniramine maleate; acetaminophen] 15•30•2•500 mg

Comtrex Multi-Symptom Cold & Flu Relief Liqui-Gels (capsules) OTC *antitussive; decongestant; antihistamine; analgesic* [dextromethorphan hydrobromide; phenylpropanolamine HCl; chlorpheniramine maleate; acetaminophen] 15•12.5•2•500 mg

Comtrex Non-Drowsy caplets OTC *antitussive; decongestant; analgesic* [dextromethorphan hydrobromide; pseudoephedrine HCl; acetaminophen] 15•30•500 mg

Comvax IM injection ℞ *infant (1½–15 months) vaccine for H. influenzae and hepatitis B* [Hemophilus b purified capsular polysaccharide; *Neisseria meningitidis* OMPC; hepatitis B virus vaccine] 7.5•125•5 µg/0.5 mL

Conceive Ovulation Predictor 5-day test kit for professional use *in vitro diagnostic aid to predict ovulation time*

Conceive Pregnancy test kit for home use OTC *in vitro diagnostic aid for urine pregnancy test*

Concentrated Cleaner solution OTC *cleaning solution for rigid gas permeable contact lenses*

Conceptrol Contraceptive Inserts vaginal suppositories OTC *spermicidal contraceptive* [nonoxynol 9] 150 mg

Conceptrol Disposable Contraceptive vaginal gel OTC *spermicidal contraceptive* [nonoxynol 9] 4%

Condrin-LA sustained-release capsules (discontinued 1995) ℞ *decongestant; antihistamine* [phenylpropanolamine HCl; chlorpheniramine maleate] 75•12 mg

Condylox solution, gel ℞ *topical antimitotic for external genital and perianal warts* [podofilox] 0.5%

cone flower, purple *medicinal herb* [see: echinacea]

conessine INN

conessine hydrobromide [see: conessine]

Conex syrup OTC *decongestant; expectorant* [phenylpropanolamine HCl; guaifenesin] 12.5•100 mg/5 mL

Conex with Codeine syrup ℞ *narcotic antitussive; decongestant; expectorant* [codeine phosphate; phenylpropanolamine HCl; guaifenesin] 10•12.5•100 mg/5 mL

confectioner's sugar [see: sugar, confectioner's]

Confide test kit for home use OTC *in vitro diagnostic aid for HIV in the blood*

congazone sodium [see: Congo red]

Congespirin for Children chewable tablets (discontinued 1995) OTC *decongestant; analgesic* [phenylephrine HCl; acetaminophen] 1.25•81 mg

Congess JR capsules ℞ *decongestant; expectorant* [pseudoephedrine HCl; guaifenesin] 60•125 mg

Congess SR sustained-release capsules ℞ *decongestant; expectorant* [pseudoephedrine HCl; guaifenesin] 120•250 mg

Congestac caplets OTC *decongestant; expectorant* [pseudoephedrine HCl; guaifenesin] 60•400 mg

Congestant tablets (name changed to Improved Congestant in 1995)

Congestant D tablets OTC *decongestant; antihistamine; analgesic* [phenylpropanolamine HCl; chlorpheniramine maleate; acetaminophen] 12.5•2•325 mg

Congestion Relief tablets OTC *nasal decongestant* [pseudoephedrine HCl] 30, 60 mg

Congestion Relief, Children's liquid OTC *nasal decongestant* [pseudoephedrine HCl] 30 mg/5 mL

Congo red USP

conorfone INN *analgesic* [also: conorphone HCl]

conorfone HCl [see: conorphone HCl]

conorphone HCl USAN *analgesic* [also: conorfone]

CONPADRI; CONPADRI-I (cyclophosphamide, Oncovin, L-phenylalanine mustard, Adriamycin) *chemotherapy protocol*

Conray; Conray 30; Conray 43 injection ℞ *radiopaque contrast medium* [iothalamate meglumine (47% iodine)] 600 mg/mL (282 mg/mL); 300 mg/mL (141 mg/mL); 430 mg/mL (202 mg/mL)

Conray 325 injection (discontinued 1999) ℞ *radiopaque contrast medium* [iothalamate sodium (59.9% iodine)] 543 mg/mL (325 mg/mL)

Conray 400 injection ℞ *radiopaque contrast medium* [iothalamate sodium (59.9% iodine)] 668 mg/mL (400 mg/mL)

Consonar ℞ *investigational reversible/ selective MAO inhibitor, type A* [brofaromine]

Constilac syrup ℞ *laxative* [lactulose] 10 g/15 mL

Constulose syrup ℞ *laxative* [lactulose] 10 g/15 mL

consumptive's weed *medicinal herb* [see: yerba santa]

Contac 12 Hour sustained-release capsules, sustained-release caplets OTC *decongestant; antihistamine* [phenylpropanolamine HCl; chlorpheniramine maleate] 75•8 mg; 75•12 mg

Contac Cough & Chest Cold liquid OTC *antitussive; decongestant; expectorant; analgesic* [dextromethorphan hydrobromide; pseudoephedrine HCl; guaifenesin; acetaminophen; alcohol 10%] 5•15•50•125 mg/5 mL

Contac Cough & Sore Throat liquid OTC *antitussive; analgesic* [dextromethorphan hydrobromide; acetaminophen; alcohol 10%] 5•125 mg/5 mL

Contac Day & Night Allergy/Sinus daytime caplets + nighttime caplets OTC *decongestant; analgesic; (antihistamine/sleep aid added nighttime)* [pseudoephedrine HCl; acetaminophen; (diphenhydramine HCl added nighttime)] 60•650 mg daytime; 60•650•50 mg nighttime

Contac Day & Night Cold & Flu daytime caplets + nighttime caplets OTC *decongestant; analgesic; (antitussive added daytime; antihistamine/sleep aid added nighttime)* [pseudoephedrine HCl; acetaminophen; (dextromethorphan hydrobromide added daytime; diphenhydramine HCl added nighttime)] 60•650•30 mg daytime; 60•650•50 mg nighttime

Contac Non-Drowsy Formula Sinus tablets, caplets (discontinued 1995) OTC *decongestant; analgesic; antipyretic* [pseudoephedrine HCl; acetaminophen] 30•500 mg

Contac Severe Cold & Flu Formula caplets (discontinued 1995) OTC *antitussive; decongestant; antihistamine; analgesic* [dextromethorphan hydrobromide; phenylpropanolamine HCl; chlorpheniramine maleate; acetaminophen] 15•12.5•2•500 mg

Contac Severe Cold & Flu Hot Medicine powder (discontinued 1995) OTC *antitussive; decongestant; antihistamine; analgesic* [dextromethorphan hydrobromide; pseudoephedrine HCl; chlorpheniramine maleate; acetaminophen] 20•60•4•650 mg/packet

Contac Severe Cold & Flu Nighttime liquid OTC *antitussive; decongestant; antihistamine; analgesic* [dextromethorphan hydrobromide; pseudoephedrine HCl; chlorpheniramine maleate; acetaminophen; alcohol 18.5%] 5•10•0.67•167 mg/5 mL

Contac-C Cold Care Formula ⒸⒶⓃ (U.S. product: Contac Severe Cold & Flu Formula) caplets OTC *antitussive; decongestant; antihistamine; analgesic* [dextromethorphan hydrobromide; phenylpropanolamine HCl; chlorpheniramine maleate; acetaminophen] 15•12.5•2•500 mg

conteben [see: thioacetazone; thiacetazone]

ConTE-Pak-4 IV injection ℞ *intravenous nutritional therapy* [multiple trace elements (metals)] ±

Contigen urethral injection ℞ *treatment for stress urinary incontinence* [collagen implant, purified]

Contramid ℞ *investigational (Phase III) controlled-release solid oral form of a racemic albuterol bronchodilator for asthma and COPD* [levalbuterol]

Contrin capsules ℞ *hematinic* [ferrous fumarate; cyanocobalamin; ascorbic acid; intrinsic factor concentrate; folic acid] 110 mg•15 μg•75 mg•240 mg•0.5 mg

Control timed-release capsules OTC *diet aid* [phenylpropanolamine HCl] 75 mg

ControlPak (trademarked packaging form) *tamper-resistant unit-dose package*

Contuss liquid ℞ *decongestant; expectorant* [phenylpropanolamine HCl;

phenylephrine HCl; guaifenesin; alcohol 5%] 20•5•100 mg/5 mL

conval lily *medicinal herb* [see: lily of the valley]

Convallaria majalis *medicinal herb* [see: lily of the valley]

conventional (typical) antipsychotics *a class of dopamine receptor antagonists with a higher affinity to the D_2 than D_1 receptors and little affinity to the nondopaminergic receptors; high incidence of extrapyramidal side effects (EPS)* [compare to: novel (atypical) antipsychotics]

Convolvulus sepium *medicinal herb* [see: hedge bindweed]

convulsion root; convulsion weed *medicinal herb* [see: fit root]

ConXn *investigational (Phase II/III) for scleroderma* [relaxin H2, recombinant human]

Conyza canadensis *medicinal herb* [see: horseweed]

Cooper's regimen *chemotherapy protocol* [see: CMFVP]

COP [see: creatinolfosfate]

COP (cyclophosphamide, Oncovin, prednisone) *chemotherapy protocol*

COP 1 (copolymer 1) [see: glatiramer acetate]

COPA (Cytoxin, Oncovin, prednisone, Adriamycin) *chemotherapy protocol*

COPA-BLEO (cyclophosphamide, Oncovin, prednisone, Adriamycin, bleomycin) *chemotherapy protocol*

COPAC (CCNU, Oncovin, prednisone, Adriamycin, cyclophosphamide) *chemotherapy protocol*

Copaxone powder for subcu injection *℞ immunomodulator for relapsing-remitting multiple sclerosis (orphan)* [glatiramer acetate] 20 mg

COPB (cyclophosphamide, Oncovin, prednisone, bleomycin) *chemotherapy protocol*

COP-BLAM (cyclophosphamide, Oncovin, prednisone, bleomy-

cin, Adriamycin, Matulane) *chemotherapy protocol*

COP-BLEO (cyclophosphamide, Oncovin, prednisone, bleomycin) *chemotherapy protocol*

Cope tablets OTC *analgesic; antipyretic; anti-inflammatory; antacid* [aspirin; caffeine; magnesium hydroxide; aluminum hydroxide] 421•32•50•25 mg

COPE (cyclophosphamide, Oncovin, Platinol, etoposide) *chemotherapy protocol*

Cophene No. 2 sustained-release capsules *℞ decongestant; antihistamine* [pseudoephedrine HCl; chlorpheniramine maleate] 120•12 mg

Cophene XP liquid *℞ narcotic antitussive; decongestant; expectorant* [hydrocodone bitartrate; pseudoephedrine HCl; guaifenesin; alcohol 12.5%] 5•60•200 mg/5 mL

Cophene-B subcu or IM injection (discontinued 1997) *℞ antihistamine for anaphylaxis* [brompheniramine maleate] 10 mg/mL

Cophene-X capsules *℞ antitussive; decongestant; expectorant* [carbetapentane citrate; phenylephrine HCl; phenylpropanolamine HCl; potassium guaiacolsulfonate] 20•10•10•45 mg

copolymer 1 (COP 1) [see: glatiramer acetate]

copovithane BAN

COPP (CCNU, Oncovin, procarbazine, prednisone) *chemotherapy protocol*

COPP (cyclophosphamide, Oncovin, procarbazine, prednisone) *chemotherapy protocol*

copper *element (Cu)*

copper chloride dihydrate [see: cupric chloride]

copper gluconate (copper D-gluconate) USP *trace mineral supplement*

copper sulfate pentahydrate [see: cupric sulfate]

copper 10-undecenoate [see: copper undecylenate]

copper undecylenate USAN

copperhead snake antivenin [see: antivenin (Crotalidae) polyvalent]

Coptis trifolia medicinal herb [see: gold thread]

Co-Pyronil 2 Pulvules (capsules) OTC decongestant; antihistamine [pseudo-ephedrine HCl; chlorpheniramine maleate] 60•4 mg

CoQ10 [see: coenzyme Q10]

Coracin ophthalmic ointment (discontinued 1995) ℞ topical ophthalmic corticosteroidal anti-inflammatory; antibiotic [hydrocortisone acetate; neomycin sulfate; bacitracin zinc; polymyxin B sulfate] 1%•0.5%•400 U/g•10 000 U/g

coral (*Goniopora* **spp.;** *Porite* **spp.)** natural material used as a substrate for bone grafts and fractures and in reconstructive surgery

coral root (*Corallorhiza odontorhiza***)** medicinal herb for diaphoresis, fever, insomnia, and sedation

coral snake antivenin [see: antivenin (Micrurus fulvius)]

corbadrine INN adrenergic; vasoconstrictor [also: levonordefrin]

Cordarone tablets, IV infusion ℞ antiarrhythmic for acute ventricular tachycardia and fibrillation (orphan) [amiodarone HCl] 200 mg; 50 mg/mL

Cordase injection ℞ investigational (Phase II) treatment for Dupuytren's disease [collagenase]

Cordox ℞ investigational asthma treatment [fructose-1,6-diphosphate]

Cordox ℞ investigational (Phase III) cytoprotective agent for the vaso-occlusive episodes of sickle cell disease

Cordran ointment, lotion, tape ℞ topical corticosteroidal anti-inflammatory [flurandrenolide] 0.025%, 0.05%; 0.05%; 4 μg/cm²

Cordran SP cream ℞ topical corticosteroidal anti-inflammatory [flurandrenolide] 0.025%, 0.05%

Coreg Tiltab (film-coated tablets) ℞ antihypertensive; α- and β-blocker for congestive heart failure [carvedilol] 3.125, 6.25, 12.5, 25 mg

Corgard tablets ℞ antihypertensive; antianginal; β-blocker [nadolol] 20, 40, 80, 120, 160 mg

coriander (*Coriandrum sativum***)** seed medicinal herb used as antispasmodic, appetizer, carminative, and stomachic

coriander oil NF

Coricidin tablets OTC antihistamine; analgesic [chlorpheniramine maleate; acetaminophen] 2•325 mg

Coricidin D; Coricidin Sinus Headache tablets OTC decongestant; antihistamine; analgesic [phenylpropanolamine HCl; chlorpheniramine maleate; acetaminophen] 12.5•2•325 mg; 12.5•2•500 mg

corkwood tree (*Duboisia myoporoides***)** leaves medicinal herb used as a central nervous system stimulant and in homeopathic therapy for eye disorders; not generally regarded as safe and effective as it contains scopolamine and related alkaloids, which may be fatal in high doses

Corlopam IV infusion ℞ rapid-acting vasodilator for in-hospital management of severe hypertension [fenoldopam mesylate] 10 mg/mL

Cormax ointment ℞ topical corticosteroidal anti-inflammatory [clobetasol propionate] 0.05%

cormed [see: nikethamide]

cormetasone INN topical anti-inflammatory [also: cormethasone acetate]

cormetasone acetate [see: cormethasone acetate]

cormethasone acetate USAN topical anti-inflammatory [also: cormetasone]

corn, turkey medicinal herb [see: turkey corn]

corn cockle (*Agrostemma githago***)** seeds and root medicinal herb for cancer, edema, exanthema, hemorrhoids, jaundice, and worms; also used as an emmenagogue and expectorant, and in homeopathic remedies for gastritis and paralysis; not generally regarded as safe and effective as it is extremely poisonous

Corn Huskers lotion OTC moisturizer; emollient

corn oil NF *solvent; caloric replacement*

corn silk (stigmata maidis) *medicinal herb* [see: Indian corn]

cornflower (*Centaurea cyanus*) plant *medicinal herb for conjunctivitis, corneal ulcers and other eye disorders and for nervous disorders and poisonous bites and stings*

corpse plant *medicinal herb* [see: fit root]

corpus luteum extract [see: progesterone]

Corque cream R̞ *topical corticosteroidal anti-inflammatory; antifungal; antibacterial* [hydrocortisone; clioquinol] 1%•3%

Correctol tablets OTC *stimulant laxative* [bisacodyl] 5 mg

Correctol tablets (discontinued 1996) OTC *stimulant laxative; stool softener* [yellow phenolphthalein; docusate sodium] 65•100 mg

Correctol Extra Gentle soft gel capsules OTC *stool softener* [docusate sodium] 100 mg

CortaGel OTC *topical corticosteroidal anti-inflammatory* [hydrocortisone] 1%

Cortaid cream, ointment OTC *topical corticosteroidal anti-inflammatory* [hydrocortisone acetate] 1%

Cortaid lotion (discontinued 1997) OTC *topical corticosteroidal anti-inflammatory* [hydrocortisone acetate] 1%

Cortaid pump spray OTC *topical corticosteroidal anti-inflammatory* [hydrocortisone] 1%

Cortaid Faststick roll-on stick OTC *topical corticosteroidal anti-inflammatory* [hydrocortisone; alcohol 55%] 1%

Cortaid Intensive Therapy cream OTC *topical corticosteroidal anti-inflammatory* [hydrocortisone] 1%

Cortaid with Aloe cream, ointment OTC *topical corticosteroidal anti-inflammatory* [hydrocortisone acetate] 0.5%

Cortatrigen Modified ear drops, otic suspension R̞ *topical corticosteroidal anti-inflammatory; antibiotic* [hydrocortisone; neomycin sulfate; polymyxin B sulfate] 1%•5 mg•10 000 U per mL

Cort-Dome cream R̞ *topical corticosteroidal anti-inflammatory* [hydrocortisone] 0.5%, 1% ⊘ Cortone

Cort-Dome High Potency rectal suppositories R̞ *corticosteroidal anti-inflammatory* [hydrocortisone acetate] 25 mg

Cortef tablets, oral suspension R̞ *corticosteroid; anti-inflammatory* [hydrocortisone] 5, 10, 20 mg; 10 mg/5 mL

Cortef Feminine Itch cream OTC *topical corticosteroidal anti-inflammatory* [hydrocortisone acetate] 0.5%

Cortenema retention enema R̞ *corticosteroid for ulcerative colitis* [hydrocortisone] 100 mg/60 mL ⊘ quart enema

cortenil [see: desoxycorticosterone acetate]

cortexolone [see: cortodoxone]

Cortic ear drops R̞ *topical corticosteroidal anti-inflammatory; topical anesthetic; bacteriostatic* [hydrocortisone; pramoxine HCl; chloroxylenol] 10•10•1 mg/mL

Corticaine anorectal cream (discontinued 1995) OTC *topical corticosteroidal anti-inflammatory; local anesthetic* [hydrocortisone acetate; dibucaine] 0.5%•0.5%

Corticaine cream OTC *topical corticosteroidal anti-inflammatory* [hydrocortisone acetate] 0.5%

corticorelin ovine triflutate USAN, INN *corticotropin-releasing hormone; diagnostic aid for Cushing syndrome and adrenocortical insufficiency (orphan)*

corticosteroids *a class of anti-inflammatory drugs*

corticotrophin INN, BAN *adrenocorticotropic hormone; corticosteroid; anti-inflammatory; diagnostic aid* [also: corticotropin]

corticotrophin-zinc hydroxide INN *adrenocorticotropic hormone; corticosteroid; anti-inflammatory; diagnostic aid* [also: corticotropin zinc hydroxide]

corticotropin USP *adrenocorticotropic hormone; corticosteroid; anti-inflam-*

matory; diagnostic aid [also: cortico-trophin] 40 U/vial injection

corticotropin, repository USP *adreno-corticotropic hormone; corticosteroid; anti-inflammatory; diagnostic aid*

corticotropin tetracosapeptide [see: cosyntropin]

corticotropin zinc hydroxide USP *adrenocorticotropic hormone; cortico-steroid; anti-inflammatory; diagnostic aid* [also: corticotrophin-zinc hydroxide]

corticotropin-releasing factor *inves-tigational (Phase I/II, orphan) agent for peritumoral brain edema*

Cortifoam intrarectal foam aerosol R̥ *corticosteroid for ulcerative proctitis* [hydrocortisone acetate] 90 mg/dose

Cortin cream R̥ *topical corticosteroidal anti-inflammatory; antifungal; anti-bacterial* [hydrocortisone; clioquinol] ⨂ Cotrim

cortisol [see: hydrocortisone]

cortisol 21-acetate [see: hydrocorti-sone acetate]

cortisol 21-butyrate [see: hydrocorti-sone butyrate]

cortisol 21-cyclopentanepropionate [see: hydrocortisone cypionate]

cortisol cyclopentylpropionate [see: hydrocortisone cypionate]

cortisol 21-valerate [see: hydrocorti-sone valerate]

cortisone INN, BAN *corticosteroid; anti-inflammatory* [also: cortisone acetate] ⨂ Cortizone

cortisone acetate USP *corticosteroid; anti-inflammatory* [also: cortisone] 5, 10, 25 mg oral

Cortisporin cream R̥ *topical cortico-steroidal anti-inflammatory; antibiotic* [hydrocortisone acetate; neomycin sulfate; polymyxin B sulfate] 0.5%•0.5%•10 000 U per g

Cortisporin eye drop suspension R̥ *top-ical ophthalmic corticosteroidal anti-inflammatory; antibiotic* [hydrocorti-sone; neomycin sulfate; polymyxin B sulfate] 1%•0.35%•10 000 U per mL

Cortisporin ointment R̥ *topical cortico-steroidal anti-inflammatory; antibiotic* [hydrocortisone; neomycin sulfate; bacitracin zinc; polymyxin B sulfate] 1%•0.5%•400 U•5000 U per g

Cortisporin ophthalmic ointment R̥ *topical ophthalmic corticosteroidal anti-inflammatory; antibiotic* [hydrocorti-sone; neomycin sulfate; bacitracin zinc; polymyxin B sulfate] 1%• 0.35%•400 U/g•10 000 U/g

Cortisporin Otic ear drops, otic sus-pension R̥ *topical corticosteroidal anti-inflammatory; antibiotic* [hydrocorti-sone; neomycin sulfate; polymyxin B sulfate] 1%•5 mg•10 000 U per mL

Cortisporin-TC ear drop suspension R̥ *topical corticosteroidal anti-inflamma-tory; antibiotic; surface-active synergist* [hydrocortisone acetate; neomycin sulfate; colistin sulfate; thonzonium bromide] 10•3.3•3•0.5 mg/mL

cortisuzol INN

cortivazol USAN, INN *corticosteroid; anti-inflammatory*

Cortizone for Kids cream OTC *topical corticosteroidal anti-inflammatory* [hydrocortisone] 0.5%

Cortizone-5 ointment, cream OTC *top-ical corticosteroidal anti-inflammatory* [hydrocortisone] 0.5%; 1% ⨂ corti-sone

Cortizone-10 ointment OTC *topical corticosteroidal anti-inflammatory* [hydrocortisone] 1%

cortodoxone USAN, INN, BAN *anti-inflammatory*

Cortone Acetate tablets, intra-articu-lar or intralesional injection (dis-continued 1998) R̥ *corticosteroid; anti-inflammatory* [cortisone acetate] 25 mg; 50 mg/mL ⨂ Cort-Dome

Cortrosyn powder for injection R̥ *multiple sclerosis; infantile spasms; diagnostic aid for adrenal function* [cosyntropin] 0.25 mg

Corvert IV infusion R̥ *antiarrhythmic for atrial fibrillation/flutter* [ibutilide fumarate] 0.1 mg/mL

corydalis (*Corydalis cava*) root *medicinal herb used as an antispasmodic, hypnotic, and antiparkinsonian*

Corydalis formosa medicinal herb [see: turkey corn]

Corynanthe johimbe medicinal herb [see: yohimbe]

Corzide 40/5; Corzide 80/5 tablets ℞ *antihypertensive; β-blocker; diuretic* [nadolol; bendroflumethiazide] 40•5 mg; 80•5 mg

Cosmegen powder for IV injection ℞ *antibiotic antineoplastic for melanomas, sarcomas, testicular and trophoblastic tumors* [dactinomycin] 0.5 mg

cosmoline [see: petrolatum]

Cosopt eye drops ℞ *topical carbonic anhydrase inhibitor and beta-blocker for glaucoma* [dorzolamide HCl; timolol maleate] 2%•0.5%

cosyntropin USAN *adrenocorticotropic hormone; diagnostic aid for adrenal function* [also: tetracosactide; tetracosactrin]

cotarnine chloride NF

cotarnine HCl [see: cotarnine chloride]

Cotazym capsules ℞ *digestive enzymes; antacid* [lipase; protease; amylase; calcium carbonate] 8000 U•30 000 U•30 000 U•25 mg

Cotazym-S capsules containing enteric-coated spheres ℞ *digestive enzymes* [lipase; protease; amylase] 5000•20 000•20 000 U

cotinine INN *antidepressant* [also: cotinine fumarate]

cotinine fumarate USAN *antidepressant* [also: cotinine]

Cotridin ⓒᴬᴺ syrup ℞ *narcotic antitussive; decongestant; antihistamine* [codeine phosphate; pseudoephedrine HCl; triprolidine HCl] 2•6•0.4 mg/mL

Cotridin Expectorant ⓒᴬᴺ oral solution ℞ *narcotic antitussive; decongestant; antihistamine* [codeine phosphate; pseudoephedrine HCl; triprolidine HCl; guaifenesin] 2•6•0.4•20 mg/mL

Cotrim; Cotrim D.S. tablets ℞ *anti-infective; antibacterial* [trimethoprim; sulfamethoxazole] 80•400 mg; 160•800 mg ② Cortin

Cotrim Pediatric oral suspension ℞ *anti-infective; antibacterial* [trimethoprim; sulfamethoxazole] 40•200 mg/5 mL

co-trimoxazole BAN [also: trimethoprim + sulfamethoxazole] ② clotrimazole

cotriptyline INN

cotton, purified USP *surgical aid*

cottonseed oil NF *solvent*

cottonweed medicinal herb [see: milkweed]

Co-Tuss V liquid ℞ *narcotic antitussive; expectorant* [hydrocodone bitartrate; guaifenesin] 5•100 mg

couch grass (*Agropyron repens*) rhizomes, roots, and stems *medicinal herb for blood cleansing, cystitis, diabetes, jaundice, kidney problems, upper respiratory tract inflammation with mucous discharge, rheumatism, and urinary infections*

Cough syrup OTC *antitussive; decongestant; expectorant* [dextromethorphan hydrobromide; phenylephrine HCl; guaifenesin] 10•5•100 mg/5 mL

Cough Formula liquid OTC *antitussive; antihistamine* [dextromethorphan hydrobromide; chlorpheniramine maleate; alcohol 10%] 15•2 mg/5 mL

Cough Formula with Decongestant liquid OTC *antitussive; decongestant* [dextromethorphan hydrobromide; pseudoephedrine HCl; alcohol 10%] 10•20 mg/5 mL

coughroot medicinal herb [see: birthroot]

coughweed medicinal herb [see: life root]

coughwort medicinal herb [see: coltsfoot]

Cough-X lozenges OTC *antitussive; topical oral anesthetic* [dextromethorphan hydrobromide; benzocaine] 5•2 mg

Coulter HIV-1 p24 Antigen Assay test for professional use *in vitro diagnostic aid for HIV in the blood*

Coumadin tablets, powder for IV injection ℞ *coumarin-derivative anticoagulant* [warfarin sodium] 1, 2, 2.5, 3, 4, 5, 6, 7.5, 10 mg; 2 mg ② Kemadrin

coumafos INN [also: coumaphos]
coumamycin INN *antibacterial* [also: coumermycin]
coumaphos BAN [also: coumafos]
coumarin NF *anticoagulant; investigational (orphan) for renal cell carcinoma*
coumarins *a class of anticoagulants that interfere with vitamin K-dependent clotting factors*
coumazoline INN
coumermycin USAN *antibacterial* [also: coumamycin]
coumermycin sodium USAN *antibacterial*
coumetarol INN [also: cumetharol]
counterirritants *a class of agents that produce superficial irritation in one part of the body to relieve irritation in another part*
Covangesic tablets OTC *decongestant; antihistamine; analgesic* [phenylpropanolamine HCl; phenylephrine HCl; chlorpheniramine maleate; pyrilamine maleate; acetaminophen] 12.5•7.5•2•12.5•275 mg
covatin HCl [see: captodiame HCl]
Covera-HS film-coated, extended-release tablets ℞ *antihypertensive; antianginal; antiarrhythmic; calcium channel blocker* [verapamil HCl] 180, 240 mg ② Provera
Coviracil ℞ *investigational (Phase I/II) antiviral for HIV* [emtricitabine]
cow cabbage *medicinal herb* [see: masterwort; white pond lily]
cow parsnip *medicinal herb* [see: masterwort]
cowslip (Caltha palustris) *plant medicinal herb used as an analgesic, antispasmodic, diaphoretic, diuretic, expectorant, and rubefacient*
cowslip, Jerusalem *medicinal herb* [see: lungwort]
COX-2 (cyclooxygenase-2) inhibitors *a class of nonsteroidal anti-inflammatory drugs (NSAIDs) for osteoarthritis, rheumatoid arthritis, acute pain, and primary dysmenorrhea*
Cozaar film-coated tablets ℞ *antihypertensive; angiotensin II receptor*

antagonist [losartan potassium] 25, 50, 100 mg
CP (chlorambucil, prednisone) *chemotherapy protocol*
CP (cyclophosphamide, Platinol) *chemotherapy protocol*
CP (cyclophosphamide, prednisone) *chemotherapy protocol*
CPB (cyclophosphamide, Platinol, BCNU) *chemotherapy protocol*
CPB-1011 *investigational (Phase III) treatment for idiopathic thrombocytopenic purpura (ITP)*
CPC (cyclophosphamide, Platinol, carboplatin) *chemotherapy protocol*
CPC-111 *investigational (Phase III) cardioprotective agent used in coronary artery bypass graft surgery; investigational (Phase II) for pain during sickle cell crisis*
CPM (CCNU, procarbazine, methotrexate) *chemotherapy protocol*
CPOB (cyclophosphamide, prednisone, Oncovin, bleomycin) *chemotherapy protocol*
CPT-11 (camptothecin-11) [see: irinotecan]
CPX *investigational (Phase II) protein repair therapy for cystic fibrosis*
^{51}Cr [see: albumin, chromated Cr 51 serum]
^{51}Cr [see: chromic chloride Cr 51]
^{51}Cr [see: chromic phosphate Cr 51]
^{51}Cr [see: sodium chromate Cr 51]
cramp bark (Viburnum opulus) bark and berries *medicinal herb for asthma, convulsions, cramps, heart palpitations, hypertension, hysteria, leg cramps, nervousness, spasm, and urinary disorders*
crampweed *medicinal herb* [see: cinquefoil]
cranberry (Vaccinium edule; V. erythrocarpum; V. macrocarpon; V. oxycoccos; V. vitis) fruit *medicinal herb for bladder, kidney, and urinary tract infections; also used to decrease the rate of urine degradation and odor formation in incontinent patients*
cranesbill; spotted cranesbill *medicinal herb* [see: alum root]

Crataegus laevigata; C. monogyna; C. oxyacantha medicinal herb [see: hawthorn]

crawley; crawley root medicinal herb [see: coral root]

CRDS (curdlan sulfate) [q.v.]

Creamy Tar shampoo OTC *antiseborrheic; antipsoriatic; antipruritic; antibacterial* [coal tar] 7.32%

creatinolfosfate INN

Creon capsules containing enteric-coated microspheres ℞ *digestive enzymes* [pancreatin; lipase; protease; amylase] 300 mg•8000 U•13 000 U•30 000 U

Creon 10; Creon 20 capsules containing enteric-coated microspheres ℞ *digestive enzymes* [lipase; amylase; protease] 10 000•33 200•37 500 U; 20 000•66 400•75 000 U

creosote carbonate USP

Creo-Terpin liquid OTC *antitussive* [dextromethorphan hydrobromide; alcohol 25%] 10 mg/15 mL

cresol NF *disinfectant*

cresotamide INN

cresoxydiol [see: mephenesin]

crestomycin sulfate [see: paromomycin sulfate]

Cresylate ear drops ℞ *antibacterial; antifungal* [m-cresyl acetate; chlorobutanol; alcohol] 25%•25%•1%

cresylic acid [see: cresol]

crilanomer INN

crilvastatin USAN, INN *antihyperlipidemic*

Crinone vaginal gel ℞ *progestin replacement or supplementation for assisted reproductive technology (ART) treatment* [progesterone] 8%

crisnatol INN *antineoplastic* [also: crisnatol mesylate]

crisnatol mesylate USAN *antineoplastic* [also: crisnatol]

Criticare HN ready-to-use liquid OTC *enteral nutritional therapy* [lactose-free formula]

Crixivan capsules ℞ *antiviral; HIV protease inhibitor* [indinavir sulfate] 200, 333, 400 mg

crobefate INN *combining name for radicals or groups*

croconazole INN

crocus, autumn medicinal herb [see: autumn crocus]

Crocus sativus medicinal herb [see: saffron]

crofilcon A USAN *hydrophilic contact lens material*

Crolom eye drops ℞ *mast cell stabilizer; ocular antiallergic and antiviral for vernal keratoconjunctivitis (orphan)* [cromolyn sodium] 4%

cromacate INN *combining name for radicals or groups*

cromakalim INN, BAN

Cro-Man-Zin tablets OTC *mineral supplement* [chromium; manganese; zinc] 0.2•5•25 mg

cromesilate INN *combining name for radicals or groups*

cromitrile INN *antiasthmatic* [also: cromitrile sodium]

cromitrile sodium USAN *antiasthmatic* [also: cromitrile]

cromoglicic acid INN *prophylactic antiasthmatic* [also: cromolyn sodium; cromoglycic acid]

cromoglycic acid BAN *prophylactic antiasthmatic* [also: cromolyn sodium; cromoglicic acid]

cromolyn sodium USAN, USP *anti-inflammatory; mast cell stabilizer for prophylactic treatment of allergy, asthma, and bronchospasm; treatment for mastocytosis and vernal keratoconjunctivitis (orphan)* [also: cromoglicic acid; cromoglycic acid] 20 mg/2 mL inhalation

Cronassial orphan status withdrawn 1996 [gangliosides, sodium salts]

cronetal [see: disulfiram]

cronidipine INN

cropropamide INN, BAN

croscarmellose INN *tablet disintegrant* [also: croscarmellose sodium]

croscarmellose sodium USAN, NF *tablet disintegrant* [also: croscarmellose]

crosfumaril [see: hemoglobin crosfumaril]

crospovidone NF *tablet excipient*
cross-linked carboxymethylcellulose sodium [now: croscarmellose sodium]
cross-linked carmellose sodium [see: croscarmellose sodium]
CroTab ℞ *investigational (orphan) treatment of Crotalidae snake bites* [antivenin (Crotalidae) polyvalent (ovine) Fab]
crotaline antivenin [see: antivenin (Crotalidae) polyvalent]
crotamiton USP, INN, BAN *scabicide*
crotetamide INN [also: crotethamide]
crotethamide BAN [also: crotetamide]
crotoniazide INN
crotonylidenisoniazid [see: crotoniazide]
crotoxyfos BAN
crowfoot *medicinal herb* [see: alum root; buttercup]
crowfoot buttercup; acrid crowfoot; cursed crowfoot; marsh crowfoot; meadow crowfoot; tall crowfoot; water crowfoot *medicinal herb* [see: buttercup]
crown, priest's *medicinal herb* [see: dandelion]
crude tuberculin [see: tuberculin, old]
Cruex cream, aerosol powder OTC *topical antifungal* [undecylenic acid; zinc undecylenate] 20% total; 19% total
Cruex powder OTC *topical antifungal* [calcium undecylenate] 10%
crufomate USAN, INN, BAN *veterinary anthelmintic*
cryofluorane INN *aerosol propellant* [also: dichlorotetrafluoroethane]
Cryptaz ℞ *investigational (NDA filed, orphan) anti-infective for AIDS-related cryptosporidial diarrhea (NDA withdrawn 1998)* [nitazoxanide]
cryptenamine acetates
Crypto-LA slide test for professional use *in vitro diagnostic aid for Cryptococcus neoformans antigens*
Cryptosporidium parvum bovine colostrum IgG concentrate *investigational (orphan) for Cryptosporidium-induced diarrhea in immunocompromised patients*

crystal violet [see: gentian violet]
crystallized trypsin [see: trypsin, crystallized]
Crystamine IM or subcu injection ℞ *antianemic; vitamin B$_{12}$ supplement* [cyanocobalamin] 1000 μg/mL
Crysti 1000 IM or subcu injection ℞ *antianemic; vitamin B$_{12}$ supplement* [cyanocobalamin] 1000 μg/mL
Crysticillin 300 A.S.; Crysticillin 600 A.S. IM injection (discontinued 1998) ℞ *natural penicillin antibiotic* [penicillin G procaine] 300 000 U/mL; 600 000 U/1.2 mL dose
Crystodigin tablets ℞ *cardiac glycoside to increase cardiac output; antiarrhythmic* [digitoxin] 0.05, 0.1 mg
crystografin [see: meglumine diatrizoate]
^{131}Cs [see: cesium chloride Cs 131]
C-Solve OTC *lotion base*
CSP (cellulose sodium phosphate) [q.v.]
CT (cisplatin, Taxol) *chemotherapy protocol*
CT (cytarabine, thioguanine) *chemotherapy protocol*
CT-3 *investigational anti-inflammatory*
CTAB (cetyltrimethyl ammonium bromide)
CTCb (cyclophosphamide, thiotepa, carboplatin) *chemotherapy protocol*
CTH (ceramide trihexosidase) [q.v.]
CTLA4-Ig *investigational humanized monoclonal antibody for psoriasis, organ transplant rejection, and autoimmune disorders*
CTP-37 *investigational theraccine for metastatic colorectal cancer*
C/T/S topical solution ℞ *topical antibiotic for acne* [clindamycin phosphate] 10 mg/mL
Ctx-Plat (cyclophosphamide, Platinol) *chemotherapy protocol*
^{64}Cu [see: cupric acetate Cu 64]
cubeb *(Piper cubeba)* unripe berries *medicinal herb used as an antiseptic, antisyphilitic, carminative, diuretic, expectorant, stimulant, and stomachic*

cucurbita (*Cucurbita maxima; C. moschata; C. pepa*) seeds *medicinal herb for prophylaxis, immobilizing, and aiding in the expulsion of intestinal worms and parasites; also used in prostate gland disorders*

Culturette 10 Minute Group A Strep ID slide test *for professional use in vitro diagnostic test for Group A streptococcal antigens in throat swabs* [latex agglutination test]

Culver's physic *medicinal herb* [see: Culver's root]

Culver's root (*Varonicastrum virginicum*) *medicinal herb for blood cleansing, diarrhea, and liver and stomach disorders*

cumetharol BAN [also: coumetarol]

cumin (*Cuminum cyminum; C. odorum*) seeds and oil *medicinal herb for gastric cancer; also used as an antioxidant*

cupric acetate Cu 64 USAN *radioactive agent*

cupric chloride USP *dietary copper supplement*

cupric sulfate USP *antidote to phosphorus; dietary copper supplement* 0.4, 2 mg/mL injection

Cuprimine capsules ℞ *metal chelating agent for rheumatoid arthritis, Wilson's disease, and cystinuria* [penicillamine] 125, 250 mg

cuprimyxin USAN, INN *veterinary antibacterial; antifungal*

cuproxoline INN, BAN

Curaçao aloe *medicinal herb* [see: aloe]

curare [see: tubocurarine chloride]

Curcuma domestica; C. longa *medicinal herb* [see: turmeric]

curdlan sulfate (CRDS) *investigational (Phase II) antiviral for HIV*

cure-all *medicinal herb* [see: lemon balm]

curium *element* (Cm)

curled dock; curly dock *medicinal herb* [see: yellow dock]

curled mint *medicinal herb* [see: peppermint]

curls, blue *medicinal herb* [see: woundwort]

Curosurf ℞ *investigational (orphan) for infant respiratory distress syndrome of prematurity* [pulmonary surfactant replacement, porcine]

curral [see: diallylbarbituric acid]

currant (*Ribes nigrum; R. rubrum*) leaves and fruit *medicinal herb used as a diaphoretic and diuretic*

Curretab tablets ℞ *progestin for secondary amenorrhea, abnormal uterine bleeding, and endometrial hyperplasia* [medroxyprogesterone acetate] 10 mg

custard apple *medicinal herb* [see: pawpaw]

Cūtar Bath Oil Emulsion OTC *antipsoriatic; antiseborrheic; antipruritic; emollient* [coal tar] 7.5%

Cūtemol cream OTC *moisturizer; emollient* [allantoin]

Cuticura ointment (discontinued 1995) OTC *topical acne treatment* [sulfur; phenol; oxyquinoline] 0.5% • 0.1% • 0.05%

Cuticura Medicated Soap bar OTC *therapeutic skin cleanser* [triclocarban] 1%

Cutivate cream, ointment ℞ *topical corticosteroidal anti-inflammatory* [fluticasone propionate] 0.05%; 0.005%

CV (cisplatin, VePesid) *chemotherapy protocol*

CVA (cyclophosphamide, vincristine, Adriamycin) *chemotherapy protocol*

CVA-BMP; CVA + BMP (cyclophosphamide, vincristine, Adriamycin, BCNU, methotrexate, procarbazine) *chemotherapy protocol*

CVAD; C-VAD (cyclophosphamide, vincristine, Adriamycin, dexamethasone) *chemotherapy protocol*

CVB (CCNU, vinblastine, bleomycin) *chemotherapy protocol*

CVBD (CCNU, bleomycin, vinblastine, dexamethasone) *chemotherapy protocol*

CVD (cisplatin, vinblastine, dacarbazine) *chemotherapy protocol*

CVEB (cisplatin, vinblastine, etoposide, bleomycin) *chemotherapy protocol*

CVI (carboplatin, VePesid, ifosfamide [with mesna rescue]) *chemotherapy protocol* [also: VIC]

CVM (cyclophosphamide, vincristine, methotrexate) *chemotherapy protocol*

CVP (cyclophosphamide, vincristine, prednisone) *chemotherapy protocol*

CVPP (CCNU, vinblastine, procarbazine, prednisone) *chemotherapy protocol*

CVPP (cyclophosphamide, Velban, procarbazine, prednisone) *chemotherapy protocol*

CVPP-CCNU (cyclophosphamide, vinblastine, procarbazine, prednisone, CCNU) *chemotherapy protocol*

CVT-124 *investigational (Phase II) for treatment of edema associated with congestive heart failure*

CVT-313 *investigational agent for preventing restenosis*

CVT-510 *investigational (Phase I) selective adenosine A1 receptor agonist for atrial arrhythmias*

CY-1503 *investigational (Phase III, orphan) adjunct to surgery for congenital heart defects in newborns; investigational (orphan) for postischemic pulmonary reperfusion edema (all clinical trials discontinued 1999)*

CY-1899 *investigational (orphan) for chronic active hepatitis B*

CY-2301 *investigational (Phase I) vaccine for HIV*

cyacetacide INN [also: cyacetazide]

cyacetazide BAN [also: cyacetacide]

CyADIC (cyclophosphamide, Adriamycin, DIC) *chemotherapy protocol*

cyamemazine INN

cyamepromazine [see: cyamemazine]

cyanamide JAN [also: calcium carbimide]

cyani *medicinal herb* [see: cornflower]

Cyanide Antidote Package ℞ *emergency treatment of cyanide poisoning* [sodium nitrite; sodium thiosulfate; amyl nitrite inhalant] 300 mg•12.5 g•0.3 mL

cyanoacetohydrazide [see: cyacetazide]

cyanocobalamin USP, INN, BAN, JAN *vitamin B₁₂; hematopoietic* 25, 50, 100, 250, 500, 1000 μg oral; 100, 1000 μg/mL injection

cyanocobalamin (⁵⁷Co) INN *pernicious anemia test; radioactive agent* [also: cyanocobalamin Co 57]

cyanocobalamin (⁵⁸Co) INN

cyanocobalamin (⁶⁰Co) INN *pernicious anemia test; radioactive agent* [also: cyanocobalamin Co 60]

cyanocobalamin Co 57 USAN, USP *pernicious anemia test; radioactive agent* [also: cyanocobalamin (⁵⁷Co)]

cyanocobalamin Co 60 USAN, USP *pernicious anemia test; radioactive agent* [also: cyanocobalamin (⁶⁰Co)]

Cyanoject IM or subcu injection ℞ *antianemic; vitamin B₁₂ supplement* [cyanocobalamin] 1000 μg/mL

cyclacillin USAN, USP *antibacterial* [also: ciclacillin]

cyclamate calcium NF

cyclamic acid USAN, BAN *non-nutritive sweetener (banned in the U.S.)*

cyclamide [see: glycyclamide]

Cyclan capsules (discontinued 1997) ℞ *peripheral vasodilator; vascular smooth muscle relaxant* [cyclandelate] 200, 400 mg

cyclandelate INN, BAN, JAN *peripheral vasodilator; vascular smooth muscle relaxant*

cyclarbamate INN, BAN

cyclazocine USAN, INN *analgesic*

cyclazodone INN

cyclexanone INN

cyclic propylene carbonate [see: propylene carbonate]

cyclindole USAN *antidepressant* [also: ciclindole]

Cyclinex-1 powder OTC *formula for infants with urea cycle disorders or gyrate atrophy*

Cyclinex-2 powder OTC *enteral nutritional therapy for urea cycle disorders* *or gyrate atrophy* [multiple essential amino acids]

cycliramine INN *antihistamine* [also: cycliramine maleate]

cycliramine maleate USAN *antihistamine* [also: cycliramine]

cyclizine USP, INN, BAN *antihistamine; antiemetic; anticholinergic; motion sickness relief*

cyclizine HCl USP, BAN *antiemetic*

cyclizine lactate USP, BAN *antinauseant*

cyclobarbital NF, INN [also: cyclobarbitone]

cyclobarbital calcium NF

cyclobarbitone BAN [also: cyclobarbital]

cyclobendazole USAN *anthelmintic* [also: ciclobendazole]

cyclobenzaprine INN *skeletal muscle relaxant* [also: cyclobenzaprine HCl]

cyclobenzaprine HCl USAN, USP *skeletal muscle relaxant* [also: cyclobenzaprine] 10 mg oral

cyclobutoic acid INN

cyclobutyrol INN

cyclocarbothiamine [see: cycotiamine]

Cyclocort ointment, cream, lotion ℞ *topical corticosteroidal anti-inflammatory* [amcinonide] 0.1%

cyclocoumarol BAN

cyclocumarol [see: cyclocoumarol]

α-cyclodextrin [see: alfadex]

Cyclofed Pediatric syrup ℞ *pediatric narcotic antitussive, decongestant, and expectorant* [codeine phosphate; pseudoephedrine HCl; guaifenesin; alcohol 6%] 10•30•100 mg/5 mL

cyclofenil INN, BAN

cyclofilcon A USAN *hydrophilic contact lens material*

cycloguanil embonate INN, BAN *antimalarial* [also: cycloguanil pamoate]

cycloguanil pamoate USAN *antimalarial* [also: cycloguanil embonate]

Cyclogyl Drop-Tainers (eye drops) ℞ *cycloplegic; mydriatic* [cyclopentolate HCl] 0.5%, 1%, 2%

cyclohexanehexol [see: inositol]

cyclohexanesulfamate dihydrate [see: sodium cyclamate]

cyclohexanesulfamic acid *(banned in the U.S.)* [see: cyclamic acid]

cycloheximide USAN *antipsoriatic* [also: cicloheximide]

p-cyclohexylhydratropic acid [see: hexaprofen]

N-cyclohexyllinoleamide [see: clinolamide]

4-cyclohexyloxybenzoate [see: cyclomethycaine]

1-cyclohexylpropyl carbamate [see: procymate]

N-cyclohexylsulfamic acid *(banned in the U.S.)* [see: cyclamic acid]

cyclomenol INN

cyclomethicone NF *wetting agent*

cyclomethycaine INN, BAN *local anesthetic* [also: cyclomethycaine sulfate]

cyclomethycaine sulfate USP *local anesthetic* [also: cyclomethycaine]

Cyclomydril Drop-Tainers (eye drops) ℞ *cycloplegic; mydriatic* [cyclopentolate HCl; phenylephrine HCl] 0.2%•1%

cyclonium iodide [see: oxapium iodide]

cyclooxygenase-2 (COX-2) inhibitors *a class of investigational anti-inflammatory drugs*

cyclopentamine INN, BAN [also: cyclopentamine HCl]

cyclopentamine HCl USP [also: cyclopentamine]

cyclopentaphene [see: cyclarbamate]

cyclopenthiazide USAN, INN, BAN *antihypertensive*

cyclopentolate INN, BAN *ophthalmic anticholinergic* [also: cyclopentolate HCl]

cyclopentolate HCl USP *ophthalmic anticholinergic; mydriatic; cycloplegic* [also: cyclopentolate] 1% eye drops

8-cyclopentyl 1,3-dipropylxanthine *investigational (orphan) for cystic fibrosis*

cyclophenazine HCl USAN *antipsychotic* [also: ciclofenazine]

cyclophosphamide USP, INN, BAN, JAN *nitrogen mustard-type alkylating antineoplastic; immunosuppressive*

cycloplegics *a class of drugs that paralyze the ciliary muscles of the eye*

cyclopolydimethylsiloxane [see: cyclomethicone]

cyclopregnol INN

cycloprolol BAN *antiadrenergic (β-receptor)* [also: cicloprolol HCl; cicloprolol]

cyclopropane USP, INN *inhalation general anesthetic*

Cyclo-Prostin ℞ *investigational (orphan) vasodilator for primary pulmonary hypertension* [epoprostenol]

cyclopyrronium bromide INN

cycloserine (L-cycloserine) USP, INN, BAN, JAN *bacteriostatic; tuberculosis retreatment; investigational (orphan) for Gaucher's disease*

Cyclospasmol capsules (discontinued 1997) ℞ *peripheral vasodilator; vascular smooth muscle relaxant* [cyclandelate] 200, 400 mg

Cyclospasmol ⓐ film-coated tablets ℞ *peripheral vasodilator; vascular smooth muscle relaxant* [cyclandelate] 200 mg

cyclosporin BAN *immunosuppressive* [also: cyclosporine; ciclosporin]

cyclosporin A [now: cyclosporine]

cyclosporine USAN, USP *immunosuppressive for transplants, rheumatoid arthritis, and psoriasis; investigational (orphan) for Sjögren's keratoconjunctivitis sicca and corneal melting syndrome* [also: ciclosporin; cyclosporin]

CycloTech (trademarked delivery device) *provides premeasured doses of oral liquids and records dosing times*

cyclothiazide USAN, USP, INN, BAN *diuretic; antihypertensive*

cyclovalone INN

cycobemin [see: cyanocobalamin]

Cycofed Pediatric syrup ℞ *narcotic antitussive; decongestant; expectorant* [codeine phosphate; pseudoephedrine HCl; guaifenesin; alcohol 6%] 10•30•100 mg

cycotiamine INN

cycrimine INN, BAN [also: cycrimine HCl]

cycrimine HCl USP [also: cycrimine]

Cycrin tablets ℞ *progestin for secondary amenorrhea, abnormal uterine bleeding, and endometrial hyperplasia* [medroxyprogesterone acetate] 2.5, 5, 10 mg

cyfluthrin BAN

cyhalothrin BAN

cyheptamide USAN, INN *anticonvulsant*

cyheptropine INN

CyHOP (cyclophosphamide, Halotestin, Oncovin, prednisone) *chemotherapy protocol*

Cyklokapron tablets, IV injection ℞ *systemic hemostatic; orphan status withdrawn 1996* [tranexamic acid] 500 mg; 100 mg/mL

Cylert tablets, chewable tablets ℞ *CNS stimulant for attention deficit hyperactivity disorders (ADHD)* [pemoline] 18.75, 37.5, 75 mg; 37.5 mg

Cylex; Cylex Sugar-Free throat lozenges OTC *topical oral anesthetic; antiseptic* [benzocaine; cetylpyridinium chloride] 15•5 mg

Cylexin ℞ *investigational (Phase III, orphan) adjunct to surgery for congenital heart defects in newborns; investigational (orphan) for postischemic pulmonary reperfusion edema (all clinical trials discontinued 1999)* [CY-1503 (code name—generic name not yet assigned)]

Cymbopogon citratus *medicinal herb* [see: lemongrass]

Cymbopogon nardus; C. winterianus *medicinal herb* [see: citronella]

cymemoxine [see: cimemoxin]

Cynara scolymus *medicinal herb* [see: artichoke]

cynarine INN

Cyomin IM or subcu injection ℞ *antianemic; vitamin B$_{12}$ supplement* [cyanocobalamin] 1000 μg/mL

cypenamine INN, BAN *antidepressant* [also: cypenamine HCl]

cypenamine HCl USAN *antidepressant* [also: cypenamine]

cypionate USAN, BAN *combining name for radicals or groups* [also: cipionate]

Cyplex *investigational (Phase II) platelet alternative* [infusible platelet membranes]

cypothrin USAN *veterinary insecticide*

cyprazepam USAN, INN *sedative*

cyprenorphine INN, BAN

cyprenorphine HCl [see: cyprenorphine]

Cypripedium pubescens medicinal herb [see: lady's slipper]

cyprodemanol [see: cyprodenate]

cyprodenate INN

cyproheptadine INN, BAN *piperidine antihistamine; antipruritic* [also: cyproheptadine HCl]

cyproheptadine HCl USP, JAN *piperidine antihistamine; antipruritic* [also: cyproheptadine] 4 mg oral; 2 mg/5 mL oral

cyprolidol INN *antidepressant* [also: cyprolidol HCl]

cyprolidol HCl USAN *antidepressant* [also: cyprolidol]

cyproquinate USAN *coccidiostat for poultry* [also: ciproquinate]

cyproterone INN, BAN *antiandrogen* [also: cyproterone acetate]

cyproterone acetate USAN *antiandrogen; orphan status withdrawn 1996* [also: cyproterone]

cyproximide USAN *antipsychotic; antidepressant* [also: ciproximide]

cyren A [see: diethylstilbestrol]

cyren B [see: diethylstilbestrol dipropionate]

cyromazine INN, BAN

Cystadane powder for oral solution ℞ *electrolyte replenisher for homocystinuria (orphan)* [betaine HCl] 1 g

Cystagon capsules ℞ *antiurolithic for nephropathic cystinosis (orphan)* [cysteamine bitartrate] 50, 150 mg

cystamin [see: methenamine]

cysteamine USAN, BAN *antiurolithic for nephropathic cystinosis (orphan)* [also: mercaptamine]

cysteamine bitartrate *antiurolithic for nephropathic cystinosis (orphan)*

cysteamine HCl USAN *antiurolithic; investigational (orphan) for corneal cystine crystal accumulation in cystinosis patients*

cysteine (L-cysteine) INN *nonessential amino acid; symbols: Cys, C; investigational (orphan) for erythropoietic protoporphyria photosensitivity* [also: cysteine HCl]

cysteine HCl (L-cysteine HCl) USP *nonessential amino acid* [also: cysteine] 50 mg/mL injection

L-cysteine HCl monohydrate [see: cysteine HCl]

Cystex tablets ℞ *urinary antibiotic; analgesic; acidifier* [methenamine; sodium salicylate; benzoic acid] 162•162.5•32 mg

cystic fibrosis gene therapy *investigational (orphan) for cystic fibrosis*

cystic fibrosis transmembrane conductance regulator (CFTR) *investigational (orphan) for cystic fibrosis*

cystic fibrosis transmembrane conductance regulator, recombinant adenovirus (AdGV-CFTR) *investigational (orphan) for cystic fibrosis*

cystine (L-cystine) USAN *amino acid*

Cysto-Conray; Cysto-Conray II intracavitary instillation ℞ *radiopaque contrast medium for urological imaging* [iothalamate meglumine (47% iodine)] 430 mg/mL (202 mg/mL); 172 mg/mL (81 mg/mL)

cystogen [see: methenamine]

Cystografin; Cystografin Dilute intracavitary instillation ℞ *radiopaque contrast medium for urological imaging* [diatrizoate meglumine (46.67% iodine)] 300 mg/mL (141 mg/mL); 180 mg/mL (85 mg/mL)

Cystospaz tablets ℞ *GI antispasmodic; anticholinergic* [hyoscyamine sulfate] 0.15 mg

Cystospaz-M timed-release capsules ℞ *GI antispasmodic; anticholinergic* [hyoscyamine sulfate] 0.375 mg

CYT-103-Y-90 *investigational for ovarian cancer; orphan status withdrawn 1998*

CYTABOM (cytarabine, bleomycin, Oncovin, mechlorethamine) *chemotherapy protocol*

Cytadren tablets ℞ *adrenal steroid inhibitor; antisteroidal antineoplastic for corticotropin-producing tumors* [aminoglutethimide] 250 mg

cytarabine USAN, USP, INN, BAN *antimetabolite antineoplastic for various leukemias* 100, 500, 1000, 2000 mg injection ⑨ vidarabine

cytarabine, liposomal *antimetabolite antineoplastic for lymphomatous neoplastic meningitis (orphan)*

cytarabine HCl USAN *antiviral*

Cytisus scoparius medicinal herb [see: broom]

CytoGam IV infusion ℞ *adjunct to organ transplants from CMV seropositive donor to CMV seronegative recipient (orphan)* [cytomegalovirus immune globulin, solvent/detergent treated] 50 mg/mL

CytoImplant ℞ *investigational (orphan) for pancreatic cancer* [blood mononuclear cells, allogenic peripheral]

Cytolex cream ℞ *investigational (NDA filed) broad-spectrum antibiotic for impetigo and diabetic foot ulcers* [pexiganan acetate] 1%

cytolin *investigational (Phase I/II) monoclonal antibody for AIDS*

cytomegalovirus immune globulin, human *prevention of primary cytomegalovirus in organ transplants in immunocompromised patients (orphan)*

cytomegalovirus immune globulin intravenous (CMV-IGIV) & ganciclovir sodium *investigational (orphan) for cytomegalovirus pneumonia in bone marrow transplant patients*

Cytomel tablets ℞ *thyroid hormone* [liothyronine sodium] 5, 25, 50 µg

cytoprotective agents *a class of drugs that provide prophylaxis against the side effects of antineoplastic agents*

Cytosar-U powder for subcu, intrathecal or IV injection ℞ *antimetabolite antineoplastic for various leukemias* [cytarabine] 100, 500, 1000, 2000 mg/vial

cytosine arabinoside (ara-C) [see: cytarabine]

cytosine arabinoside HCl [now: cytarabine HCl]

Cytosol liquid ℞ *sterile irrigant* [physiological irrigating solution]

CytoTab ℞ *investigational (Phase I) antibody for use in renal transplantation*

Cytotec tablets ℞ *prevention of NSAID-induced gastric ulcers* [misoprostol] 100, 200 µg

cytotoxic lymphocyte maturation factor [see: edodekin alfa]

Cytovene capsules ℞ *antiviral for cytomegalovirus (CMV); investigational (Phase I/II) for AIDS prophylaxis* [ganciclovir] 250, 500 mg

Cytovene powder for IV infusion ℞ *antiviral for cytomegalovirus (CMV); investigational (Phase I/II) for AIDS prophylaxis* [ganciclovir sodium] 500 mg/vial

Cytoxan tablets, powder for IV injection ℞ *nitrogen mustard-type alkylating antineoplastic for multiple leukemias, lymphomas, blastomas, sarcomas and organ cancers* [cyclophosphamide] 25, 50 mg; 100 mg

Cytra-2 solution ℞ *urinary alkalizing agent* [sodium citrate; citric acid] 500•334 mg/5 mL

Cytra-3 syrup ℞ *urinary alkalinizing agent* [potassium citrate; sodium citrate; citric acid] 550•500•334 mg/5 mL

Cytra-K oral solution ℞ *urinary alkalizing agent* [potassium citrate; citric acid] 1100•334 mg/5 mL

Cytra-LC solution ℞ *urinary alkalizing agent* [potassium citrate; sodium citrate; citric acid] 550•500•334 mg/5 mL

CY-VA-DACT (Cytoxin, vincristine, Adriamycin, dactinomycin) *chemotherapy protocol*

CYVADIC; CY-VA-DIC; CyVADIC (cyclophosphamide, vincristine, Adriamycin, DIC) *chemotherapy protocol*

CYVMAD (cyclophosphamide, vincristine, methotrexate, Adriamycin, DTIC) *chemotherapy protocol*

D (vitamin D) [q.v.]

D-2.5-W; D-5-W; D-10-W; D-20-W; D-25-W; D-30-W; D-40-W; D-50-W; D-60-W; D-70-W ℞ *intravenous nutritional therapy* [dextrose]

D₂ (vitamin D₂) [see: ergocalciferol]

D-2163 *investigational (Phase I) anticancer agent*

D₃ (vitamin D₃) [see: cholecalciferol]

d4T [see: stavudine]

D.A. chewable tablets ℞ *decongestant; antihistamine; anticholinergic* [phenylephrine HCl; chlorpheniramine maleate; methscopolamine nitrate] 10•2•1.25 mg

DA (daunorubicin, ara-C) *chemotherapy protocol*

D.A. II tablets ℞ *decongestant; antihistamine; anticholinergic* [phenylephrine HCl; chlorpheniramine maleate; methscopolamine nitrate] 10•4•1.25 mg

DAA (dihydroxyaluminum aminoacetate) [q.v.]

DAB₃₈₉ IL-2 fusion toxin [now: denileukin diftitox]

dacarbazine USAN, USP, INN, BAN *antineoplastic for metastatic malignant melanoma and Hodgkin's disease* ② Dicarbosil; procarbazine

dacemazine INN

dacisteine INN

dacliximab USAN, INN *immunosuppressant monoclonal antibody for organ and bone marrow transplants (orphan)*

Dacplat ℞ *investigational (orphan) alkylating antineoplastic for ovarian and colorectal cancers* [oxaliplatin]

Dacriose ophthalmic solution OTC *extraocular irrigating solution* [sterile isotonic solution]

dactinomycin USAN, USP, BAN *antibiotic antineoplastic* [also: actinomycin D]

dacuronium bromide INN, BAN

DADDS (diacetyl diaminodiphenylsulfone) [see: acedapsone]

dagapamil INN

Daily Care ointment (name changed to Desitin Creamy in 1997)

Daily Vitamins liquid OTC *vitamin supplement* [multiple vitamins] ±

Daily-Vite with Iron & Minerals tablets OTC *vitamin/mineral/iron supplement* [multiple vitamins & minerals; iron; folic acid; biotin] ±•18•0.4•± mg

Dairy Ease chewable tablets OTC *digestive aid for lactose intolerance* [lactase enzyme] 3300 U

daisy, wild *medicinal herb* [see: wild daisy]

Daisy 2 test kit for home use (discontinued 1995) OTC *in vitro diagnostic aid for urine pregnancy test*

Dakin solution [see: sodium hypochlorite]

Dakrina eye drops (discontinued 1998) OTC *ophthalmic moisturizer/lubricant* [vitamin A palmitate; polyvinyl alcohol] 350 IU•0.6%

DAL (daunorubicin, ara-C, L-asparaginase) *chemotherapy protocol*

Dalacin ⒸⒶⓃ (U.S. product: Cleocin) vaginal cream ℞ *lincosamide antibiotic for bacterial vaginosis* [clindamycin phosphate] 2% (100 mg/5 g dose)

Dalacin C ⒸⒶⓃ (U.S. product: Cleocin) capsules ℞ *lincosamide antibiotic* [clindamycin HCl] 150, 300 mg

Dalacin C ⒸⒶⓃ (U.S. product: Cleocin Pediatric) granules for oral solution ℞ *lincosamide antibiotic* [clindamycin palmitate HCl] 75 mg/5 mL

Dalacin C Phosphate ⒸⒶⓃ (U.S. product: Cleocin Phosphate) IV infusion, IM injection ℞ *lincosamide antibiotic; treatment for AIDS-related Pneumocystis carinii pneumonia* [clindamycin phosphate] 150 mg/mL

Dalacin T ⒸⒶⓃ (U.S. product: Cleocin T) topical solution ℞ *topical antibiotic for acne* [clindamycin phosphate]

Dalalone intra-articular, intralesional, soft tissue, or IM injection ℞ *cortico-*

steroid; anti-inflammatory [dexamethasone sodium phosphate] 4 mg/mL

Dalalone D.P. intra-articular, soft tissue, or IM injection R̸ corticosteroid; anti-inflammatory [dexamethasone acetate] 16 mg/mL

Dalalone L.A. intralesional, intra-articular, soft tissue, or IM injection R̸ corticosteroid; anti-inflammatory [dexamethasone acetate] 8 mg/mL

dalanated insulin [see: insulin, dalanated]

dalbraminol INN

daledalin INN antidepressant [also: daledalin tosylate]

daledalin tosylate USAN antidepressant [also: daledalin]

dalfopristin USAN, INN streptogramin antibiotic bacteriostatic to gram-positive infections

dalfopristin & quinupristin two streptogramin antibiotics that are synergistically bactericidal to gram-positive infections; investigational (NDA filed) for pneumonia

Dalgan IV, subcu or IM injection R̸ narcotic agonist-antagonist analgesic [dezocine] 5, 10, 15 mg/mL

Dallergy tablets, sustained-release caplets, syrup R̸ decongestant; antihistamine; anticholinergic [phenylephrine HCl; chlorpheniramine maleate; methscopolamine nitrate] 10•4•1.25 mg; 20•8•2.5 mg; 10•2•0.625 mg/5 mL

Dallergy-D syrup OTC decongestant; antihistamine [phenylephrine HCl; chlorpheniramine maleate] 5•2 mg/5 mL

Dallergy-JR sustained-release capsules R̸ pediatric decongestant and antihistamine [pseudoephedrine HCl; brompheniramine maleate] 60•6 mg

Dalmane capsules R̸ benzodiazepine sedative; hypnotic; sometimes abused as a street drug [flurazepam HCl] 15, 30 mg ☒ Dialume

dalteparin sodium USAN, INN, BAN a low molecular weight heparin-type anticoagulant and antithrombotic for prevention of deep vein thrombosis

(DVT), unstable angina, and myocardial infarction

daltroban USAN, INN immunosuppressive

Damason-P tablets R̸ narcotic analgesic [hydrocodone bitartrate; aspirin] 5•500 mg

dambose [see: inositol]

dametralast INN

damiana (Turnera aphrodisiaca; T. diffusa; T. microphylla) leaves medicinal herb for bed-wetting, bronchitis, emphysema, headache, hormonal imbalance, hot flashes, menopause, and Parkinson's disease; also used as an aphrodisiac

damotepine INN

D-Amp capsules (discontinued 1997) R̸ aminopenicillin antibiotic [ampicillin] 500 mg

danaparoid sodium USAN, BAN glycosaminoglycan anticoagulant and antithrombotic to prevent deep vein thrombosis (DVT)

danazol USAN, USP, INN, BAN anterior pituitary suppressant; gonadotropin inhibitor for endometriosis 200 mg oral

dandelion (Leontodon taraxacum; Taraxacum officinale) leaves and root medicinal herb for anemia, analgesia, blisters, blood cleansing, blood glucose regulation, constipation, diaphoresis, dyspepsia, edema, endurance, gallbladder disease, hypertension, and liver disorders

daniplestim USAN treatment for chemotherapy-induced bone marrow suppression

daniquidone BAN

danitamon [see: menadione]

danitracen INN

Danocrine capsules R̸ gonadotropin inhibitor for endometriosis, fibrocystic breast disease, and hereditary angioedema [danazol] 50, 100, 200 mg

danofloxacin INN veterinary antibacterial [also: danofloxacin mesylate]

danofloxacin mesylate USAN veterinary antibacterial [also: danofloxacin]

danosteine INN

danshen (Salvia miltiorrhiza) medicinal herb for abdominal pain, bruises, circulatory problems, insomnia, menstrual irregularity, and stroke; also used as an aid in granulation of wounds

danthron USP, BAN (withdrawn from market by FDA) [also: dantron] ⊉ Dantrium

Dantrium capsules, powder for IV injection ℞ skeletal muscle relaxant [dantrolene sodium] 25, 50, 100 mg; 20 mg/vial (0.32 mg/mL) ⊉ danthron

dantrolene USAN, INN, BAN skeletal muscle relaxant

dantrolene sodium USAN, BAN skeletal muscle relaxant

dantron INN (withdrawn from market by FDA) [also: danthron]

Dapa tablets, capsules (discontinued 1997) OTC analgesic; antipyretic [acetaminophen] 325 mg; 500 mg

Dapacin Cold capsules OTC decongestant; antihistamine; analgesic [phenylpropanolamine HCl; chlorpheniramine maleate; acetaminophen] 12.5•2•325 mg

Daphne mezereum medicinal herb [see: mezereon]

dapiprazole INN α-adrenergic blocker; miotic; neuroleptic [also: dapiprazole HCl]

dapiprazole HCl USAN α-adrenergic blocker; miotic; neuroleptic [also: dapiprazole]

dapsone USAN, USP, BAN bactericidal; leprostatic; herpetiform dermatitis suppressant; investigational (orphan) for Pneumocystis carinii and toxoplasmosis

dapsone & trimethoprim investigational for Pneumocystis carinii pneumonia; orphan status withdrawn 1998

daptazole [see: amiphenazole]

daptomycin USAN, INN, BAN investigational (Phase III) antibiotic

Daranide tablets ℞ carbonic anhydrase inhibitor; diuretic [dichlorphenamide] 50 mg ⊉ Daraprim

Daraprim tablets ℞ antimalarial; toxoplasmosis treatment adjunct [pyrimethamine] 25 mg ⊉ Daranide

darbufelone mesylate USAN anti-inflammatory; antiarthritic; cyclo-oxygenase inhibitor; 5-lipoxygenase inhibitor

darenzepine INN

darglitazone sodium USAN oral hypoglycemic

Daricon tablets (discontinued 1997) ℞ adjunctive therapy for peptic ulcer [oxyphencyclimine HCl] 10 mg ⊉ Darvon

darodipine USAN, INN antihypertensive; bronchodilator; vasodilator

Darvocet-N 50; Darvocet-N 100 tablets ℞ narcotic analgesic [propoxyphene napsylate; acetaminophen] 50•325 mg; 100•650 mg ⊉ Darvon-N

Darvon Pulvules (capsules) ℞ narcotic analgesic [propoxyphene HCl] 65 mg ⊉ Daricon

Darvon Compound-65 Pulvules (capsules) ℞ narcotic analgesic [propoxyphene HCl; aspirin; caffeine] 65•389•32.4 mg

Darvon-N film-coated tablets ℞ narcotic analgesic [propoxyphene napsylate] 100 mg

Dasin capsules (discontinued 1995) OTC analgesic; antipyretic; anti-inflammatory; antispasmodic; emetic [aspirin; caffeine; atropine sulfate; ipecac] 130•8•0.13•3 mg

DAT (daunorubicin, ara-C, thioguanine) chemotherapy protocol [also: DCT; TAD]

datelliptium chloride INN

Datura stramonium medicinal herb [see: jimsonweed]

daturine hydrobromide [see: hyoscyamine hydrobromide]

DATVP (daunorubicin, ara-C, thioguanine, vincristine, prednisone) chemotherapy protocol

Daucus carota medicinal herb [see: carrot]

daunomycin [see: daunorubicin HCl]

daunorubicin (DNR) INN, BAN anthracycline antibiotic antineoplastic [also: daunorubicin HCl] ⊉ doxorubicin

daunorubicin citrate, liposomal anthracycline antibiotic antineoplastic for advanced HIV-related Kaposi sarcoma (orphan)

daunorubicin HCl USAN, USP, JAN *anthracycline antibiotic antineoplastic* [also: daunorubicin] ② doxorubicin

DaunoXome IV infusion ℞ *antibiotic antineoplastic for advanced AIDS-related Kaposi sarcoma (orphan)* [daunorubicin citrate, liposomal] 2 mg/mL

DAV (daunorubicin, ara-C, VePesid) *chemotherapy protocol*

DAVA (desacetyl vinblastine amide) [see: vindesine]

DAVH (dibromodulcitol, Adriamycin, vincristine, Halotestin) *chemotherapy protocol*

davitamon [see: menadione]

Dayalets Filmtabs (film-coated tablets) OTC *vitamin supplement* [multiple vitamins; folic acid] ± •0.4 mg

Dayalets + Iron Filmtabs (film-coated tablets) OTC *vitamin/iron supplement* [multiple vitamins; ferrous sulfate; folic acid] ± •18•0.4 mg

Daypro film-coated caplets ℞ *nonsteroidal anti-inflammatory drug (NSAID) for osteoarthritis and rheumatoid arthritis* [oxaprozin] 600 mg

DayQuil LiquiCaps (soft gel capsules), liquid OTC *antitussive; decongestant; expectorant; analgesic* [dextromethorphan hydrobromide; pseudoephedrine HCl; guaifenesin; acetaminophen] 10•30•100•250 mg; 3.3•10•33.3•108.3 mg/5 mL

DayQuil Allergy Relief 4 Hour tablets OTC *decongestant; antihistamine* [phenylpropanolamine HCl; brompheniramine maleate] 25•4 mg

DayQuil Allergy Relief 12 Hour extended-release tablets OTC *decongestant; antihistamine* [phenylpropanolamine HCl; brompheniramine maleate] 75•12 mg

DayQuil Sinus Pressure & Congestion Relief caplets (discontinued 1997) OTC *decongestant* [phenylpropanolamine HCl; guaifenesin] 25•200 mg

DayQuil Sinus Pressure & Pain Relief caplets OTC *decongestant; anal-*

gesic; antipyretic [pseudoephedrine HCl; acetaminophen] 30•500 mg

Dayto Himbin tablets ℞ *no FDA-approved uses; sympatholytic; mydriatic; aphrodisiac* [yohimbine HCl] 5.4 mg

Dayto Sulf vaginal cream ℞ *broad-spectrum bacteriostatic* [sulfathiazole; sulfacetamide; sulfabenzamide] 3.42%•2.86%•3.7%

dazadrol INN *antidepressant* [also: dazadrol maleate]

dazadrol maleate USAN *antidepressant* [also: dazadrol]

Dazamide tablets ℞ *carbonic anhydrase inhibitor diuretic; treatment for acute mountain sickness* [acetazolamide] 250 mg

dazepinil INN *antidepressant* [also: dazepinil HCl]

dazepinil HCl USAN *antidepressant* [also: dazepinil]

dazidamine INN

dazmegrel USAN, INN, BAN *thromboxane synthetase inhibitor*

dazolicine INN

dazopride INN *peristaltic stimulant* [also: dazopride fumarate]

dazopride fumarate USAN *peristaltic stimulant* [also: dazopride]

dazoquinast INN

dazoxiben INN, BAN *antithrombotic* [also: dazoxiben HCl]

dazoxiben HCl USAN *antithrombotic* [also: dazoxiben]

DBED (dibenzylethylenediamine dipenicillin G) [see: penicillin G benzathine]

DBM (dibromomannitol) [see: mitobronitol]

DC softgels OTC *stool softener* [docusate calcium] 240 mg

DC (daunorubicin, cytarabine) *chemotherapy protocol*

D&C Brown No. 1 (drugs & cosmetics) [see: resorcin brown]

DCA (desoxycorticosterone acetate) [q.v.]

DCF (2′-deoxycoformycin) [see: pentostatin]

DCL (descarboethoxyloratadine) [q.v.]

DCMP (daunorubicin, cytarabine, mercaptopurine, prednisone) *chemotherapy protocol*

DCPM (daunorubicin, cytarabine, prednisone, mercaptopurine) *chemotherapy protocol*

DCT (daunorubicin, cytarabine, thioguanine) *chemotherapy protocol* [also: DAT; TAD]

DCV (DTIC, CCNU, vincristine) *chemotherapy protocol*

DDAVP tablets, nasal spray, rhinal tube, subcu or IV injection ℞ *posterior pituitary hormone for hemophilia A, von Willebrand's disease (orphan), central diabetes insipidus, and nocturnal enuresis* [desmopressin acetate] 0.1, 0.2 mg; 10 μg/dose; 0.1 mg/mL; 15 μg/mL

DDAVP (1-deamino-8-D-arginine-vasopressin) [see: desmopressin acetate]

DDC; ddC (dideoxycytidine) [see: zalcitabine]

o,p'-DDD [now: mitotane]

DDI; ddI (dideoxyinosine) [see: didanosine]

DDP; cis-DDP (diamminedichloroplatinum) [see: cisplatin]

DDS (diaminodiphenylsulfone) [now: dapsone]

DDT (dichlorodiphenyltrichloroethane) [see: chlorophenothane]

DDVP (dichlorovinyl dimethyl phosphate) [see: dichlorvos]

DEA (diethanolamine) [q.v.]

deacetyllanatoside C [see: deslanoside]

deadly nightshade *medicinal herb* [see: belladonna]

deadly nightshade leaf [see: belladonna extract]

deal pine *medicinal herb* [see: white pine]

1-deamino-8-D-arginine-vasopressin (DDAVP) [see: desmopressin acetate]

deanil INN *combining name for radicals or groups*

deanol BAN [also: deanol aceglumate]

deanol aceglumate INN [also: deanol]

deanol acetamidobenzoate

deba [see: barbital]

deboxamet INN

Debrisan beads, paste ℞ *debrider and cleanser for wet wounds* [dextranomer]

debrisoquin sulfate USAN *antihypertensive* [also: debrisoquine]

debrisoquine INN, BAN *antihypertensive* [also: debrisoquin sulfate]

Debrox ear drops OTC *agent to emulsify and disperse ear wax* [carbamide peroxide] 6.5%

Decadron tablets, elixir ℞ *corticosteroid; anti-inflammatory* [dexamethasone] 0.5, 0.75, 1.5, 4 mg; 0.5 mg/5 mL ② Decaderm; Percodan

Decadron Phosphate cream (discontinued 1998) ℞ *topical corticosteroidal anti-inflammatory* [dexamethasone sodium phosphate] 0.1%

Decadron Phosphate intra-articular, intralesional, soft tissue or IM injection ℞ *corticosteroid; anti-inflammatory* [dexamethasone sodium phosphate] 4 mg/mL

Decadron Phosphate IV injection ℞ *corticosteroid; anti-inflammatory* [dexamethasone sodium phosphate] 24 mg/mL

Decadron Phosphate Ocumeter (eye drops), ophthalmic ointment ℞ *topical ophthalmic corticosteroidal anti-inflammatory* [dexamethasone sodium phosphate] 0.1%; 0.05%

Decadron with Xylocaine soft tissue injection ℞ *corticosteroid; anti-inflammatory* [dexamethasone sodium phosphate; lidocaine HCl] 4•10 mg/mL

Decadron-LA intralesional, intra-articular, soft tissue, or IM injection ℞ *corticosteroid; anti-inflammatory* [dexamethasone acetate] 8 mg/mL

Deca-Durabolin IM injection ℞ *anabolic steroid for anemia of renal insufficiency; sometimes abused as a street drug* [nandrolone decanoate] 50, 100, 200 mg/mL

Decagen tablets OTC *vitamin/mineral/iron supplement* [multiple vitamins &

minerals; iron; folic acid; biotin] ± •
18 mg•0.4 mg•30 µg

Decaject intra-articular, intralesional,
soft tissue, or IM injection ℞ *corticosteroid; anti-inflammatory* [dexamethasone sodium phosphate] 4 mg/mL

Decaject-L.A. intralesional, intra-articular, soft tissue, or IM injection
℞ *corticosteroid; anti-inflammatory*
[dexamethasone acetate] 8 mg/mL

DECAL (dexamethasone, etoposide, cisplatin, ara-C, L-asparaginase) *chemotherapy protocol*

decamethonium bromide USP, INN
[also: decamethonium iodide]

decamethonium iodide BAN [also:
decamethonium bromide]

Decapeptyl injection ℞ *antineoplastic;
orphan status withdrawn 1996* [triptorelin pamoate]

decapinol [see: delmopinol]

Decaspray aerosol (discontinued
1996) ℞ *topical corticosteroidal anti-inflammatory* [dexamethasone] 0.04%

decavitamin USP

Decholin tablets OTC *laxative; hydrocholeretic* [dehydrocholic acid] 250 mg

decicain [see: tetracaine HCl]

decil INN *combining name for radicals
or groups*

decimemide INN

decitabine USAN, INN, BAN *antineoplastic*

decitropine INN

declaben [now: lodelaben]

declenperone USAN, INN *veterinary
sedative*

Declomycin capsules, film-coated tablets ℞ *broad-spectrum antibiotic* [demeclocycline HCl] 150 mg; 150, 300 mg

decloxizine INN

Decofed syrup OTC *nasal decongestant*
[pseudoephedrine HCl] 30 mg/5 mL

Decohistine DH liquid ℞ *narcotic
antitussive; decongestant; antihistamine*
[codeine phosphate; pseudoephedrine HCl; chlorpheniramine maleate;
alcohol 5.8%] 10•30•2 mg/5 mL

decominol INN

Deconamine tablets, syrup ℞ *decongestant; antihistamine* [pseudoephed-

rine HCl; chlorpheniramine maleate] 60•4 mg; 30•2 mg/5 mL

Deconamine CX tablets, liquid ℞
*narcotic antitussive; decongestant;
expectorant* [hydrocodone bitartrate;
pseudoephedrine HCl; guaifenesin]
5•30•300 mg; 5•60•200 mg/5 mL

Deconamine SR sustained-release
capsules ℞ *decongestant; antihistamine* [pseudoephedrine HCl; chlorpheniramine maleate] 120•8 mg

Decongestabs sustained-release tablets ℞ *decongestant; antihistamine*
[phenylpropanolamine HCl; phenylephrine HCl; chlorpheniramine
maleate; phenyltoloxamine citrate]
40•10•5•15 mg

Decongestant sustained-release tablets ℞ *decongestant; antihistamine*
[phenylpropanolamine HCl; phenylephrine HCl; chlorpheniramine
maleate; phenyltoloxamine citrate]
40•10•5•15 mg

Decongestant tablets OTC *decongestant; antihistamine; analgesic* [phenylephrine HCl; chlorpheniramine maleate; acetaminophen] 5•2•325 mg

Decongestant Expectorant liquid ℞
*narcotic antitussive; decongestant;
expectorant* [codeine phosphate;
pseudoephedrine HCl; guaifenesin;
alcohol 7.5%] 10•30•100 mg/5 mL

Decongestant S.R. sustained-release
tablets (discontinued 1995) ℞
decongestant; antihistamine [phenylpropanolamine HCl; phenylephrine
HCl; chlorpheniramine maleate;
phenyltoloxamine citrate] 40•10•
5•15 mg

Deconhist L.A. sustained-release tablets ℞ *decongestant; antihistamine;
anticholinergic* [phenylpropanolamine
HCl; phenylephrine HCl; chlorpheniramine maleate; hyoscyamine
sulfate; atropine sulfate; scopolamine
hydrobromide] 50•25•8•0.19•
0.04•0.01 mg

Deconomed SR sustained-release
capsules ℞ *decongestant; antihista-*

mine [pseudoephedrine HCl; chlorpheniramine maleate] 120•8 mg

Deconsal II sustained-release tablets ℞ *decongestant; expectorant* [pseudoephedrine HCl; guaifenesin] 60•600 mg ② Deconal

Deconsal Pediatric syrup (discontinued 1998) ℞ *narcotic antitussive; decongestant; expectorant* [codeine phosphate; pseudoephedrine HCl; guaifenesin; alcohol 6%] 10•30•100 mg ② Deconal

Deconsal Sprinkle sustained-release capsules ℞ *decongestant; expectorant* [phenylephrine HCl; guaifenesin] 10•300 mg ② Deconal

decoquinate USAN, INN, BAN *coccidiostat for poultry*

dectaflur USAN, INN *dental caries prophylactic*

Decylenes ointment OTC *topical antifungal* [undecylenic acid; zinc undecylenate]

deditonium bromide INN

Deep-Down Rub OTC *topical analgesic; counterirritant* [methyl salicylate; menthol; camphor] 15%•5%•0.5%

deer musk (*Moschus moschiferus*) *natural remedy in ancient Chinese medicine; reported to have antianginal, antibacterial, antihistaminic, antiinflammatory, CNS-depressant, and stimulant activity in clinical studies*

deerberry *medicinal herb* [see: holly; squaw vine; wintergreen]

DEET (diethyltoluamide) [q.v.]

DeFed-60 tablets OTC *nasal decongestant* [pseudoephedrine HCl] 60 mg

Defen-LA sustained-release tablets ℞ *decongestant; expectorant* [pseudoephedrine HCl; guaifenesin] 60•600 mg

deferoxamine USAN, INN *iron-chelating agent* [also: desferrioxamine]

deferoxamine & dextran *investigational (orphan) for acute iron poisoning*

deferoxamine HCl USAN

deferoxamine mesylate USAN, USP *antidote to iron poisoning; iron-chelat-*

ing agent [also: desferrioxamine mesylate]

defibrotide INN, BAN *investigational (orphan) for thrombotic thrombocytopenic purpura*

Definity ℞ *investigational (NDA filed) ultrasound contrast medium* [perflutren]

deflazacort USAN, INN, BAN *antiinflammatory*

defosfamide INN

defungit sodium salt [see: bensuldazic acid]

Defy eye drops ℞ *topical ophthalmic antibiotic* [tobramycin] 0.3%

Degas chewable tablets OTC *antiflatulent* [simethicone] 80 mg

Degest 2 eye drops OTC *topical ophthalmic decongestant and vasoconstrictor* [naphazoline HCl] 0.012%

Dehist subcu or IM injection (discontinued 1997) ℞ *antihistamine for anaphylaxis* [brompheniramine maleate] 10 mg/mL

DEHOP (diethylhomospermine) [q.v.]

DEHSPM (diethylhomospermine) [q.v.]

dehydrated alcohol [see: alcohol, dehydrated]

dehydrex *investigational (orphan) for recurrent corneal erosion*

dehydroacetic acid NF *preservative*

dehydroandrosterone [see: prasterone]

dehydrocholate sodium USP [also: sodium dehydrocholate]

7-dehydrocholesterol, activated [now: cholecalciferol]

dehydrocholic acid USP, INN, BAN, JAN *choleretic; laxative* 250 mg oral

dehydrocholin [see: dehydrocholic acid]

dehydroemetine INN, BAN, DCF *investigational anti-infective for amebiasis and amebic dysentery*

dehydroepiandrosterone (DHEA) *natural hormone precursor; investigational (Phase III, orphan) for systemic lupus erythematosus (SLE)*

dehydroepiandrosterone sulfate (DHEAS) *investigational (Phase II) injectable antiasthmatic*

dehydroepiandrosterone sulfate sodium *investigational (orphan) for re-epithelialization of serious burns and skin graft donor sites*

Del Aqua-5; Del Aqua-10 gel ℞ *topical keratolytic for acne* [benzoyl peroxide] 5%; 10%

Deladiol-40 IM injection (discontinued 1996) ℞ *estrogen replacement therapy for postmenopausal disorders; antineoplastic for prostate cancer* [estradiol valerate in oil] 40 mg/mL

Deladumone IM injection (discontinued 1995) ℞ *estrogen/androgen for menopausal vasomotor symptoms* [estradiol valerate; testosterone enanthate] 4•90 mg/mL

delanterone INN

Delaprem (commercially available in several foreign countries) ℞ *investigational (NDA filed) tocolytic and bronchodilator* [hexoprenaline sulfate]

delapril INN *antihypertensive; angiotensin-converting enzyme inhibitor* [also: delapril HCl]

delapril HCl USAN *antihypertensive; angiotensin-converting enzyme inhibitor* [also: delapril]

Delatestryl IM injection ℞ *androgen replacement for delayed puberty or breast cancer; sometimes abused as a street drug* [testosterone enanthate] 200 mg/mL

delavirdine INN *antiviral; non-nucleoside reverse transcriptase inhibitor (NNRTI) for HIV and AIDS* [also: delavirdine mesylate]

delavirdine mesylate USAN *antiviral; investigational (Phase III) non-nucleoside reverse transcriptase inhibitor (NNRTI) for HIV and AIDS* [also: delavirdine]

delayed-release aspirin [see: aspirin]

Delcap (trademarked dosage form) *unit dispensing cap*

Delcort cream OTC *topical corticosteroidal anti-inflammatory* [hydrocortisone] 0.5%, 1% ⧉ Dilacor

delequamine INN α_2 *adrenoreceptor antagonist for sexual dysfunction* [also: delequamine HCl]

delequamine HCl USAN α_2 *adrenoreceptor antagonist for sexual dysfunction* [also: delequamine]

delergotrile INN

Delestrogen IM injection ℞ *estrogen replacement therapy for postmenopausal disorders; antineoplastic for prostatic cancer* [estradiol valerate in oil] 10, 20, 40 mg/mL

delfantrine INN

delfaprazine INN

Delfen Contraceptive vaginal foam OTC *spermicidal contraceptive* [nonoxynol 9] 12.5%

delmadinone INN, BAN *progestin; antiandrogen; antiestrogen* [also: delmadinone acetate]

delmadinone acetate USAN *progestin; antiandrogen; antiestrogen* [also: delmadinone]

delmetacin INN

delmopinol INN

Del-Mycin topical solution ℞ *topical antibiotic for acne* [erythromycin] 2%

delnav [see: dioxathion]

delorazepam INN

deloxolone INN

m-**delphene** [see: diethyltoluamide]

delprostenate INN, BAN

Delsym sustained-action liquid OTC *antitussive* [dextromethorphan polistirex] 30 mg/5 mL

Delta-Cortef tablets ℞ *corticosteroid; anti-inflammatory* [prednisolone] 5 mg

deltacortone [see: prednisone]

Delta-D tablets OTC *vitamin supplement* [cholecalciferol (vitamin D_3)] 400 IU

deltafilcon A USAN *hydrophilic contact lens material*

deltafilcon B USAN *hydrophilic contact lens material*

delta-1-hydrocortisone [see: prednisolone]

Deltasone tablets ℞ *corticosteroid; anti-inflammatory* [prednisone] 2.5, 5, 10, 20, 50 mg

delta-9-tetrahydrocannabinol (THC) [see: dronabinol]

delta-9-THC (tetrahydrocannabinol) [see: dronabinol]

Delta-Tritex cream, ointment ℞ *topical corticosteroidal anti-inflammatory* [triamcinolone acetonide] 0.1%

Deltavac vaginal cream ℞ *broad-spectrum antibiotic; antiseptic; vulnerary* [sulfanilamide; aminacrine HCl; allantoin] 15%•0.2%•2%

deltibant USAN *bradykinin antagonist for treatment of systemic inflammatory response syndrome*

deltra-stab [see: prednisolone]

Del-Vi-A capsules ℞ *vitamin deficiency therapy* [vitamin A] 50 000 IU

Demadex tablets, IV injection ℞ *antihypertensive; loop diuretic* [torsemide] 5, 10, 20, 100 mg; 10 mg/mL

Demazin Repetabs (repeat-action tablets), syrup OTC *decongestant; antihistamine* [phenylpropanolamine HCl; chlorpheniramine maleate] 25•4 mg; 12.5•2 mg/5 mL

dembrexine INN, BAN

dembroxol [see: dembrexine]

demecarium bromide USP, INN, BAN *antiglaucoma agent; reversible cholinesterase inhibitor miotic*

demeclocycline USP, BAN *tetracycline antibiotic*

demeclocycline HCl USP, BAN *tetracycline antibiotic; antirickettsial*

demecolcine INN, BAN

demecycline USAN, INN *antibacterial*

demegestone INN

demekastigmine bromide [see: demecarium bromide]

demelverine INN

Demerol HCl IV or IM injection (discontinued 1999) ℞ *narcotic analgesic; also abused as a street drug* [meperidine HCl] 50, 100 mg/mL

Demerol HCl tablets, syrup ℞ *narcotic analgesic; also abused as a street*

drug [meperidine HCl] 50, 100 mg; 50 mg/5 mL

demetacin [see: delmetacin]

11-demethoxyreserpine [see: deserpidine]

demethylchlortetracycline (DMCT) [now: demeclocycline]

demethylchlortetracycline HCl [see: demeclocycline HCl]

N-demethylcodeine [see: norcodeine]

demexiptiline INN

Demi-Regroton tablets ℞ *antihypertensive; diuretic* [chlorthalidone; reserpine] 25•0.125 mg

democonazole INN

Demolin liniment OTC *topical analgesic* [methyl salicylate; camphor; racemic menthol; mustard oil] ⊘ Demulen

demoxepam USAN, INN *minor tranquilizer*

demoxytocin INN

Demser capsules ℞ *antihypertensive for pheochromocytoma* [metyrosine] 250 mg

demulcents *a class of agents that soothe irritated or abraded tissues, particularly mucous membranes*

Demulen 1/35; Demulen 1/50 tablets ℞ *monophasic oral contraceptive* [ethynodiol diacetate; ethinyl estradiol] 1 mg•35 µg; 1 mg•50 µg ⊘ Demerol; Demolin

denatonium benzoate USAN, NF, INN, BAN *alcohol denaturant; flavoring agent*

denaverine INN

Denavir cream ℞ *nucleoside analogue antiviral for herpes labialis* [penciclovir] 1%

denbufylline INN, BAN

denileukin diftitox USAN, INN *antineoplastic for cutaneous T-cell lymphoma (CTCL) (orphan); investigational agent for various malignant diseases and autoimmune disorders* [previously known as DAB$_{389}$ IL-2 fusion toxin]

denipride INN

denofungin USAN *antifungal; antibacterial*

denopamine INN

Denorex shampoo OTC *antiseborrheic; antipsoriatic; antipruritic; antibacterial* [coal tar; menthol; alcohol] 9%•1.5•7.5%; 12.5%•1.5%•10.4%

denpidazone INN

Denquel toothpaste OTC *tooth desensitizer* [potassium nitrate] 5%

dental antiformin [see: antiformin, dental]

dental-type silica [see: silica, dental-type]

Dentipatch transmucosal patch ℞ *mucous membrane anesthetic* [lidocaine HCl] 23, 46.1 mg

Dent's Lotion-Jel lotion/gel OTC *topical oral anesthetic* [benzocaine]

Dent's Toothache Gum; Dent's Toothache Drops OTC *topical oral anesthetic* [benzocaine]

denyl sodium [see: phenytoin sodium]

denzimol INN

deodorants *a class of agents that mask undesirable or offensive odors* [also called: antibromics]

2′-deoxycoformycin (DCF) [see: pentostatin]

deoxycorticosterone acetate [see: desoxycorticosterone acetate]

deoxycorticosterone pivalate [see: desoxycorticosterone pivalate]

deoxycortolone pivalate BAN *salt-regulating adrenocortical steroid* [also: desoxycorticosterone pivalate]

deoxycortone BAN *salt-regulating adrenocortical steroid* [also: desoxycorticosterone acetate; desoxycortone]

2′-deoxycytidine *investigational (orphan) host-protective agent in acute myelogenous leukemia*

deoxyephedrine HCl [see: methamphetamine HCl]

12-deoxyerythromycin [see: berythromycin]

deoxynojirimycin (DNJ) *investigational (Phase II) antiviral for AIDS and ARC*

deoxyribonuclease, recombinant human (rhDNase) [see: dornase alfa]

deoxyribonucleic acid (DNA)

15-deoxyspergualin trihydrochloride [now: gusperimus trihydrochloride]

Depacin capsules OTC *analgesic; antipyretic* [acetaminophen] 325 mg

Depacin Cold Capsules OTC *decongestant; antihistamine; analgesic* [phenylpropanolamine HCl; chlorpheniramine maleate; acetaminophen]

Depacon IV infusion ℞ *anticonvulsant* [valproate sodium] 500 mg/5 mL

Depade tablets ℞ *narcotic antagonist for opiate dependence or overdose (orphan) and alcoholism* [naltrexone HCl] 50 mg

Depakene capsules ℞ *anticonvulsant* [valproic acid] 250 mg

Depakene syrup ℞ *anticonvulsant* [valproate sodium] 250 mg/5 mL

Depakote delayed-release tablets ℞ *anticonvulsant; antipsychotic for manic episodes of a bipolar disorder; migraine prophylaxis* [divalproex sodium] 125, 250, 500 mg

Depakote sprinkle capsules ℞ *anticonvulsant* [divalproex sodium] 125 mg

depAndro 100; depAndro 200 IM injection ℞ *androgen replacement for delayed puberty or breast cancer* [testosterone cypionate] 100 mg/mL; 200 mg/mL

depAndrogyn IM injection ℞ *estrogen/androgen for menopausal vasomotor symptoms* [estradiol cypionate; testosterone cypionate] 2•50 mg/mL

Depen titratable tablets ℞ *metal chelating agent for rheumatoid arthritis, Wilson's disease, and cystinuria* [penicillamine] 250 mg

depepsen [see: sodium amylosulfate]

depGynogen IM injection ℞ *estrogen replacement therapy for postmenopausal disorders* [estradiol cypionate in oil] 5 mg/mL

Depitol tablets (discontinued 1998) ℞ *anticonvulsant; analgesic for trigeminal neuralgia; antipsychotic* [carbamazepine] 200 mg

depMedalone 40; depMedalone 80 intralesional, soft tissue, and IM injection ℞ *corticosteroid; anti-*

inflammatory; immunosuppressant [methylprednisolone acetate] 40 mg/mL; 80 mg/mL

DepoCyt sustained-release intrathecal injection ℞ *antineoplastic for neoplastic meningitis (NM) arising from solid tumors or non-Hodgkin's lymphoma (orphan)* [cytarabine, liposomal]

Depo-Estradiol Cypionate IM injection ℞ *estrogen replacement therapy for postmenopausal disorders* [estradiol cypionate in oil] 5 mg/mL

DepoGen IM injection ℞ *estrogen replacement therapy for postmenopausal disorders* [estradiol cypionate in oil] 5 mg/mL

Depoject intralesional, soft tissue, and IM injection ℞ *corticosteroid; anti-inflammatory; immunosuppressant* [methylprednisolone acetate] 40, 80 mg/mL

Depo-Medrol intralesional, soft tissue, and IM injection ℞ *corticosteroid; anti-inflammatory; immunosuppressant* [methylprednisolone acetate] 20, 40, 80 mg/mL

DepoMorphine ℞ *investigational (Phase II) sustained-release, encapsulated formulation to treat severe postsurgical pain* [morphine sulfate]

Deponit transdermal patch ℞ *antianginal; vasodilator* [nitroglycerin] 16, 32 mg

Depopred-40; Depopred-80 intralesional, soft tissue, and IM injection ℞ *corticosteroid; anti-inflammatory; immunosuppressant* [methylprednisolone acetate] 40 mg/mL; 80 mg/mL

Depo-Provera IM injection ℞ *hormonal antineoplastic adjunct for metastatic endometrial and renal carcinoma; long-term injectable contraceptive* [medroxyprogesterone acetate] 150, 400 mg/mL

Depotest 100; Depotest 200 IM injection ℞ *androgen replacement for delayed puberty or breast cancer* [testosterone cypionate] 100 mg/mL; 200 mg/mL

Depo-Testadiol IM injection ℞ *estrogen/androgen for menopausal vasomotor symptoms* [estradiol cypionate; testosterone cypionate] 2•50 mg/mL

Depotestogen IM injection ℞ *estrogen/androgen for menopausal vasomotor symptoms* [estradiol cypionate; testosterone cypionate] 2•50 mg/mL

Depo-Testosterone IM injection ℞ *androgen replacement for delayed puberty or breast cancer; sometimes abused as a street drug* [testosterone cypionate] 100, 200 mg/mL

depramine INN [also: balipramine]

deprenyl (L-deprenyl) [see: selegiline HCl]

depreotide USAN *radiopharmaceutical imaging agent for lung cancer; investigational (NDA filed) for malignant melanoma and neuroendocrine tumors*

depressants *a class of agents that reduce functional activity and vital energy in general by producing muscular relaxation and diaphoresis*

deprodone INN, BAN

Deproic ⒸⒶⓃ (U.S. product: Depakene) capsules, syrup ℞ *anticonvulsant* [valproic acid] 250, 500 mg; 250 mg/5 mL

Deproist Expectorant with Codeine liquid ℞ *narcotic antitussive; decongestant; expectorant* [codeine phosphate; pseudoephedrine HCl; guaifenesin; alcohol 8.2%] 10•30•100 mg/5 mL

Deprol tablets (discontinued 1995) ℞ *psychotherapeutic agent; anxiolytic* [meprobamate; benactyzine HCl] 400•1 mg

deprostil USAN, INN *gastric antisecretory*

deptropine INN, BAN

deptropine citrate [see: deptropine]

depurants; depuratives *a class of agents that purify or cleanse the system, particularly the blood* [also called: pellants]

dequalinium chloride INN, BAN

Dequasine tablets OTC *dietary supplement* [multiple minerals & amino acids; vitamin C] ±•200 mg

deracoxib USAN *COX-2 inhibitor anti-inflammatory and analgesic for osteoarthritis and rheumatoid arthritis*

Derifil tablets OTC *systemic deodorant for ostomy, breath, and body odors* [chlorophyllin] 100 mg

Derma Comb cream ℞ *topical corticosteroidal anti-inflammatory; antifungal* [triamcinolone acetonide; nystatin]

Derma Viva lotion OTC *moisturizer; emollient*

Dermabase OTC *cream base*

Dermabet cream ℞ *topical corticosteroidal anti-inflammatory* [betamethasone valerate]

Dermabond liquid OTC *topical skin adhesive for closing surgical incisions and traumatic lacerations*

Dermacoat aerosol OTC *topical local anesthetic* [benzocaine] 4.5%

Dermacort cream, lotion ℞ *topical corticosteroidal anti-inflammatory* [hydrocortisone] 1% ② DermiCort

DermaFlex gel OTC *topical local anesthetic* [lidocaine] 2.5%

Dermagraft; Dermagraft-TC (approved for marketing in the UK) ℞ *investigational (NDA filed) fully human skin replacement or temporary wound covering for partial-thickness burns; investigational for diabetic foot ulcers*

Dermal-Rub balm OTC *counterirritant* [methyl salicylate; camphor; racemic manthol; cajuput oil]

Dermamycin cream, spray OTC *topical antihistamine* [diphenhydramine HCl] 2%

Derma-Pax lotion OTC *topical antihistamine; antiseptic; antipruritic* [pyrilamine maleate; chlorpheniramine maleate; alcohol 35%] 0.44%•0.06%

Dermarest gel OTC *topical antihistamine; antifungal* [diphenhydramine HCl; resorcinol] 2%•2%

Dermarest Dricort Creme OTC *topical corticosteroidal anti-inflammatory* [hydrocortisone acetate] 1%

Dermarest Plus gel, spray OTC *topical antihistamine; analgesic; counterirri-*

tant [diphenhydramine HCl; menthol] 2%•1%

Dermasept Antifungal liquid spray OTC *antifungal; antiseptic; anesthetic; astringent* [tolnaftate; tannic acid; zinc chloride; benzocaine; methylbenzethonium HCl; undecylenic acid; alcohol 58.54%] 1.017%•6.098%•5.081%•2.032%•3.049%•5.081%

Dermasil lotion OTC *bath emollient*

Derma-Smoothe/FS oil ℞ *topical corticosteroidal anti-inflammatory; emollient* [fluocinolone acetonide] 0.01%

dermatan sulfate [see: danaparoid sodium]

dermatol [see: bismuth subgallate]

Dermatop cream ℞ *topical corticosteroidal anti-inflammatory* [prednicarbate] 0.1%

Dermatophytin shallow subcu or intradermal injection (discontinued 1996) ℞ *diagnosis and treatment of Trichophyton-induced skin infections* [Trichophyton extract] 5 mL (undiluted or 1:30)

Dermatophytin "O" shallow subcu or intradermal injection (discontinued 1996) ℞ *diagnosis and treatment of oidiomycin (Candida)-induced infections* [Candida albicans skin test antigen] 5 mL (undiluted or 1:100)

Derm-Cleanse liquid OTC *soap-free therapeutic skin cleanser*

DermiCort cream, lotion OTC *topical corticosteroidal anti-inflammatory* [hydrocortisone] ② Dermacort

Dermol HC anorectal cream, anorectal ointment ℞ *topical corticosteroidal anti-inflammatory* [hydrocortisone] 1%, 2.5%; 1%

Dermolate Anti-Itch cream OTC *topical corticosteroidal anti-inflammatory* [hydrocortisone] 0.5%

Dermolin liniment OTC *topical analgesic; counterirritant; antiseptic* [methyl salicylate; camphor; racemic menthol; mustard oil; alcohol 8%]

Dermoplast aerosol spray, lotion OTC *topical local anesthetic; analgesic*

[benzocaine; menthol] 20%•0.5%; 8%•0.5%

Dermovan OTC *cream base*

Dermoxyl gel (discontinued 1995) OTC *topical keratolytic for acne* [benzoyl peroxide] 2.5%, 5%, 10%

Dermprotective Factor (DPF) (trademarked ingredient) *aromatic syrup* [eriodictyon]

Dermtex HC with Aloe cream OTC *topical corticosteroidal anti-inflammatory* [hydrocortisone] 0.5%

Dermuspray aerosol spray ℞ *topical enzyme for wound debridement* [trypsin; peruvian balsam] 0.1•72.5 mg/0.82 mL

derpanicate INN

DES (diethylstilbestrol) [q.v.]

desacetyl vinblastine amide (DAVA) [see: vindesine]

desacetyl-lanatoside C [see: deslanoside]

desaglybuzole [see: glybuzole]

desamino-oxytocin [see: demoxytocin]

desaspidin INN

descarboethoxyloratadine (DCL) *investigational antihistamine for allergy*

desciclovir USAN, INN *antiviral*

descinolone INN *corticosteroid; anti-inflammatory* [also: descinolone acetonide]

descinolone acetonide USAN *corticosteroid; anti-inflammatory* [also: descinolone]

Desenex foam, soap OTC *topical antifungal* [undecylenic acid] 10%

Desenex powder, aerosol powder, ointment, cream OTC *topical antifungal* [undecylenic acid; zinc undecylenate] 25% total

Desenex spray liquid (discontinued 1998) OTC *topical antifungal* [tolnaftate] 1%

Desenex, Prescription Strength cream OTC *topical antifungal* [clotrimazole] 1%

Desenex, Prescription Strength spray liquid, spray powder OTC *topical antifungal* [miconazole nitrate] 2%

Desenex Antifungal cream OTC *topical antifungal* [miconazole nitrate] 2%

deserpidine INN, BAN *antihypertensive; peripheral antiadrenergic; rauwolfia derivative* ⑨ desipramine

desert herb; desert tea *medicinal herb* [see: ephedra]

Desert Pure Calcium film-coated tablets OTC *calcium supplement* [calcium carbonate; vitamin D] 500 mg•125 IU

Desferal powder for IM, IV, or subcu injection ℞ *adjunct treatment for iron intoxication or overload* [deferoxamine mesylate] 500 mg ⑨ Disophrol

desferrioxamine BAN *iron-chelating agent* [also: deferoxamine]

desferrioxamine mesylate BAN *antidote to iron poisoning; iron-chelating agent* [also: deferoxamine mesylate]

desflurane USAN, INN *inhalation general anesthetic*

desglugastrin INN

desipramine INN, BAN *tricyclic antidepressant* [also: desipramine HCl] ⑨ deserpidine

desipramine HCl USAN, USP *tricyclic antidepressant* [also: desipramine] 10, 25, 50, 75, 100, 150 mg oral

desirudin USAN *anticoagulant; thrombin inhibitor* [recombinant hirudin]

Desitin ointment OTC *moisturizer; emollient; astringent; antiseptic* [cod liver oil; zinc oxide]

Desitin Creamy ointment OTC *topical diaper rash treatment* [zinc oxide] 10%

Desitin with Zinc Oxide powder OTC *topical diaper rash treatment* [zinc oxide; corn starch] 10%•88.2%

deslanoside USP, INN, BAN *cardiotonic; cardiac glycoside*

desloratadine USAN *investigational (Phase III) histamine H_1 receptor antagonist for allergic rhinitis (active metabolite of loratadine)*

deslorelin USAN, INN *LHRH agonist; investigational (orphan) for central precocious puberty*

desmethylmoramide INN

desmophosphamide [see: defosfamide]

desmopressin INN, BAN *posterior pitu-itary antidiuretic hormone (ADH)* [also: desmopressin acetate]

desmopressin acetate USAN *posterior pituitary antidiuretic hormone for hemophilia A, von Willebrand's disease (orphan), and nocturnal enuresis* [also: desmopressin] 4 μg/mL injection

desocriptine INN

Desogen tablets ℞ *monophasic oral contraceptive* [desogestrel; ethinyl estradiol] 0.15 mg•30 μg

desogestrel USAN, INN, BAN *progestin*

desolone [see: deprodone]

desomorphine INN, BAN

desonide USAN, INN, BAN *topical corticosteroidal anti-inflammatory* 0.05% topical

DesOwen ointment, cream, lotion ℞ *topical corticosteroidal anti-inflammatory* [desonide] 0.05%

desoximetasone USAN, USP, INN *topical corticosteroidal anti-inflammatory* [also: desoxymethasone] 0.05%, 0.25% topical ⧈ dexamethasone

desoxycholic acid *increases secretion of bile acids*

desoxycorticosterone acetate (DCA; DOCA) USP *salt-regulating adrenocortical steroid* [also: desoxycortone; deoxycortone]

desoxycorticosterone pivalate USP *salt-regulating adrenocortical steroid* [also: deoxycortolone pivalate]

desoxycorticosterone trimethylace-tate USP

desoxycortone INN *salt-regulating adrenocortical steroid* [also: desoxycorticosterone acetate; deoxycortone]

l-desoxyephedrine *nasal decongestant*

desoxyephedrine HCl [see: metham-phetamine HCl]

desoxymethasone BAN *topical corticosteroidal anti-inflammatory* [also: desoximetasone]

Desoxyn Gradumets (sustained-release tablets), tablets ℞ *CNS stimulant; sometimes abused as a street drug* [methamphetamine HCl] 5, 10, 15 mg; 5 mg ⧈ digitoxin; digoxin

desoxyribonuclease [see: fibrinolysin & desoxyribonuclease]

Despec liquid ℞ *decongestant; expectorant* [phenylephrine HCl; phenyl-propanolamine HCl; guaifenesin] 20•5•100 mg/5 mL

Desquam-E; Desquam-E 5; Desquam-E 10 gel ℞ *topical keratolytic for acne* [benzoyl peroxide] 2.5%; 5%; 10%

Desquam-X 2.5 gel (discontinued 1995) ℞ *topical keratolytic for acne* [benzoyl peroxide] 2.5%

Desquam-X 5; Desquam-X 10 gel ℞ *topical keratolytic for acne* [benzoyl peroxide] 5%; 10%

Desquam-X 5 Wash; Desquam-X 10 Wash liquid ℞ *topical keratolytic for acne* [benzoyl peroxide] 5%; 10%

de-Stat solution (discontinued 1995) OTC *cleaning/soaking solution for hard contact lenses*

de-Stat 3; de-Stat 4 solution OTC *cleaning/disinfecting/soaking solution for rigid gas permeable contact lenses*

destradiol [see: estradiol]

63-desulfohirudin [see: desirudin]

Desyrel film-coated tablets, Dividose (multiple-scored tablets) ℞ *antidepressant used for panic disorders, aggressive behavior, alcoholism, and cocaine withdrawal* [trazodone HCl] 50, 100 mg; 150, 300 mg

DET (diethyltryptamine) [q.v.]

detajmium bitartrate INN

Detane gel OTC *topical local anesthetic* [benzocaine] 7.5%

detanosal INN

Detect-A-Strep slide tests for professional use *in vitro diagnostic aid for streptococcal antigens in throat swabs*

Detecto-Seal (trademarked packaging form) *tamper-resistant parenteral package*

deterenol INN *ophthalmic adrenergic* [also: deterenol HCl]

deterenol HCl USAN *ophthalmic adrenergic* [also: deterenol]

detergents *a class of agents that cleanse wounds and sores*

detigon HCl [see: chlophedianol HCl]

detirelix INN *luteinizing hormone-releasing hormone (LHRH) antagonist* [also: detirelix acetate]

detirelix acetate USAN *luteinizing hormone-releasing hormone (LHRH) antagonist* [also: detirelix]

detomidine INN, BAN *veterinary analgesic; sedative* [also: detomidine HCl]

detomidine HCl USAN *veterinary analgesic; sedative* [also: detomidine]

detorubicin INN

detralfate INN

Detrol film-coated tablets ℞ *muscarinic receptor antagonist for urinary frequency, urgency, and incontinence* [tolterodine tartrate] 1, 2 mg

detrothyronine INN

Detrusitol (European name for U.S. product Detrol)

Detussin liquid ℞ *narcotic antitussive; decongestant* [hydrocodone bitartrate; pseudoephedrine HCl; alcohol 5%] 5•60 mg/5 mL

Detussin Expectorant liquid ℞ *narcotic antitussive; decongestant; expectorant* [hydrocodone bitartrate; pseudoephedrine HCl; guaifenesin; alcohol] 5•60•200 mg/5 mL

deuterium oxide USAN *radioactive agent*

devapamil INN

devazepide USAN *cholecystokinin antagonist*

devil's bones *medicinal herb* [see: wild yam]

devil's claw (Harpagophytum procumbens) root *medicinal herb for arrhythmias, arteriosclerosis, arthritis, blood cleansing, diabetes, hypertension, liver disease, lowering cholesterol, rheumatism, stomach disorders, and strengthening bladder and kidneys*

devil's club (Echinopanax horridum; Fatsia horrida; Oplopanax horridus; Panax horridum) cambium and stem *medicinal herb for arthritis, burns and cuts, colds, cough, fever, inducing vomiting and bowel evacuation, pneumonia, and tuberculosis*

devil's dung *medicinal herb* [see: asafetida]

devil's eye *medicinal herb* [see: henbane]

devil's fuge *medicinal herb* [see: mistletoe]

devil's shrub *medicinal herb* [see: Siberian ginseng]

Devrom chewable tablets OTC *systemic deodorizer for ostomy and incontinence odors* [bismuth subgallate] 200 mg

dewberry *medicinal herb* [see: blackberry]

Dex4 Glucose chewable tablets OTC *glucose elevating agent* [glucose] ⁴

dexa [see: dexamethasone]

Dexacidin eye drop suspension, ophthalmic ointment ℞ *topical ophthalmic corticosteroidal anti-inflammatory; antibiotic* [dexamethasone; neomycin sulfate; polymyxin B sulfate] 0.1%•0.35%•10 000 U/mL; 0.1%•0.35%•10 000 U/g

Dexacort Phosphate Respihaler (oral inhalation aerosol) ℞ *corticosteroid for bronchial asthma* [dexamethasone sodium phosphate] 84 μg/dose

Dexacort Phosphate Turbinaire (nasal inhalation aerosol) ℞ *intranasal corticosteroidal anti-inflammatory* [dexamethasone sodium phosphate; alcohol 2%] 84 μg/dose

Dexafed Cough syrup OTC *antitussive; decongestant; expectorant* [dextromethorphan hydrobromide; phenylephrine HCl; guaifenesin] 10•5•100 mg/5 mL

Dexameth tablets ℞ *corticosteroid; anti-inflammatory* [dexamethasone] 0.5, 0.75, 1.5, 4 mg

dexamethasone USP, INN, BAN *corticosteroidal anti-inflammatory* 0.25, 0.5, 0.75, 1, 1.5, 2, 4, 6 mg oral; 0.5 mg/5 mL oral; 0.5 mg/0.5 mL oral ☑ desoximetasone

dexamethasone acefurate USAN, INN *corticosteroidal anti-inflammatory*

dexamethasone acetate USAN, USP, BAN *corticosteroidal anti-inflammatory* 8 mg/mL injection

dexamethasone dipropionate USAN *corticosteroidal anti-inflammatory*

dexamethasone sodium phosphate USP, BAN *corticosteroid; anti-inflammatory* 0.05%, 0.1% eye drops; 4, 10 mg/mL injection

dexamfetamine INN *CNS stimulant* [also: dextroamphetamine; dexamphetamine]

dexamisole USAN, INN *antidepressant*

dexamphetamine BAN *CNS stimulant* [also: dextroamphetamine; dexamfetamine]

dexanabinol *investigational treatment for ulcerative colitis, inflammatory bowel disease (IBD), and AIDS-wasting syndrome*

dexanabinol *nonpsychotropic synthetic analog of marijuana; investigational (Phase II) for severe head trauma*

Dexaphen S.A. sustained-release tablets R *decongestant; antihistamine* [pseudoephedrine sulfate; dexbrompheniramine maleate] 120•6 mg

Dexasone intra-articular, intralesional, soft tissue, or IM injection R *corticosteroid; anti-inflammatory* [dexamethasone sodium phosphate] 4 mg/mL

Dexasone L.A. intralesional, intra-articular, soft tissue, or IM injection R *corticosteroid; anti-inflammatory* [dexamethasone acetate] 8 mg/mL

Dexasporin eye drop suspension (discontinued 1995) R *topical ophthalmic corticosteroidal anti-inflammatory; antibiotic* [dexamethasone; neomycin sulfate; polymyxin B sulfate] 0.1%•0.35%•10 000 U/mL

Dexasporin ophthalmic ointment R *topical ophthalmic corticosteroidal anti-inflammatory; antibiotic* [dexamethasone; neomycin sulfate; polymyxin B sulfate] 0.1%•0.35%•10 000 U/g

Dexatrim extended-release tablets, timed-release capsules OTC *diet aid* [phenylpropanolamine HCl] 75 mg

Dexatrim plus Vitamin C timed-release capsules OTC *diet aid* [phenylpropanolamine HCl; vitamin C] 75•180 mg

Dexatrim Plus Vitamins timed-release caplets (diet aid) + caplets (vitamins) (discontinued 1998) OTC *diet aid + vitamin/mineral/iron supplement* [(phenylpropanolamine HCl; vitamin C) + (multiple vitamins/minerals; iron; folic acid; biotin)] (75•60 mg) + (± •18•0.4•0.03 mg)

Dexatrim Pre-Meal timed-release capsules OTC *diet aid* [phenylpropanolamine HCl] 25 mg

dexbrompheniramine INN, BAN *antihistamine* [also: dexbrompheniramine maleate]

dexbrompheniramine maleate USP *antihistamine* [also: dexbrompheniramine]

Dexchlor extended-release tablets (discontinued 1997) R *antihistamine* [dexchlorpheniramine maleate] 4, 6 mg

dexchlorpheniramine INN *alkylamine antihistamine* [also: dexchlorpheniramine maleate]

dexchlorpheniramine maleate USP *alkylamine antihistamine* [also: dexchlorpheniramine] 4, 6 mg oral

dexclamol INN *sedative* [also: dexclamol HCl]

dexclamol HCl USAN *sedative* [also: dexclamol]

Dexedrine Spansules (sustained-release capsules), tablets R *amphetamine; CNS stimulant; widely abused as a street drug* [dextroamphetamine sulfate] 5, 10, 15 mg; 5 mg ⑦ dextran

dexetimide USAN, INN, BAN *anticholinergic*

dexetozoline INN

dexfenfluramine INN, BAN *anorexiant; appetite suppressant; serotonin reuptake inhibitor* [also: dexfenfluramine HCl]

dexfenfluramine HCl USAN *anorexiant; appetite suppressant; serotonin reuptake inhibitor* [also: dexfenfluramine]

DexFerrum IV or IM injection R *hematinic* [iron dextran] 50 mg/mL

dexibuprofen USAN, INN *analgesic; cyclooxygenase inhibitor; anti-inflammatory*

dexibuprofen lysine USAN *analgesic; cyclooxygenase inhibitor; anti-inflammatory* [also: dexibuprofen]

deximafen USAN, INN *antidepressant*

dexindoprofen INN

Dexiron ⓒ (U.S. product: DexFerrum) IM injection ℞ *hematinic* [iron dextran] 50 mg/mL

dexivacaine USAN, INN *anesthetic*

dexlofexidine INN

dexmedetomidine USAN, INN, BAN *investigational (NDA filed) tranquilizer*

dexnorgestrel acetime [now: norgestimate]

Dexone intra-articular, intralesional, soft tissue, or IM injection ℞ *corticosteroid; anti-inflammatory* [dexamethasone sodium phosphate] 4 mg/mL

Dexone tablets ℞ *corticosteroid; anti-inflammatory* [dexamethasone] 0.5, 0.75, 1.5, 4 mg

Dexone LA intralesional, intra-articular, soft tissue, or IM injection ℞ *corticosteroid; anti-inflammatory* [dexamethasone acetate] 8 mg/mL

dexormaplatin USAN, INN *antineoplastic*

dexoxadrol INN *CNS stimulant; analgesic* [also: dexoxadrol HCl]

dexoxadrol HCl USAN *CNS stimulant; analgesic* [also: dexoxadrol]

dexpanthenol USAN, USP, INN, BAN *cholinergic; antipruritic; postoperative prophylaxis for paralytic ileus* 250 mg/mL injection

dexpemedolac USAN *analgesic*

dexpropranolol HCl USAN *antiarrhythmic; antiadrenergic (β-receptor)* [also: dexpropranolol]

dexproxibutene INN

dexrazoxane USAN, INN, BAN *cardioprotectant for doxorubicin-induced cardiomyopathy (orphan); chelates intracellular iron*

dexsecoverine INN

dexsotalol HCl USAN *class III antiarrhythmic*

dextilidine INN

dextran INN, BAN *blood flow adjuvant; plasma volume extender* [also: dextran 40] ② Dexedrine; dextrin

dextran, high molecular weight [see: dextran 70]

dextran, low molecular weight [see: dextran 40]

dextran 1 *monovalent hapten for prevention of dextran-induced anaphylactic reactions*

dextran 40 USAN *blood flow adjuvant; plasma volume extender* [also: dextran] 10% injection

dextran 70 USAN *plasma volume extender; viscosity-increasing agent* 6% injection

dextran 75 USAN *plasma volume extender; viscosity-increasing agent* 6% injection

dextran & deferoxamine *investigational (orphan) for acute iron poisoning*

dextran sulfate *investigational (Phase II) antiviral for HIV and AIDS; investigational (orphan) inhalant for cystic fibrosis*

dextran sulfate, sodium salt, aluminum complex [see: detralfate]

dextran sulfate sodium *investigational (orphan) for AIDS*

dextranomer INN, BAN *wound debrider/cleanser*

dextrates USAN, NF *tablet binder and diluent*

dextriferron NF, INN, BAN

dextrin NF, BAN *suspending agent; tablet binder and diluent* ② dextran

dextroamphetamine USAN *CNS stimulant; widely abused as a street drug, which causes strong psychic dependence* [also: dexamfetamine; dexamphetamine]

dextroamphetamine phosphate USP *CNS stimulant*

dextroamphetamine saccharate *CNS stimulant*

dextroamphetamine sulfate USP *CNS stimulant; widely abused as a street drug, which causes psychic dependence* 5, 10, 15 mg oral

dextrobrompheniramine maleate [see: dexbrompheniramine maleate]

dextrochlorpheniramine maleate [see: dexchlorpheniramine maleate]

dextrofemine INN

dextromethorphan USP, INN, BAN *antitussive*

dextromethorphan hydrobromide USP, BAN *antitussive* 10 mg/5 mL oral

dextromethorphan polistirex USAN *antitussive*

dextromoramide INN, BAN

dextromoramide tartrate [see: dextromoramide]

dextro-pantothenyl alcohol [see: dexpanthenol]

dextropropoxiphene chloride [see: propoxyphene HCl]

dextropropoxyphene INN, BAN *narcotic analgesic* [also: propoxyphene HCl]

dextropropoxyphene HCl BAN [also: propoxyphene HCl]

dextrorphan INN, BAN *adjunct to vasospastic therapy; investigational glutamate receptor antagonist for neurodegenerative disorders* [also: dextrorphan HCl]

dextrorphan HCl USAN *adjunct to vasospastic therapy; investigational glutamate receptor antagonist for neurodegenerative disorders* [also: dextrorphan]

dextrose USP *fluid and nutrient replenisher; parenteral antihypoglycemic*

5% Dextrose and Electrolyte #48; 5% Dextrose and Electrolyte #75; 10% Dextrose and Electrolyte #48 IV infusion ℞ *intravenous nutritional/electrolyte therapy* [combined electrolyte solution; dextrose]

dextrose excipient NF *tablet excipient*

50% Dextrose with Electrolyte Pattern A (or N) IV infusion ℞ *intravenous nutritional/electrolyte therapy* [combined electrolyte solution; dextrose]

Dextrostat tablets ℞ *amphetamine; CNS stimulant* [dextroamphetamine sulfate] 5 mg

Dextrostix reagent strips for home use OTC *in vitro diagnostic aid for blood glucose*

dextrothyronine [see: detrothyronine]

dextrothyroxine BAN *antihyperlipidemic* [also: dextrothyroxine sodium]

dextrothyroxine sodium USAN, USP, INN *antihyperlipidemic* [also: dextrothyroxine]

dexverapamil INN *investigational adjunct to chemotherapy*

Dey-Dose (delivery system) *nebulizer*

Dey-Lute (delivery system) *nebulizer*

Dey-Pak Sodium Chloride 0.45% & 0.9% solution OTC *for respiratory therapy and tracheal lavage* [sodium chloride] 0.45%; 0.9%

Dey-Pak Sodium Chloride 3% & 10% solution ℞ *for inducing sputum production for specimen collection* [sodium chloride] 3%; 10%

Dey-Vial Sodium Chloride 0.9% solution OTC *for respiratory therapy and tracheal lavage* [sodium chloride] 0.9%

dezaguanine USAN, INN *antineoplastic*

dezaguanine mesylate USAN *antineoplastic*

dezinamide USAN, INN *anticonvulsant*

dezocine USAN, INN *narcotic analgesic*

DFMO (difluoromethylornithine) [see: eflornithine]

DFMO (difluoromethylornithine) HCl [see: eflornithine HCl]

DFMO-MGBG (eflornithine, mitoguazone) *chemotherapy protocol* [also see: DFMO; MGBG]

DFP (diisopropyl flurophosphate) [see: isoflurophate]

DFV (DDP, fluorouracil, VePesid) *chemotherapy protocol*

DGH-3515 *antagonist to the long-term euphoriant effects of JEK-554* [q.v.]

DHA (docosahexaenoic acid) [see: doconexent]

DHAP (dexamethasone, high-dose ara-C, Platinol) *chemotherapy protocol*

DHC Plus capsules ℞ *narcotic analgesic* [dihydrocodeine bitartrate; acetaminophen; caffeine] 16•356.4•30 mg

DHE (dihydroergotamine) [see: dihydroergotamine mesylate]

D.H.E. 45 IV or IM injection ℞ *migraine prophylaxis or treatment* [dihydroergotamine mesylate] 1 mg/mL

DHEA (dehydroepiandrosterone) [q.v.]

DHPG (dihydroxy propoxymethyl guanine) [see: ganciclovir]

DHS Tar liquid shampoo, gel shampoo OTC *antiseborrheic; antipsoriatic; antipruritic; antibacterial* [coal tar] 0.5%

DHS Zinc shampoo OTC *antiseborrheic; antibacterial; antifungal* [pyrithione zinc] 2%

DHT tablets, Intensol (concentrated oral solution) ℞ *vitamin D₁ therapy for tetany* [dihydrotachysterol] 0.125, 0.2, 0.4 mg; 0.2 mg/mL

DHT (dihydrotachysterol) [q.v.]

DHT (dihydrotestosterone) [see: androstanolone; stanolone]

DI (doxorubicin, ifosfamide [with mesna rescue]) *chemotherapy protocol*

Diab II ℞ *investigational treatment for type 2 diabetes*

Diaβeta (or DiaBeta) tablets ℞ *sulfonylurea antidiabetic* [glyburide] 1.25, 2.5, 5 mg

Diabetic Tussin liquid OTC *antitussive; decongestant; expectorant* [dextromethorphan hydrobromide; phenylephrine HCl; guaifenesin] 10•5• 100 mg/5 mL

Diabetic Tussin DM liquid OTC *antitussive; expectorant* [dextromethorphan hydrobromide; guaifenesin] 10•100 mg/5 mL

Diabetic Tussin EX liquid OTC *expectorant* [guaifenesin] 100 mg/5 mL

Diabinese tablets ℞ *sulfonylurea antidiabetic* [chlorpropamide] 100, 250 mg

diacerein INN

diacetamate INN, BAN

diacetolol INN, BAN *antiadrenergic (β-receptor)* [also: diacetolol HCl]

diacetolol HCl USAN *antiadrenergic (β-receptor)* [also: diacetolol]

diacetoxyphenylisatin [see: oxyphenisatin acetate]

diacetoxyphenyloxindol [see: oxyphenisatin acetate]

diacetrizoate sodium [see: diatrizoate sodium]

diacetyl diaminodiphenylsulfone (DADDS) [see: acedapsone]

diacetylated monoglycerides NF *plasticizer*

diacetylcholine chloride [see: succinylcholine chloride]

diacetyl-dihydroxydiphenylisatin [see: oxyphenisatin acetate]

diacetyldioxphenylisatin [see: oxyphenisatin acetate]

diacetylmorphine HCl USP *(heroin; banned in USA)* [also: diamorphine]

diacetylmorphine salts *(heroin; banned in USA)*

diacetylsalicylic acid [see: dipyrocetyl]

diacetyltannic acid [see: acetyltannic acid]

diacetylthiamine [see: acetiamine]

diagniol [see: sodium acetrizoate]

diallybarbituric acid [see: allobarbital]

diallylbarbituric acid [now: allobarbital]

diallylnortoxiferene dichloride [see: alcuronium chloride]

diallymal [see: allobarbital]

Dialose tablets OTC *stool softener* [docusate sodium] 100 mg

Dialose Plus tablets, capsules OTC *stimulant laxative; stool softener* [yellow phenolphthalein; docusate sodium] 65•100 mg

Dialpak (trademarked packaging form) *reusable patient compliance package for oral contraceptives*

Dialume capsules ℞ *antacid* [aluminum hydroxide gel] 500 mg ⊠ Dalmane

Dialyte Pattern LM solution ℞ *peritoneal dialysis solution* [multiple electrolytes; dextrose] 1.5%• ±, 2.5%• ±, 4.5%• ±

dia-mer-sulfonamides (sulfadiazine & sulfamerazine) [q.v.]

diamethine [see: dimethyltubocurarinium chloride; dimethyltubocurarine]

diamfenetide INN [also: diamphenethide]

Diamine T.D. timed-release tablets (discontinued 1997) ℞ *antihistamine* [brompheniramine maleate] 8, 12 mg

diaminedipenicillin G [see: penicillin G benzathine]

diaminodiphenylsulfone (DDS) [now: dapsone]

3,4-diaminopyridine *investigational (orphan) for Lambert-Eaton myasthenic syndrome*

*cis-***diamminedichloroplatinum (DDP)** [see: cisplatin]

diammonium phosphate [see: ammonium phosphate]

diamocaine INN, BAN *local anesthetic* [also: diamocaine cyclamate]

diamocaine cyclamate USAN *local anesthetic* [also: diamocaine]

diamorphine BAN *(heroin; banned in USA)* [also: diacetylmorphine HCl]

Diamox powder for IV injection ℞ *carbonic anhydrase inhibitor diuretic; antiglaucoma; anticonvulsant; treatment for acute mountain sickness* [acetazolamide sodium] 500 mg

Diamox tablets, Sequels (sustained-release capsules) ℞ *carbonic anhydrase inhibitor diuretic; antiglaucoma; anticonvulsant; treatment for acute mountain sickness* [acetazolamide] 125, 250 mg; 500 mg

diamphenethide BAN [also: diamfenetide]

diampromide INN, BAN

diampron [see: amicarbalide]

diamthazole BAN [also: dimazole]

diamthazole dihydrochloride [see: diamthazole]

Diane-35 ⒸⒶ sugar-coated tablets ℞ *antiandrogen/estrogen for severe acne in women* [cyproterone acetate; ethinyl estradiol] 2•0.035 mg

Dianeal Peritoneal Dialysis Solution with 1.1% Amino Acids ℞ *investigational (orphan) nutritional supplement for continuous ambulatory peritoneal dialysis patients*

diapamide USAN *diuretic; antihypertensive* [also: tiamizide]

Diaparene Baby cream OTC *topical diaper rash treatment*

Diaparene Cornstarch Baby powder OTC *topical diaper rash treatment* [corn starch; aloe]

Diaparene Diaper Rash ointment OTC *topical diaper rash treatment* [zinc oxide]

Diaper Guard ointment OTC *topical diaper rash treatment* [dimethicone; vitamins A, D, and E; zinc oxide] 1%•±•?

Diaper Rash ointment OTC *topical diaper rash treatment* [zinc oxide]

diaphene [see: dibromsalan]

diaphenylsulfone [see: dapsone]

diaphoretics *a class of agents that promote profuse perspiration* [also called: sudorifics]

Diapid nasal spray ℞ *pituitary antidiuretic hormone for diabetes insipidus* [lypressin] 50 U/mL

Diar-Aid tablets OTC *antidiarrheal; GI adsorbent* [loperamide HCl] 2 mg

diarbarone INN

Diascan reagent strips for home use OTC *in vitro diagnostic aid for blood glucose*

DiaScreen reagent strips for professional use ℞ *in vitro diagnostic aid for multiple disease markers in the urine*

Diasorb tablets, liquid OTC *antidiarrheal; GI adsorbent* [activated attapulgite] 750 mg; 750 mg/5 mL

Diastat rectal gel in a disposable applicator ("pediatric" and "adult" refer to the length of the applicator tip) ℞ *benzodiazepine anticonvulsant for acute repetitive seizures (orphan)* [diazepam] 2.5, 5, 10 mg (pediatric); 10, 15, 20 mg (adult)

Diastix reagent strips for home use OTC *in vitro diagnostic aid for urine glucose*

diathymosulfone INN

diatrizoate meglumine USP *oral/parenteral radiopaque contrast medium (46.67% iodine)* [also: meglumine diatrizoate] 76% injection

diatrizoate methylglucamine [see: diatrizoate meglumine]

diatrizoate sodium USP *oral/rectal/parenteral radiopaque contrast medium (59.87% iodine)* [also: sodium amidotrizoate; sodium diatrizoate]

diatrizoate sodium I 125 USAN *radioactive agent*

diatrizoate sodium I 131 USAN *radioactive agent*

diatrizoic acid USAN, USP, BAN *radiopaque contrast medium* [also: amidotrizoic acid]

diaveridine USAN, INN, BAN *antibacterial*

diazacholesterol dihydrochloride [see: azacosterol HCl]

Diazemuls Ⓒ emulsified IV injection ℞ *benzodiazepine sedative; anxiolytic; anticonvulsant; skeletal muscle relaxant* [diazepam] 5 mg/mL

diazepam USAN, USP, INN, BAN, JAN *benzodiazepine anxiolytic; anticonvulsant; sedative; skeletal muscle relaxant; investigational (orphan) for acute repetitive seizures; also abused as a street drug* 2, 5, 10 mg oral; 1, 5 mg/mL oral; 5 mg/mL injection

diazinon BAN [also: dimpylate]

diaziquone USAN, INN *antineoplastic*

diazoxide USAN, USP, INN, BAN *emergency antihypertensive; vasodilator; glucose-elevating agent*

dibasic calcium phosphate [see: calcium phosphate, dibasic]

dibasic potassium phosphate [see: potassium phosphate, dibasic]

dibasic sodium phosphate [see: sodium phosphate, dibasic]

dibasol [see: bendazol]

dibazol [see: bendazol]

dibekacin INN, BAN

dibemethine INN

dibencil [see: penicillin G benzathine]

dibencozide [see: cobamamide]

Dibent IM injection ℞ *GI antispasmodic* [dicyclomine HCl] 10 mg/mL

dibenthiamine [see: bentiamine]

dibenzathione [see: sulbentine]

dibenzepin INN, BAN *antidepressant* [also: dibenzepin HCl]

dibenzepin HCl USAN *antidepressant* [also: dibenzepin]

dibenzodiazepines *a class of novel (atypical) antipsychotic agents*

dibenzothiazepines *a class of novel (atypical) antipsychotic agents*

dibenzothiazine [see: phenothiazine]

dibenzothiophene USAN *keratolytic*

dibenzoxazepines *a class of dopamine receptor antagonists with antipsychotic, hypotensive, antiemetic, antispasmodic, and antihistaminic activity*

dibenzoyl peroxide [see: benzoyl peroxide]

dibenzoylthiamin [see: bentiamine]

dibenzthion [see: sulbentine]

dibenzylethylenediamine dipenicillin G (DBED) [see: penicillin G benzathine]

Dibenzyline capsules ℞ *antihypertensive for pheochromocytoma* [phenoxybenzamine HCl] 10 mg

N,N-dibenzylmethylamine [see: dibemethine]

dibromodulcitol [see: mitolactol]

dibromohydroxyquinoline [see: broxyquinoline]

dibromomannitol (DBM) [see: mitobronitol]

dibromopropamidine BAN [also: dibrompropamidine]

dibrompropamidine INN [also: dibromopropamidine]

dibromsalan USAN, INN *disinfectant*

dibrospidium chloride INN

dibucaine USP *topical local anesthetic* [also: cinchocaine] 1% topical

dibucaine HCl USP *local anesthetic* [also: cinchocaine HCl]

dibudinate INN *combining name for radicals or groups*

dibunate INN *combining name for radicals or groups*

dibuprol INN

dibupyrone INN, BAN

dibusadol INN

dibutoline sulfate

DIC (dimethyl imidazole carboxamide) [see: dacarbazine]

Dical CapTabs (capsule-shaped tablets) OTC *dietary supplement* [dibasic calcium phosphate; vitamin D] 117 mg (Ca)•90 mg (P)•133 IU

dicalcium phosphate [see: calcium phosphate, dibasic]

Dical-D tablets, chewable wafers OTC *dietary supplement* [dibasic calcium phosphate; vitamin D] 117 mg

(Ca)•90 mg (P)•133 IU; 232 mg
(Ca)•180 mg (P)•200 IU

dicarbine INN

Dicarbosil chewable tablets (discontinued 1998) OTC *antacid* [calcium carbonate] 500 mg ② dacarbazine

dicarfen INN

dichlofenthion BAN

dichloralantipyrine [see: dichloralphenazone]

dichloralphenazone (chloral hydrate & phenazone) BAN *mild sedative*

dichloralpyrine [see: dichloralphenazone]

dichloramine-T NF

dichloranilino imidazolin [see: clonidine HCl]

dichloren [see: mechlorethamine HCl]

dichlorisone INN

dichlorisone acetate [see: dichlorisone]

dichlormethazanone [see: dichlormezanone]

dichlormezanone INN

dichloroacetate sodium *orphan status withdrawn 1996*

dichloroacetic acid *strong keratolytic/cauterant* ② Bichloracetic acid '

dichlorodifluoromethane NF *aerosol propellant; topical refrigerant anesthetic*

dichlorodiphenyl trichloroethane (DDT) [see: chlorophenothane]

dichlorometaxylenol [see: dichloroxylenol]

dichloromethane [see: methylene chloride]

dichlorophen INN, BAN

dichlorophenarsine INN, BAN [also: dichlorophenarsine HCl]

dichlorophenarsine HCl USP [also: dichlorophenarsine]

dichlorotetrafluoroethane NF *aerosol propellant; topical refrigerant anesthetic* [also: cryofluorane]

dichlorovinyl dimethyl phosphate (DDVP) [see: dichlorvos]

dichloroxylenol INN, BAN

dichlorphenamide USP, BAN *carbonic anhydrase inhibitor; diuretic* [also: diclofenamide]

dichlorvos USAN, INN, BAN *anthelmintic*

dichysterol [see: dihydrotachysterol]

diciferron INN

dicirenone USAN, INN *hypotensive; aldosterone antagonist*

Dick test (scarlet fever streptococcus toxin)

diclazuril USAN, INN, BAN *coccidiostat for poultry; investigational for cryptosporidiosis in AIDS*

diclofenac INN, BAN *antiarthritic; nonsteroidal anti-inflammatory drug (NSAID); analgesic* [also: diclofenac potassium]

diclofenac potassium USAN *antiarthritic; nonsteroidal anti-inflammatory drug (NSAID); analgesic* [also: diclofenac] 25, 50, 75 mg oral

diclofenac potassium & hyaluronate sodium *investigational (Phase III) topical treatment for actinic keratosis; clinical trials as a topical analgesic discontinued 1996*

diclofenac sodium USAN, JAN *antiarthritic; analgesic; nonsteroidal anti-inflammatory drug (NSAID); ocular treatment for cataract extraction* 25, 50, 75 mg oral; 0.1% eye drops

diclofenamide INN *carbonic anhydrase inhibitor* [also: dichlorphenamide]

diclofensine INN

diclofibrate [see: simfibrate]

diclofurime INN

diclometide INN

diclonixin INN

dicloralurea USAN, INN *veterinary food additive*

Diclotec Ⓐ suppositories ℞ *nonsteroidal anti-inflammatory drug (NSAID); antiarthritic; analgesic* [diclofenac sodium] 50, 100 mg

dicloxacillin USAN, INN, BAN *penicillinase-resistant penicillin antibiotic*

dicloxacillin sodium USAN, USP, BAN *penicillinase-resistant penicillin antibiotic* 250, 500 mg oral

dicobalt edetate INN, BAN

dicolinium iodide INN

dicophane BAN [also: chlorophenothane; clofenotane]

dicoumarin [see: dicumarol]

dicoumarol INN *coumarin-derivative anticoagulant* [also: dicumarol]

dicresulene INN

Dictamnus albus medicinal herb [see: fraxinella]

dicumarol USAN, USP *coumarin-derivative anticoagulant* [also: dicoumarol] 25 mg oral ⑨ Demerol

dicyclomine BAN *anticholinergic* [also: dicyclomine HCl; dicycloverine]

dicyclomine HCl USP *GI antispasmodic; anticholinergic* [also: dicycloverine; dicyclomine] 10, 20 mg oral; 10 mg/5 mL oral; 10 mg/mL injection

dicycloverine INN *anticholinergic* [also: dicyclomine HCl; dicyclomine]

dicycloverine HCl [see: dicyclomine HCl]

dicysteine [see: cystine]

didanosine USAN, INN, BAN *antiviral for AIDS*

didehydrodideoxythymidine [see: stavudine]

Di-Delamine gel, spray OTC *topical antihistamine; bacteriostatic* [diphenhydramine HCl; tripelennamine HCl] 1%•0.5%•

dideoxycytidine (DDC; ddC) [see: zalcitabine]

dideoxyinosine (DDI; ddI) [see: didanosine]

Didrex tablets ℞ *anorexiant* [benzphetamine HCl] 25, 50 mg

Didro-Kit (Italian name for U.S. product Didronel)

Didronel IV infusion ℞ *bisphosphonate bone resorption inhibitor for hypercalcemia of malignancy (orphan)* [etidronate disodium] 300 mg/ampule

Didronel tablets ℞ *bisphosphonate bone resorption inhibitor for Paget's disease and heterotopic ossification* [etidronate disodium] 200, 400 mg

didrovaltrate INN

didroxane [see: dichlorophen]

dieldrin INN, BAN

dielytra; choice dielytra *medicinal herb* [see: turkey corn]

diemal [see: barbital]

dienestrol USP, INN *estrogen* [also: dienoestrol]

dienoestrol BAN *estrogen* [also: dienestrol]

dienogest INN

Diet Ayds candy OTC *decrease taste perception of sweetness* [benzocaine] 6 mg

dietamiphylline [see: etamiphyllin]

dietamiverine HCl [see: bietamiverine HCl]

diethadione INN, BAN

diethanolamine NF *alkalizing agent*

diethazine INN, BAN

diethazine HCl [see: diethazine]

diethyl phthalate NF *plasticizer*

diethylamine p-aminobenzenestibonate [see: stibosamine]

3-diethylaminobutyranilide [see: octacaine]

diethylbarbiturate monosodium [see: barbital sodium]

diethylbarbituric acid [see: barbital]

diethylcarbamazine INN, BAN *anthelmintic for Bancroft's filariasis, onchocerciasis, tropical eosinophilia, and loiasis* [also: diethylcarbamazine citrate]

diethylcarbamazine citrate USP *anthelmintic for Bancroft's filariasis, onchocerciasis, tropical eosinophilia, and loiasis* [also: diethylcarbamazine]

diethylcarbamazine dihydrogen citrate [see: diethylcarbamazine citrate]

diethyldithiocarbamate *investigational (Phase II/III, orphan) immunomodulator for HIV and AIDS*

diethyldixanthogen [see: dixanthogen]

diethylenediamine citrate [see: piperazine citrate]

diethylenetriaminepentaacetic acid (DTPA) [see: pentetic acid]

diethylhomospermine (DEHOP; DEHSPM) *investigational (Phase II) agent for AIDS-associated, uncontrolled, refractory diarrhea*

N,N-diethyllysergamide [see: lysergide]

diethylmalonylurea [see: barbital]

diethylmalonylurea sodium [see: barbital sodium]

N,N-diethylnicotinamide [see: nikethamide]

diethylnorspermine *investigational (Phase I) anticancer agent*

diethylpropion BAN *anorexiant; CNS stimulant* [also: diethylpropion HCl; amfepramone] 75 mg oral

diethylpropion HCl USP *anorexiant; CNS stimulant* [also: amfepramone; diethylpropion] 25 mg oral

diethylstilbestrol (DES) USP, INN *hormonal antineoplastic for inoperable prostatic and breast cancer* [also: stilboestrol] 1, 5 mg oral

diethylstilbestrol diphosphate USP *hormonal antineoplastic* [also: fosfestrol]

diethylstilbestrol dipropionate NF

p-diethylsulfamoylbenzoic acid [see: etebenecid; ethebenecid]

diethylthiambutene INN, BAN

diethyltoluamide (DEET) USP, BAN *arthropod repellent*

diethyltryptamine (DET) *a hallucinogenic street drug closely related to dimethyltryptamine (DMT), but prepared synthetically*

N,N-diethylvanillamide [see: ethamivan]

dietifen INN

dietroxine [see: diethadione]

Dieutrim T.D. timed-release capsules OTC *diet aid; decrease perception of sweetness* [phenylpropanolamine HCl; benzocaine] 75•9 mg

diexanthogen [see: dixanthogen]

difebarbamate INN

difemerine INN [also: difemerine HCl]

difemerine HCl [also: difemerine]

difemetorex INN

difenamizole INN

difencloxazine INN

difencloxazine HCl [see: difencloxazine]

difenidol INN *antiemetic; antivertigo* [also: diphenidol]

difenoximide INN *antiperistaltic* [also: difenoximide HCl]

difenoximide HCl USAN *antiperistaltic* [also: difenoximide]

difenoxin USAN, INN, BAN *antiperistaltic*

difenoxin HCl *antiperistaltic*

difetarsone INN, BAN

difeterol INN

Differin solution, gel ℞ *synthetic retinoid analog for acne* [adapalene] 0.1%

diflorasone INN, BAN *topical corticosteroidal anti-inflammatory* [also: diflorasone diacetate]

diflorasone diacetate USAN, USP *topical corticosteroidal anti-inflammatory* [also: diflorasone]

difloxacin INN *anti-infective; DNA gyrase inhibitor* [also: difloxacin HCl]

difloxacin HCl USAN *anti-infective; DNA gyrase inhibitor* [also: difloxacin]

difluanazine INN *CNS stimulant* [also: difluanine HCl]

difluanazine HCl [see: difluanine HCl]

difluanine HCl USAN *CNS stimulant* [also: difluanazine]

Diflucan tablets, powder for oral suspension, IV infusion ℞ *systemic antifungal* [fluconazole] 50, 100, 150, 200 mg; 10, 40 mg/mL; 2 mg/mL

diflucortolone USAN, INN, BAN *corticosteroid; anti-inflammatory*

diflucortolone pivalate USAN *corticosteroid; anti-inflammatory*

diflumidone INN, BAN *anti-inflammatory* [also: diflumidone sodium]

diflumidone sodium USAN *anti-inflammatory* [also: diflumidone]

diflunisal USAN, USP, INN, BAN *anti-inflammatory; analgesic; antipyretic; antiarthritic; antirheumatic* 250, 500 mg oral

difluoromethylornithine (DFMO) [see: eflornithine]

difluoromethylornithine HCl [see: eflornithine HCl]

difluprednate USAN, INN *anti-inflammatory*

difolliculin [see: estradiol benzoate]

diftalone USAN, INN *anti-inflammatory*

digalloyl trioleate USAN

Di-Gel liquid OTC *antacid; antiflatulent* [aluminum hydroxide; magnesium hydroxide; simethicone] 200•200•20 mg/5 mL

Di-Gel, Advanced Formula chewable tablets OTC *antacid; antiflatulent* [magnesium hydroxide; calcium carbonate; simethicone] 128•280•20 mg

Digepepsin dual-coated tablets ℞ *digestive enzymes* [pancreatin; pepsin; bile salts] 300•250•150 mg

digestants; digestives *a class of agents that promote or aid in digestion*

Digestozyme tablets ℞ *digestive enzymes; laxative; choleretic* [pancreatin; pepsin; dehydrocholic acid] 300•250•25 mg

Digibind powder for IV injection ℞ *antidote to digoxin/digitoxin overdose (orphan); investigational (orphan) for other cardiac glycoside intoxication* [digoxin immune Fab (ovine)] 38 mg/vial

Digidote ℞ *antidote to digoxin/digitoxin overdose (orphan); investigational (orphan) for other cardiac glycoside intoxication* [digoxin immune Fab (ovine)]

digitalis USP *cardiotonic*

Digitalis ambigua; D. ferriginea; D. grandiflora; D. lanata; D. lutea; D. purpurea medicinal herb [see: foxglove]

digitalis glycosides *a class of cardiovascular drugs that increase the force of cardiac contractions* [also called: cardiac glycosides]

digitoxin USP, INN, BAN *cardiotonic; cardiac glycoside* ⃰ Desoxyn; digoxin

digitoxin, acetyl [see: acetyldigitoxin]

α-digitoxin monoacetate [see: acetyldigitoxin]

digitoxoside [see: digitoxin]

digolil INN *combining name for radicals or groups*

digoxin USP, INN, BAN *cardiotonic; cardiac glycoside antiarrhythmic* 0.125, 0.25, 0.5 mg oral, 0.05 mg/mL oral, 0.15 mg/mL injection ⃰ Desoxyn; digitoxin

digoxin antibody [see: digoxin immune Fab]

digoxin immune Fab (ovine) *antidote to digoxin/digitoxin intoxication (orphan); investigational (orphan) for other cardiac glycoside intoxication*

dihematoporphyrin ethers *orphan status withdrawn 1996*

dihexyverine INN *anticholinergic* [also: dihexyverine HCl]

dihexyverine HCl USAN *anticholinergic* [also: dihexyverine]

Dihistine DH liquid OTC *narcotic antitussive; decongestant; antihistamine* [codeine phosphate; pseudoephedrine HCl; chlorpheniramine maleate; alcohol] 10•30•2 mg/5 mL

Dihistine Expectorant liquid ℞ *narcotic antitussive; decongestant; expectorant* [codeine phosphate; pseudoephedrine HCl; guaifenesin; alcohol] 10•30•100 mg/5 mL

dihydan soluble [see: phenytoin sodium]

dihydralazine INN, BAN

dihydralazine sulfate [see: dihydralazine]

5,6-dihydro-5-azacytidine *investigational (orphan) for malignant mesothelioma*

dihydrobenzthiazide [see: hydrobentizide]

dihydrocodeine INN, BAN *analgesic* [also: dihydrocodeine bitartrate]

dihydrocodeine bitartrate USP *analgesic* [also: dihydrocodeine]

dihydrocodeinone bitartrate [see: hydrocodone bitartrate]

dihydroergocornine [see: ergoloid mesylates]

dihydroergocristine [see: ergoloid mesylates]

dihydroergocryptine [see: ergoloid mesylates]

dihydroergotamine (DHE) INN, BAN *antiadrenergic; anticoagulant; ergot alkaloid for rapid control of migraines* [also: dihydroergotamine mesylate; dihydroergotamine mesilate]

dihydroergotamine mesilate JAN *antiadrenergic; anticoagulant; ergot alkaloid for rapid control of migraines* [also: dihydroergotamine mesylate; dihydroergotamine]

dihydroergotamine mesylate USAN, USP *antiadrenergic; anticoagulant;*

ergot alkaloid for rapid control of migraines [also: dihydroergotamine; dihydroergotamine mesilate]

dihydroergotamine methanesulfonate [see: dihydroergotamine mesylate]

dihydroergotoxine mesylate [now: ergoloid mesylates]

dihydroergotoxine methanesulfonate [now: ergoloid mesylates]

dihydroethaverine [see: drotaverine]

dihydrofollicular hormone [see: estradiol]

dihydrofolliculine [see: estradiol]

dihydrogenated ergot alkaloids [now: ergoloid mesylates]

dihydrohydroxycodeinone [see: oxycodone]

dihydrohydroxycodeinone HCl [see: oxycodone HCl]

6-dihydro-6-iminopurine [see: adenine]

dihydroindolones *a class of dopamine receptor antagonists with conventional (typical) antipsychotic activity* [also called: indolones]

dihydroisoperparine [see: drotaverine]

dihydromorphinone HCl [now: hydromorphone HCl]

dihydroneopine [see: dihydrocodeine bitartrate]

dihydropyridines *a class of calcium channel blockers*

dihydrostreptomycin (DST) INN *antibacterial* [also: dihydrostreptomycin sulfate]

dihydrostreptomycin sulfate USP *antibacterial* [also: dihydrostreptomycin]

dihydrostreptomycin-streptomycin [see: streptoduocin]

dihydrotachysterol (DHT) USP, INN, BAN, JAN *vitamin D$_1$; calcium regulator for tetany and hypoparathyroidism* 0.125, 0.2, 0.4 mg oral; 0.2 mg/mL oral

dihydrotestosterone (DHT) *investigational (orphan) for AIDS-wasting syndrome* [see: androstanolone; stanolone]

dihydrotheelin [see: estradiol]

dihydroxy(stearato)aluminum [see: aluminum monostearate]

dihydroxy propoxymethyl guanine (DHPG) [see: gancyclovir]

dihydroxyacetone *skin darkener for vitiligo and hypopigmented areas*

dihydroxyaluminum aminoacetate (DAA) USP *antacid*

dihydroxyaluminum sodium carbonate USP *antacid*

dihydroxyanthranol [see: anthralin]

dihydroxyanthraquinone *(withdrawn from market)* [see: danthron]

1,25-dihydroxycholecalciferol [see: calcitriol]

24,25-dihydroxycholecalciferol *investigational (orphan) for uremic osteodystrophy*

dihydroxyestrin [see: estradiol]

dihydroxyfluorane [see: fluorescein]

dihydroxyphenylalanine (DOPA) [see: levodopa]

dihydroxyphenylisatin [see: oxyphenisatin acetate]

dihydroxyphenyloxindol [see: oxyphenisatin acetate]

dihydroxyprogesterone acetophenide [see: algestone acetophenide]

dihydroxypropyl theophylline [see: dyphylline]

diiodobuphenine [see: bufeniode]

diiodohydroxyquin [now: iodoquinol]

diiodohydroxyquinoline INN, BAN *antiamebic* [also: iodoquinol]

diisopromine INN

diisopromine HCl [see: diisopromine]

diisopropanolamine NF *alkalizing agent*

diisopropyl flurophosphate (DFP) [see: isoflurophate]

diisopropyl flurophosphonate [see: isoflurophate]

diisopropyl phosphorofluoridate [see: isoflurophate]

2,6-diisopropylphenol [see: propofol]

Dilacor XR sustained-release capsules ℞ *antihypertensive; antianginal; antiarrhythmic; calcium channel blocker* [diltiazem HCl] 120, 180, 240 mg ② Delcort

Dilantin Infatabs (chewable tablets) ℞ *hydantoin anticonvulsant* [phenytoin] 50 mg ② Milontin; Mylanta; Xalatan

Dilantin IV or IM injection (discontinued 1996) ℞ *hydantoin anticonvulsant* [phenytoin sodium] 50 mg/mL ☒ Milontin; Mylanta; Xalatan

Dilantin Kapseals (capsules) ℞ *hydantoin anticonvulsant* [phenytoin sodium] 30, 100 mg ☒ Milontin; Mylanta; Xalatan

Dilantin with Phenobarbital Kapseals (capsules) (discontinued 1996) ℞ *hydantoin anticonvulsant; sedative* [phenytoin sodium; phenobarbital] 100•16, 100•32 mg ☒ Milontin; Mylanta; Xalatan

Dilantin-30 Pediatric oral suspension (discontinued 1996) ℞ *hydantoin anticonvulsant* [phenytoin] 30 mg/5 mL ☒ Milontin; Mylanta; Xalatan

Dilantin-125 oral suspension ℞ *hydantoin anticonvulsant* [phenytoin] 125 mg/5 mL ☒ Milontin; Mylanta; Xalatan

Dilatrate-SR sustained-release capsules ℞ *antianginal; vasodilator* [isosorbide dinitrate] 40 mg

Dilaudid tablets, oral liquid, subcu or IM injection, suppositories ℞ *narcotic analgesic; widely abused as a street drug* [hydromorphone HCl] 1, 2, 4, 8 mg; 5 mg/5 mL; 1, 2, 4 mg/mL; 3 mg

Dilaudid Cough syrup ℞ *narcotic antitussive; expectorant* [hydromorphone HCl; guaifenesin; alcohol 5%] 1•100 mg/5 mL

Dilaudid-HP subcu or IM injection ℞ *narcotic analgesic* [hydromorphone HCl] 10 mg/mL (250 mg/vial)

dilazep INN

dilevalol INN, BAN *antihypertensive; antiadrenergic (β-receptor)* [also: dilevalol HCl]

dilevalol HCl USAN, JAN *antihypertensive; antiadrenergic (β-receptor)* [also: dilevalol]

dilithium carbonate [see: lithium carbonate]

dill *(Anethum graveolens)* fruit and seed *medicinal herb used as an aro-*

matic, carminative, diaphoretic, stimulant, and stomachic

dilmefone INN

Dilocaine injection ℞ *injectable local anesthetic* [lidocaine HCl] 1%, 2%

Dilor tablets, elixir, IM injection ℞ *antiasthmatic; bronchodilator* [dyphylline] 200 mg; 160 mg/15 mL; 250 mg/mL

Dilor 400 tablets ℞ *antiasthmatic; bronchodilator* [dyphylline] 400 mg

Dilor-G tablets, liquid ℞ *antiasthmatic; bronchodilator; expectorant* [dyphylline; guaifenesin] 200•200 mg; 300•300 mg/15 mL

diloxanide INN, BAN, DCF

diloxanide furoate *investigational antiinfective for amebiasis (available only from the Centers for Disease Control and Prevention)*

diltiazem INN, BAN *coronary vasodilator; calcium channel blocker; antianginal; antihypertensive* [also: diltiazem HCl]

diltiazem HCl USAN, USP, JAN *coronary vasodilator; calcium channel blocker; antianginal; antihypertensive; antiarrhythmic* [also: diltiazem] 30, 60, 90, 120 mg oral; 5 mg/mL injection

diltiazem malate USAN *coronary vasodilator; calcium channel blocker; antianginal; antihypertensive; antiarrhythmic*

diluted acetic acid [see: acetic acid, diluted]

diluted alcohol [see: alcohol, diluted]

diluted hydrochloric acid [see: hydrochloric acid, diluted]

diluted sodium hypochlorite [see: sodium hypochlorite, diluted]

dimabefylline INN

Dimacol caplets OTC *antitussive; decongestant; expectorant* [dextromethorphan hydrobromide; pseudoephedrine HCl; guaifenesin] 10•30•100 mg ☒ dimercaprol

dimantine INN *anthelmintic* [also: dymanthine HCl]

dimantine HCl INN [also: dymanthine HCl]

Dimaphen tablets, Release-Tabs (timed-release tablets), elixir OTC *decongestant; antihistamine* [phenylpropanolamine HCl; brompheniramine maleate] 25•4 mg; 75•12 mg; 12.5•2 mg/5 mL

dimazole INN [also: diamthazole]

dimazole dihydrochloride [see: dimazole; diamthazole]

dimecamine INN

dimecolonium iodide INN

dimecrotic acid INN

dimedrol [see: diphenhydramine HCl]

dimefadane USAN, INN *analgesic*

dimefilcon A USAN *hydrophilic contact lens material*

dimefline INN, BAN *respiratory stimulant* [also: dimefline HCl]

dimefline HCl USAN *respiratory stimulant* [also: dimefline]

dimefocon A USAN *hydrophobic contact lens material*

dimekolin [see: dimecolonium iodide]

dimelazine INN

dimelin [see: dimecolonium iodide]

dimemorfan INN

dimenhydrinate USP, INN, BAN *antiemetic; anticholinergic; antivertigo; motion sickness prophylaxis* 50 mg oral; 12.5 mg/4 mL oral; 50 mg/mL injection ☒ diphenhydramine

dimenoxadol INN [also: dimenoxadole]

dimenoxadole BAN [also: dimenoxadol]

dimepheptanol INN, BAN

dimepranol INN *immunomodulator* [also: dimepranol acedoben]

dimepranol acedoben USAN *immunomodulator* [also: dimepranol]

dimepregnen INN, BAN

dimepropion BAN [also: metamfepramone]

dimeprozan INN

dimeprozinum [see: dimeprozan]

dimercaprol USP, INN *antidote to arsenic, gold and mercury poisoning; lead poisoning adjunct; chelating agent* ☒ Dimacol

dimercaptopropanol [see: dimercaprol]

2,3-dimercaptosuccinic acid (DMSA) [see: succimer]

dimesna INN

dimesone INN, BAN

Dimetabs tablets ℞ *anticholinergic; antiemetic; antivertigo agent; motion sickness preventative* [dimenhydrinate] 50 mg ☒ Dimetane; Dimetapp

dimetacrine INN

dimetamfetamine INN

Dimetane elixir (discontinued 1996) OTC *antihistamine* [brompheniramine maleate] 2 mg/5 mL ☒ Dimetabs

Dimetane Extentabs (long-acting tablets) (discontinued 1997) OTC *antihistamine* [brompheniramine maleate] 12 mg ☒ Dimetabs

Dimetane Decongestant caplets, elixir OTC *decongestant; antihistamine* [phenylephrine HCl; brompheniramine maleate] 10•4 mg; 5•2 mg/5 mL

Dimetane-DC Cough syrup ℞ *narcotic antitussive; decongestant; antihistamine* [codeine phosphate; phenylpropanolamine HCl; brompheniramine maleate; alcohol 0.95%] 10•12.5•2 mg/5 mL

Dimetane-DX Cough syrup ℞ *antitussive; decongestant; antihistamine* [dextromethorphan hydrobromide; pseudoephedrine HCl; brompheniramine maleate; alcohol 0.95%] 10•30•2 mg/5 mL

Dimetapp tablets, Extentabs (long-acting tablets), elixir OTC *decongestant; antihistamine* [phenylpropanolamine HCl; brompheniramine maleate] 25•4 mg; 75•12 mg; 12.5•2 mg/5 mL ☒ Dimetabs

Dimetapp 4-Hour Liqui-Gels (liquid-filled capsules) OTC *decongestant; antihistamine* [phenylpropanolamine HCl; brompheniramine maleate] 25•4 mg

Dimetapp Allergy liqui-gels OTC *antihistamine* [brompheniramine maleate] 4 mg

Dimetapp Cold & Allergy chewable tablets, quick-dissolve tablets OTC *pediatric decongestant and antihistamine* [phenylpropanolamine HCl; brompheniramine maleate] 6.25•1 mg

Dimetapp Cold & Flu caplets OTC *decongestant; antihistamine; analgesic*

[phenylpropanolamine HCl; brompheniramine maleate; acetaminophen] 12.5•2•500 mg

Dimetapp DM elixir OTC *antitussive; decongestant; antihistamine* [dextromethorphan hydrobromide; phenylpropanolamine HCl; brompheniramine maleate] 10•12.5•2 mg/5 mL

Dimetapp Sinus caplets OTC *decongestant; analgesic* [pseudoephedrine HCl; ibuprofen] 30•200 mg

dimethadione USAN, INN *anticonvulsant*

dimethazan

dimethazine [see: mebolazine]

dimethicone USAN, NF, BAN *lubricant and hydrophobing agent; soft tissue prosthetic aid* [also: dimeticone] ⑨ cimetidine

dimethicone 350 USAN *soft tissue prosthetic aid*

dimethindene BAN *antihistamine* [also: dimethindene maleate; dimetindene]

dimethindene maleate USP *antihistamine* [also: dimetindene; dimethindene]

dimethiodal sodium INN

dimethisoquin BAN [also: dimethisoquin HCl; quinisocaine]

dimethisoquin HCl USAN [also: quinisocaine; dimethisoquin]

dimethisterone USAN, NF, INN, BAN *progestin*

dimetholizine INN

dimethothiazine BAN *serotonin inhibitor* [also: fonazine mesylate; dimetotiazine]

dimethoxanate INN, BAN

dimethoxanate HCl [see: dimethoxanate]

2,5-dimethoxy-4-methylamphetamine (DOM) *a hallucinogenic street drug derived from amphetamine, popularly called STP*

dimethoxyphenyl penicillin sodium [see: methicillin sodium]

dimethpyridene maleate [see: dimethindene maleate]

dimethyl ketone [see: acetone]

dimethyl phthalate USP

dimethyl polysiloxane [see: dimethicone]

dimethyl sulfoxide (DMSO) USAN, USP, INN *solvent; topical anti-inflammatory for symptomatic relief of interstitial cystitis; investigational (orphan) for traumatic brain coma; investigational (orphan) topical treatment for extravasation of cytotoxic drugs* [also: dimethyl sulphoxide]

dimethyl sulphoxide BAN *topical anti-inflammatory; solvent* [also: dimethyl sulfoxide]

dimethyl triazeno imidazole carboxamide (DIC; DTIC) [see: dacarbazine]

dimethylaminophenazone [see: aminopyrine]

dimethylcysteine [see: penicillamine]

dimethylglycine HCl

dimethylhexestrol [see: methestrol]

1,5-dimethylhexylamine [see: octodrine]

5,5-dimethyl-2,4-oxazolidinedione (DMO) [see: dimethadione]

dimethyloxyquinazine [see: antipyrine]

o,α-dimethylphenethylamine [see: ortetamine]

dimethylsiloxane polymers [see: dimethicone]

dimethylthiambutene INN, BAN

dimethyltryptamine (DMT) *hallucinogenic street drug derived from a plant native to South America and the West Indies*

dimethyltubocurarine BAN [also: dimethyltubocurarinium chloride]

dimethyltubocurarine iodide [see: metocurine iodide]

dimethyltubocurarinium chloride INN [also: dimethyltubocurarine]

dimethylxanthine [see: theophylline]

dimeticone INN *lubricant and hydrophobing agent; soft tissue prosthetic aid* [also: dimethicone]

dimetindene INN *antihistamine* [also: dimethindene maleate; dimethindene]

dimetindene maleate [see: dimethindene maleate]

dimetipirium bromide INN
dimetofrine INN
dimetotiazine INN *serotonin inhibitor*
[also: fonazine mesylate; dimethothi-
azine]
dimetridazole INN, BAN
dimevamide INN
dimevamide sulfate [see: dimevamide]
diminazene INN, BAN
dimoxamine HCl USAN *memory adjuvant*
dimoxaprost INN
dimoxyline INN
dimpylate INN [also: diazinon]
dinaline INN
Dinate IV or IM injection ℞ *anticholinergic; antiemetic; antivertigo agent;
motion sickness preventative* [dimen-
hydrinate] 50 mg/mL
dinazafone INN
diniprofylline INN
dinitolmide INN, BAN
dinitrotoluamide [see: dinitolmide]
dinoprost USAN, INN, BAN *oxytocic;
prostaglandin*
dinoprost trometamol BAN *oxytocic;
prostaglandin* [also: dinoprost tro-
methamine]
dinoprost tromethamine USAN *oxytocic; prostaglandin-type abortifacient*
[also: dinoprost trometamol]
dinoprostone USAN, INN, BAN *oxytocic
for induction of labor; prostaglandin-type
abortifacient; cervical ripening agent*
dinsed USAN, INN *coccidiostat for poultry*
Diocto liquid, syrup OTC *stool softener*
[docusate sodium] 150 mg/15 mL; 60
mg/15 mL
Diocto-C syrup OTC *stimulant laxative;
stool softener* [casanthranol; docusate
sodium] 30•60 mg/15 mL
Diocto-K capsules OTC *stool softener*
[docusate potassium] 100 mg
Diocto-K Plus capsules OTC *stimulant
laxative; stool softener* [casanthranol;
docusate potassium] 30•100 mg
Dioctolose Plus capsules OTC *stimulant laxative; stool softener* [casanthra-
nol; docusate potassium] 30•100 mg

dioctyl calcium sulfosuccinate
[now: docusate calcium]
dioctyl potassium sulfosuccinate
[now: docusate potassium]
**dioctyl sodium sulfosuccinate
(DSS)** [now: docusate sodium]
Diodex ⊕ (U.S. product: Decadron
Phosphate) eye drops ℞ *topical ophthalmic corticosteroidal anti-inflammatory* [dexamethasone sodium phos-
phate] 0.1%
diodone INN [also: iodopyracet]
Dioeze capsules OTC *stool softener* [doc-
usate sodium] 250 mg
diohippuric acid I 125 USAN *radioactive agent*
diohippuric acid I 131 USAN *radioactive agent*
diolamine USAN, INN *combining name
for radicals or groups*
diolostene [see: methandriol]
dionin [see: ethylmorphine HCl]
Dionosil Oily suspension for intratracheal use (discontinued 1999) ℞
radiopaque contrast medium [propylio-
done in peanut oil (56.7% iodine)]
60% (34%)
diophyllin [see: aminophylline]
Dioscorea villosa medicinal herb [see:
wild yam]
diosmin INN
Diostate D tablets OTC *dietary supplement* [calcium; phosphorus; vitamin
D] 114 mg•88 mg•133 IU
diotyrosine I 125 USAN *radioactive agent*
diotyrosine I 131 USAN *radioactive agent*
Dioval XX; Dioval 40 IM injection
(discontinued 1998) ℞ *estrogen
replacement therapy for postmenopausal disorders; antineoplastic for prostatic cancer* [estradiol valerate in oil]
20 mg/mL; 40 mg/mL
Diovan capsules ℞ *antihypertensive;
angiotensin II receptor antagonist* [val-
sartan] 80, 160 mg
Diovan HCT tablets ℞ *antihypertensive; angiotensin II receptor antagonist;
diuretic* [valsartan; hydrochlorothia-
zide] 80•12.5, 160•12.5 mg
dioxadilol INN

dioxadrol INN *antidepressant* [also: dioxadrol HCl]

dioxadrol HCl USAN *antidepressant* [also: dioxadrol]

***d*-dioxadrol HCl** [see: dexoxadrol HCl]

dioxamate INN, BAN

dioxaphetyl butyrate INN, BAN

dioxathion BAN [also: dioxation]

dioxation INN [also: dioxathion]

dioxethedrin INN

dioxethedrin HCl [see: dioxethedrin]

dioxifedrine INN

dioxindol [see: oxyphenisatin acetate]

dioxyanthranol [see: anthralin]

dioxyanthraquinone (*withdrawn from market*) [see: danthron]

dioxybenzone USAN, USP, INN *ultraviolet screen*

dipalmitoylphosphatidylcholine (DPPC) [see: colfosceril palmitate]

diparcol HCl [see: diethazine HCl]

dipegyl [see: niacinamide]

dipenicillin G [see: penicillin G benzathine]

dipenine bromide BAN [also: diponium bromide]

Dipentum capsules ℞ *anti-inflammatory for ulcerative colitis* [olsalazine sodium] 250 mg

diperodon USP, INN, BAN *topical anesthetic*

diperodon HCl *topical anesthetic*

diphemanil methylsulfate USP *anticholinergic* [also: diphemanil metilsulfate; diphemanil methylsulphate]

diphemanil methylsulphate BAN *anticholinergic* [also: diphemanil methylsulfate; diphemanil metilsulfate]

diphemanil metilsulfate INN *anticholinergic* [also: diphemanil methylsulfate; diphemanil methylsulphate]

Diphen AF liquid OTC *antihistamine* [diphenhydramine HCl] 6.25 mg/5 mL

Diphen Cough syrup OTC *antihistamine; antitussive* [diphenhydramine HCl; alcohol 5%] 12.5 mg/5 mL

diphenadione USP, INN, BAN

diphenan INN

diphenatil [see: diphemanil methylsulfate]

diphenchloxazine HCl [see: difencloxazine HCl]

diphenesenic acid [see: xenyhexenic acid]

Diphenhist caplets, softgels, liquid OTC *antihistamine* [diphenhydramine HCl] 25 mg; 25 mg; 12.5 mg/5 mL

diphenhydramine INN, BAN *ethanolamine antihistamine; anticholinergic; antiparkinsonian; motion sickness relief* [also: diphenhydramine citrate] ⑨ dimenhydrinate

Diphenhydramine 50 capsules OTC *antihistamine* [diphenhydramine HCl] 50 mg

diphenhydramine citrate USP *ethanolamine antihistamine; anticholinergic; antiparkinsonian; motion sickness relief* [also: diphenhydramine]

diphenhydramine HCl USP, BAN *ethanolamine antihistamine; antitussive; motion sickness preventative; sleep aid* 25, 50 mg oral; 12.5 mg/5 mL oral; 50 mg/mL injection

diphenhydramine theoclate [see: dimenhydrinate]

diphenidol USAN, BAN *antiemetic; antivertigo* [also: difenidol]

diphenidol HCl USAN *antiemetic*

diphenidol pamoate USAN *antiemetic*

diphenmethanil methylsulfate [see: diphemanil methylsulfate]

diphenoxylate INN, BAN *antiperistaltic* [also: diphenoxylate HCl]

diphenoxylate HCl USP *antiperistaltic* [also: diphenoxylate]

diphenylacetylindandione [see: diphenadione]

diphenylalkylamines *a class of calcium channel blockers*

Diphenylan Sodium capsules ℞ *anticonvulsant* [phenytoin sodium] 30, 100 mg ⑨ Diphenylin

diphenylbutazone [see: phenylbutazone]

diphenylbutylpiperidines [see: phenylbutylpiperidines]

diphenylhydantoin [now: phenytoin]

diphenylhydantoin sodium [now: phenytoin sodium]

diphenylisatin [see: oxyphenisatin]

diphenylpyraline INN, BAN *antihistamine* [also: diphenylpyraline HCl]

diphenylpyraline HCl USP *antihistamine* [also: diphenylpyraline]

diphetarsone [see: difetarsone]

diphexamide iodomethylate [see: buzepide metiodide]

diphosphonic acid [see: etidronic acid]

diphosphopyridine nucleotide (DPN) [now: nadide]

diphosphoric acid, tetrasodium salt [see: sodium pyrophosphate]

diphosphothiamin [see: co-carboxylase]

diphoxazide INN

diphtheria antitoxin USP *passive immunizing agent* [also: diphtheria toxoid] 500 U/mL injection

diphtheria equine antitoxin *investigational passive immunizing agent (available only from the Centers for Disease Control and Prevention)*

diphtheria & tetanus toxoids, adsorbed (DT; Td) USP *active immunizing agent* 2•2, 2•5, 2•10, 6.6•5, 7.5•7.5, 10•5, 12.5•5, 15•10 LfU/0.5 mL injection

diphtheria & tetanus toxoids & acellular pertussis vaccine (DTaP) *active immunizing agent*

diphtheria & tetanus toxoids & pertussis vaccine (DTP) USP *active immunizing agent*

diphtheria & tetanus toxoids & whole-cell pertussis vaccine (DTwP) *active immunizing agent* 6.5•5•4, 10•5.5•4 LfU/0.5 mL injection

diphtheria toxin, diagnostic [now: diphtheria toxin for Schick test]

diphtheria toxin, inactivated diagnostic [now: Schick test control]

diphtheria toxin for Schick test USP *dermal diphtheria immunity test*

diphtheria toxoid USP *active immunizing agent* [also: diphtheria antitoxin]

diphtheria toxoid, adsorbed USP *active immunizing agent* 15 LfU/0.5 mL injection

dipipanone INN, BAN

dipipanone HCl [see: dipipanone]

dipiproverine INN

dipiproverine HCl [see: dipiproverine]

dipivalyl epinephrine (DPE) [now: dipivefrin]

dipivefrin USAN *ophthalmic adrenergic* [also: dipivefrine]

dipivefrin HCl USP *topical antiglaucoma agent* 0.1% eye drops

dipivefrine INN, BAN *ophthalmic adrenergic* [also: dipivefrin]

diponium bromide INN [also: dipenine bromide]

dipotassium carbonate [see: potassium carbonate]

dipotassium clorazepate INN *benzodiazepine anxiolytic; minor tranquilizer; anticonvulsant adjunct; alcohol withdrawal aid* [also: clorazepate dipotassium]

dipotassium hydrogen phosphate [see: potassium phosphate, dibasic]

dipotassium phosphate [see: potassium phosphate, dibasic]

dipotassium pyrosulfite [see: potassium metabisulfite]

diprafenone INN

diprenorphine INN, BAN

Diprivan emulsion for IV ℞ *general anesthetic* [propofol] 10 mg/mL

diprobutine INN, BAN

diprofene INN

diprogulic acid INN

diproleandomycin INN

Diprolene ointment, gel, lotion ℞ *topical corticosteroidal anti-inflammatory* [betamethasone dipropionate, augmented] 0.05%

Diprolene AF cream ℞ *topical corticosteroidal anti-inflammatory* [betamethasone dipropionate, augmented] 0.05%

diprophylline INN, BAN *bronchodilator* [also: dyphylline]

dipropylacetic acid [see: valproic acid]

2-dipropylaminoethyl diphenylthioacetate [see: diprofene]

1,1-dipropylbutylamine [see: diprobutine]

diproqualone INN

Diprosone ointment, cream, lotion, aerosol ℞ *topical corticosteroidal antiinflammatory* [betamethasone dipropionate] 0.05%; 0.05%; 0.05%; 0.1%

diproteverine INN, BAN

diprothazine [see: dimelazine]

diprotrizoate sodium USP [also: sodium diprotrizoate]

diproxadol INN

Dipteryx odorata; D. oppositifolia medicinal herb [see: tonka bean]

dipyridamole USAN, USP, INN, BAN *coronary vasodilator; platelet aggregation inhibitor; diagnostic aid for coronary artery function* 25, 50, 75 mg oral

dipyrithione USAN, INN *antibacterial; antifungal*

dipyrocetyl INN

dipyrone USAN, BAN *analgesic; antipyretic* [also: metamizole sodium]

Dirame ℞ *investigational (Phase III) narcotic agonist-antagonist analgesic for moderate to severe pain* [propiram fumarate]

dirithromycin USAN, INN, BAN *macrolide antibiotic*

disaccharide tripeptide glycerol dipalmitoyl *investigational (orphan) for pulmonary and hepatic metastases of colorectal adenocarcinoma and osteosarcoma; investigational (Phase II, orphan) for Ewing sarcoma*

Disalcid film-coated tablets, capsules ℞ *analgesic; antipyretic; anti-inflammatory; antirheumatic* [salsalate] 500, 750 mg; 500 mg

disalicylic acid [see: salsalate]

Disanthrol capsules OTC *stimulant laxative; stool softener* [casanthranol; docusate sodium] 30•100 mg

Dis-Co Pack (trademarked packaging form) *unit-dose package*

discutients *a class of agents that cause a dispersal or disappearance of a pathological condition, such as a tumor*

disinfectants *a class of agents that inhibit the growth and development of micro-organisms, usually on an inanimate surface, without necessarily killing them* [see also: antiseptics; germicides]

Disinfecting Solution OTC *chemical disinfecting solution for soft contact lenses*

Disipal ⊛ film-coated tablets ℞ *anticholinergic; antiparkinsonian* [orphenadrine HCl] 50 mg

disiquonium chloride USAN, INN *antiseptic*

Disket (trademarked dosage form) *dispersible tablet*

Diskhaler (trademarked device) *inhalation powder dispenser* [used with a Rotadisk]

Diskus (trademarked device) *inhalation powder dispenser*

Disobrom sustained-release tablets ℞ *decongestant; antihistamine* [pseudoephedrine sulfate; dexbrompheniramine maleate] 120•6 mg

disobutamide USAN, INN *antiarrhythmic*

disodium carbenicillin [see: carbenicillin disodium]

disodium carbonate [see: sodium carbonate]

disodium cefotetan [see: cefotetan disodium]

disodium chromate [see: sodium chromate]

disodium clodronate *investigational (orphan) for hypercalcemia of malignancy* [also: clodronate disodium]

disodium clodronate tetrahydrate *investigational (orphan) for increased bone resorption due to malignancy*

disodium cromoglycate (DSC; DSCG) [see: cromolyn sodium]

disodium dihydrogen methylenediphosphonate [see: medronate disodium]

disodium edathamil [see: edathamil disodium]

disodium edetate BAN *metal-chelating agent* [also: edetate disodium]

disodium ethylenediamine tetraacetate [see: edetate disodium]

disodium hydrogen phosphate [see: sodium phosphate]

disodium hydrogen phosphate heptahydrate [see: sodium phosphate, dibasic]

disodium hydrogen phosphate hydrate [see: sodium phosphate, dibasic]

(disodium) methylene diphosphonate (MDP) [now: medronate disodium]

disodium phosphate [see: sodium phosphate, dibasic]

disodium phosphate heptahydrate [see: sodium phosphate]

disodium phosphonoacetate monohydrate [see: fosfonet sodium]

disodium phosphorofluoridate [see: sodium monofluorophosphate]

disodium pyrosulfite [see: sodium metabisulfite]

disodium silibinin dihemisuccinate *orphan status withdrawn 1997*

disodium sulfate decahydrate [see: sodium sulfate]

disodium thiosulfate pentahydrate [see: sodium thiosulfate]

disofenin USAN, INN, BAN *carrier agent in diagnostic tests*

disogluside INN

Disolan capsules OTC *stimulant laxative; stool softener* [phenolphthalein; docusate sodium] 65•100 mg

Disolan Forte capsules OTC *stimulant/bulk laxative; stool softener* [casanthranol; carboxymethylcellulose sodium; docusate sodium] 30•400•100 mg

Disonate capsules, syrup, liquid OTC *stool softener* [docusate sodium] 100, 240 mg; 60 mg/15 mL; 150 mg/15 mL

Disophrol tablets, Chronotabs (sustained-action tablets) OTC *decongestant; antihistamine* [pseudoephedrine sulfate; dexbrompheniramine maleate] 60•2 mg; 120•6 mg ② Desferal; disoprofol; Stilphostrol

Disoplex capsules OTC *bulk laxative; stool softener* [carboxymethylcellulose sodium; docusate sodium] 400•100 mg

disoprofol [see: propofol] ② Disophrol

disopromine HCl [see: diisopromine HCl]

disopyramide USAN, INN, BAN *antiarrhythmic*

disopyramide phosphate USAN, USP, BAN *antiarrhythmic* 100, 150 mg oral

Disotate IV infusion ℞ *chelating agent for hypercalcemia and ventricular arrhythmias due to digitalis toxicity* [edetate disodium] 150 mg/mL

disoxaril USAN, INN *antiviral*

Di-Spaz capsules, IM injection ℞ *GI antispasmodic* [dicyclomine HCl] 10 mg; 10 mg/mL

Dispenserpak (trademarked packaging form) *unit-of-use package*

dispersible cellulose BAN *tablet and capsule diluent* [also: cellulose, microcrystalline]

Dispertab (trademarked dosage form) *delayed-release tablet*

Dispette (trademarked delivery system) *disposable pipette*

Dispos-a-Med (trademarked delivery form) *solution for inhalation*

distaquaine [see: penicillin V]

distigmine bromide INN, BAN

disulergine INN

disulfamide INN [also: disulphamide]

disulfiram USP, INN, BAN *deterrent to alcohol consumption* 250, 500 mg oral

disulfurous acid, dipotassium salt [see: potassium metabisulfite]

disulfurous acid, disodium salt [see: sodium metabisulfite]

disulphamide BAN [also: disulfamide]

disuprazole INN

Dital slow-release capsules ℞ *anorexiant; CNS stimulant* [phendimetrazine tartrate] 105 mg

ditazole INN

ditekiren USAN *antihypertensive; renin inhibitor*

ditercalinium chloride INN

dithiazanine BAN [also: dithiazanine iodide]

dithiazanine iodide USP, INN [also: dithiazanine]

dithranol INN, BAN *topical antipsoriatic* [also: anthralin]

204. D.I.T.I.-2

D.I.T.I.-2 vaginal cream ℞ *broad-spectrum antibiotic; antiseptic; vulnerary* [sulfanilamide; aminacrine HCl; allantoin] 15%•0.2%•2%
ditiocarb sodium INN
ditiomustine INN
ditolamide INN
ditophal INN, BAN
Ditropan tablets, syrup ℞ *urinary antispasmodic* [oxybutynin chloride] 5 mg; 5 mg/5 mL ② Intropin
Ditropan XL extended-release tablets ℞ *anticholinergic and urinary antispasmodic for urge urinary incontinence and frequency* [oxybutynin chloride] 5, 10, 15 mg
Diucardin tablets ℞ *diuretic; antihypertensive* [hydroflumethiazide] 50 mg
Diupres-250; Diupres-500 tablets (discontinued 1996) ℞ *antihypertensive* [chlorothiazide; reserpine] 250• 0.125 mg; 500•0.125 mg
Diurese tablets ℞ *diuretic; antihypertensive* [trichlormethiazide] 4 mg
diuretics *a class of agents that stimulate increased excretion of urine*
Diurigen tablets ℞ *diuretic* [chlorothiazide] 500 mg
Diuril tablets, oral suspension ℞ *diuretic* [chlorothiazide] 250, 500 mg; 250 mg/5 mL
Diutensen-R tablets ℞ *antihypertensive* [methyclothiazide; reserpine] 2.5•0.1 mg ② Salutensin
divabuterol INN
divalproex sodium USAN *anticonvulsant; antipsychotic for manic episodes; migraine prophylaxis* [also: valproate semisodium; semisodium valproate]
divanilliden cyclohexanone [see: cyclovalone]
divaplon INN
Divide-Tab (trademarked dosage form) *scored tablet*
Dividose (trademarked dosage form) *multiple-scored tablets*
diviminol [see: viminol]
divinyl ether [see: vinyl ether]
divinyl oxide [see: vinyl ether]

dixamone bromide [see: methantheline bromide]
dixanthogen INN
dixarit [see: clonidine]
Dizac emulsified IV injection (discontinued 1999) ℞ *benzodiazepine sedative; anxiolytic; anticonvulsant; skeletal muscle relaxant* [diazepam] 5 mg/mL
dizatrifone INN
Dizmiss chewable tablets OTC *anticholinergic; antivertigo agent; motion sickness preventative* [meclizine HCl] 25 mg
dizocilpine INN *neuroprotective; NMDA (N-methyl-D-aspartate) antagonist* [also: dizocilpine maleate]
dizocilpine maleate USAN *neuroprotective; NMDA (N-methyl-D-aspartate) antagonist* [also: dizocilpine]
dizocilpine maleate & citicoline *investigational (Phase III) neuroprotective treatment for stroke*
D-Lay (trademarked dosage form) *timed-release tablet*
DM Cough Syrup OTC *antitussive* [dextromethorphan hydrobromide]
DMC (dactinomycin, methotrexate, cyclophosphamide) *chemotherapy protocol*
DMCT (demethylchlortetracycline) [see: demeclocycline]
DML lotion OTC *moisturizer; emollient*
DML Forte cream OTC *moisturizer; emollient*
DMO (dimethyl oxazolidinedione) [see: dimethadione]
DMP 450 *investigational (Phase I/II) second-generation protease inhibitor for HIV*
DMP 504 *investigational (Phase III) hydrogel bile acid sequestrant (BAS) for lowering serum cholesterol*
DMP 777 *investigational (orphan) for management of cystic fibrosis lung disease*
DMP-115 *investigational (Phase III) ultrasound contrast medium*
d-MPH (d-methylphenidate HCl) [q.v.]
DMSA (dimercaptosuccinic acid) [see: succimer]
DMSO (dimethyl sulfoxide) [q.v.]

DMT (dimethyltryptamine) *street drug* [q.v.]

DNA (deoxyribonucleic acid)

DNA polymerase [see: reverse transcriptase inhibitors; non-nucleoside reverse transcriptase inhibitors]

DNase (recombinant human deoxyribonuclease I) [see: dornase alfa]

DNJ (deoxynojirimycin) [q.v.]

DNR (daunorubicin) [q.v.]

Doak Tar bath oil, lotion, shampoo OTC *topical antipsoriatic; antiseborrheic; antiseptic* [coal tar] 0.8%; 2%; 1.2%, 3%

Doak Tar Distillate liquid OTC *topical antipsoriatic; antiseborrheic; antiseptic* [coal tar] 40%

Doak Tar Oil liquid OTC *topical antipsoriatic; antiseborrheic; antiseptic* [coal tar] 2%

Doan's Pills caplets OTC *analgesic; antirheumatic* [magnesium salicylate] 325, 500 mg

Doan's P.M. caplets OTC *analgesic; antirheumatic; antihistaminic sleep aid* [magnesium salicylate; diphenhydramine HCl] 500•25 mg

DOAP (daunorubicin, Oncovin, ara-C, prednisone) *chemotherapy protocol*

dobupride INN

dobutamine USAN, INN, BAN *cardiotonic; vasopressor for shock* ② dopamine

dobutamine HCl USAN, USP, BAN *cardiotonic; vasopressor for shock* 12.5 mg/mL injection

dobutamine lactobionate USAN *cardiotonic*

dobutamine tartrate USAN *cardiotonic*

Dobutrex IV infusion ℞ *vasopressor for cardiac shock* [dobutamine HCl] 12.5 mg/mL

DOCA (desoxycorticosterone acetate) [q.v.]

docarpamine INN

docebenone USAN, INN *5-lipoxygenase inhibitor*

docetaxel USAN, INN *antineoplastic for advanced or metastatic breast cancer; analog to paclitaxel*

dock, curled; curly dock; narrow dock; sour dock *medicinal herb* [see: yellow dock]

dock, patience; sweet dock *medicinal herb* [see: bistort]

doconazole USAN, INN *antifungal*

doconexent INN *omega-3 marine triglyceride*

docosahexaenoic acid (DHA) [see: doconexent]

n-docosanol *investigational (NDA filed) topical treatment of oral herpes simplex type 1*

docosil INN *combining name for radicals or groups*

Doctar shampoo OTC *antiseborrheic; antipsoriatic; antipruritic; antibacterial* [coal tar] 0.5%

Docucal-P softgels OTC *stimulant laxative; stool softener* [phenolphthalein; docusate calcium] 65•60 mg

docusate calcium USAN, USP *stool softener* 240 mg oral

docusate potassium USAN, USP *stool softener*

docusate sodium USAN, USP, BAN *stool softener; surfactant/wetting agent* [also: sodium dioctyl sulfosuccinate] 50, 100, 250 mg oral; 50, 60 mg/15 mL oral;

dodecafluoropentane [see: perflenapent]

dodeclonium bromide INN

2-dodecylisoquinolinium bromide [see: lauryl isoquinolinium bromide]

dofamium chloride INN, BAN

dofetilide USAN, INN, BAN *antiarrhythmic; potassium channel blocker*

dofosfate INN *combining name for radicals or groups*

dog grass *medicinal herb* [see: couch grass]

dog poison (Aethusa cynapium) plant *medicinal herb used as an antispasmodic and emetic in homeopathic remedies; not generally regarded as safe and effective as ingestion may be fatal*

dogbane (Apocynum androsaemifolium) root *medicinal herb used as a* *cathartic, diuretic, emetic, expectorant, stimulant, and sudorific*

dogwood, black; black alder dogwood *medicinal herb* [see: buckthorn; cascara sagrada]

DOK capsules, syrup, liquid OTC *stool softener* [docusate sodium] 100, 250 mg; 60 mg/15 mL; 150 mg/15 mL

Dolacet capsules ℞ *narcotic analgesic* [hydrocodone bitartrate; acetaminophen] 5•500 mg

Dolanex elixir (discontinued 1997) OTC *analgesic; antipyretic* [acetaminophen] 325 mg/5 mL

dolantal [see: meperidine HCl]

dolantin [see: meperidine HCl]

dolasetron INN *antiemetic; antimigraine; selective serotonin 5-HT₃ receptor antagonist* [also: dolasetron mesylate]

dolasetron mesylate USAN *antiemetic; antimigraine; selective serotonin 5-HT₃ receptor antagonist* [also: dolasetron]

Dolene capsules (discontinued 1999) ℞ *narcotic analgesic* [propoxyphene HCl; acetaminophen] 65 mg

Dolfen tablets ℞ *narcotic analgesic* [hydrocodone bitartrate; acetaminophen]

doliracetam INN

Dolobid film-coated tablets ℞ *analgesic; antiarthritic; antirheumatic; antiinflammatory; antipyretic* [diflunisal] 250, 500 mg

dolomite *nutritional supplement; source of calcium and magnesium*

Dolomite tablets OTC *mineral supplement* [calcium; magnesium] 130•78 mg

Dolophine HCl tablets, subcu or IM injection ℞ *narcotic analgesic; narcotic addiction detoxicant; often abused as a street drug* [methadone HCl] 5, 10 mg; 10 mg/mL

Dolorac cream OTC *topical analgesic* [capsaicin] 0.025%

dolosal [see: meperidine HCl]

Dolsed sugar-coated tablets ℞ *urinary antibiotic; analgesic; antispasmodic; acidifier* [methenamine; phenyl salicylate; atropine sulfate; methylene blue;

hyoscyamine sulfate; benzoic acid] 40.8•18.1•0.03•5.4•0.03•4.5 mg

dolvanol [see: meperidine HCl]

DOM (2,5-dimethoxy-4-methylamphetamine) *a hallucinogenic street drug derived from amphetamine, popularly called STP*

domazoline INN *anticholinergic* [also: domazoline fumarate]

domazoline fumarate USAN *anticholinergic* [also: domazoline]

Domeboro powder packets, effervescent tablets OTC *astringent wet dressing (modified Burow solution)* [aluminum sulfate; calcium acetate]

Domeboro Otic [see: Otic Domeboro]

Dome-Paste medicated gauze bandage OTC *protection and support of extremities* [zinc oxide; calamine; gelatin]

domestrol [see: diethylstilbestrol]

domibrom [see: domiphen bromide]

domiodol USAN, INN *mucolytic*

domiphen bromide USAN, BAN *topical anti-infective*

domipizone INN

Domol Bath and Shower Oil OTC *bath emollient*

domoprednate INN

domoxin INN

domperidone USAN, INN, BAN, JAN *antiemetic for diabetic gastroparesis and chronic gastritis*

Donatussin drops ℞ *pediatric decongestant, antihistamine, and expectorant* [phenylephrine HCl; chlorpheniramine maleate; guaifenesin] 2•1•20 mg/mL

Donatussin syrup ℞ *antitussive; decongestant; antihistamine; expectorant* [dextromethorphan hydrobromide; phenylephrine HCl; chlorpheniramine maleate; guaifenesin] 7.5•10•2•100 mg/5 mL

Donatussin DC syrup ℞ *narcotic antitussive; decongestant; expectorant* [hydrocodone bitartrate; phenylephrine HCl; guaifenesin] 2.5•7.5•50 mg/5 mL

donepezil HCl USAN *reversible acetyl-cholinesterase (AChE) inhibitor; cognition adjuvant for Alzheimer's dementia*
donetidine USAN, INN, BAN *antagonist to histamine H₂ receptors*
dong quai *(Angelica polymorpha; A. sinensis; A. dahurica) root medicinal herb for allergies, anemia, blood cleansing, constipation, female hormonal problems, hypertension, internal bleeding, menopausal symptoms, nourishing brain, and ulcers; not generally regarded as safe and effective as it contains coumarins and safrole*
Donnagel chewable tablets, liquid OTC *antidiarrheal; GI adsorbent* [attapulgite] 600 mg; 600 mg/15 mL ② Donnatal
Donnamar tablets ℞ *GI antispasmodic; anticholinergic* [hyoscyamine sulfate] 0.125 mg
Donnamor elixir (discontinued 1995) ℞ *GI antispasmodic; anticholinergic; sedative* [atropine sulfate; scopolamine hydrobromide; hyoscyamine hydrobromide; phenobarbital] 0.0194•0.0065•0.1037•16.2 mg/5 mL
Donnapine tablets (discontinued 1995) ℞ *GI antispasmodic; anticholinergic; sedative* [atropine sulfate; scopolamine hydrobromide; hyoscyamine hydrobromide; phenobarbital] 0.0194•0.0065•0.1037•16.2 mg
Donna-Sed elixir ℞ *GI antispasmodic; anticholinergic; sedative* [atropine sulfate; scopolamine hydrobromide; hyoscyamine hydrobromide; phenobarbital] 0.0194•0.0065•0.1037•16.2 mg/5 mL
Donnatal capsules & tablets, elixir, Extentabs (extended-release tablets) ℞ *GI antispasmodic; anticholinergic; sedative* [atropine sulfate; scopolamine hydrobromide; hyoscyamine sulfate; phenobarbital] 0.0194•0.0065•0.1037•16.2 mg; 0.0194•0.0065•0.1037•16.2 mg/5 mL; 0.0582•0.0195•0.3111•48.6 mg ② Donnagel

Donnatal No. 2 tablets ℞ *GI antispasmodic; anticholinergic; sedative* [atropine sulfate; scopolamine hydrobromide; hyoscyamine sulfate; phenobarbital] 0.0194•0.0065•0.1037•32.4 mg
Donnazyme tablets ℞ *digestive enzymes* [pancreatin; lipase; protease; amylase] 500 mg•1000 U•12 500 U•12 500 U ② Entozyme
DOPA (dihydroxyphenylalanine) [see: levodopa]
L-dopa [see: levodopa]
dopamantine USAN, INN *antiparkinsonian*
dopamine INN, BAN *adrenergic; vasopressor for shock* [also: dopamine HCl] ② dobutamine; Dopram
dopamine HCl USAN, USP *adrenergic; vasopressor for shock* [also: dopamine] 40, 80, 160 mg/mL injection
dopamine HCl in 5% dextrose *adrenergic; vasopressor for shock* 80, 160, 320 mg/100 mL injection
dopaminergics *a class of antiparkinsonian agents that affect the dopamine neurotransmitters in the brain*
Dopar capsules ℞ *dopamine precursor; antiparkinsonian* [levodopa] 100, 250, 500 mg ② Dopram
Dopascan injection *investigational diagnostic imaging aid for dopamine and serotonin transporter sites* [iometopane I 123]
dopexamine USAN, INN, BAN *cardiovascular agent*
dopexamine HCl USAN, BAN *cardiovascular agent*
Dopram IV injection or infusion ℞ *CNS stimulant; analeptic; adjunct to postanesthesia "stir-up"* [doxapram HCl] 20 mg/mL ② dopamine; Dopar
dopropidil INN
doqualast INN
Doral tablets ℞ *sedative; hypnotic* [quazepam] 7.5, 15 mg
dorastine INN *antihistamine* [also: dorastine HCl]
dorastine HCl USAN *antihistamine* [also: dorastine]

Dorcol Children's Cold Formula
liquid OTC *pediatric decongestant and antihistamine* [pseudoephedrine HCl; chlorpheniramine maleate] 15•1 mg/5 mL

Dorcol Children's Cough syrup OTC *pediatric antitussive, decongestant, and expectorant* [dextromethorphan hydrobromide; pseudoephedrine HCl; guaifenesin] 5•15•50 mg/5 mL

Dorcol Children's Decongestant liquid OTC *nasal decongestant* [pseudoephedrine HCl] 15 mg/5 mL

Dorcol Children's Fever & Pain Reducer liquid (discontinued 1997) OTC *analgesic; antipyretic* [acetaminophen] 160 mg/5 mL

doreptide INN

doretinel USAN, INN *antikeratinizing agent*

Dormarex 2 tablets OTC *antihistaminic sleep aid; motion sickness preventative* [diphenhydramine HCl] 50 mg

dormethan [see: dextromethorphan hydrobromide]

Dormin caplets, capsules OTC *antihistaminic sleep aid* [diphenhydramine HCl] 25 mg

dormiral [see: phenobarbital]

dormonal [see: barbital]

dornase alfa USAN, INN *reduces respiratory viscoelasticity of sputum in cystic fibrosis (orphan)*

Doryx capsules ℞ *tetracycline antibiotic* [doxycycline hyclate] 100 mg

dorzolamide HCl USAN *topical carbonic anhydrase inhibitor for glaucoma*

DOS softgels OTC *stool softener* [docusate sodium] 100, 250 mg

Dosalax syrup OTC *stimulant laxative* [senna concentrate; alcohol 7%] ≗

Dosa-Trol Pack (trademarked dosage form) *unit-of-use package*

Dosepak (trademarked dosage form) *unit-of-use package*

dosergoside INN

Dosette (trademarked dosage form) *injectable unit-of-use system (vials, ampules, syringes, etc.)*

Dospan (trademarked form) *controlled-release tablets*

Dostinex tablets ℞ *dopamine agonist for hyperprolactinemia; investigational treatment for Parkinson's disease and gynecologic disorders* [cabergoline] 0.5 mg

dosulepin INN *antidepressant* [also: dothiepin HCl; dothiepin; dosulepin HCl]

dosulepin HCl JAN *antidepressant* [also: dothiepin HCl; dosulepin; dothiepin]

dotarizine INN

dotefonium bromide INN

dothiepin BAN *antidepressant* [also: dothiepin HCl; dosulepin; dosulepin HCl]

dothiepin HCl USAN *antidepressant* [also: dosulepin; dothiepin; dosulepin HCl]

Double Ice ArthriCare [see: ArthriCare, Double Ice]

Double-Action Toothache Kit tablets + liquid OTC *analgesic; topical oral anesthetic* [(acetaminophen) + (benzocaine; alcohol 74%)] (325 mg) + (≗)

Dovonex cream, ointment, scalp solution ℞ *topical antipsoriatic* [calcipotriene] 0.005%

doxacurium chloride USAN, INN, BAN *nondepolarizing neuromuscular blocker; muscle relaxant; adjunct to anesthesia*

doxaminol INN

doxapram INN, BAN *respiratory stimulant* [also: doxapram HCl]

doxapram HCl USAN, USP *respiratory stimulant; analeptic* [also: doxapram] 20 mg/mL injection

doxaprost USAN, INN *bronchodilator*

doxate [see: docusate sodium]

doxazosin INN, BAN *antihypertensive; α_1-adrenergic blocker; treatment for benign prostatic hyperplasia* [also: doxazosin mesylate]

doxazosin mesylate USAN *antihypertensive; α_1-adrenergic blocker; treatment for benign prostatic hyperplasia* [also: doxazosin]

doxefazepam INN

doxenitoin INN

doxepin INN, BAN *tricyclic antidepressant; anxiolytic; topical antihistamine* [also: doxepin HCl] ② Doxidan; Loxitane

doxepin HCl USAN, USP *tricyclic antidepressant; anxiolytic; topical antihistamine* [also: doxepin] 10, 25, 50, 75, 100, 150 mg oral; 10 mg/mL oral

doxercalciferol *serum calcium regulator for elevated idiopathic parathyroid hormone levels in dialysis patients*

doxibetasol INN [also: doxybetasol]

Doxidan capsules OTC *stimulant laxative; stool softener* [phenolphthalein; docusate calcium] 65•60 mg ② doxepin

doxifluridine INN, JAN *investigational antineoplastic*

Doxil IV injection ℞ *anthracycline antibiotic antineoplastic for Kaposi sarcoma and ovarian cancer; investigational (NDA filed) for prostate cancer* [doxorubicin HCl, liposome-encapsulated] 20 mg/vial

doxofylline USAN, INN *bronchodilator*

doxorubicin USAN, INN, BAN *anthracycline antibiotic antineoplastic* ② daunorubicin

doxorubicin HCl USP *anthracycline antibiotic antineoplastic* 10, 20, 50 mg, 2 mg/mL injection

doxorubicin HCl, liposome-encapsulated (LED) *anthracycline antibiotic antineoplastic for Kaposi sarcoma and ovarian cancer; investigational (NDA filed) for prostate cancer*

doxpicodin HCl [now: doxpicomine HCl]

doxpicomine INN *analgesic* [also: doxpicomine HCl]

doxpicomine HCl USAN *analgesic* [also: doxpicomine]

Doxy 100; Doxy 200 powder for IV injection ℞ *tetracycline antibiotic* [doxycycline hyclate] 100 mg; 200 mg

Doxy Caps capsules ℞ *tetracycline antibiotic* [doxycycline hyclate] 100 mg

doxybetasol BAN [also: doxibetasol]

Doxychel Hyclate capsules, tablets, powder for IV injection ℞ *tetracycline antibiotic* [doxycycline hyclate] 50, 100 mg; 50, 100 mg; 100, 200 mg

doxycycline USAN, USP, INN, BAN *antibiotic; antirickettsial; malaria prophylaxis*

doxycycline calcium USP *antibiotic; antiprotozoal*

doxycycline fosfatex USAN, BAN *antibiotic*

doxycycline hyclate USP *antibiotic* 50, 100 mg oral; 100, 200 mg/vial injection

doxylamine INN, BAN *antihistamine* [also: doxylamine succinate]

doxylamine succinate USP *antihistamine; sleep aid* [also: doxylamine]

DPE (dipivalyl epinephrine) [now: dipivefrin]

DPF [see: Dermprotective Factor]

DPN (diphosphopyridine nucleotide) [now: nadide]

DPPC (dipalmitoylphosphatidylcholine) [see: colfosceril palmitate]

Dr. Brown's Home Drug Testing System OTC *in vitro diagnostic aid for detection of multiple illicit drugs in the urine*

Dr. Caldwell Senna Laxative liquid OTC *stimulant laxative* [senna concentrate] 33.3 mg/mL

Dr. Dermi-Heal ointment OTC *vulnerary; antipruritic; astringent* [allantoin; zinc oxide; peruvian balsam] 1%• ² • ²

Dr. Scholl's Advanced Pain Relief Corn Removers; Dr. Scholl's Callus Removers; Dr Scholl's Clear Away; Dr. Scholl's Corn Removers medicated discs OTC *topical keratolytic* [salicylic acid in a rubber-based vehicle] 40%

Dr. Scholl's Athlete's Foot powder, spray powder, spray liquid OTC *topical antifungal* [tolnaftate] 1%

Dr. Scholl's Clear Away OneStep; Dr. Scholl's OneStep Corn Removers medicated strips OTC *topical keratolytic* [salicylic acid in a rubber-based vehicle] 40%

Dr. Scholl's Corn/Callus Remover liquid OTC *topical keratolytic* [salicylic acid in flexible collodion] 17%

Dr. Scholl's Cracked Heel Relief cream OTC *topical local anesthetic; antiseptic* [lidocaine HCl; benzalkonium chloride] 2%•0.13%

Dr. Scholl's Moisturizing Corn Remover Kit medicated discs + cushions + moisturizing cream OTC *topical keratolytic* [salicylic acid in a rubber-based vehicle] 40%

Dr. Scholl's Tritin powder, spray powder OTC *topical antifungal* [tolnaftate] 1%

Dr. Scholl's Wart Remover Kit liquid + adhesive pads OTC *topical keratolytic* [salicylic acid in flexible collodion] 17%

draflazine USAN *cardioprotectant*

dragée (French for "sugar plum") *a sugar-coated pill or medicated confection* [pronounced "drah zhá"]

dragon's claw, scaly *medicinal herb* [see: coral root]

dragonwort *medicinal herb* [see: bistort]

Dramamine liquid ℞ *antinauseant; antiemetic; antivertigo agent; motion sickness preventative* [dimenhydrinate] 15.62 mg/5 mL

Dramamine tablets, chewable tablets, liquid OTC *antinauseant; antiemetic; antivertigo agent; motion sickness preventative* [dimenhydrinate] 50 mg; 50 mg; 12.5 mg/4 mL

Dramamine, Children's liquid OTC *antinauseant; antiemetic; antivertigo agent; motion sickness preventative* [dimenhydrinate; alcohol 5%] 12.5 mg/5 mL

Dramamine II tablets OTC *anticholinergic; antihistamine; antivertigo agent; motion sickness preventative* [meclizine HCl] 25 mg

Dramanate IV or IM injection ℞ *antinauseant; antiemetic; antivertigo agent; motion sickness preventative* [dimenhydrinate] 50 mg/mL ⊉ Dommanate

dramarin [see: dimenhydrate]

dramedilol INN

Dramilin IV or IM injection ℞ *antinauseant; antiemetic; antivertigo agent; motion sickness preventative* [dimenhydrinate] 50 mg/mL

Dramoject IV or IM injection (discontinued 1996) ℞ *antinauseant; antiemetic; antivertigo agent; motion sickness preventative* [dimenhydrinate] 50 mg/mL

dramyl [see: dimenhydrate]

draquinolol INN

drazidox INN

Drepanol ℞ *investigational (orphan) for prophylactic treatment of sickle cell disease* [OM 401 (code name—generic name not yet assigned)]

dribendazole USAN, INN *anthelmintic*

dricol [see: amidephrine]

Dri/Ear ear drops OTC *antibacterial; antifungal* [boric acid] 2.75%

dried aluminum hydroxide gel [see: aluminum hydroxide gel, dried]

dried basic aluminum carbonate [see: aluminum carbonate, basic]

dried ferrous sulfate [see: ferrous sulfate, dried]

dried yeast [see: yeast, dried]

drinidene USAN, INN *analgesic*

Drisdol capsules ℞ *vitamin deficiency therapy* [ergocalciferol (vitamin D_2)] 50 000 IU

Drisdol Drops OTC *vitamin supplement* [ergocalciferol (vitamin D_2)] 8000 IU/mL

Dristan nasal spray OTC *nasal decongestant; antihistamine* [phenylephrine HCl; pheniramine maleate] 0.5%•0.2%

Dristan 12-Hr. nasal spray OTC *nasal decongestant* [oxymetazoline HCl] 0.05%

Dristan Allergy caplets (discontinued 1995) OTC *decongestant; antihistamine* [pseudoephedrine HCl; brompheniramine maleate] 60•4 mg

Dristan Cold caplets OTC *decongestant; analgesic; antipyretic* [pseudoephedrine HCl; acetaminophen] 30•500 mg

Dristan Cold, Maximum Strength caplets OTC *decongestant; antihista-*

mine; *analgesic* [pseudoephedrine HCl; brompheniramine maleate; acetaminophen] 30•2•500 mg

Dristan Cold & Flu powder (discontinued 1995) OTC *antitussive; decongestant; antihistamine; analgesic* [dextromethorphan hydrobromide; pseudoephedrine HCl; chlorpheniramine maleate; acetaminophen] 20•60•4•500 mg/packet

Dristan Cold Multi-Symptom Formula tablets OTC *decongestant; antihistamine; analgesic* [phenylephrine HCl; chlorpheniramine maleate; acetaminophen] 5•2•325 mg

Dristan Juice Mix-In powder (discontinued 1995) OTC *antitussive; decongestant; analgesic* [dextromethorphan hydrobromide; pseudoephedrine HCl; acetaminophen] 20•60•500 mg/packet

Dristan Saline Spray OTC *nasal moisturizer* [sodium chloride (saline solution)]

Dristan Sinus caplets OTC *decongestant; analgesic* [pseudoephedrine HCl; ibuprofen] 30•200 mg

Drithocreme; Drithocreme HP 1%; Dritho-Scalp cream ℞ *topical antipsoriatic* [anthralin] 0.1%, 0.25%, 0.5%; 1%; 0.5%

Drixomed sustained-release tablets ℞ *decongestant; antihistamine* [pseudoephedrine sulfate; dexbrompheniramine maleate] 120•6 mg

Drixoral syrup OTC *decongestant; antihistamine* [pseudoephedrine sulfate; brompheniramine maleate] 30•2 mg/5 mL

Drixoral Allergy Sinus extended-release tablets (name changed to Drixoral Plus in 1996)

Drixoral Cold & Allergy sustained-action tablets OTC *decongestant; antihistamine* [pseudoephedrine sulfate; dexbrompheniramine maleate] 120•6 mg

Drixoral Cold & Flu; Drixoral Plus extended-release tablets OTC *decongestant; antihistamine; analgesic* [pseudoephedrine sulfate; dexbromphen-

iramine maleate; acetaminophen] 60•3•500 mg

Drixoral Cough & Congestion Liquid Caps (capsules) OTC *antitussive; decongestant* [dextromethorphan hydrobromide; pseudoephedrine HCl] 30•60 mg

Drixoral Cough Liquid Caps (liquid-filled capsules) (discontinued 1998) OTC *antitussive* [dextromethorphan hydrobromide] 30 mg

Drixoral Cough & Sore Throat Liquid Caps (liquid-filled capsules) OTC *antitussive; analgesic* [dextromethorphan hydrobromide; acetaminophen] 15•325 mg

Drixoral Non-Drowsy Formula extended-release tablets OTC *nasal decongestant* [pseudoephedrine sulfate] 120 mg

Drize sustained-release capsules ℞ *decongestant; antihistamine* [phenylpropanolamine HCl; chlorpheniramine maleate] 75•12 mg

drobuline USAN, INN *antiarrhythmic*

drocarbil NF

drocinonide USAN, INN *anti-inflammatory*

droclidinium bromide INN

drocode [see: dihydrocodeine]

drofenine INN

droloxifene INN *investigational (Phase III) antineoplastic for breast cancer; investigational (Phase III) antiestrogen for postmenopausal osteoporosis*

droloxifene citrate USAN *antineoplastic; antiestrogen*

drometrizole USAN, INN *ultraviolet screen*

dromostanolone propionate USAN, USP *antineoplastic* [also: drostanolone]

dronabinol USAN, USP, INN *antiemetic for chemotherapy; appetite stimulant in AIDS patients (orphan)*

drop chalk [see: calcium carbonate]

dropberry *medicinal herb* [see: Solomon's seal]

Drop-Dose (trademarked delivery system) *prefilled eye drop dispenser*

dropempine INN

droperidol USAN, USP, INN, BAN *general anesthetic; antiemetic; antipsychotic*

Dropperettes (delivery system) *pre-filled droppers*

droprenilamine USAN, INN *coronary vasodilator*

dropropizine INN, BAN

Drop-Tainers (trademarked dosage form) *prefilled eye drop dispenser*

drospirenone USAN *oral contraceptive; aldosterone antagonist*

drostanolone INN, BAN *antineoplastic* [also: dromostanolone propionate]

drotaverine INN

drotebanol INN, BAN

Drotic ear drops ℞ *topical corticosteroidal anti-inflammatory; antibiotic* [hydrocortisone; neomycin sulfate; polymyxin B sulfate] 1% • 5 mg • 10 000 U per mL

droxacin INN *antibacterial* [also: droxacin sodium]

droxacin sodium USAN *antibacterial* [also: droxacin]

droxicainide INN

droxicam INN

droxidopa INN

droxifilcon A USAN *hydrophilic contact lens material*

droxinavir HCl USAN *antiviral; HIV-1 protease inhibitor*

droxypropine INN, BAN

Dry Eye Therapy eye drops (discontinued 1998) OTC *ophthalmic moisturizer/lubricant* [glycerin] 0.3%

Dry Eyes eye drops OTC *ophthalmic moisturizer/lubricant* [polyvinyl alcohol] 1.4%

Dry Eyes ophthalmic ointment OTC *ocular moisturizer/lubricant* [white petrolatum; mineral oil]

Dryopteris filix-mas medicinal herb [see: aspidium]

Dryox 2.5; Dryox 5; Dryox 10; Dryox 20 gel OTC *topical keratolytic for acne* [benzoyl peroxide] 2.5%; 5%; 10%; 20%

Dryox 10S 5; Dryox 20S 10 gel OTC *topical keratolytic for acne* [benzoyl peroxide; sulfur] 10% • 5%; 20% • 10%

Dryox Wash 5; Dryox Wash 10 liquid OTC *topical keratolytic for acne* [benzoyl peroxide] 5%; 10%

Drysol solution ℞ *astringent for hyperhidrosis* [aluminum chloride] 20%

Drytergent liquid OTC *soap-free therapeutic skin cleanser*

Drytex lotion OTC *topical keratolytic cleanser for acne* [salicylic acid; acetone; isopropyl alcohol] 2 • 10% • 40%

DSC; DSCG (disodium cromoglycate) [see: cromolyn sodium]

DSMC Plus capsules OTC *stimulant laxative; stool softener* [casanthranol; docusate potassium] 30 • 100 mg

D-S-S capsules OTC *stool softener* [docusate sodium] 100 mg

DSS (dioctyl sodium sulfosuccinate) [now: docusate sodium]

D-S-S Plus capsules (discontinued 1997) OTC *stimulant laxative; stool softener* [casanthranol; docusate sodium] 30 • 100 mg

DST (dihydrostreptomycin) [q.v.]

DT; Td (diphtheria & tetanus [toxoids]) *the designation DT (or TD) denotes the pediatric vaccine; Td denotes the adult vaccine* [see: diphtheria & tetanus toxoids, adsorbed]

DTaP (diphtheria & tetanus [toxoids] & acellular pertussis [vaccine]) [q.v.]

DTIC (dimethyl triazeno imidazole carboxamide) [see: dacarbazine]

DTIC-ACTD; DTIC-ACT-D (DTIC, actinomycin D) *chemotherapy protocol*

DTIC-Dome IV injection ℞ *antineoplastic for metastatic malignant melanoma and Hodgkin's disease* [dacarbazine] 10 mg/mL

DTP (diphtheria & tetanus [toxoids] & pertussis [vaccine]) [q.v.]

DTPA (diethylenetriaminepentaacetic acid) [see: pentetic acid]

DTPA (diethylenetriaminepentaacetic acid) technetium (^{99m}Tc), human serum albumin [see: technetium Tc 99m pentetate]

DTwP (diphtheria & tetanus [tox-oids] & whole-cell pertussis [vac-cine]) [q.v.]

Duadacin capsules OTC *decongestant; antihistamine; analgesic* [phenylpropa-nolamine HCl; chlorpheniramine maleate; acetaminophen] 12.5•2•325 mg

duazomycin USAN, INN *antineoplastic*

duazomycin A [see: duazomycin]

duazomycin B [see: azotomycin]

duazomycin C [see: ambomycin]

Duboisia myoporoides medicinal herb [see: corkwood]

duck's foot *medicinal herb* [see: man-drake]

ducodal [see: oxycodone]

Dulcagen enteric-coated tablets OTC *stimulant laxative* [bisacodyl] 5 mg

Dulcagen suppositories OTC *stimulant laxative* [bisacodyl] 10 mg

Dulcet (trademarked dosage form) *chewable tablet*

Dulcolax enteric-coated tablets OTC *stimulant laxative* [bisacodyl] 5 mg

Dulcolax suppositories OTC *stimulant laxative* [bisacodyl] 10 mg

Dulcolax Bowel Prep Kit 4 enteric-coated tablets + 1 suppository OTC *pre-procedure bowel evacuant* [bisaco-dyl] 5 mg; 10 mg

Dull-C powder OTC *vitamin supplement* [ascorbic acid] 4 g/tsp.

dulofibrate INN

duloxetine INN *antidepressant* [also: duloxetine HCl]

duloxetine HCl USAN *antidepressant* [also: duloxetine]

dulozafone INN

dumorelin INN

duneryl [see: phenobarbital]

Duocet tablets ℞ *narcotic analgesic* [hydrocodone bitartrate; acetamino-phen] 5•500 mg

Duo-Cyp IM injection ℞ *estrogen/androgen for menopausal vasomotor symptoms* [estradiol cypionate; tes-tosterone cypionate] 2•50 mg/mL

DuoDerm CGF; DuoDerm Extra Thin; DuoDerm Hydroactive adhesive dressings OTC *occlusive wound dressing* [hydrocolloid gel]

DuoDerm Hydroactive paste, gran-ules OTC *wound dressing* [hydrocol-loid gel] 30 g; 5 g

DuoFilm liquid OTC *topical keratolytic* [salicylic acid in flexible collodion] 17%

DuoFilm transdermal patch OTC *topi-cal keratolytic* [salicylic acid in a rub-ber-based vehicle] 40%

Duo-Medihaler inhalation aerosol (discontinued 1997) ℞ *bronchodila-tor* [isoproterenol HCl; phenyleph-rine bitartrate] 0.16•0.24 mg/dose

duometacin INN

duomycin [see: chlortetracycline HCl]

duoperone INN *neuroleptic* [also: duo-perone fumarate]

duoperone fumarate USAN *neurolep-tic* [also: duoperone]

DuoPlant gel ℞ *topical keratolytic* [sali-cylic acid in flexible collodion] 17%

duotal [see: guaiacol carbonate]

Duo-Trach Kit pre-filled syringe with cannula ℞ *injectable local anesthetic* [lidocaine HCl] 4%

Duotrate; Duotrate 45 sustained-release capsules (discontinued 1995) ℞ *antianginal; vasodilator* [pentaery-thritol tetranitrate] 30 mg; 45 mg

Duphalac syrup ℞ *laxative* [lactulose] 10 g/15 mL

Duplex liquid OTC *soap-free therapeu-tic skin cleanser* [sodium lauryl sul-fate] 15%

Duplex T shampoo OTC *antiseborrheic; antipsoriatic; antipruritic; antibacterial* [coal tar] 10%

duponol [see: sodium lauryl sulfate]

dupracetam INN

Durabolin IM injection ℞ *anabolic steroid for metastatic breast cancer in women; also abused as a street drug* [nandrolone phenpropionate] 25, 50 mg/mL

Duracaps (dosage form) *sustained-release capsules*

DURAcare solution (discontinued 1995) OTC *surfactant cleaning solution for soft contact lenses*

DURAcare II solution OTC *surfactant cleaning solution for soft contact lenses*

Duraclon continuous epidural infusion ℞ *central analgesic; adjunct to opioid analgesics for severe cancer pain (orphan)* [clonidine HCl] 100 μg/mL

Duract capsules (discontinued 1998) ℞ *long-acting nonsteroidal anti-inflammatory drug (NSAID); analgesic; antipyretic* [bromfenac sodium] 25 mg

Dura-Estrin IM injection (discontinued 1996) ℞ *hormone replacement therapy for postmenopausal disorders* [estradiol cypionate in oil] 5 mg/mL

DuraGen ℞ *resorbable graft matrix to repair the dura mater following brain surgery or traumatic injury*

Duragen-20; Duragen-40 IM injection (discontinued 1996) ℞ *estrogen replacement therapy for postmenopausal disorders; antineoplastic for prostatic cancer* [estradiol valerate in oil] 20 mg/mL; 40 mg/mL

Duragesic-25; Duragesic-50; Duragesic-75; Duragesic-100 transdermal patch ℞ *narcotic analgesic* [fentanyl] 25 μg/hr.; 50 μg/hr.; 75 μg/hr.; 100 μg/hr.

Dura-Gest capsules ℞ *decongestant; expectorant* [phenylephrine HCl; phenylpropanolamine HCl; guaifenesin] 45•5•200 mg

Duralex sustained-release capsules ℞ *decongestant; antihistamine* [pseudoephedrine HCl; chlorpheniramine maleate] 120•8 mg

Duralith ⊛ (U.S. product: Lithobid) sustained-release tablets ℞ *antipsychotic for manic episodes* [lithium carbonate] 300 mg

Duralone-40; Duralone-80 intralesional, soft tissue, and IM injection ℞ *corticosteroid; anti-inflammatory; immunosuppressant* [methylprednisolone acetate] 40 mg/mL; 80 mg/mL

Duralutin IM injection (discontinued 1996) ℞ *progestin for amenorrhea,* metrorrhagia, and dysfunctional uterine bleeding [hydroxyprogesterone caproate in oil] 250 mg/mL

Duramist Plus nasal spray OTC *nasal decongestant* [oxymetazoline HCl] 0.05%

Duramorph IV, subcu or IM injection ℞ *narcotic analgesic* [morphine sulfate] 0.5, 1 mg/mL

duramycin *investigational (orphan) for cystic fibrosis*

Duranest; Duranest MPF injection ℞ *injectable local anesthetic* [etidocaine HCl] 1%

Duranest; Duranest MPF injection ℞ *injectable local anesthetic* [etidocaine; epinephrine] 1%•1:200 000, 1.5%•1:200 000

Duranest HCl injection (name changed to Duranest in 1995)

durapatite USAN *prosthetic aid* [also: calcium phosphate, tribasic; hydroxyapatite]

DuraSite (delivery system) *polymer-based eye drops*

Dura-Tab (trademarked dosage form) *sustained-release tablet*

Dura-Tap/PD prolonged-action capsule ℞ *pediatric decongestant and antihistamine* [pseudoephedrine HCl; chlorpheniramine maleate] 60•4 mg

Duratears Naturale ophthalmic ointment OTC *ocular moisturizer/lubricant* [white petrolatum; mineral oil; lanolin]

Duratest 100; Duratest 200 IM injection ℞ *androgen replacement for delayed puberty or breast cancer* [testosterone cypionate] 100 mg/mL; 200 mg/mL

Duratestrin IM injection ℞ *estrogen/androgen for menopausal vasomotor symptoms* [estradiol cypionate; testosterone cypionate] 2•50 mg/mL

Durathate-200 IM injection ℞ *androgen replacement for delayed puberty or breast cancer* [testosterone enanthate] 200 mg/mL

Duration nasal spray OTC *nasal decongestant* [oxymetazoline HCl] 0.05%

Duratuss long-acting film-coated tablets ℞ *decongestant; expectorant* [pseudoephedrine HCl; guaifenesin] 120•600 mg

Duratuss HD elixir ℞ *narcotic antitussive; decongestant; expectorant* [hydrocodone bitartrate; pseudoephedrine HCl; guaifenesin] 2.5•30•100 mg/5 mL

Duratuss-G film-coated tablets ℞ *expectorant* [guaifenesin] 1.2 g

Dura-Vent long-acting tablets ℞ *decongestant; expectorant* [phenylpropanolamine HCl; guaifenesin] 75•600 mg

Dura-Vent/A continuous-release capsule ℞ *decongestant; antihistamine* [phenylpropanolamine HCl; chlorpheniramine maleate] 75•10 mg

Dura-Vent/DA sustained-release tablets ℞ *decongestant; antihistamine; anticholinergic* [phenylephrine HCl; chlorpheniramine maleate; methscopolamine nitrate] 20•8•2.5 mg

Duricef capsules, tablets, powder for oral suspension ℞ *cephalosporin antibiotic* [cefadroxil] 500 mg; 1000 mg; 125, 250, 500 mg/5 mL

DUROS implant ℞ *investigational (Phase III) hormonal antineoplastic for the palliative treatment of advanced prostate cancer* [leuprolide acetate]

dusting powder, absorbable USP *surgical glove lubricant*

dutasteride USAN *5α-reductase inhibitor for benign prostatic hyperplasia*

Dutonin (British name for U.S. product Serzone)

Duvoid tablets ℞ *cholinergic urinary stimulant for postsurgical and postpartum urinary retention* [bethanechol chloride] 10, 25, 50 mg

DV vaginal cream (discontinued 1996) ℞ *estrogen replacement therapy for postmenopausal disorders* [dienestrol] 0.01%

DVB (DDP, vindesine, bleomycin) *chemotherapy protocol*

DVP (daunorubicin, vincristine, prednisone) *chemotherapy protocol*

DVPL-ASP (daunorubicin, vincristine, prednisone, L-asparaginase) *chemotherapy protocol*

dwarf ginseng (Panax trifolius) *medicinal herb* [see: ginseng]

dwarf palm; dwarf palmetto *medicinal herb* [see: saw palmetto]

dwarf sumach *medicinal herb* [see: sumach]

Dwelle eye drops (discontinued 1998) OTC *ocular moisturizer/lubricant*

Dyazide capsules ℞ *antihypertensive; diuretic* [triamterene; hydrochlorothiazide] 37.5•25 mg ② thiazides; Tiazac

Dycill capsules ℞ *penicillinase-resistant penicillin antibiotic* [dicloxacillin sodium] 250, 500 mg

dyclocaine BAN *topical anesthetic* [also: dyclonine HCl; dyclonine]

Dyclone solution ℞ *anesthetic prior to upper GI and respiratory endoscopies* [dyclonine HCl] 0.5%, 1%

dyclonine INN *topical anesthetic* [also: dyclonine HCl; dyclocaine]

dyclonine HCl USP *topical anesthetic* [also: dyclonine; dyclocaine]

dydrogesterone USAN, USP, INN, BAN *progestin*

dyer's broom (Genista tinctoria) flowering twigs *medicinal herb used as an aperient, diuretic, stimulant, and vasoconstrictor*

dyer's bugloss *medicinal herb* [see: henna (Alkanna)]

dyer's saffron *medicinal herb* [see: safflower]

dyer's weed *medicinal herb* [see: goldenrod]

Dyflex-200 tablets (discontinued 1996) ℞ *antiasthmatic; bronchodilator* [dyphylline] 200 mg

Dyflex-G tablets ℞ *antiasthmatic; bronchodilator; expectorant* [dyphylline; guaifenesin] 200•200 mg

dyflos BAN *antiglaucoma agent; irreversible cholinesterase inhibitor miotic* [also: isoflurophate]

Dy-G oral liquid ℞ *antiasthmatic; bronchodilator; expectorant* [dyphylline; guaifenesin] 100•100 mg/5 mL

dylate [see: clonitrate]

Dyline-GG tablets, liquid ℞ *antiasthmatic; bronchodilator; expectorant* [dyphylline; guaifenesin] 200•200 mg; 300•300 mg/15 mL

dymanthine HCl USAN *anthelmintic* [also: dimantine HCl]

Dymelor tablets ℞ *sulfonylurea antidiabetic* [acetohexamide] 250, 500 mg ⚕ Demerol; Pamelor

Dymenate IV or IM injection ℞ *antinauseant; antiemetic; antivertigo; motion sickness preventative* [dimenhydrinate] 50 mg/mL

Dynabac enteric-coated tablets ℞ *once-daily macrolide antibiotic for respiratory and dermatological infections* [dirithromycin] 250 mg

Dynacin capsules ℞ *tetracycline antibiotic* [minocycline HCl] 50, 75, 100 mg

DynaCirc capsules ℞ *antihypertensive; dihydropyridine calcium channel blocker* [isradipine] 2.5, 5 mg

DynaCirc CR controlled-release tablets ℞ *once-daily antihypertensive; dihydropyridine calcium channel blocker* [isradipine] 5, 10 mg

dynacoryl [see: nikethamide]

Dynafed; Dynafed Plus tablets OTC *decongestant; analgesic; antipyretic* [pseudoephedrine HCl; acetaminophen] 30•500 mg

Dynafed Asthma Relief tablets OTC *decongestant; expectorant* [ephedrine HCl; guaifenesin] 25•200 mg

Dynafed E.X. tablets OTC *analgesic; antipyretic* [acetaminophen] 500 mg

Dynafed IB tablets OTC *nonsteroidal anti-inflammatory drug (NSAID); antiarthritic; analgesic* [ibuprofen] 200 mg

Dynafed Jr., Children's chewable tablets OTC *analgesic; antipyretic* [acetaminophen] 80 mg

Dynafed Pseudo tablets OTC *nasal decongestant* [pseudoephedrine HCl] 60 mg

Dyna-Hex Skin Cleanser; Dyna-Hex 2 Skin Cleanser liquid OTC *broad-spectrum antimicrobial; germicidal* [chlorhexidine gluconate; alcohol 4%] 4%; 2%

dynamine *investigational (orphan) for Lambert-Eaton myasthenic syndrome and Charcot-Marie-Tooth disease*

Dynapen capsules, powder for oral suspension ℞ *penicillinase-resistant penicillin antibiotic* [dicloxacillin sodium] 125, 250, 500 mg; 62.5 mg/5 mL

dynarsan [see: acetarsone]

Dynospheres M-035 ℞ *investigational imaging agent for MRI* [ferristene]

dyphylline USP *bronchodilator* [also: diprophylline] 200, 400 mg oral

Dyphylline-GG elixir OTC *antiasthmatic; bronchodilator; expectorant* [dyphylline; guaifenesin] 100•100 mg/15 mL

Dyprotex pads OTC *topical diaper rash treatment* [zinc oxide; dimethicone] 40%•2.5%

Dyrenium capsules ℞ *antihypertensive; potassium-sparing diuretic* [triamterene] 50, 100 mg ⚕ Pyridium

Dyrexan-OD sustained-release capsules ℞ *anorexiant; CNS stimulant* [phendimetrazine tartrate] 105 mg

Dysport ℞ *blepharospasm and strabismus of dystonia (orphan); investigational (orphan) for pediatric cerebral palsy and cervical dystonia* [botulinum toxin, type A]

dysprosium *element (Dy)*

DZAPO (daunorubicin, azacitidine, ara-C, prednisone, Oncovin) *chemotherapy protocol*

E2III transdermal patch ℞ *investigational (NDA filed) 7-day patch for hormone replacement therapy* [estrogen]

E-200; E-400; E-1000 softgels OTC *vitamin supplement* [vitamin E] 147 mg; 400 IU; 1000 IU

E25 *investigational (Phase III) monoclonal antibody for allergic asthma*

E5 MAb [now: edobacomab]

EACA (epsilon-aminocaproic acid) [see: aminocaproic acid]

EAP (etoposide, Adriamycin, Platinol) *chemotherapy protocol*

ear, lion's *medicinal herb* [see: motherwort]

Ear-Dry ear drops OTC *antibacterial; antifungal* [boric acid] 2.75%

Ear-Eze ear drops ℞ *topical corticosteroidal anti-inflammatory; antibiotic* [hydrocortisone; neomycin sulfate; polymyxin B sulfate] 1%•5 mg• 10 000 U per mL

EarSol ear drops OTC *antiseptic* [alcohol] 44%

EarSol-HC ear drops OTC *topical corticosteroidal anti-inflammatory; antiseptic* [hydrocortisone; alcohol 44%] 1%

earthnut oil [see: peanut oil]

Easprin enteric-coated delayed-release tablets ℞ *analgesic; antipyretic; anti-inflammatory; antirheumatic* [aspirin] 975 mg

Easter giant *medicinal herb* [see: bistort]

Easy A1C fingerstick test kit for home use OTC *in vitro diagnostic aid for glycated hemoglobin levels*

EasyInjector (trademarked device) *self-injector*

E-Base delayed-release enteric-coated caplets and tablets ℞ *macrolide antibiotic* [erythromycin] 333, 500 mg

ebastine USAN, INN *antihistamine*

ebiratide INN

ebrotidine INN

ebselen INN

EC (etoposide, carboplatin) *chemotherapy protocol*

ecadotril USAN, INN *antihypertensive*

ecamsule USAN *UVA sunscreen*

ecarazine [see: todralazine]

ecastolol INN

Ecee Plus tablets OTC *vitamin/mineral supplement* [vitamins C and E; zinc sulfate; magnesium sulfate] 100• 165•80•70 mg

echinacea (Echinacea angustifolia; E. purpurea; E. pallida) root *medicinal herb for anemia, blood diseases, blood poisoning, boils, dizziness, immune system stimulation, lymph disorders, promoting wound healing, prostate disorders, skin infections, and snake bites*

Echinopanax horridum *medicinal herb* [see: devil's club]

ECHO (etoposide, cyclophosphamide, hydroxydaunomycin, Oncovin) *chemotherapy protocol*

EchoGen emulsion ℞ *investigational (NDA filed) ultrasound contrast agent for stress cardiography and transrectal prostate imaging* [perflenapent; perflisopent] 85%•15%

echothiophate iodide USP *antiglaucoma agent; irreversible cholinesterase inhibitor miotic* [also: ecothiopate iodide]

Echovist (CAN) *intrauterine suspension* ℞ *ultrasound contrast medium for gynecological imaging* [galactose]

ecipramidil INN

eclanamine INN *antidepressant* [also: eclanamine maleate]

eclanamine maleate USAN *antidepressant* [also: eclanamine]

eclazolast USAN, INN *antiallergic; mediator release inhibitor*

EC-Naprosyn enteric-coated delayed-release tablets ℞ *nonsteroidal anti-inflammatory drug (NSAID); antiarthritic; analgesic* [naproxen] 375, 500 mg

ecogramostim BAN

E-Complex-600 capsules OTC *dietary supplement* [vitamin E] 600 IU

ecomustine INN

econazole USAN, INN, BAN *antifungal*

econazole nitrate USAN, USP, BAN *antifungal*

Econo B & C caplets OTC *vitamin supplement* [multiple B vitamins; vitamin C] ± •300 mg

Econopred; Econopred Plus Drop-Tainers (eye drop suspension) ℞ *topical ophthalmic corticosteroidal anti-inflammatory* [prednisolone acetate] 0.125%; 1%

ecopipam HCl USAN *selective dopamine receptor antagonist for addiction*

ecostigmine iodide [see: echothiophate iodide]

ecothiopate iodide INN, BAN *antiglaucoma agent; irreversible cholinesterase inhibitor miotic* [also: echothiophate iodide]

Ecotrin enteric-coated tablets, enteric-coated caplets OTC *analgesic; antipyretic; anti-inflammatory; antiarthritic* [aspirin] 325, 500 mg ② Edecrin

Ecotrin Adult Low Strength enteric-coated tablets OTC *analgesic; antipyretic; anti-inflammatory; antiarthritic* [aspirin] 81 mg

ectylurea BAN

Ed A·Hist long-acting capsules, liquid ℞ *decongestant; antihistamine* [phenylephrine HCl; chlorpheniramine maleate] 20•8 mg; 10•4 mg/5 mL

edamine [see: ethylenediamine]

EDAP (etoposide, dexamethasone, ara-C, Platinol) *chemotherapy protocol*

edathamil [now: edetate calcium disodium]

edathamil calcium disodium [now: edetate calcium disodium]

edathamil disodium [now: edetate disodium]

edatrexate USAN, INN *antineoplastic; methotrexate analog*

Edecrin tablets ℞ *antihypertensive; loop diuretic* [ethacrynic acid] 25, 50 mg ② Ecotrin; Ethaquin

Edecrin Sodium powder for IV injection ℞ *antihypertensive; loop diuretic* [ethacrynate sodium] 50 mg

edelfosine INN

edetate calcium disodium USAN, USP *heavy metal chelating agent for lead poisoning* [also: sodium calcium edetate; sodium calciumedetate; calcium disodium edetate]

edetate dipotassium USAN *chelating agent*

edetate disodium USP *chelating agent; preservative; antioxidant* [also: disodium edetate] 150 mg/mL injection

edetate sodium USAN *chelating agent*

edetate trisodium USAN *chelating agent*

edetic acid NF, INN, BAN *chelating agent*

edetol USAN, INN *alkalizing agent*

Edex injection, pre-filled cartridges ℞ *vasodilator for erectile dysfunction* [alprostadil] 5, 10, 20, 40 μg/mL; 10, 20, 40 μg/mL

edifolone INN *antiarrhythmic* [also: edifolone acetate]

edifolone acetate USAN *antiarrhythmic* [also: edifolone]

Ed-In-Sol drops OTC *hematinic* [ferrous sulfate (source of iron)] 75 mg/0.6 mL (15 mg/0.6 mL)

edisilate INN *combining name for radicals or groups* [also: edisylate]

edisylate USAN, BAN *combining name for radicals or groups* [also: edisilate]

edithamil [see: edetate ...]

edobacomab USAN *antiendotoxin monoclonal antibody for gram-negative sepsis; clinical trials discontinued 1997*

edodekin alfa USAN *antiasthmatic; investigational (Phase I) immunomodulator for HIV; investigational (orphan) for renal cell carcinoma* [previously: interleukin 12 (IL-12)]

edogestrone INN, BAN

edoxudine USAN, INN *antiviral*

edrecolomab USAN *monoclonal antibody; antineoplastic adjuvant*

edrofuradene [see: nifurdazil]

Edronax (commercially available in England) ℞ *investigational (NDA filed) fast-acting selective norepinephrine reuptake inhibitor for depression* [reboxetine]

edrophone chloride [see: edrophonium chloride]

edrophonium chloride USP, INN, BAN *cholinergic/anticholinesterase muscle stimulant; antidote to curare; myasthenia gravis diagnostic aid*

Ed-Spaz tablets ℞ *GI antispasmodic; anticholinergic* [hyoscyamine sulfate] 0.125 mg

EDTA (ethylenediaminetetraacetic acid) [see: edetate disodium]

EDTA calcium [see: edetate calcium disodium]

ED-TLC; ED Tuss HC liquid ℞ *narcotic antitussive; decongestant; antihistamine* [hydrocodone bitartrate; phenylephrine HCl; chlorpheniramine maleate] 1.67•5•2 mg/5 mL; 2.5•10•4 mg/5 mL

E.E.S. granules for oral suspension ℞ *macrolide antibiotic* [erythromycin ethylsuccinate] 200 mg/5 mL

EES (erythromycin ethylsuccinate) [q.v.]

E.E.S. 200 oral suspension ℞ *macrolide antibiotic* [erythromycin ethylsuccinate] 200 mg/5 mL

E.E.S. 400 film-coated tablets, oral suspension ℞ *macrolide antibiotic* [erythromycin ethylsuccinate] 400 mg; 400 mg/5 mL

EF-27 *investigational agent to reduce chemotherapy side effects (clinical trials discontinued 1998)*

Efamol PMS soft gel capsules OTC *dietary supplement* [multiple vitamins & amino acids]

efaroxan INN, BAN

efavirenz *antiviral non-nucleoside reverse transcriptase inhibitor (NNRTI) for HIV*

Efed II capsules OTC *decongestant* [phenylpropanolamine HCl]

efegatran sulfate USAN *antithrombotic*

efetozole INN

Effer-K effervescent tablets ℞ *potassium supplement* [potassium bicarbonate; potassium citrate] 25 mEq

Effervescent Potassium effervescent tablets ℞ *potassium supplement* [potassium bicarbonate; potassium citrate] 25 mEq

Effexor tablets ℞ *antidepressant* [venlafaxine HCl] 25, 37.5, 50, 75, 100 mg

Effexor XR extended-release capsules ℞ *once-daily antidepressant and anxiolytic* [venlafaxine HCl] 37.5, 75, 150 mg

Efidac/24 extended-release tablets OTC *nasal decongestant* [pseudoephedrine HCl] 240 mg

Efidac/24 Chlorpheniramine extended-release tablets OTC *antihistamine* [chlorpheniramine maleate] 16 mg

Eflone eye drop suspension ℞ *topical ophthalmic corticosteroidal anti-inflammatory* [fluorometholone acetate] 0.1%

eflornithine INN, BAN *antineoplastic; antiprotozoal* [also: eflornithine HCl]

eflornithine HCl USAN *antiprotozoal for Trypanosoma brucei gambiense (sleeping sickness) infection (orphan); investigational (Phase III) antineoplastic for bladder cancer* [also: eflornithine]

efloxate INN

eflumast INN

Efodine ointment OTC *broad-spectrum antimicrobial* [povidone-iodine] 1%

eformoterol fumarate BAN *bronchodilator* [also: formoterol; formoterol fumarate]

EFP (etoposide, fluorouracil, Platinol) *chemotherapy protocol*

efrotomycin USAN, INN, BAN *veterinary growth stimulant*

Efudex cream, topical solution ℞ *antimetabolite antineoplastic for actinic keratoses and basal cell carcinomas* [fluorouracil] 5%; 2%, 5%

EGF-Genistein *investigational antineoplastic for breast cancer*

egtazic acid USAN, INN *pharmaceutic aid*

Egyptian privet *medicinal herb* [see: henna (Lawsonia)]

Egyptian thorn *medicinal herb* [see: acacia]

EHDP (ethane hydroxydiphosphonate) [see: etidronate disodium]

Ehrlich 594 [see: acetarsone]

Ehrlich 606 [see: arsphenamine]

eicosapentaenoic acid (EPA) [see: icosapent]

8 in 1 (Medrol, vincristine, CCNU, procarbazine, hydroxyurea, cisplatin, ara-C, cyclophosphamide) *chemotherapy protocol*

8 in 1 (Medrol, vincristine, CCNU, procarbazine, hydroxyurea, cisplatin, ara-C, dacarbazine) *chemotherapy protocol*

8-MOP capsules ℞ *systemic psoralens for repigmentation of idiopathic vitiligo; used to increase tolerance to sunlight and enhance pigmentation* [methoxsalen] 10 mg

einsteinium *element (Es)*

eIPV (enhanced, inactivated polio vaccine) [see: poliovirus vaccine, enhanced inactivated]

elacridar HCl USAN *chemotherapy potentiator; multi–drug-resistance inhibitor*

ELA-Max cream OTC *topical local anesthetic* [lidocaine] 4%

elantrine USAN, INN *anticholinergic*

elanzepine INN

Elase powder, ointment (discontinued 1999) ℞ *topical enzyme for biochemical debridement* [fibrinolysin; desoxyribonuclease] 25•15 000 U; 1•666.6 U/g

Elase-Chloromycetin ointment (discontinued 1999) ℞ *topical enzyme for biochemical debridement; antibiotic* [fibrinolysin; desoxyribonuclease; chloramphenicol] 1 U•666.6 U•10 mg per g

elastofilcon A USAN *hydrophilic contact lens material*

Elavil film-coated tablets, IM injection ℞ *tricyclic antidepressant* [amitriptyline HCl] 10, 25, 50, 75, 100, 150 mg; 10 mg/mL ⊉ Aldoril; Eldepryl; Enovil; Equanil; Mellaril

elbanizine INN

elcatonin INN, JAN *investigational (orphan) intrathecal treatment of intractable pain*

eldacimibe USAN *antihyperlipidemic; antiatherosclerotic; AcylCoA transferase (ACAT) inhibitor*

Eldecort cream (discontinued 1995) ℞ *topical corticosteroidal anti-inflammatory* [hydrocortisone] 2.5%

Eldepryl capsules ℞ *dopaminergic antiparkinsonian (orphan)* [selegiline HCl] 5 mg ⊉ Aldoril; Elavil; Enovil; Equanil; Mellaril

elder flower; elderberry (*Sambucus canadensis*; *S. ebulus*; *S. nigra*; *S. racemosa*) berries and flowers *medicinal herb for allergies, asthma, bronchitis, colds, constipation, edema, fever, hay fever, pneumonia, and sinus congestion; also used topically as an astringent*

Eldercaps capsules ℞ *vitamin/mineral supplement* [multiple vitamins & minerals; folic acid] ± • 1 mg

Eldertonic liquid OTC *vitamin/mineral supplement* [multiple B vitamins & minerals; alcohol 13.5%] ±

eldexomer INN

Eldisine ℞ *investigational (NDA filed) antineoplastic for leukemia, melanoma, breast and lung cancers* [vindesine sulfate]

Eldopaque; Eldopaque-Forte cream OTC *hyperpigmentation bleaching agent; sunscreen* [hydroquinone in a sunblock base] 2%; 4%

Eldoquin; Eldoquin-Forte Sunbleaching cream OTC *hyperpigmentation bleaching agent* [hydroquinone] 2%; 4%

elecampane (*Inula helenium*) root *medicinal herb for chronic bronchitis and cough*

electrocortin [see: aldosterone]

eledoisin INN

Eleutherococcus senticosus *medicinal herb* [see: Siberian ginseng]

ELF (etoposide, leucovorin [rescue], fluorouracil) *chemotherapy protocol*

elfazepam USAN, INN *veterinary appetite stimulant*

elfdock; elfwort *medicinal herb* [see: elecampane]

elgodipine INN

Elimite cream ℞ *pediculicide for lice; scabicide* [permethrin] 5%

eliprodil INN *investigational treatment for ischemic stroke*

Elixomin elixir ℞ *antiasthmatic; bronchodilator* [theophylline] 80 mg/15 mL

Elixophyllin capsules, elixir ℞ *antiasthmatic; bronchodilator* [theophylline] 100, 200 mg; 80 mg/15 mL

Elixophyllin GG liquid ℞ *antiasthmatic; bronchodilator; expectorant* [theophylline; guaifenesin] 100•100 mg/15 mL

Elixophyllin-KI elixir ℞ *antiasthmatic; bronchodilator; expectorant* [theophylline; potassium iodide] 80• 130 mg/15 mL

ellagic acid INN

Elliott's B solution *investigational (orphan) intrathecal chemotherapy diluent*

elliptinium acetate INN, BAN

elm, American; Indian elm; moose elm; red elm; rock elm; sweet elm; winged elm *medicinal herb* [see: slippery elm]

Elmiron capsules ℞ *urinary tract anti-inflammatory and analgesic for interstitial cystitis (orphan)* [pentosan polysulfate sodium] 100 mg

elmustine INN

elnadipine INN

Elocon ointment, cream, lotion ℞ *topical corticosteroidal anti-inflammatory* [mometasone furoate] 0.1%

E-Lor film-coated tablets (discontinued 1995) ℞ *narcotic analgesic* [propoxyphene HCl; acetaminophen] 65•650 mg

Eloxatin ℞ *investigational (orphan) alkylating antineoplastic for ovarian and colorectal cancers* [oxaliplatin]

elsamitrucin USAN, INN *antineoplastic*

Elspar powder for IV or IM injection ℞ *antineoplastic adjunct for acute lymphocytic leukemia* [asparaginase] 10 000 IU

eltanolone INN *investigational IV anesthetic*

eltenac INN

eltoprazine INN

Eltroxin tablets ℞ *thyroid hormone* [levothyroxine sodium] 50, 75, 100, 125, 150, 200, 300 μg

elucaine USAN, INN *gastric anticholinergic*

Elymus repens *medicinal herb* [see: couch grass]

elziverine INN

EMA (estramustine L-alanine) [q.v.]

EMA 86 (etoposide, mitoxantrone, ara-C) *chemotherapy protocol*

EMACO (etoposide, methotrexate, actinomycin D, cyclophosphamide, Oncovin) *chemotherapy protocol*

Emadine eye drops ℞ *topical antihistamine for allergic conjunctivitis* [emedastine difumarate] 0.05%

embinal [see: barbital sodium]

embonate INN, BAN *combining name for radicals or groups* [also: pamoate]

embramine INN, BAN

embramine HCl [see: embramine]

Embutane ℞ *veterinary anesthetic; veterinary euthanasia* [embutramide]

embutramide USAN, INN, BAN *veterinary anesthetic; veterinary euthanasia*

Emcyt capsules ℞ *nitrogen mustard-type alkylating antineoplastic for metastatic or progressive prostatic carcinoma* [estramustine phosphate sodium] 140 mg

Emdogain ℞ *investigational enamel matrix protein for wound healing*

Emecheck liquid (discontinued 1998) OTC *antinauseant; antiemetic* [phosphorated carbohydrate solution (glucose, fructose, and phosphoric acid)]

emedastine INN *ophthalmic antihistamine* [also: emedastine difumarate]

emedastine difumarate USAN, JAN *ophthalmic antihistamine* [also: emedastine]

emepronium bromide INN, BAN

emepronium carrageenate BAN

Emergent-Ez Kit *carry-kit for medical personnel* [multiple drugs and devices for emergencies]

Emersal emulsion ℞ *topical antipsoriatic; antiseborrheic* [ammoniated mercury; salicylic acid] 5%•2.5%

emetic herb; emetic weed *medicinal herb* [see: lobelia]

emetics *a class of agents that induce vomiting*

emetine BAN *antiamebic* [also: emetine HCl] ☑ Emetrol

emetine bismuth iodide [see: emetine HCl]

emetine HCl USP *amebicide* [also: emetine]

Emetrol solution OTC *antinauseant; antiemetic* [phosphorated carbohydrate solution (fructose, dextrose, and phosphoric acid)] 1.87 g•1.87 g•21.5 mg ☑ emetine

Emgel gel ℞ *topical antibiotic for acne* [erythromycin] 2%

emiglitate INN, BAN

emilium tosilate INN *antiarrhythmic* [also: emilium tosylate]

emilium tosylate USAN *antiarrhythmic* [also: emilium tosilate]

Eminase powder for IV injection ℞ *thrombolytic enzyme for acute myocardial infarction* [anistreplase] 30 U/vial

Emitasol intranasal ℞ *investigational antiemetic for chemotherapy* [metoclopramide HCl]

emitefur USAN *antineoplastic for stomach, colorectal, breast, pancreatic, and non-small cell lung cancers*

Emko; Emko Pre-Fil vaginal foam OTC *spermicidal contraceptive* [nonoxynol 9] 8%

EMLA cream, adhesive disc ℞ *topical local anesthetic* [lidocaine; prilocaine] 2.5%•2.5%

emmenagogues *a class of agents that induce or increase menstruation*

Emollia lotion OTC *moisturizer; emollient*

emollients *a class of dermatological agents that soften and soothe the skin*

emonapride INN

emopamil INN

emorfazone INN

Empirin tablets OTC *analgesic; antipyretic; anti-inflammatory; antirheumatic* [aspirin] 325 mg

Empirin with Codeine No. 3 & No. 4 tablets ℞ *narcotic analgesic; sometimes abused as a street drug* [codeine phosphate; aspirin] 30•325 mg; 60•325 mg

emtricitabine USAN *investigational (Phase I/II) antiviral for HIV and hepatitis B*

emtryl [see: dimetridazole]

emu oil *natural remedy for arthritis pain, hair loss prevention, and chronic skin disorders*

emulsifying wax [see: wax, emulsifying]

Emulsoil emulsion OTC *stimulant laxative* [castor oil] 95%

E-Mycin enteric-coated tablets ℞ *macrolide antibiotic* [erythromycin] 250, 333 mg

emylcamate INN, BAN

Enable ℞ *investigational (NDA filed) anti-inflammatory for rheumatoid arthritis and osteoarthritis* [tenidap]

enadoline INN *analgesic* [also: enadoline HCl]

enadoline HCl USAN *analgesic; investigational (orphan) for severe head injury* [also: enadoline]

enalapril INN, BAN *antihypertensive; angiotensin-converting enzyme (ACE) inhibitor* [also: enalapril maleate]

enalapril maleate USAN, USP *antihypertensive; angiotensin-converting enzyme (ACE) inhibitor* [also: enalapril]

enalaprilat USAN, USP, INN, BAN *antihypertensive; angiotensin-converting enzyme (ACE) inhibitor*

enalkiren USAN, INN *antihypertensive; renin inhibitor*

enallynymal sodium [see: methohexital sodium]

enantate INN *combining name for radicals or groups* [also: enanthate]

enanthate USAN, USP, BAN *combining name for radicals or groups* [also: enantate]

Enbrel powder for subcu injection ℞ *soluble tumor necrosis factor receptor (sTNFR) inhibitor for rheumatoid arthritis and juvenile rheumatoid arthritis (JRA); investigational (NDA filed) for congestive heart failure* [etanercept] 25 mg ☑ Incel

enbucrilate INN, BAN

encainide INN, BAN *antiarrhythmic* [also: encainide HCl]

encainide HCl USAN *antiarrhythmic* [also: encainide]

Encare vaginal suppositories OTC *spermicidal contraceptive* [nonoxynol 9] 2.27%

En-Cebrin Pulvules (capsules) OTC *vitamin/mineral/iron supplement* [multiple vitamins & minerals; iron]

enciprazine INN, BAN *minor tranquilizer* [also: enciprazine HCl]

enciprazine HCl USAN *minor tranquilizer* [also: enciprazine]

enclomifene INN [also: enclomiphene]

enclomiphene USAN [also: enclomifene]

encyprate USAN, INN *antidepressant*

End Lice liquid OTC *pediculicide for lice* [pyrethrins; piperonyl butoxide] 0.3%•3%

Endafed sustained-release capsules ℞ *decongestant; antihistamine* [pseudoephedrine HCl; brompheniramine maleate] 120•12 mg

Endagen-HD liquid ℞ *narcotic antitussive; decongestant; antihistamine* [hydrocodone bitartrate; phenylephrine HCl; chlorpheniramine maleate] 1.67•5•2 mg/5 mL

Endal timed-release tablets ℞ *decongestant; expectorant* [phenylephrine HCl; guaifenesin] 20•300 mg ② Intal

Endal Expectorant syrup ℞ *narcotic antitussive; decongestant; expectorant* [codeine phosphate; phenylpropanolamine HCl; guaifenesin; alcohol 5%] 10•12.5•100 mg/5 mL

Endal-HD; Endal-HD Plus liquid ℞ *narcotic antitussive; decongestant; antihistamine* [hydrocodone bitartrate; phenylephrine HCl; chlorpheniramine maleate] 1.7•5•2 mg/5 mL; 2.5•5•2 mg/5 mL

Endep film-coated tablets (discontinued 1996) ℞ *tricyclic antidepressant* [amitriptyline HCl] 10, 50, 75, 100, 150 mg

endiemal [see: metharbital]

endive *medicinal herb* [see: chicory]

endive, white; wild endive *medicinal herb* [see: dandelion]

endixaprine INN

endobenzyline bromide

endocaine [see: pyrrocaine]

Endocet tablets ℞ *narcotic analgesic* [oxycodone HCl; acetaminophen] 5•325 mg

endolate [see: meperidine HCl]

Endolor capsules ℞ *analgesic; sedative* [acetaminophen; caffeine; butalbital] 325•40•50 mg

endomide INN

endomycin

endothelin-1 receptor antagonists *a class of antihypertensives that block the action of endothelin-1, a vascular vasoconstrictor more potent than angiotensin II*

endralazine INN, BAN *antihypertensive* [also: endralazine mesylate]

endralazine mesylate USAN *antihypertensive* [also: endralazine]

Endrate IV infusion ℞ *chelating agent for hypercalcemia and ventricular arrhythmias due to digitalis toxicity* [edetate disodium] 150 mg/mL

endrisone INN *topical ophthalmic anti-inflammatory* [also: endrysone]

endrysone USAN *topical ophthalmic anti-inflammatory* [also: endrisone]

Enduret (trademarked dosage form) *prolonged-action tablet*

Enduron tablets ℞ *diuretic; antihypertensive* [methyclothiazide] 5 mg ② Imuran; Inderal

Enduronyl; Enduronyl Forte tablets ℞ *antihypertensive* [methyclothiazide; deserpidine] 5•0.25 mg; 5•0.5 mg ② Inderal

Enecat concentrated rectal suspension ℞ *radiopaque contrast medium for gastrointestinal imaging* [barium sulfate] 5%

enefexine INN

Ener-B nasal gel OTC *vitamin supplement* [cyanocobalamin] 400 μg

enestebol INN

Enfamil liquid, powder OTC *total or supplementary infant feeding*

Enfamil Human Milk Fortifier powder OTC *supplement to breast milk*

Enfamil LactoFree liquid, liquid concentrate, powder OTC *hypoallergenic infant formula* [milk-based formula, lactose free] 946 mL; 384 mL; 397 g

Enfamil Next Step liquid, powder OTC *total or supplementary infant feeding*

Enfamil Premature Formula liquid OTC *total or supplementary infant feeding*

Enfamil with Iron liquid, powder OTC *total or supplementary infant feeding*

enfenamic acid INN

enflurane USAN, USP, INN, BAN *inhalation general anesthetic* 125, 250 mL

Engerix-B adult IM injection, pediatric IM injection ℞ *active immunizing agent for hepatitis B and D* [hepatitis B virus vaccine, recombinant] 20 μg/mL, 10 μg/0.5 mL

English elm (*Ulmus campestris*) *medicinal herb* [see: slippery elm]

English hawthorn *medicinal herb* [see: hawthorn]

English ivy (*Hedera helix*) leaves *medicinal herb used as an antispasmodic and antiexanthematous agent*

English oak (*Quercus robur*) *medicinal herb* [see: white oak]

English valerian *medicinal herb* [see: valerian]

English walnut (*Juglans regia*) leaves *medicinal herb used as an astringent*

englitazone INN *antidiabetic* [also: englitazone sodium]

englitazone sodium USAN *antidiabetic* [also: englitazone]

enhanced, inactivated polio vaccine (eIPV) [see: poliovirus vaccine, enhanced inactivated]

Enhancer oral suspension ℞ *radiopaque contrast medium for gastrointestinal imaging* [barium sulfate] 98%

enhexymal [see: hexobarbital]

eniclobrate INN

enilconazole USAN, INN, BAN *antifungal*

enilospirone INN

eniluracil USAN *antineoplastic potentiator for fluorouracil; uracil reductase inhibitor*

enisoprost USAN, INN *antiulcerative; orphan status withdrawn 1996*

enisoprost & cyclosporine *orphan status withdrawn 1996*

Enisyl tablets OTC *dietary amino acid supplement* [L-lysine] 334, 500 mg

Enlon IV or IM injection ℞ *myasthenia gravis treatment; antidote to curare overdose* [edrophonium chloride] 10 mg/mL

Enlon Plus IV or IM injection ℞ *muscle stimulant; neuromuscular blocker antagonist* [edrophonium chloride; atropine sulfate] 10•0.14 mg

enloplatin USAN, INN *antineoplastic*

enocitabine INN

enofelast USAN, INN *antiasthmatic*

enolicam INN *anti-inflammatory; antirheumatic* [also: enolicam sodium]

enolicam sodium USAN *anti-inflammatory; antirheumatic* [also: enolicam]

Enomine capsules ℞ *decongestant; expectorant* [phenylpropanolamine HCl; phenylephrine HCl; guaifenesin] 45•5•200 mg

Enovid tablets (discontinued 1997) ℞ *estrogen/progestin combination for hypermenorrhea or endometriosis* [mestranol; norethynodrel] 75 μg•5 mg; 150 μg•9.85 mg

Enovil IM injection (discontinued 1996) ℞ *tricyclic antidepressant* [amitriptyline HCl] 10 mg/mL ② Aldoril; Elavil; Eldepryl; Equanil; Mellaril

enoxacin USAN, INN, BAN, JAN *broad-spectrum fluoroquinolone antibiotic*

enoxamast INN

enoxaparin BAN *a low molecular weight heparin-type anticoagulant and antithrombotic for the prevention of deep vein thrombosis (DVT), unstable angina, and myocardial infarction* [also: enoxaparin sodium]

enoxaparin sodium USAN, INN *a low molecular weight heparin-type anticoagulant and antithrombotic for the prevention of deep vein thrombosis*

(DVT), unstable angina, and myocardial infarction [also: enoxaparin]

enoximone USAN, INN, BAN cardiotonic

enoxolone INN, BAN

enphenemal [see: mephobarbital]

enpiprazole INN, BAN

enpiroline INN antimalarial [also: enpiroline phosphate]

enpiroline phosphate USAN antimalarial [also: enpiroline]

enprazepine INN

enprofen [now: furaprofen]

enprofylline USAN, INN bronchodilator

enpromate USAN, INN antineoplastic

enprostil USAN, INN, BAN investigational antisecretory and antiulcerative for acute peptic ulcers

enramycin INN

enrofloxacin USAN, INN, BAN veterinary antibacterial

Enseal (trademarked dosage form) enteric-coated tablet

Ensure liquid, powder OTC enteral nutritional therapy [lactose-free formula]

Ensure pudding OTC enteral nutritional therapy [milk-based formula] 150 g

Ensure Glucerna beverage, bars OTC diabetic nutritional supplements/snacks

Ensure High Calcium ready-to-use liquid OTC enteral nutritional therapy for postmenopausal women

Ensure High Protein ready-to-use liquid OTC enteral nutritional therapy [lactose-free formula] 237 mL

Ensure HN; Ensure with Fiber ready-to-use liquid OTC enteral nutritional therapy [lactose-free formula]

Ensure Plus; Ensure Plus HN liquid OTC enteral nutritional therapy [lactose-free formula]

E.N.T. sustained-release tablets (discontinued 1997) R̞ decongestant; antihistamine [phenylpropanolamine HCl; brompheniramine maleate] 75•12 mg

EN-tab (trademarked dosage form) enteric-coated tablet

entacapone USAN investigational (NDA filed) COMT inhibitor for Parkinson's disease

enteramine [see: serotonin]

Entero-Test; Entero-Test Pediatric string capsules for professional use in vitro diagnostic aid for GI disorders

Entertainer's Secret Throat Relief spray OTC saliva substitute

Entex capsules, liquid R̞ decongestant; expectorant [phenylephrine HCl; phenylpropanolamine HCl; guaifenesin] 5•45•200 mg; 5•20•100 mg/5 mL

Entex LA long-acting tablets R̞ decongestant; expectorant [phenylpropanolamine HCl; guaifenesin] 75•400 mg

Entex PSE prolonged-action tablets R̞ decongestant; expectorant [pseudoephedrine HCl; guaifenesin] 60•120 mg

Entocort Ⓒᴬᴺ tablets for rectal suspension R̞ steroidal anti-inflammatory for bowel disease [budesonide]

Entri-Pak (dosage form) liquid-filled pouch

Entrition 0.5 liquid OTC enteral nutritional therapy [lactose-free formula]

Entrition HN Entri-Pak (liquid-filled pouch) OTC enteral nutritional therapy [lactose-free formula]

Entrobar oral suspension (with Entrocel diluent) R̞ radiopaque contrast medium for gastrointestinal imaging [barium sulfate; (methylcellulose diluent)] 50% (500 mL)

entsufon INN detergent [also: entsufon sodium]

entsufon sodium USAN detergent [also: entsufon]

Entuss Expectorant liquid R̞ narcotic antitussive; expectorant [hydrocodone bitartrate; potassium guaiacolsulfonate] 5•300 mg/5 mL

Entuss Expectorant tablets R̞ narcotic antitussive; expectorant [hydrocodone bitartrate; guaifenesin] 5•300 mg

Entuss-D liquid R̞ narcotic antitussive; decongestant [hydrocodone bitartrate; pseudoephedrine HCl] 5•30 mg/5 mL

Entuss-D tablets R̞ narcotic antitussive; decongestant; expectorant [hydrocodone bitartrate; pseudoephedrine HCl; guaifenesin] 5•30•300 mg

Entuss-D Jr. liquid ℞ *pediatric narcotic antitussive, decongestant, and expectorant* [hydrocodone bitartrate; pseudoephedrine HCl; guaifenesin; alcohol 5%] 2.5•30•100 mg/5 mL

Enuclene eye drops OTC *cleaning, wetting and lubricating agent for artificial eyes* [tyloxapol] 0.25%

Enulose syrup ℞ *prevent and treat portal-systemic encephalopathy* [lactulose] 10 g/15 mL

enviomycin INN

enviradene USAN, INN *antiviral*

Enviro-Stress slow-release tablets OTC *vitamin/mineral supplement* [multiple vitamins & minerals; folic acid] ≐•0.4 mg

enviroxime USAN, INN *antiviral*

Enzone cream ℞ *topical corticosteroidal anti-inflammatory; local anesthetic* [hydrocortisone acetate; pramoxine HCl] 1%•1%

Enzymatic Cleaner for Extended Wear tablets OTC *enzymatic cleaner for soft contact lenses* [pork pancreatin]

Enzyme chewable tablets OTC *digestive enzymes* [amylase; protease; lipase; cellulase] 30•6•2•25 mg

EP (etoposide, Platinol) *chemotherapy protocol*

EPA capsules OTC *dietary supplement* [omega-3 fatty acids] 1000 mg

EPA (eicosapentaenoic acid) [see: icosapent]

epalrestat INN *investigational treatment for diabetic neuropathy*

epanolol INN, BAN

eperezolid USAN *antibacterial*

eperisone INN

epervudine INN

ephedra (*Ephedra* spp.) plant *medicinal herb for asthma, blood cleansing, bronchitis, bursitis, chills, colds, edema, fever, flu, headache, kidney disorders, nasal congestion, and venereal disease*

ephedrine USP, BAN *sympathomimetic bronchodilator; nasal decongestant;*

vasopressor for shock ② Appedrine; aprindine

ephedrine HCl USP, BAN *sympathomimetic bronchodilator; nasal decongestant; vasopressor for shock*

ephedrine sulfate USP *sympathomimetic bronchodilator; nasal decongestant; vasopressor for acute hypotensive shock* [also: ephedrine sulphate] 25 mg oral; 50 mg/mL injection

ephedrine sulphate BAN *sympathomimetic bronchodilator; nasal decongestant* [also: ephedrine sulfate]

ephedrine tannate *sympathomimetic bronchodilator; nasal decongestant*

EPI-2010 *investigational for asthma*

Epi-C concentrated oral suspension ℞ *radiopaque contrast medium for gastrointestinal imaging* [barium sulfate] 150%

epicainide INN

epicillin USAN, INN, BAN *antibacterial*

epicriptine INN

epidermal growth factor, human *investigational (orphan) for acceleration of corneal regeneration*

epiestriol INN [also: epioestriol]

Epifoam aerosol foam ℞ *topical corticosteroidal anti-inflammatory; local anesthetic* [hydrocortisone acetate; pramoxine] 1%•1%

Epifrin eye drops ℞ *topical antiglaucoma agent* [epinephrine HCl] 0.5%, 1%, 2% ② epinephrine; EpiPen

Epiject ⚘ (U.S. product: Depacon) IV infusion ℞ *anticonvulsant* [valproate sodium] 100 mg/mL

EpiLeukin ℞ *investigational (Phase III) treatment for malignant melanoma*

epilin [see: dietifen]

E-Pilo-1; E-Pilo-2; E-Pilo-4; E-Pilo-6 eye drops ℞ *topical antiglaucoma agent* [pilocarpine HCl; epinephrine bitartrate] 1%•1%; 2%•1%; 4%•1%; 6%•1%

E-Pilo-3 eye drops (discontinued 1995) ℞ *topical antiglaucoma agent* [pilocarpine HCl; epinephrine bitartrate] 3%•1%

Epilyt lotion concentrate OTC *moisturizer; emollient*

epimestrol USAN, INN, BAN *anterior pituitary activator*

Epinal eye drops ℞ *topical antiglaucoma agent* [epinephryl borate] 0.5%, 1% ⊠ Epitol

epinastine INN

epinephran [see: epinephrine]

epinephrine USP, INN *vasoconstrictor; sympathomimetic bronchodilator; topical antiglaucoma agent; vasopressor for shock* [also: adrenaline] 1:1000, 1:10 000 (1, 0.1 mg/mL) injection ⊠ Epifrin

epinephrine bitartrate USP *sympathomimetic bronchodilator; ophthalmic adrenergic; topical antiglaucoma agent*

epinephrine borate *topical antiglaucoma agent*

epinephrine & cisplatin *investigational (Phase II) injectable gel for inoperable primary liver cancer*

epinephrine HCl *sympathomimetic bronchodilator; nasal decongestant; topical antiglaucoma agent; vasopressor for shock* 0.1% eye drops; 1:1000, 1:2000, 1:10 000 (1, 0.5, 0.1 mg/mL) injection

Epinephrine Pediatric subcu injection ℞ *bronchodilator for bronchial asthma or bronchospasm; vasopressor for shock* [epinephrine HCl] 1:100 000 (0.01 mg/mL)

epinephryl borate USAN, USP *adrenergic; topical antiglaucoma agent*

epioestriol BAN [also: epiestriol]

EpiPen; EpiPen Jr. auto-injector (automatic IM injection device) ℞ *emergency treatment of anaphylaxis; vasopressor for shock* [epinephrine] 1:1000 (1 mg/mL); 1:2000 (0.5 mg/mL) ⊠ Epifrin

epipropidine USAN, INN *antineoplastic*

epirizole USAN, INN *analgesic; anti-inflammatory*

epiroprim INN

epirubicin INN, BAN *anthracycline antibiotic antineoplastic* [also: epirubicin HCl]

epirubicin HCl USAN, JAN *anthracycline antibiotic antineoplastic* [also: epirubicin]

epitetracycline HCl USP *antibacterial*

epithiazide USAN, BAN *antihypertensive; diuretic* [also: epitizide]

epithioandrostanol [see: epitiostanol]

epitiostanol INN

epitizide INN *antihypertensive; diuretic* [also: epithiazide]

Epitol tablets ℞ *anticonvulsant; analgesic for trigeminal neuralgia; antipsychotic* [carbamazepine] 200 mg ⊠ Epinal

Epival ✪ (U.S. product: Depakote) enteric-coated tablets ℞ *anticonvulsant; antipsychotic for manic episodes of a bipolar disorder* [divalproex sodium] 125, 250, 500 mg

Epivir film-coated tablets, oral solution ℞ *antiviral nucleoside reverse transcriptase inhibitor for HIV* [lamivudine] 150 mg; 10 mg/mL

Epivir-HBV film-coated tablets, oral solution ℞ *antiviral nucleoside reverse transcriptase inhibitor for hepatitis B virus (HBV)* [lamivudine] 100 mg; 5 mg/mL

eplerenone USAN *aldosterone receptor antagonist for congestive heart failure, hypertension, and cirrhosis*

EPlus tablets OTC *vitamin supplement* [multiple vitamins; lemon bioflavonoids]

EPO (epoetin alfa) [q.v.]

EPO (evening primrose oil) [see: evening primrose]

EPOCH (etoposide, prednisone, Oncovin, cyclophosphamide, Halotestin) *chemotherapy protocol*

epoetin alfa (EPO) USAN, INN, BAN, JAN *hematinic for anemia of chronic renal failure, HIV, and chemotherapy (orphan); to reduce blood transfusions in surgery*

epoetin beta USAN, INN, BAN, JAN *antianemic; hematinic; investigational (orphan) for anemia of end-stage renal disease*

Epogen IV or subcu injection ℞ *stimulates RBC production; for anemia of chronic renal failure, HIV, or chemotherapy (orphan)* [epoetin alfa] 2000, 3000, 4000, 10 000, 20 000 U/mL ⊠ "amp and gent" (ampicillin & gentamicin)

epoprostenol USAN, INN *platelet aggregation inhibitor; investigational (orphan) vasodilator for primary pulmonary hypertension*

epoprostenol sodium USAN, BAN *platelet aggregation inhibitor and vasodilator for hypertension*

epostane USAN, INN, BAN *interceptive*

epoxytropine tropate methylbromide [see: methscopolamine bromide]

Eppy/N 1%; Eppy/N 2% eye drops (discontinued 1995) ℞ *topical antiglaucoma agent* [epinephrine borate] 1%; 2%

eprazinone INN

Eprex (name changed to Procrit in 1997)

eprinomectin USAN *veterinary antiparasitic*

epristeride USAN, INN, BAN *alpha reductase inhibitor for benign prostatic hypertrophy*

Epromate tablets (discontinued 1995) ℞ *analgesic; antipyretic; anti-inflammatory; anxiolytic* [aspirin; meprobamate] 325•200 mg

eprosartan USAN *antihypertensive (angiotensin II blocker)*

eprosartan mesylate USAN *antihypertensive (angiotensin II blocker)*

eprovafen INN

eproxindine INN

eprozinol INN

epsikapron [see: aminocaproic acid]

epsilon-aminocaproic acid (EACA) [see: aminocaproic acid]

epsiprantel INN, BAN

Epsom salt [see: magnesium sulfate]

e.p.t. Quick Stick test stick for home use OTC *in vitro diagnostic aid for urine pregnancy test*

eptaloprost INN

eptamestrol [see: etamestrol]

eptaprost [see: eptaloprost]

eptastatin sodium [see: pravastatin sodium]

eptastigmine INN *investigational treatment for Alzheimer's disease*

eptazocine INN

eptifibatide *glycoprotein (GP) IIb/IIIa receptor antagonist; platelet aggregation inhibitor for acute coronary syndrome, unstable angina, myocardial infarction, and cardiac surgery*

Epulor liquid OTC *enteral nutritional therapy* [milk-based formula]

Equagesic tablets ℞ *analgesic; antipyretic; anti-inflammatory; anxiolytic* [aspirin; meprobamate] 325•200 mg

Equalactin chewable tablets OTC *bulk laxative; antidiarrheal* [calcium polycarbophil] 625 mg

Equanil tablets ℞ *anxiolytic* [meprobamate] 200, 400 mg ☒ Aldoril; Elavil; Eldepryl; Enovil; Mellaril

Equazine M tablets (discontinued 1995) ℞ *analgesic; antipyretic; anti-inflammatory; anxiolytic* [aspirin; meprobamate] 325•200 mg

Equilet chewable tablets OTC *antacid* [calcium carbonate] 500 mg

equilin USP *estrogen*

Equipoise *brand name for boldenone undecylenate, a veterinary anabolic steroid abused as a street drug*

Equisetum arvens *medicinal herb* [see: horsetail]

Eramycin film-coated tablets (discontinued 1998) ℞ *macrolide antibiotic* [erythromycin stearate] 250 mg

erbium *element (Er)*

erbulozole USAN, INN *antineoplastic adjunct*

erbumine USAN, INN, BAN *combining name for radicals or groups*

Ercaf tablets ℞ *migraine-specific vasoconstrictor* [ergotamine tartrate; caffeine] 1•100 mg

erdosteine INN

Erechtites hieracfolia *medicinal herb* [see: pilewort]

Ergamisol tablets ℞ *biological response modifier; antineoplastic adjunct for colon cancer* [levamisole HCl] 50 mg

ergocalciferol USP, INN, BAN, JAN *vitamin D_2; antirachitic* 50 000 IU (1.25 mg) oral

ergoloid mesylates USAN, USP *cognition adjuvant for age-related mental* *capacity decline* [also: co-dergocrine mesylate] 0.5, 1 mg oral

Ergomar sublingual tablets ℞ *migraine treatment; vasoconstrictor* [ergotamine tartrate] 2 mg

ergometrine INN, BAN *oxytocic for induction of labor* [also: ergonovine maleate]

ergonovine maleate USP *oxytocic for induction of labor* [also: ergometrine]

Ergoset once-daily tablets ℞ *investigational (NDA filed) dopamine agonist for hypoglycemic control in type 2 diabetes; investigational (Phase II/III) treatment for clinical obesity* [bromocriptine mesylate]

Ergostat sublingual tablets (discontinued 1996) ℞ *migraine-specific vasoconstrictor* [ergotamine tartrate] 2 mg

ergosterol, activated [see: ergocalciferol]

ergot (*Claviceps purpurea***)** dried sclerotia *medicinal herb used as an abortifacient, emmenagogue, hemostatic, oxytocic, and vasoconstrictor; source of ergotamine and LSD*

ergot alkaloids [see: ergoloid mesylates]

ergotamine INN, BAN *migraine-specific analgesic* [also: ergotamine tartrate]

ergotamine tartrate USP *migraine-specific analgesic* [also: ergotamine]

Ergotrate Maleate IM or IV injection ℞ *oxytocic for the induction of labor and prevention of postpartum and postabortal hemorrhage* [ergonovine maleate] 0.2 mg/mL

Ergotrate Maleate tablets (discontinued 1995) ℞ *oxytocic for the induction of labor and prevention of postpartum and postabortal hemorrhage* [ergonovine maleate] 0.2 mg

ericolol INN

Eridium tablets (discontinued 1996) ℞ *urinary analgesic* [phenazopyridine HCl] 100 mg

Erigeron canadensis medicinal herb [see: fleabane; horseweed]

eriodictyon NF

Eriodictyon californicum medicinal herb [see: yerba santa]

eritrityl tetranitrate INN *coronary vasodilator* [also: erythrityl tetranitrate]

erizepine INN

E-R-O Ear Drops OTC *agent to emulsify and disperse ear wax* [carbamide peroxide] 6.5%

erocainide INN

errhines *a class of agents that promote nasal discharge or secretion*

ersofermin USAN, INN *wound healing agent; transglutaminase inhibitor for the treatment of scar tissue*

Erwinase ℞ *investigational (orphan) antineoplastic for acute lymphocytic leukemia* [erwinia L-asparaginase]

erwinia L-asparaginase *investigational (orphan) antineoplastic for acute lymphocytic leukemia*

ERYC delayed-release capsules containing enteric-coated pellets ℞ *macrolide antibiotic* [erythromycin] 250 mg ⧉ ara-C

Erycette topical solution ℞ *topical antibiotic for acne* [erythromycin] 2% ⧉ Aricept

EryDerm 2% topical solution ℞ *topical antibiotic for acne* [erythromycin] 2%

Erygel gel ℞ *topical antibiotic for acne* [erythromycin; alcohol 92%] 2%

Erymax topical solution ℞ *topical antibiotic for acne* [erythromycin] 2%

Eryngium aquaticum medicinal herb [see: water eryngo]

EryPed chewable tablets, drops ℞ *macrolide antibiotic* [erythromycin ethylsuccinate] 200 mg; 100 mg/2.5 mL

EryPed granules for oral suspension (discontinued 1998) ℞ *macrolide antibiotic* [erythromycin ethylsuccinate] 400 mg/5 mL

EryPed 200; EryPed 400 oral suspension ℞ *macrolide antibiotic* [erythromycin ethylsuccinate] 200 mg/5 mL; 400 mg/5 mL

Ery-Sol topical solution (discontinued 1995) ℞ *topical antibiotic for acne* [erythromycin] 2%

Ery-Tab enteric-coated delayed-release tablets ℞ *macrolide antibiotic* [erythromycin] 250, 333, 500 mg

erythorbic acid

Erythra-Derm topical solution ℞ *topical antibiotic for acne* [erythromycin] 2%

Erythraea centaurium medicinal herb [see: centaury]

erythrityl tetranitrate USAN, USP *coronary vasodilator; antianginal* [also: eritrityl tetranitrate]

Erythrocin powder for IV injection ℞ *macrolide antibiotic* [erythromycin lactobionate] 500, 1000 mg/vial

Erythrocin Stearate Filmtabs (film-coated tablets) ℞ *macrolide antibiotic* [erythromycin stearate] 250, 500 mg

erythrol tetranitrate [now: erythrityl tetranitrate]

erythromycin USP, INN, BAN *macrolide antibiotic* 250, 500 mg oral; 2% topical; 5 mg/g topical ⊠ clarithromycin

erythromycin 2′-acetate octadecanoate [see: erythromycin acistrate]

erythromycin 2′-acetate stearate [see: erythromycin acistrate]

erythromycin acistrate USAN, INN *macrolide antibiotic*

erythromycin B [see: berythromycin]

erythromycin estolate USAN, USP, BAN *macrolide antibiotic* 250 mg oral; 125, 250 mg/5 mL oral

erythromycin ethyl succinate BAN *macrolide antibiotic* [also: erythromycin ethylsuccinate]

erythromycin ethylcarbonate USP *macrolide antibiotic*

erythromycin ethylsuccinate (EES) USP *macrolide antibiotic* [also: erythromycin ethyl succinate] 400 mg oral; 200, 400 mg/5 mL oral;

erythromycin gluceptate USP *macrolide antibiotic*

erythromycin glucoheptonate [see: erythromycin gluceptate]

erythromycin lactobionate USP *macrolide antibiotic* 500, 1000 mg/vial injection

erythromycin lauryl sulfate, propionyl [now: erythromycin estolate]

erythromycin monoglucoheptonate [see: erythromycin gluceptate]

erythromycin octadecanoate [see: erythromycin stearate]

erythromycin 2′-propanoate [see: erythromycin propionate]

erythromycin propionate USAN *macrolide antibiotic*

erythromycin 2′-propionate dodecyl sulfate [see: erythromycin estolate]

erythromycin propionate lauryl sulfate [now: erythromycin estolate]

erythromycin salnacedin USAN *macrolide antibiotic for acne vulgaris*

erythromycin stearate USP, BAN *macrolide antibiotic* 250, 500 mg oral

erythromycin stinoprate INN *macrolide antibiotic*

Erythronium americanum medicinal herb [see: adder's tongue]

erythropoietin, gene-activated (GA-EPO) *investigational (Phase III) agent for anemia of renal failure*

erythropoietin, recombinant human (rEPO) [see: epoetin alfa; epoetin beta]

erythrosine sodium USP *dental disclosing agent*

Eryzole granules for oral suspension ℞ *antibiotic* [erythromycin ethylsuccinate; sulfisoxazole acetyl] 200• 600 mg/5 mL

esafloxacin INN

esaprazole INN

Esclim transdermal patch ℞ *estrogen replacement therapy for postmenopausal disorders* [estradiol] 25, 37.5, 50, 75, 100 μg/day

esculamine INN

eseridine INN

eserine [see: physostigmine]

Eserine Salicylate eye drops (discontinued 1995) ℞ *topical antiglaucoma agent; reversible cholinesterase inhibitor miotic* [physostigmine salicylate] 0.5%

Eserine Sulfate ophthalmic ointment (discontinued 1999) ℞ *topical antiglaucoma agent; reversible cholinesterase inhibitor miotic* [physostigmine sulfate] 0.25%

esflurbiprofen INN, BAN

Esgic tablets, capsules ℞ *analgesic; sedative* [acetaminophen; caffeine; butalbital] 325•40•50 mg

Esgic-Plus tablets ℞ *analgesic; sedative* [acetaminophen; caffeine; butalbital] 500•40•50 mg

ESHAP (etoposide, Solu-Medrol, high-dose ara-C, Platinol) *chemotherapy protocol*

ESHAP-MINE (alternating cycles of ESHAP and MINE) *chemotherapy protocol*

Esidrix tablets ℞ *antihypertensive; diuretic* [hydrochlorothiazide] 25, 50, 100 mg ⊡ Lasix

esilate INN *combining name for radicals or groups* [also: esylate]

Esimil tablets ℞ *antihypertensive; diuretic* [hydrochlorothiazide; guanethidine monosulfate] 25•10 mg ⊡ Estinyl; Isomil

Eskalith capsules, tablets ℞ *antipsychotic for manic episodes* [lithium carbonate] 300 mg

Eskalith CR controlled-release tablets ℞ *antipsychotic for manic episodes* [lithium carbonate] 450 mg

esmolol INN, BAN *antihypertensive; antiadrenergic (β-receptor)* [also: esmolol HCl]

esmolol HCl USAN *antihypertensive; antiarrhythmic; antiadrenergic (β-receptor)* [also: esmolol]

E-Solve OTC *lotion base*

esorubicin INN *antineoplastic* [also: esorubicin HCl]

esorubicin HCl USAN *antineoplastic* [also: esorubicin]

Esotérica Dry Skin Treatment lotion OTC *moisturizer; emollient*

Esotérica Facial; Esotérica Fortified; Esotérica Sunscreen cream OTC *hyperpigmentation bleaching agent; sunscreen* [hydroquinone; padimate O; oxybenzone] 2%•3.3%•2.5%

Esotérica Regular; Esotérica Sensitive Skin Formula cream OTC *hyperpigmentation bleaching agent* [hydroquinone] 2%; 1.5%

Esotérica Soap OTC *bath emollient*

Espotabs tablets (discontinued 1998) OTC *stimulant laxative* [yellow phenolphthalein] 97.2 mg

esproquin HCl USAN *adrenergic* [also: esproquine]

esproquine INN *adrenergic* [also: esproquin HCl]

Essential Protein powder OTC *oral protein supplement* [soy protein]

Estar gel OTC *topical antipsoriatic; antiseborrheic* [coal tar] 5%

estazolam USAN, INN *hypnotic* 1, 2 mg oral

Ester-C Plus capsules OTC *dietary supplement* [vitamin C; calcium; multiple bioflavonoids; rutin] 500•62•45•5 mg

Ester-C Plus, Extra Potency tablets OTC *dietary supplement* [vitamin C; calcium; multiple bioflavonoids; rutin] 1000•125•250•25 mg

Ester-C Plus Multi-Mineral capsules OTC *dietary supplement* [vitamin C; multiple minerals; multiple bioflavonoids; rutin] 425•±•75•5 mg

esterified estrogens [see: estrogens, esterified]

esterifilcon A USAN *hydrophilic contact lens material*

estilben [see: diethylstilbestrol dipropionate]

Estinyl tablets ℞ *estrogen replacement therapy for postmenopausal disorders; palliative therapy for inoperable prostate and breast cancers* [ethinyl estradiol] 0.02, 0.05, 0.5 mg ⊡ Esimil

Estivin II eye drops (discontinued 1995) OTC *topical ophthalmic decongestant and vasoconstrictor* [naphazoline HCl] 0.012%

estolate INN *combining name for radicals or groups*

estomycin sulfate [see: paromomycin sulfate]

Estrace tablets ℞ *estrogen replacement therapy for postmenopausal disorders; palliative therapy for prostate and metastatic breast cancers* [estradiol] 0.5, 1, 2 mg

Estrace vaginal cream ℞ *estrogen replacement for postmenopausal atrophic vaginitis* [estradiol] 0.1 mg/g

Estra-D IM injection (discontinued 1996) ℞ *estrogen replacement therapy for postmenopausal disorders* [estradiol cypionate in oil] 5 mg/mL

Estraderm transdermal patch ℞ *estrogen replacement therapy for postmenopausal disorders* [estradiol] 50, 100 μg/day ⅻ Estradurin

estradiol USP, INN *estrogen replacement therapy for postmenopausal disorders; palliative therapy for prostate and metastatic breast cancers* [also: oestradiol] 0.5, 1, 2 mg oral

estradiol benzoate USP, INN, JAN [also: oestradiol benzoate]

estradiol 17-cyclopentanepropionate [see: estradiol cypionate]

estradiol cypionate USP *estrogen replacement therapy for postmenopausal disorders* 5 mg/mL injection (in oil)

estradiol dipropionate NF, JAN

estradiol enanthate USAN *estrogen*

estradiol hemihydrate *topical estrogen therapy for atrophic vaginitis*

estradiol 17-heptanoate [see: estradiol enanthate]

estradiol monobenzoate [see: estradiol benzoate]

estradiol 17-nicotinate 3-propionate [see: estrapronicate]

estradiol phosphate polymer [see: polyestradiol phosphate]

estradiol 17-undecanoate [see: estradiol undecylate]

estradiol undecylate USAN, INN *estrogen*

estradiol valerate USP, INN, JAN *estrogen replacement; hormonal antineoplastic for prostatic carcinoma* [also: oestradiol valerate] 20, 40 mg/mL IM injection

Estra-L 20 IM injection (discontinued 1998) ℞ *estrogen replacement therapy for postmenopausal disorders; palliative therapy for inoperable prostate cancer* [estradiol valerate in oil] 20 mg/mL

Estra-L 40 IM injection ℞ *estrogen replacement therapy for postmenopausal disorders; antineoplastic for prostatic cancer* [estradiol valerate in oil] 40 mg/mL

estramustine USAN, INN, BAN *nitrogen mustard-type alkylating antineoplastic*

estramustine phosphate sodium USAN, BAN, JAN *nitrogen mustard-type alkylating antineoplastic for prostate cancer*

estrapronicate INN

Estrasorb cream, transdermal patch ℞ *investigational (Phase II) hormone replacement therapy for postmenopausal symptoms* [estrogen]

Estratab tablets ℞ *estrogen replacement therapy for postmenopausal disorders; palliative therapy for inoperable prostate and breast cancers* [esterified estrogens] 0.3, 0.625, 2.5 mg ⅻ Ethatab

Estratest; Estratest H.S. sugar-coated tablets ℞ *estrogen/androgen for menopausal vasomotor symptoms* [esterified estrogens; methyltestosterone] 1.25•2.5 mg; 0.625•1.25 mg

Estra-Testrin IM injection (discontinued 1995) ℞ *estrogen/androgen for menopausal vasomotor symptoms* [estradiol valerate; testosterone enanthate] 4•90 mg/mL

estrazinol INN *estrogen* [also: estrazinol hydrobromide]

estrazinol hydrobromide USAN *estrogen* [also: estrazinol]

Estrinex (name changed to Fareston upon release in 1998)

Estring vaginal ring ℞ *three-month estrogen replacement for postmenopausal atrophic vaginitis* [estradiol] 2 mg (7.5 μg/day)

estriol USP *estrogen* [also: estriol succinate; oestriol succinate]

estriol succinate INN *estrogen* [also: estriol; oestriol succinate]

estrobene [see: diethylstilbestrol]

estrobene DP [see: diethylstilbestrol dipropionate]

Estro-Cyp IM injection (discontinued 1998) ℞ *hormone replacement therapy* for *postmenopausal disorders* [estradiol cypionate in oil] 5 mg/mL

estrofurate USAN, INN *estrogen*

Estrogenic Substance Aqueous IM injection (discontinued 1998) ℞ *estrogen replacement therapy for postmenopausal disorders; palliative therapy for prostate and breast cancers* [estrone and other estrogens] 2 mg/mL

estrogenic substances, conjugated [see: estrogens, conjugated]

estrogenine [see: diethylstilbestrol]

estrogens *a class of female sex hormones that includes estradiol, estrone, and estriol, also used as an antineoplastic*

estrogens, conjugated USP, JAN *estrogen replacement therapy for postmenopausal disorders; palliative therapy for prostate and metastatic breast cancers*

estrogens, esterified USP *estrogen replacement therapy for postmenopausal disorders; palliative therapy for inoperable prostate and breast cancers*

Estroject-L.A. IM injection (discontinued 1995) ℞ *hormone for estrogen replacement therapy* [estradiol cypionate in oil] 5 mg/mL

estromenin [see: diethylstilbestrol]

estrone USP, INN *estrogen replacement therapy for postmenopausal disorders; palliative therapy for prostate and breast cancers* [also: oestrone]

Estrone 5 IM injection (discontinued 1998) ℞ *estrogen replacement therapy for postmenopausal disorders; palliative therapy for prostate and breast cancers* [estrone] 5 mg/mL

Estrone Aqueous IM injection ℞ *estrogen replacement therapy for postmenopausal disorders; palliative therapy for prostate and breast cancers* [estrone] 5 mg/mL

estrone hydrogen sulfate [see: estrone sodium sulfate]

estrone sodium sulfate

Estrophasic (trademarked/patented dosing regimen) *gradual estrogen intake with steady progestin intake*

estropipate USP *estrogen replacement therapy for postmenopausal disorders* 0.75, 1.5, 3, 6 mg oral

Estrostep 21 tablets ℞ *triphasic oral contraceptive* [norethindrone acetate; ethinyl estradiol] Phase 1: 1 mg•20 µg; Phase 2: 1 mg•30 µg; Phase 3: 1 mg•35 µg

Estrostep Fe tablets ℞ *triphasic oral contraceptive with iron* [norethindrone acetate; ethinyl estradiol; ferrous fumarate] Phase 1: 1 mg•20 µg•75 mg; Phase 2: 1 mg•30 µg•75 mg; Phase 3: 1 mg•35 µg•75 mg; Counters: 0•0•75 mg (iron only)

Estrovis tablets (discontinued 1996) ℞ *estrogen replacement therapy for postmenopausal disorders* [quinestrol] 100 µg

esuprone INN

esylate USAN, BAN *combining name for radicals or groups* [also: esilate]

etabenzarone INN

etabonate USAN, INN *combining name for radicals or groups*

etacepride INN

etacrynic acid INN, JAN *antihypertensive; loop diuretic* [also: ethacrynic acid]

etafedrine INN, BAN *adrenergic* [also: etafedrine HCl]

etafedrine HCl USAN *adrenergic* [also: etafedrine]

etafenone INN

etafilcon A USAN *hydrophilic contact lens material*

etamestrol INN

etaminile INN

etamiphyllin INN [also: etamiphylline]

etamiphyllin methesculetol [see: metescufylline]

etamiphylline BAN [also: etamiphyllin]

etamivan INN *central and respiratory stimulant* [also: ethamivan]

etamocycline INN

etamsylate INN *hemostatic* [also: ethamsylate]

etanercept USAN *soluble tumor necrosis factor receptor (sTNFR) inhibitor for rheumatoid arthritis; investigational (NDA filed) for congestive heart failure*

etanidazole USAN, INN *antineoplastic; hypoxic cell radiosensitizer*

etanterol INN

etaperazine [see: perphenazine]

etaqualone INN

etarotene USAN, INN *keratolytic*

etasuline INN

etazepine INN

etazolate INN *antipsychotic* [also: etazolate HCl]

etazolate HCl USAN *antipsychotic* [also: etazolate]

etebenecid INN [also: ethebenecid]

etenzamide BAN [also: ethenzamide]

eterobarb USAN, INN, BAN *anticonvulsant*

etersalate INN

ethacridine INN [also: ethacridine lactate; acrinol] ⊇ ethacrynic

ethacridine lactate [also: ethacridine; acrinol]

ethacrynate sodium USAN, USP *antihypertensive; loop diuretic*

ethacrynic acid USAN, USP, BAN *antihypertensive; loop diuretic* [also: etacrynic acid] ⊇ ethacridine

ethambutol INN, BAN *bacteriostatic; primary tuberculostatic* [also: ethambutol HCl]

ethambutol HCl USAN, USP *bacteriostatic; primary tuberculostatic* [also: ethambutol]

ethamivan USAN, USP, BAN *central and respiratory stimulant* [also: etamivan]

Ethamolin IV injection ℞ *sclerosing agent for bleeding esophageal varices (orphan)* [ethanolamine oleate] 5%

ethamsylate USAN, BAN *hemostatic* [also: etamsylate]

ethanol JAN *topical anti-infective/antiseptic; astringent; solvent; a widely abused "legal street drug" used to produce euphoria* [also: alcohol]

ethanol, dehydrated JAN *antidote* [also: alcohol, dehydrated]

ethanolamine oleate USAN *sclerosing agent for bleeding esophageal varices (orphan)* [also: monoethanolamine oleate]

ethanolamines *a class of antihistamines that includes diphenhydramine HCl and clemastine fumarate*

Ethaquin tablets (discontinued 1996) ℞ *peripheral vasodilator* [ethaverine HCl] 100 mg ⊇ Edecrin

Ethatab tablets (discontinued 1996) ℞ *peripheral vasodilator* [ethaverine HCl] 100 mg ⊇ Estratab

ethaverine INN *peripheral vasodilator*

ethaverine HCl *peripheral vasodilator* [see: ethaverine]

Ethavex-100 tablets (discontinued 1996) ℞ *peripheral vasodilator* [ethaverine HCl] 100 mg

ethchlorvynol USP, INN, BAN *sedative; hypnotic*

ethebenecid BAN [also: etebenecid]

ethenzamide INN, JAN [also: etenzamide]

ether USP *inhalation anesthetic*

ethiazide INN, BAN

ethidium bromide [see: homidium bromide]

ethinamate USP, INN, BAN *sedative; hypnotic* ⊇ ethionamide

ethinyl estradiol USP *estrogen replacement therapy for postmenopausal disorders; palliative therapy for inoperable prostate and breast cancers; investigational (orphan) for Turner syndrome* [also: ethinylestradiol; ethinyloestradiol]

ethinylestradiol INN *estrogen replacement therapy for postmenopausal disorders; palliative therapy for inoperable prostate and breast cancers* [also: ethinyl estradiol; ethinyloestradiol]

ethinyloestradiol BAN *estrogen replacement therapy for postmenopausal disorders; palliative therapy for inoperable prostate and breast cancers* [also: ethinyl estradiol; ethinylestradiol]

ethiodized oil USP *parenteral radiopaque contrast medium (37% iodine)*

ethiodized oil (^{131}I) INN *antineoplastic; radioactive agent* [also: ethiodized oil I 131]

ethiodized oil I 131 USAN *antineoplastic; radioactive agent* [also: ethiodized oil (^{131}I)]

Ethiodol intracavitary instillation R̥ *radiopaque contrast medium for lymphography and gynecological imaging* [ethiodized oil (37% iodine)] 1284 mg/mL (475 mg/mL) ② ethynodiol

ethiofos [now: amifostine]

ethionamide USAN, USP, INN, BAN *bacteriostatic; tuberculosis retreatment* ② ethinamate

ethisterone NF, INN, BAN

Ethmozine film-coated tablets R̥ *antiarrhythmic* [moricizine HCl] 200, 250, 300 mg

ethodryl [see: diethylcarbamazine citrate]

ethoglucid BAN [also: etoglucid]

ethoheptazine BAN [also: ethoheptazine citrate]

ethoheptazine citrate NF, INN [also: ethoheptazine]

ethohexadiol USP

ethomoxane INN, BAN

ethomoxane HCl [see: ethomoxane]

ethonam nitrate USAN *antifungal* [also: etonam]

ethopabate BAN

ethopropazine BAN *anticholinergic; antiparkinsonian* [also: ethopropazine HCl; profenamine]

ethopropazine HCl USP *anticholinergic; antiparkinsonian* [also: profenamine; ethopropazine]

ethosalamide BAN [also: etosalamide]

ethosuximide USAN, USP, INN, BAN *anticonvulsant* 250 mg/5 mL oral

ethotoin USP, INN, BAN *hydantoin anticonvulsant*

ethoxarutine [see: ethoxazorutoside]

ethoxazene HCl USAN *analgesic* [also: etoxazene]

ethoxazorutoside INN

ethoxyacetanilide (*withdrawn from market*) [see: phenacetin]

o-**ethoxybenzamide** [see: ethenzamide; etenzamide]

ethoxzolamide USP

Ethrane liquid for vaporization R̥ *inhalation general anesthetic* [enflurane]

ethybenztropine USAN, BAN *anticholinergic* [also: etybenzatropine]

ethyl acetate NF *solvent*

ethyl alcohol (EtOH; ETOH) [now: alcohol; ethanol]

ethyl aminobenzoate (ethyl *p*-aminobenzoate) JAN *topical anesthetic; nonprescription diet aid* [also: benzocaine]

ethyl 2-benzimidazolecarbamate [see: lobendazole]

ethyl N-benzylcyclopropanecarbamate [see: encyprate]

ethyl biscoumacetate NF, INN, BAN

ethyl biscumacetate [see: ethyl biscoumacetate]

ethyl carbamate [now: urethane]

ethyl carfluzepate INN

ethyl cartrizoate INN

ethyl chloride USP *topical local anesthetic; topical vapo-coolant*

ethyl dibunate USAN, INN, BAN *antitussive*

ethyl dirazepate INN

ethyl ether [see: ether]

ethyl *p*-fluorophenyl sulfone [see: fluoresone]

ethyl *p*-hydroxybenzoate [see: ethylparaben]

ethyl loflazepate INN

ethyl nitrite NF

ethyl oleate NF *vehicle*

ethyl oxide [see: ether]

ethyl vanillin NF *flavoring agent*

ethylcellulose NF *tablet binder*

ethylchlordiphene [see: etofamide]

ethyldicoumarol [see: ethyl biscoumacetate]

ethylene NF *inhalation general anesthesia*

ethylene distearate [see: glycol distearate]

ethylenediamine USP, JAN

ethylenediaminetetraacetate [see: edetate disodium]

ethylenediaminetetraacetic acid (EDTA) [see: edetate disodium]

N,N-ethylenediarsanilic acid [see: difetarsone]

**ethylenedinitrilotetraacetate diso-
dium** [see: edetate disodium]

ethylestrenol USAN, INN *anabolic steroid; also abused as a street drug* [also:
ethyloestrenol; ethylnandrol]

ethylhexanediol [see: ethohexadiol]

2-ethylhexyl diphenyl phosphate
[see: octicizer]

ethylhydrocupreine HCl NF

ethylmethylthiambutene INN, BAN

ethylmorphine BAN [also: ethylmorphine HCl]

ethylmorphine HCl NF [also: ethyl-
morphine]

ethylnandrol JAN *anabolic steroid; also
abused as a street drug* [also: ethylestrenol; ethyloestrenol]

ethylnorepinephrine HCl USP *sympathomimetic bronchodilator*

ethyloestradiol BAN *estrogen* [also:
ethinyl estradiol]

ethyloestrenol BAN *anabolic steroid;
also abused as a street drug* [also: ethylestrenol; ethylnandrol]

ethylpapaverine HCl [see: ethaverine HCl]

ethylparaben NF *antifungal agent*

ethylphenacemide [see: pheneturide]

ethylstibamine [see: stibosamine]

2-ethylthioisonicotinamide [see:
ethionamide]

ethynerone USAN, INN *progestin*

ethynodiol BAN *progestin* [also: ethynodiol diacetate; etynodiol] ⑤
Ethiodol

ethynodiol diacetate USAN, USP *progestin* [also: etynodiol; ethynodiol]

5-ethynyluracil [see: enaluracil]

Ethyol powder for IV infusion ℞
*chemoprotective agent for cisplatin and
paclitaxel chemotherapy (orphan);
radioprotective agent; investigational
(orphan) for cyclophosphamide rescue*
[amifostine] 500 mg/vial

ethypicone INN

ethypropymal sodium [see: probarbital sodium]

etibendazole USAN, INN *anthelmintic*

eticlopride INN

eticyclidine INN

etidocaine USAN, INN, BAN *injectable
local anesthetic*

etidocaine HCl *injectable local anesthetic*

etidronate disodium USAN, USP *bisphosphonate bone resorption inhibitor
for Paget's disease, heterotopic ossification, and hypercalcemia of malignancy
(orphan)*

etidronate monosodium

etidronate sodium *(this term is used
only when the form of sodium cannot
be more accurately identified)*

etidronate tetrasodium

etidronate trisodium

etidronic acid USAN, INN, BAN *calcium
regulator*

etifelmine INN

etifenin USAN, INN, BAN *diagnostic aid*

etifoxin BAN [also: etifoxine]

etifoxine INN [also: etifoxin]

etilamfetamine INN

etilefrine INN

etilefrine pivalate INN

etintidine INN *antagonist to histamine
H_2 receptors* [also: etintidine HCl]

etintidine HCl USAN *antagonist to histamine H_2 receptors* [also: etintidine]

etiocholanedione *investigational
(orphan) for aplastic anemia and
Prader-Willi syndrome*

etipirium iodide INN

etiproston INN

etiracetam INN

etiroxate INN

etisazole INN, BAN

etisomicin INN, BAN

etisulergine INN

etizolam INN

etobedolum [see: etonitazene]

etocarlide INN

etocrilene INN *ultraviolet screen* [also:
etocrylene]

etocrylene USAN *ultraviolet screen*
[also: etocrilene]

etodolac USAN, INN, BAN *antiarthritic;
nonsteroidal anti-inflammatory drug
(NSAID); analgesic* [also: etodolic
acid] 400 mg oral

etodolic acid INN *antiarthritic; nonsteroidal anti-inflammatory drug (NSAID); analgesic* [also: etodolac]

etodroxizine INN

etofamide INN

etofenamate USAN, INN, BAN *analgesic; anti-inflammatory*

etofenprox INN

etofibrate INN

etoformin INN *antidiabetic* [also: etoformin HCl]

etoformin HCl USAN *antidiabetic* [also: etoformin]

etofuradine INN

etofylline INN

etofylline clofibrate INN *antihyperlipoproteinemic* [also: theofibrate]

etoglucid INN [also: ethoglucid]

EtOH; ETOH (ethyl alcohol) [now: alcohol]

etolorex INN

etolotifen INN

etoloxamine INN

etomidate USAN, INN, BAN *rapid-acting nonbarbiturate general anesthetic; hypnotic*

etomidoline INN

etomoxir INN

etonam INN *antifungal* [also: ethonam nitrate]

etonam nitrate [see: ethonam nitrate]

etonitazene INN, BAN

etonogestrel USAN, INN *progestin*

etoperidone INN *antidepressant* [also: etoperidone HCl]

etoperidone HCl USAN *antidepressant* [also: etoperidone]

etophylate [see: acepifylline]

Etopophos powder for IV injection ℞ *antineoplastic for testicular and small cell lung cancers* [etoposide phosphate diethanolate] 119.3 mg/vial

etoposide USAN, INN, BAN *antineoplastic* 20, 30 mg/mL injection

etoposide phosphate USAN *antineoplastic*

etoprindole INN

etoprine USAN *antineoplastic*

etorphine INN, BAN

etosalamide INN [also: ethosalamide]

etoxadrol INN *anesthetic* [also: etoxadrol HCl]

etoxadrol HCl USAN *anesthetic* [also: etoxadrol]

etoxazene INN *analgesic* [also: ethoxazene HCl]

etoxazene HCl [see: ethoxazene HCl]

etoxeridine INN, BAN

etozolin USAN, INN *diuretic*

etrabamine INN

Etrafon; Etrafon 2-10; Etrafon-A; Etrafon-Forte tablets ℞ *conventional (typical) antipsychotic; antidepressant* [perphenazine; amitriptyline HCl] 2•25 mg; 2•10 mg; 4•10 mg; 4•25 mg

etretin [see: acitretin]

etretinate USAN, INN, BAN, JAN *systemic antipsoriatic; retinoic acid analog*

etryptamine INN, BAN *CNS stimulant* [also: etryptamine acetate]

etryptamine acetate USAN *CNS stimulant* [also: etryptamine]

etybenzatropine INN *anticholinergic* [also: ethybenztropine]

etymemazine INN

etymemazine HCl [see: etymemazine]

etynodiol INN *progestin* [also: ethynodiol diacetate; ethynodiol]

etyprenaline [see: isoetharine]

eucaine HCl NF

Eucalyptamint ointment, gel OTC *topical analgesic; counterirritant; antiseptic* [menthol; eucalyptus oil] 16%•⅛; 8%•⅛

eucalyptol USAN *topical bacteriostatic antiseptic/germicidal*

eucalyptus (Eucalyptus globulus) oil *medicinal herb for bronchitis, lung disorders, neuralgia, and skin sores*

eucalyptus oil NF *topical antiseptic*

eucatropine INN, BAN *ophthalmic anticholinergic* [also: eucatropine HCl]

eucatropine HCl USP *ophthalmic anticholinergic* [also: eucatropine]

Eucerin cream, lotion OTC *moisturizer; emollient*

Eucerin OTC *cream base*

Eucerin Plus lotion OTC *moisturizer; emollient* [sodium lactate; urea] 5%• 5%

eucodal [see: oxycodone]

Eudal-SR sustained-release tablets ℞ *decongestant; expectorant* [pseudoephedrine HCl; guaifenesin] 120• 400 mg

euflavine [see: acriflavine]

Euflex Ⓒⓐⓝ (U.S. product: Eulexin) tablets ℞ *antiandrogen antineoplastic adjunct to metastatic prostate cancer* [flutamide] 250 mg

Eugenia caryophyllata medicinal herb [see: cloves]

Eugenia pimenta medicinal herb [see: allspice]

eugenol USP *dental analgesic*

Euglucon Ⓒⓐⓝ (U.S. product: DiaBeta) tablets ℞ *sulfonylurea antidiabetic* [glyburide] 2.5, 5 mg

eukadol [see: oxycodone]

Eulexin capsules ℞ *antiandrogen antineoplastic adjunct to metastatic prostate cancer* [flutamide] 125 mg

Euonymus atropurpureus medicinal herb [see: wahoo]

Eupatorium cannabinum medicinal herb [see: hemp agrimony]

Eupatorium perfoliatum medicinal herb [see: boneset]

Eupatorium purpureum medicinal herb [see: queen of the meadow]

Euphorbia poinsettia; E. pulcherrima medicinal herb [see: poinsettia]

euphoretics; euphoriants; euphoragens *a class of agents that produce euphoria*

Euphrasia officinalis; E. rostkoviana; E. strica medicinal herb [see: eyebright]

euprocin INN *topical anesthetic* [also: euprocin HCl]

euprocin HCl USAN *topical anesthetic* [also: euprocin]

euquinine [see: quinine ethylcarbonate]

Eurax cream, lotion ℞ *scabicide; antipruritic* [crotamiton] 10% ▣ Serax; Urex

European alder; European black alder; European buckthorn *medicinal herb* [see: buckthorn]

European aspen *medicinal herb* [see: black poplar]

europium *element (Eu)*

EVA (etoposide, vinblastine, Adriamycin) *chemotherapy protocol*

Evacet ℞ *investigational (NDA filed) antibiotic antineoplastic for metastatic breast cancer* [doxorubicin, liposomal]

Evac-Q-Kit oral solution + 2 tablets + 2 suppositories OTC *pre-procedure bowel evacuant* [Evac-Q-Mag (q.v.); Evac-Q-Tabs (q.v.); Evac-Q-Sert (q.v.)] ▣ Evac-Q-Kwik

Evac-Q-Kwik suppositories OTC *stimulant laxative* [bisacodyl] 10 mg ▣ Evac-Q-Kit

Evac-Q-Kwik Kit oral solution + 2 tablets + 1 suppository OTC *pre-procedure bowel evacuant* [Evac-Q-Mag (q.v.); Evac-Q-Tabs (q.v.); Evac-Q-Kwik suppository (q.v.)]

Evac-Q-Mag carbonated oral solution OTC *laxative* [magnesium citrate; citric acid; potassium citrate]

Evac-Q-Sert suppositories OTC *laxative* [sodium bicarbonate; potassium bitartrate]

Evac-Q-Tabs tablets OTC *stimulant laxative* [phenolphthalein] 130 mg

Evac-U-Gen chewable tablets (discontinued 1998) OTC *stimulant laxative* [yellow phenolphthalein] 97.2 mg

Evac-U-Lax chewable wafers (discontinued 1998) OTC *stimulant laxative* [phenolphthalein] 80 mg

Evalose syrup ℞ *laxative* [lactulose] 10 g/15 mL

evandamine INN

Evans blue USP *diagnostic aid for blood volume* [also: azovan blue] 5 mL injection

evening primrose (Oenothera biennis) bark, leaves, oil *medicinal herb for cardiovascular health, hypertension, mastalgia, multiple sclerosis, nerves, obesity, premenstrual syndrome, prostate disorders, rheumatoid arthritis, and skin disorders*

everlasting (Anaphalis margaritacea; Gnaphalium polycephalum; G.

uliginosum) plant *medicinal herb used as an astringent, diaphoretic, febrifuge, pectoral, vermifuge, and vulnerary*

Everone 200 IM injection ℞ *androgen replacement for delayed puberty or breast cancer* [testosterone enanthate] 200 mg/mL

E-Vista IM injection (discontinued 1997) ℞ *anxiolytic; minor tranquilizer* [hydroxyzine HCl] 50 mg/mL

Evista film-coated tablets ℞ *selective estrogen receptor modulator (SERM) for the prevention of postmenopausal osteoporosis* [raloxifene HCl] 60 mg ② Avita

E-Vitamin ointment OTC *emollient* [vitamin E] 30 mg/g

E-Vitamin Succinate capsules OTC *vitamin supplement* [vitamin E] 165, 330 mg

E-VMAC (escalated methotrexate, vinblastine, Adriamycin, cisplatin) *chemotherapy protocol*

E-VMAC (escalated methotrexate, vinblastine, Adriamycin, cyclophosphamide) *chemotherapy protocol*

Exact liquid OTC *topical keratolytic cleanser for acne* [salicylic acid] 2%

Exact vanishing cream OTC *topical keratolytic for acne* [benzoyl peroxide] 5%

exalamide INN

exametazime USAN, INN, BAN *regional cerebral perfusion imaging aid*

exaprolol INN *antiadrenergic (β-receptor)* [also: exaprolol HCl]

exaprolol HCl USAN *antiadrenergic (β-receptor)* [also: exaprolol]

Excedrin caplets, tablets, geltabs OTC *analgesic; antipyretic; anti-inflammatory* [acetaminophen; aspirin; caffeine] 250•250•65 mg

Excedrin, Sinus tablets, caplets OTC *decongestant; analgesic; antipyretic* [pseudoephedrine HCl; acetaminophen] 30•500 mg

Excedrin Dual, Aspirin Free film-coated caplets OTC *analgesic; antipyretic; antacid* [acetaminophen; calcium carbonate; magnesium car-

bonate; magnesium oxide] 500• 111•64•30 mg

Excedrin Extra Strength; Aspirin Free Excedrin caplets, geltabs OTC *analgesic; antipyretic* [acetaminophen; caffeine] 500•65 mg

Excedrin IB tablets, caplets (discontinued 1995) OTC *nonsteroidal anti-inflammatory drug (NSAID); antiarthritic; analgesic* [ibuprofen] 200 mg

Excedrin Migraine tablets OTC *analgesic for relief of mild-to-moderate migraine headache pain* [acetaminophen; aspirin; caffeine] 250•250•65 mg

Excedrin P.M. liquid, liquigels OTC *antihistaminic sleep aid; analgesic* [diphenhydramine HCl; acetaminophen] 50• 1000 mg/30 mL; 25•500 mg

Excedrin P.M. tablets, caplets, geltabs OTC *antihistaminic sleep aid; analgesic* [diphenhydramine citrate; acetaminophen] 38•500 mg

Excita Extra premedicated condom OTC *spermicidal/barrier contraceptive* [nonoxynol 9] 8%

Exelderm solution ℞ *topical antifungal* [sulconazole nitrate] 1%

Exelon ℞ *investigational (NDA filed) acetylcholinesterase inhibitor for Alzheimer's disease* [rivastigmine tartrate]

exemestane INN *investigational (orphan) hormonal antineoplastic for metastatic breast cancer*

exepanol INN

Exgest LA long-acting tablets ℞ *decongestant; expectorant* [phenylpropanolamine HCl; guaifenesin] 75•400 mg

Ex-Histine syrup ℞ *decongestant; antihistamine; anticholinergic* [phenylephrine HCl; chlorpheniramine maleate; methscopolamine bromide] 10• 2•1.25 mg

Exidine Skin Cleanser; Exidine-2 Scrub; Exidine-4 Scrub liquid OTC *broad-spectrum antimicrobial; germicidal* [chlorhexidine gluconate; alcohol 4%] 4%; 2%; 4%

exifone INN

exiproben INN

exisulind *investigational (Phase III, orphan) for familial adenomatous polyposis (FAP; also known as adenomatous polyposis coli, or APC); investigational (Phase II/III) for prostate cancer*

Ex-Lax tablets, chocolated chewable tablets OTC *stimulant laxative* [sennosides] 15, 25 mg; 15 mg

Ex-Lax Extra Gentle Pills tablets (discontinued 1997) OTC *stimulant laxative; stool softener* [phenolphthalein; docusate sodium] 65•75 mg

Ex-Lax Gentle Nature tablets (discontinued 1997) OTC *stimulant laxative* [sennosides] 20 mg

Ex-Lax Maximum Relief; Ex-Lax Unflavored tablets (discontinued 1997) OTC *stimulant laxative* [yellow phenolphthalein] 135 mg; 90 mg

Ex-Lax Stool Softener caplets OTC *stool softener* [docusate sodium] 100 mg

Exna tablets ℞ *diuretic; antihypertensive* [benzthiazide] 50 mg

Exocaine Medicated Rub; Exocaine Plus Rub OTC *counterirritant* [methyl salicylate] 25%; 30%

Exosurf ℞ *investigational (orphan) for adult respiratory distress syndrome (ARDS)* [colfosceril palmitate]

Exosurf Neonatal powder for injection, intratracheal suspension ℞ *pulmonary surfactant for hyaline membrane disease and respiratory distress syndrome (orphan)* [colfosceril palmitate] 108 mg

expectorants *a class of drugs that promote the ejection of mucus from the respiratory tract*

Expidet (trademarked dosage form) *fast-dissolving dose*

Exsel lotion/shampoo ℞ *antiseborrheic; antifungal* [selenium sulfide] 2.5%

exsiccated sodium arsenate [see: sodium arsenate, exsiccated]

Extencap (trademarked dosage form) *extended-release capsule*

extended insulin zinc [see: insulin zinc, extended]

Extendryl chewable tablets, syrup ℞ *decongestant; antihistamine; anticholin-*ergic [phenylephrine HCl; chlorpheniramine maleate; methscopolamine nitrate] 10•2•1.25 mg; 10•2•1.25 mg/5 mL

Extendryl JR sustained-release capsules ℞ *pediatric decongestant, antihistamine, and anticholinergic* [phenylephrine HCl; chlorpheniramine maleate; methscopolamine nitrate] 10•4•1.25 mg

Extendryl SR sustained-release capsules ℞ *decongestant; antihistamine; anticholinergic* [phenylephrine HCl; chlorpheniramine maleate; methscopolamine nitrate] 20•8•2.5 mg

Extentab (trademarked dosage form) *extended-release tablet*

Extra Action Cough syrup OTC *antitussive; expectorant* [dextromethorphan hydrobromide; guaifenesin; alcohol 1.4%] 10•100 mg/5 mL

"Extra Strength" products [see under product name]

Extraneal Peritoneal Dialysis Solution ℞ *investigational (orphan) for end-stage renal disease* [icodextrin] 7.5%

eye balm; eye root *medicinal herb* [see: goldenseal]

Eye Drops OTC *topical ophthalmic decongestant and vasoconstrictor* [tetrahydrozoline HCl] 0.05%

Eye Irrigating Solution OTC *extraocular irrigating solution* [sterile isotonic solution]

Eye Irrigating Wash OTC *extraocular irrigating solution* [sterile isotonic solution]

Eye Scrub solution OTC *eyelid cleanser for blepharitis or contact lenses*

Eye Stream ophthalmic solution OTC *extraocular irrigating solution* [sterile isotonic solution]

Eye Wash ophthalmic solution OTC *extraocular irrigating solution* [sterile isotonic solution]

eyebright (*Euphrasia officinalis; E. rostkoviana; E. strica*) *plant medicinal herb for blood cleansing, cataracts, colds, conjunctivitis, eye disorders and infections, and stimulating liver func-*

tion; *not generally regarded as safe and effective for topical ophthalmic use*

Eye-Lube-A eye drops OTC *ophthalmic moisturizer/lubricant* [glycerin] 0.25%

Eye-Sed eye drops OTC *ophthalmic astringent* [zinc sulfate] 0.25%

Eyesine eye drops OTC *topical ophthalmic decongestant and vasoconstrictor* [tetrahydrozoline HCl] 0.05%

EZ Detect test kit for home use OTC *in vitro diagnostic aid for fecal occult blood*

EZ Detect test kit for home use (discontinued 1995) OTC *in vitro diagnostic aid for urine occult blood*

EZ Detect Strep-A swab test for professional use (discontinued 1995) *in vitro diagnostic aid for streptococci*

Ezide tablets ℞ *antihypertensive; diuretic* [hydrochlorothiazide] 50 mg

1+1-F Creme ℞ *topical corticosteroidal anti-inflammatory; antifungal; antibacterial; local anesthetic* [hydrocortisone; clioquinol; pramoxine] 1%•3%•1%

¹⁸F [see: fludeoxyglucose F 18]

¹⁸F [see: sodium fluoride F 18]

FABRase ℞ *investigational (orphan) enzyme replacement therapy for Fabry's disease* [alpha-galactosidase A]

FAC (fluorouracil, Adriamycin, cyclophosphamide) *chemotherapy protocol*

FAC-LEV (fluorouracil, Adriamycin, Cytoxin, levamisole) *chemotherapy protocol*

FAC-M (fluorouracil, Adriamycin, cyclophosphamide, methotrexate) *chemotherapy protocol*

Fact Plus test kit for home use OTC *in vitro diagnostic aid for urine pregnancy test*

factor II (prothrombin)

factor III [see: thromboplastin]

factor VIIa, recombinant *coagulant for hemophilia A and B (orphan); investigational (orphan) for von Willebrand's disease*

factor VIII [see: antihemophilic factor]

factor VIII (rDNA) BAN *blood coagulating factor*

factor VIII fraction BAN *blood coagulating factor*

factor VIII SQ, recombinant *investigational (orphan) for long-term hemophilia A treatment or for surgical procedures*

factor IX complex USP *systemic hemostatic; antihemophilic for hemophilia B (orphan)* [also: factor IX fraction]

factor IX fraction BAN *systemic hemostatic; antihemophilic* [also: factor IX complex]

factor XIII, plasma-derived *investigational (orphan) for congenital factor XIII deficiency*

factor XIII, recombinant *orphan status withdrawn 1996*

Factrel powder for subcu or IV injection ℞ *gonadotropin releasing hormone* [gonadorelin HCl] 100, 500 μg

fadrozole INN *antineoplastic; aromatase inhibitor* [also: fadrozole HCl]

fadrozole HCl USAN *antineoplastic; aromatase inhibitor* [also: fadrozole]

falintolol INN

falipamil INN

false foxglove *medicinal herb* [see: feverweed]

false unicorn (Chamaelirium luteum) root *medicinal herb used for amenorrhea, morning sickness, and preventing miscarriages; also used for colic, cough, and digestive, kidney, and prostate problems; emetic in high doses*

false valerian *medicinal herb* [see: life root]

false vervain *medicinal herb* [see: blue vervain]

FAM (fluorouracil, Adriamycin, mitomycin) *chemotherapy protocol*

FAM-CF (fluorouracil, Adriamycin, mitomycin, citrovorum factor) *chemotherapy protocol*

famciclovir USAN, INN, BAN *antiviral for herpes simplex and zoster*

FAME; FAMe (fluorouracil, Adriamycin, MeCCNU) *chemotherapy protocol*

Family Tabs tablets (discontinued 1995) OTC *vitamin supplement* [multiple vitamins; folic acid] $\pm \bullet 0.4$ mg

Familytabs with Calcium, Iron & Zinc tablets (discontinued 1995) OTC *vitamin/mineral supplement* [multiple vitamins; calcium carbonate; ferrous fumarate; zinc oxide]

Familytabs with Iron tablets (discontinued 1995) OTC *vitamin/iron supplement* [multiple vitamins; iron]

famiraprinium chloride INN

FAMMe (fluorouracil, Adriamycin, mitomycin, MeCCNU) *chemotherapy protocol*

famotidine USAN, USP, INN, BAN *histamine H_2 antagonist for gastric ulcers*

famotine INN *antiviral* [also: famotine HCl]

famotine HCl USAN *antiviral* [also: famotine]

fampridine USAN, INN *investigational (orphan) for multiple sclerosis and spinal cord injury*

famprofazone INN, BAN

FAM-S (fluorouracil, Adriamycin, mitomycin, streptozocin) *chemotherapy protocol*

FAMTX (fluorouracil, Adriamycin, methotrexate [with leucovorin rescue]) *chemotherapy protocol*

Famvir film-coated tablets R̸ *antiviral for acute herpes zoster and genital herpes infections and suppression of recurrent episodes* [famciclovir] 125, 250, 500 mg

fananserin USAN *antipsychotic; antischizophrenic; dopamine D_2 and serotonin $5\text{-}HT_2$ receptor antagonist*

fanetizole INN, BAN *immunoregulator* [also: fanetizole mesylate]

fanetizole mesylate USAN *immunoregulator* [also: fanetizole]

Fansidar tablets R̸ *antimalarial* [sulfadoxine; pyrimethamine] $500 \bullet 25$ mg

fanthridone BAN *antidepressant* [also: fantridone HCl; fantridone]

fantridone INN *antidepressant* [also: fantridone HCl; fanthridone]

fantridone HCl USAN *antidepressant* [also: fantridone; fanthridone]

FAP (fluorouracil, Adriamycin, Platinol) *chemotherapy protocol*

Farbee with Vitamin C caplets OTC *vitamin supplement* [multiple B vitamins; vitamin C] $\pm \bullet 300$ mg

Fareston tablets R̸ *antiestrogen antineoplastic for estrogen-receptive metastatic breast cancer in postmenopausal women (orphan); investigational (orphan) for desmoid tumors* [toremifene citrate] 60 mg

farnesil INN *combining name for radicals or groups*

fasiplon INN

Faspak (trademarked form) *flexible plastic bag*

Fastin capsules R̸ *anorexiant; CNS stimulant* [phentermine HCl] 30 mg

Fast-Trak (trademarked delivery system) *quick-loading syringe*

fat, hard NF *suppository base*

fat emulsion, intravenous *parenteral essential fatty acid replacement*

Father John's Medicine Plus liquid OTC *antitussive; decongestant; antihistamine; expectorant* [dextromethorphan hydrobromide; phenylephrine HCl; chlorpheniramine maleate; guaifenesin; ammonium chloride] $7.5 \bullet 2.5 \bullet 1 \bullet 30 \bullet 83.3$ mg/5 mL

Fatsia horrida medicinal herb [see: devil's club]

fazadinium bromide INN, BAN

fazarabine USAN, INN *antineoplastic*

5-FC (5-fluorocytosine) [see: flucytosine]

FCAP (fluorouracil, cyclophosphamide, Adriamycin, Platinol) *chemotherapy protocol*

FCE (fluorouracil, cisplatin, etoposide) *chemotherapy protocol*

F-CL (fluorouracil, leucovorin calcium [rescue]) *chemotherapy protocol* [also: FU/LV]

FCP (fluorouracil, cyclophosphamide, prednisone) *chemotherapy protocol*

FD&C Red No. 2 (Food, Drug & Cosmetic Act) [see: amaranth]

FD&C Red No. 3 (Food, Drug & Cosmetic Act) [see: erythrosine sodium]

F-ddA (fluorodideoxyadenosine) [see: lodenosine]

^{18}FDG (fludeoxyglucose) [see: fludeoxyglucose F 18]

FDP (fructose-1,6-diphosphate) [q.v.]

Fe^{50} (or Fe50) extended-release caplets OTC *hematinic* [ferrous sulfate, dried (source of iron)] 160 mg (50 mg)

^{59}Fe [see: ferric chloride Fe 59]

^{59}Fe [see: ferric citrate (^{59}Fe)]

^{59}Fe [see: ferrous citrate Fe 59]

^{59}Fe [see: ferrous sulfate Fe 59]

febantel USAN, INN, BAN *veterinary anthelmintic*

febarbamate INN

febricides *a class of agents that relieve or reduce fever* [also called: antifebriles; antipyretics; antithermics; febrifuges]

febrifuges *a class of agents that relieve or reduce fever* [also called: antifebriles; antipyretics; antithermics; febricides]

febuprol INN

febuverine INN

FEC (fluorouracil, epirubicin, cyclophosphamide) *chemotherapy protocol*

feclemine INN

feclobuzone INN

FED (fluorouracil, etoposide, DDP) *chemotherapy protocol*

Fedahist tablets OTC *decongestant; antihistamine* [pseudoephedrine HCl; chlorpheniramine maleate] 60•4 mg

Fedahist Timecaps (timed-release capsules), Gyrocaps (extended-release capsules) R *decongestant; antihistamine* [pseudoephedrine HCl; chlorpheniramine maleate] 120•8 mg; 65•10 mg

Fedahist Expectorant pediatric drops (discontinued 1995) OTC *decongestant; expectorant* [pseudoephedrine HCl; guaifenesin] 7.5•40 mg/mL

Fedahist Expectorant syrup (discontinued 1998) OTC *decongestant; expectorant* [pseudoephedrine HCl; guaifenesin] 20•200 mg/5 mL

fedotozine INN *investigational kappa selective opioid agonist for irritable bowel syndrome*

fedrilate INN

Feen-A-Mint chewable tablets, gum (discontinued 1997) OTC *stimulant laxative* [yellow phenolphthalein] 97.2 mg

Feen-A-Mint chocolated chewable tablets (discontinued 1997) OTC *stimulant laxative* [yellow phenolphthalein] 65 mg

Feen-A-Mint tablets OTC *stimulant laxative* [bisacodyl] 5 mg

Feen-A-Mint Pills tablets OTC *stimulant laxative; stool softener* [phenolphthalein; docusate sodium] 65•100 mg

Feiba VH Immuno IV injection or drip R *antihemophilic to correct factor VIII deficiency and coagulation deficiency* [anti-inhibitor coagulant complex, vapor heated and freeze-dried] (each bottle is labeled with dosage)

felbamate USAN, INN *anticonvulsant; adjunctive therapy for Lennox-Gastaut syndrome (orphan)*

Felbatol tablets, oral suspension (the FDA and the manufacturer strongly caution against its use due to adverse side effects) R *anticonvulsant; adjunctive therapy for Lennox-Gastaut syndrome (orphan)* [felbamate] 400, 600 mg; 600 mg/5 mL

felbinac USAN, INN, BAN *anti-inflammatory*

Feldene capsules ℞ *nonsteroidal antiinflammatory drug (NSAID); antiarthritic* [piroxicam] 10, 20 mg

felipyrine INN

felodipine USAN, INN, BAN *vasodilator; antihypertensive; calcium channel blocker*

felonwood; felonwort *medicinal herb* [see: bittersweet nightshade]

felvizumab USAN *monoclonal antibody for prophylaxis and treatment of respiratory syncytial virus (RSV)*

felypressin USAN, INN, BAN *vasoconstrictor*

Fem-1 tablets OTC *analgesic; antiinflammatory; diuretic* [acetaminophen; pamabrom] 500•25 mg

female fern *(Polypodium vulgare)* root *medicinal herb used as an anthelmintic, cholagogue, demulcent, and purgative*

female regulator *medicinal herb* [see: life root]

Femara film-coated tablets ℞ *hormonal antineoplastic/aromatase inhibitor for advanced breast cancer in postmenopausal women* [letrozole] 2.5 mg

FemCal tablets OTC *calcium supplement* [calcium carbonate; vitamin D; multiple minerals] 250 mg•100 IU• ±

FemCare vaginal cream, tablets (discontinued 1996) OTC *antifungal* [clotrimazole] 1%; 100 mg

Femcet capsules ℞ *analgesic; sedative* [acetaminophen; caffeine; butalbital] 325•40•50 mg

Fem-Etts tablets (discontinued 1997) OTC *analgesic; anti-inflammatory; diuretic* [acetaminophen; pamabrom] 325•25 mg

Femicine vaginal suppositories (discontinued 1998) OTC *for vaginal irritations, itching, and burning* [pulsatilla 28x]

Femidine Douche solution (discontinued 1995) OTC *antiseptic/germicidal; vaginal cleanser and deodorizer* [povidone-iodine]

Femilax tablets OTC *stimulant laxative; stool softener* [phenolphthalein; docusate sodium] 65•100 mg

Feminique Disposable Douche solution OTC *antiseptic; antifungal; vaginal cleanser and deodorizer; acidity modifier* [sodium benzoate; sorbic acid; lactic acid]

Feminique Disposable Douche solution OTC *vaginal cleanser and deodorizer; acidity modifier* [vinegar (acetic acid)]

Femiron tablets OTC *hematinic* [ferrous fumarate (source of iron)] 63 mg (20 mg) ⟲ Remeron

Femiron Multi-Vitamins and Iron tablets OTC *vitamin/iron supplement* [multiple vitamins; ferrous fumarate; folic acid] ±•20•0.4 mg

Femizol-M vaginal cream OTC *antifungal* [miconazole nitrate] 2%

femoxetine INN

FemPatch transdermal patch ℞ *estrogen replacement therapy for postmenopausal disorders* [estradiol] 25 μg/day

Femstat vaginal cream (discontinued 1995) ℞ *antifungal* [butoconazole nitrate] 2%

Femstat 3; FemStat One vaginal cream in prefilled applicator OTC *antifungal* [butoconazole nitrate] 2%

fenabutene INN

fenacetinol INN

fenaclon INN

fenadiazole INN

fenaftic acid INN

fenalamide USAN, INN *smooth muscle relaxant*

fenalcomine INN

fenamifuril INN

fenamisal INN *antibacterial; tuberculostatic* [also: phenyl aminosalicylate]

fenamole USAN, INN *anti-inflammatory*

fenaperone INN

fenarsone [see: carbarsone]

fenasprate [see: benorilate]

fenbendazole USAN, INN, BAN *anthelmintic*

fenbenicillin INN [also: phenbenicillin]

fenbufen USAN, INN, BAN *anti-inflammatory*

fenbutrazate INN [also: phenbutrazate]

fencamfamin INN, BAN

fencamfamin HCl [see: fencamfamin]

fencarbamide INN *anticholinergic* [also: phencarbamide]

fenchlorphos BAN *systemic insecticide* [also: ronnel; fenclofos]

fencilbutirol USAN, INN *choleretic*

fenclexonium metilsulfate INN

fenclofenac USAN, INN, BAN *anti-inflammatory*

fenclofos INN *systemic insecticide* [also: ronnel; fenchlorphos]

fenclonine USAN, INN *serotonin inhibitor*

fenclorac USAN, INN *anti-inflammatory*

fenclozic acid INN, BAN

fendiline INN

fendizoate INN *combining name for radicals or groups*

fendosal USAN, INN, BAN *anti-inflammatory*

feneritrol INN

Fenesin sustained-release tablets ℞ *expectorant* [guaifenesin] 600 mg

Fenesin DM tablets ℞ *antitussive; expectorant* [dextromethorphan hydrobromide; guaifenesin] 30•600 mg

fenestrel USAN, INN *estrogen*

fenethazine INN

fenethylline BAN *CNS stimulant* [also: fenethylline HCl; fenetylline]

fenethylline HCl USAN *CNS stimulant* [also: fenetylline; fenethylline]

fenetradil INN

fenetylline INN *CNS stimulant* [also: fenethylline HCl; fenethylline]

fenflumizole INN

fenfluramine INN, BAN *anorexiant; CNS depressant* [also: fenfluramine HCl]

fenfluramine HCl USAN *anorexiant; CNS depressant* [also: fenfluramine]

fenfluthrin INN, BAN

fengabine USAN, INN, BAN *mood regulator*

fenharmane INN

fenimide USAN, INN, BAN *antipsychotic*

feniodium chloride INN

fenipentol INN

fenirofibrate INN

fenisorex USAN, INN, BAN *anorectic*

fenleuton USAN *5-lipoxygenase inhibitor*

fenmetozole INN *antidepressant; narcotic antagonist* [also: fenmetozole HCl]

fenmetozole HCl USAN *antidepressant; narcotic antagonist* [also: fenmetozole]

fenmetramide USAN, INN, BAN *antidepressant*

fennel (Anethum foeniculum; Foeniculum officinale; F. vulgare) seeds *medicinal herb for colic, gas, intestinal problems, promoting expectoration, stimulating lactation and menses, and sedation in children*

fennel oil NF

fenobam USAN, INN *sedative*

fenocinol INN

fenoctimine INN *gastric antisecretory* [also: fenoctimine sulfate]

fenoctimine sulfate USAN *gastric antisecretory* [also: fenoctimine]

fenofibrate INN, BAN *antihyperlipidemic for hypertriglyceridemia*

fenoldopam INN, BAN *vasodilator for hypertensive emergencies; dopamine agonist* [also: fenoldopam mesylate]

fenoldopam mesylate USAN *vasodilator for hypertensive emergencies; dopamine agonist* [also: fenoldopam]

fenoprofen USAN, INN, BAN *nonsteroidal anti-inflammatory drug (NSAID); analgesic*

fenoprofen calcium USAN, USP, BAN *antiarthritic; nonsteroidal anti-inflammatory drug (NSAID); analgesic* 200, 300, 600 mg oral

fenoterol USAN, INN, BAN *bronchodilator* [also: fenoterol hydrobromide]

fenoterol hydrobromide JAN *bronchodilator* [also: fenoterol]

fenoverine INN

fenoxazol [see: pemoline]

fenoxazoline INN

fenoxazoline HCl [see: fenoxazoline]

fenoxedil INN

fenoxypropazine INN [also: phenoxypropazine]

fenozolone INN

fenpentadiol INN

fenperate INN

fenpipalone USAN, INN *anti-inflammatory*

fenpipramide INN, BAN

fenpiprane INN, BAN

fenpiprane HCl [see: fenpiprane]

fenpiverinium bromide INN

fenprinast INN *bronchodilator; antiallergic* [also: fenprinast HCl]

fenprinast HCl USAN *bronchodilator; antiallergic* [also: fenprinast]

fenproporex INN

fenprostalene USAN, INN, BAN *luteolysin*

fenquizone USAN, INN *diuretic*

fenretinide USAN, INN *investigational (Phase III) retinoid cancer chemopreventative*

fenspiride INN *bronchodilator; antiadrenergic (α-receptor)* [also: fenspiride HCl]

fenspiride HCl USAN *bronchodilator; antiadrenergic (α-receptor)* [also: fenspiride]

fentanyl INN, BAN *narcotic analgesic; also abused as a street drug* [also: fentanyl citrate] ☒ Sentinel

fentanyl citrate USAN, USP, JAN *narcotic analgesic; also abused as a street drug* [also: fentanyl] 0.05 mg/mL injection

Fentanyl Oralet lozenges ℞ *oral transmucosal narcotic analgesic for anesthesia premedication* [fentanyl citrate] 100, 200, 300, 400 μg

fenthion BAN

fentiazac USAN, INN, BAN *anti-inflammatory*

fenticlor USAN, INN, BAN *topical anti-infective*

fenticonazole INN, BAN *antifungal* [also: fenticonazole nitrate]

fenticonazole nitrate USAN *antifungal* [also: fenticonazole]

fentonium bromide INN

fenugreek (Trigonella foenum-graecum) seeds *medicinal herb for boils, bronchial secretions, cellulitis, diabetes, hypercholesterolemia, kidney stones, lung infections, promoting expectoration, stomach irritation, and tuberculosis*

fenyramidol INN *analgesic; skeletal muscle relaxant* [also: phenyramidol HCl]

fenyripol INN *skeletal muscle relaxant* [also: fenyripol HCl]

fenyripol HCl USAN *skeletal muscle relaxant* [also: fenyripol]

Feocyte prolonged-action tablets ℞ *hematinic* [ferrous fumarate; ferrous gluconate; ferrous sulfate; liver, desiccated; vitamins B_6, B_{12}, and C; folic acid] 110 mg (total iron)•15 mg•2 mg•50 μg•100 mg•0.8 mg

Fe-O.D. timed-release tablets (discontinued 1998) OTC *hematinic* [ferrous fumarate; ascorbic acid] 100•500 mg

Feosol caplets OTC *hematinic* [carbonyl iron] 50 mg

Feosol elixir OTC *hematinic* [ferrous sulfate (source of iron)] 220 mg/5 mL (44 mg/5 mL) ☒ Feostat; Fer-In-Sol; Festal

Feosol tablets OTC *hematinic* [ferrous sulfate, dried (source of iron)] 200 mg (65 mg)

Feosol timed-release capsules (discontinued 1998) OTC *hematinic* [ferrous sulfate, dried (source of iron)] 159 mg (50 mg)

Feostat chewable tablets, suspension, drops OTC *hematinic* [ferrous fumarate (source of iron)] 100 mg (33 mg); 100 mg/5 mL (33 mg/5 mL); 45 mg/0.6 mL (15 mg/0.6 mL) ☒ Feosol

fepentolic acid INN

fepitrizol INN

fepradinol INN

feprazone INN, BAN

fepromide INN

feprosidnine INN

Ferancee chewable tablets (discontinued 1998) OTC *hematinic* [ferrous fumarate; ascorbic acid] 67•150 mg

Ferancee-HP film-coated tablets (discontinued 1998) OTC *hematinic* [ferrous fumarate; ascorbic acid] 110•600 mg

Feratab tablets OTC *hematinic* [ferrous sulfate, dried (source of iron)] 187 mg (60 mg)

Fer-gen-sol drops OTC *hematinic* [ferrous sulfate (source of iron)] 75 mg/0.6 mL (15 mg/0.6 mL)

Fergon elixir (discontinued 1998) OTC *hematinic* [ferrous gluconate (source of iron)] 300 mg/5 mL (34 mg/5 mL)

Fergon tablets OTC *hematinic* [ferrous gluconate (source of iron)] 240 mg (27 mg)

Fergon Plus caplets (discontinued 1995) ℞ *hematinic* [ferrous gluconate; vitamin B$_{12}$; intrinsic factor concentrate; ascorbic acid] 58 mg• 0.5 U•75 mg

Feridex IV injection ℞ *contrast agent for MRI of the liver* [ferumoxides] (11.2 mg iron)

Fer-In-Sol capsules (discontinued 1997) OTC *hematinic* [ferrous sulfate, dried (source of iron)] 190 mg (60 mg) ▣ Feosol

Fer-In-Sol drops, syrup OTC *hematinic* [ferrous sulfate (source of iron)] 75 mg/0.6 mL (15 mg/0.6 mL); 90 mg/5 mL (18 mg/5 mL)

Fer-Iron drops OTC *hematinic* [ferrous sulfate (source of iron)] 75 mg/0.6 mL (15 mg/0.6 mL)

fermium *element (Fm)*

fern; fern brake *medicinal herb* [see: buckhorn brake; female fern]

fern, flowering; king's fern; water fern *medicinal herb* [see: buckhorn brake]

fern-leaved foxglove *medicinal herb* [see: feverweed]

Ferocyl sustained-release tablets (discontinued 1998) OTC *hematinic* [ferrous fumarate; docusate sodium] 150•100 mg

Fero-Folic-500 controlled-release Filmtabs (film-coated tablets) ℞ *hematinic* [ferrous sulfate; ascorbic acid; folic acid] 105•500•0.8 mg

Fero-Grad-500 controlled-release Filmtabs (film-coated tablets) OTC *hematinic* [iron (from ferrous sulfate); sodium ascorbate] 105•500 mg

Fero-Gradumet timed-release Filmtabs (film-coated tablets) (discontinued 1998) OTC *hematinic* [ferrous sulfate (source of iron)] 525 mg (105 mg)

Ferospace capsules (discontinued 1998) OTC *hematinic* [ferrous sulfate (source of iron)] 250 mg (50 mg)

Ferotrinsic capsules ℞ *hematinic* [ferrous fumarate; cyanocobalamin; ascorbic acid; intrinsic factor concentrate; folic acid] 110 mg•15 μg• 75 mg•240 mg•0.5 mg

Ferralet tablets (discontinued 1998) OTC *hematinic* [ferrous gluconate (source of iron)] 320 mg (37 mg)

Ferralet Plus tablets OTC *hematinic* [ferrous gluconate; cyanocobalamin; ascorbic acid; folic acid] 46 mg•25 μg•400 mg•0.8 mg

Ferralet S.R. sustained-release tablets (discontinued 1998) OTC *hematinic* [ferrous gluconate (source of iron)] 320 mg (37 mg)

Ferralyn Lanacaps (timed-release capsules) (discontinued 1998) OTC *hematinic* [ferrous sulfate, dried (source of iron)] 250 mg (50 mg)

Ferra-TD timed-release capsules (discontinued 1998) OTC *hematinic* [ferrous sulfate, dried (source of iron)] 250 mg (50 mg)

Ferretts tablets (discontinued 1997) OTC *hematinic* [ferrous fumarate] 325 mg

ferric ammonium citrate NF

ferric ammonium sulfate

ferric cacodylate NF

ferric chloride

ferric chloride Fe 59 USAN *radioactive agent*

ferric citrate (^{59}Fe) INN

ferric citrochloride NF

ferric fructose USAN, INN *hematinic*

ferric glycerophosphate NF

ferric hypophosphite NF

ferric oxide NF *coloring agent*

ferric oxide, red NF

ferric oxide, yellow NF

ferric pyrophosphate, soluble NF

ferric subsulfate NF

ferricholinate [see: ferrocholinate]

ferriclate calcium sodium USAN *hematinic* [also: calcium sodium ferriclate]

ferristene USAN *paramagnetic imaging agent for MRI*

Ferrlecit IV infusion ℞ *hematinic for iron deficiency of chronic hemodialysis with erythropoietin therapy* [sodium ferric gluconate] 62.5 mg/5 mL

Ferro Dok TR timed-release capsules (discontinued 1998) OTC *hematinic* [ferrous fumarate; docusate sodium] 150•100 mg

ferrocholate [see: ferrocholinate]

ferrocholinate INN

Ferro-Docusate T.R. timed-release capsules (discontinued 1998) OTC *hematinic* [ferrous fumarate; docusate sodium] 150•100 mg

Ferro-DSS S.R. timed-release capsules (discontinued 1998) OTC *hematinic* [ferrous fumarate; docusate sodium] 150•100 mg

Ferromar sustained-release caplets OTC *hematinic* [ferrous fumarate; vitamin C] 201.5•200 mg

ferropolimaler INN

Ferro-Sequels timed-release tablets OTC *hematinic* [ferrous fumarate; docusate sodium] 50• ⚥ mg

ferrotrenine INN

ferrous citrate Fe 59 USAN, USP *radioactive agent*

ferrous fumarate USP *hematinic (33% elemental iron)* 200, 325 mg oral

ferrous gluconate USP *hematinic (11.6% elemental iron)* 325 mg oral

ferrous lactate NF

ferrous orotate JAN

ferrous sulfate USP, JAN *hematinic (20% elemental iron)* 250, 325 mg oral; 220 mg/5 mL oral; 75 mg/0.6 mL oral

ferrous sulfate, dried USP *hematinic (30% elemental iron)*

ferrous sulfate, exsiccated [see: ferrous sulfate, dried]

ferrous sulfate Fe 59 USAN *radioactive agent*

Fertinex subcu injection ℞ *follicle-stimulating hormone (FSH); ovulation stimulant for polycystic ovary disease (orphan) and assisted reproductive technologies (ART); investigational*

(orphan) for spermatogenesis in hormone-deficient males [urofollitropin] 75, 150 IU

fertirelin INN, BAN *veterinary gonadotropin-releasing hormone* [also: fertirelin acetate]

fertirelin acetate USAN *veterinary gonadotropin-releasing hormone* [also: fertirelin]

ferucarbotran USAN *superparamagnetic diagnostic aid*

Ferula assafoetida; F. foetida; F. rubricaulis medicinal herb [see: asafetida; asafoetida]

ferumoxides USAN *diagnostic aid for magnetic resonance imaging of the liver*

ferumoxsil USAN *oral MRI contrast medium for upper GI tract imaging*

ferumoxtran-10 USAN *superparamagnetic diagnostic aid*

Fetal Fibronectin Test kit for professional use *in vitro diagnostic aid for fetal fibronectin in vaginal secretions at 24–34 weeks, a predictor of preterm delivery*

fetal neural cells [see: neural cells, porcine fetal]

fetid hellebore (*Helleborus foetidus*) [see: hellebore]

fetid hellebore (*Helleborus foetidus*) [see: hellebore]

fetoxilate INN *smooth muscle relaxant* [also: fetoxylate HCl; fetoxylate]

fetoxylate BAN *smooth muscle relaxant* [also: fetoxylate HCl; fetoxilate]

fetoxylate HCl USAN *smooth muscle relaxant* [also: fetoxilate; fetoxylate]

fever root *medicinal herb* [see: coral root]

fever twig *medicinal herb* [see: bittersweet nightshade]

Feverall, Children's; Infant's Feverall; Junior Feverall suppositories OTC *analgesic; antipyretic* [acetaminophen] 120 mg; 80 mg; 325 mg

Feverall, Children's; Junior Feverall Sprinkle Caps (powder) OTC *analgesic; antipyretic* [acetaminophen] 80 mg; 160 mg ② Fiberall

feverbush *medicinal herb* [see: winterberry]

feverfew (*Chrysanthemum parthenium; Leucanthemum parthenium; Pyrethrum parthenium; Tanacetum parthenium*) leaves and flowers *medicinal herb used as an aspirin substitute for chills, colds, fever, inflammation, and migraine and sinus headache*

feverweed (*Gerardia pedicularia*) plant *medicinal herb used as an antiseptic, diaphoretic, febrifuge, and sedative*

fexicaine INN, DCF

Fexicam ⓒ suppositories ℞ *nonsteroidal anti-inflammatory drug (NSAID) for rheumatoid arthritis, osteoarthritis, ankylosing spondylitis, and primary dysmenorrhea* [piroxicam] 20 mg

fexinidazole INN

fexofenadine HCl USAN *second-generation piperidine antihistamine*

fezatione INN

fezolamine INN *antidepressant* [also: fezolamine fumarate]

fezolamine fumarate USAN *antidepressant* [also: fezolamine]

FGN-1 *investigational (Phase III, orphan) for familial adenomatous polyposis (FAP; also known as adenomatous polyposis coli, or APC)* [now: exisulind]

fiacitabine (FIAC) USAN, INN *antiviral; investigational (Phase I/II) for HIV and AIDS*

fialuridine (FIAU) USAN, INN *antiviral; investigational (Phase II) for HIV; investigational (orphan) for chronic active hepatitis B*

Fiberall chewable tablets OTC *bulk laxative; antidiarrheal* [calcium polycarbophil] 1250 mg ⓓ Feverall

Fiberall powder, wafers OTC *bulk laxative* [psyllium hydrophilic mucilloid] 3.4 g/tsp.; 3.4 g

FiberCon film-coated tablets OTC *bulk laxative; antidiarrheal* [calcium polycarbophil] 500 mg

Fiberlan liquid OTC *enteral nutritional therapy* [lactose-free formula]

Fiber-Lax tablets OTC *bulk laxative; antidiarrheal* [calcium polycarbophil] 625 mg

FiberNorm tablets OTC *bulk laxative; antidiarrheal* [calcium polycarbophil] 625 mg

Fiblast ℞ *investigational (Phase II/III) basic fibroblast growth factor (bFGF) for stroke and coronary artery disease* [trafermin]

fibracillin INN

Fibrad powder (discontinued 1997) OTC *oral dietary fiber supplement* [pea, oat and sugar beet fiber] 7 g total fiber per serving

fibrin INN

fibrinase [see: factor XIII]

fibrinogen (^{125}I) INN [also: fibrinogen I 125]

fibrinogen, human USP *investigational (orphan) to control bleeding in fibrinogen-deficient patients*

fibrinogen I 125 USAN *vascular patency test; radioactive agent* [also: fibrinogen (^{125}I)]

fibrinoligase [see: factor XIII]

fibrinolysin, human INN [also: plasmin]

fibrinolysin & desoxyribonuclease *topical enzymes for necrotic tissue debridement*

fibrin-stabilizing factor (FSF) [see: factor XIII]

fibroblast growth factor, basic (bFGF) [see: ersofermin]

fibroblast interferon [now: interferon beta]

Fibrogammin P ℞ *investigational (orphan) for congenital factor XIII deficiency* [factor XIII, plasma-derived]

fibronectin *investigational (orphan) for nonhealing corneal ulcers or epithelial defects*

Ficus carica medicinal herb [see: fig]

50% Dextrose with Electrolyte Pattern A (or N) IV infusion ℞ *intravenous nutritional/electrolyte therapy* [combined electrolyte solution; dextrose]

fig (*Ficus carica*) fruit *medicinal herb used as a demulcent, emollient, and laxative*

figwort (*Scrophularia nodosa*) leaves, stems, and roots *medicinal herb for* *abrasions, athlete's foot, cradle cap, fever, impetigo, restlessness, skin diseases, and skin tumors*

filaminast USAN *selective phosphodiesterase IV inhibitor for asthma*

filenadol INN

filgrastim USAN, INN, BAN *hematopoietic stimulant for severe chronic neutropenia (orphan); investigational (Phase III, orphan) cytokine for CMV retinitis of AIDS*

filgrastim & methionyl stem cell factor, recombinant human *investigational adjunct to myelosuppressive or myeloablative therapy; orphan status withdrawn 1998*

Filibon tablets (discontinued 1995) OTC *vitamin/calcium/iron supplement* [multiple vitamins; calcium; iron; folic acid] $\pm \bullet 125 \bullet 18 \bullet 0.4$ mg

Filibon F.A.; Filibon Forte tablets (discontinued 1995) ℞ *vitamin/calcium/iron supplement* [multiple vitamins; calcium; iron; folic acid] $\pm \bullet$ $250 \bullet 45 \bullet 1$ mg; $300 \bullet 45 \bullet 1$ mg

Filipendula ulmaria medicinal herb [see: meadowsweet]

filipin USAN, INN *antifungal*

Filmix ℞ *investigational (orphan) neurosonographic contrast medium for intracranial tumors* [microbubble contrast agent]

Filmlok (trademarked dosage form) *film-coated tablet*

Filmseal (trademarked dosage form) *film-coated tablet*

Filmtabs (trademarked dosage form) *film-coated tablets*

FIME (fluorouracil, ICRF-159, MeCCNU) *chemotherapy protocol*

Finac lotion OTC *topical acne treatment* [salicylic acid; isopropyl alcohol] $2\% \bullet 22.5\%$

Finajet; Finaplix *brand names for trenbolone acetate, a European veterinary anabolic steroid abused as a street drug*

finasteride USAN, INN, BAN *α-reductase inhibitor; androgen hormone inhibitor for benign prostatic hypertension and androgenic alopecia in men*

finger leaf *medicinal herb* [see: cinquefoil]

Fiogesic tablets OTC *decongestant; antihistamine; analgesic* [phenylpropanolamine HCl; pheniramine maleate; pyrilamine maleate; aspirin]

Fiorgen PF tablets (discontinued 1998) ℞ *analgesic; sedative* [aspirin; caffeine; butalbital] $325 \bullet 40 \bullet 50$ mg

Fioricet tablets ℞ *analgesic; sedative* [acetaminophen; caffeine; butalbital] $325 \bullet 40 \bullet 50$ mg ② Lorcet

Fioricet with Codeine capsules ℞ *narcotic analgesic; sedative* [codeine phosphate; acetaminophen; caffeine; butalbital] $30 \bullet 325 \bullet 40 \bullet 50$ mg

Fiorinal tablets, capsules ℞ *analgesic; sedative* [aspirin; caffeine; butalbital] $325 \bullet 40 \bullet 50$ mg ② Florinef

Fiorinal with Codeine capsules ℞ *narcotic analgesic; sedative* [codeine phosphate; aspirin; caffeine; butalbital] $30 \bullet 325 \bullet 40 \bullet 50$ mg

Fiorpap tablets ℞ *analgesic; sedative* [acetaminophen; caffeine; butalbital] $325 \bullet 40 \bullet 50$ mg

Fiortal capsules ℞ *analgesic; sedative* [aspirin; caffeine; butalbital] $325 \bullet 40 \bullet 50$ mg

fipexide INN

fire ant venom allergenic extract *investigational (orphan) skin test and immunotherapy for fire ant reactions*

fireweed *medicinal herb* [see: pilewort]

First Choice reagent strips for home use OTC *in vitro diagnostic aid for blood glucose*

First Response test stick for home use OTC *in vitro diagnostic aid for urine pregnancy test*

First Response Ovulation Predictor test kit for home use OTC *in vitro diagnostic aid to predict ovulation time*

fisalamine [see: mesalamine]

fit root (*Monotropa uniflora*) *medicinal herb used as an antispasmodic, febrifuge, nervine, and sedative*

5 + 2 protocol (cytarabine, daunorubicin) *chemotherapy protocol*

5 + 2 protocol (cytarabine, mito-xantrone) *chemotherapy protocol*

5-ALA HCl; ALA [see: aminolevu-linic acid HCl]

5% Alcohol and 5% Dextrose in Water; 10% Alcohol and 5% Dextrose in Water IV infusion ℞ *for caloric replacement and rehydration* [dextrose; alcohol] 5%•5%; 10%•5%

5 Benzagel; 10 Benzagel gel ℞ *topical keratolytic for acne* [benzoyl peroxide] 5%; 10%

5% Dextrose and Electrolyte #48; 5% Dextrose and Electrolyte #75; 10% Dextrose and Electrolyte #48 IV infusion ℞ *intravenous nutritional/electrolyte therapy* [combined electrolyte solution; dextrose]

5% Travert and Electrolyte No. 2; 10% Travert and Electrolyte No. 2 IV infusion ℞ *intravenous nutritional/electrolyte therapy* [combined electrolyte solution; invert sugar (50% dextrose + 50% fructose)]

520C9x22 [see: bispecific antibody 520C9x22]

five-finger grass; five fingers *medicinal herb* [see: cinquefoil]

five-fingers root *medicinal herb* [see: ginseng]

5G1.1-SC *investigational (Phase I/II) C5 complement inhibitor for rheumatoid arthritis; investigational (Phase II) for cardiopulmonary bypass during coronary artery bypass graft surgery*

5-HT (5-hydroxytryptamine) [see: serotonin]

5-HT₃ (hydroxytryptamine) receptor antagonists *a class of antiemetic and antinauseant agents used primarily after emetogenic cancer chemotherapy* [also called: selective serotonin 5-HT₃ blockers]

5-HTP (5-hydroxytryptophan) [see: L-5 hydroxytryptophan]

FK-565 *investigational (Phase I) immunomodulator for cancer and HIV*

FL (flutamide, leuprolide acetate) *chemotherapy protocol*

FLAC (fluorouracil, leucovorin [rescue], Adriamycin, cyclophosphamide) *chemotherapy protocol*

flag, sweet; myrtle flag *medicinal herb* [see: calamus]

flag lily; poison flag; water flag *medicinal herb* [see: blue flag]

Flagyl film-coated tablets, capsules ℞ *antibiotic; antiprotozoal; amebicide* [metronidazole] 250, 500 mg; 375 mg

Flagyl ER film-coated extended-release tablets ℞ *once-daily antibiotic for bacterial vaginosis* [metronidazole] 750 mg

Flagyl IV powder for injection ℞ *antibiotic; antiprotozoal; amebicide* [metronidazole HCl] 500 mg

Flagyl IV RTU (ready-to-use) injection ℞ *antibiotic; antiprotozoal; amebicide* [metronidazole] 500 mg/100 mL

flamenol INN

Flanders Buttocks ointment OTC *topical diaper rash treatment* [zinc oxide; peruvian balsam]

flannel flower *medicinal herb* [see: mullein]

FLAP (fluorouracil, leucovorin [rescue], Adriamycin, Platinol) *chemotherapy protocol*

Flarex Drop-Tainers (eye drop suspension) ℞ *topical ophthalmic corticosteroidal anti-inflammatory* [fluorometholone acetate] 0.1%

Flatulex drops OTC *antiflatulent* [simethicone] 40 mg/0.6 mL

Flatulex tablets OTC *adsorbent; detoxicant; antiflatulent* [activated charcoal; simethicone] 250•80 mg

flavamine INN

flavine [see: acriflavine HCl]

flavivirus vaccine, chimeric *investigational vaccine*

flavodic acid INN

flavodilol INN *antihypertensive* [also: flavodilol maleate]

flavodilol maleate USAN *antihypertensive* [also: flavodilol]

flavonoid [see: troxerutin]

Flavons-500 tablets OTC *dietary supplement* [citrus bioflavonoids and hesperidin complex] 500 mg

Flavorcee chewable tablets OTC *vitamin supplement* [ascorbic acid] 100, 250, 500 mg

flavoxate INN, BAN *smooth muscle relaxant; urinary antispasmodic* [also: flavoxate HCl]

flavoxate HCl USAN *smooth muscle relaxant; urinary antispasmodic* [also: flavoxate]

Flaxedil IV (discontinued 1996) ℞ *neuromuscular blocker* [gallamine triethiodide] 20 mg/mL ② Flexeril

flaxseed *(Linum usitatissimum) medicinal herb for arthritis, autoimmune diseases, colds, constipation, cough, heart disease, lowering cholesterol levels, skin disorders, and urinary tract infections*

flazalone USAN, INN, BAN *anti-inflammatory*

FLe (fluorouracil, levamisole) *chemotherapy protocol*

flea seed; fleawort *medicinal herb* [see: plantain]

fleabane; horseweed *(Erigeron canadensis)* plant *medicinal herb used as an astringent, diuretic, and hemostatic*

fleawort; flea seed *medicinal herb* [see: plantain]

flecainide INN, BAN *antiarrhythmic* [also: flecainide acetate]

flecainide acetate USAN *antiarrhythmic* [also: flecainide]

Fleet Babylax rectal liquid OTC *hyperosmolar laxative* [glycerin] 4 mL/dose

Fleet Bisacodyl Enema; Fleet Bisacodyl Prep rectal liquid OTC *stimulant laxative* [bisacodyl] 10 mg/30 mL; 10 mg/packet

Fleet Enema rectal liquid OTC *saline laxative* [monobasic sodium phosphate; dibasic sodium phosphate] 7•19 g/118 mL

Fleet Flavored Castor Oil emulsion OTC *stimulant laxative* [castor oil] 67%

Fleet Laxative enteric-coated tablets OTC *stimulant laxative* [bisacodyl] 5 mg

Fleet Laxative suppositories OTC *stimulant laxative* [bisacodyl] 10 mg

Fleet Medicated Wipes cleansing pads OTC *moisturizer and cleanser for external rectal/vaginal areas; astringent; antiseptic; antifungal* [hamamelis water; glycerin; alcohol] 50%•10%•7%

Fleet Mineral Oil Enema rectal liquid OTC *lubricant laxative* [mineral oil]

Fleet Pain Relief anorectal wipes OTC *topical local anesthetic* [pramoxine HCl; glycerin] 1%•12%

Fleet Phospho-Soda oral solution OTC *buffered saline laxative* [monobasic sodium phosphate; dibasic sodium phosphate] 18•48 g/100 mL

Fleet Prep Kits No. 1 to No. 6 OTC *pre-procedure bowel evacuant* [other Fleet products in combination kits]

Fleet Relief anorectal ointment (discontinued 1995) OTC *hemorrhoidal astringent; protectant* [zinc oxide; white petrolatum; mineral oil]

Fleet Relief Anesthetic Hemorrhoidal ointment (discontinued 1995) OTC *topical local anesthetic* [pramoxine HCl] 1%

FLEP (fluorouracil, leucovorin, etoposide, Platinol) *chemotherapy protocol*

flerobuterol INN

fleroxacin USAN, INN *antibacterial*

flesinoxan INN *investigational antidepressant and anxiolytic*

flestolol INN *antiadrenergic (β-receptor)* [also: flestolol sulfate]

flestolol sulfate USAN *antiadrenergic (β-receptor)* [also: flestolol]

fletazepam USAN, INN, BAN *skeletal muscle relaxant*

Fletcher's Castoria liquid OTC *stimulant laxative* [senna concentrate] 33.3 mg/mL

fleur-de-lis *medicinal herb* [see: blue flag]

Flex-all 454 gel OTC *topical analgesic; antipruritic; counterirritant; topical local anesthetic* [menthol; methyl salicylate] 16%• ②

Flexaphen capsules ℞ *skeletal muscle relaxant; analgesic* [chlorzoxazone; acetaminophen] 250•300 mg

Flex-Care Especially for Sensitive Eyes solution OTC *chemical disinfecting solution for soft contact lenses* [note: soft contact indication different from RGP contact indication for same product]

Flex-Care Especially for Sensitive Eyes solution OTC *disinfecting/wetting/soaking solution for rigid gas permeable contact lenses* [note: RGP contact indication different from soft contact indication for same product]

Flexeril film-coated tablets R *skeletal muscle relaxant* [cyclobenzaprine HCl] 10 mg ⊉ Flaxedil

Flexoject IV or IM injection R *skeletal muscle relaxant* [orphenadrine citrate] 30 mg/mL

Flexon IV or IM injection R *skeletal muscle relaxant* [orphenadrine citrate] 30 mg/mL

FlexPack HP test for professional use *diagnostic aid for serum IgG antibodies to H. pylori (for peptic ulcers)*

Flextra-DS tablets OTC *analgesic; antipyretic; antihistamine* [acetaminophen; phenyltoloxamine citrate] 500•50 mg

flibanserin USAN *antidepressant*

Flintstones Children's; Flintstones Plus Calcium; Flintstones Plus Extra C Children's chewable tablets OTC *vitamin supplement* [multiple vitamins; folic acid] ≟•0.3 mg

Flintstones Complete chewable tablets OTC *vitamin/mineral/iron supplement* [multiple vitamins & minerals; iron; folic acid; biotin] ≟•18 mg•0.4 mg•40 μg

Flintstones Plus Iron chewable tablets OTC *vitamin/iron supplement* [multiple vitamins; iron; folic acid] ≟•15•0.3 mg

Flo-Coat oral/rectal suspension R *radiopaque contrast medium for gastrointestinal imaging* [barium sulfate] 100%

Flocor R *investigational (Phase III, orphan) coagulation inhibitor for sickle cell crisis; investigational (orphan) for*

severe burns, and vasospasm following cerebral aneurysm repair

floctafenine USAN, INN, BAN *analgesic*

Flolan IV infusion R *platelet aggregation inhibitor; investigational (orphan) vasodilator for primary pulmonary hypertension* [epoprostenol] 0.5, 1.5 mg

Flomax capsules R $α_1$ *antagonist for benign prostatic hypertrophy (BPH)* [tamsulosin HCl] 0.4 mg ⊉ Slow-Mag; Zomig

flomoxef INN

Flonase nasal spray R *corticosteroidal anti-inflammatory for seasonal or perennial rhinitis* [fluticasone propionate] 50 μg/dose

Flo-Pack (trademarked packaging form) *vial for IV drip*

flopropione INN

florantyrone INN, BAN

flordipine USAN, INN *antihypertensive*

floredil INN

Florentine iris *medicinal herb* [see: orris root]

floretione [see: fluoresone]

florfenicol USAN, INN, BAN *veterinary antibacterial*

Florical capsules, tablets OTC *calcium/fluoride supplement* [calcium carbonate; sodium fluoride] 364•8.3 mg

Florida Sunburn Relief lotion OTC *topical analgesic; antipruritic; counterirritant* [phenol; camphor; menthol; benzyl alcohol] 0.4%•0.2%•0.15%•3%

florifenine INN

Florinef Acetate tablets R *adrenocortical insufficiency in Addison's disease* [fludrocortisone acetate] 0.1 mg ⊉ Fiorinal

Florone cream, ointment R *topical corticosteroidal anti-inflammatory* [diflorasone diacetate] 0.05%

Florone E cream R *topical corticosteroidal anti-inflammatory; emollient* [diflorasone diacetate] 0.05%

floropipamide [now: pipamperone]

floropipeton [see: propyperone]

Floropryl ophthalmic ointment (discontinued 1995) R *antiglaucoma* agent; irreversible cholinesterase inhibitor miotic [isoflurophate] 0.025%

Florvite drops ℞ pediatric vitamin supplement and dental caries preventative [multiple vitamins; sodium fluoride] ≛•0.25, ≛•0.5 mg/mL

Florvite; Florvite Half Strength chewable tablets ℞ pediatric vitamin supplement and dental caries preventative [multiple vitamins; sodium fluoride; folic acid] ≛•1•0.3 mg; ≛• 0.5•0.3 mg

Florvite + Iron drops ℞ pediatric vitamin/iron supplement and dental caries preventative [multiple vitamins & minerals; sodium fluoride; ferrous sulfate] ≛•0.25•10, ≛•0.5•10 mg/mL

Florvite + Iron; Half Strength Florvite + Iron chewable tablets ℞ pediatric vitamin/iron supplement and dental caries preventative [multiple vitamins & minerals; sodium fluoride; ferrous sulfate; folic acid] ≛• 1•12•0.3 mg; ≛•0.5•12•0.3 mg

flosequinan USAN, INN, BAN antihypertensive; vasodilator

flotrenizine INN

Flovent metered dose inhaler, Rotadisk (inhalation powder) ℞ corticosteroidal antiasthmatic [fluticasone propionate] 44, 110, 220 μg/dose; 50, 100, 250 μg/dose

floverine INN

flower velure medicinal herb [see: coltsfoot]

flower-de-luce medicinal herb [see: blue flag]

floxacillin USAN antibacterial [also: flucloxacillin]

floxacrine INN

Floxin film-coated tablets, UroPak (3-day supply), IV injection ℞ broad-spectrum fluoroquinolone antibiotic [ofloxacin] 200, 300, 400 mg; 6 tablets × 200 mg; 200, 400 mg

Floxin Otic ear drops ℞ broad-spectrum fluoroquinolone antibiotic [ofloxacin] 3 mg/mL

floxuridine USAN, USP, INN antimetabolic antineoplastic for GI adenocarcinoma metastatic to the liver

FLT (fluorothymidine) [q.v.]

Flu, Cold & Cough Medicine powder for oral solution OTC antitussive; decongestant; antihistamine; analgesic [dextromethorphan hydrobromide; pseudoephedrine HCl; chlorpheniramine maleate; acetaminophen] 20• 60•4•500 mg/packet

Flu OIA (Optical ImmunoAssay) test for professional use rapid (less than 20 minutes) diagnostic aid for influenza A and B in sputum, nasal aspirate, or nasopharyngeal swab

fluacizine INN

flualamide INN

fluanisone INN, BAN

fluazacort USAN, INN anti-inflammatory

flubanilate INN CNS stimulant [also: flubanilate HCl]

flubanilate HCl USAN CNS stimulant [also: flubanilate]

flubendazole USAN, INN, BAN antiprotozoal

flubenisolone [see: betamethasone]

flubepride INN

flubuperone [see: melperone]

flucarbril INN

flucetorex INN

flucindole USAN, INN antipsychotic

fluciprazine INN

fluclorolone acetonide INN, BAN corticosteroid; anti-inflammatory [also: flucloronide]

flucloronide USAN corticosteroid; anti-inflammatory [also: fluclorolone acetonide]

flucloxacillin INN, BAN antibacterial [also: floxacillin]

fluconazole USAN, INN, BAN broad-spectrum systemic fungistatic

flucrilate INN tissue adhesive [also: flucrylate]

flucrylate USAN tissue adhesive [also: flucrilate]

flucytosine USAN, USP, INN, BAN fungicidal

fludalanine USAN, INN antibacterial

Fludara powder for IV injection ℞ antineoplastic for chronic lymphocytic leukemia and non-Hodgkin's lymphoma (orphan) [fludarabine phosphate] 50 mg

fludarabine INN antimetabolic antineoplastic [also: fludarabine phosphate]

fludarabine phosphate USAN antineoplastic for chronic lymphocytic leukemia and non-Hodgkin's lymphoma (orphan) [also: fludarabine]

fludazonium chloride USAN, INN topical anti-infective

fludeoxyglucose (^{18}F) INN diagnostic aid; radioactive agent [also: fludeoxyglucose F 18]

fludeoxyglucose F 18 USAN, USP diagnostic aid; radioactive agent [also: fludeoxyglucose (^{18}F)]

fludiazepam INN

fludorex USAN, INN anorectic; antiemetic

fludoxopone INN

fludrocortisone INN, BAN salt-regulating adrenocortical steroid; mineralocorticoid [also: fludrocortisone acetate]

fludrocortisone acetate USP salt-regulating adrenocortical steroid; mineralocorticoid [also: fludrocortisone]

fludroxicortide [see: flurandrenolide]

fludroxycortide INN topical corticosteroid [also: flurandrenolide; flurandrenolone]

flufenamic acid USAN, INN, BAN anti-inflammatory

flufenisal USAN, INN analgesic

flufosal INN

flufylline INN

flugestone INN, BAN progestin [also: flurogestone acetate]

flugestone acetate [see: flurogestone acetate]

Fluimucil ℞ investigational (Phase I) immunomodulator for HIV and AIDS [acetylcysteine]

fluindarol INN

fluindione INN

Flumadine film-coated tablets, syrup ℞ antiviral; prophylaxis and treatment for influenza A virus [rimantadine HCl] 100 mg; 50 mg/5 mL

flumazenil USAN, INN, BAN benzodiazepine antagonist/antidote

flumazepil [see: flumazenil]

flumecinol INN investigational (orphan) for neonatal hyperbilirubinemia

flumedroxone INN, BAN

flumequine USAN, INN, BAN antibacterial

flumeridone USAN, INN, BAN antiemetic

flumetasone INN corticosteroid; anti-inflammatory [also: flumethasone]

flumethasone USAN, BAN topical corticosteroidal anti-inflammatory [also: flumetasone]

flumethasone pivalate USAN, USP, BAN topical corticosteroidal anti-inflammatory

flumethiazide INN, BAN

flumethrin BAN

flumetramide USAN, INN skeletal muscle relaxant

flumexadol INN

flumezapine USAN, INN, BAN antipsychotic; neuroleptic

fluminorex USAN, INN anorectic

FluMist ℞ investigational (NDA filed) intranasal influenza virus vaccine

flumizole USAN, INN anti-inflammatory

flumoxonide USAN, INN adrenocortical steroid

flunamine INN

flunarizine INN, BAN vasodilator; investigational (orphan) for alternating hemiplegia [also: flunarizine HCl]

flunarizine HCl USAN vasodilator [also: flunarizine]

flunidazole USAN, INN antiprotozoal

flunisolide USAN, USP, INN, BAN corticosteroidal anti-inflammatory for chronic asthma and rhinitis

flunisolide acetate USAN anti-inflammatory

flunitrazepam USAN, INN, BAN, JAN benzodiazepine sedative and hypnotic; also abused as a "date rape" street drug

flunixin USAN, INN, BAN anti-inflammatory; analgesic

flunixin meglumine USAN anti-inflammatory; analgesic

flunoprost INN

flunoxaprofen INN

fluocinolide [now: fluocinonide]

fluocinolone BAN *topical corticosteroidal anti-inflammatory* [also: fluocinolone acetonide]

fluocinolone acetonide USAN, USP, INN *topical corticosteroidal anti-inflammatory* [also: fluocinolone] 0.01%, 0.025% topical

fluocinonide USAN, USP, INN, BAN *topical corticosteroidal anti-inflammatory* 0.05% topical

fluocortin INN *anti-inflammatory* [also: fluocortin butyl]

fluocortin butyl USAN, BAN *anti-inflammatory* [also: fluocortin]

fluocortolone USAN, INN, BAN *corticosteroid; anti-inflammatory*

fluocortolone caproate USAN *corticosteroid; anti-inflammatory*

Fluogen IM injection, Steri-Vials, Steri-Dose (disposable syringes) ℞ *flu vaccine* [influenza split-virus vaccine] 0.5 mL/dose

Fluonex cream ℞ *topical corticosteroidal anti-inflammatory* [fluocinonide] 0.05%

Fluonid topical solution ℞ *topical corticosteroidal anti-inflammatory* [fluocinolone acetonide] 0.01%

fluopromazine BAN *antipsychotic* [also: triflupromazine]

Fluoracaine eye drops ℞ *topical ophthalmic anesthetic; corneal disclosing agent* [proparacaine HCl; fluorescein sodium] 0.5%•0.25%

fluoracizine [see: fluacizine]

fluorescein USP, BAN, JAN *ophthalmic diagnostic aid*

fluorescein, soluble [now: fluorescein sodium]

fluorescein sodium USP, BAN, JAN *ophthalmic diagnostic aid* 2% eye drops

fluorescein sodium & proparacaine HCl *corneal disclosing agent; topical ophthalmic anesthetic* 0.25%•0.5%

Fluorescite antecubital venous injection ℞ *ophthalmic diagnostic agent* [fluorescein sodium] 10%, 25%

Fluoresoft eye drops ℞ *diagnostic aid in fitting contact lenses* [fluorexon] 0.35%

fluoresone INN

Fluorets ophthalmic strips OTC *corneal disclosing agent* [fluorescein sodium] 1 mg

fluorexon *diagnosis and fitting aid for contact lenses*

fluorhydrocortisone acetate [see: fludrocortisone acetate]

Fluoride tablets OTC *dental caries preventative* [sodium fluoride] 2.21 mg

Fluoride Loz lozenges ℞ *topical dental caries preventative* [sodium fluoride] 2.21 mg

Fluorigard oral rinse OTC *topical dental caries preventative* [sodium fluoride; alcohol 6%] 0.05%

Fluori-Methane spray ℞ *topical vapocoolant anesthetic* [trichloromonofluoromethane; dichlorodifluoromethane] 85%•15%

fluorine *element (F)*

fluorine F 18 fluorodeoxyglucose [see: fludeoxyglucose F 18]

Fluorinse oral rinse ℞ *topical dental caries preventative* [sodium fluoride] 0.2%

Fluor-I-Strip; Fluor-I-Strip A.T. ophthalmic strips ℞ *corneal disclosing agent* [fluorescein sodium] 9 mg; 1 mg

Fluoritab chewable tablets, drops ℞ *dental caries preventative* [sodium fluoride] 1.1, 2.2 mg; 0.55 mg/drop

fluormethylprednisolone [see: dexamethasone]

5-fluorocytosine (5-FC) [see: flucytosine]

fluorodeoxyglucose F 18 [see: fludeoxyglucose F 18]

fluorodideoxyadenosine (F-ddA) [see: lodenosine]

fluorometholone USP, INN, BAN *topical ophthalmic corticosteroidal anti-inflammatory* 0.1% eye drops

fluorometholone acetate USAN *topical ophthalmic corticosteroidal anti-inflammatory*

Fluor-Op eye drop suspension ℞ *topical ophthalmic corticosteroidal anti-inflammatory* [fluorometholone] 0.1%

Fluoroplex cream, topical solution ℞ *antimetabolite antineoplastic for actinic* keratoses and basal cell carcinomas [fluorouracil] 1%

fluoroquinolones *a class of synthetic, broad-spectrum, antimicrobial, bactericidal antibiotics*

fluorosalan USAN *disinfectant* [also: flusalan]

fluorothymidine (FLT) *investigational (Phase II) antiviral for HIV and AIDS*

fluorouracil (5-FU) USAN, USP, INN, BAN *antimetabolite antineoplastic for colorectal, breast, stomach, and pancreatic cancers; investigational (Phase III) microsponge delivery system for actinic keratosis* 50 mg/mL injection

fluorouracil & interferon alfa-2a *investigational (orphan) for esophageal and advanced colorectal carcinoma*

fluorouracil & leucovorin *antineoplastic for metastatic colorectal cancer (orphan)*

fluoruridine deoxyribose [see: floxuridine]

Fluosol *emulsion for intracoronary perfusion (discontinued 1995)* ℞ *myocardial oxygenation during PTCA* [intravascular perfluorochemical (PFC) emulsion] 20%

fluostigmine [see: isoflurophate]

Fluothane *liquid for vaporization* ℞ *inhalation general anesthetic* [halothane]

fluotracen INN *antipsychotic; antidepressant* [also: fluotracen HCl]

fluotracen HCl USAN *antipsychotic; antidepressant* [also: fluotracen]

fluoxetine USAN, INN, BAN *selective serotonin reuptake inhibitor (SSRI) for depression, obsessive-compulsive disorder, and bulimia nervosa*

fluoxetine HCl USAN *selective serotonin reuptake inhibitor (SSRI) for depression, obsessive-compulsive disorder, and bulimia nervosa*

fluoximesterone [see: fluoxymesterone]

Flu-Oxinate *eye drops* ℞ *topical ophthalmic anesthetic; corneal disclosing agent* [benoxinate HCl; fluorescein sodium] 0.4% • 0.25%

fluoxiprednisolone [see: triamcinolone]

fluoxymesterone USP, INN, BAN *oral androgen; hormonal antineoplastic for female breast cancer* 10 mg oral

fluparoxan INN, BAN *antidepressant* [also: fluparoxan HCl]

fluparoxan HCl USAN *antidepressant* [also: fluparoxan]

flupenthixol BAN *thioxanthene antipsychotic* [also: flupentixol]

flupentixol INN *thioxanthene antipsychotic* [also: flupenthixol]

fluperamide USAN, INN *antiperistaltic*

fluperlapine INN

fluperolone INN, BAN *corticosteroid; anti-inflammatory* [also: fluperolone acetate]

fluperolone acetate USAN *corticosteroid; anti-inflammatory* [also: fluperolone]

fluphenazine INN, BAN *phenothiazine antipsychotic* [also: fluphenazine enanthate]

fluphenazine decanoate *phenothiazine antipsychotic; prolonged parenteral neuroleptic therapy* 25 mg/mL injection

fluphenazine enanthate USP *phenothiazine antipsychotic; prolonged parenteral neuroleptic therapy* [also: fluphenazine]

fluphenazine HCl USP, BAN *phenothiazine antipsychotic* 1, 2.5, 5, 10 mg oral; 5 mg/mL oral; 2.5 mg/mL injection

flupimazine INN

flupirtine INN, BAN *analgesic* [also: flupirtine maleate]

flupirtine maleate USAN *analgesic* [also: flupirtine]

flupranone INN

fluprazine INN

fluprednidene INN, BAN

fluprednisolone USAN, NF, INN, BAN *corticosteroid; anti-inflammatory*

fluprednisolone valerate USAN *corticosteroid; anti-inflammatory*

fluprofen INN, BAN

fluprofylline INN

fluproquazone USAN, INN, BAN *analgesic*

fluprostenol INN, BAN *prostaglandin* [also: fluprostenol sodium]

fluprostenol sodium USAN *prostaglandin* [also: fluprostenol]

fluquazone USAN, INN *anti-inflammatory*

Flura tablets ℞ *dental caries preventative* [sodium fluoride] 2.2 mg

fluracil [see: fluorouracil]

fluradoline INN *analgesic* [also: fluradoline HCl]

fluradoline HCl USAN *analgesic* [also: fluradoline]

Flura-Drops ℞ *dental caries preventative* [sodium fluoride] 0.55 mg/drop

Flura-Loz lozenges ℞ *topical dental caries preventative* [sodium fluoride] 2.2 mg

flurandrenolide USAN, USP *topical corticosteroid* [also: fludroxycortide; flurandrenolone] 0.05% topical

flurandrenolone BAN *topical corticosteroid* [also: flurandrenolide; fludroxycortide]

flurantel INN

Flurate eye drops ℞ *topical ophthalmic anesthetic; corneal disclosing agent* [benoxinate HCl; fluorescein sodium] 0.4%•0.25%

flurazepam INN, BAN *anticonvulsant; hypnotic; muscle relaxant; sedative; also abused as a street drug* [also: flurazepam HCl]

flurazepam HCl USAN, USP *anticonvulsant; hypnotic; muscle relaxant; sedative; also abused as a street drug* [also: flurazepam] 15, 30 mg oral

flurbiprofen USAN, USP, INN, BAN *antiarthritic; nonsteroidal anti-inflammatory drug (NSAID); analgesic* 50, 100 mg oral

flurbiprofen sodium USP *prostaglandin synthesis inhibitor; antimiotic; ophthalmic nonsteroidal anti-inflammatory drug (NSAID)* 0.03% eye drops

Fluress eye drops ℞ *topical ophthalmic anesthetic; corneal disclosing agent* [benoxinate HCl; fluorescein sodium] 0.4%•0.25%

fluretofen USAN, INN *anti-inflammatory; antithrombotic*

flurfamide [now: flurofamide]

flurithromycin INN

flurocitabine USAN, INN *antineoplastic*

Fluro-Ethyl aerosol spray ℞ *topical refrigerant anesthetic* [ethyl chloride; dichlorotetrafluoroethane] 25%•75%

flurofamide USAN, INN *urease enzyme inhibitor*

flurogestone acetate USAN *progestin* [also: flugestone]

Flurosyn ointment, cream ℞ *topical corticosteroidal anti-inflammatory* [fluocinolone acetonide] 0.025%; 0.01, 0.025%

flurothyl USAN, USP, BAN *CNS stimulant* [also: flurotyl]

flurotyl INN *CNS stimulant* [also: flurothyl]

fluroxene USAN, NF, INN *inhalation anesthetic*

fluroxyspiramine [see: spiramide]

flusalan INN *disinfectant* [also: fluorosalan]

FluShield IM injection, Tubex (cartridge-needle unit) ℞ *flu vaccine* [influenza purified split-virus vaccine] 0.5 mL/dose

flusoxolol INN, BAN

fluspiperone USAN, INN *antipsychotic*

fluspirilene USAN, INN, BAN *diphenylbutylpiperidine antipsychotic*

flutamide USAN, INN, BAN *antiandrogen antineoplastic for prostatic carcinoma*

flutazolam INN

flutemazepam INN

Flutex ointment, cream ℞ *topical corticosteroidal anti-inflammatory* [triamcinolone acetonide] 0.025%, 0.1%, 0.5%

flutiazin USAN, INN *veterinary anti-inflammatory*

fluticasone INN, BAN *corticosteroidal anti-inflammatory for chronic asthma or rhinitis* [also: fluticasone propionate]

fluticasone propionate USAN *corticosteroidal anti-inflammatory for chronic asthma or rhinitis* [also: fluticasone]

flutizenol INN

flutomidate INN

flutonidine INN

flutoprazepam INN

flutrimazole INN

flutroline USAN, INN *antipsychotic*

flutropium bromide INN

fluvastatin INN, BAN *HMG-CoA reductase inhibitor for hypercholesterolemia and atherosclerosis* [also: fluvastatin sodium]

fluvastatin sodium USAN *HMG-CoA reductase inhibitor for hypercholesterolemia and atherosclerosis* [also: fluvastatin]

Fluvirin IM injection, prefilled syringes ℞ *flu vaccine* [influenza purified surface antigen] 0.5 mL/dose

fluvoxamine INN, BAN *selective serotonin reuptake inhibitor (SSRI) for obsessive-compulsive disorder* [also: fluvoxamine maleate]

fluvoxamine maleate USAN *selective serotonin reuptake inhibitor (SSRI) for obsessive-compulsive disorder; investigational (Phase III) for depression and panic disorder* [also: fluvoxamine]

flux root *medicinal herb* [see: pleurisy root]

fluzinamide USAN, INN *anticonvulsant*

Fluzone IM injection, prefilled syringes ℞ *flu vaccine* [influenza split-virus or whole-virus vaccine] 0.5 mL/dose

fluzoperine INN

flytrap *medicinal herb* [see: dogbane]

FML; FML Forte eye drop suspension ℞ *topical ophthalmic corticosteroidal anti-inflammatory* [fluorometholone] 0.1%; 0.25%

FML S.O.P. ophthalmic ointment ℞ *topical ophthalmic corticosteroidal anti-inflammatory* [fluorometholone] 0.1%

FML-S eye drop suspension ℞ *topical ophthalmic corticosteroidal anti-inflammatory; antibiotic* [fluorometholone; sulfacetamide sodium] 0.1%•10%

FMS (fluorouracil, mitomycin, streptozocin) *chemotherapy protocol*

FMV (fluorouracil, MeCCNU, vincristine) *chemotherapy protocol*

FNC (fluorouracil, Novantrone, cyclophosphamide) *chemotherapy protocol* [also: CFM; CNF]

FNM (fluorouracil, Novantrone, methotrexate) *chemotherapy protocol*

foal's foot *medicinal herb* [see: coltsfoot]

FOAM (fluorouracil, Oncovin, Adriamycin, mitomycin) *chemotherapy protocol*

Foamicon chewable tablets OTC *antacid* [aluminum hydroxide; magnesium trisilicate] 80•20 mg

focofilcon A USAN *hydrophilic contact lens material*

fodipir USAN *excipient*

Foeniculum officinale; F. vulgare *medicinal herb* [see: fennel]

fohy030 gene *investigational gene that encodes the protein melastatin, a metastasis suppressor in malignant melanoma*

Foille spray OTC *topical local anesthetic; antiseptic* [benzocaine; chloroxylenol] 5%•0.63%

Foille Medicated First Aid ointment, aerosol spray OTC *topical local anesthetic; antiseptic* [benzocaine; chloroxylenol] 5%•0.1%; 5%•0.6%

Foille Plus aerosol spray OTC *topical local anesthetic; antiseptic* [benzocaine; chloroxylenol; alcohol 57.33%] 5%•0.6%

folacin [see: folic acid] ℞ Fulvicin

folate [see: folic acid]

folate sodium USP

Folergot-DF tablets ℞ *GI anticholinergic; sedative; analgesic* [belladonna alkaloids; phenobarbital; ergotamine tartrate] 0.2•40•0.6 mg

folescutol INN

Folex PFS powder for IV or IM injection ℞ *antimetabolite antineoplastic for leukemia; systemic antipsoriatic; antirheumatic* [methotrexate sodium] 25 mg/mL

folic acid USP, INN, BAN *vitamin B_c; vitamin M; hematopoietic* 0.4, 0.8, 1 mg oral; 5 mg/mL injection

folinate-SF calcium [see: leucovorin calcium]

folinic acid [see: leucovorin calcium]

follicle-stimulating hormone (FSH) BAN [also: menotropins]

follidrin [see: estradiol benzoate]

Follistim subcu or IM injection ℞ *recombinant follicle-stimulating hor-*

mone (FSH) for the induction of ovulation [follitropin beta] 75 IU

follitropin alfa INN *recombinant follicle-stimulating hormone (FSH) for the induction of ovulation*

follitropin beta INN *recombinant follicle-stimulating hormone (FSH) for the induction of ovulation*

follotropin [see: menotropins]

Follow-Up [see: Carnation Follow-Up]

Follutein powder for IM injection (discontinued 1995) ℞ *hormone for prepubertal cryptorchidism and hypogonadism; ovulation stimulant* [chorionic gonadotropin] 1000 U/mL

Foloxatine ℞ *investigational (orphan) alkylating antineoplastic for ovarian and colorectal cancers* [oxaliplatin]

Foltrin capsules ℞ *hematinic* [ferrous fumarate; cyanocobalamin; ascorbic acid; intrinsic factor concentrate; folic acid] 110 mg•15 μg•75 mg•240 mg•0.5 mg

Folvite IM injection ℞ *antianemic* [folic acid] 5 mg/mL

fomepizole USAN, INN *antidote; alcohol dehydrogenase inhibitor for methanol or ethylene glycol poisoning (orphan)*

FOMI; FOMi (fluorouracil, Oncovin, mitomycin) *chemotherapy protocol*

fomidacillin INN, BAN

fominoben INN [also: fominoben HCl]

fominoben HCl JAN [also: fominoben]

fomivirsen sodium *antisense drug for AIDS-related CMV retinitis*

fomocaine INN, BAN

fonatol [see: diethylstilbestrol]

fonazine mesylate USAN *serotonin inhibitor* [also: dimetotiazine; dimethothiazine]

fontarsol [see: dichlorophenarsine HCl]

fopirtoline INN

Foradil Ⓐ encapsulated powder for inhalation ℞ *twice-daily bronchodilator for asthma (investigational (NDA filed) in the USA)* [formoterol fumarate]

Forane liquid for vaporization ℞ *inhalation general anesthetic* [isoflurane]

forasartan USAN *antihypertensive; CHF treatment; angiotensin II receptor antagonist*

foreign colombo *medicinal herb* [see: colombo]

forfenimex INN

formaldehyde solution USP *disinfectant; anhidrotic*

Formalyde-10 spray ℞ *for hyperhidrosis and bromhidrosis* [formaldehyde] 10%

formebolone INN, BAN

formetamide [see: formetorex]

formetorex INN

formidacillin [see: fomidacillin]

forminitrazole INN, BAN

formocortal USAN, INN, BAN *corticosteroid; anti-inflammatory*

formoterol INN *bronchodilator* [also: eformoterol; formoterol fumarate]

formoterol fumarate USAN, JAN *investigational (NDA filed) twice-daily bronchodilator for asthma* [also: formoterol; eformoterol fumarate]

Formula 44 Cough Control Disks; Formula 44 Cough Silencers lozenges OTC *antitussive; topical oral anesthetic* [dextromethorphan hydrobromide; benzocaine] 5•1.25 mg; 2.5•1 mg

Formula 405 cleansing bar OTC *therapeutic skin cleanser*

Formula B tablets ℞ *vitamin supplement* [multiple B vitamins; vitamin C; folic acid] ±•500•0.5 mg

Formula B Plus tablets ℞ *vitamin/mineral/iron supplement* [multiple vitamins & minerals; ferrous fumarate; folic acid; biotin] ±•27•0.8•0.15 mg

Formula Q capsules (discontinued 1996) OTC *prevention and treatment of nocturnal leg cramps* [quinine sulfate] 65 mg

Formula VM-2000 tablets OTC *dietary supplement* [multiple vitamins & minerals; multiple amino acids; iron; folic acid; biotin] ±•5 mg•0.2 mg•50 μg

4'-formylacetanilide thiosemicarbazone [see: thioacetazone; thiacetazone]

foropafant INN

forskolin [see: colforsin]

Forta Drink powder OTC *enteral nutritional therapy* [lactose-free formula]

Forta Shake powder OTC *enteral nutritional therapy* [milk-based formula]

Fortaz powder or frozen premix for IV or IM injection ℞ *cephalosporin antibiotic* [ceftazidime] 0.5, 1, 2, 6 g

Forte L.I.V. IM injection ℞ *antianemic* [ferrous gluconate; multiple B vitamins; procaine]

Fortel Home Ovulation Test kit for home use (discontinued 1995) OTC *in vitro diagnostic aid to predict ovulation time*

Fortel Midstream test stick for professional use *in vitro diagnostic aid for urine pregnancy test*

Fortel Plus test kit for home use OTC *in vitro diagnostic aid for urine pregnancy test*

Fortical ℞ *investigational (Phase III) calcium regulator for hypercalcemia, Paget's disease, and postmenopausal osteoporosis* [calcitonin (salmon), recombinant]

fortimicin A [now: astromicin sulfate]

Fortovase capsules ℞ *antiviral protease inhibitor for HIV* [saquinavir] 200 mg

40 winks capsules OTC *antihistaminic sleep aid* [diphenhydramine HCl] 50 mg

Fosamax tablets ℞ *bisphosphonate bone resorption inhibitor for postmenopausal and corticosteroid-induced osteoporosis and Paget's disease* [alendronate sodium] 5, 10, 40 mg

fosarilate USAN, INN *antiviral*

fosazepam USAN, INN, BAN *hypnotic*

foscarnet sodium USAN, INN, BAN *antiviral for cytomegalovirus (CMV) and various herpes viruses (HSV-1, HSV-2)*

Foscavir IV injection ℞ *antiviral for cytomegalovirus (CMV) retinitis and herpes simplex virus (HSV) infections in immunocompromised patients* [foscarnet sodium] 24 mg/mL

Foscavir topical ℞ *investigational (Phase I) antiviral for herpes simplex infections in AIDS* [foscarnet sodium]

foscolic acid INN

fosenazide INN

fosenopril sodium [see: fosinopril sodium]

fosfestrol INN, BAN *antineoplastic; estrogen* [also: diethylstilbestrol diphosphate]

fosfocreatinine INN

fosfomycin USAN, INN, BAN *antibacterial* [also: fosfomycin calcium; fosfomycin sodium]

fosfomycin calcium JAN *antibacterial* [also: fosfomycin; fosfomycin sodium]

fosfomycin sodium JAN *antibacterial* [also: fosfomycin; fosfomycin calcium]

fosfomycin tromethamine USAN *broad-spectrum bactericidal antibiotic for urinary tract infections*

fosfonet sodium USAN, INN *antiviral*

fosfosal INN

Fosfree tablets OTC *vitamin/iron supplement* [multiple vitamins; iron] ≛•29 mg

fosinopril INN, BAN *antihypertensive; angiotensin-converting enzyme (ACE) inhibitor* [also: fosinopril sodium]

fosinopril sodium USAN *antihypertensive; angiotensin-converting enzyme (ACE) inhibitor* [also: fosinopril]

fosinoprilat USAN, INN *antihypertensive*

fosmenic acid INN

fosmidomycin INN

fosphenytoin INN *hydantoin anticonvulsant* [also: fosphenytoin sodium]

fosphenytoin sodium USAN *hydantoin anticonvulsant for grand mal status epilepticus (orphan)* [also: fosphenytoin]

fospirate USAN, INN *veterinary anthelmintic*

fosquidone USAN, INN, BAN *antineoplastic*

fostedil USAN, INN *vasodilator; calcium channel blocker*

Fostex cleansing bar OTC *topical keratolytic for acne* [benzoyl peroxide] 10% ② pHisoHex

Fostex 10% BPO gel OTC *topical keratolytic for acne* [benzoyl peroxide] 10%

Fostex 10% Wash liquid OTC *topical keratolytic for acne* [benzoyl peroxide] 10%

Fostex Acne Cleansing cream OTC *topical keratolytic for acne* [salicylic acid] 2%

Fostex Acne Medication Cleansing bar OTC *medicated cleanser for acne* [salicylic acid] 2%

Fostex Medicated Cleansing Shampoo OTC *antiseborrheic; keratolytic* [sulfur; salicylic acid] 2%•2%

fostriecin INN *antineoplastic* [also: fostriecin sodium]

fostriecin sodium USAN *antineoplastic* [also: fostriecin]

Fostril lotion OTC *topical acne treatment* [sulfur; zinc oxide]

fotemustine INN, BAN

fo-ti; ho-shou-wu *(Polygonum multiflorum)* root *medicinal herb for atherosclerosis, blood cleansing, constipation, improving liver and kidney function, insomnia, malaria, muscle aches, TB, and weak bones; also used to increase fertility, prevent aging, and promote longevity*

Fototar cream OTC *topical antipsoriatic; antiseborrheic* [coal tar] 2%

fotretamine INN

Fouchet's reagent (solution)

4 Hair softgel capsules OTC *vitamin/mineral/iron supplement* [multiple vitamins & minerals; iron; folic acid; biotin] ± •2.5•33.3•0.25 mg

4 Nails softgel capsules OTC *vitamin/mineral/calcium/iron supplement* [multiple vitamins & minerals; calcium; iron; folic acid; biotin] ± •167•3•0.333•0.0083 mg

4-Way Cold tablets (discontinued 1995) OTC *decongestant; antihistamine; analgesic* [phenylpropanolamine HCl; chlorpheniramine maleate; acetaminophen] 12.5•2•325 mg

4-Way Fast Acting nasal spray OTC *nasal decongestant; antihistamine* [phenylephrine HCl; naphazoline HCl; pyrilamine maleate] 0.5%•0.05%•0.2%

4-Way Long Lasting nasal spray OTC *nasal decongestant* [oxymetazoline HCl] 0.05%

4B5 antibody *investigational (Phase I) fully human monoclonal antibody for immunotherapy in melanoma patients*

Fourneau 309 (available only from the Centers for Disease Control) R *antiparasitic for African trypanosomiasis and onchocerciasis* [suramin sodium]

foxglove *(Digitalis ambigua; D. ferriginea; D. grandiflora; D. lanata; D. lutea; D. purpurea)* leaves *medicinal herb for asthma, burns, congestive heart failure, edema, promoting wound healing, and sedation; not generally regarded as safe and effective for children as ingestion can be fatal*

foxglove, American; false foxglove; fern-leaved foxglove *medicinal herb* [see: feverweed]

foxtail *medicinal herb* [see: club moss]

frabuprofen INN

Fractar (trademarked ingredient) OTC *antipsoriatic; antiseborrheic* [crude coal tar]

Fragaria vesca *medicinal herb* [see: strawberry]

Fragmin deep subcu injection, prefilled syringes R *anticoagulant/antithrombotic for prevention of deep vein thrombosis (DVT) after abdominal or hip replacement surgery, unstable angina, and myocardial infarction* [dalteparin sodium] 2500, 5000, 10 000 IU/0.2 mL (16, 32, 64 mg/0.2 mL)

framycetin INN, BAN *anti-infective wound dressing*

francium *element* (Fr)

Frangula purshiana *medicinal herb* [see: cascara sagrada]

frankincense *(Boswellia serrata)* leaves and bark *medicinal herb for anaphylaxis, arthritis, asthma, blood cleansing, bronchial disorders, dysentery, rheumatism, skin ailments, ulcers, and wound healing*

fraxinella *(Dictamnus albus)* root, plant, and seed *medicinal herb used as*

an anthelmintic, diuretic, emmenagogue, expectorant, and febrifuge

Fraxiparine ⓒ subcu injection, prefilled syringes ℞ anticoagulant/anti-
thrombotic for prevention of deep vein
thrombosis (DVT) after surgery and
clotting during hemodialysis
[nadroparin calcium] 9500 IU/mL;
0.2, 0.3, 0.4, 0.6, 0.8, 1 mL

**FreAmine III 3% (8.5%) with Elec-
trolytes** IV infusion ℞ total parenteral nutrition (8.5% only); peripheral
parenteral nutrition (both) [multiple
essential and nonessential amino
acids; electrolytes]

**FreAmine III 8.5%; FreAmine III
10%** IV infusion ℞ total parenteral
nutrition; peripheral parenteral nutrition [multiple essential and nonessential amino acids]

FreAmine HBC 6.9% IV infusion ℞
nutritional therapy for high metabolic
stress [multiple branched-chain
essential and nonessential amino
acids; electrolytes]

Free & Clear shampoo OTC soap-free
therapeutic cleanser

Freedavite tablets OTC vitamin/min-
eral/iron supplement [multiple vitamins & minerals; ferrous fuma-
rate6400.2] ± ● 10 mg

Freedox solution ℞ investigational
(Phase III) lazaroid for subarachnoid
hemorrhage, ischemic stroke, spinal cord
and head injury [tirilazad mesylate]

Freezone liquid OTC topical keratolytic
[salicylic acid in a collodion-like
vehicle] 13.6%

frentizole USAN, INN, BAN immunoregulator

fringe tree (Chionanthus virginica)
bark medicinal herb used as an aperient, diuretic, febrifuge, and tonic

Frisium ℞ investigational benzodiazepine
tranquilizer; anxiolytic [clobazam]

fronepidil INN

frost plant; frost weed; frostwort
medicinal herb [see: rock rose]

frovatriptan succinate USAN investigational (NDA filed) $5\text{-}HT_{1B/1D}$ agonist for acute treatment of migraine

froxiprost INN

fructose (D-fructose) USP nutrient;
caloric replacement [also: levulose]

fructose-1,6-diphosphate (FDP)
investigational asthma treatment; investigational (orphan) for vaso-occlusive
episodes of sickle cell disease

Fruity Chews chewable tablets OTC
vitamin supplement [multiple vitamins; folic acid] ± ● 0.3 mg

Fruity Chews with Iron chewable
tablets OTC vitamin/iron supplement
[multiple vitamins; iron; folic acid]
± ● 12 ● 0.3 mg

frusemide BAN antihypertensive; loop
diuretic [also: furosemide]

FS Shampoo ℞ topical corticosteroidal
anti-inflammatory; antiseborrheic [fluo-
cinolone acetonide] 0.01%

FSF (fibrin-stabilizing factor) [see:
factor XIII]

FSH (follicle-stimulating hormone)
[see: menotropins]

ftalofyne INN veterinary anthelmintic
[also: phthalofyne]

ftaxilide INN

FTC investigational (Phase I/II) anti-
HIV agent

ftivazide INN

ftormetazine INN

ftorpropazine INN

5-FU (5-fluorouracil) [see: fluorouracil]

fubrogonium iodide INN

fuchsin, basic USP topical antibacterial/
antifungal

Fucus versiculosus medicinal herb [see:
kelp]

FUDR powder for intra-arterial infusion ℞ antimetabolic antineoplastic for
GI adenocarcinoma metastatic to the
liver [floxuridine] 500 mg

**FUDR; FUdR (5-fluorouracil deoxy-
ribonucleoside)** [see: floxuridine]

fuge, devil's medicinal herb [see: mis-
tletoe]

Ful-Glo ophthalmic strips ℞ *corneal disclosing agent* [fluorescein sodium] 0.6 mg

fulmicoton [see: pyroxylin]

FU/LV (fluorouracil, leucovorin calcium [rescue]) *chemotherapy protocol* [also: F-CL]

Fulvicin P/G tablets ℞ *systemic antifungal* [griseofulvin (ultramicrosize)] 125, 165, 250, 330 mg ☑ folacin; Furacin

Fulvicin U/F tablets ℞ *systemic antifungal* [griseofulvin (microsize)] 250, 500 mg

FUM (fluorouracil, methotrexate) *chemotherapy protocol*

fumagillin INN, BAN

Fumaria officinalis medicinal herb [see: fumitory]

fumaric acid NF *acidifier*

Fumasorb tablets (discontinued 1998) OTC *hematinic* [ferrous fumarate (source of iron)] 200 mg (66 mg)

Fumatinic sustained-release capsules ℞ *hematinic* [ferrous fumarate; cyanocobalamin; ascorbic acid; folic acid] 90 mg•15 μg•100 mg•1 mg

Fumerin sugar-coated tablets (discontinued 1998) OTC *hematinic* [ferrous fumarate (source of iron)] 195 mg (64 mg)

fumitory (*Fumaria officinalis*) plant *medicinal herb for cardiovascular disorders, constipation, eczema, edema, and hepatobiliary disorders*

fumoxicillin USAN, INN *antibacterial*

Funduscein-10; Funduscein-25 antecubital venous injection ℞ *ophthalmic diagnostic agent* [fluorescein sodium] 10%; 25%

Fungatin cream OTC *topical antifungal* [tolnaftate]

fungicidin [see: nystatin]

fungimycin USAN *antifungal*

Fungi-Nail liquid OTC *topical antifungal; keratolytic; anesthetic* [resorcinol; salicylic acid; chloroxylenol; benzocaine; alcohol 50%] 1%•2%•2%•0.5%

Fungizone cream, lotion, ointment ℞ *topical antifungal* [amphotericin B] 3%

Fungizone oral suspension ℞ *systemic antifungal; "swish and swallow" treatment for oral candidiasis* [amphotericin B] 100 mg/mL

Fungizone powder for IV infusion ℞ *systemic polyene antifungal* [amphotericin B deoxycholate] 50 mg/vial

Fung-O liquid OTC *topical keratolytic* [salicylic acid] 17%

Fungoid cream, solution ℞ *topical antifungal* [clotrimazole] 1%

Fungoid solution (became OTC and name changed to Fungoid AF in 1997) ℞ *topical antifungal* [undecylenic acid] 25%

Fungoid tincture OTC *topical antifungal* [miconazole nitrate] 2%

Fungoid AF solution OTC *topical antifungal* [undecylenic acid] 25%

Fungoid-HC cream ℞ *topical corticosteroidal anti-inflammatory; antipruritic; antifungal; antibacterial* [miconazole nitrate; hydrocortisone] 2%•1%

fuprazole INN

furacilin [see: nitrofurazone]

Furacin topical solution, cream ℞ *broad-spectrum antibacterial; adjunct to burn therapy and skin grafting* [nitrofurazone] 0.2% ☑ Fulvicin

Furacin Soluble Dressing ointment ℞ *broad-spectrum antibacterial; adjunct to burn therapy and skin grafting* [nitrofurazone] 0.2%

furacrinic acid INN, BAN

Furadantin oral suspension ℞ *urinary antibiotic* [nitrofurantoin] 25 mg/5 mL

furafylline INN

Furalan tablets ℞ *urinary antibiotic* [nitrofurantoin] 50, 100 mg

furalazine INN

furaltadone INN, BAN

Furamide (available only from the Centers for Disease Control) ℞ *investigational anti-infective for amebiasis* [diloxanide furoate]

furaprofen USAN, INN *anti-inflammatory*

furazabol INN

furazolidone USP, INN, BAN *bactericidal; antiprotozoal (Trichomonas); antidiarrheal*

furazolium chloride USAN, INN *anti-bacterial*
furazolium tartrate USAN *antibacterial*
furbucillin INN
furcloprofen INN
furegrelate INN *thromboxane synthetase inhibitor* [also: furegrelate sodium]
furegrelate sodium USAN *thromboxane synthetase inhibitor* [also: furegrelate]
furethidine INN, BAN
furfenorex INN
furfuryltrimethylammonium iodide [see: furtrethonium iodide]
furidarone INN
furmethoxadone INN
furobufen USAN, INN *anti-inflammatory*
furodazole USAN, INN *anthelmintic*
furofenac INN
furomazine INN
furosemide USAN, USP, INN, JAN *antihypertensive; loop diuretic* [also: frusemide] 20, 40, 80 mg oral; 10 mg/mL oral; 40 mg/5 mL oral; 10 mg/mL injection

furostilbestrol INN
furoxicillin [see: fumoxicillin]
Furoxone tablets, liquid ℞ *antibacterial* [furazolidone] 100 mg; 50 mg/15 mL
fursalan USAN, INN *disinfectant*
fursultiamine INN
furterene INN
furtrethonium iodide INN
furtrimethonium iodide [see: furtrethonium iodide]
fusafungine INN, BAN
fusidate sodium USAN *antibacterial*
fusidic acid USAN, INN, BAN *antibacterial*
fusidic acid, sodium salt [see: fusidate sodium]
FUVAC (5-FU, vinblastine, Adriamycin, cyclophosphamide) *chemotherapy protocol*
fuzlocillin INN, BAN
fytic acid INN
FZ (flutamide, Zoladex) *chemotherapy protocol*

⁶⁷Ga [see: gallium citrate Ga 67]
gabapentin USAN, INN *anticonvulsant; investigational (orphan) for amyotrophic lateral sclerosis*
Gabbromicina ℞ *investigational (orphan) for tuberculosis, Mycobacterium avium complex, and visceral leishmaniasis* [aminosidine]
gabexate INN
Gabitril Filmtabs (film-coated tablets) ℞ *anticonvulsant adjunct* [tiagabine HCl] 4, 12, 16, 20 mg ☑ Carbatrol
gaboxadol INN
gadobenate dimeglumine USAN *MRI diagnostic aid* [also: gadobenic acid]
gadobenic acid INN *MRI diagnostic aid* [also: gadobenate dimeglumine]
gadobutrol INN *investigational aid for MRI*

gadodiamide USAN, INN, BAN *parenteral MRI contrast medium*
gadolinium *element (Gd)*
gadolinium texaphyrin (Gd-Tex) *investigational (Phase I/II) radiation sensitizer for brain metastases*
Gadolite oral suspension ℞ *investigational diagnostic aid*
gadopenamide INN
gadopentetate dimeglumine USAN *parenteral MRI contrast medium* [also: gadopentetic acid]
gadopentetic acid INN, BAN *parenteral MRI contrast medium* [also: gadopentetate dimeglumine]
gadoteric acid INN
gadoteridol USAN, INN, BAN *MRI contrast medium*

gadoversetamide USAN, INN *MRI contrast medium for brain, head, and spine imaging*

gadoxanum USAN *gadolinium-xanthan gum complex; diagnostic aid*

gadozelite USAN *gadolinium zeolite complex; diagnostic aid*

GA-EPO (gene-activated erythropoietin) [see: erythropoietin, gene-activated]

gaiactamine [see: guaiactamine]

gaietamine [see: guaiactamine]

galactagogues *a class of agents that promote or increase the flow of breast milk* [also called: lactagogues]

galactochitosan *investigational immune system stimulant and anticancer therapy*

galactose *ultrasound contrast medium*

galamustine INN

galangal (*Alpinia galanga; A. officinarum*) *rhizomes medicinal herb for diuresis, fungal infections, gas, hypertension, tumors, ulcers, and worms; also used as an antiplatelet agent*

galantamine INN *investigational (Phase III) cognition enhancer for Alzheimer's disease*

galantamine hydrobromide *cognition enhancer*

galanthamine [see: galantamine]

Galardin ℞ *investigational (orphan) matrix metalloproteinase (MMP) inhibitor for corneal ulcers* [ilomastat]

galdansetron INN, BAN *antiemetic* [also: galdansetron HCl]

galdansetron HCl USAN *antiemetic* [also: galdansetron]

Galeopsis tetrahit *medicinal herb* [see: hemp nettle]

Galium aparine; G. verum *medicinal herb* [see: bedstraw]

Galium odoratum *medicinal herb* [see: sweet woodruff]

gallamine BAN *neuromuscular blocker* [also: gallamine triethiodide]

gallamine triethiodide USP, INN *neuromuscular blocker; muscle relaxant* [also: gallamine]

gallamone triethiodide [see: gallamine triethiodide]

gallic acid NF

gallic acid, bismuth basic salt [see: bismuth subgallate]

gallium *element (Ga)*

gallium (⁶⁷Ga) citrate INN *radiopaque contrast medium; radioactive agent* [also: gallium citrate Ga 67]

gallium citrate Ga 67 USAN, USP *radiopaque contrast medium; radioactive agent* [also: gallium (⁶⁷Ga) citrate]

gallium nitrate USAN *bone resorption inhibitor for hypercalcemia of malignancy (orphan)*

gallium nitrate nonahydrate [see: gallium nitrate]

gallopamil INN, BAN

gallotannic acid [see: tannic acid]

gallstone solubilizing agents *a class of drugs that dissolve gallstones*

galosemide INN

galtifenin INN

Galzin capsules ℞ *copper blocking/complexing agent for Wilson's disease (orphan)* [zinc acetate] 25, 50 mg

Gamastan IM injection (discontinued 1996) ℞ *passive immunizing agent* [immune globulin] 2, 10 mL ☒ Garamycin

gamfexine USAN, INN *antidepressant*

Gamimune N IV infusion ℞ *passive immunizing agent for HIV, ITP, and BMT; infection prophylaxis in pediatric HIV (orphan); investigational (orphan) for myocarditis and juvenile rheumatoid arthritis* [immune globulin] 5%, 10%

gamma benzene hexachloride [now: lindane]

gamma globulin [see: globulin, immune]

gamma hydroxybutyrate (GHB) *a CNS depressant used as an anesthetic in some countries, produced and abused as a "date rape" street drug in the U.S.; investigational (orphan) for narcolepsy, cataplexy, sleep paralysis, and hypnagogic hallucinations* [the sodium salt is medically known as sodium oxybate]

gamma oryzanol; gamma-oz *medicinal herb* [see: rice bran oil]

Gammagard S/D freeze-dried powder for IV infusion R *passive immunizing agent for HIV, idiopathic thrombocytopenic purpura (ITP), B-cell chronic lymphocytic leukemia, and Kawasaki syndrome* [immune globulin, solvent/detergent treated] 50 mg/mL

gamma-hydroxybutyrate sodium [see: sodium oxybate]

gamma-linolenic acid (GLA) *investigational (orphan) for juvenile rheumatoid arthritis*

gammaphos [now: ethiofos]

Gammar IM injection (discontinued 1996) R *immunizing agent* [immune globulin] 2, 10 mL

Gammar-IV powder for IV infusion (replaced with Gammar-P IV in 1996; P is for "pasteurized") R *immunizing agent* [immune globulin] 5%

Gammar-P IV powder for IV infusion R *passive immunizing agent and immunomodulator for HIV* [immune globulin, pasteurized] 5%

gamma-vinyl GABA (gamma-aminobutyric acid) [see: vigabatrin]

gamolenic acid INN, BAN

Gamulin Rh IM injection R *obstetric Rh factor immunity suppressant* [Rh$_0$(D) immune globulin] 300 μg

ganaxolone USAN *neuroactive steroid; investigational (orphan) for infantile spasms; investigational (Phase II) for migraine and adult epilepsy*

ganciclovir USAN, INN, BAN *antiviral; ocular implant for cytomegalovirus retinitis (orphan); investigational (Phase I/II) for HIV prophylaxis* [also: ganciclovir sodium]

ganciclovir sodium USAN *antiviral* [also: ganciclovir]

ganciclovir sodium & cytomegalovirus immune globulin intravenous (CMV-IGIV) *investigational (orphan) for cytomegalovirus pneumonia in bone marrow transplant patients*

ganglefene INN

gangliosides, sodium salts *orphan status withdrawn 1996*

ganirelix INN *gonad-stimulating principle* [also: ganirelix acetate]

ganirelix acetate USAN *gonad-stimulating principle* [also: ganirelix]

Ganite IV infusion R *bone resorption inhibitor for hypercalcemia of malignancy (orphan)* [gallium nitrate] 25 mg/mL

Gantanol tablets R *broad-spectrum sulfonamide bacteriostatic* [sulfamethoxazole] 500 mg

Gantrisin eye drops (discontinued 1995) R *ophthalmic bacteriostatic* [sulfisoxazole diolamine] 4% ② Gantanol

Gantrisin pediatric suspension (discontinued 1996) R *broad-spectrum bacteriostatic* [sulfisoxazole acetyl] 500 mg/5 mL

Gantrisin tablets (discontinued 1996) R *broad-spectrum bacteriostatic* [sulfisoxazole] 500 mg

gapicomine INN

gapromidine INN

Garamicina (Mexican name for U.S. product Garamycin)

Garamycin cream, ointment R *topical antibiotic* [gentamicin sulfate] 0.1% ② Gamastan; kanamycin; Terramycin; Theramycin

Garamycin eye drops, ophthalmic ointment R *topical ophthalmic antibiotic* [gentamicin sulfate] 3 mg/mL; 3 mg/g

Garamycin intrathecal injection (discontinued 1998) R *aminoglycoside antibiotic* [gentamicin sulfate] 2 mg/mL

Garamycin IV or IM injection R *aminoglycoside antibiotic* [gentamicin sulfate] 40 mg/mL

Garamycin Pediatric IV or IM injection (discontinued 1998) R *aminoglycoside antibiotic* [gentamicin sulfate] 10 mg/mL

garcinia (Garcinia cambogia) fruit *medicinal herb for appetite suppressant, thermogenesis, and weight control*

garden nightshade *medicinal herb* [see: bittersweet nightshade]

garden patience *medicinal herb* [see: yellow dock]

Gardrin R *investigational treatment for acute peptic ulcers* [enprostil]

Garfield; Garfield Plus Extra C
chewable tablets OTC *vitamin supplement* [multiple vitamins; folic acid]
±•0.3 mg

Garfield Complete with Minerals
chewable tablets OTC *vitamin/mineral/iron supplement* [multiple vitamins & minerals; iron; folic acid; biotin] ±•18•0.4•0.04 mg

Garfield Plus Iron chewable tablets OTC *vitamin/iron supplement* [multiple vitamins; iron; folic acid] ±•15•0.3 mg

garget *medicinal herb* [see: pokeweed]

garlic (Allium sativum) bulb *medicinal herb for asthma, cancer immunity, diabetes, digestive disorders, ear infections, flatulence, hypercholesterolemia, hypertension, and infectious diseases*

gas gangrene antitoxin, pentavalent

gas gangrene antitoxin, polyvalent
[see: gas gangrene antitoxin, pentavalent]

Gas Permeable Daily Cleaner solution OTC *cleaning solution for rigid gas permeable contact lenses*

Gas Relief chewable tablets, drops OTC *antiflatulent* [simethicone] 80, 125 mg; 40 mg/0.6 mL

Gas-Ban tablets OTC *antacid; antiflatulent* [calcium carbonate; simethicone] 300•40 mg

Gas-Ban DS liquid OTC *antacid; antiflatulent* [aluminum hydroxide; magnesium hydroxide; simethicone] 400•400•40 mg/5 mL

gastric acid inhibitors [see: proton pump inhibitors]

gastric mucin BAN

Gastrimmune ℞ *investigational (Phase III) synthetic peptide vaccine for gastrointestinal cancers*

Gastroccult slide test for professional use *in vitro diagnostic aid for gastric occult blood*

Gastrocrom capsules (discontinued 1999) ℞ *mastocytosis treatment (orphan)* [cromolyn sodium] 100 mg

Gastrocrom oral solution ℞ *mastocytosis treatment (orphan); investigational*

prophylactic treatment for food allergies [cromolyn sodium] 100 mg/5 mL

Gastrografin oral solution ℞ *radiopaque contrast medium for gastrointestinal imaging* [diatrizoate meglumine; diatrizoate sodium (48.29% total iodine)] 660•100 mg/mL (367 mg/mL)

GastroMARK oral suspension ℞ *MRI contrast medium for upper GI tract imaging* [ferumoxsil] 175 μg iron/mL

Gastrosed drops, tablets ℞ *GI antispasmodic; anticholinergic* [hyoscyamine sulfate] 0.125 mg/mL; 0.125 mg

Gastro-Test string capsules for professional use *in vitro diagnostic aid for GI disorders*

Gastrozepine ℞ *investigational (NDA filed) treatment for peptic ulcers* [pirenzepine HCl]

Gas-X chewable tablets, softgels OTC *antiflatulent* [simethicone] 80, 125 mg; 125 mg

gatifloxacin USAN *investigational (NDA filed) broad-spectrum fluoroquinolone antibiotic*

gaultheria oil [see: methyl salicylate]

Gaultheria procumbens *medicinal herb* [see: wintergreen]

gauze, absorbent USP *surgical aid*

gauze, petrolatum USP *surgical aid*

gauze bandage [see: bandage, gauze]

gavestinel USAN *N-methyl-D-aspartate (NMDA) receptor antagonist for stroke*

Gaviscon liquid OTC *antacid* [aluminum hydroxide; magnesium carbonate] 31.7•119.3 mg/5 mL

Gaviscon; Gaviscon-2 chewable tablets OTC *antacid* [aluminum hydroxide; magnesium trisilicate] 80•20 mg; 160•40 mg

Gaviscon Relief Formula chewable tablets, liquid OTC *antacid* [aluminum hydroxide; magnesium carbonate] 160•105 mg; 254•237.5 mg/5 mL

G-CSF (granulocyte colony-stimulating factor) [see: filgrastim]

Gd-Tex (gadolinium texaphyrin) [q.v.]

gedocarnil INN *investigational treatment of central nervous system disorders*

Gee-Gee tablets OTC *expectorant* [guaifenesin] 200 mg

gefarnate INN, BAN

gelatin NF *encapsulating, suspending, binding and coating agent*

gelatin film, absorbable USP *topical local hemostat for surgery*

gelatin powder, absorbable *topical local hemostat for surgery*

gelatin solution, special intravenous [see: polygeline]

gelatin sponge, absorbable USP *topical local hemostat for surgery*

gelcaps (dosage form) *soft gelatin capsules*

Gelfilm; Gelfilm Ophthalmic ℞ *topical local hemostat for surgery* [absorbable gelatin film]

Gelfoam powder ℞ *topical local hemostat for surgery* [absorbable gelatin powder] ② Ger-O-Foam

Gelfoam sponge, packs, dental packs, prostatectomy cones ℞ *topical local hemostat for surgery* [absorbable gelatin sponge] ② Ger-O-Foam

Gel-Kam gel ℞ *topical dental caries preventative* [stannous fluoride] 0.4%

Gelpirin tablets OTC *analgesic; antipyretic; anti-inflammatory* [acetaminophen; aspirin, buffered; caffeine] 125•240•32 mg

Gelpirin-CCF tablets OTC *decongestant; antihistamine; analgesic; expectorant* [phenylpropanolamine HCl; chlorpheniramine maleate; acetaminophen; guaifenesin] 12.5•1•325•25 mg

Gelseal (trademarked dosage form) *soft gelatin capsule*

gelsemium *(Bignonia sempervirens; Gelsemium nitidum; G. sempervirens)* plant *medicinal herb for asthma, neuralgia, and respiratory disorders; not generally regarded as safe and effective as it is highly toxic*

gelsolin, recombinant human *investigational (orphan) for respiratory symptoms of cystic fibrosis and bronchiectasis*

Gel-Tin gel OTC *topical dental caries preventative* [stannous fluoride] 0.4%

Gelusil chewable tablets OTC *antacid; antiflatulent* [aluminum hydroxide; magnesium hydroxide; simethicone] 200•200•25 mg

Gelusil liquid (discontinued 1996) OTC *antacid; antiflatulent* [aluminum hydroxide; magnesium hydroxide; simethicone] 200•200•25 mg/5 mL

GEM-231 *investigational (Phase I) anticancer agent for treatment of solid tumors*

GEM-92 tablets ℞ *investigational mixed backbone antisense compound for AIDS and HIV infection*

gemazocine INN

gemcadiol USAN, INN *antihyperlipoproteinemic*

gemcitabine USAN, INN, BAN *antimetabolite antineoplastic*

gemcitabine HCl USAN *antineoplastic for advanced or metastatic pancreatic and non-small cell lung cancers*

Gemcor film-coated tablets ℞ *antihyperlipidemic for hypercholesterolemia* [gemfibrozil] 600 mg

gemeprost USAN, INN, BAN *prostaglandin*

gemfibrozil USAN, USP, INN, BAN *antihyperlipidemic for hypertriglyceridemia and coronary heart disease* 600 mg oral

Gemzar powder for IV infusion ℞ *antineoplastic for advanced or metastatic pancreatic and non-small cell lung cancers* [gemcitabine HCl] 20 mg/mL

Genabid timed-release capsules (discontinued 1997) ℞ *peripheral vasodilator; smooth muscle relaxant for cerebral, myocardial, and peripheral ischemias* [papaverine HCl] 150 mg

Genac tablets OTC *decongestant; antihistamine* [pseudoephedrine HCl; triprolidine HCl] 60•2.5 mg

Genacol tablets OTC *antitussive; decongestant; antihistamine; analgesic* [dextromethorphan hydrobromide; phenylpropanolamine HCl; chlorpheniramine maleate; acetaminophen] 10•30•2•325 mg

Genagesic tablets (discontinued 1995) ℞ *narcotic analgesic* [propoxyphene HCl; acetaminophen] 65•650 mg

Genahist capsules, tablets (discontinued 1997) ℞ *antihistamine* [diphenhydramine HCl] 25 mg; 25 mg

Genahist liquid OTC *antihistamine* [diphenhydramine HCl] 12.5 mg/5 mL

Gen-Allerate tablets OTC *antihistamine* [chlorpheniramine maleate] 4 mg

Genamin Cold syrup OTC *decongestant; antihistamine* [phenylpropanolamine HCl; chlorpheniramine maleate] 6.25•1 mg/5 mL

Genapap tablets, caplets OTC *analgesic; antipyretic* [acetaminophen] 325, 500 mg; 500 mg

Genapap, Children's chewable tablets, elixir OTC *analgesic; antipyretic* [acetaminophen] 80 mg; 160 mg/5 mL

Genapap, Infants' drops OTC *analgesic; antipyretic* [acetaminophen] 100 mg/mL

Genaphed tablets OTC *nasal decongestant* [pseudoephedrine HCl] 30 mg

Genasal nasal spray OTC *nasal decongestant* [oxymetazoline HCl] 0.05%

Genasoft Plus softgels OTC *stimulant laxative; stool softener* [casanthranol; docusate sodium] 30•100 mg

Genaspor cream OTC *topical antifungal* [tolnaftate] 1%

Genatap elixir OTC *decongestant; antihistamine* [phenylpropanolamine HCl; brompheniramine maleate] 12.5•2 mg/5 mL ⊚ Genapap

Genaton chewable tablets OTC *antacid* [aluminum hydroxide; magnesium trisilicate] 80•20 mg

Genaton liquid OTC *antacid* [aluminum hydroxide; magnesium carbonate] 31.7•137.3 mg/5 mL

Genaton, Extra Strength chewable tablets OTC *antacid* [aluminum hydroxide; magnesium carbonate] 160•105 mg

Genatuss syrup OTC *expectorant* [guaifenesin; alcohol 3.5%] 100 mg/5 mL

Genatuss DM syrup OTC *antitussive; expectorant* [dextromethorphan hydrobromide; guaifenesin] 10•100 mg/5 mL

Gen-bee with C caplets OTC *vitamin supplement* [multiple B vitamins; vitamin C] ≐•300 mg

Gencalc 600 film-coated tablets OTC *calcium supplement* [calcium carbonate] 1.5 g

Gencold sustained-release capsules OTC *decongestant; antihistamine* [phenylpropanolamine HCl; chlorpheniramine maleate] 75•8 mg

Gendecon tablets OTC *decongestant; antihistamine; analgesic* [phenylephrine HCl; chlorpheniramine maleate; acetaminophen] 5•2•325 mg

Gendex 75 IV infusion ℞ *plasma volume expander for shock due to hemorrhage, burns, or surgery* [dextran 75] 6%

Genebs tablets, caplets OTC *analgesic; antipyretic* [acetaminophen] 325, 500 mg; 500 mg

Generet-500 timed-release tablets OTC *hematinic* [ferrous sulfate; multiple B vitamins; sodium ascorbate] 105•≐•500 mg ⊚ Gentap

Generix-T tablets OTC *vitamin/mineral/ iron supplement* [multiple vitamins & minerals; iron] ≐•15 mg

GenESA computer-controlled IV infusion device ("GenESA System") ℞ *cardiac stressor for diagnosis of coronary artery disease* [arbutamine HCl] 0.05 mg/mL

Genevax-HIV-Px ℞ *investigational (Phase I/II) vaccine for HIV*

Geneye eye drops OTC *topical ophthalmic decongestant and vasoconstrictor* [tetrahydrozoline HCl] 0.05%

Geneye AC Allergy Formula eye drops (discontinued 1997) OTC *topical ophthalmic decongestant and astringent* [tetrahydrozoline HCl; zinc sulfate] 0.05%•0.25%

Geneye Extra eye drops OTC *topical ophthalmic decongestant, vasoconstrictor, and lubricant* [tetrahydrozoline HCl; polytheylene glycol 400] 0.05%•1%

Genista tinctoria *medicinal herb* [see: dyer's broom]

Genistein [see: EGF-Genistein]

Genite liquid OTC *antitussive; decongestant; antihistamine; analgesic* [dextromethorphan hydrobromide; pseudoephedrine HCl; doxylamine succinate; acetaminophen; alcohol 25%] 5•10•1.25•167 mg/5 mL

Gen-K powder ℞ *potassium supplement* [potassium chloride] 20 mEq/packet

genophyllin [see: aminophylline]

Genoptic eye drops ℞ *topical ophthalmic antibiotic* [gentamicin sulfate] 3 mg/mL

Genoptic S.O.P. ophthalmic ointment ℞ *topical ophthalmic antibiotic* [gentamicin sulfate] 3 mg/g

Genora 0.5/35; Genora 1/35 tablets ℞ *monophasic oral contraceptive* [norethindrone; ethinyl estradiol] 0.5 mg•35 μg; 1 mg•35 μg

Genora 1/50 tablets ℞ *monophasic oral contraceptive* [norethindrone; mestranol] 1 mg•50 μg

Genotonorm (name changed to Genotropin upon release in 1995)

Genotropin powder for subcu injection ℞ *growth hormone for children or adults with congenital or endogenous growth hormone deficiency, children with Turner syndrome or renal-induced growth failure, or AIDS-wasting syndrome* (orphan) [somatropin] 1.5, 5.8 mg (4, 15 IU) per mL

Genpril film-coated tablets, film-coated caplets OTC *nonsteroidal anti-inflammatory drug (NSAID); antiarthritic; analgesic* [ibuprofen] 200 mg

Genprin tablets OTC *analgesic; antipyretic; anti-inflammatory; antirheumatic* [aspirin] 325 mg

Gensan tablets OTC *analgesic; antipyretic; anti-inflammatory* [aspirin; caffeine] 400•32 mg

Gentacidin eye drops, ophthalmic ointment ℞ *topical ophthalmic antibiotic* [gentamicin sulfate] 3 mg/mL; 3 mg/g

Gentak eye drops, ophthalmic ointment ℞ *topical ophthalmic antibiotic* [gentamicin sulfate] 3 mg/mL; 3 mg/g

gentamicin BAN *aminoglycoside antibiotic* [also: gentamicin sulfate] ② Jenamicin; kanamycin

gentamicin sulfate USAN, USP *aminoglycoside antibiotic* [also: gentamicin] 3 mg/mL eye drops; 3 mg/g topical; 0.1% topical; 10, 40 mg/mL injection

gentamicin sulfate, liposomal *investigational* (orphan) *for disseminated Mycobacterium avium-intracellulare infection*

gentamicin-impregnated polymethyl methacrylate (PMMA) beads *investigational* (orphan) *for chronic osteomyelitis*

gentian (Gentiana lutea) root *medicinal herb for aiding digestion, appetite stimulation, arthritis, hysteria, jaundice, liver disorders, and sore throat*

gentian violet USP *topical anti-infective/antifungal* [also: methylrosanilinium chloride] 1%, 2%

gentisic acid ethanolamide NF *complexing agent*

Gentlax granules OTC *stimulant laxative* [senna concentrate] 326 mg/tsp.

Gentlax S tablets OTC *stimulant laxative; stool softener* [docusate sodium; sennosides] 50•8.6 mg

Gentran 40 IV injection ℞ *plasma volume expander for shock due to hemorrhage, burns, or surgery* [dextran 40] 10%

Gentran 70 IV infusion ℞ *plasma volume expander for shock due to hemorrhage, burns, or surgery* [dextran 70] 6%

Gentran 75 IV infusion (discontinued 1996) ℞ *plasma volume expander for shock due to hemorrhage, burns, or surgery* [dextran 75] 6%

Gentz anorectal wipes (discontinued 1995) OTC *topical local anesthetic; astringent* [pramoxine HCl; alcloxa; hamamelis water; propylene glycol] 1%•0.2%•50%•10%

Genvir ℞ *investigational* (Phase III) *controlled-release form for acute genital herpes* [acyclovir]

Genvite tablets OTC *antianemic* [ferrous fumarate; multiple vitamins]

Gen-Xene tablets R *anxiolytic; minor tranquilizer; anticonvulsant adjunct; alcohol withdrawal aid* [chlorazepate dipotassium] 3.75, 7.5, 15 mg

Geocillin film-coated tablets R *extended-spectrum penicillin antibiotic* [carbenicillin indanyl sodium] 382 mg

gepefrine INN

gepirone INN *tranquilizer; anxiolytic; antidepressant* [also: gepirone HCl]

gepirone HCl USAN *tranquilizer; anxiolytic; antidepressant* [also: gepirone]

Geranium maculatum medicinal herb [see: alum root]

2-geranylhydroquinone [see: geroquinol]

Gerardia pedicularia medicinal herb [see: feverweed]

Geravim elixir OTC *vitamin/mineral supplement* [multiple B vitamins & minerals] ±

Geravite elixir OTC *geriatric vitamin supplement* [multiple B vitamins] ±

Gerber Baby Formula with Iron liquid, powder (discontinued 1997) OTC *total or supplementary infant feeding*

Gerber Baby Low Iron Formula liquid, powder OTC *total or supplementary infant feeding*

Gerber Soy Formula liquid (discontinued 1997) OTC *hypoallergenic infant formula* [soy protein formula]

Gerber Soy Formula powder OTC *hypoallergenic infant formula* [soy protein formula]

Geref powder for IV injection R *diagnostic aid for pituitary function; treatment for growth hormone deficiency (orphan), anovulation, and AIDS-related weight loss* [sermorelin acetate] 50 μg

Geridium tablets (discontinued 1997) R *urinary analgesic* [phenazopyridine HCl] 100, 200 mg

Gerimal sublingual tablets, tablets R *cognition adjuvant for age-related mental capacity decline* [ergoloid mesylates] 0.5, 1 mg; 1 mg

Gerimed film-coated tablets OTC *geriatric vitamin/mineral supplement* [multiple vitamins & minerals] ±

Geriot film-coated tablets OTC *hematinic; vitamin/mineral supplement* [carbonyl iron; multiple vitamins & minerals; folic acid; biotin] 50 mg• ±•0.4 mg•45 μg

Geriplex-FS Kapseals (capsules) (discontinued 1995) OTC *geriatric dietary supplement* [multiple vitamins & minerals] ±

Geritol Complete tablets OTC *vitamin/mineral/iron supplement* [multiple vitamins & minerals; ferrous fumarate; folic acid; biotin] ±•18 mg• 0.4 mg•45 μg

Geritol Extend caplets OTC *vitamin/mineral/iron supplement* [multiple vitamins & minerals; ferrous fumarate; folic acid] ±•10•0.2 mg

Geritol Tonic liquid OTC *hematinic* [ferric pyrophosphate; multiple B vitamins; alcohol 12%] 18• ± mg/15 mL

Geritonic liquid OTC *hematinic* [ferric ammonium citrate; liver fraction 1; multiple B vitamins & minerals; alcohol 20%] 105•375• ± mg/15 mL

Gerivite liquid OTC *geriatric vitamin/mineral supplement* [multiple B vitamins & minerals; alcohol 18%] ±

Gerivites tablets OTC *hematinic; vitamin/mineral supplement* [ferrous sulfate; multiple vitamins & minerals; folic acid] 50• ±•0.4 mg

German valerian medicinal herb [see: valerian]

Germanin (available only from the Centers for Disease Control) R *antiparasitic for African trypanosomiasis and onchocerciasis* [suramin sodium]

germanium element (Ge)

germicides a class of agents that destroy micro-organisms [see also: antiseptics; disinfectants]

geroquinol INN

Geroton Forte liquid OTC *geriatric vitamin/mineral supplement* [multiple B vitamins & minerals; alcohol 13.5%] ±

gesarol [see: chlorophenothane]
gestaclone USAN, INN *progestin*
gestadienol INN
gestanin [see: allyloestrenol]
gestodene USAN, INN, BAN *progestin*
gestonorone caproate USAN, INN *progestin* [also: gestronol]
gestrinone USAN, INN *progestin*
gestronol BAN *progestin* [also: gestonorone caproate]
Get Better Bear Sore Throat Pops OTC *throat emollient and protectant* [pectin] 19 mg
Gets-It liquid OTC *topical keratolytic* [salicylic acid; zinc chloride; alcohol 28%]
gevotroline INN *antipsychotic* [also: gevotroline HCl]
gevotroline HCl USAN *antipsychotic* [also: gevotroline]
Gevrabon liquid OTC *vitamin/mineral supplement* [multiple B vitamins & minerals; alcohol 18%] ±
Gevral tablets OTC *vitamin/mineral/iron supplement* [multiple vitamins & minerals; ferrous fumarate; folic acid] ±•18 mg•0.4 mg
Gevral Protein powder OTC *oral protein supplement* [calcium caseinate; sucrose]
Gevral T film-coated tablets (discontinued 1995) OTC *vitamin/mineral/iron supplement* [ferrous fumarate; multiple vitamins & minerals; folic acid] 27•±•0.4 mg
G-F 20 [see: hylan G-F 20]
GG-Cen capsules OTC *expectorant* [guaifenesin] 200 mg
GHB (gamma hydroxybutyrate) *a CNS depressant used as an anesthetic in some countries, produced and abused as a "date rape" street drug in the U.S.* [the sodium salt is medically known as sodium oxybate]
GHRF; GH-RF (growth hormone-releasing factor) [q.v.]
Gilead, balm of *medicinal herb* [see: balm of Gilead]
ginger (Zingiber officinale) root *medicinal herb for childhood diseases, colds, colic, dizziness, fever, flu, gas*

pains, headache, indigestion, morning sickness, nausea, poor circulation, toothache, and vestibular disorders
ginger, wild *medicinal herb* [see: wild ginger]
ginkgo (Ginkgo biloba) leaves *medicinal herb for Alzheimer's disease, antioxidant, anxiety, asthma, attention deficit disorders, chilblains, cerebral insufficiency, dementia, dizziness, memory loss, poor circulation, Raynaud's disease, stroke, and tinnitus*
ginseng (Panax spp.) root *medicinal herb for age spots, blood diseases, depression, hemorrhage, increasing endurance and longevity, and stress; also used as an aphrodisiac* [also see: Siberian ginseng]
ginseng, blue; yellow ginseng *medicinal herb* [see: blue cohosh]
giparmen INN
giractide INN
girisopam INN
gitalin NF [also: gitalin amorphous]
gitalin amorphous INN [also: gitalin]
gitaloxin INN
gitoformate INN
gitoxin 16-formate [see: gitaloxin]
gitoxin pentaacetate [see: pengitoxin]
GLA (gamma-linolenic acid)
glacial acetic acid [see: acetic acid, glacial]
glafenine INN, DCF, JAN
Glandosane oral spray OTC *saliva substitute*
glaphenine [see: glafenine]
glatiramer acetate USAN *immunomodulator for relapsing-remitting multiple sclerosis (orphan)* [formerly known as copolymer 1]
Glauber salt [see: sodium sulfate]
glaucarubin
Glaucon Drop-Tainers (eye drops) ℞ *topical antiglaucoma agent* [epinephrine HCl] 1%, 2%
GlaucTabs tablets ℞ *carbonic anhydrase inhibitor for glaucoma* [methazolamide] 25, 50 mg
glaze, pharmaceutical NF *tablet-coating agent*

glaziovine INN

glemanserin USAN, INN *anxiolytic*

gleptoferron USAN, INN, BAN *veterinary hematinic*

Gliadel wafers ℞ *nitrosourea-type alkylating antineoplastic cerebral implants for excised brain tumors (orphan)* [carmustine in a polifeprosan 20 carrier] 7.7 mg

gliamilide USAN, INN *antidiabetic*

glibenclamide INN, BAN *sulfonylurea antidiabetic* [also: glyburide]

glibornuride USAN, INN, BAN *antidiabetic*

glibutimine INN

glicaramide INN

glicetanile INN *antidiabetic* [also: glicetanile sodium]

glicetanile sodium USAN *antidiabetic* [also: glicetanile]

gliclazide INN, BAN *sulfonylurea antidiabetic*

glicondamide INN

glidazamide INN

gliflumide USAN, INN *antidiabetic*

glimepiride USAN, INN, BAN *sulfonylurea antidiabetic*

glipentide [see: glisentide]

glipizide USAN, INN, BAN *sulfonylurea antidiabetic* 5, 10 mg oral

gliquidone INN, BAN

glisamuride INN

glisentide INN

glisindamide INN

glisolamide INN

glisoxepide INN, BAN

globin zinc insulin INN [also: insulin, globin zinc]

globulin, immune USP *passive immunizing agent for HIV, ITP, B-cell CLL, and BMT; infection prophylaxis in pediatric HIV (orphan); investigational (orphan) for myocarditis and juvenile rheumatoid arthritis*

globulin, immune human serum [now: globulin, immune]

Glossets (trademarked form) *sublingual or rectal administration*

gloxazone USAN, INN, BAN *veterinary anaplasmodastat*

gloximonam USAN, INN *antibacterial*

GlucaGen Diagnostic Kit injection ℞ *to inhibit GI tract movement during radiographic procedures* [glucagon, recombinant] 1 mg

GlucaGen Emergency Kit injection ℞ *emergency treatment for hypoglycemic crisis* [glucagon, recombinant] 1 mg

glucagon USP, INN, BAN *antidiabetic; glucose elevating agent; diagnostic aid for GI imaging*

Glucagon Diagnostic Kit IM or IV injection ℞ *to inhibit GI tract movement during radiographic procedures* [glucagon, recombinant] 1 mg (1 U)

Glucagon Emergency Kit subcu, IM, or IV injection ℞ *emergency treatment for hypoglycemic crisis* [glucagon, recombinant] 1 mg (1 U)

glucalox INN [also: glycalox]

glucametacin INN

D-**glucaric acid, calcium salt tetrahydrate** [see: calcium saccharate]

gluceptate USAN, USP, INN, BAN *combining name for radicals or groups*

gluceptate sodium USAN *pharmaceutic aid*

Glucerna ready-to-use liquid OTC *enteral nutritional therapy for abnormal glucose tolerance*

D-**glucitol** [see: sorbitol]

D-**glucitol hexanicotinate** [see: sorbinicate]

β-**glucocerebrosidase, macrophage-targeted** [see: alglucerase]

glucocerebrosidase, recombinant retroviral vector *investigational (orphan) enzyme replacement for types I, II, or III Gaucher's disease*

glucocerebrosidase-β-glucosidase [see: alglucerase]

glucocorticoids *a class of adrenal cortical steroids that modify the body's immune response*

Glucofilm reagent strips for home use OTC *in vitro diagnostic aid for blood glucose*

glucoheptonic acid, calcium salt [see: calcium gluceptate]

glucomannan (*Amorphophallus konjac*) root *medicinal herb for constipa-*

tion, *diverticular disease, hemorrhoids, hypercholesterolemia, and obesity; not generally regarded as safe and effective for diabetics as it may result in altered insulin requirements or hypoglycemia*

Glucometer Encore; Glucometer Elite reagent strips for home use OTC *in vitro diagnostic aid for blood glucose*

D-**gluconic acid, calcium salt** [see: calcium gluconate]

D-**gluconic acid, magnesium salt** [see: magnesium gluconate]

D-**gluconic acid, monopotassium salt** [see: potassium gluconate]

D-**gluconic acid, monosodium salt** [see: sodium gluconate]

Glucophage film-coated tablets ℞ *biguanide antidiabetic* [metformin HCl] 500, 850 mg

β-D-**glucopyranuronamide** [see: glucuronamide]

glucosamine USAN, INN *pharmaceutic aid*

glucosamine sulfate *natural remedy for osteoarthritis*

d-**glucose** [see: dextrose]

glucose, liquid NF *tablet binder and coating agent; antihypoglycemic; diagnostic aid for diabetes* ② Glutose

Glucose & Ketone Urine Test reagent strips (discontinued 1995) *in vitro diagnostic aid for multiple urine products*

d-**glucose monohydrate** [see: dextrose]

glucose oxidase

glucose polymers *caloric replacement*

Glucose-40 ophthalmic ointment (discontinued 1999) ℞ *corneal edema-reducing agent* [glucose] 40%

Glucostix reagent strips for home use OTC *in vitro diagnostic aid for blood glucose*

glucosulfamide INN

glucosulfone INN

glucosylceramidase [see: alglucerase]

Glucotrol tablets ℞ *sulfonylurea antidiabetic* [glipizide] 5, 10 mg

Glucotrol XL extended-release tablets ℞ *sulfonylurea antidiabetic* [glipizide] 5, 10 mg

glucurolactone INN

glucuronamide INN, BAN

Glukor powder for IM injection (discontinued 1995) ℞ *hormone for prepubertal cryptorchidism and hypogonadism; ovulation stimulant* [chorionic gonadotropin] 200 U/mL

glunicate INN

gluside [see: saccharin]

gluside, soluble [see: saccharin sodium]

glusoferron INN

glutamic acid (L-glutamic acid) USAN, INN *nonessential amino acid; symbols: Glu, E 340,* 500 mg oral

glutamic acid HCl *gastric acidifier*

glutamine (L-glutamine) *nonessential amino acid; symbols: Gln, Q* [see: levoglutamide]

glutamine & somatropin *investigational (orphan) for GI malabsorption due to short bowel syndrome*

glutaral USAN, USP, INN *disinfectant*

glutaraldehyde [see: glutaral]

Glutarex-1 powder OTC *formula for infants with glutaric aciduria type I*

Glutarex-2 powder OTC *enteral nutritional therapy for glutaric aciduria type I*

glutasin [see: glutamic acid HCl]

L-**glutathione, reduced** *investigational (orphan) for AIDS-related cachexia*

glutaurine INN

glutethimide USP, INN, BAN *sedative; sometimes abused as a street drug* 250, 500 mg oral

Glutofac tablets OTC *vitamin/mineral supplement* [multiple vitamins & minerals] ±

Glutose gel OTC *glucose elevating agent* [glucose] 40% ② glucose

Glyate syrup OTC *expectorant* [guaifenesin; alcohol 3.5%] 100 mg/5 mL

glyburide USAN *sulfonylurea antidiabetic* [also: glibenclamide] 1.25, 1.5, 2.5, 3, 4.5, 5, 6 mg oral

glybutamide [see: carbutamide]

glybuthiazol INN

glybuthizol [see: glybuthiazol]

glybuzole INN

glycalox BAN [also: glucalox]

glycerides oleiques polyoxyethylenes [see: peglicol 5 oleate]

glycerin USP *humectant; solvent; osmotic diuretic; laxative; emollient/protectant; ophthalmic moisturizer* [also: glycerol]

glycerol INN *humectant; solvent; osmotic diuretic; laxative; emollient/protectant; monoctanoin component D* [also: glycerin]

glycerol, iodinated USAN, BAN *(disapproved for use as an expectorant in 1991)*

glycerol 1-decanoate *monoctanoin component B* [see: monoctanoin]

glycerol 1,2-dioctanoate *monoctanoin component C* [see: monoctanoin]

glycerol 1-octanoate *monoctanoin component A* [see: monoctanoin]

glycerol phosphate, manganese salt [see: manganese glycerophosphate]

glyceryl behenate NF *tablet and capsule lubricant*

glyceryl borate [see: boroglycerin]

glyceryl guaiacolate [now: guaifenesin]

glyceryl monostearate NF *emulsifying agent*

glyceryl triacetate [now: triacetin]

glyceryl trierucate *investigational (orphan) for adrenoleukodystrophy* [also: glyceryl trioleate]

glyceryl trinitrate BAN *coronary vasodilator* [also: nitroglycerin]

glyceryl trioleate *investigational (orphan) for adrenoleukodystrophy* [also: glyceryl trierucate]

glycerylaminophenaquine [see: glafenine]

Glyceryl-T capsules, liquid ℞ *antiasthmatic; bronchodilator; expectorant* [theophylline; guaifenesin] 150•90 mg; 150•90 mg/15 mL

glycinato dihydroxyaluminum hydrate [see: dihydroxyaluminum aminoacetate]

glycine USP, INN *nonessential amino acid; urologic irrigant; symbols: Gly, G* [also: aminoacetic acid] 1.5%

glycine aluminum-zirconium complex [see: aluminum zirconium tetrachlorohydrex gly; aluminum zirconium trichlorohydrex gly]

Glycine max medicinal herb [see: soy]

glyclopyramide INN

glycobiarsol USP, INN [also: bismuth glycollylarsanilate]

glycocholate sodium [see: sodium glycocholate]

glycocoll [see: glycine]

Glycofed tablets OTC *decongestant; expectorant* [pseudoephedrine HCl; guaifenesin] 30•100 mg

glycol distearate USAN *thickening agent*

glycolic acid *mild exfoliant and keratolytic*

p-**glycolophenetidide** [see: fenacetinol]

glycopeptides *a class of antibiotic antineoplastics*

glycophenylate [see: mepenzolate bromide]

glycoprotein (GP) IIb/IIIa receptor antagonists *a class of platelet aggregation inhibitors for acute coronary syndrome, unstable angina, myocardial infarction, and cardiac surgery*

glycopyrrolate USAN, USP *GI antispasmodic; peptic ulcer adjunct* [also: glycopyrronium bromide] 0.2 mg/mL injection

glycopyrrone bromide [see: glycopyrrolate]

glycopyrronium bromide INN, BAN *anticholinergic* [also: glycopyrrolate]

glycosaminoglycans *a class of anticoagulants used for the prophylaxis of postoperative deep vein thrombosis (DVT)*

glycosides, cardiac *a class of cardiovascular drugs that increase the force of cardiac contractions* [also called: digitalis glycosides]

Glycotuss tablets OTC *expectorant* [guaifenesin] 100 mg ⧉ Glytuss

Glycotuss-dM tablets OTC *antitussive; expectorant* [dextromethorphan hydrobromide; guaifenesin] 10•100 mg

glycyclamide INN, BAN

glycyrrhetinic acid [see: enoxolone]

glycyrrhiza NF

Glycyrrhiza glabra; G. palidiflora; G. uralensis medicinal herb [see: licorice]

glydanile sodium [now: glicetanile sodium]

glyhexamide USAN, INN *antidiabetic*

glyhexylamide [see: metahexamide]

Glylorin ℞ *investigational (Phase III, orphan) for non-bullous congenital ichthyosiform erythroderma* [monolaurin]

glymidine BAN *antidiabetic* [also: glymidine sodium]

glymidine sodium USAN, INN *antidiabetic* [also: glymidine]

glymol [see: mineral oil]

Glynase PresTabs (micronized tablets) ℞ *sulfonylurea antidiabetic* [glyburide] 1.5, 3, 6 mg

glyoctamide USAN, INN *antidiabetic*

Gly-Oxide oral solution OTC *oral anti-inflammatory and anti-infective* [carbamide peroxide] 10%

glyparamide USAN *antidiabetic*

glyphylline [see: dyphylline]

glypinamide INN

Glypressin ℞ *investigational (orphan) for bleeding esophageal ulcers* [terlipressin]

glyprothiazol INN

glyprothizol [see: glyprothiazol]

Glyset tablets ℞ *antidiabetic agent for type 2 diabetes; α-glucosidase inhibitor that delays the digestion of dietary carbohydrates* [miglitol] 25, 50, 100 mg

glysobuzole INN [also: isobuzole]

Glytuss film-coated tablets OTC *expectorant* [guaifenesin] 200 mg ② Glycotuss

GM-CSF (granulocyte-macrophage colony-stimulating factor) [see: regramostim; sargramostim; molgramostim]

GMK *investigational (Phase III) GM2 ganglioside protein vaccine for malignant melanoma*

G-myticin cream, ointment ℞ *topical antibiotic* [gentamicin sulfate] 1 mg

Gnaphalium polycephalum; G. uliginosum medicinal herb [see: everlasting]

goatweed *medicinal herb* [see: St. John's wort]

Go-Evac powder for oral solution ℞ *pre-procedure bowel evacuant* [polyethylene glycol-electrolyte solution; electrolytes] 59 g/L

gold *element (Au)*

gold Au 198 USAN, USP *antineoplastic; liver imaging aid; radioactive agent*

gold sodium thiomalate USP *antirheumatic (50% gold)* [also: sodium aurothiomalate] 50 mg/mL injection

gold sodium thiosulfate NF [also: sodium aurotiosulfate]

gold thioglucose [see: aurothioglucose]

gold thread (*Coptis trifolia*) root *medicinal herb used as an antiphlogistic, bitter tonic, and sedative*

golden senecio *medicinal herb* [see: life root]

goldenrod (*Solidago nemoralis; S. odora; S. virgaurea*) leaves and flowering tops *medicinal herb used as an astringent, carminative, diaphoretic, diuretic, and stimulant*

goldenseal (*Hydrastis canadensis*) rhizome and root *medicinal herb used as an antibiotic and antiseptic and for internal bleeding, colon inflammation, eye infections, liver disorders, menorrhagia, mouth sores, muscular pain, sciatic pain, and vaginitis*

GoLYTELY powder for oral solution ℞ *pre-procedure bowel evacuant* [polyethylene glycol-electrolyte solution]

gonacrine [see: acriflavine]

Gonadimmune *investigational anti-gonadotropin-releasing hormone for prostate, breast, and endometrial cancer and endometriosis*

gonadorelin INN, BAN *gonad-stimulating principle* [also: gonadorelin acetate]

gonadorelin acetate USAN *gonad-stimulating principle for hypothalamic amenorrhea (orphan); diagnostic aid for fertility* [also: gonadorelin]

gonadorelin HCl USAN *gonad-stimulating principle*

gonadotrophin, chorionic INN, BAN *gonad-stimulating principle* [also: gonadotropin, chorionic]

gonadotrophin, serum INN

gonadotropin, chorionic USP *gonad-stimulating principle* [also: gonadotrophin, chorionic] 500, 1000, 2000 U/mL injection

gonadotropin, serum [see: gonadotrophin, serum]

gonadotropin-releasing hormone analogs *a class of hormonal antineoplastics*

gonadotropins *a class of hormones that stimulate the ovaries, including follicle-stimulating hormone and luteinizing hormone*

Gonak ophthalmic solution OTC *gonioscopic examination aid* [hydroxypropyl methylcellulose] 2.5% ☑ Gonic

Gonal-F subcu injection ℞ *recombinant follicle-stimulating hormone (FSH) for induction of ovulation* [follitropin alfa] 75, 150 IU

Gonic powder for IM injection ℞ *hormone for prepubertal cryptorchidism and hypogonadism; ovulation stimulant* [chorionic gonadotropin] 1000 U/mL ☑ Gonak

Goniopora **spp.** *natural material* [see: coral]

Gonioscopic Prism Solution Drop-Tainers (eye drops) OTC *agent for bonding gonioscopic prisms to eye* [hydroxyethyl cellulose]

Goniosol ophthalmic solution OTC *gonioscopic examination aid* [hydroxypropyl methylcellulose] 2.5%

Gonodecten Test Kit tube test for professional use (discontinued 1995) *in vitro diagnostic aid for Neisseria gonorrhoeae*

Gonozyme Diagnostic reagent kit for professional use *in vitro diagnostic aid for Neisseria gonorrhoeae*

GoodStart [see: Carnation GoodStart]

Goody's Headache powder OTC *analgesic; antipyretic; anti-inflammatory* [acetaminophen; aspirin; caffeine] 250•520•32.5 mg/dose

goose grass *medicinal herb* [see: bedstraw; cinquefoil]

goose hair; gosling weed *medicinal herb* [see: bedstraw]

Gordobalm OTC *topical analgesic; counterirritant; antiseptic* [methyl salicylate; menthol; camphor; alcohol 16%]

Gordochom solution ℞ *topical antifungal; antiseptic* [undecylenic acid; chloroxylenol] 25%•3%

Gordofilm liquid ℞ *topical keratolytic* [salicylic acid in flexible collodion] 16.7%

Gordogesic Creme OTC *counterirritant* [methyl salicylate] 10%

Gordon's Urea 40% cream ℞ *for removal of dystrophic nails* [urea] 40%

Gormel Creme OTC *moisturizer; emollient; keratolytic* [urea] 20%

goserelin USAN, INN, BAN *hormonal antineoplastic for prostate and breast cancer; luteinizing hormone-releasing hormone (LHRH) agonist* [also: goserelin acetate]

goserelin acetate JAN *hormonal antineoplastic for prostatic carcinoma, breast cancer, and endometriosis; luteinizing hormone-releasing hormone (LHRH) agonist* [also: goserelin]

gosling weed; goose grass; goose hair *medicinal herb* [see: bedstraw]

gossypol (*Gossypium* spp.) *seed oil medicinal herb for male and female contraception; not generally regarded as safe and effective as male sterility may be irreversible; investigational for metastatic endometrial carcinoma; investigational antiviral/interferon inducer for AIDS; investigational (orphan) for adrenal cortex cancer*

gotu kola (*Centella asiatica; Hydrocotyle asiatica*) *entire plant medicinal herb for abscesses, hypertension, contraception, leprosy, nervous breakdown, physical and mental fatigue, promoting wound healing, and rheumatism*

goutberry *medicinal herb* [see: blackberry]

govafilcon A USAN *hydrophilic contact lens material*

GP IIb/IIIa inhibitors [see: glycoprotein (GP) IIb/IIIa receptor antagonists]

gp100 adenoviral gene therapy *investigational (orphan) for metastatic melanoma*

gp120 (glycoprotein 120) antigens *investigational (Phase II) antiviral vaccine for HIV prophylaxis* [also: AIDS vaccine]

gp160 (glycoprotein 160) antigens *investigational (orphan) antiviral (therapeutic, Phase II) and vaccine (preventative, Phase I) for HIV and AIDS*

GP-500 tablets ℞ *decongestant; expectorant* [pseudoephedrine HCl; guaifenesin] 120•500 mg

GPI-1046 *investigational neurotrophic agent for treatment of Parkinson's disease*

GPI-5000 *investigational for stroke*

grace, herb of *medicinal herb* [see: rue]

Gradumet (trademarked dosage form) *controlled-release tablet*

graftskin *a living, bilayered skin construct for diabetic foot ulcers and pressure sores (the epidermal layer is living human keratinocytes; the dermal layer is living human fibroblasts)*

gramicidin USP, INN *antibacterial antibiotic*

gramicidin S INN

Graminis rhizoma *medicinal herb* [see: couch grass]

granisetron USAN, INN, BAN *antiemetic*

granisetron HCl USAN $5\text{-}HT_3$ *receptor antagonist; antiemetic/antinauseant for chemotherapy*

Granulderm aerosol spray ℞ *topical enzyme for wound debridement* [trypsin; peruvian balsam] 0.1•72.5 mg/0.82 mL

Granulex aerosol spray ℞ *topical enzyme for wound debridement* [trypsin; peruvian balsam] 0.1•72.5 mg/0.82 mL

granulocyte colony-stimulating factor (G-CSF), recombinant [see: filgrastim]

granulocyte-macrophage colony-stimulating factor (GM-CSF) [see: regramostim; sargramostim; molgramostim]

GranuMed aerosol spray ℞ *topical enzyme for wound debridement* [trypsin; peruvian balsam] 0.1•72.5 mg/0.82 mL

grape, bear's *medicinal herb* [see: uva ursi]

grape, Rocky Mountain; wild Oregon grape *medicinal herb* [see: Oregon grape]

grape seed (Vitis coigetiae; V. vinifera) *oil medicinal herb for dental caries; also used as a dietary source of essential fatty acids and tocopherols*

grape seed extract *natural free radical scavenger for inflammatory collagen disease and peripheral vascular disease; contains 92%–95% procyanidolic oligomers (PCOs)*

grapefruit (Citrus paradisi) *medicinal herb for potassium replacement; the pectin is used to help reduce cholesterol and promote regression of atherosclerosis*

grass burdock *medicinal herb* [see: burdock]

grass myrtle *medicinal herb* [see: calamus]

Gratiola officinalis *medicinal herb* [see: hedge hyssop]

gravelroot *medicinal herb* [see: queen of the meadow]

graybeard tree *medicinal herb* [see: fringe tree]

great wild valerian *medicinal herb* [see: valerian]

greater celandine *medicinal herb* [see: celandine]

green broom; greenweed *medicinal herb* [see: dyer's broom]

green hellebore (Veratrum viride) *medicinal herb* [see: hellebore]

green soap [see: soap, green]

green tea (Camellia sinensis) *leaves medicinal herb used as an antihyperlipidemic, antimicrobial, antineoplastic, and antioxidant; also used to promote longevity by attenuating severe fatal diseases*

greenweed; green broom *medicinal herb* [see: dyer's broom]

grepafloxacin INN *broad-spectrum fluoroquinolone antibiotic*

grepafloxacin HCl USAN *broad-spectrum fluoroquinolone antibiotic*

GRF1-44 *investigational (Phase III) human growth hormone releasing factor* *in slow-release implant form for growth disorders*

Grifola frondosa *medicinal herb* [see: maitake mushrooms]

Grifulvin V tablets, oral suspension ℞ *systemic antifungal* [griseofulvin (microsize)] 250, 500 mg; 125 mg/5 mL

Grindelia squarrosa *medicinal herb* [see: gum weed]

Grisactin; Grisactin 250 capsules (discontinued 1996) ℞ *systemic antifungal* [griseofulvin (microsize)] 125 mg; 250 mg

Grisactin 500 tablets ℞ *systemic antifungal* [griseofulvin (microsize)] 500 mg

Grisactin Ultra tablets ℞ *systemic antifungal* [griseofulvin (ultramicrosize)] 125, 250, 330 mg

griseofulvin USP, INN, BAN *systemic antifungal* 165, 330 mg oral

Gris-PEG film-coated tablets ℞ *systemic antifungal* [griseofulvin (ultramicrosize)] 125, 250 mg

ground apple *medicinal herb* [see: chamomile]

ground berry *medicinal herb* [see: wintergreen]

ground holly *medicinal herb* [see: pipsissewa]

ground lemon *medicinal herb* [see: mandrake]

ground lily *medicinal herb* [see: birthroot]

ground raspberry *medicinal herb* [see: goldenseal]

ground squirrel pea *medicinal herb* [see: twin leaf]

ground thistle *medicinal herb* [see: carline thistle]

growth hormone, human (hGH) [see: somatropin]

growth hormone, human recombinant (rhGH) with insulin-like growth factor, human recombinant (rhIGF) *investigational (Phase II) cytokine for AIDS wasting syndrome*

growth hormone-releasing factor (GHRF; GH-RF) *investigational (orphan) for inadequate endogenous growth hormone in children*

GS 393 *investigational (Phase I/II) antiviral for HIV* [also: PMEA]

GS 4104 *investigational (NDA filed) oral neuraminidase inhibitor for treatment and prevention of viral influenza*

G-strophanthin [see: ouabain]

guabenxan INN

guacetisal INN

guafecainol INN

guaiac

guaiacol NF

guaiacol carbonate NF

guaiacol glyceryl ether [see: guaifenesin]

guaiactamine INN

guaiapate USAN, INN *antitussive*

guaiazulene soluble [see: sodium guaiazulene]

guaietolin INN

Guaifed syrup OTC *decongestant; expectorant* [pseudoephedrine HCl; guaifenesin] 30•200 mg

Guaifed timed-release capsules ℞ *decongestant; expectorant* [pseudoephedrine HCl; guaifenesin] 120•250 mg

Guaifed-PD timed-release capsules ℞ *pediatric decongestant and expectorant* [pseudoephedrine HCl; guaifenesin] 60•300 mg

guaifenesin USAN, USP, INN *expectorant* [also: guaiphenesin] 100 mg/5 mL oral ☑ guanfacine

guaifenesin & codeine phosphate *expectorant; antitussive; narcotic analgesic* 300•10 mg oral; 100•10 mg/5 mL oral

Guaifenesin DAC liquid OTC *narcotic antitussive; decongestant; expectorant* [codeine phosphate; pseudoephedrine HCl; guaifenesin; alcohol 1.9%] 10•30•100 mg

guaifenesin & hydrocodone bitartrate *expectorant; antitussive* 100•5 mg/5 mL oral

Guaifenex liquid ℞ *decongestant; expectorant* [phenylpropanolamine HCl; phenylephrine HCl; guaifenesin] 20•5•100 mg/5 mL

Guaifenex DM extended-release tablets ℞ *antitussive; expectorant* [dextromethorphan hydrobromide; guaifenesin] 30•600 mg

Guaifenex LA extended-release tablets ℞ *expectorant* [guaifenesin] 600 mg

Guaifenex PPA 75 extended-release tablets ℞ *decongestant; expectorant* [phenylpropanolamine HCl; guaifenesin] 75•600 mg

Guaifenex PSE 60; Guaifenex PSE 120; Guaifenex Rx DM extended-release tablets ℞ *decongestant; expectorant* [pseudoephedrine HCl; guaifenesin] 60•600 mg; 120•600 mg; 60•600 mg

Guaifenex Rx extended-release tablets (AM and PM) ℞ *decongestant; expectorant* [pseudoephedrine HCl + guaifenesin (AM); guaifenesin (PM)] 60•600 mg; 600 mg

guaifylline INN *bronchodilator; expectorant* [also: guaithylline]

GuaiMAX-D extended-release tablets ℞ *decongestant; expectorant* [pseudoephedrine HCl; guaifenesin] 120•600 mg

guaimesal INN

Guaipax sustained-release tablets ℞ *decongestant; expectorant* [phenylpropanolamine HCl; guaifenesin] 75•400 mg

guaiphenesin BAN *expectorant* [also: guaifenesin]

guaisteine INN

Guaitab tablets OTC *decongestant; expectorant* [pseudoephedrine HCl; guaifenesin] 60•400 mg

Guaitex capsules, liquid ℞ *decongestant; expectorant* [phenylephrine HCl; phenylpropanolamine HCl; guaifenesin] 5•45•200 mg; 5•20•100 mg/5 mL

Guaitex LA sustained-release tablets ℞ *decongestant; expectorant* [phenylpropanolamine HCl; guaifenesin] 75•400 mg

Guaitex PSE tablets ℞ *decongestant; expectorant* [pseudoephedrine HCl; guaifenesin] 120•500 mg

guaithylline USAN *bronchodilator; expectorant* [also: guaifylline]

Guaivent capsules ℞ *decongestant; expectorant* [pseudoephedrine HCl; guaifenesin] 120•250 mg

Guaivent PD capsules ℞ *pediatric decongestant and expectorant* [pseudoephedrine HCl; guaifenesin] 60•300 mg

Guai-Vent/PSE sustained-release tablets ℞ *decongestant; expectorant* [pseudoephedrine HCl; guaifenesin] 120•600 mg

guamecycline INN, BAN

guanabenz USAN, INN *centrally acting antiadrenergic antihypertensive*

guanabenz acetate USAN, USP, JAN *centrally acting antiadrenergic antihypertensive* 4, 8 mg oral

guanacline INN, BAN *antihypertensive* [also: guanacline sulfate]

guanacline sulfate USAN *antihypertensive* [also: guanacline]

guanadrel INN *antihypertensive* [also: guanadrel sulfate]

guanadrel sulfate USAN, USP *antihypertensive* [also: guanadrel]

guanatol HCl [see: chloroguanide HCl]

guanazodine INN

guancidine INN *antihypertensive* [also: guancydine]

guancydine USAN *antihypertensive* [also: guancidine]

guanethidine INN, BAN *antihypertensive* [also: guanethidine monosulfate] ⊡ guanidine

guanethidine monosulfate USAN, USP *antihypertensive; investigational (orphan) for reflex sympathetic dystrophy and causalgia* [also: guanethidine]

guanethidine sulfate USAN, USP, JAN *antihypertensive*

guanfacine INN, BAN *antihypertensive; antiadrenergic* [also: guanfacine HCl] ⊡ guaifenesin

guanfacine HCl USAN *antihypertensive; antiadrenergic* [also: guanfacine] 1, 2 mg oral

guanidine HCl *cholinergic muscle stimulant* 125 mg oral ⊡ guanethidine

guanisoquin sulfate USAN *antihypertensive* [also: guanisoquine]

guanisoquine INN *antihypertensive* [also: guanisoquin sulfate]

guanoclor INN, BAN *antihypertensive* [also: guanoclor sulfate]

guanoclor sulfate USAN *antihypertensive* [also: guanoclor]

guanoctine INN *antihypertensive* [also: guanoctine HCl]

guanoctine HCl USAN *antihypertensive* [also: guanoctine]

guanoxabenz USAN, INN *antihypertensive*

guanoxan INN, BAN *antihypertensive* [also: guanoxan sulfate]

guanoxan sulfate USAN *antihypertensive* [also: guanoxan]

guanoxyfen INN *antihypertensive; antidepressant* [also: guanoxyfen sulfate]

guanoxyfen sulfate USAN *antihypertensive; antidepressant* [also: guanoxyfen]

guar gum NF *tablet binder and disintegrant*

guarana *(Paullinia cupana; P. sorbilis)* seed paste *medicinal herb for dysentery, malaria, and weight reduction*

guaranine [see: caffeine]

guggul *(Commiphora mukul)* plant *medicinal herb for hypercholesterolemia and for arthritis and weight reduction in Ayurvedic medicine*

GuiaCough CF liquid OTC *antitussive; decongestant; expectorant* [dextromethorphan hydrobromide; phenylpropanolamine HCl; guaifenesin; alcohol 4.75%] 10•12.5•100 mg/5 mL

GuiaCough PE syrup OTC *decongestant; expectorant* [pseudoephedrine HCl; guaifenesin; alcohol 1.4%] 30•100 mg/5 mL

Guiatex LA tablets ℞ *decongestant; expectorant* [phenylpropanolamine HCl; guaifenesin] 75•400 mg

Guiatex PSE tablets ℞ *decongestant; expectorant* [pseudoephedrine HCl; guaifenesin] 120•500 mg

Guiatuss syrup OTC *expectorant* [guaifenesin] 100 mg/5 mL ⊇ Guiatussin

Guiatuss AC syrup ℞ *narcotic antitussive; expectorant* [codeine phosphate; guaifenesin; alcohol] 10•100 mg/5 mL

Guiatuss CF liquid OTC *antitussive; decongestant; expectorant* [dextromethorphan hydrobromide; phenylpropanolamine HCl; guaifenesin; alcohol 4.75%] 10•12.5•100 mg/5 mL

Guiatuss DAC liquid ℞ *narcotic antitussive; decongestant; expectorant* [codeine phosphate; pseudoephedrine HCl; guaifenesin; alcohol] 10•30•100 mg/5 mL

Guiatuss DM liquid OTC *antitussive; expectorant* [dextromethorphan hydrobromide; guaifenesin] 10•100 mg/5 mL

Guiatuss PE liquid OTC *decongestant; expectorant* [pseudoephedrine HCl; guaifenesin; alcohol 1.4%] 30•100 mg/5 mL

Guiatussin DAC syrup ℞ *narcotic antitussive; decongestant; expectorant* [codeine phosphate; pseudoephedrine HCl; guaifenesin; alcohol 1.6%] 10•30•100 mg/5 mL ⊇ Guiatuss

Guiatussin with Codeine Expectorant liquid ℞ *narcotic antitussive; expectorant* [codeine phosphate; guaifenesin; alcohol 3.5%] 10•100 mg/5 mL

Guiatussin with Dextromethorphan liquid OTC *antitussive; expectorant* [dextromethorphan hydrobromide; guaifenesin; alcohol 1.4%] 15•100 mg/5 mL

Guipax tablets ℞ *decongestant; expectorant* [phenylpropanolamine HCl; guaifenesin]

gum Arabic *medicinal herb* [see: acacia]

gum arabic [see: acacia]

gum ivy *medicinal herb* [see: English ivy]

gum myrrh tree *medicinal herb* [see: myrrh]

gum plant *medicinal herb* [see: comfrey; yerba santa]

gum senegal [see: acacia]

gum tree, hemlock *medicinal herb* [see: hemlock]

gum weed *(Grindelia squarrosia)* flowering top and leaves *medicinal herb for asthma, bronchitis, bladder* infection, poison ivy and oak, and psoriasis and other skin disorders

guncotton, soluble [see: pyroxylin]

gusperimus INN *immunosuppressant; investigational (orphan) for acute renal graft rejection* [also: gusperimus trihydrochloride; gusperimus HCl]

gusperimus HCl JAN *immunosuppressant* [also: gusperimus trihydrochloride; gusperimus]

gusperimus trihydrochloride USAN *immunosuppressant* [also: gusperimus; gusperimus HCl]

Gustase tablets OTC *digestive enzymes* [amylase; protease; cellulase] 30•6•2 mg

Gustase Plus tablet R *digestive enzymes; sedative* [amylase; protease; cellulase; homatropine methylbromide; phenobarbital] 30•6•2•2.5•8 mg

gutta percha USP *dental restoration agent*

GVAX R *investigational (Phase I/II) theraccine for prostate cancer*

G-Well lotion, shampoo R *pediculicide for lice; scabicide* [lindane] 1%

gymnema (Gymnema melicida; G. sylvestre) leaves and roots *medicinal herb for diabetes, hyperactivity, and hypoglycemia*

Gynecort 5 cream (discontinued 1997) OTC *topical corticosteroidal anti-inflammatory* [hydrocortisone acetate] 0.5%

Gynecort 10 (name changed to Gynecort Female Creme in 1997)

Gynecort Female Creme cream OTC *topical corticosteroidal anti-inflammatory* [hydrocortisone acetate] 1%

Gyne-Lotrimin combination pack (name changed to Gyne-Lotrimin 7 in 1999)

Gyne-Lotrimin vaginal inserts, vaginal cream OTC *antifungal* [clotrimazole] 100 mg; 1%

Gyne-Lotrimin 3 vaginal inserts, combination pack (vaginal inserts + cream) OTC *antifungal* [clotrimazole] 100, 200 mg; 100 mg + 1%, 200 mg + 1%

Gyne-Lotrimin 7 combination pack (vaginal inserts + cream) OTC *antifungal* [clotrimazole] 100 mg + 1%

Gyne-Moistrin vaginal gel (discontinued 1998) OTC *lubricant* [propylene glycol]

gynergon [see: estradiol]

Gyne-Sulf vaginal cream R *broadspectrum bacteriostatic* [sulfathiazole; sulfacetamide; sulfabenzamide] 3.42%•2.86%•3.7%

gynoestryl [see: estradiol]

Gynogen L.A. 20 IM injection R *estrogen replacement therapy for postmenopausal disorders; antineoplastic for prostatic cancer* [estradiol valerate in oil] 20 mg/mL

Gynogen L.A. 40 IM injection (discontinued 1996) R *estrogen replacement therapy for postmenopausal disorders; antineoplastic for prostatic cancer* [estradiol valerate in oil] 40 mg/mL

Gynol II Contraceptive vaginal gel, vaginal jelly OTC *spermicidal contraceptive (for use with a diaphragm)* [nonoxynol 9] 2%; 3%

Gynostemma pentaphyllum *medicinal herb* [see: jiaogulan]

Gynovite Plus tablets OTC *vitamin/ mineral/calcium/iron supplement* [multiple vitamins & minerals; calcium; iron; folic acid; biotin] ≛•83•3•0.067•≛ mg

Gy-Pak (trademarked packaging form) *unit-of-issue package*

gypsy weed *medicinal herb* [see: speedwell]

Gyrocap (trademarked dosage form) *timed-release capsule*

H₁ blockers *a class of antihistamines* [also called: histamine H₁ antagonists]

²H (deuterium) [see: deuterium oxide]

H₂ blockers *a class of gastrointestinal antisecretory agents* [also called: histamine H₂ antagonists]

H₂¹⁵O [see: water O 15]

³H (tritium) [see: tritiated water]

Habitrol transdermal patch ℞ *smoking deterrent; nicotine withdrawal aid* [nicotine] 17.5, 35, 52.5 mg

hachimycin INN, BAN

HAD (hexamethylmelamine, Adriamycin, DDP) *chemotherapy protocol*

hafnium *element (Hf)*

Hair Booster Vitamin tablets OTC *vitamin/mineral/iron supplement* [multiple B vitamins & minerals; iron; folic acid] ±•18•0.4 mg

halarsol [see: dichlorophenarsine HCl]

halazepam USAN, USP, INN, BAN *anxiolytic; sedative*

halazone USP, INN *disinfectant; water purifier*

Halazone tablets (discontinued 1996) OTC *water purifier*

halcinonide USAN, USP, INN, BAN *topical corticosteroidal anti-inflammatory*

Halcion tablets ℞ *benzodiazepine sedative; hypnotic* [triazolam] 0.125, 0.25 mg

Haldol oral concentrate, IM injection ℞ *conventional (typical) antipsychotic; antidyskinetic for Tourette syndrome* [haloperidol lactate] 2 mg/mL; 5 mg/mL ☐ Halenol; Halog

Haldol tablets ℞ *conventional (typical) antipsychotic; antidyskinetic for Tourette syndrome* [haloperidol] 0.5, 1, 2, 5, 10, 20 mg

Haldol Decanoate 50; Haldol Decanoate 100 long-acting IM injection ℞ *conventional (typical) antipsychotic* [haloperidol decanoate] 50 mg/mL; 100 mg/mL

Halenol, Children's liquid OTC *analgesic; antipyretic* [acetaminophen] 160 mg/5 mL

Halercol capsules OTC *vitamin supplement* [multiple vitamins]

haletazole INN [also: halethazole]

halethazole BAN [also: haletazole]

Haley's M·O liquid OTC *laxative* [magnesium hydroxide; mineral oil] 900 mg•3.75 mL per 15 mL

Halfan tablets ℞ *antimalarial (orphan)* [halofantrine HCl] 250 mg

Halfprin; Halfprin 81 enteric-coated tablets OTC *analgesic; antipyretic; anti-inflammatory; antirheumatic* [aspirin] 165 mg; 81 mg

Hall's Plus lozenges OTC *topical oral analgesic; counterirritant; mild local anesthetic; antiseptic* [menthol] 10 mg

Hall's Sugar Free Mentho-Lyptus lozenges OTC *topical oral analgesic; counterirritant; mild local anesthetic; antiseptic* [menthol; eucalyptus oil] 5•2.8, 6•2.8 mg

Halls Zinc Defense lozenges OTC *topical anti-infective to relieve sore throat* [zinc acetate] 5 mg

hallucinogens *a class of agents that induce hallucinations*

halobetasol propionate USAN *topical corticosteroidal anti-inflammatory* [also: ulobetasol]

halocarban INN *disinfectant* [also: cloflucarban]

halocortolone INN

halocrinic acid [see: brocrinat]

halofantrine INN, BAN *antimalarial* [also: halofantrine HCl]

halofantrine HCl USAN *antimalarial (orphan)* [also: halofantrine]

Halofed tablets OTC *nasal decongestant* [pseudoephedrine HCl] 30, 60 mg

halofenate USAN, INN, BAN *antihyperlipoproteinemic; uricosuric*

halofuginone INN, BAN *antiprotozoal* [also: halofuginone hydrobromide]

halofuginone hydrobromide USAN *antiprotozoal* [also: halofuginone]

Halog ointment, cream, solution ℞ *topical corticosteroidal anti-inflamma-*

tory [halcinonide] 0.1%; 0.025%, 0.1%; 0.1% ⊠ Haldol

Halog-E cream ℞ *topical corticosteroidal anti-inflammatory; emollient* [halcinonide] 0.1%

halometasone INN

halonamine INN

halopemide USAN, INN *antipsychotic*

halopenium chloride INN, BAN

haloperidol USAN, USP, INN, BAN *butyrophenone antipsychotic; antidyskinetic for Tourette syndrome* 0.5, 1, 2, 5, 10, 20 mg oral

haloperidol decanoate USAN, BAN *butyrophenone antipsychotic*

Haloperidol LA ⊛ (U.S. product: Haldol Decanoate) long-acting IM injection ℞ *conventional (typical) antipsychotic* [haloperidol decanoate] 50, 100 mg/mL

haloperidol lactate *butyrophenone antipsychotic; antidyskinetic for Tourette syndrome* 2 mg/mL oral; 5 mg/mL injection

halopone chloride [see: halopenium chloride]

halopredone INN *topical anti-inflammatory* [also: halopredone acetate]

halopredone acetate USAN *topical anti-inflammatory* [also: halopredone]

haloprogesterone USAN, INN *progestin*

haloprogin USAN, USP, INN, JAN *antibacterial; antifungal*

halopyramine BAN [also: chloropyramine]

Halotestin tablets ℞ *androgenic hormone for male hypogonadism and female breast cancer* [fluoxymesterone] 2, 5, 10 mg ⊠ Halotex; Halotussin

Halotex cream, solution ℞ *topical antifungal* [haloprogin] 1% ⊠ Halotestin

halothane USP, INN, BAN *inhalation general anesthetic*

Halotussin syrup OTC *expectorant* [guaifenesin; alcohol 3.5%] 100 mg/5 mL ⊠ Halotestin

Halotussin-DM liquid, sugar-free liquid OTC *antitussive; expectorant* [dextromethorphan hydrobromide; guaifenesin] 10•100 mg/5 mL

haloxazolam INN

haloxon INN, BAN

halquinol BAN *topical anti-infective* [also: halquinols]

halquinols USAN *topical anti-infective* [also: halquinol]

Haltran tablets OTC *nonsteroidal anti-inflammatory drug (NSAID); antiarthritic; analgesic* [ibuprofen] 200 mg

HAM (hexamethylmelamine, Adriamycin, melphalan) *chemotherapy protocol*

HAM (hexamethylmelamine, Adriamycin, methotrexate) *chemotherapy protocol*

Hamamelis virginiana *medicinal herb* [see: witch hazel]

hamamelis water *medicinal herb* [see: witch hazel]

hamycin USAN, INN *antifungal*

hard fat [see: fat, hard]

hardock *medicinal herb* [see: burdock]

hareburr *medicinal herb* [see: burdock]

Harpagophytum procumbens *medicinal herb* [see: devil's claw]

hashish (*Cannabis sativa*) *euphoric/hallucinogenic street drug made from the resin of the flowering tops of the cannabis plant*

Havrix IM injection, prefilled syringe ℞ *immunization against hepatitis A virus (HAV)* [hepatitis A vaccine, inactivated] 720 ELISA units (EL.U.)/0.5 mL (pediatric), 1440 EL.U./mL (adult)

haw *medicinal herb* [see: hawthorn]

Hawaiian Tropic Cool Aloe with I.C.E. gel OTC *topical local anesthetic; analgesic; counterirritant* [lidocaine; menthol] 2•2

hawthorn (*Crataegus laevigata; C. monogyna; C. oxyacantha*) flowers, leaves, and berries *medicinal herb for angina pectoris, arrhythmias, arteriosclerosis, enlarged heart, high or low blood pressure, hypoglycemia, palpitations, and tachycardia; also used as an antiseptic*

Hayfebrol liquid OTC *decongestant; antihistamine* [pseudoephedrine

HCl; chlorpheniramine maleate] 30•2 mg/5 mL

hazel, snapping; hazelnut *medicinal herb* [see: witch hazel]

H-BIG IM injection ℞ *hepatitis B immunizing agent* [hepatitis B immune globulin] 4, 5 mL

H-BIG IV injection *investigational (orphan) prophylaxis against hepatitis B reinfection in liver transplant patients* [hepatitis B immune globulin]

HBIG (hepatitis B immune globulin) [q.v.]

HBY097 *investigational (Phase II) nonnucleoside reverse transcriptase inhibitor (NNRTI) for HIV*

1% HC ointment ℞ *topical corticosteroidal anti-inflammatory* [hydrocortisone] 1%

HC (hydrocortisone) [q.v.]

4-HC (4-hydroperoxycyclophosphamide) [q.v.]

HC Derma-Pax liquid OTC *topical corticosteroidal anti-inflammatory; antihistamine; antiseptic* [hydrocortisone; pyrilamine maleate; chlorpheniramine maleate; chlorobutanol] 0.5%•0.44%•0.06%•25%

HCA (hydrocortisone acetate) [q.v.]

H-CAP (hexamethylmelamine, cyclophosphamide, Adriamycin, Platinol) *chemotherapy protocol*

hCG (human chorionic gonadotropin) [see: gonadotropin, chorionic]

HCG-nostick test kit for professional use (discontinued 1995) *in vitro diagnostic aid for urine pregnancy test* [sol particle immunoassay (SPIA)]

HCP-30 *investigational (Phase I) vaccine for HIV*

HCT (hydrochlorothiazide) [q.v.]

HCTZ (hydrochlorothiazide) [q.v.]

HD 85 oral/rectal suspension ℞ *radiopaque contrast medium for gastrointestinal imaging* [barium sulfate] 85%

HD 200 Plus powder for oral suspension ℞ *radiopaque contrast medium for gastrointestinal imaging* [barium sulfate] 98%

HDCV (human diploid cell vaccine) [see: rabies vaccine]

HDMTX (high-dose methotrexate [with leucovorin rescue]) *chemotherapy protocol*

HDMTX-CF (high-dose methotrexate, citrovorum factor) *chemotherapy protocol*

HDMTX/LV (high-dose methotrexate, leucovorin [rescue]) *chemotherapy protocol*

HDPEB (high-dose PEB protocol) *chemotherapy protocol* [see: PEB]

HD-VAC (high-dose [methotrexate], vinblastine, Adriamycin, cisplatin) *chemotherapy protocol*

Head & Shoulders cream shampoo, lotion shampoo OTC *antiseborrheic; antibacterial; antifungal* [pyrithione zinc] 1%

Head & Shoulders Dry Scalp shampoo OTC *antiseborrheic; antibacterial; antifungal* [pyrithione zinc] 1%

Head & Shoulders Intensive Treatment Dandruff Shampoo OTC *antiseborrheic* [selenium sulfide] 1%

heal-all *medicinal herb* [see: figwort; stone root; woundwort]

healing herb *medicinal herb* [see: comfrey]

Healon; Healon GV intraocular injection ℞ *viscoelastic agent for ophthalmic surgery* [hyaluronate sodium] 10 mg/mL; 14 mg/mL

Healon Yellow intraocular injection ℞ *viscoelastic agent for ophthalmic surgery; diagnostic agent* [hyaluronate sodium; fluorescein sodium] 10• 0.005 mg/mL

heart, mother's; shepherd's heart *medicinal herb* [see: shepherd's purse]

Heartline enteric-coated tablets OTC *analgesic; antipyretic; anti-inflammatory; antirheumatic* [aspirin] 81 mg

heather (Calluna vulgaris) flowering shoots *medicinal herb used as an antiseptic, cholagogue, diaphoretic, diuretic, expectorant, and vasoconstrictor*

heavy liquid petrolatum [see: mineral oil]

heavy water (D₂O) [see: deuterium oxide]

Heb Cream Base (discontinued 1998) OTC *cream base*

Hectorol soft capsules ℞ *serum calcium regulator for idiopathic hyperparathyroidism in dialysis patients with end-stage renal disease* [doxercalciferol] 2.5 μg

hedaquinium chloride INN, BAN

Hedeoma pulegeoides medicinal herb [see: pennyroyal]

Hedera helix medicinal herb [see: English ivy]

hedge bindweed (Convolvulus sepium) flowering plant and roots *medicinal herb used as a cholagogue, febrifuge, and purgative*

hedge garlic (Sisymbrium alliaria) *medicinal herb* [see: garlic]

hedge hyssop (Gratiola officinalis) plant *medicinal herb used as a cardiac, diuretic, purgative, and vermifuge*

hedge-burs *medicinal herb* [see: bedstraw]

"hedgehog" proteins *a class of novel human proteins that induce the formation of regenerative tissue*

Heet Liniment OTC *counterirritant; topical antiseptic* [methyl salicylate; camphor; capsaicin; alcohol 70%] 15%•3.6%•0.025%

hefilcon A USAN *hydrophilic contact lens material*

hefilcon B USAN *hydrophilic contact lens material*

hefilcon C USAN *hydrophilic contact lens material*

helenien [see: xantofyl palmitate]

Helianthemum canadense medicinal herb [see: rock rose]

helicon [see: aspirin]

Helidac 14-day dose-pack ℞ *combination treatment for active duodenal ulcer with H. pylori infection* [bismuth subsalicylate (chewable tablets); metronidazole (tablets); tetracycline HCl (capsules)] 262.4 mg; 250 mg; 500 mg

heliomycin INN

heliox *helium-oxygen mixture used for respiratory distress* (usually an 80%•20% mix)

Helistat sponge ℞ *topical local hemostat for surgery* [absorbable collagen sponge]

helium USP *diluent for gases; element (He)*

Helixate powder for IV injection ℞ *antihemophilic to correct coagulation deficiency* [antihemophilic factor VIII, recombinant] 250, 500, 1000 IU

hellebore (Helleborus spp.; Veratrum spp.) rhizome *medicinal herb used as an antihypertensive; not generally regarded as safe and effective for internal consumption due to toxicity*

Helleborus species medicinal herb [see: hellebore]

helmet flower *medicinal herb* [see: aconite; sandalwood; skullcap]

helmet pod *medicinal herb* [see: twin leaf]

Hem Fe capsules (discontinued 1996) ℞ *hematinic* [ferrous fumarate; cyanocobalamin; ascorbic acid; docusate sodium] 100 mg•5 μg•125 mg•25 mg

HEMA (2-hydroxyethyl methacrylate) *contact lens material*

Hemabate IM injection ℞ *prostaglandin-type abortifacient; for postpartum uterine bleeding* [carboprost tromethamine] 250 μg/mL

Hema-Check slide tests for home use OTC *in vitro diagnostic aid for fecal occult blood*

Hema-Combistix reagent strips *in vitro diagnostic aid for multiple urine products*

Hemaseel HMN ℞ *investigational (Phase III) fibrin sealant for surgery*

Hemaspan timed-release tablets OTC *hematinic* [iron (from ferrous fumarate); ascorbic acid; docusate sodium] 110•200•20 mg

HemAssist *investigational (Phase III) blood substitute for perfusion deficit disorders and blood loss from severe trauma* [hemoglobin crosfumaril]

Hemastix reagent strips for professional use *in vitro diagnostic aid for urine occult blood*

Hematest reagent tablets for professional use *in vitro diagnostic aid for fecal occult blood*

hematinics *a class of iron-containing agents for the prevention and treatment of iron-deficiency anemia*

hematopoietics *a class of antianemic agents that promote the formation of red blood cells*

heme arginate *investigational (orphan) for acute symptomatic porphyria and myelodysplastic syndrome*

HemeSelect Collection kit for home use *in vitro diagnostic aid for fecal occult blood* [for use with HemeSelect Reagent kit]

HemeSelect Reagent kit for professional use *in vitro diagnostic aid for fecal occult blood* [for use with HemeSelect Collection kit]

Hemex ℞ *investigational (orphan) for acute porphyric syndromes* [hemin; zinc mesoporphyrin]

hemiacidrin [see: citric acid, glucono-delta-lactone & magnesium carbonate]

hemin *enzyme inhibitor for acute intermittent porphyria (AIP), porphyria variegata, and hereditary coproporphyria (orphan)*

hemin & zinc mesoporphyrin *investigational (orphan) for acute porphyric syndromes*

hemlock *(Tsuga canadensis)* bark *medicinal herb used as an astringent, diaphoretic, and diuretic*

Hemocaine anorectal ointment (discontinued 1995) OTC *topical anesthetic; vasoconstrictor; astringent* [diperodon HCl; pyrilamine maleate; phenylephrine HCl; bismuth subcarbonate; zinc oxide] 0.25%•0.1%•0.25%•0.2%•5%

Hemoccult slide tests for professional use, test tape for professional use *in vitro diagnostic aid for fecal occult blood*

Hemoccult II slide tests for professional use *in vitro diagnostic aid for fecal occult blood*

Hemoccult II Dispenserpak; Hemoccult II Dispenserpak Plus slide tests for home use OTC *in vitro diagnostic aid for fecal occult blood*

Hemoccult SENSA; Hemoccult II SENSA slide tests for professional use *in vitro diagnostic aid for fecal occult blood*

Hemocitrate *investigational (orphan) adjunct to leukapheresis procedures* [sodium citrate]

Hemocyte IM injection (discontinued 1995) ℞ *hematinic* [ferrous gluconate; multiple B vitamins; procaine HCl] 3 mg/mL•±•2%

Hemocyte tablets OTC *hematinic* [ferrous fumarate (source of iron)] 324 mg (106 mg)

Hemocyte Plus elixir ℞ *hematinic* [polysaccharide-iron complex; multiple B vitamins & minerals; folic acid] 12•±•0.33 mg

Hemocyte Plus tablets ℞ *hematinic* [ferrous fumarate; multiple B vitamins & minerals; sodium ascorbate; folic acid] 106•±•200•1 mg

Hemocyte-F tablets ℞ *hematinic* [ferrous fumarate; folic acid] 106•1 mg

Hemocyte-V IM injection (discontinued 1995) ℞ *hematinic* [ferrous gluconate; multiple B vitamins] 3.6•± mg/mL

Hemofil M IV injection ℞ *antihemophilic to correct coagulation deficiency* [antihemophilic factor VIII] 10, 20, 30 mL

hemoglobin, recombinant human (rHb1.1) *investigational agent for chronic anemia*

hemoglobin crosfumaril USAN, INN *investigational (Phase III) blood substitute for perfusion deficit disorders and blood loss due to severe trauma*

Hemokine *investigational progenitor cell stimulator for neutropenia and thrombocytopenia* [muplestim]

Hemolink ℞ *investigational (Phase III) human blood substitute for surgery and chronic anemia associated with kidney failure*

Hemonyne IV infusion ℞ *antihemophilic to correct factor IX deficiency (Christmas disease)* [coagulation factors II, VII, IX, and X, heat treated] 20, 40 mL

Hemopad fiber ℞ *topical hemostatic aid in surgery* [microfibrillar collagen hemostat]

Hemophilus b conjugate vaccine *active bacterin for Haemophilus influenzae type b*

Hemopure ℞ *investigational (Phase III) blood substitute*

Hemorid for Women cream OTC *topical local anesthetic and vasoconstrictor for hemorrhoids* [pramoxine HCl; phenylephrine HCl] 1%•0.25%

Hemorid for Women lotion OTC *topical emollient and protectant for hemorrhoids* [mineral oil; petrolatum; glycerin]

Hemorid for Women rectal suppositories OTC *vasoconstrictor and astringent for hemorrhoids* [zinc oxide; phenylephrine HCl] 11%•0.25%

Hemorrhoidal HC rectal suppositories ℞ *corticosteroidal anti-inflammatory for hemorrhoids* [hydrocortisone acetate] 25 mg

hemostatics *a class of therapeutic blood modifiers that arrest the flow of blood* [see also: astringents; styptics]

Hemotene fiber ℞ *topical hemostatic aid in surgery* [microfibrillar collagen hemostat] 1 g

hemp *medicinal herb* [see: marijuana]

hemp agrimony (Eupatorium cannabinum) plant *medicinal herb used as a cholagogue, diaphoretic, diuretic, emetic, expectorant, and purgative*

hemp nettle (Galeopsis tetrahit) plant *medicinal herb used as an astringent, diuretic, and expectorant*

Hem-Prep anorectal ointment, rectal suppositories OTC *temporary relief of hemorrhoidal symptoms; topical vasoconstrictor; astringent* [phenylephrine HCl; zinc oxide] 0.025%•11%; 0.25%•11%

Hemril Uniserts (rectal suppositories) OTC *temporary relief of hemorrhoidal symptoms* [bismuth subgallate; bismuth resorcin compound; benzyl benzoate; peruvian balsam; zinc oxide] 2.25%•1.75%•1.2%•1.8%•11%

Hemril-HC Uniserts (suppositories) ℞ *corticosteroidal anti-inflammatory for hemorrhoids* [hydrocortisone acetate] 25 mg

henbane (Hyoscyamus niger) plant *medicinal herb used as an anodyne, antispasmodic, calmative, and narcotic; primarily used externally because of its high toxicity*

heneicosafluorotripropylamine [see: perfluamine]

henna (Alkanna tinctoria) root *medicinal herb used as an astringent, antibiotic, and cosmetic dye; not generally regarded as safe and effective*

henna (Lawsonia inermis) leaves *medicinal herb used as an astringent*

HEOD (hexachloro-epoxy-octahydro-dimethanonaphthalene) [see: dieldrin]

Hepagene ℞ *investigational (NDA filed) hepatitis B vaccine and treatment for chronic carriers*

Hepandrin ℞ *anabolic steroid for weight gain; investigational (orphan) for muscular dystrophy, AIDS-wasting syndrome, and alcoholic hepatitis; also abused as a street drug* [oxandrolone]

heparin BAN *anticoagulant; antithrombotic* [also: heparin calcium]

heparin, 2-0-desulfated *investigational (orphan) for cystic fibrosis*

heparin calcium USP *anticoagulant; antithrombotic* [also: heparin]

Heparin Lock Flush solution ℞ IV *flush for catheter patency (not therapeutic)* [heparin sodium] 10, 100 U/mL

heparin sodium USP, INN, BAN *anticoagulant; antithrombotic* 1000, 2000, 2500, 5000, 7500, 10 000, 20 000, 40 000 U/mL injection

heparin sodium & sodium chloride 0.45% *anticoagulant; antithrombotic* 12 500 U•250 mL, 25 000 U•250 mL, 25 000 U•500 mL

heparin sodium & sodium chloride 0.9% *anticoagulant; antithrombotic* 1000 U•500 mL, 2000 U•1000 mL

heparin sulfate [see: danaparoid sodium]

heparin whole blood [see: blood, whole]

heparinase 1 *investigational (Phase III) agent for the reversal of heparin-induced anticoagulation*

heparinase III *investigational cardio-protective agent*

HepatAmine IV infusion ℞ *nutritional therapy for hepatic failure and hepatic encephalopathy* [multiple branched-chain essential and nonessential amino acids; electrolytes]

hepatica (*Hepatica acutiloba; H. triloba*) *leaves and flowers medicinal herb used as a diuretic and pectoral*

Hepatic-Aid II Instant Drink powder OTC *enteral nutritional treatment for chronic liver disease* [multiple branched chain amino acids]

hepatics *a class of agents that affect the liver (a term used in folk medicine)*

hepatitis A vaccine, inactivated *active immunizing agent for the hepatitis A virus (HAV)*

hepatitis B immune globulin (HBIG) USP *passive immunizing agent; investigational (orphan) prophylaxis against hepatitis B reinfection in liver transplant patients*

hepatitis B surface antigen [see: hepatitis B virus vaccine, inactivated]

hepatitis B virus vaccine, inactivated USP *active immunizing agent for hepatitis B and D*

hepatitis C vaccine *investigational (Phase I) immunizing agent for hepatitis C*

Hep-B-Gammagee IM injection (discontinued 1996) ℞ *hepatitis B immunizing agent* [hepatitis B immune globulin] 5 mL

Hep-Forte capsules OTC *geriatric dietary supplement* [multiple vitamins & food products; folic acid; biotin] ± • 60• ≟ μg

Hep-Lock; Hep-Lock U/P solution ℞ *IV flush for catheter patency (not therapeutic)* [heparin sodium] 10, 100 U/mL

HEPP (H-chain ε [IgE] pentapeptide) [see: pentigetide]

hepronicate INN

heptabarb INN [also: heptabarbitone]

heptabarbital [see: heptabarb; heptabarbitone]

heptabarbitone BAN [also: heptabarb]

Heptalac syrup ℞ *laxative* [lactulose] 10 g/15 mL

heptaminol INN, BAN

heptaminol HCl [see: heptaminol]

2-heptanamine [see: tuaminoheptane]

2-heptanamine sulfate [see: tuaminoheptane sulfate]

heptaverine INN

heptolamide INN

Heptovir ⒸⒶⓃ (U.S. product: Epivir-HBV) ℞ *antiviral nucleoside reverse transcriptase inhibitor for hepatitis B virus (HBV)* [lamivudine]

Heptuna Plus capsules (discontinued 1995) ℞ *hematinic* [ferrous sulfate; multiple vitamins & minerals; intrinsic factor concentrate] 100• ± • ± •150•25 mg

hepzidine INN

HER2 (human epidermal growth factor receptor 2) MAb [see: trastuzumab]

Heracleum lanatum medicinal herb [see: masterwort]

herb of grace *medicinal herb* [see: rue]

Herbal Laxative tablets OTC *stimulant laxative* [senna leaves; cascara sagrada bark] 125•20 mg

HercepTest test kit ℞ *diagnostic aid for the HER2 protein, used to screen patients who may benefit from treatment with Herceptin*

Herceptin powder for IV infusion ℞ *anti-HER2 monoclonal antibody for metastatic breast cancer; investigational*

(NDA filed) for ovarian and female genital tract cancers [trastuzumab] 440 mg

Hercules woundwort *medicinal herb* [see: woundwort]

heroin *potent narcotic analgesic street drug which is highly addictive; banned in the U.S.* [medically known as diacetylmorphine HCl and diamorphine]

heroin HCl *(banned in the USA)* [see: diacetylmorphine HCl]

Herpecin-L lip balm OTC *vulnerary; sunblock* [allantoin; padimate O]

herpes simplex virus gene *investigational (orphan) for primary and metastatic brain tumors*

Herpetrol tablets OTC *dietary supplement; claimed to prevent and treat herpes simplex infections* [L-lysine; multiple vitamins; zinc]

Herplex eye drops (discontinued 1997) R *ophthalmic antiviral* [idoxuridine] 0.1%

Herrick Lacrimal Plug R *blocks the puncta and canaliculus to eliminate tear loss in keratitis sicca* [silicone plug]

HES (hydroxyethyl starch) [see: hetastarch]

Hespan IV infusion R *plasma volume expander for shock due to hemorrhage, burns, surgery* [hetastarch] 6 g/100 mL ☒ Histatan

hesperidin

hesperidin methyl chalcone [see: bioflavonoids]

hetacillin USAN, USP, INN, BAN *antibacterial*

hetacillin potassium USAN, USP *antibacterial*

hetaflur USAN, INN, BAN *dental caries prophylactic*

hetastarch USAN, BAN *plasma volume extender* [also: hydroxyethylstarch] 6% in normal saline

heteronium bromide USAN, INN, BAN *anticholinergic*

Hetrazan tablets (available for compassionate use only) R *anthelmintic for Bancroft's filariasis, onchocerciasis, tropical eosinophilia, and loiasis* [diethylcarbamazine citrate] 50 mg

hexaammonium molybdate tetrahydrate [see: ammonium molybdate]

Hexabrix injection R *radiopaque contrast medium* [ioxaglate meglumine; ioxaglate sodium (54.3% total iodine)] 393•196 mg/mL (320 mg/mL)

HexaCAF; Hexa-CAF (hexamethylmelamine, cyclophosphamide, amethopterin, fluorouracil) *chemotherapy protocol*

hexacarbacholine bromide INN [also: carbolonium bromide]

hexachlorane [see: lindane]

hexachlorocyclohexane [see: lindane]

hexachlorophane BAN *topical anti-infective; detergent* [also: hexachlorophene]

hexachlorophene USP, INN *topical anti-infective; detergent* [also: hexachlorophane]

hexacyclonate sodium INN

hexacyprone INN

hexadecanoic acid, methylethyl ester [see: isopropyl palmitate]

hexadecanol [see: cetyl alcohol]

hexadecylamine hydrofluoride [see: hetaflur]

hexadecylpyridinium chloride [see: cetylpyridinium chloride]

hexadecyltrimethylammonium bromide [see: cetrimonium bromide]

hexadecyltrimethylammonium chloride [see: cetrimonium chloride]

2,4-hexadienoic acid, potassium salt [see: potassium sorbate]

hexadiline INN

hexadimethrine bromide INN, BAN

hexadiphane [see: prozapine]

Hexadrol tablets, elixir R *corticosteroid; anti-inflammatory* [dexamethasone] 1.5, 4 mg; 0.5 mg/5 mL ☒ Hexalol

Hexadrol Phosphate intra-articular, intralesional, soft tissue, or IM injection R *corticosteroid; anti-inflammatory* [dexamethasone sodium phosphate] 4, 10, 20 mg/mL

hexadylamine [see: hexadiline]

hexafluorenium bromide USAN, USP *skeletal muscle relaxant; succinyl-*

choline synergist [also: hexafluronium bromide]

hexafluorodiethyl ether [see: flurothyl]

hexaflurone bromide [see: hexafluorenium bromide]

hexafluronium bromide INN *skeletal muscle relaxant; succinylcholine synergist* [also: hexafluorenium bromide]

Hexalen capsules ℞ *antineoplastic for advanced ovarian adenocarcinoma (orphan)* [altretamine] 50 mg ⑦ Hexalol

hexamarium bromide [see: distigmine bromide]

hexametazime BAN

hexamethone bromide [see: hexamethonium bromide]

hexamethonium bromide INN, BAN

hexamethylenamine [now: methenamine]

hexamethylenamine mandelate [see: methenamine mandelate]

hexamethylenetetramine [see: methenamine]

hexamethylmelamine (HMM; HXM) [see: altretamine]

hexamidine INN

hexamine hippurate BAN *urinary antibacterial* [also: methenamine hippurate]

hexamine mandelate [see: methenamine mandelate]

hexapradol INN

hexaprofen INN, BAN

hexapropymate INN, BAN

hexasonium iodide INN

Hexastat (name changed to Hexalen upon marketing approval in 1995)

hexavitamin USP

Hexavitamin tablets OTC *vitamin supplement* [multiple vitamins] ±

hexcarbacholine bromide INN [also: carbolonium bromide]

hexedine USAN, INN *antibacterial*

hexemal [see: cyclobarbital]

hexestrol NF, INN

hexetidine BAN

hexicide [see: lindane]

hexinol [see: cyclomenol]

hexobarbital USP, INN

hexobarbital sodium NF

hexobendine USAN, INN, BAN *vasodilator*

hexocyclium methylsulfate *peptic ulcer adjunct* [also: hexocyclium metilsulfate; hexocyclium methylsulphate]

hexocyclium methylsulphate BAN [also: hexocyclium methylsulfate; hexocyclium metilsulfate]

hexocyclium metilsulfate INN [also: hexocyclium methylsulfate; hexocyclium methylsulphate]

hexoprenaline INN, BAN *tocolytic; bronchodilator* [also: hexoprenaline sulfate]

hexoprenaline sulfate USAN, JAN *tocolytic; bronchodilator* [also: hexoprenaline]

hexopyrimidine [see: hexetidine]

hexopyrrolate [see: hexopyrronium bromide]

hexopyrronium bromide INN

Hextend ℞ *investigational (NDA filed) blood plasma volume expander for surgical blood loss*

hexydaline [see: methenamine mandelate]

hexylcaine INN *local anesthetic* [also: hexylcaine HCl]

hexylcaine HCl USP *local anesthetic* [also: hexylcaine]

hexylene glycol NF *humectant; solvent*

hexylresorcinol USP *anthelmintic; topical antiseptic*

1-hexyltheobromine [see: pentifylline]

H-F Gel ℞ *investigational (orphan) emergency treatment for hydrofluoric acid burns* [calcium gluconate]

hFSH (human follicle-stimulating hormone) [now: menotropins]

HFZ (homofenazine) [q.v.]

^{197}**Hg** [see: chlormerodrin Hg 197]

^{197}**Hg** [see: merisoprol acetate Hg 197]

^{197}**Hg** [see: merisoprol Hg 197]

^{203}**Hg** [see: chlormerodrin Hg 203]

^{203}**Hg** [see: merisoprol acetate Hg 203]

hGH (human growth hormone) [see: somatropin]

HGP-30W *investigational (Phase II) vaccine for HIV*

hibenzate INN *combining name for radicals or groups* [also: hybenzate]

Hibiclens sponge/brush OTC *broad-spectrum antimicrobial; germicidal* [chlorhexidine gluconate; alcohol 4%] 4%

Hibiclens Antiseptic/AntiMicrobial Skin Cleanser liquid OTC *broad-spectrum antimicrobial; germicidal* [chlorhexidine gluconate; alcohol 4%] 4%

hibiscus (*Hibiscus sabdariffa* and other species) flowers and leaves *medicinal herb for cancer, edema, heart problems and nervous disorders; also used topically as an emollient; not generally regarded as safe and effective*

Hibistat Germicidal Hand Rinse liquid OTC *broad-spectrum antimicrobial; germicidal* [chlorhexidine gluconate; alcohol 70%] 0.5%

Hibistat Towelette OTC *broad-spectrum antimicrobial; germicidal* [chlorhexidine gluconate; alcohol 70%] 0.5%

HibTITER IM injection ℞ *Haemophilus influenzae type b (HIB) vaccine* [Hemophilus b conjugate vaccine] 0.5 mL

Hi-Cal VM nutrition bar OTC *enteral nutritional therapy for HIV and AIDS*

Hi-Cor 1.0; Hi-Cor 2.5 cream ℞ *topical corticosteroidal anti-inflammatory* [hydrocortisone] 1%; 2.5%

HIDA (hepatoiminodiacetic acid) [see: lidofenin]

HiDAC (high-dose ara-C) *chemotherapy protocol*

Hieracium pilosella medicinal herb [see: mouse ear]

high angelica *medicinal herb* [see: angelica]

high molecular weight dextran [see: dextran 70]

high osmolar contrast media (HOCM) *a class of older radiopaque agents that have a high osmolar concentration of iodine (the contrast agent), which corresponds to a higher incidence of adverse reactions* [also called: ionic contrast media]

High Potency N-Vites tablets OTC *vitamin supplement* [multiple B vitamins; vitamin C] ≛•500 mg

High Potency Tar gel shampoo OTC *antiseborrheic; antipsoriatic; antipruritic; antibacterial* [coal tar] 25%

hilafilcon A USAN *hydrophilic contact lens material*

hillberry *medicinal herb* [see: wintergreen]

Himalayan ginseng (*Panax pseudoginseng*) *medicinal herb* [see: ginseng]

hindheel *medicinal herb* [see: tansy]

hini *medicinal herb* [see: Culver's root]

hioxifilcon A USAN *hydrophilic contact lens material*

Hipotest tablets OTC *dietary supplement* [multiple vitamins & minerals; multiple food products; calcium; iron; biotin] ≛•53.5•50•0.001 mg

Hi-Po-Vites tablets OTC *dietary supplement* [multiple vitamins & minerals; multiple food products; iron; folic acid; biotin] ≛•6•0.4•1 mg

Hiprex tablets ℞ *urinary antibiotic* [methenamine hippurate] 1 g

Hirudo medicinalis natural treatment [see: leeches]

Hirulog ℞ *investigational (NDA filed) antithrombotic for DVT and unstable angina, and to prevent reocclusion in MI and angioplasty* [bivalirudin]

Hismanal tablets (discontinued 1999) ℞ *nonsedating antihistamine* [astemizole] 10 mg

Histagesic Modified tablets OTC *decongestant; antihistamine; analgesic* [phenylephrine HCl; chlorpheniramine maleate; acetaminophen] 10•4•324 mg

Histaject subcu or IM injection (discontinued 1996) ℞ *antihistamine for anaphylaxis* [brompheniramine maleate] 10 mg/mL

Histalet syrup ℞ *decongestant; antihistamine* [pseudoephedrine HCl; chlorpheniramine maleate] 45•3 mg/5 mL

Histalet Forte tablets ℞ *decongestant; antihistamine* [phenylpropanolamine HCl; phenylephrine HCl; chlorpheniramine maleate; pyrilamine maleate] 50•10•4•25 mg

Histalet X tablets, syrup ℞ *deconges-tant; expectorant* [pseudoephedrine HCl; guaifenesin] 120•400 mg; 45•200 mg/5 mL

Histamic sustained-release capsules ℞ *decongestant; antihistamine* [phenyl-propanolamine HCl; phenylephrine HCl; chlorpheniramine maleate; phenyltoloxamine citrate]

histamine dihydrochloride USAN

histamine H₁ antagonists *a class of antihistamines* [also called: H₁ blockers]

histamine H₂ antagonists *a class of antihistamines* [also called: H₂ blockers]

histamine phosphate USP *gastric secretory stimulant; diagnostic aid for pheochromocytoma*

histantin [see: chlorcyclizine HCl]

histapyrrodine INN

Histatab Plus tablets OTC *decongestant; antihistamine* [phenylephrine HCl; chlorpheniramine maleate] 5•2 mg

Hista-Vadrin tablets ℞ *decongestant; antihistamine* [phenylpropanolamine HCl; phenylephrine HCl; chlor-pheniramine maleate] 40•5•6 mg

Histerone 100 IM injection ℞ *andro-gen replacement for delayed puberty or breast cancer* [testosterone] 100 mg/mL

histidine (L-histidine) USAN, USP, INN *amino acid (essential in infants and in renal failure, nonessential other-wise); symbols: His, H*

histidine monohydrochloride NF

495-L-histidineglucosylceramidase [see: imiglucerase]

Histine DM syrup ℞ *antitussive; decon-gestant; antihistamine* [dextromethor-phan hydrobromide; phenylpropa-nolamine HCl; brompheniramine maleate] 10•12.5•2 mg/5 mL

Histinex HC syrup ℞ *narcotic antitus-sive; decongestant; antihistamine* [hydrocodone bitartrate; phenyleph-rine HCl; chlorpheniramine male-ate] 2•5•2 mg/5 mL

Histinex PV syrup ℞ *narcotic antitus-sive; decongestant; antihistamine* [hydrocodone bitartrate; pseudo-

ephedrine HCl; chlorpheniramine maleate] 2.5•30•2 mg/5 mL

Histolyn-CYL intradermal injection ℞ *diagnostic aid for histoplasmosis* [histo-plasmin (mycelial derivative)] 1:100

histoplasmin USP *dermal histoplasmosis test; Histoplasma capsulatum cultures in mycelial or yeast lysate form* 1:100 injection (yeast lysate form)

Histor-D syrup ℞ *decongestant; antihis-tamine* [phenylephrine HCl; chlor-pheniramine maleate; alcohol 2%] 5•2 mg/5 mL

Histor-D Timecelles (sustained-release capsules) (discontinued 1995) ℞ *decongestant; antihistamine; anticholin-ergic* [phenylephrine HCl; chlor-pheniramine maleate; methscopo-lamine nitrate] 20•8•2.5 mg

Histosal tablets OTC *decongestant; anti-histamine; analgesic* [phenylpropanol-amine HCl; pyrilamine maleate; acetaminophen; caffeine] 20•12.5•324•30 mg

histrelin USAN, INN *LHRH agonist; investigational (orphan) for acute inter-mittent porphyria, hereditary copropor-phyria, and variegate porphyria*

histrelin acetate *LHRH agonist; cen-tral precocious puberty treatment (orphan)*

Histussin D oral liquid ℞ *narcotic antitussive; decongestant* [hydroco-done bitartrate; pseudoephedrine HCl] 5•60 mg/5 mL

Histussin HC syrup ℞ *narcotic antitus-sive; decongestant; antihistamine* [hydrocodone bitartrate; phenyleph-rine HCl; chlorpheniramine male-ate] 2.5•5•2 mg/5 mL

HIV immune globulin (HIVIG) *investigational (Phase III, orphan) immunomodulator for AIDS and maternal/fetal HIV transfer*

HIV immunotherapeutic (HIV-IT); HIV therapeutic *investigational (Phase II) gene therapy for HIV; inves-tigational (Phase I–III) antiviral for symptomatic HIV*

HIV protease inhibitors *a class of antivirals that block HIV replication*
HIV vaccine [see: AIDS vaccine]
HIV-1 LA test [see: Recombigen HIV-1 LA]
HIV-1 peptide vaccine *investigational (Phase I) vaccine for HIV*
HIVAB HIV-1 EIA; HIVAB HIV-1/ HIV-2 EIA; HIVAB HIV-2 EIA reagent kit for professional use *in vitro diagnostic aid for HIV antibodies* [enzyme immunoassay (EIA)]
HIVAG-1 reagent kit for professional use *in vitro diagnostic aid for HIV antibodies* [enzyme immunoassay (EIA)]
hive vine *medicinal herb* [see: squaw vine]
Hi-Vegi-Lip tablets OTC *digestive enzymes* [pancreatin; lipase; protease; amylase] 2400 mg•4800 U•60 000 U•60 000 U
Hivid film-coated tablets ℞ *antiviral for advanced HIV infection and AIDS (orphan)* [zalcitabine] 0.375, 0.75 mg
HIV-IG ℞ *investigational (Phase III, orphan) immunomodulator for AIDS and maternal/fetal HIV transfer* [HIV immune globulin]
HIV-neutralizing antibodies *orphan status withdrawn 1997*
HK-Cardiosol *investigational heart preservation solution*
HMB (homatropine methylbromide) [q.v.]
HMDP (hydroxymethylene diphosphonate) [see: oxidronic acid]
hMG (human menopausal gonadotropin) [see: menotropins]
HMG-CoA (3-hydroxy-3-methylglutaryl-coenzyme A) reductase inhibitors *a class of antihyperlipidemics that reduce serum LDL, VLDL, and triglycerides, but increase HDL* [also called: "statins"]
HMM (hexamethylmelamine) [see: altretamine]
HMR-3480 *investigational anti-inflammatory agent*

HMS eye drop suspension ℞ *corticosteroidal anti-inflammatory* [medrysone] 1%
HN₂ (nitrogen mustard) [see: mechlorethamine HCl]
hNGF (human nerve growth factor) [see: nerve growth factor]
HNK-20 *investigational (Phase III) monoclonal IgA antibody for respiratory syncytial virus (RSV) infections in infants; investigational (Phase III) nose drops for prevention of viral pneumonia in infants*
HOAP-BLEO (hydroxydaunomycin, Oncovin, ara-C, prednisone, bleomycin) *chemotherapy protocol*
hoarhound *medicinal herb* [see: horehound]
hock heal *medicinal herb* [see: woundwort]
hog apple *medicinal herb* [see: mandrake; noni]
hogweed *medicinal herb* [see: broom; masterwort]
Hold DM; Children's Hold lozenges OTC *antitussive* [dextromethorphan hydrobromide] 5 mg
holly *(Ilex aquifolium; I. opaca; I. vomitoria)* leaves and berries *medicinal herb used as a CNS stimulant and emetic; not generally regarded as safe and effective*
holly, ground *medicinal herb* [see: pipsissewa]
holly bay *medicinal herb* [see: magnolia]
holly-leaved barberry; holly mahonia *medicinal herb* [see: Oregon grape]
holmium *element (Ho)*
holy thistle; blessed cardus *medicinal herb* [see: blessed thistle]
homarylamine INN
homatropine BAN *ophthalmic anticholinergic* [also: homatropine hydrobromide]
homatropine hydrobromide USP *ophthalmic anticholinergic; cycloplegic; mydriatic* [also: homatropine] 5% eye drops

296   homatropine methylbromide

homatropine methylbromide USP, INN, BAN *anticholinergic*

Home Access; Home Access Express test kit for home use OTC *in vitro diagnostic aid for HIV in the blood*

Home Access Hepatitis C Check test kit for home use OTC *in vitro diagnostic aid for hepatitis C in the blood*

homidium bromide INN, BAN

Hominex-1 powder OTC *formula for infants with homocystinuria or hypermethioninemia*

Hominex-2 powder OTC *enteral nutritional therapy for homocystinuria or hypermethioninemia*

homochlorcyclizine INN, BAN

homofenazine (HFZ) INN

homomenthyl salicylate [now: homosalate]

homopipramol INN

homosalate USAN, INN *ultraviolet screen*

4-homosulfanilamide [see: mafenide]

homprenorphine INN, BAN

honey *natural remedy used as an antibacterial and wound healing agent and as a gargle to promote expectoration; not generally regarded as safe and effective for infants because of possible Clostridium botulinum contamination*

honeybee venom *natural remedy* [see: bee venom]

honeybloom *medicinal herb* [see: dogbane]

hoodwart *medicinal herb* [see: skullcap]

HOP (hydroxydaunomycin, Oncovin, prednisone) *chemotherapy protocol*

hopantenic acid INN

hops (Humulus lupulus) *flower medicinal herb for aiding digestion, appetite stimulation, bronchitis, cystitis, delirium, edema, headache, hyperactivity, insomnia, intestinal cramps, menstrual disorders, nervousness, pain, excessive sexual desire, and TB*

hoquizil INN *bronchodilator* [also: hoquizil HCl]

hoquizil HCl USAN *bronchodilator* [also: hoquizil]

Hordeum vulgare *medicinal herb* [see: barley]

horehound (Marrubium vulgare) *plant medicinal herb for asthma, colds and cough, croup, inducing diaphoresis and diuresis, intestinal parasites, lung disorders, promoting expectoration, and respiratory disorders*

horse chestnut (Aesculus californica; A. glabra; A. hippocastanum) *leaves and nuts medicinal herb for arthritis, colds and congestion, hemorrhoids, rheumatism, and varicose veins; not generally regarded as safe and effective for internal use as it is highly toxic*

horse-elder; horseheal *medicinal herb* [see: elecampane]

horsefoot; horsehoof *medicinal herb* [see: coltsfoot]

horsemint (Monarda punctata) *leaves and flowering tops medicinal herb used as a cardiac, carminative, diaphoretic, diuretic, emmenagogue, stimulant, and sudorific*

horseradish (Armoracia lapathiofolia; A. rusticana) *root medicinal herb for appetite stimulation, colic, cough, edema, expelling afterbirth, hay fever, poor circulation, sciatic pain, sinus disorders, and skin and internal tumors; also used as a vermifuge*

horsetail (Equisetum arvens) *plant medicinal herb for bladder disorders, brittle nails, glandular disorders, internal bleeding, nosebleeds, poor circulation, tuberculosis, and urinary disorders*

horseweed; fleabane (Erigeron canadensis) *plant medicinal herb used as an astringent, diuretic, and hemostatic*

ho-shou-wu; fo-ti (Polygonum multiflorum) *root medicinal herb for atherosclerosis, blood cleansing, constipation, improving liver and kidney function, insomnia, malaria, muscle aches, TB, and weak bones; also used to increase fertility, prevent aging, and promote longevity*

H.P. Acthar Gel IM or subcu injectable gel ℞ *corticosteroid; anti-inflammatory* [corticotropin repository] 40, 80 U/mL

HP-3 *investigational (Phase II) treatment for cystic fibrosis and chronic obstructive pulmonary disease*

HP-4 *investigational (Phase II) treatment for benign prostatic hyperplasia*

HPMCP (hydroxypropyl methylcellulose phthalate) [q.v.]

HPMPC (3-hydroxy-2-phosphonomethoxypropyl cytosine [dihydrate]) [see: cidofovir]

H-R Lubricating vaginal jelly OTC *lubricant* [hydroxypropyl methylcellulose]

5-HT (5-hydroxytryptamine) [see: serotonin]

HT (human thrombin) [see: thrombin]

HT; 3-HT (3-hydroxytyramine) [see: dopamine]

5-HTP (5-hydroxytryptophan) [see: L-5 hydroxytryptophan]

H-Tuss-D liquid ℞ *narcotic antitussive; decongestant* [hydrocodone bitartrate; pseudoephedrine HCl; alcohol 5%] 5•60 mg/5 mL

HU-1124 *investigational (Phase II) monoclonal antibody for the treatment for psoriasis*

Hu23F2G *investigational (Phase II) cell adhesion inhibitor for ischemic stroke, acute myocardial infarction, and trauma-induced hemorrhagic shock*

huckleberry *medicinal herb* [see: bilberry]

Humalog subcu injection, prefilled syringe cartridges ℞ *insulin analog for diabetes* [insulin lispro, human (rDNA)] 100 U/mL; 1.5 mL

human acid alpha-glucosidase *investigational (orphan) for glycogen storage disease type II*

human albumin [see: albumin, human]

human amniotic fluid-derived surfactant [see: surfactant, human amniotic fluid derived]

human antihemophilic factor [see: antihemophilic factor]

human chorionic gonadotropin (hCG) [see: gonadotropin, chorionic]

human complement receptor [see: complement receptor type I, soluble recombinant human]

human cytomegalovirus immune globulin [see: cytomegalovirus immune globulin, human]

human diploid cell vaccine (HDCV) [see: rabies vaccine]

human epidermal growth factor [see: epidermal growth factor, human]

human fibrinogen [see: fibrinogen, human]

human fibrinolysin [see: fibrinolysin, human]

human follicle-stimulating hormone (hFSH) [now: menotropins]

human growth hormone (hGH) JAN *growth hormone* [also: somatropin]

human growth hormone, recombinant (rhGH) [see: somatropin]

human growth hormone releasing factor [see: growth hormone-releasing factor]

human immunodeficiency virus (HIV-1) immune globulin (HIVIG) [see: HIV immune globulin]

human insulin [see: insulin, human]

human luteinizing hormone, recombinant & menotropins *investigational for chronic anovulation due to hypogonadotropic hypogonadism; orphan status withdrawn 1998*

human menopausal gonadotropin (hMG) [see: menotropins]

human nerve growth factor (hNGF) [see: nerve growth factor]

human respiratory syncytial virus immune globulin [see: respiratory syncytial virus immune globulin, human]

human serum albumin diethylenetriaminepentaacetic acid (DTPA) technetium (^{99m}Tc) JAN *radioactive agent* [also: technetium Tc 99m pentetate]

human superoxide dismutase (SOD) [see: superoxide dismutase, human]

human T-cell inhibitor [see: muromonab-CD3]

human T-cell lymphotrophic virus type III (HTLV-III) [now: human immunodeficiency virus (HIV)]

Human T-Lymphotropic Virus Type I EIA reagent kit for professional use *in vitro diagnostic aid for HTLV I antibody in serum or plasma* [enzyme immunoassay (EIA)]

Humate-P IV injection ℞ *antihemophilic for von Willebrand's disease (orphan)* [antihemophilic factor VIII] 2̲

Humatin capsules ℞ *aminoglycoside antibiotic; amebicide* [paromomycin sulfate] 250 mg

Humatrope powder for subcu or IM injection ℞ *growth hormone for adults or children with congenital or endogenous growth hormone deficiency, children with Turner syndrome or renal-induced growth failure, or AIDS-wasting syndrome (orphan)* [somatropin] 5 mg (15 IU) per vial

Humegon powder for IM injection ℞ *ovulation stimulant for women; spermatogenesis stimulant for men* [menotropins] 75, 150 IU

Humibid DM sustained-release tablets ℞ *antitussive; expectorant* [dextromethorphan hydrobromide; guaifenesin] 30•600 mg

Humibid DM Sprinkle sustained-release capsules ℞ *antitussive; expectorant* [dextromethorphan hydrobromide; guaifenesin] 15•300 mg

Humibid L.A. sustained-release tablets ℞ *expectorant* [guaifenesin] 600 mg

Humibid Sprinkle sustained-release capsules ℞ *expectorant* [guaifenesin] 300 mg

HuMist nasal mist OTC *nasal moisturizer* [sodium chloride (saline solution)] 0.65%

Humorphan H.P. (name changed to Numorphan HP in 1996)

Humorsol Ocumeter (eye drops) ℞ *antiglaucoma agent; reversible cholinesterase inhibitor miotic* [demecarium bromide] 0.125%, 0.25%

Humulin 30/70 ⒸⒶ (U.S. product: Humulin 70/30) subcu injection, prefilled syringe cartridges OTC *antidiabetic* [insulin; isophane insulin] 100 U/mL; 1.5 mL

Humulin 50/50 subcu injection (prefilled cartridges available in Canada) OTC *antidiabetic* [isophane human insulin (rDNA); human insulin (rDNA)] 100 U/mL; 1.5 mL

Humulin 70/30 subcu injection, prefilled syringe cartridges OTC *antidiabetic* [isophane human insulin (rDNA); human insulin (rDNA)] 100 U/mL; 1.5 mL

Humulin L subcu injection OTC *antidiabetic* [human insulin zinc (rDNA)] 100 U/mL

Humulin N subcu injection, prefilled syringe cartridges OTC *antidiabetic* [isophane human insulin (rDNA)] 100 U/mL; 1.5 mL

Humulin R ⒸⒶ (U.S. product: Regular Iletin I) subcu injection OTC *antidiabetic* [human insulin (recombinant)] 100 U/mL; 1.5 mL

Humulin U Ultralente subcu injection OTC *antidiabetic* [extended human insulin zinc (rDNA)] 100 U/mL

Humulin-U ⒸⒶ (U.S. product: Humulin U Ultralente) subcu injection OTC *antidiabetic* [extended insulin zinc] 100 U/mL

Humulus lupulus medicinal herb [see: hops]

hurr-burr medicinal herb [see: burdock]

Hurricaine spray, liquid, gel OTC *mucous membrane anesthetic* [benzocaine] 20%

HXM (hexamethylmelamine) [see: altretamine]

Hyacne ℞ investigational (Phase III) acne treatment

Hyalgan intra-articular injection ℞ *viscoelastic lubricant and "shock absorber" for osteoarthritis and temporomandibular joint syndrome* [hyaluronate sodium] 20 mg/2 mL

hyalosidase INN, BAN

hyaluronate sodium USAN, JAN *ophthalmic surgical aid; treatment for osteoarthritis and TMJ syndrome; vet-*

erinary synovitis agent [also: hyaluronic acid]

hyaluronate sodium & diclofenac potassium *investigational (Phase III) topical treatment for actinic keratosis; clinical trials as a topical analgesic discontinued 1996*

hyaluronic acid BAN *ophthalmic surgical aid; treatment for osteoarthritis and TMJ syndrome; veterinary synovitis agent* [also: hyaluronate sodium]

hyaluronidase USP, INN, BAN *dispersion aid; absorption facilitator*

hyaluronoglucosaminidase [see: hyalosidase]

hyamate [see: buramate]

Hyanalgese-D ℞ *investigational (Phase III) topical NSAID analgesic for cystitis; clinical trials discontinued 1996* [hyaluronate sodium; diclofenac potassium]

hybenzate USAN *combining name for radicals or groups* [also: hibenzate]

Hybolin Decanoate-50; Hybolin Decanoate-100 IM injection ℞ *anabolic steroid for anemia of renal insufficiency* [nandrolone decanoate] 50 mg/mL; 100 mg/mL

Hybolin Improved IM injection ℞ *anabolic steroid for metastatic breast cancer in women* [nandrolone phenpropionate] 50 mg/mL

Hybri-CEAker *orphan status withdrawn 1997* [indium In 111 altumomab pentetate]

Hycamtin powder for IV injection ℞ *antineoplastic/topoisomerase I inhibitor for ovarian and small cell lung cancers* [topotecan HCl] 4 mg/vial

hycanthone USAN, INN *antischistosomal*

hycanthone mesylate *antischistosomal*

hyclate INN *combining name for radicals or groups*

HyClinda ℞ *investigational (Phase III) antibiotic delivery system* [clindamycin]

HycoClear Tuss syrup ℞ *narcotic antitussive; expectorant* [hydrocodone bitartrate; guaifenesin] 5•100 mg/5 mL

Hycodan tablets, syrup ℞ *narcotic antitussive; anticholinergic* [hydroco-

done bitartrate; homatropine methylbromide] 5•1.5 mg; 5•1.5 mg/5 mL ⅔ Hycomine; Vicodin

Hycomine syrup, pediatric syrup ℞ *narcotic antitussive; decongestant* [hydrocodone bitartrate; phenylpropanolamine HCl] 5•25 mg/5 mL; 2.5•12.5 mg/5 mL ⅔ Byclomine; Hycodan; Vicodin

Hycomine Compound tablets ℞ *narcotic antitussive; decongestant; antihistamine; analgesic* [hydrocodone bitartrate; phenylephrine HCl; chlorpheniramine maleate; acetaminophen; caffeine] 5•10•2•250•30 mg

Hycort cream, ointment ℞ *topical corticosteroidal anti-inflammatory* [hydrocortisone] 1%

Hycotuss Expectorant syrup ℞ *narcotic antitussive; expectorant* [hydrocodone bitartrate; guaifenesin; alcohol 10%] 5•100 mg/5 mL

hydantoins *a class of anticonvulsants*

Hydeltrasol IV, IM injection ℞ *corticosteroid; anti-inflammatory* [prednisolone sodium phosphate] 20 mg/mL

Hydeltra-T.B.A. intra-articular, intralesional, or soft tissue injection (discontinued 1997) ℞ *corticosteroid; anti-inflammatory* [prednisolone tebutate] 20 mg/mL

Hydergine sublingual tablets, tablets, liquid ℞ *cognition adjuvant for age-related mental capacity decline* [ergoloid mesylates] 0.5, 1 mg; 1 mg; 1 mg/mL ⅔ Hydramine

Hydergine LC liquid capsules ℞ *cognition adjuvant for age-related mental capacity decline* [ergoloid mesylates] 1 mg

hydracarbazine INN

hydragogues *a class of purgatives that produce abundant watery discharge from the bowels*

hydralazine INN, BAN *antihypertensive; peripheral vasodilator* [also: hydralazine HCl]

hydralazine HCl USP, JAN *antihypertensive; peripheral vasodilator* [also:

hydralazine] 10, 25, 50, 100 mg oral; 20 mg/mL injection

hydralazine polistirex USAN *antihypertensive*

Hydramyn syrup (discontinued 1997) ℞ *antihistamine; antitussive* [diphenhydramine HCl; alcohol 5%] 12.5 mg/5 mL ② Hydramine; Hytramyn

hydrangea (*Hydrangea arborescens*) leaves and root *medicinal herb for arthritis, bladder infections, gallstones, gonorrhea, gout, kidney stones, rheumatism, and urinary disorders*

Hydrap-ES tablets ℞ *antihypertensive; vasodilator; diuretic* [hydrochlorothiazide; reserpine; hydralazine HCl] 15•0.1•25 mg

hydrargaphen INN, BAN

hydrastine USP

hydrastine HCl USP

hydrastinine HCl NF

Hydrastis canadensis medicinal herb [see: goldenseal]

Hydrate IV or IM injection ℞ *antinauseant; antiemetic; antivertigo; motion sickness preventative* [dimenhydrinate] 50 mg/mL

Hydrazide 25/25; Hydrazide 50/50 capsules (discontinued 1995) ℞ *antihypertensive; vasodilator; diuretic* [hydrochlorothiazide; hydralazine HCl] 25•25 mg; 50•50 mg

hydrazinecarboximidamide monohydrochloride [see: pimagedine HCl]

hydrazinoxane [see: domoxin]

Hydrea capsules ℞ *antineoplastic for melanoma, ovarian carcinoma, and myelocytic leukemia; sickle cell anemia treatment (orphan)* [hydroxyurea] 500 mg

Hydrisea lotion OTC *moisturizer; emollient* [Dead Sea salts]

Hydrisinol cream, lotion OTC *moisturizer; emollient*

Hydro Cobex IM injection ℞ *antianemic; vitamin B₁₂ supplement* [hydroxocobalamin] 1000 μg/mL

hydrobentizide INN

Hydrobexan IM injection (discontinued 1995) ℞ *antianemic; vitamin B₁₂ supplement* [hydroxocobalamin] 1000 μg/mL

hydrobutamine [see: butidrine]

Hydrocare Cleaning and Disinfecting solution OTC *chemical disinfecting solution for soft contact lenses*

Hydrocare Preserved Saline solution OTC *rinsing/storage solution for soft contact lenses* [sodium chloride (preserved saline solution)]

Hydrocet capsules ℞ *narcotic analgesic* [hydrocodone bitartrate; acetaminophen] 5•500 mg

hydrochloric acid NF *acidifying agent*

hydrochloric acid, diluted NF *acidifying agent*

hydrochlorothiazide (HCT; HCTZ) USP, INN, BAN *antihypertensive; diuretic* 25, 50, 100 mg oral; 50 mg/5 mL oral; 100 mg/mL oral

hydrocholeretics *a class of gastrointestinal drugs that exert laxative effects and increase volume and water content of bile actions*

Hydrocil Instant powder OTC *bulk laxative* [psyllium hydrophilic mucilloid] 3.5 g/scoop or packet

hydrocodone INN, BAN *antitussive* [also: hydrocodone bitartrate]

hydrocodone bitartrate USAN, USP *antitussive* [also: hydrocodone]

hydrocodone bitartrate & acetaminophen *antitussive; analgesic* 7.5•650, 10•650 mg oral

hydrocodone bitartrate & guaifenesin *antitussive; expectorant* 5•100 mg/5 mL oral

Hydrocodone Compound syrup ℞ *narcotic antitussive; anticholinergic* [hydrocodone bitartrate; homatropine hydrobromide] 5•1.5 mg/5 mL

Hydrocodone CP; Hydrocodone HD oral liquid ℞ *narcotic antitussive; decongestant; antihistamine* [hydrocodone bitartrate; phenylephrine HCl; chlorpheniramine maleate] 2.5•5•2 mg/5 mL; 1.67•5•2 mg/5 mL

Hydrocodone GF syrup ℞ *narcotic antitussive; expectorant* [hydrocodone bitartrate; guaifenesin] 5•100 mg/5 mL

Hydrocodone PA syrup, pediatric syrup ℞ *narcotic antitussive; decongestant* [hydrocodone bitartrate; phenylpropanolamine HCl] 5•25 mg/5 mL; 2.5•12.5 mg/5 mL

hydrocodone polistirex USAN *antitussive*

hydrocolloid gel *dressings for wet wounds*

Hydrocort cream ℞ *topical corticosteroidal anti-inflammatory* [hydrocortisone] 2.5%

hydrocortamate INN

hydrocortamate HCl [see: hydrocortamate]

hydrocortisone (HC) USP, INN, BAN *corticosteroid; anti-inflammatory* 5, 10, 20 mg oral; 0.5%, 1%, 2.5% topical

hydrocortisone aceponate INN *corticosteroid; anti-inflammatory*

hydrocortisone acetate (HCA) USP, BAN *corticosteroid; anti-inflammatory* 25, 50 mg/mL injection

hydrocortisone buteprate USAN *topical corticosteroidal anti-inflammatory*

hydrocortisone butyrate BAN *topical corticosteroidal anti-inflammatory* [also: hydrocortisone probutate]

hydrocortisone cyclopentylpropionate *corticosteroid; anti-inflammatory* [see: hydrocortisone cypionate]

hydrocortisone cypionate USP *corticosteroid; anti-inflammatory*

hydrocortisone hemisuccinate USP *corticosteroid; anti-inflammatory*

hydrocortisone probutate USAN, USP *topical corticosteroidal anti-inflammatory* [also: hydrocortisone buteprate]

hydrocortisone sodium phosphate USP, BAN *corticosteroid; anti-inflammatory*

hydrocortisone sodium succinate USP, BAN *corticosteroid; anti-inflammatory*

hydrocortisone valerate USAN, USP *topical corticosteroidal anti-inflammatory* 0.2% topical

Hydrocortone tablets ℞ *corticosteroid; anti-inflammatory* [hydrocortisone] 10, 20 mg

Hydrocortone Acetate intralesional, intra-articular, or soft tissue injection ℞ *corticosteroid; anti-inflammatory* [hydrocortisone acetate] 25, 50 mg/mL

Hydrocortone Phosphate IV, subcu, or IM injection ℞ *corticosteroid; anti-inflammatory* [hydrocortisone sodium phosphate] 50 mg/mL

Hydrocotyle asiatica *medicinal herb* [see: gotu kola]

Hydrocream Base OTC *cream base*

Hydro-Crysti 12 IM injection ℞ *antianemic; vitamin B_{12} supplement* [hydroxocobalamin] 1000 μg/mL

HydroDIURIL tablets ℞ *antihypertensive; diuretic* [hydrochlorothiazide] 25, 50, 100 mg

hydrofilcon A USAN *hydrophilic contact lens material*

hydroflumethiazide USP, INN, BAN *antihypertensive; diuretic* 50 mg oral

hydrofluoric acid *dental caries prophylactic*

hydrogen *element (H)*

hydrogen peroxide USP *topical anti-infective*

hydrogen tetrabromoaurate [see: bromauric acid]

hydrogenated ergot alkaloids [now: ergoloid mesylates]

hydrogenated vegetable oil [see: vegetable oil, hydrogenated]

Hydrogesic capsules ℞ *narcotic analgesic* [hydrocodone bitartrate; acetaminophen] 5•500 mg

hydromadinone INN

Hydromet syrup ℞ *narcotic antitussive; anticholinergic* [hydrocodone bitartrate; homatropine methylbromide] 5•1.5 mg/5 mL

hydromorphinol INN, BAN

hydromorphone INN, BAN *narcotic analgesic; widely abused as a street drug* [also: hydromorphone HCl]

hydromorphone HCl USP *narcotic analgesic; widely abused as a street drug* [also: hydromorphone] 2, 4, 8 mg oral; 5 mg/5 mL oral; 3 mg rectal; 1, 2, 4, 10 mg/mL injection

hydromorphone sulfate

Hydromox tablets ℞ *diuretic; antihypertensive* [quinethazone] 50 mg

Hydropane syrup (name changed to Hydrocodone Compound in 1995)

Hydro-Par tablets ℞ *antihypertensive; diuretic* [hydrochlorothiazide] 25, 50 mg

Hydropel ointment OTC *skin protectant* [silicone; hydrophobic starch derivative] 30%•10%

Hydrophed tablets ℞ *antiasthmatic; bronchodilator; decongestant; antihistamine* [theophylline; ephedrine sulfate; hydroxyzine HCl] 130•25•10 mg

Hydrophilic OTC *ointment base*

hydrophilic ointment [see: ointment, hydrophilic]

hydrophilic petrolatum [see: petrolatum, hydrophilic]

Hydropres-25 tablets (discontinued 1996) ℞ *antihypertensive; diuretic* [hydrochlorothiazide; reserpine] 25•0.125 mg

Hydropres-50 tablets ℞ *antihypertensive; diuretic* [hydrochlorothiazide; reserpine] 50•0.125 mg

hydroquinone USP *hyperpigmentation bleaching agent* 3%, 4% topical

Hydro-Serp tablets ℞ *antihypertensive; diuretic* [hydrochlorothiazide; reserpine] 50•0.125 mg

Hydroserpine #1; Hydroserpine #2 tablets ℞ *antihypertensive; diuretic* [hydrochlorothiazide; reserpine] 25•0.125 mg; 50•0.125 mg

Hydrosine 25, Hydrosine 50 tablets ℞ *antihypertensive; diuretic* [hydrochlorothiazide; reserpine]

HydroStat IR tablets (discontinued 1999) ℞ *narcotic analgesic* [hydromorphone HCl] 1, 2, 3, 4 mg

hydrotalcite INN, BAN

HydroTex cream ℞ *topical corticosteroidal anti-inflammatory* [hydrocortisone] 0.5%

hydroxamethocaine BAN [also: hydroxytetracaine]

hydroxidione sodium succinate [see: hydroxydione sodium succinate]

hydroxindasate INN

hydroxindasol INN

hydroxizine chloride [see: hydroxyzine HCl]

hydroxocobalamin USAN, USP, INN, BAN, JAN *vitamin B₁₂; hematopoietic* [also: hydroxocobalamin acetate] 1 mg/mL injection

hydroxocobalamin acetate JAN *vitamin B₁₂; hematopoietic* [also: hydroxocobalamin]

hydroxocobalamin & sodium thiosulfate *investigational (orphan) for severe acute cyanide poisoning*

hydroxocobemine [see: hydroxocobalamin]

3-hydroxy-2-phosphonomethoxypropyl cytosine (HPMPC) dihydrate [see: cidofovir]

N-hydroxyacetamide [see: acetohydroxamic acid]

4′-hydroxyacetanilide [see: acetaminophen]

4′-hydroxyacetanilide salicylate [see: acetaminosalol]

hydroxyamfetamine INN *ophthalmic adrenergic; mydriatic* [also: hydroxyamphetamine hydrobromide; hydroxyamphetamine]

hydroxyamphetamine BAN *ophthalmic adrenergic; mydriatic* [also: hydroxyamphetamine hydrobromide; hydroxyamfetamine]

hydroxyamphetamine hydrobromide USP *ophthalmic adrenergic/vasoconstrictor; mydriatic* [also: hydroxyamfetamine; hydroxyamphetamine]

hydroxyapatite BAN *prosthetic aid* [also: durapatite; calcium phosphate, tribasic]

2-hydroxybenzamide [see: salicylamide]

2-hydroxybenzoic acid [see: salicylic acid]

o-hydroxybenzyl alcohol [see: salicyl alcohol]

hydroxybutanedioic acid [see: malic acid]

4-hydroxybutanoic acid, sodium salt [see: sodium oxybate]

hydroxybutyrate sodium, gamma
[see: sodium oxybate]

hydroxycarbamide INN *antineoplastic*
[also: hydroxyurea]

hydroxychloroquine INN, BAN *antimalarial; lupus erythematosus suppressant* [also: hydroxychloroquine sulfate]

hydroxychloroquine sulfate USP *antimalarial; antirheumatic; lupus erythematosus suppressant* [also: hydroxychloroquine] 200 mg oral

25-hydroxycholecalciferol [see: calcifediol]

hydroxycincophene [see: oxycinchophen]

hydroxydaunomycin [see: doxorubicin]

14-hydroxydihydromorphine [see: hydromorphinol]

hydroxydione sodium succinate INN, BAN

hydroxyethyl cellulose NF *suspending and viscosity-increasing agent; ophthalmic aid*

2-hydroxyethyl methacrylate (HEMA) *contact lens material*

hydroxyethyl starch (HES) [see: hetastarch]

hydroxyethylstarch JAN *plasma volume extender* [also: hetastarch]

hydroxyhexamide

hydroxylapatite [see: durapatite; calcium phosphate, tribasic]

hydroxymagnesium aluminate [see: magaldrate]

hydroxymesterone [see: medrysone]

hydroxymethylene diphosphonate (HMDP) [see: oxidronic acid]

hydroxymethylgramicidin [see: methocidin]

N-hydroxynaphthalimide diethyl phosphate [see: naftalofos]

hydroxypethidine INN, BAN

hydroxyphenamate USAN *minor tranquilizer* [also: oxyfenamate]

N-4-hydroxyphenylretinamide [see: fenretinide]

hydroxyprocaine INN, BAN

hydroxyprogesterone INN, BAN *progestin for amenorrhea, metrorrhagia,* *and dysfunctional uterine bleeding* [also: hydroxyprogesterone caproate]

hydroxyprogesterone caproate USP, INN, JAN *progestin for amenorrhea, metrorrhagia, and dysfunctional uterine bleeding* [also: hydroxyprogesterone] 125, 250 mg/mL IM injection (in oil)

2-hydroxypropanoic acid, calcium salt, hydrate [see: calcium lactate]

hydroxypropyl cellulose NF *topical protectant; emulsifying and coating agent* [also: hydroxypropylcellulose]

hydroxypropyl methylcellulose USP *suspending and viscosity-increasing agent; ophthalmic moisturizer and surgical aid* [also: hypromellose; hydroxypropylmethylcellulose]

hydroxypropyl methylcellulose 1828 USP

hydroxypropyl methylcellulose phthalate (HPMCP) NF *tablet-coating agent* [also: hydroxypropylmethylcellulose phthalate]

hydroxypropyl methylcellulose phthalate 200731 NF *tablet-coating agent*

hydroxypropyl methylcellulose phthalate 220824 NF *tablet-coating agent*

hydroxypropylcellulose JAN *topical protectant; emulsifying and coating agent* [also: hydroxypropyl cellulose]

hydroxypropylmethylcellulose JAN *suspending and viscosity-increasing agent; ophthalmic surgical aid* [also: hydroxypropyl methylcellulose; hypromellose]

hydroxypropylmethylcellulose phthalate JAN *tablet-coating agent* [also: hydroxypropyl methylcellulose phthalate]

hydroxypyridine tartrate INN

hydroxyquinoline *topical antiseptic*

4'-hydroxysalicylanilide [see: osalmid]

hydroxystearin sulfate NF

hydroxystenozole INN

hydroxystilbamidine INN, BAN *antileishmanial* [also: hydroxystilbamidine isethionate]

hydroxystilbamidine isethionate
USP *antileishmanial* [also: hydroxystil-
bamidine]

hydroxysuccinic acid [see: malic acid]

hydroxytetracaine INN [also: hydrox-
amethocaine]

hydroxytoluic acid INN, BAN

5-hydroxytryptamine₁ (5-HT₁) [see:
serotonin]

**5-hydroxytryptamine₃ (5-HT₃)
receptor antagonists** *a class of antinauseant and antiemetic agents used
primarily after emetogenic cancer chemotherapy*

5-hydroxytryptophan (5-HTP) [see:
L-5 hydroxytryptophan]

3-hydroxytyramine (HT; 3-HT)
[see: dopamine]

hydroxyurea USAN, USP, BAN *antimetabolite antineoplastic; sickle cell anemia treatment (orphan); investigational
adjunctive therapy for HIV* [also:
hydroxycarbamide] 500 mg oral

hydroxyzine INN, BAN *anxiolytic;
minor tranquilizer; antiemetic; piperazine antihistamine; antipruritic* [also:
hydroxyzine HCl]

hydroxyzine HCl USP *anxiolytic; minor
tranquilizer; antiemetic; piperazine antihistamine; antipruritic* [also: hydroxy-
zine] 10, 25, 50 mg oral; 10 mg/5 mL
oral; 25, 50 mg/mL injection

hydroxyzine pamoate USP *anxiolytic;
minor tranquilizer; antiemetic; piperazine antihistamine; antipruritic* 25, 50,
100 mg oral

Hygenic Cleansing anorectal pads
OTC *moisturizer and cleanser for external rectal/vaginal areas; astringent*
[witch hazel] 50%

Hygroton tablets ℞ *antihypertensive;
diuretic* [chlorthalidone] 25, 50, 100
mg ⃞ Regroton

Hylagel Uro ℞ *investigational (Phase
I) hylan B gel tissue augmentation
agent for the treatment of urge urinary
incontinence*

hylan G-F 20 *hylan gel-fluid polymer
mixture for osteoarthritis and TMJ syndrome*

Hylorel tablets ℞ *antihypertensive*
[guanadrel sulfate] 10, 25 mg

Hylutin IM injection ℞ *progestin for
amenorrhea, metrorrhagia, and dysfunctional uterine bleeding* [hydroxy-
progesterone caproate in oil] 125,
250 mg/mL

hymecromone USAN, INN *choleretic*

hyoscine hydrobromide BAN *GI
antispasmodic; prevent motion sickness; cycloplegic; mydriatic* [also: scopolamine hydrobromide]

hyoscine methobromide BAN *anticholinergic* [also: methscopolamine
bromide]

hyoscyamine (L-hyoscyamine) USP,
BAN *anticholinergic; urinary antispasmodic*

hyoscyamine hydrobromide USP *GI
antispasmodic; anticholinergic*

hyoscyamine sulfate USP *GI/urinary
antispasmodic; anticholinergic* [also:
hyoscyamine sulphate] 0.375 mg
oral; 0.125 mg/mL oral

hyoscyamine sulphate BAN *GI antispasmodic; anticholinergic* [also: hyoscyamine sulfate]

Hyoscyamus niger *medicinal herb* [see:
henbane]

Hyosophen tablets, elixir ℞ *GI antispasmodic; anticholinergic; sedative*
[atropine sulfate; scopolamine
hydrobromide; hyoscyamine hydrobromide; phenobarbital] 0.0194•
0.0065•0.1037•16.2 mg; 0.0194•
0.0065•0.1037•16.2 mg/5 mL

**Hypaque Meglumine 30%;
Hypaque Meglumine 60%** injection ℞ *radiopaque contrast medium*
[diatrizoate meglumine (46.67%
iodine)] 300 mg/mL (141 mg/mL);
600 mg/mL (282 mg/mL)

Hypaque Sodium oral/rectal solution, powder for oral/rectal solution
℞ *radiopaque contrast medium for gastrointestinal imaging* [diatrizoate
sodium (59.87% iodine)] 416.7 mg
(249 mg); 1002 mg (600 mg)

Hypaque Sodium 20% intracavitary
instillation ℞ *radiopaque contrast*

medium for urological imaging [diatrizoate sodium (59.87% iodine)] 200 mg/mL (120 mg/mL)

Hypaque Sodium 25%; Hypaque Sodium 50% injection ℞ *radiopaque contrast medium* [diatrizoate sodium (46.67% iodine)] 250 mg/mL (150 mg/mL); 500 mg/mL (300 mg/mL)

Hypaque-76 injection ℞ *radiopaque contrast medium* [diatrizoate meglumine; diatrizoate sodium (48.7% total iodine)] 660•100 mg/mL (370 mg/mL)

Hypaque-Cysto intracavitary instillation ℞ *radiopaque contrast medium for urological imaging* [diatrizoate meglumine (46.67% iodine)] 300 mg/mL (141 mg/mL)

Hypaque-M 75; Hypaque-M 90 injection (discontinued 1999) ℞ *radiopaque contrast medium* [diatrizoate meglumine; diatrizoate sodium (51.1% total iodine)] 50%•25% (38.3%); 60%•30% (46%)

Hyperab IM injection ℞ *rabies prophylaxis* [rabies immune globulin] 150 IU/mL

HyperHep IM injection ℞ *hepatitis B immunizing agent* [hepatitis B immune globulin] 0.5, 1, 5 mL ⊡ Hyper-Tet; Hyperstat

hypericin *investigational (Phase I) antiviral for HIV and AIDS*

Hypericum perforatum *medicinal herb* [see: St. John's wort]

Hyperlyte; Hyperlyte CR; Hyperlyte R IV admixture ℞ *intravenous electrolyte therapy* [combined electrolyte solution]

Hypermune RSV ℞ *preventative for respiratory syncytial virus (RSV) infections in high-risk infants (orphan); investigational (orphan) treatment for RSV* [respiratory syncytial virus immune globulin (RSV-IG)]

Hyperstat IV injection ℞ *vasodilator for hypertensive emergency* [diazoxide] 15 mg/mL ⊡ Hyper-Tet; HyperHep; Nitrostat

Hyper-Tet IM injection ℞ *tetanus immunizing agent* [tetanus immune globulin] 250 U ⊡ HyperHep; Hyperstat

Hyphed syrup ℞ *narcotic antitussive; decongestant; antihistamine* [hydrocodone bitartrate; pseudoephedrine HCl; chlorpheniramine maleate; alcohol ≟%] 2.5•30•2 mg/5 mL

Hy-Phen tablets ℞ *narcotic analgesic* [hydrocodone bitartrate; acetaminophen] 5•500 mg

hyphylline [see: dyphylline]

hypnogene [see: barbital]

hypnotics *a class of agents that induce sleep*

hypochlorous acid, sodium salt [see: sodium hypochlorite]

β-hypophamine [see: vasopressin]

α-hypophamine [see: oxytocin]

hypophosphorous acid NF *antioxidant*

Hyporet (trademarked delivery system) *prefilled disposable syringe*

HypoTears ophthalmic ointment OTC *ocular moisturizer/lubricant* [white petrolatum; mineral oil]

HypoTears; HypoTears PF eye drops OTC *ophthalmic moisturizer/lubricant* [polyvinyl alcohol] 1%

HypRho-D; HypRho-D Mini-Dose IM injection ℞ *obstetric Rh factor immunity suppressant* [$Rh_0(D)$ immune globulin] 300 μg; 50 μg

Hyprogest 250 IM injection (discontinued 1997) ℞ *progestin for amenorrhea, metrorrhagia, and dysfunctional uterine bleeding* [hydroxyprogesterone caproate in oil] 250 mg/mL

hyprolose [see: hydroxypropyl cellulose]

hypromellose INN, BAN *suspending and viscosity-increasing agent* [also: hydroxypropyl methylcellulose; hydroxypropylmethylcellulose]

Hyrexin-50 injection ℞ *antihistamine; motion sickness preventative; sleep aid; antiparkinsonian* [diphenhydramine HCl] 50 mg/mL

Hyskon uterine infusion ℞ *hysteroscopy aid* [dextran 70; dextrose] 32%•10%

Hysone cream OTC *topical corticosteroidal anti-inflammatory; antifungal; antibacterial* [hydrocortisone; clioquinol] 10•30 mg/g

hyssop *(Hyssopus officinalis)* leaves *medicinal herb for chronic hay fever, congestion, cough, lung ailments, promoting expectoration, and sore throat*

hyssop, hedge *medicinal herb* [see: hedge hyssop]

hyssop, Indian; wild hyssop *medicinal herb* [see: blue vervain]

hyssop, prairie *medicinal herb* [see: wild hyssop]

Hytakerol capsules R *vitamin D₁ therapy for tetany and hypoparathyroidism* [dihydrotachysterol] 0.125 mg

Hytinic capsules, elixir OTC *hematinic* [polysaccharide-iron complex] 150 mg; 100 mg/5 mL

Hytinic IM injection R *hematinic* [ferrous gluconate; multiple B vitamins; procaine HCl] 3 mg/mL• ± •2%

Hytone cream, lotion, ointment R *topical corticosteroidal anti-inflammatory* [hydrocortisone] 1%, 2.5%; 1%, 2.5%; 2.5% 🔲 Vytone

Hytone 1% ointment, spray R *topical corticosteroidal anti-inflammatory* [hydrocortisone] 1%

Hytrin soft capsules R *antihypertensive (α-blocker); treatment for benign prostatic hyperplasia (BPH)* [terazosin HCl] 1, 2, 5, 10 mg

Hytrin 🇨🇦 tablets R *antihypertensive (α-blocker); treatment for benign prostatic hyperplasia (BPH)* [terazosin HCl] 1, 2, 5, 10 mg

Hytuss tablets OTC *expectorant* [guaifenesin] 100 mg

Hytuss 2X capsules OTC *expectorant* [guaifenesin] 200 mg

Hyzaar film-coated tablets R *antihypertensive; angiotensin II receptor antagonist; diuretic* [losartan potassium; hydrochlorothiazide] 50•12.5, 100•25 mg

Hyzine-50 IM injection (discontinued 1998) R *anxiolytic; antiemetic* [hydroxyzine HCl] 50 mg/mL

I

¹²³**I** [see: iodohippurate sodium I 123]
¹²³**I** [see: sodium iodide I 123]
¹²⁵**I** [see: albumin, iodinated I 125 serum]
¹²⁵**I** [see: diatrizoate sodium I 125]
¹²⁵**I** [see: diohippuric acid I 125]
¹²⁵**I** [see: diotyrosine I 125]
¹²⁵**I** [see: fibrinogen I 125]
¹²⁵**I** [see: insulin I 125]
¹²⁵**I** [see: iodohippurate sodium I 125]
¹²⁵**I** [see: iodopyracet I 125]
¹²⁵**I** [see: iomethin I 125]
¹²⁵**I** [see: iothalamate sodium I 125]
¹²⁵**I** [see: liothyronine I 125]
¹²⁵**I** [see: oleic acid I 125]
¹²⁵**I** [see: povidone I 125]
¹²⁵**I** [see: rose bengal sodium I 125]
¹²⁵**I** [see: sodium iodide I 125]
¹²⁵**I** [see: thyroxine I 125]

¹²⁵**I** [see: triolein I 125]
¹³¹**I** [see: albumin, aggregated iodinated I 131 serum]
¹³¹**I** [see: albumin, iodinated I 131 serum]
¹³¹**I** [see: diatrizoate sodium I 131]
¹³¹**I** [see: diohippuric acid I 131]
¹³¹**I** [see: diotyrosine I 131]
¹³¹**I** [see: ethiodized oil I 131]
¹³¹**I** [see: insulin I 131]
¹³¹**I** [see: iodipamide sodium I 131]
¹³¹**I** [see: iodoantipyrine I 131]
¹³¹**I** [see: iodocholesterol I 131]
¹³¹**I** [see: iodohippurate sodium I 131]
¹³¹**I** [see: iodopyracet I 131]
¹³¹**I** [see: iomethin I 131]
¹³¹**I** [see: iothalamate sodium I 131]
¹³¹**I** [see: iotyrosine I 131]
¹³¹**I** [see: liothyronine I 131]

¹³¹I [see: macrosalb (¹³¹I)]
¹³¹I [see: oleic acid I 131]
¹³¹I [see: povidone I 131]
¹³¹I [see: rose bengal sodium I 131]
¹³¹I [see: sodium iodide I 131]
¹³¹I [see: thyroxine I 131]
¹³¹I [see: tolpovidone I 131]
¹³¹I [see: triolein I 131]

Iamin ℞ *investigational (Phase II) immunostimulating gel for peptic ulcers, surgical wound repair, venous leg ulcers, and bone healing* [prezatide copper acetate]

IB-367 *investigational topical antimicrobial compound*

ibacitabine INN

ibafloxacin USAN, INN, BAN *antibacterial*

ibandronate sodium USAN *bone resorption inhibitor for postmenopausal osteoporosis, metastatic bone disease, hypercalcemia of malignancy, and Paget's disease*

ibazocine INN

IBC (isobutyl cyanoacrylate) [see: bucrylate]

Iberet; Iberet-500 controlled-release Filmtabs (film-coated tablets) OTC *hematinic* [ferrous sulfate; multiple B vitamins; sodium ascorbate] 105•±•150 mg; 105•±•500 mg

Iberet; Iberet-500 liquid OTC *hematinic* [ferrous sulfate; multiple B vitamins] 78.75•± mg/15 mL

Iberet-Folic-500 controlled-release Filmtabs (film-coated tablets) ℞ *hematinic* [ferrous sulfate; multiple B vitamins; sodium ascorbate; folic acid] 105•±•500•0.8 mg

iboga (Tabernanthe iboga) *euphoric/hallucinogenic street drug, the root of which is chewed or chopped into a fine powder and mixed with other drugs; doses high enough to induce hallucinations are also most likely to cause death*

ibopamine USAN, INN, BAN *peripheral dopaminergic agent; vasodilator*

ibrotal [see: ibrotamide]

ibrotamide INN

Ibu film-coated tablets ℞ *nonsteroidal anti-inflammatory drug (NSAID);*

antiarthritic; analgesic [ibuprofen] 400, 600, 800 mg

ibudilast INN

ibufenac USAN, INN, BAN *analgesic; anti-inflammatory*

Ibuprin tablets OTC *nonsteroidal anti-inflammatory drug (NSAID); antiarthritic; analgesic* [ibuprofen] 200 mg

ibuprofen USAN, USP, INN, BAN *antiarthritic; nonsteroidal anti-inflammatory drug (NSAID); analgesic; investigational (orphan) IV treatment for patent ductus arteriosus* 200, 300, 400, 600, 800 mg oral; 100 mg/5 mL oral; 40 mg/mL oral

ibuprofen aluminum USAN *anti-inflammatory*

ibuprofen piconol USAN *topical anti-inflammatory*

Ibuprohm caplets, tablets OTC *nonsteroidal anti-inflammatory drug (NSAID); antiarthritic; analgesic* [ibuprofen] 200 mg

Ibuprohm tablets ℞ *nonsteroidal anti-inflammatory drug (NSAID); antiarthritic; analgesic* [ibuprofen] 400 mg

ibuproxam INN

Ibu-Tab film-coated tablets (discontinued 1996) OTC *nonsteroidal anti-inflammatory drug (NSAID); antiarthritic; analgesic* [ibuprofen] 200 mg

Ibu-Tab film-coated tablets (discontinued 1996) ℞ *nonsteroidal anti-inflammatory drug (NSAID); antiarthritic; analgesic* [ibuprofen] 400, 600, 800 mg

ibutamoren mesylate USAN *growth hormone for congenital growth hormone deficiency, musculoskeletal impairment, and hip fractures*

ibuterol INN

ibutilide INN *antiarrhythmic* [also: ibutilide fumarate]

ibutilide fumarate USAN *antiarrhythmic for atrial fibrillation/flutter* [also: ibutilide]

ibuverine INN

ibylcaine chloride [see: butethamine HCl]

IC-351 *investigational (Phase II) agent for erectile dysfunction*

ICAPS timed-release tablets OTC *vitamin/mineral supplement* [multiple vitamins & minerals] ≛

ICAPS Plus tablets OTC *vitamin/mineral supplement* [multiple vitamins & minerals] ≛

icatibant acetate USAN *antiasthmatic*

ICE (ifosfamide [with mesna rescue], carboplatin, etoposide) *chemotherapy protocol* [also: MICE]

Iceland moss (*Cetraria islandica*) plant *medicinal herb for anemia, bronchitis, hay fever, congestion, cough, digestive disorders, and lung disorders*

ichthammol USP, BAN *topical anti-infective* 10%, 20%

iclazepam INN

icodextrin INN, BAN *investigational (orphan) peritoneal dialysis agent for end stage renal disease*

icopezil maleate USAN *acetylcholinesterase inhibitor; cognition adjuvant for Alzheimer's disease*

icosapent INN *omega-3 marine triglyceride*

icospiramide INN

icotidine USAN *antagonist to histamine H_1 and H_2 receptors*

ictasol USAN *disinfectant*

Ictotest reagent tablets for professional use *in vitro diagnostic aid for bilirubin in the urine*

Icy Hot balm, cream, stick OTC *topical analgesic; counterirritant* [methyl salicylate; menthol] 29%•7.6%; 30%•10%; 30%•10%

Idamycin powder for IV injection ℞ *anthracycline antibiotic antineoplastic for acute myelogenous and other leukemias (orphan); investigational (orphan) for pediatric use* [idarubicin HCl] 5, 10, 20 mg

Idamycin PFS powder for IV injection ℞ *anthracycline antibiotic antineoplastic for acute myelogenous and other leukemias (orphan); investigational (orphan) for pediatric use* [idarubicin HCl] 1 mg/mL

idarubicin INN, BAN *anthracycline antibiotic antineoplastic* [also: idarubicin HCl]

idarubicin HCl USAN, INN *anthracycline antibiotic antineoplastic for acute myelogenous and other leukemias (orphan); investigational (orphan) for pediatric use* [also: idarubicin]

idaverine INN

idazoxan INN, BAN

idebenone INN, JAN *investigational treatment for Alzheimer's disease*

IDEC-131 *investigational (Phase I) anti-gp39 monoclonal antibody for systemic lupus erythematosus (SLE)*

IDEC-CE9.1 *investigational (Phase III) anti-CD4 antibody for rheumatoid arthritis* [also: SB-210396]

IDEC-Y2B8 *investigational radioimmunotherapy for refractory non-Hodgkin's B-cell lymphoma*

idenast INN

Identi-Dose (trademarked dosage form) *unit dose package*

idoxifene USAN *antihormone antineoplastic; osteoporosis treatment; estrogen receptor antagonist for hormone replacement therapy*

idoxuridine (IDU) USAN, USP, INN, BAN, JAN *ophthalmic antiviral; investigational (orphan) for nonparenchymatous sarcomas*

idralfidine INN

idrobutamine [see: butidrine]

idrocilamide INN

idropranolol INN

IDU (idoxuridine) [q.v.]

IE (ifosfamide [with mesna rescue], etoposide) *chemotherapy protocol*

ifenprodil INN

ifetroban USAN *antithrombotic; anti-ischemic; antivasospastic*

ifetroban sodium USAN *antithrombotic; anti-ischemic; antivasospastic*

Ifex powder for IV injection ℞ *nitrogen mustard-type alkylating antineoplastic for testicular cancer (orphan); investigational (orphan) for bone and soft tissue sarcomas* [ifosfamide] 1, 3 g

IFN (interferon) [q.v.]

IFN-alpha 2 (interferon alfa-2) [see: interferon alfa-2b, recombinant]

ifosfamide USAN, USP, INN, BAN *nitrogen mustard-type alkylating antineoplastic for testicular cancer (orphan); investigational (orphan) for bone and soft tissue sarcomas*
IfoVP (ifosfamide [with mesna rescue], VePesid) *chemotherapy protocol*
ifoxetine INN
IG (immune globulin) [see: globulin, immune]
IgE pentapeptide [see: pentigetide]
Igel 56 *hydrophilic contact lens material* [hefilcon C]
IGF-1 (insulin-like growth factor-1) [now: mecasermin]
IGF-BP3 complex *investigational (Phase II) treatment for muscle degradation following severe burns and hip fracture surgery*
IgG 1 [see: immunoglobulin G 1]
IGIV (immune globulin intravenous) [see: globulin, immune]
igmesine HCl USAN *sigma receptor ligand antidepressant*
IL-1, IL-2, etc. [see: interleukin-1, interleukin-2, etc.]
IL-1R (interleukin-1 receptor) [q.v.]
IL-2 (interleukin-2) [see: aldesleukin; teceleukin; celmoleukin]
IL-2 fusion toxin *investigational (Phase I/II) agent for HIV*
IL-4R (interleukin-4 receptor) [q.v.]
IL-13-PE38QQR protein *investigational novel chimeric human protein for kidney cancer therapy*
ilepcimide USAN, INN *anticonvulsant; investigational (orphan) for drug-resistant generalized tonic-clonic epilepsy*
Iletin (U.S. products) [see under: Regular, NPH, Lente, and Ultralente]
Iletin ⓒⒶⓃ (U.S. product: Lente Iletin I) subcu injection OTC *antidiabetic* [insulin zinc (beef-pork)] 100 U/mL
Iletin ⓒⒶⓃ (U.S. product: Regular Iletin I) subcu injection OTC *antidiabetic* [insulin (beef-pork)] 100 U/mL
Iletin NPH ⓒⒶⓃ (U.S. product: NPH Iletin I) subcu injection OTC *antidiabetic* [insulin (beef-pork)] 100 U/mL

Iletin II ⓒⒶⓃ (U.S. product: Lente Iletin II) subcu injection OTC *antidiabetic* [insulin zinc (pork)] 100 U/mL
Iletin II ⓒⒶⓃ (U.S. product: Regular Iletin II) subcu injection OTC *antidiabetic* [insulin (pork)] 100 U/mL
Iletin II NPH ⓒⒶⓃ (U.S. product: NPH Iletin II) subcu injection OTC *antidiabetic* [insulin (pork)] 100 U/mL
Ilex aquifolium; I. opaca; I. vomitoria medicinal herb [see: holly]
Ilex paraguariensis medicinal herb [see: yerba maté]
Ilex verticillata medicinal herb [see: winterberry]
Illicium anisatum; I. verum medicinal herb [see: star anise]
ilmofosine USAN, INN *antineoplastic*
ilomastat USAN *matrix metalloproteinase (MMP) inhibitor for corneal ulcers, inflammation, and cancers*
ilonidap USAN, INN *anti-inflammatory*
Ilopan IM injection, IV infusion ℞ *postoperative ileus prophylactic* [dexpanthenol] 250 mg/mL
Ilopan-Choline tablets ℞ *antiflatulent for splenic flexure syndrome* [dexpanthenol; choline bitartrate] 50•25 mg
iloperidone USAN, INN *investigational (Phase III) novel antipsychotic for schizophrenia*
iloprost INN, BAN *prostacyclin analog for cardiovascular disorders; orphan status withdrawn 1996*
Ilosone tablets, Pulvules (capsules), oral suspension ℞ *macrolide antibiotic* [erythromycin estolate] 500 mg; 250 mg; 125, 250 mg/5 mL ⑫ inosine
Ilotycin ophthalmic ointment ℞ *topical ophthalmic antibiotic* [erythromycin] 5 mg/g
Ilotycin Gluceptate IV injection ℞ *macrolide antibiotic* [erythromycin gluceptate] 1 g/vial
Ilozyme tablets ℞ *digestive enzymes* [lipase; protease; amylase] 11 000•30 000•30 000 U
I-L-X elixir OTC *hematinic* [ferrous gluconate; liver concentrate 1:20; multiple B vitamins] 70•98• ± mg/15 mL

I-L-X B$_{12}$ caplets OTC *hematinic* [carbonyl iron; liver, desiccated; multiple B vitamins; ascorbic acid] 37.5 • 130 • ± • 120 mg

I-L-X B$_{12}$ elixir OTC *hematinic* [ferric ammonium citrate; liver fraction 1; multiple B vitamins] 102 • 98 • ± mg/15 mL

imafen INN *antidepressant* [also: imafen HCl]

imafen HCl USAN *antidepressant* [also: imafen]

Imagent GI oral liquid Ŗ *oral GI contrast agent for MRI and x-ray imaging* [perflubron] 200 mL

Imagent US Ŗ *investigational imaging agent for cardiac ultrasound procedures*

Imager ac rectal suspension Ŗ *radiopaque contrast medium for gastrointestinal imaging* [barium sulfate] 100%

imanixil INN

imazodan INN *cardiotonic* [also: imazodan HCl]

imazodan HCl USAN *cardiotonic* [also: imazodan]

imcarbofos USAN, INN *veterinary anthelmintic*

imciromab INN *antimyosin monoclonal antibody* [also: imciromab pentetate]

imciromab pentetate USAN, BAN *antimyosin monoclonal antibody; investigational (orphan) diagnostic aid for myocarditis and cardiac transplant rejection* [also: imciromab]

Imdur extended-release tablets Ŗ *antianginal; vasodilator* [isosorbide mononitrate] 30, 60, 120 mg

imexon INN *investigational (orphan) for multiple myeloma*

IMF (ifosfamide [with mesna rescue], methotrexate, fluorouracil) *chemotherapy protocol*

imiclopazine INN

imidapril INN, BAN

imidazole carboxamide [see: dacarbazine]

imidazole salicylate INN

imidecyl iodine USAN *topical anti-infective*

imidocarb INN, BAN *antiprotozoal (Babesia)* [also: imidocarb HCl]

imidocarb HCl USAN *antiprotozoal (Babesia)* [also: imidocarb]

imidoline INN *antipsychotic* [also: imidoline HCl]

imidoline HCl USAN *antipsychotic* [also: imidoline]

imidurea NF *antimicrobial*

imiglucerase USAN, INN *glucocerebrosidase enzyme replacement for types I, II, and III Gaucher's disease (orphan)*

Imigran (foreign name for U.S. product Imitrex)

imiloxan INN *antidepressant* [also: imiloxan HCl]

imiloxan HCl USAN *antidepressant* [also: imiloxan]

iminophenimide INN

iminostilbene [see: carbamazepine]

imipemide [now: imipenem]

imipenem USAN, USP, INN, BAN, JAN *carbapenem antibiotic*

imipramine INN, BAN *tricyclic antidepressant* [also: imipramine HCl] ☑ Imferon; Norpramin; trimipramine

imipramine HCl USP *tricyclic antidepressant; treatment for childhood enuresis* [also: imipramine] 10, 25, 50 mg oral ☑ Imferon; Norpramin; trimipramine

imipramine pamoate *tricyclic antidepressant* ☑ Imferon; Norpramin; trimipramine

imipraminoxide INN

imiquimod USAN, INN *immunomodulator for external genital and perianal warts*

imirestat INN

Imitrex film-coated tablets, nasal spray Ŗ *vascular serotonin 5-HT$_1$ receptor agonist for migraine headache* [sumatriptan succinate] 25, 50 mg (100 mg available in Canada); 5, 20 mg

Imitrex subcu injection in vials, prefilled syringes, or STATdose kits (two prefilled syringes) Ŗ *vascular serotonin 5-HT$_1$ receptor agonist for migraine and cluster headaches* [sumatriptan succinate] 12 mg/mL

ImmTher Ŗ *investigational (orphan) immunostimulant for pulmonary and*

hepatic metastases of colorectal adenocarcinoma and osteosarcoma; investigational (Phase II, orphan) for Ewing sarcoma [disaccharide tripeptide glycerol dipalmitoyl]

ImmuCyst Ⓒ (U.S. product: Thera-Cys) powder for intravesical instillation ℞ *antineoplastic for urinary bladder cancer* [BCG vaccine, live] 81 mg

ImmuDyn *investigational (orphan) agent to increase platelet count in immune thrombocytopenic purpura* [*Pseudomonas aeruginosa* purified extract]

Immun-Aid powder OTC *enteral nutritional therapy for immunocompromised patients*

immune globulin (IG) [see: globulin, immune]

immune globulin intramuscular [see: globulin, immune]

immune globulin intravenous (IGIV) [see: globulin, immune]

immune globulin intravenous pentetate USAN *radiodiagnostic imaging agent for inflammation and infection* [also: indium In 111 IGIV pentetate]

immune serum globulin (ISG) [see: globulin, immune]

Immunex CRP test kit for professional use *in vitro diagnostic aid for C-reactive protein (CRP) in blood to diagnose inflammatory conditions* [latex agglutination test]

Immuno-C ℞ *investigational (Phase II, orphan) treatment of cryptosporidiosis in immunocompromised patients* [*Cryptosporidium parvum* bovine colostrum IgG concentrate]

immunoglobulin G 1 (mouse monoclonal 7E11-C5.3 antihuman prostatic carcinoma cell) disulfide [see: capromab pendetide]

immunoglobulin G 1 (mouse monoclonal ZCE025 antihuman antigen CEA) disulfide [see: indium In 111 altumomab pentetate; altumomab]

immunosuppressants *a class of drugs used to suppress the immune response,* *used primarily after organ transplantation surgery*

Immupath *orphan status withdrawn 1997* [HIV-neutralizing antibodies]

ImmuRAID-AFP ℞ *investigational (orphan) for diagnostic aid for AFP-producing tumors, hepatoblastoma, and hepatocellular carcinoma* [technetium Tc 99m murine MAb to human alpha-fetoprotein (AFP)]

ImmuRAID-hCG ℞ *investigational (orphan) for diagnostic aid for hCG-producing tumors* [technetium Tc 99m murine MAb to human chorionic gonadotropin (hCG)]

ImmuRAID-LL2 (name changed to LymphoScan in 1996)

ImmuRAIT-LL2 ℞ *investigational (orphan) treatment for B-cell leukemia and lymphoma* [iodine I 131 murine MAb IgG$_2$a to B cell]

Imodium capsules ℞ *antidiarrheal* [loperamide HCl] 2 mg

Imodium Ⓒ quick-dissolving lingual tablets OTC *antidiarrheal* [loperamide HCl] 2 mg

Imodium A-D caplets, liquid OTC *antidiarrheal* [loperamide HCl] 1 mg; 1 mg/5 mL

Imogam IM injection ℞ *rabies prophylaxis* [rabies immune globulin] 150 IU/mL

imolamine INN, BAN

Imovane Ⓒ tablets ℞ *sedative; hypnotic* [zopiclone] 7.5 mg

Imovax intradermal (ID) injection, IM injection ℞ *rabies prophylaxis* [rabies vaccine (HDCV)] 0.25 IU/0.1 mL; 2.5 IU/mL

imoxiterol INN

impacarzine INN

Impact ready-to-use liquid OTC *enteral nutritional therapy* [lactose-free formula]

Impact Rubella slide test for professional use *in vitro diagnostic aid for detection of rubella virus antibodies in serum* [latex agglutination test]

Impatiens balsamina; I. biflora; I. capensis medicinal herb [see: jewelweed]

IMPE [see: etipirium iodide]

impromidine INN, BAN *gastric secretion indicator* [also: impromidine HCl]

impromidine HCl USAN *gastric secretion indicator* [also: impromidine]

improsulfan INN

Improved Analgesic ointment OTC *topical analgesic; counterirritant* [methyl salicylate; menthol] 18.3%•16%

Improved Congestant tablets OTC *antihistamine; analgesic* [chlorpheniramine maleate; acetaminophen] 2•325 mg

Imreg-1 ℞ *investigational (Phase III) immunomodulator for HIV*

imuracetam INN

Imuran IV injection ℞ *immunosuppressant for organ transplantation and rheumatoid arthritis* [azathioprine sodium] 100 mg ⊡ Enduron; Imferon

Imuran tablets ℞ *immunosuppressant for organ transplantation and rheumatoid arthritis* [azathioprine] 50 mg

Imuthiol ℞ *investigational (Phase II/III, orphan) immunomodulator for HIV and AIDS* [diethyldithiocarbamate]

Imuvert ℞ *investigational (orphan) for primary brain malignancies* [*Serratia marcescens* extract (polyribosomes)]

^{111}**In** [see: indium In 111 altumomab pentetate]

^{111}**In** [see: indium In 111 imciromab pentetate]

^{111}**In** [see: indium In 111 murine anti-CEA monoclonal antibody]

^{111}**In** [see: indium In 111 murine monoclonal antibody]

^{111}**In** [see: indium In 111 oxyquinoline]

^{111}**In** [see: indium In 111 pentetate]

^{111}**In** [see: indium In 111 pentetreotide]

^{111}**In** [see: indium In 111 satumomab pendetide]

^{111}**In** [see: pentetate indium disodium In 111]

^{113m}**In** [see: indium chlorides In 113m]

inactivated mumps vaccine [see: mumps virus vaccine, inactivated]

inactivated poliomyelitis vaccine (IPV) [see: poliovirus vaccine, inactivated]

inactivated poliovirus vaccine (IPV) [see: poliovirus vaccine, inactivated]

inaperisone INN

Inapsine IV or IM injection ℞ *general anesthetic; antiemetic* [droperidol] 2.5 mg/mL

Incel ℞ *investigational (Phase II) multi-drug-resistance inhibitor for prostate and ovarian cancers* [biricodar dicitrate] ⊡ Enbrel

Incremin with Iron syrup (discontinued 1995) OTC *hematinic* [ferric pyrophosphate; multiple B vitamins; lysine; alcohol 0.75%] 90• ≛ •900 mg/15 mL

indacrinic acid [see: indacrinone]

indacrinone USAN, INN *antihypertensive; diuretic*

indalpine INN, BAN

indanazoline INN

indanediones *a class of anticoagulants that interfere with vitamin K–dependent clotting factors*

indanidine INN

indanorex INN

indapamide USAN, INN, BAN *antihypertensive; diuretic* 1.25, 2.5 mg oral

indatraline INN

indecainide INN *antiarrhythmic* [also: indecainide HCl]

indecainide HCl USAN *antiarrhythmic* [also: indecainide]

indeloxazine INN *antidepressant* [also: indeloxazine HCl]

indeloxazine HCl USAN *antidepressant* [also: indeloxazine]

indenolol INN, BAN

Inderal tablets, IV injection ℞ *antianginal; antihypertensive; antiarrhythmic; β-blocker; migraine preventative* [propranolol HCl] 10, 20, 40, 60, 80 mg; 1 mg/mL ⊡ Enduron; Enduronyl; Inderide

Inderal LA long-acting capsules ℞ *antianginal; antihypertensive; antiarrhythmic; β-blocker; migraine preventative* [propranolol HCl] 60, 80, 120, 160 mg

Inderide 40/25; Inderide 80/25 tablets ℞ *antihypertensive; β-blocker; diuretic* [propranolol HCl; hydrochlorothiazide] 40•25 mg; 80•25 mg ⑨ Inderal

Inderide LA 80/50; Inderide LA 120/50; Inderide LA 160/50 long-acting capsules ℞ *antihypertensive; β-blocker; diuretic* [propranolol HCl; hydrochlorothiazide] 80•50 mg; 120•50 mg; 160•50 mg

Indian apple *medicinal herb* [see: mandrake]

Indian arrow; Indian arrow wood *medicinal herb* [see: wahoo]

Indian bark *medicinal herb* [see: magnolia]

Indian bay *medicinal herb* [see: laurel]

Indian corn (Zea mays) styles (silk) *medicinal herb used as an analgesic, diuretic, demulcent, and litholytic*

Indian cress (Tropaeolum majus) flowers, leaves, and seeds *medicinal herb used as an antiseptic and expectorant*

Indian elm *medicinal herb* [see: slippery elm]

Indian frankincense *medicinal herb* [see: frankincense]

Indian hemp *medicinal herb* [see: marijuana]

Indian hyssop *medicinal herb* [see: blue vervain]

Indian paint, red *medicinal herb* [see: bloodroot]

Indian paint, yellow *medicinal herb* [see: goldenseal]

Indian pipe *medicinal herb* [see: fit root]

Indian plant *medicinal herb* [see: bloodroot; goldenseal]

Indian poke (Veratrum viride) *medicinal herb* [see: hellebore]

Indian root *medicinal herb* [see: spikenard; wahoo]

Indian shamrock *medicinal herb* [see: birthroot]

Indian tobacco *medicinal herb* [see: lobelia]

indigo (Indigofera spp.) plant *medicinal herb for fever, hemorrhoids, inducing emesis, inflammation, liver cleansing, ovarian and stomach cancer, pain, scorpion bites, and worms; not generally regarded as safe and effective*

indigo, wild *medicinal herb* [see: wild indigo]

indigo carmine BAN *cystoscopy aid* [also: indigotindisulfonate sodium]

indigotindisulfonate sodium USP *cystoscopy aid* [also: indigo carmine]

indinavir USAN *antiviral; HIV-1 protease inhibitor*

indinavir sulfate USAN *antiviral; HIV-1 protease inhibitor*

indium *element (In)*

indium (¹¹¹In) diethylenetriamine pentaacetate JAN *radionuclide cisternography aid; radioactive agent* [also: indium In 111 pentetate]

indium chlorides In 113m USAN, USP *radioactive agent*

indium In 111 altumomab pentetate USAN *radiodiagnostic monoclonal antibody for colorectal carcinoma; anticarcinoembryonic antigen; orphan status withdrawn 1997* [also: altumomab]

indium In 111 antimelanoma antibody XMMME-0001-DTPA [see: antimelanoma antibody]

indium In 111 CYT-103 [now: indium In 111 satumomab pendetide]

indium In 111 IGIV pentetate *radiodiagnostic imaging agent for inflammation and infection* [also: immune globulin intravenous pentetate]

indium In 111 imciromab pentetate *radioactive diagnostic aid for cardiac imaging*

indium In 111 murine anti-CEA MAb type ZCE 025 *orphan status withdrawn 1997*

indium In 111 murine MAb (2B8-MXDTPA) & yttrium Y 90 murine MAb (2B8-MXDTPA) *investigational (orphan) for non-Hodgkin's B-cell lymphoma*

indium In 111 murine MAb Fab to myosin [now: imciromab pentetate]

indium In 111 oxyquinoline USAN, USP *radioactive agent; diagnostic aid*

indium In 111 pentetate USP *radionuclide cisternography aid; radioactive agent* [also: indium (¹¹¹In) diethylenetriamine pentaacetate]

indium In 111 pentetreotide USAN *radioactive imaging agent for SPECT scans of neuroendocrine tumors*

indium In 111 satumomab pendetide USAN *radiodiagnostic imaging aid for ovarian (orphan) and colorectal carcinoma* [also: satumomab]

indobufen INN

indocate INN

Indochron E-R extended-release tablets ℞ *nonsteroidal anti-inflammatory drug (NSAID); antiarthritic; analgesic* [indomethacin] 75 mg

Indocin capsules, oral suspension, suppositories ℞ *nonsteroidal anti-inflammatory drug (NSAID); antiarthritic; analgesic* [indomethacin] 25, 50 mg; 25 mg/5 mL; 50 mg ☑ Lincocin; Minocin

Indocin I.V. powder for IV injection ℞ *prostaglandin synthesis inhibitor for neonatal closure of patent ductus arteriosus* [indomethacin sodium trihydrate] 1 mg

Indocin SR sustained-release capsules ℞ *nonsteroidal anti-inflammatory drug (NSAID); antiarthritic; analgesic* [indomethacin] 75 mg

indocyanine green USP, JAN *cardiac output test; hepatic function test; ophthalmic angiography*

indolapril INN *antihypertensive* [also: indolapril HCl]

indolapril HCl USAN *antihypertensive* [also: indolapril]

indolidan USAN, INN, BAN *cardiotonic*

indolones *a class of dopamine receptor antagonists with conventional (typical) antipsychotic activity* [also called: dihydroindolones]

indometacin INN, JAN *nonsteroidal anti-inflammatory drug (NSAID); antiarthritic; analgesic* [also: indomethacin]

indometacin farnecil JAN *nonsteroidal anti-inflammatory drug (NSAID); antiarthritic; analgesic* [also: indomethacin]

indomethacin USAN, USP, BAN *nonsteroidal anti-inflammatory drug (NSAID); antiarthritic; analgesic* [also: indometacin; indometacin farnecil] 25, 50, 75 mg oral; 25 mg/5 mL oral

indomethacin sodium USAN *anti-inflammatory*

indomethacin sodium trihydrate *neonatal closure of patent ductus arteriosus*

indopanolol INN

indopine INN

indoprofen USAN, INN, BAN *analgesic; anti-inflammatory*

indoramin USAN, INN, BAN *antihypertensive*

indoramin HCl USAN, BAN *antihypertensive*

indorenate INN *antihypertensive* [also: indorenate HCl]

indorenate HCl USAN *antihypertensive* [also: indorenate]

indoxole USAN, INN *antipyretic; anti-inflammatory*

indriline INN *CNS stimulant* [also: indriline HCl]

indriline HCl USAN *CNS stimulant* [also: indriline]

inductin [see: diphoxazide]

Infalyte oral solution OTC *electrolyte replacement* [sodium, potassium, and chloride electrolytes]

Infanrix IM injection ℞ *immunization against diphtheria, tetanus, and pertussis* [diphtheria & tetanus toxoids & acellular pertussis (DTaP) vaccine] 25 Lf•10 Lf•25 μg per 0.5 mL

Infasurf intratracheal suspension ℞ *prophylaxis for respiratory distress syndrome (RDS) in premature infants* [calfactant] 6 mL

Infatab (trademarked dosage form) *pediatric chewable tablet*

InFeD IV or IM injection ℞ *hematinic* [iron dextran] 50 mg/mL

Infergen subcu injection, SingleJect (prefilled syringe) ℞ *consensus interferon for the treatment of chronic hepatitis C* [interferon alfacon-1] 9, 15 μg

Inflamase Mild; Inflamase Forte eye drops ℞ *topical ophthalmic corticosteroidal anti-inflammatory* [prednisolone sodium phosphate] 0.125%; 1%

infliximab *anti-inflammatory; anti-TNFα monoclonal antibody for Crohn's disease (orphan); investiga-*

tional (Phase III) for rheumatoid arthritis

influenza purified surface antigen [see: influenza split-virus vaccine]

influenza split-virus vaccine *subcategory of influenza virus vaccine*

influenza subvirion vaccine [see: influenza split-virus vaccine]

influenza vaccine, intranasal *investigational (Phase III) delivery form for the vaccine*

influenza virus vaccine USP *active immunizing agent for influenza* [1999/2000 season: A/Beijing/262/95 (H1N1), A/Sydney/5/97 (H3N2), & B/Yamanashi/166/98 virus strains]

influenza whole-virus vaccine *subcategory of influenza virus vaccine*

infraRUB cream OTC *topical analgesic; counterirritant* [methyl salicylate; menthol] 35% • 10%

Infumorph concentrate for continuous microinfusion ℞ *narcotic analgesic; intraspinal microinfusion for intractable chronic pain (orphan)* [morphine sulfate] 10, 25 mg/mL

Infurfer ⒸⒶⓃ (U.S. product: InFeD) IV or IM injection ℞ *hematinic* [iron dextran] 50 mg/mL

infusible platelet membranes *investigational platelet alternative*

INGN-201 *investigational (Phase I/II) adenoviral-p53 gene therapy for various cancers* [also: adenoviral p53 gene; p53 adenoviral gene]

INH (isonicotinic acid hydrazide) [see: isoniazid]

Inhal-Aid (trademarked form) *portable inhalation device*

inhalants *a class of street drugs that include nitrous oxide, volatile nitrites, and petroleum distillates* [see: nitrous oxide; volatile nitrites; petroleum distillate inhalants]

Inhibace (commercially available in Latin America) ℞ *antihypertensive; ACE inhibitor (approved by the FDA, but not being marketed by the manufacturer)* [cilazapril]

inicarone INN

Inject-all (trademarked delivery system) *prefilled disposable syringe*

Inlay-Tab (trademarked dosage form) *tablets with contrasting inlay*

InnoGel Plus gel packs + comb OTC *pediculicide for lice* [pyrethrins; piperonyl butoxide technical] 0.3% • 3%

Innohep ℞ *investigational low molecular weight heparin for thrombosis* [tinzaparin sodium]

Innovar injection ℞ *narcotic analgesic; major tranquilizer* [fentanyl citrate; droperidol] 0.05 • 2.5 mg/mL

Inocor IV injection ℞ *vasodilator for congestive heart failure* [amrinone lactate] 5 mg/mL

inocoterone INN *anti-acne* [also: inocoterone acetate]

inocoterone acetate USAN *anti-acne* [also: inocoterone]

inosine INN, JAN ② Ilosone

inosine pranobex BAN, JAN *investigational antiviral/immunomodulator for AIDS; investigational (orphan) for subacute sclerosing panencephalitis*

inosiplex [now: inosine pranobex]

inositol NF *dietary lipotropic supplement* 250, 500, 650 mg oral

inositol niacinate USAN *peripheral vasodilator* [also: inositol nicotinate]

inositol nicotinate INN, BAN *peripheral vasodilator* [also: inositol niacinate]

inotropes *a class of drugs that affect the force or energy of muscle contractions*

Inpersol; Inpersol-LM solution (discontinued 1996) ℞ *peritoneal dialysis solution* [multiple electrolytes; dextrose] ± • 1.5%, ± • 2.5%, ± • 4.5%

inprochone [see: inproquone]

inproquone INN, BAN

INS-1 *investigational (Phase II) treatment for type 2 diabetes*

INSH (isonicotinoyl-salicylidene-hydrazine) [see: salinazid]

InspirEase (trademarked form) *portable inhalation device*

Insta-Glucose gel OTC *glucose elevating agent* [glucose] 40%

insulin USP, JAN *antidiabetic* ② inulin

insulin, biphasic INN, BAN *antidiabetic*

insulin, biphasic isophane BAN *antidiabetic*

insulin, dalanated USAN, INN *antidiabetic*

insulin, globin zinc USP [also: globin zinc insulin]

insulin, isophane USP, BAN, INN, JAN *antidiabetic*

insulin, neutral USAN, JAN *antidiabetic* [also: neutral insulin]

insulin, NPH (neutral protamine Hagedorn) [see: insulin, isophane]

insulin, protamine zinc (PZI) USP *antidiabetic* [also: insulin zinc protamine; protamine zinc insulin]

insulin argine INN *antidiabetic*

insulin aspart USAN, INN *antidiabetic; investigational (NDA filed) rapid-acting insulin analog*

insulin defalan INN *antidiabetic*

insulin glargine INN *antidiabetic; investigational long-acting, once-daily basal insulin*

insulin human USAN, USP, INN, BAN, JAN *antidiabetic*

insulin human, isophane USP *antidiabetic*

insulin human zinc USP *antidiabetic*

insulin human zinc, extended USP *antidiabetic*

insulin I 125 USAN *radioactive agent*

insulin I 131 USAN *radioactive agent*

insulin lispro USAN, INN, BAN *antidiabetic*

Insulin Reaction gel OTC *glucose elevating agent* [glucose] 40%

insulin zinc USP, INN, BAN, JAN *antidiabetic*

insulin zinc, extended USP *antidiabetic* [also: insulin zinc suspension (crystalline)]

insulin zinc, prompt USP *antidiabetic* [also: insulin zinc suspension (amorphous)]

insulin zinc protamine JAN *antidiabetic* [also: insulin, protamine zinc; protamine zinc insulin]

insulin zinc suspension (amorphous) INN, BAN, JAN *antidiabetic* [also: insulin zinc, prompt]

insulin zinc suspension (crystalline) INN, BAN, JAN *antidiabetic* [also: insulin zinc, extended]

insulin-like growth factor-1, recombinant human (rhIGF-) [now: mecasermin]

Intal encapsulated powder for inhalation (discontinued 1995) ℞ *anti-inflammatory/mast cell stabilizer for the prophylaxis of asthma and bronchospasm* [cromolyn sodium] 20 mg ⏸ Endal

Intal solution for nebulization, aerosol spray ℞ *anti-inflammatory; mast cell stabilizer for prophylactic treatment of allergy, asthma, and bronchospasm* [cromolyn sodium] 20 mg/ampule; 800 μg/dose ⏸ Endal

Integra (commercially available in 21 countries) *investigational artificial skin*

Integrilin IV injection ℞ *GP IIb/IIIa platelet aggregation inhibitor for acute coronary syndrome, unstable angina, myocardial infarction, and cardiac surgery* [eptifibatide] 0.75, 2 mg/mL

Intensol (trademarked form) *concentrated oral solution*

α-2-interferon [see: interferon alfa-2b, recombinant]

interferon, fibroblast [now: interferon beta]

interferon, leukocyte [now: interferon alfa-n3]

interferon α2b [see: interferon alfa-2b]

interferon αA [see: interferon alfa-2a]

interferon alfa JAN

interferon alfa (BALL-1) JAN

interferon alfa-2a (IFN-αA) USAN, INN, BAN, JAN *antineoplastic/antiviral for hairy cell leukemia and Kaposi sarcoma (orphan); hepatitis C treatment; investigational (orphan) for chronic myelogenous leukemia and renal cell carcinoma*

interferon alfa-2a & fluorouracil *investigational (orphan) for esophageal carcinoma and advanced colorectal cancer*

interferon alfa-2a & teceleukin *investigational (orphan) for metastatic*

renal cell carcinoma and metastatic
malignant melanoma

interferon alfa-2b (IFN-α2) USAN,
INN, BAN *antineoplastic for various
cancers and AIDS-related Kaposi sarcoma (orphan); antiviral for chronic
hepatitis B and C; adjunctive therapy
for malignant melanoma; investigational (Phase I/II) cytokine for AIDS*

interferon alfacon-1 USAN *bioengi-
neered consensus interferon for the
treatment of chronic hepatitis C*

interferon alfa-n1 USAN, INN, BAN
*antineoplastic; biological response mod-
ifier for chronic hepatitis C (orphan);
investigational (Phase III) cytokine for
HIV; investigational (orphan) for
human papillomavirus in severe respiratory papillomatosis*

interferon alfa-n3 USAN *antineoplastic; antiviral; investigational (Phase
III) cytokine for HIV, AIDS, ARC,
and hepatitis C*

interferon beta (IFN-B) BAN, JAN *antineoplastic; antiviral; immunomodulator*

interferon beta-1a USAN *immunomodulator for relapsing multiple sclerosis
(orphan); investigational (orphan) for
non-A, non-B hepatitis, Kaposi sarcoma, and various other cancers*

interferon beta-1b USAN *immunomodulator for relapsing-remitting multiple
sclerosis (orphan); investigational
(Phase II/III) cytokine for AIDS;
investigational (Phase III) for atopic
dermatitis*

interferon gamma-1a JAN

interferon gamma-1b USAN, INN,
BAN *antineoplastic; antiviral; immunoregulator for chronic granulomatous
disease (orphan); investigational
(orphan) for renal cell carcinoma and
severe congenital osteopetrosis*

interferon gamma-2a [see: interferon
gamma-1b]

α-interferons [see: interferon alfa-n1
and -n3]

**interleukin-1 alpha, recombinant
human** *orphan status withdrawn 1996*

interleukin-1 beta *investigational antineoplastic for melanoma; investigational liposome-encapsulated formulation for influenza A*

interleukin-1 receptor (IL-1R) *investigational treatment for rheumatoid
arthritis, sepsis, graft vs. host disease,
AML, asthma, and allergy*

interleukin-1 receptor, soluble *investigational (Phase I) antiviral for HIV*

**interleukin-1 receptor antagonist,
recombinant human** [now: ana-
kinra]

**interleukin-2, liposome-encapsu-
lated recombinant** *investigational
(orphan) for brain, central nervous system, kidney, and pelvic cancers*

interleukin-2, recombinant (IL-2)
[see: aldesleukin; teceleukin; celmo-
leukin]

interleukin-2 PEG [see: PEG-inter-
leukin-2]

**interleukin-2 receptor (IL-2R)
fusion protein** *investigational (NDA
filed) for cutaneous T-cell lymphoma
(CTCL); investigational (Phase II) for
other lymphomas and leukemias*

interleukin-3, recombinant human
*investigational (Phase I) cytokine for
HIV with cytopenia; investigational
adjunct to bone marrow transplants;
orphan status withdrawn 1996*

**interleukin-3, recombinant human
& sargramostim** *orphan status withdrawn 1996*

interleukin-4 receptor (IL-4R)
*investigational (Phase II) treatment for
allergy, asthma, transplant rejection,
and infectious diseases*

**interleukin-6, recombinant human
(rhIL-6)** *investigational (Phase III)
bone marrow/platelet stimulant adjunct
for chemotherapy*

**interleukin-11, recombinant
human (rhIL-11)** *platelet growth
factor for thrombocytopenia of chemotherapy or radiation (orphan)* [also:
oprelvekin]

interleukin-12 (IL-12) [see: edodekin alfa]

intermedine INN

Interquim ℞ *investigational treatment for stroke and head trauma* [citicoline sodium]

intoplicine INN *investigational (Phase I) antineoplastic and topoisomerase I and II inhibitor*

Intrachol ℞ *investigational (orphan) for choline deficiency of long-term parenteral nutrition* [choline chloride]

IntraDose injectable gel ℞ *investigational (Phase II) alkylating antineoplastic for inoperable primary liver cancer* [cisplatin; epinephrine]

Intralipid 10%; Intralipid 20% IV infusion ℞ *nutritional therapy* [fat emulsion]

IntraSite gel OTC *wound dressing* [graft T starch copolymer] 2%

intravascular perfluorochemical emulsion *synthetic blood oxygen carrier for PTCA*

intravenous fat emulsion [see: fat emulsion, intravenous]

intravenous immunoglobulin (IVIG) *investigational IV solution of concentrated antibodies for AIDS*

intrazole USAN, INN *anti-inflammatory*

intrifiban [now: eptifibatide]

intrinsic factor concentrate *antianemic to enhance the body's utilization of vitamin B_{12}*

intriptyline INN *antidepressant* [also: intriptyline HCl]

intriptyline HCl USAN *antidepressant* [also: intriptyline]

Introlan Half-Strength liquid OTC *enteral nutritional therapy* [lactose-free formula]

Introlite liquid OTC *enteral nutritional therapy* [lactose-free formula]

Intron A subcu or IM injection ℞ *antineoplastic for hairy cell leukemia, non-Hodgkin's lymphoma, and Kaposi sarcoma (orphan); antiviral for chronic hepatitis B and C; investigational (Phase I/II) cytokine for AIDS* [interferon alfa-2b] 3, 5, 10, 18, 25, 50 million IU/vial

Intropaste oral paste ℞ *radiopaque contrast medium for esophageal imaging* [barium sulfate] 70%

Intropin IV injection ℞ *vasopressor for cardiac, pulmonary, traumatic, septic, or renal shock* [dopamine HCl] 40, 80, 160 mg/mL ② Ditropan; Isoptin

Inula helenium medicinal herb [see: elecampane]

inulin USP *diagnostic aid for renal function* 100 mg/mL injection ② insulin

invenol [see: carbutamide]

Inversine tablets ℞ *antihypertensive* [mecamylamine HCl] 2.5 mg

invert sugar [see: sugar, invert]

Invicorp intracavernosal injection ℞ *investigational (NDA filed) treatment for organic-based erectile dysfunction* [vasoactive intestinal polypeptide; phentolamine mesylate]

Invirase capsules (this product is being replaced by Fortovase) ℞ *antiviral protease inhibitor for HIV* [saquinavir mesylate] 200 mg

iobenguane (^{131}I) INN *radioactive agent* [also: iobenguane I 131]

iobenguane I 123 USP *radioactive agent*

iobenguane I 131 USAN *radioactive agent* [also: iobenguane (^{131}I)]

iobenguane sulfate I 123 USAN *radiopharmaceutical diagnostic aid for adrenomedullary disorders and neuroendocrine tumors*

iobenguane sulfate I 131 USAN *diagnostic aid for pheochromocytoma (orphan)*

iobenzamic acid USAN, INN, BAN *radiopaque contrast medium for cholecystography*

Iobid DM sustained-release tablets ℞ *antitussive; expectorant* [dextromethorphan hydrobromide; guaifenesin] 30•600 mg

iobutoic acid INN

iocanlidic acid I 123 USAN *cardiac diagnostic aid*

Iocare Balanced Salt ophthalmic solution OTC *intraocular irrigating solution* [sodium chloride (balanced saline solution)]

iocarmate meglumine USAN *radiopaque contrast medium* [also: meglumine iocarmate]

iocarmic acid USAN, INN, BAN *radiopaque contrast medium*

iocetamic acid USAN, USP, INN, BAN *oral radiopaque contrast medium for cholecystography (62% iodine)*

Iocon shampoo OTC *antiseborrheic; antipsoriatic; antipruritic; antibacterial* [coal tar; alcohol]

Iodal HD liquid ℞ *narcotic antitussive; decongestant; antihistamine* [hydrocodone bitartrate; phenylephrine HCl; chlorpheniramine maleate] 1.67•5•2 mg/5 mL

iodamide USAN, INN, BAN *radiopaque contrast medium*

iodamide meglumine USAN *radiopaque contrast medium*

iodecimol INN

iodecol [see: iodecimol]

iodenosine *investigational (Phase I) anti-HIV agent*

iodetryl INN

Iodex; Iodex-P ointment OTC *broad-spectrum antimicrobial* [povidone-iodine] 4.7%; 10%

Iodex with Methyl Salicylate salve OTC *counterirritant; topical anti-infective* [methyl salicylate; iodine; oil of wintergreen] ≟•4.7%•4.8%

iodinated (¹²⁵I) human serum albumin INN *radioactive agent; blood volume test* [also: albumin, iodinated I 125 serum]

iodinated (¹³¹I) human serum albumin INN, JAN *radioactive agent; intrathecal imaging agent; blood volume test* [also: albumin, iodinated I 131 serum]

iodinated glycerol [see: glycerol, iodinated]

iodinated I 125 albumin [see: albumin, iodinated I 125]

iodinated I 131 aggregated albumin [see: albumin, iodinated I 131 aggregated]

iodinated I 131 albumin [see: albumin, iodinated I 131]

iodine USP *broad-spectrum topical anti-infective; element (I)* 2% topical

iodine I 123 murine MAb to alpha-fetoprotein (AFP) *investigational (orphan) diagnostic aid for AFP-producing tumors, hepatocellular carcinoma, and hepatoblastoma*

iodine I 123 murine MAb to human chorionic gonadotropin (hCG) *investigational (orphan) diagnostic aid for hCG-producing tumors*

iodine I 131 6B-iodomethyl-19-norcholesterol *investigational (orphan) for adrenal cortical imaging*

iodine I 131 Lym-1 MAb *investigational (Phase III, orphan) treatment for non-Hodgkin's B-cell lymphoma*

iodine I 131 metaiodobenzylguanidine sulfate [now: iobenguane sulfate I 131]

iodine I 131 murine MAb IgG₂a to B cell *investigational (orphan) for B-cell leukemia and lymphoma*

iodine I 131 murine MAb to alpha-fetoprotein (AFP) *investigational (orphan) treatment for AFP-producing tumors, hepatocellular carcinoma, and hepatoblastoma*

iodine I 131 murine MAb to human chorionic gonadotropin (hCG) *investigational (orphan) treatment for hCG-producing tumors*

iodine I 131 radiolabeled B1 MAb *investigational (orphan) for non-Hodgkin's B-cell lymphoma*

iodine I 131 tositumomab *investigational (Phase III) treatment for low-grade non-Hodgkin's lymphoma*

iodipamide USP, BAN *parenteral radiopaque contrast medium* [also: adipiodone]

iodipamide meglumine USP, BAN *parenteral radiopaque contrast medium (49.42% iodine)* [also: adipiodone meglumine]

iodipamide methylglucamine [see: iodipamide meglumine]

iodipamide sodium USP *parenteral radiopaque contrast medium*

iodipamide sodium I 131 USAN *radioactive agent*

iodisan [see: prolonium iodide]

iodixanol USAN, INN, BAN *parenteral radiopaque contrast medium (49.1% iodine)*

iodized oil NF

iodoalphionic acid NF [also: pheniodol sodium]

iodoantipyrine I 131 USAN *radioactive agent*

iodobehenate calcium NF

iodobenzylguaninine sulfate I 123 [see: iobenguane sulfate I 123]

iodocetylic acid (^{123}I) INN *diagnostic aid* [also: iodocetylic acid I 123]

iodocetylic acid I 123 USAN *diagnostic aid* [also: iodocetylic acid (^{123}I)]

iodochlorhydroxyquin [now: clioquinol]

iodocholesterol (^{131}I) INN *radioactive agent* [also: iodocholesterol I 131]

iodocholesterol I 131 USAN *radioactive agent* [also: iodocholesterol (^{131}I)]

iodoform NF

iodohippurate sodium I 123 USAN, USP *renal function test; radioactive agent*

iodohippurate sodium I 125 USAN *radioactive agent*

iodohippurate sodium I 131 USAN, USP *renal function test; radioactive agent* [also: sodium iodohippurate (^{131}I)]

iodohydroxyquin [see: clioquinol]

iodol USP

iodomethamate sodium NF

Iodo-Pak IV injection ℞ *intravenous nutritional therapy* [sodium iodide]

iodopanoic acid [see: iopanoic acid]

Iodopen IV injection ℞ *intravenous nutritional therapy* [sodium iodide] 118 μg/mL

iodophthalein, soluble [now: iodophthalein sodium]

iodophthalein sodium NF, INN

iodopyracet NF [also: diodone]

iodopyracet I 125 USAN *radioactive agent*

iodopyracet I 131 USAN *radioactive agent*

iodoquinol USAN, USP *amebicide; antimicrobial* [also: diiodohydroxyquinoline]

iodothiouracil INN, BAN

iodothymol [see: thymol iodide]

Iodotope capsules, oral solution ℞ *radioactive agent for hyperthyroidism and thyroid carcinoma* [sodium iodide I 131] 1–50 mCi; 7.05 mCi/mL

iodoxamate meglumine USAN, BAN *radiopaque contrast medium*

iodoxamic acid USAN, INN, BAN *radiopaque contrast medium*

iodoxyl [see: iodomethamate sodium]

Iofed extended-release capsules ℞ *decongestant; antihistamine* [pseudoephedrine HCl; brompheniramine maleate] 120•12 mg

Iofed PD extended-release capsules ℞ *pediatric decongestant and antihistamine* [pseudoephedrine HCl; brompheniramine maleate] 60•6 mg

iofendylate INN *radiopaque contrast medium* [also: iophendylate]

iofetamine (^{123}I) INN *diagnostic aid; radioactive agent* [also: iofetamine HCl I 123]

iofetamine HCl I 123 USAN *diagnostic aid; radioactive agent* [also: iofetamine (^{123}I)]

Iofoam (trademarked form) *foaming skin cleanser*

IoGen ℞ *investigational (Phase II) oral treatment for fibrocystic breast disease*

ioglicic acid USAN, INN, BAN *radiopaque contrast medium*

ioglucol USAN, INN *radiopaque contrast medium*

ioglucomide USAN, INN *radiopaque contrast medium*

ioglunide INN

ioglycamic acid USAN, INN, BAN *radiopaque contrast medium for cholecystography*

iogulamide USAN *radiopaque contrast medium*

iohexol USAN, INN, BAN *parenteral radiopaque contrast medium (46.36% iodine)*

Iohist D elixir ℞ *decongestant; antihistamine* [phenylpropanolamine HCl;

phenyltoloxamine citrate; pyrilamine maleate; pheniramine maleate] 25•4•4•4 mg/5 mL

Iohist DM syrup ℞ *antitussive; decongestant; antihistamine* [dextromethorphan hydrobromide; phenylpropanolamine HCl; brompheniramine maleate] 10•12.5•2 mg/5 mL

iolidonic acid INN

iolixanic acid INN

iomeglamic acid INN

iomeprol USAN, INN, BAN *radiopaque contrast medium*

iomethin I 125 USAN *neoplasm test; radioactive agent* [also: iometin (^{125}I)]

iomethin I 131 USAN *neoplasm test; radioactive agent* [also: iometin (^{131}I)]

iometin (^{125}I) INN *neoplasm test; radioactive agent* [also: iomethin I 125]

iometin (^{131}I) INN *neoplasm test; radioactive agent* [also: iomethin I 131]

iometopane I 123 USAN *diagnostic imaging aid for dopamine and serotonin transporter sites*

iomorinic acid INN

Ionamin capsules ℞ *anorexiant; CNS stimulant* [phentermine HCl resin complex] 15, 30 mg

Ionax foam OTC *medicated cleanser for acne* [benzalkonium chloride]

Ionax Astringent Skin Cleanser liquid OTC *topical keratolytic cleanser for acne* [salicylic acid; isopropyl alcohol]

Ionax Scrub OTC *abrasive medicated cleanser for acne* [benzalkonium chloride]

ionic contrast media *a class of older radiopaque agents that, in general, have a high osmolar concentration of iodine (the contrast agent), which corresponds to a higher incidence of adverse reactions* [also called: high osmolar contrast media (HOCM)]

Ionil shampoo OTC *antiseborrheic; keratolytic; antiseptic* [salicylic acid; benzalkonium chloride]

Ionil Plus shampoo OTC *antiseborrheic; keratolytic* [salicylic acid] 2%

Ionil T shampoo OTC *antiseborrheic; antipsoriatic; keratolytic; antiseptic*

[coal tar; salicylic acid; benzalkonium chloride]

Ionil-T Plus shampoo OTC *antiseborrheic; antipsoriatic; antipruritic; antibacterial* [coal tar] 2%

ionphylline [see: aminophylline]

iopamidol USAN, USP, INN, BAN *parenteral radiopaque contrast medium (49% iodine)*

iopanoic acid USP, INN, BAN *oral radiopaque contrast medium for cholecystography (66.68% iodine)*

iopentol USAN, INN, BAN *radiopaque contrast medium*

Iophen tablets, elixir, drops ℞ *expectorant* [iodinated glycerol] 30 mg; 60 mg/5 mL; 50 mg/mL

Iophen-C liquid ℞ *narcotic antitussive; expectorant* [codeine phosphate; iodinated glycerol] 10•30 mg/5 mL

Iophen-DM liquid ℞ *antitussive; expectorant* [dextromethorphan hydrobromide; iodinated glycerol] 10•30 mg/5 mL

iophendylate USP, BAN *radiopaque contrast medium* [also: iofendylate]

iophenoic acid INN [also: iophenoxic acid]

iophenoxic acid USP [also: iophenoic acid]

Iophylline elixir ℞ *antiasthmatic; bronchodilator; expectorant* [theophylline; iodinated glycerol] 120•30 mg/15 mL

Iopidine Drop-Tainer (eye drops) ℞ *topical sympathomimetic antiglaucoma agent* [apraclonidine HCl] 0.5%, 1%

ioprocemic acid USAN, INN *radiopaque contrast medium*

iopromide USAN, INN, BAN *parenteral radiopaque contrast medium (39% iodine)*

iopronic acid USAN, INN, BAN *radiopaque contrast medium for cholecystography*

iopydol USAN, INN, BAN *radiopaque contrast medium for bronchography*

iopydone USAN, INN, BAN *radiopaque contrast medium for bronchography*

Iosal II extended-release tablets ℞
decongestant; expectorant [pseudo-
ephedrine HCl; guaifenesin] 60•600
mg

iosarcol INN

iosefamic acid USAN, INN *radiopaque
contrast medium*

ioseric acid USAN, INN *radiopaque contrast medium*

iosimide INN

iosulamide INN *radiopaque contrast
medium* [also: iosulamide meglumine]

iosulamide meglumine USAN *radiopaque contrast medium* [also: iosula-
mide]

iosulfan blue *parenteral radiopaque
contrast medium for lymphography*

iosumetic acid USAN, INN *radiopaque
contrast medium*

iotalamic acid INN *radiopaque contrast
medium* [also: iothalamic acid]

iotasul USAN, INN *radiopaque contrast
medium*

iotetric acid USAN, INN *radiopaque
contrast medium*

iothalamate meglumine USP *parenteral radiopaque contrast medium
(47% iodine)* [also: meglumine
iothalamate]

iothalamate sodium USP *parenteral
radiopaque contrast medium (59.9%
iodine)* [also: sodium iothalamate]

iothalamate sodium I 125 USAN
radioactive agent [also: sodium iotalamate (^{125}I)]

iothalamate sodium I 131 USAN
radioactive agent [also: sodium iotalamate (^{131}I)]

iothalamic acid USP, BAN *radiopaque
contrast medium* [also: iotalamic acid]

iothiouracil sodium

iotranic acid INN

iotriside INN

iotrizoic acid INN

iotrol [now: iotrolan]

iotrolan USAN, INN, BAN *parenteral
radiopaque contrast medium*

iotroxic acid USAN, INN, BAN *radiopaque contrast medium*

Iotussin HC syrup ℞ *narcotic antitussive; decongestant; antihistamine*
[hydrocodone bitartrate; phenylephrine HCl; chlorpheniramine male-
ate] 2.5•5•2 mg/5 mL

iotyrosine I 131 USAN *radioactive agent*

ioversol USAN, INN, BAN *parenteral radiopaque contrast medium (47.3% iodine)*

ioxabrolic acid INN

ioxaglate meglumine USAN *radiopaque contrast medium* [also: meglumine ioxaglate]

ioxaglate sodium USAN *radiopaque
contrast medium* [also: sodium
ioxaglate]

ioxaglic acid USAN, INN, BAN *radiopaque contrast medium*

ioxilan USAN, INN *diagnostic aid*

ioxitalamic acid INN

ioxotrizoic acid USAN, INN *radiopaque
contrast medium*

iozomic acid INN

ipazilide fumarate USAN *antiarrhythmic*

ipecac USP *emetic*

ipecac, milk *medicinal herb* [see: birthroot; dogbane]

ipecac, powdered USP

ipexidine INN *dental caries prophylactic*
[also: ipexidine mesylate]

ipexidine mesylate USAN, INN *dental
caries prophylactic* [also: ipexidine]

IPL-423 *investigational agent for rheumatoid arthritis*

IPL-576 *investigational phospholipase
A2 inhibitor*

ipodate calcium USP *oral radiopaque
contrast medium for cholecystography
(61.7% iodine)*

ipodate sodium USAN, USP *oral radiopaque contrast medium for cholecystography (61.4% iodine)* [also: sodium
ipodate; sodium iopodate]

IPOL subcu injection ℞ *poliomyelitis
vaccine* [poliovirus vaccine, inacti-
vated] 0.5 mL

Ipomoea pandurata *medicinal herb* [see:
wild jalap]

Ipomoea violacea **(morning glory)**
seeds *contain lysergic acid amide,
chemically similar to LSD, which pro-*

duces hallucinations when ingested as a street drug [see also: LSD]

ipragratine INN

ipramidil INN

Ipran tablets ℞ *antianginal; antihypertensive; antiarrhythmic; β-blocker; migraine preventative* [propranolol HCl]

ipratropium bromide USAN, INN, BAN *anticholinergic bronchodilator for bronchospasm; antisecretory for rhinorrhea* 0.02% inhalation

Ipravent [see: Apo-Ipravent]

iprazochrome INN

iprazone [see: isoprazone]

ipriflavone INN

iprindole USAN, INN, BAN *antidepressant*

iprocinodine HCl USAN, BAN *veterinary antibacterial*

iproclozide INN, BAN

iprocrolol INN

iprofenin USAN *hepatic function test*

iproheptine INN

iproniazid INN, BAN

ipronidazole USAN, INN, BAN *antiprotozoal (Histomonas)*

ipropethidine [see: properidine]

iproplatin USAN, INN, BAN *antineoplastic*

iprotiazem INN

iproxamine INN *vasodilator* [also: iproxamine HCl]

iproxamine HCl USAN *vasodilator* [also: iproxamine]

iprozilamine INN

ipsalazide INN, BAN

ipsapirone INN, BAN *anxiolytic* [also: ipsapirone HCl]

ipsapirone HCl USAN *anxiolytic* [also: ipsapirone]

Ipsatol Cough Formula for Children; Ipsatol Cough Formula for Adults liquid OTC *antitussive; decongestant; expectorant* [dextromethorphan hydrobromide; phenylpropanolamine HCl; guaifenesin] 10•9•100 mg/5 mL

IPTD (isopropyl-thiadiazol) [see: glyprothiazol]

IPV (inactivated poliomyelitis vaccine) [see: poliovirus vaccine, inactivated]

IPV (inactivated poliovaccine) [see: poliovirus vaccine, inactivated]

iquindamine INN

^{192}Ir [see: iridium Ir 192]

IR-501 *investigational (Phase II) rheumatoid arthritis vaccine*

IR-502 *investigational (Phase II) T-cell receptor peptide vaccine for psoriasis*

irbesartan USAN *antihypertensive; angiotensin II receptor antagonist*

Ircon tablets OTC *hematinic* [ferrous fumarate (source of iron)] 200 mg (66 mg)

Ircon-FA tablets OTC *hematinic* [ferrous fumarate; folic acid] 82•0.8 mg

irgasan [see: triclosan]

iridium *element (Ir)*

iridium Ir 192 USAN *radioactive agent*

irindalone INN

irinotecan INN *hormonal antineoplastic/topoisomerase I inhibitor for cervical, colon, and rectal cancers* [also: irinotecan HCl]

irinotecan HCl USAN, JAN *hormonal antineoplastic/topoisomerase I inhibitor for cervical, colon, and rectal cancers* [also: irinotecan]

Iris florentina medicinal herb [see: orris root]

Iris versicolor medicinal herb [see: blue flag]

Irish broom *medicinal herb* [see: broom]

Irish moss (Chondrus crispus) *plant medicinal herb used as a demulcent*

irloxacin INN

irolapride INN

Iromin-G tablets OTC *vitamin/iron supplement* [multiple vitamins; ferrous gluconate; folic acid] ±•30•0.8 mg

iron *element (Fe)*

iron carbohydrate complex [see: polyferose]

iron dextran USP *hematinic*

iron heptonate [see: gleptoferron]

iron perchloride [see: ferric chloride]

iron polymalether [see: ferropolimaler]

iron sorbitex USAN, USP *hematinic*

Iron-Folic 500 timed-release tablets OTC *hematinic* [ferrous sulfate; multiple B vitamins; sodium ascorbate; folic acid] 105•±•500•0.8 mg

Irospan timed-release tablets, timed-release capsules OTC *hematinic* [iron (from ferrous sulfate, dried); ascorbic acid] 65•150 mg

Irrigate eye wash OTC *extraocular irrigating solution* [sterile isotonic solution]

irsogladine INN

irtemazole USAN, INN, BAN *uricosuric*

IS 5-MN (isosorbide 5-mononitrate) [see: isorbide mononitrate]

isaglidole INN

isamfazone INN

isamoltan INN

isamoxole USAN, INN, BAN *antiasthmatic*

isaxonine INN

isbogrel INN

iscador *investigational (Phase I) antiviral for HIV and AIDS*

I-Scrub solution (name changed to Eye Scrub in 1996)

isepamicin USAN, INN, BAN *aminoglycoside antibiotic*

isethionate USAN, BAN *combining name for radicals or groups* [also: isetionate]

isetionate INN *combining name for radicals or groups* [also: isethionate]

ISG (immune serum globulin) [see: globulin, immune]

ISIS 2302 *investigational (Phase II) antisense inhibitor for Crohn's disease*

ISIS 2503 *investigational (Phase I) Ha-ras selective antisense inhibitor for solid tumors*

ISIS 2922 *investigational (Phase III) antiviral for AIDS-related cytomegalovirus retinitis*

ISIS 3521 *investigational (Phase I) antisense anticancer compound*

ISIS 5132 *investigational (Phase II) anticancer agent for solid tumors*

ISIS 13312 *investigational (Phase I/II) agent for cytomegalovirus retinitis*

Ismelin tablets ℞ *antihypertensive; investigational (orphan) for reflex sympathetic dystrophy and causalgia* [guanethidine monosulfate] 25 mg ▣ Ritalin

Ismo film-coated tablets ℞ *antianginal; vasodilator* [isosorbide mononitrate] 20 mg

Ismotic solution ℞ *osmotic diuretic* [isosorbide] 45%

iso-alcoholic elixir NF

isoaminile INN, BAN

isoamyl nitrate [see: amyl nitrite]

Iso-B capsules OTC *vitamin supplement* [multiple B vitamins; folic acid; biotin] ±•200•100 μg

Iso-Bid sustained-release capsules (discontinued 1995) ℞ *antianginal; vasodilator* [isosorbide dinitrate] 40 mg

isobromindione INN

isobucaine HCl USP

isobutamben USAN, INN *topical anesthetic*

isobutane NF *aerosol propellant*

isobutyl *p*-aminobenzoate [see: isobutamben]

isobutyl α-phenylcyclohexaneglycolate [see: ibuverine]

isobutyl 2-cyanoacrylate (IBC) [see: bucrylate]

isobutyl nitrite; butyl nitrite *amyl nitrite substitutes, sold as euphoric street drugs, which produce a quick but short-lived "rush"* [see also: amyl nitrite; volatile nitrites]

***p*-isobutylhydratropohydroxamic acid** [see: ibuproxam]

isobutylhydrochlorothiazide [see: buthiazide]

isobutyramide *investigational (orphan) for sickle cell disease, beta-thalassemia syndrome, and beta-hemoglobinopathies*

isobuzole BAN [also: glysobuzole]

Isocaine HCl injection ℞ *injectable local anesthetic* [mepivacaine HCl] 3%

Isocaine HCl injection ℞ *injectable local anesthetic* [mepivacaine HCl; levonordefrin] 2%•1:20 000

Isocal liquid OTC *enteral nutritional therapy* [lactose-free formula]

Isocal HCN ready-to-use liquid OTC *enteral nutritional therapy* [lactose-free formula]

Isocal HN liquid OTC *enteral nutritional therapy* [lactose-free formula]

isocarboxazid USP, INN, BAN *antidepressant; MAO inhibitor*

Isocet tablets ℞ *analgesic; sedative* [acetaminophen; caffeine; butalbital] 325•40•50 mg

Isoclor Timesules (sustained-release capsules), tablets, liquid (discontinued 1995) OTC *decongestant; antihistamine* [pseudoephedrine HCl; chlorpheniramine maleate] 120•8 mg; 60•4 mg; 30•2 mg/5 mL

Isoclor Expectorant liquid ℞ *narcotic antitussive; decongestant; expectorant* [codeine phosphate; pseudoephedrine HCl; guaifenesin; alcohol 5%] 10•30•100 mg/5 mL

Isocom capsules ℞ *vasoconstrictor; sedative; analgesic (for migraine)* [isometheptene mucate; dichloralphenazone; acetaminophen] 65•100•325 mg

isoconazole USAN, INN, BAN *antibacterial; antifungal*

isocromil INN

Isocult for Bacteriuria culture paddles for professional use *in vitro diagnostic aid for nitrate, uropathogens, or bacteria in the urine*

Isocult for Candida culture paddles for professional use *in vitro diagnostic aid for Candida albicans in the vagina*

Isocult for N gonorrhoeae and Candida culture test for professional use OTC *in vitro diagnostic aid for gonorrhea and Candida in various specimens*

Isocult for Neisseria gonorrhoeae culture paddles for professional use *in vitro diagnostic aid for Neisseria gonorrhoeae*

Isocult for Pseudomonas aeruginosa culture test for professional use (discontinued 1995) *in vitro diagnostic aid for Pseudomonas aeruginosa in exudate or urine*

Isocult for Staphylococcus aureus culture paddles for professional use *in vitro diagnostic aid for Staphylococcus aureus in exudate*

Isocult for Streptococcal pharyngitis culture paddles for professional

use *in vitro diagnostic test for streptococcal pharyngitis in throat swabs*

Isocult for T vaginalis and Candida culture test for professional use *in vitro diagnostic aid for Trichomonas and Candida in vaginal or urethral cultures*

Isocult for Trichomonas vaginalis culture test for professional use (discontinued 1995) *in vitro diagnostic aid for Trichomonas vaginalis in urethra or vagina*

Isocult Throat Streptococci test (name changed to Isocult for Streptococcal pharyngitis in 1995)

isodapamide [see: zidapamide]

d-**isoephedrine HCl** [see: pseudoephedrine HCl]

isoetarine INN *sympathomimetic bronchodilator* [also: isoetharine]

isoethadione [see: paramethadione]

isoetharine USAN, BAN *sympathomimetic bronchodilator* [also: isoetarine]

isoetharine HCl USP, BAN *sympathomimetic bronchodilator* 1% inhalation

isoetharine mesylate USP, BAN *sympathomimetic bronchodilator*

isofezolac INN

isoflupredone INN, BAN *anti-inflammatory* [also: isoflupredone acetate]

isoflupredone acetate USAN *anti-inflammatory* [also: isoflupredone]

isoflurane USAN, USP, INN, BAN *inhalation general anesthetic*

isoflurophate USP *antiglaucoma agent; irreversible cholinesterase inhibitor miotic* [also: dyflos]

Isoject (trademarked delivery system) *prefilled disposable syringe*

Isolan liquid OTC *enteral nutritional therapy* [lactose-free formula]

isoleucine (L-isoleucine) USAN, USP, INN, JAN *essential amino acid; symbols: Ile, I*

isoleucine & leucine & valine *investigational (orphan) for hyperphenylalaninemia*

Isollyl Improved tablets, capsules (discontinued 1998) ℞ *analgesic; sedative* [aspirin; caffeine; butalbital] 325•40•50 mg

Isolyte E (G; H; M; P; R; S) with 5% Dextrose IV infusion ℞ *intravenous nutritional/electrolyte therapy* [combined electrolyte solution; dextrose]

Isolyte E; Isolyte S; Isolyte S pH 7.4 IV infusion ℞ *intravenous electrolyte therapy* [combined electrolyte solution]

Isolyte S pH 7.4 IV infusion ℞ *intravenous electrolyte therapy* [combined electrolyte solution]

isomazole INN *cardiotonic* [also: isomazole HCl]

isomazole HCl USAN *cardiotonic* [also: isomazole]

isomeprobamate [see: carisoprodol]

isomerol USAN *antiseptic*

isometamidium BAN [also: isometamidium chloride]

isometamidium chloride INN [also: isometamidium]

isomethadone INN, BAN

isomethepdrine chloride [see: isometheptene]

isometheptene INN, BAN

isometheptene HCl [see: isometheptene]

isometheptene mucate USP *cerebral vasoconstrictor; "possibly effective" for migraine headaches*

Isomil liquid, powder OTC *hypoallergenic infant food* [soy protein formula] ⊡ Esimil

Isomil DF ready-to-use liquid OTC *hypoallergenic infant food for management of diarrhea* [soy protein formula]

Isomil SF liquid OTC *hypoallergenic infant food* [soy protein formula, sucrose free]

isomylamine HCl USAN *smooth muscle relaxant*

isoniazid USP, INN, BAN *bactericidal; primary tuberculostatic* 50, 100, 300 mg oral; 50 mg/5 mL oral

isonicophen [see: aconiazide]

isonicotinic acid hydrazide (INH) [see: isoniazid]

isonicotinic acid vanillylidenehydrazide [see: ftivazide]

1-isonicotinoyl-2-salicylidenehydrazine (INSH) [see: salinazid]

isonicotinylhydrazine [see: isoniazid]

isonixin INN

isooctadecanol [see: isostearyl alcohol]

isooctadecyl alcohol [see: isostearyl alcohol]

Isopan liquid OTC *antacid* [magaldrate] 540 mg/5 mL

Isopan Plus liquid OTC *antacid; antiflatulent* [magaldrate; simethicone] 540•40 mg/5 mL

Isopap capsules ℞ *vasoconstrictor; sedative; analgesic (for migraine)* [isometheptene mucate; dichloralphenazone; acetaminophen] 65•100•325 mg

isopentyl nitrite [see: amyl nitrite]

isophenethanol [see: nifenalol]

isoprazone INN, BAN

isoprednidene INN, BAN

isopregnenone [see: dydrogesterone]

isoprenaline INN, BAN *sympathomimetic bronchodilator; vasopressor for shock* [also: isoproterenol HCl]

L-isoprenaline [see: levisoprenaline]

isoprenaline HCl [see: isoproterenol HCl]

Isoprinosine ℞ *investigational (NDA filed) antiviral/immunomodulator for AIDS; investigational (orphan) for subacute sclerosing panencephalitis* [inosine pranobex]

isoprofen INN

isopropamide iodide USP, INN, BAN *peptic ulcer adjunct*

isopropanol [see: isopropyl alcohol]

isopropicillin INN

isoproponum iodide [see: isopropamide iodide]

7-isopropoxyisoflavone [see: ipriflavone]

isopropyl alcohol USP *topical anti-infective/antiseptic; solvent*

isopropyl alcohol, rubbing USP *rubefacient*

N-isopropyl meprobamate [see: carisoprodol]

isopropyl myristate NF *emollient*

isopropyl palmitate NF *oleaginous vehicle*

isopropyl sebacate

isopropyl unoprostone *investigational (Phase III) antiglaucoma agent*

isopropylantipyrine [see: propyphenazone]

isopropylarterenol HCl [see: isoproterenol HCl]

isopropylarterenol sulfate [see: isoproterenol sulfate]

isoproterenol HCl USP *sympathomimetic bronchodilator; vasopressor for shock* [also: isoprenaline] 1:5000, 1:50 000 (0.2, 0.02 mg/mL) injection

isoproterenol sulfate USP *sympathomimetic bronchodilator*

Isoptin film-coated tablets ℞ *antianginal; antiarrhythmic; antihypertensive; calcium channel blocker* [verapamil HCl] 40, 80, 120 mg ② Intropin

Isoptin IV injection ℞ *antitachyarrhythmic; calcium channel blocker* [verapamil HCl] 5 mg/2 mL

Isoptin SR film-coated sustained-release tablets ℞ *antihypertensive; antianginal; antiarrhythmic; calcium channel blocker* [verapamil HCl] 120, 180, 240 mg

Isopto Alkaline Drop-Tainers (eye drops) (discontinued 1995) OTC *ophthalmic moisturizer/lubricant* [hydroxypropyl methylcellulose] 1%

Isopto Atropine Drop-Tainers (eye drops) ℞ *cycloplegic; mydriatic* [atropine sulfate] 0.5%, 1%

Isopto Carbachol Drop-Tainers (eye drops) ℞ *topical antiglaucoma agent; direct-acting miotic* [carbachol] 0.75%, 1.5%, 2.25%, 3%

Isopto Carpine Drop-Tainers (eye drops) ℞ *topical antiglaucoma agent; direct-acting miotic* [pilocarpine HCl] 0.25%, 0.5%, 1%, 2%, 3%, 4%, 5%, 6%, 8%, 10% ② Isopto Eserine

Isopto Cetamide Drop-Tainers (eye drops) ℞ *topical ophthalmic antibiotic* [sulfacetamide sodium] 15%

Isopto Cetapred eye drop suspension ℞ *topical ophthalmic corticosteroidal anti-inflammatory; antibiotic* [prednisolone acetate; sulfacetamide sodium] 0.25%•10%

Isopto Frin eye drops (discontinued 1995) OTC *topical ophthalmic decongestant* [phenylephrine HCl] 0.12%

Isopto Homatropine Drop-Tainers (eye drops) ℞ *cycloplegic; mydriatic* [homatropine hydrobromide] 2%, 5%

Isopto Hyoscine Drop-Tainers (eye drops) ℞ *cycloplegic; mydriatic* [scopolamine hydrobromide] 0.25%

Isopto Plain; Isopto Tears Drop-Tainers (eye drops) OTC *ophthalmic moisturizer/lubricant* [hydroxypropyl methylcellulose] 0.5%

Isordil Titradose (tablets), Tembid (sustained-release capsules and tablets), sublingual ℞ *antianginal; vasodilator* [isosorbide dinitrate] 5, 10, 20, 30, 40 mg; 40 mg; 2.5, 5, 10 mg ② Isuprel

isosorbide USAN, USP, INN, BAN *osmotic diuretic*

isosorbide dinitrate USAN, USP, INN, BAN *coronary vasodilator; antianginal* 2.5, 5, 10, 20, 30, 40 mg oral

isosorbide mononitrate USAN, INN, BAN *coronary vasodilator; antianginal* 20, 60 mg oral

Isosource; Isosource HN liquid OTC *enteral nutritional therapy* [lactose-free formula]

isospaglumic acid INN

isospirilene [see: spirilene]

isostearyl alcohol USAN *emollient; solvent*

isosulfamerazine [see: sulfaperin]

isosulfan blue USAN *lymphangiography aid* [also: sulphan blue]

isosulpride INN

Isotein HN powder OTC *enteral nutritional therapy* [lactose-free formula]

3-isothiocyanato-1-propene [see: allyl isothiocyanate]

isothiocyanic acid, allyl ester [see: allyl isothiocyanate]

isothipendyl INN, BAN

isothipendyl HCl [see: isothipendyl]

isotiquimide USAN, INN, BAN *antiulcerative*

Isotrate Timecelles (sustained-release capsules) (discontinued 1995) ℞ *antianginal; vasodilator* [isosorbide dinitrate] 40 mg

Isotrate ER extended-release tablets ℞ *antianginal; vasodilator* [isosorbide dinitrate] 60 mg

isotretinoin USAN, USP, INN, BAN *keratolytic for severe recalcitrant cystic acne*

isotretinoin anisatil USAN *keratolytic for acne vulgaris*

Isovex capsules (discontinued 1996) ℞ *peripheral vasodilator* [ethaverine HCl] 100 mg

Isovorin ℞ *chemotherapy "rescue" agent (orphan)* [L-leucovorin]

Isovue-128; Isovue-200; Isovue-250; Isovue-300; Isovue-370 injection ℞ *radiopaque contrast medium* [iopamidol (49% iodine)] 261 mg/mL (128 mg/mL); 408 mg/mL (200 mg/mL); 510 mg/mL (250 mg/mL); 612 mg/mL (300 mg/mL); 755 mg/mL (370 mg/mL)

Isovue-M 200; Isovue-M 300 intrathecal injection ℞ *radiopaque contrast medium for myelography* [iopamidol (49% iodine)] 408 mg/mL (200 mg/mL); 612 mg/mL (300 mg/mL)

isoxaprolol INN

isoxepac USAN, INN, BAN *anti-inflammatory*

isoxicam USAN, INN, BAN *nonsteroidal anti-inflammatory drug (NSAID); antiarthritic; analgesic; antipyretic*

isoxsuprine INN, BAN *peripheral vasodilator* [also: isoxsuprine HCl]

isoxsuprine HCl USP, JAN *peripheral vasodilator* [also: isoxsuprine] 10, 20 mg oral

I-Soyalac liquid OTC *hypoallergenic infant food* [soybean protein formula]

isradipine USAN, INN, BAN *antihypertensive; dihydropyridine calcium channel blocker*

isrodipine [see: isradipine]

Istin (European name for U.S. product Norvasc)

Isuprel Glossets (sublingual tablets) (discontinued 1996) ℞ *sympathomi-*

metic bronchodilator [isoproterenol HCl] 10, 15 mg

Isuprel intracardiac, IV, IM, or subcu injection ℞ *vasopressor for cardiac, hypovolemic, or septic shock; sympathomimetic bronchodilator* [isoproterenol HCl] 1:5000, 1:50 000 (0.2, 0.02 mg/mL) ⃞ Isordil

Isuprel Mistometer (metered-dose inhalation aerosol), solution for inhalation ℞ *sympathomimetic bronchodilator* [isoproterenol HCl] 103 μg/dose; 0.5% (1:200), 1% (1:100)

ISV-205 *investigational (Phase II) cyclooxygenase inhibitor for glaucoma*

ISV-208 *investigational (Phase I) ophthalmic beta blocker for elevated intraocular pressure*

itanoxone INN

itasetron USAN *anxiolytic; antidepressant; antiemetic; 5-HT$_3$ receptor antagonist*

itazigrel USAN, INN *platelet antiaggregatory agent*

itazogrel [see: itazigrel]

itchweed *(Veratrum viride) medicinal herb* [see: hellebore]

Itch-X spray, gel OTC *topical local anesthetic* [pramoxine HCl] 1%

itobarbital [see: butalbital]

itraconazole USAN, INN, BAN *systemic triazole antifungal*

itramin tosilate INN [also: itramin tosylate]

itramin tosylate BAN [also: itramin tosilate]

itrocainide INN

I-Valex-1 powder OTC *formula for infants with leucine catabolism disorder*

I-Valex-2 powder OTC *enteral nutritional therapy for leucine catabolism disorder*

Ivarest cream, lotion OTC *topical poison ivy treatment* [calamine; benzocaine] 14%•5%

ivarimod INN

Iveegam freeze-dried powder for IV infusion ℞ *passive immunizing agent for HIV and Kawasaki syndrome; investigational (orphan) for acute myo-*

carditis and juvenile rheumatoid arthritis [immune globulin] 50 mg/mL

ivermectin USAN, INN, BAN *antiparasitic; anthelmintic for strongyloidiasis and onchocerciasis*

ivermectin component B$_{1a}$

ivermectin component B$_{1b}$

IVIG (intravenous immunoglobulin) [q.v.]

Ivomec-SR (name changed to Stromectol upon marketing release in 1997)

ivoqualine INN

ivy *medicinal herb* [see: American ivy; English ivy; poison ivy]

Ivy Shield cream OTC *skin protectant*

IvyBlock OTC *topical treatment for poison ivy, poison oak, and poison sumac* [bentoquatam] 5%

Ivy-Chex spray OTC *topical poison ivy treatment* [polyvinylpyrrolidone-vinylacetate copolymers; methyl salicylate; benzalkonium chloride]

Ivy-Rid spray OTC *topical poison ivy treatment* [polyvinylpyrrolidone-vinylacetate copolymers; benzalkonium chloride]

jalap *(Ipomoea jalapa)* *medicinal herb* [see: wild jalap]

Jamaica mignonette *medicinal herb* [see: henna *(Lawsonia)*]

Jamaica pepper *medicinal herb* [see: allspice]

Jamaica sarsaparilla *medicinal herb* [see: sarsaparilla]

Jamaica sorrel *medicinal herb* [see: hibiscus]

Janimine Filmtabs (film-coated tablets) (discontinued 1996) ℞ *tricyclic antidepressant; treatment for childhood enuresis* [imipramine HCl] 10, 25, 50 mg

Japanese encephalitis (JE) virus vaccine *active immunization vaccine*

jasmine *(Jasminum officinale)* flowers *medicinal herb used as a calmative*

jaundice berry *medicinal herb* [see: barberry]

jaundice root *medicinal herb* [see: goldenseal]

java pepper *medicinal herb* [see: cubeb]

Jeffersonia diphylla *medicinal herb* [see: twin leaf]

JEK-554 *investigational (Phase III) euphoriant, emollient, and vulnerary for long-term care (clinical trials suspended 1999)* [see: DGH-3515]

Jenamicin IV or IM injection (discontinued 1998) ℞ *aminoglycoside antibiotic* [gentamicin sulfate] 40 mg/mL

Jenest-28 tablets ℞ *biphasic oral contraceptive* [norethindrone; ethinyl estradiol] Phase 1: 0.5 mg•35 μg; Phase 2: 1 mg•35 μg

Jersey tea *medicinal herb* [see: New Jersey tea]

Jerusalem cowslip; Jerusalem sage *medicinal herb* [see: lungwort]

jessamine, yellow *medicinal herb* [see: gelsemium]

Jesuit's bark *medicinal herb* [see: quinine]

Jets chewable tablets OTC *dietary supplement* [lysine; multiple vitamins] 300• ± mg

JE-VAX powder for subcu injection ℞ *active immunizing agent* [Japanese encephalitis virus vaccine] 0.5 mL

Jevity liquid OTC *enteral nutritional therapy* [lactose-free formula]

jewelweed *(Impatiens balsamina; I. biflora; I. capensis)* juice *medicinal herb for prophylaxis and treatment of poison ivy rash*

Jew's harp plant *medicinal herb* [see: birthroot]

jiaogulan (Gynostemma pentaphyllum) leaves *medicinal herb used to regulate blood pressure and strengthen the immune system, and for its adaptogenic, antihyperlipidemic, antineoplastic, antioxidant, and cardio- and cerebrovascular protective effects*

jimsonweed (Datura stramonium) leaves and flowering tops *medicinal herb used as an analgesic, antiasthmatic, antispasmodic, hypnotic, and narcotic; also abused as a street drug*

jodphthalein sodium [see: iodophthalein sodium]

joe-pye weed *medicinal herb* [see: queen of the meadow]

jofendylate [see: iophendylate]

Johnswort *medicinal herb* [see: St. John's wort]

jopanoic acid [see: iopanoic acid]

josamycin USAN, INN *antibacterial*

jotrizoic acid [see: iotrizoic acid]

JTT-501 *investigational (Phase II) insulin sensitizer for type 2 diabetes*

Juglans cinerea *medicinal herb* [see: butternut]

Juglans nigra *medicinal herb* [see: black walnut]

Juglans regia *medicinal herb* [see: English walnut]

juniper (Juniperus communis) berries *medicinal herb for arthritis, bleeding, bronchitis, colds, edema, infections, kidney infections, pancreatic disorders, uric acid build-up, urinary disorders, and water retention*

juniper, prickly (Juniperus oxycedrus) *medicinal herb* [see: juniper]

juniper tar USP *antieczematic*

Just Tears eye drops OTC *ophthalmic moisturizer/lubricant* [polyvinyl alcohol] 1.4%

K+ 8; K+ 10 film-coated extended-release tablets ℞ *potassium supplement* [potassium chloride] 8 mEq (600 mg); 10 mEq (750 mg)

K+ Care powder ℞ *potassium supplement* [potassium chloride] 15, 20, 25 mEq/packet

K+ Care ET effervescent tablets ℞ *potassium supplement* [potassium bicarbonate] 20, 25 mEq

⁴²K [see: potassium chloride K 42]

k82 ImmunoCap test kit for professional use *in vitro diagnostic aid for specific latex allergies*

Kabikinase powder for IV or intracoronary infusion ℞ *thrombolytic enzyme for lysis of thrombi and catheter clearance* [streptokinase] 250 000, 600 000, 750 000, 1 500 000 IU

Kadian polymer-coated sustained-release pellets in capsules ℞ *narcotic analgesic* [morphine sulfate] 20, 50, 100 mg

kainic acid INN

Kala tablets OTC *dietary supplement; fever blister treatment; not generally regarded as safe and effective as an antidiarrheal* [Lactobacillus acidophilus (soy-based)] 200 million U

kalafungin USAN, INN *antifungal*

kallidinogenase INN, BAN

Kalmia latifolia *medicinal herb* [see: mountain laurel]

kalmopyrin [see: calcium acetylsalicylate]

kalsetal [see: calcium acetylsalicylate]

Kaltostat; Kaltostat Fortex pads OTC *wound dressing* [calcium alginate fiber]

kalumb *medicinal herb* [see: colombo]

kanamycin INN, BAN *aminoglycoside antibiotic; tuberculosis retreatment* [also: kanamycin sulfate] ② Garamycin; gentamicin

kanamycin B [see: bekanamycin]

kanamycin sulfate USP *aminoglycoside antibiotic; tuberculosis retreatment* [also: kanamycin] 75, 500, 1000 mg/ vial injection

Kank-a liquid/film OTC *topical oral anesthetic* [benzocaine] 20%

Kantrex capsules, IV or IM injection, pediatric injection ℞ *aminoglycoside antibiotic* [kanamycin sulfate] 500 mg; 500, 1000 mg; 75 mg

Kao Lectrolyte powder for oral solution OTC *pediatric electrolyte replenisher*

Kaochlor 10%; Kaochlor S-F liquid ℞ *potassium supplement* [potassium chloride; alcohol 5%] 20 mEq/15 mL ☒ K-Lor

Kaodene Non-Narcotic liquid OTC *antidiarrheal; GI adsorbent; antacid* [kaolin; pectin; bismuth subsalicylate] 3.9 g•194.4 mg• ≗ per 30 mL ☒ codeine

Kaodene Non-Narcotic oral liquid OTC *antidiarrheal; GI adsorbent; antacid* [kaolin; pectin; bismuth subsalicylate] 130•6.48• ≗ mg/mL

kaolin USP clay *natural material used topically as an emollient and drying agent and ingested for binding gastrointestinal toxins and controlling diarrhea* ☒ Calan; Kaon

Kaon elixir ℞ *potassium supplement* [potassium gluconate] 20 mEq/15 mL ☒ Calan; kaolin

Kaon-Cl; Kaon-Cl 10 extended-release tablets ℞ *potassium supplement* [potassium chloride] 500 mg (6.7 mEq); 750 mg (10 mEq) ☒ Calan; kaolin

Kaon-Cl 20% liquid ℞ *potassium supplement* [potassium chloride; alcohol 5%] 40 mEq/15 mL ☒ Calan; kaolin

Kaopectate, Children's chewable tablets (discontinued 1995) OTC *antidiarrheal; GI adsorbent* [attapulgite] 300 mg ☒ Kapectalin

Kaopectate, Children's liquid OTC *antidiarrheal; GI adsorbent* [attapulgite] 600 mg/15 mL ☒ Kapectalin

Kaopectate II caplets OTC *antidiarrheal* [loperamide HCl] 2 mg

Kaopectate Advanced Formula oral liquid OTC *antidiarrheal; GI adsorbent* [attapulgite] 750 mg/15 mL

Kaopectate Maximum Strength caplets OTC *antidiarrheal; GI adsorbent* [attapulgite] 750 mg

Kao-Spen oral suspension OTC *GI adsorbent; antidiarrheal* [kaolin; pectin] 5.2 g•260 mg per 30 mL

Kapectolin liquid OTC *GI adsorbent; antidiarrheal* [kaolin; pectin] 90•2 g/30 mL ☒ Kaopectate

Kapseal (trademarked dosage form) *capsules sealed with a band*

karaya gum *(Sterculia tragacantha; S. urens; S. villosa) medicinal herb used as a topical astringent and bulk laxative*

Karidium tablets, chewable tablets, drops ℞ *dental caries preventative* [sodium fluoride] 2.2 mg; 2.2 mg; 0.275 mg/drop

Karigel; Karigel-N gel ℞ *topical dental caries preventative* [sodium fluoride] 1.1%

karyocyte growth factor [see: pegylated megakaryocyte growth and development factor, recombinant human]

kasal USAN *food additive*

Kasof capsules OTC *stool softener* [docusate potassium] 240 mg

Kato powder (discontinued 1995) ℞ *potassium supplement* [potassium chloride] 20 mEq/packet

kava kava *(Piper methysticum) root medicinal herb for insomnia and nervousness*

Kay Ciel liquid, powder ℞ *potassium supplement* [potassium chloride] 20 mEq/15 mL; 20 mEq/packet ☒ KCl

Kayexalate powder ℞ *potassium-removing agent for hyperkalemia* [sodium polystyrene sulfonate]

Kaylixir liquid ℞ *potassium supplement* [potassium gluconate; alcohol 5%] 20 mEq/15 mL

Kaysine injection (discontinued 1995) ℞ *treatment for varicose veins with stasis dermatitis* [adenosine phosphate] 25 mg/mL

K-C oral suspension OTC *antidiarrheal; GI adsorbent; antacid* [kaolin; pectin; bismuth subcarbonate] 5 g•260 mg• 260 mg per 30 mL

KCl (potassium chloride) [q.v.] ☑ Kay Ciel

K-Dur 10; K-Dur 20 controlled-release tablets ℞ *potassium supplement* [potassium chloride] 750 mg (10 mEq); 1500 mg (20 mEq)

kebuzone INN

Keflex pediatric drops (discontinued 1995) ℞ *cephalosporin antibiotic* [cephalexin] 100 mg/mL ☑ Keflet; Keflin

Keflex Pulvules (capsules), oral suspension ℞ *cephalosporin antibiotic* [cephalexin] 250, 500 mg; 125, 250 mg/5 mL ☑ Keflet; Keflin

Keflin, Neutral powder for IV or IM injection (discontinued 1996) ℞ *cephalosporin antibiotic* [cephalothin sodium] 1, 2 g ☑ Keflet; Keflex

Keftab tablets ℞ *cephalosporin antibiotic* [cephalexin HCl] 500 mg

Kefurox powder for IV or IM injection ℞ *cephalosporin antibiotic* [cefuroxime sodium] 0.75, 1.5, 7.5 g

Kefzol powder or frozen premix for IV or IM injection ℞ *cephalosporin antibiotic* [cefazolin sodium] 0.5, 1, 10, 20 g ☑ Cefzil

kellofylline [see: visnafylline]

kelp *(Fucus versiculosus)* plant *medicinal herb for brittle fingernails, cleaning arteries, colitis, eczema, goiter, obesity, and toning adrenal, pituitary, and thyroid glands*

kelp *(Laminaria digitata; L. japonica)* plant *medicinal herb for cervical dilation and cervical ripening*

Kemadrin tablets ℞ *anticholinergic; antiparkinsonian* [procyclidine HCl] 5 mg ☑ Coumadin

Kemsol ⓒᴬᴺ (U.S. product: Rimso-50) solution for bladder instillation ℞ *anti-inflammatory for symptomatic relief of interstitial cystitis* [dimethyl sulfoxide (DMSO)] 70%

Kenacort tablets, syrup ℞ *corticosteroid; anti-inflammatory* [triamcinolone] 4, 8 mg; 4 mg/5 mL

Kenaject-40 IM, intra-articular, intrabursal, intradermal injection ℞ *corticosteroid; anti-inflammatory* [triamcinolone acetonide] 40 mg/mL

Kenalog ointment, cream, lotion, aerosol spray ℞ *topical corticosteroidal anti-inflammatory* [triamcinolone acetonide] 0.025%, 0.1%, 0.5%; 0.025%, 0.1%, 0.5%; 0.025%, 0.1%; ♀ ☑ Ketalar

Kenalog in Orabase oral paste ℞ *topical corticosteroidal anti-inflammatory* [triamcinolone acetonide] 0.1%

Kenalog-10; Kenalog-40 IM, intra-articular, intrabursal, intradermal injection ℞ *corticosteroid; anti-inflammatory* [triamcinolone acetonide] 10 mg/mL; 40 mg/mL

Kenalog-H cream ℞ *topical corticosteroidal anti-inflammatory* [triamcinolone acetonide] 0.1%

Kendall's compound A [see: dehydrocorticosterone]

Kendall's compound B [see: corticosterone]

Kendall's compound E [see: cortisone acetate]

Kendall's compound F [see: hydrocortisone]

Kendall's desoxy compound B [see: desoxycorticosterone acetate]

Kenonel cream ℞ *topical corticosteroidal anti-inflammatory* [triamcinolone acetonide] 1%

Kenwood Therapeutic liquid OTC *vitamin/mineral supplement* [multiple vitamins & minerals] ♀

keoxifene HCl [now: raloxifene HCl]

keracyanin INN

keratinocyte growth factor-2 (KGF-2) *investigational (Phase I) vulnerary*

keratolytics *a class of agents that cause sloughing of the horny layer of the epidermis and softening of the skin*

Keri; Keri Light lotion OTC *moisturizer; emollient*

Keri Creme OTC *moisturizer; emollient*

KeriCort-10 cream OTC *topical corticosteroidal anti-inflammatory* [hydrocortisone] 1%

Kerlone tablets ℞ *antihypertensive; β-blocker* [betaxolol HCl] 10, 20 mg

kernelwort *medicinal herb* [see: figwort]

Kerodex #51 cream OTC *skin protectant for dry or oily work*

Kerodex #71 cream OTC *water repellant skin protectant for wet work*

Kestrone 5 IM injection ℞ *estrogen replacement therapy for postmenopausal disorders; palliative therapy for inoperable prostatic and breast cancer* [estrone] 5 mg/mL

Ketalar IV or IM injection ℞ *rapid-acting general anesthetic; sometimes abused as a street drug due to its "dissociative state" effects* [ketamine HCl] 10, 50, 100 mg/mL ② Kenalog

ketamine INN, BAN *a rapid-acting general anesthetic; sometimes abused as a street drug due to its "dissociative state" effects* [also: ketamine HCl]

ketamine HCl USAN, USP, JAN *a rapid-acting general anesthetic; sometimes abused as a street drug due to its "dissociative state" effects* [also: ketamine]

ketanserin USAN, INN, BAN *serotonin antagonist*

ketazocine USAN, INN *analgesic*

ketazolam USAN, INN, BAN *minor tranquilizer*

kethoxal USAN *antiviral* [also: ketoxal]

ketimipramine INN *antidepressant* [also: ketipramine fumarate]

ketimipramine fumarate [see: ketipramine fumarate]

ketipramine fumarate USAN *antidepressant* [also: ketimipramine]

7-KETO DHEA *investigational dehydroepiandrosterone (DHEA) derivative for Alzheimer's disease*

ketobemidone INN, BAN

ketocaine INN

ketocainol INN

ketocholanic acid [see: dehydrocholic acid]

ketoconazole USAN, USP, INN, BAN *broad-spectrum antifungal* 200 mg oral

ketoconazole & cyclosporine *orphan status withdrawn 1996*

Keto-Diastix reagent strips *in vitro diagnostic aid for multiple urine products*

ketohexazine [see: cetohexazine]

Ketonex-1 powder OTC *formula for infants with maple syrup urine disease*

Ketonex-2 powder OTC *enteral nutritional therapy for maple syrup urine disease (MSUD)*

ketoprofen USAN, INN, BAN *antiarthritic; nonsteroidal anti-inflammatory drug (NSAID); analgesic* 25, 50, 75, 200 mg oral

ketorfanol USAN, INN *analgesic*

ketorolac INN, BAN *analgesic; antipyretic; nonsteroidal anti-inflammatory drug (NSAID)* [also: ketorolac tromethamine]

ketorolac tromethamine USAN *analgesic; antipyretic; nonsteroidal anti-inflammatory drug (NSAID)* [also: ketorolac] 10 mg oral

Ketostix reagent strips for home use OTC *in vitro diagnostic aid for acetone (ketones) in the urine*

ketotifen INN, BAN *antihistamine; mast cell stabilizer* [also: ketotifen fumarate]

ketotifen fumarate USAN, JAN *antihistamine; mast cell stabilizer* [also: ketotifen]

ketotrexate INN

ketoxal INN *antiviral* [also: kethoxal]

Key-Plex injection ℞ *parenteral vitamin therapy* [multiple B vitamins; vitamin C] ± • 50 mg/mL

Key-Pred 25; Key-Pred 50 IM injection ℞ *corticosteroid; anti-inflammatory* [prednisolone acetate] 25 mg/mL; 50 mg/mL

Key-Pred-SP IV or IM injection ℞ *corticosteroid; anti-inflammatory* [prednisolone sodium phosphate] 20 mg/mL

K-G Elixir ℞ *potassium supplement* [potassium gluconate] 20 mEq/15 mL

KGF-2 (keratinocyte growth factor-2) [q.v.]

khellin INN

khelloside INN

Kiddy Chews chewable tablets (discontinued 1995) OTC *vitamin supple-*

ment [multiple vitamins; folic acid] ± •0.3 mg

Kiddy Chews with Iron chewable tablets (discontinued 1995) OTC *vitamin/iron supplement* [multiple vitamins; iron; folic acid] ± •15•0.3 mg

kidney root *medicinal herb* [see: queen of the meadow]

KIE syrup R *decongestant; expectorant* [ephedrine HCl; potassium iodide] 8•150 mg/5 mL

Kindercal liquid OTC *enteral nutritional therapy* [lactose-free formula]

Kinesed chewable tablets (discontinued 1995) R *GI antispasmodic; anticholinergic; sedative* [atropine sulfate; scopolamine hydrobromide; hyoscyamine hydrobromide; phenobarbital] 0.12•0.007•0.12•16 mg

Kinevac powder for IV injection R *diagnostic aid for gallbladder function* [sincalide] 1 μg/mL

king's clover *medicinal herb* [see: melilot]

king's cure *medicinal herb* [see: pipsissewa]

king's fern *medicinal herb* [see: buckhorn brake]

kininase II inhibitors [see: angiotensin-converting enzyme inhibitors]

kinnikinnik *medicinal herb* [see: uva ursi]

kitasamycin USAN, INN, BAN, JAN *antibacterial* [also: acetylkitasamycin; kitasamycin tartrate]

kitasamycin tartrate JAN *antibacterial* [also: kitasamycin; acetylkitasamycin]

KL4 surfactant *investigational (Phase II/III, orphan) for respiratory distress syndrome in adults and premature infants and meconium aspiration in newborn infants*

Klamath weed *medicinal herb* [see: St. John's wort]

Klaron lotion R *topical antibiotic for acne* [sulfacetamide sodium] 10%

KLB6; Ultra KLB6 softgels OTC *dietary supplement* [vitamin B₆; multiple food supplements] 3.5•± mg; 16.7•± mg

K-Lease extended-release capsules R *potassium supplement* [potassium chloride] 750 mg (10 mEq)

Kleen-Handz solution OTC *topical antiseptic* [ethyl alcohol] 62%

Klerist-D tablets, sustained-release capsules R *decongestant; antihistamine* [pseudoephedrine HCl; chlorpheniramine maleate] 60•4 mg; 120•8 mg

Klonopin tablets, Rx Pak (prescription package), Tel-E-Dose (unit dose package) R *anticonvulsant; investigational (orphan) for hyperexplexia (startle disease)* [clonazepam] 0.5, 1, 2 mg ② clonidine

K-Lor powder R *potassium supplement* [potassium chloride] 15, 20 mEq/packet ② Kaochlor

Klor-Con; Klor-Con/25 powder R *potassium supplement* [potassium chloride] 20 mEq/packet; 25 mEq/packet

Klor-Con 8; Klor-Con 10 film-coated extended-release tablets R *potassium supplement* [potassium chloride] 600 mg (8 mEq); 750 mg (10 mEq)

Klor-Con/EF effervescent tablets R *potassium supplement* [potassium bicarbonate; potassium citrate] 25 mEq (K)

Klorvess liquid, effervescent granules, effervescent tablets R *potassium supplement* [potassium chloride] 20 mEq/15 mL; 20 mEq/packet; 20 mEq

Klotrix film-coated controlled-release tablets R *potassium supplement* [potassium chloride] 750 mg (10 mEq) ② Liotrix

K-Lyte; K-Lyte DS effervescent tablets R *potassium supplement* [potassium bicarbonate; potassium citrate] 25 mEq; 50 mEq (K)

K-Lyte ㊖ (U.S. product: Urocit-K) effervescent tablets R *urinary alkalizer for hypocitruria* [potassium citrate] 2.5 g

K-Lyte/Cl powder R *potassium supplement* [potassium chloride] 25 mEq/dose

K-Lyte/Cl; K-Lyte/Cl 50 effervescent tablets ℞ *potassium supplement* [potassium chloride] 25 mEq; 50 mEq

KNI-272 *investigational (Phase I) antiviral for pediatric and adult HIV*

knitback; knitbone *medicinal herb* [see: comfrey]

knob grass; knob root *medicinal herb* [see: stone root]

K-Norm controlled-release capsules ℞ *potassium supplement* [potassium chloride] 750 mg (10 mEq)

knotted marjoram *medicinal herb* [see: marjoram]

knotweed *(Polygonum aviculare; P. hydropiper; P. persicaria; P. punctatum)* plant *medicinal herb used as an antiseptic, astringent, diaphoretic, diuretic, emmenagogue, rubefacient, and stimulant*

Koāte-DVI (double viral inactivation) powder for IV injection ℞ *antihemophilic to correct coagulation deficiency* [antihemophilic factor VIII, solvent/detergent and dry heat treated]

Koāte-HP powder for IV injection ℞ *antihemophilic to correct coagulation deficiency* [antihemophilic factor VIII] 250, 500, 1000, 1500 IU

Kof-Eze lozenges OTC *topical analgesic; counterirritant; mild local anesthetic* [menthol] 6 mg

KoGENate powder for IV injection ℞ *antihemophilic for treatment of hemophilia A and presurgical prophylaxis of hemophiliacs (orphan)* [antihemophilic factor VIII, recombinant] ≟

KoGENate SF ℞ *investigational (NDA filed) antihemophilic* [antihemophilic factor VIII, sucrose formulated]

KOH (potassium hydroxide) [q.v.]

kola nut *(Cola acuminata)* seed *medicinal herb used as a stimulant; natural source of caffeine*

Kolephrin caplets OTC *decongestant; antihistamine; analgesic* [pseudoephedrine HCl; chlorpheniramine maleate; acetaminophen] 30•2•325 mg

Kolephrin GG/DM liquid OTC *antitussive; expectorant* [dextromethorphan hydrobromide; guaifenesin] 10•150 mg/5 mL

Kolephrin/DM caplets OTC *antitussive; decongestant; antihistamine; analgesic* [dextromethorphan hydrobromide; pseudoephedrine HCl; chlorpheniramine maleate; acetaminophen] 10• 30•2•325 mg

kolfocon A USAN *hydrophobic contact lens material*

kolfocon B USAN *hydrophobic contact lens material*

kolfocon C USAN *hydrophobic contact lens material*

kolfocon D USAN *hydrophobic contact lens material*

Kolyum liquid ℞ *potassium supplement* [potassium gluconate; potassium chloride] 20 mEq/15 mL (K)

kombucha (yeast/bacteria/fungus symbiont) fermented tea *natural treatment for aging, cancer, intestinal disorders, and rheumatism*

Konakion IM injection (discontinued 1997) ℞ *coagulant; correct anticoagulant-induced prothrombin deficiency; vitamin K supplement* [phytonadione] 2 mg/mL

Kondon's Nasal jelly OTC *nasal decongestant* [ephedrine] 1%

Kondremul Plain emulsion OTC *emollient laxative* [mineral oil]

Kondremul with Phenolphthalein emulsion OTC *stimulant/emollient laxative* [mineral oil; phenolphthalein] 55%•150 mg/15 mL

Konsyl powder OTC *bulk laxative* [psyllium] 100%

Konsyl Fiber tablets OTC *bulk laxative; antidiarrheal* [calcium polycarbophil] 625 mg

Konsyl-D; Konsyl Orange powder OTC *bulk laxative* [psyllium hydrophilic mucilloid] 3.4 g/tbsp.

Konyne 80 IV infusion ℞ *antihemophilic to correct factor VIII (hemophilia A) and factor IX (hemophilia B; Christmas disease) deficiencies* [coagulation factors II, VII, IX, and X, heat treated] 20, 40 mL

Kophane Cough & Cold Formula liquid OTC *antitussive; decongestant; antihistamine* [dextromethorphan hydrobromide; phenylpropanolamine HCl; chlorpheniramine maleate] 10•12.5•2 mg/5 mL

Korean ginseng *(Panax ginseng; P. shin-seng) medicinal herb* [see: ginseng]

Koromex premedicated condom (discontinued 1995) OTC *spermicidal/barrier contraceptive* [nonoxynol 9] 5.6%

Koromex vaginal cream OTC *spermicidal contraceptive (for use with a diaphragm)* [octoxynol 9] 3%

Koromex vaginal foam, vaginal jelly OTC *spermicidal contraceptive* [nonoxynol 9] 12.5%; 3% ☑ Komex

Koromex Crystal Clear vaginal gel OTC *spermicidal contraceptive (for use with a diaphragm)* [nonoxynol 9] 2%

Kovitonic liquid OTC *hematinic* [ferric pyrophosphate; multiple B vitamins; lysine; folic acid] 42•±•10•0.1 mg/15 mL

K-Pek oral suspension OTC *antidiarrheal; GI adsorbent* [attapulgite] 600 mg/15 mL

K-Phen-50 injection (discontinued 1997) Rx *antihistamine; sedative; antiemetic; motion sickness relief* [promethazine HCl] 50 mg/mL

K-Phos M.F. tablets Rx *urinary acidifier* [potassium acid phosphate; sodium acid phosphate] 155•350 mg (1.1 mEq potassium, 2.9 mEq sodium)

K-Phos Neutral film-coated tablets Rx *urinary acidifier; phosphorus supplement* [sodium phosphate, dibasic; potassium phosphate, monobasic; sodium phosphate, monobasic] 852•155•130 mg (1.1 mEq potassium, 13.0 mEq sodium)

K-Phos No. 2 tablets Rx *urinary acidifier* [potassium acid phosphate; sodium acid phosphate] 305•700 mg (2.3 mEq potassium, 5.8 mEq sodium)

K-Phos Original tablets Rx *urinary acidifier* [potassium acid phosphate] 500 mg (3.7 mEq potassium)

K.P.N. tablets OTC *vitamin/mineral/calcium/iron supplement* [multiple vitamins & minerals; calcium; iron; folic acid] ±•333•11•0.27 mg

^{81m}Kr [see: krypton Kr 81m]

^{85}Kr [see: krypton clathrate Kr 85]

Kredex (European name for U.S. product Coreg)

Kronocap (trademarked dosage form) *sustained-release capsule*

Kronofed-A sustained-release capsules Rx *decongestant; antihistamine* [pseudoephedrine HCl; chlorpheniramine maleate] 120•8 mg

Kronofed-A Jr. Kronocaps (sustained-release capsules) Rx *pediatric decongestant and antihistamine* [pseudoephedrine HCl; chlorpheniramine maleate] 60•4 mg

krypton *element (Kr)*

krypton clathrate Kr 85 USAN *radioactive agent*

krypton Kr 81m USAN, USP *radioactive agent*

K-Tab film-coated extended-release tablets Rx *potassium supplement* [potassium chloride] 750 mg (10 mEq)

Kudrox oral suspension OTC *antacid* [aluminum hydroxide; magnesium hydroxide; simethicone] 500•450•40 mg/5 mL

kudzu *(Pueraria lobata; P. thunbergiana) root medicinal herb for the management of alcoholism*

Kutapressin subcu or IM injection Rx *claimed to be an anti-inflammatory for multiple dermatoses* [liver derivative complex] 25.5 mg/mL

Kutrase capsules Rx *digestive enzymes; GI antispasmodic; sedative* [amylase; protease; lipase; cellulase; hyoscyamine sulfate; phenyltoloxamine citrate] 30•6•75•2•0.0625•15 mg

Ku-Zyme capsules Rx *digestive enzymes* [amylase; protease; lipase; cellulase] 30•6•75•2 mg

Ku-Zyme HP capsules ℞ *digestive enzymes* [lipase; protease; amylase] 8000•30 000•30 000 U

K-vescent effervescent powder ℞ *potassium supplement* [potassium chloride] 20 mEq/packet

Kwelcof liquid ℞ *narcotic antitussive; expectorant* [hydrocodone bitartrate; guaifenesin] 5•100 mg/5 mL

Kwell cream, lotion, shampoo (discontinued 1996) ℞ *pediculicide for lice; scabicide* [lindane] 1%

Kwellada-P ⓒⒶⓃ (U.S. product: Elimite) lotion OTC *pediculicide for lice; scabicide* [permethrin] 5%

Kwildane lotion, shampoo ℞ *pediculicide for lice; scabicide* [lindane]

K-Y vaginal jelly OTC *lubricant* [glycerin; hydroxyethyl cellulose]

K-Y Plus vaginal gel OTC *spermicidal contraceptive (for use with a diaphragm)* [nonoxynol 9] 2.2%

kyamepromazin [see: cyamemazine]

Kybernin IV ℞ *for thrombosis and pulmonary emboli of congenital AT-III deficiency (orphan)* [antithrombin III]

Kytril film-coated tablets, IV infusion ℞ *5-HT₃ antagonist; antiemetic/antinauseant for chemotherapy and radiotherapy* [granisetron HCl] 1 mg; 1 mg/mL

L-5 hydroxytryptophan (L-5HTP) *natural precursor to serotonin; investigational (orphan) for postanoxic intention myoclonus*

LA-12 IM injection ℞ *antianemic; vitamin B_{12} supplement* [hydroxocobalamin] 1000 μg/mL

LAAM (l-acetyl-α-methadol [or] l-alpha-acetyl-methadol) [see: levomethadyl acetate]

labetalol INN, BAN *antihypertensive; antiadrenergic (α- and β-receptor)* [also: labetalol HCl]

labetalol HCl USAN, USP *antihypertensive; antiadrenergic (α- and β-receptor)* [also: labetalol] 100, 200, 300 mg oral

Labrador tea (Ledum groenlandicum; L. latifolium; L. palustre) leaves *medicinal herb for bronchial infections, cough, diarrhea, headache, kidney disorders, lung infections, malignancies, rheumatism, and sore throat*

Labstix reagent strips *in vitro diagnostic aid for multiple urine products*

Lac-Hydrin cream, lotion ℞ *moisturizer; emollient* [ammonium lactate] 12%

Lac-Hydrin Five lotion OTC *moisturizer; emollient* [lactic acid]

lacidipine USAN, INN, BAN *antihypertensive; calcium channel blocker*

Lacipil (commercially available in Europe) ℞ *investigational antihypertensive; calcium channel blocker* [lacidipine]

Lacril eye drops OTC *ophthalmic moisturizer/lubricant* [hydroxypropyl methylcellulose] 0.5%

Lacri-Lube NP; Lacri-Lube S.O.P. ophthalmic ointment OTC *ocular moisturizer/lubricant* [white petrolatum; mineral oil; lanolin]

Lacrisert ophthalmic insert OTC *ophthalmic moisturizer/lubricant* [hydroxypropyl cellulose] 5 mg

lactagogues *a class of agents that promote or increase the flow of breast milk* [also called: galactagogues]

LactAid liquid, tablets OTC *digestive aid for lactose intolerance* [lactase enzyme] 250 U/drop; 3000 U

lactalfate INN

lactase enzyme *digestive enzyme for lactose intolerance*

lactated potassic saline [see: potassic saline, lactated]

lactated Ringer's (LR) injection [see: Ringer's injection, lactated]

lactated Ringer's (LR) solution [see: Ringer's injection, lactated]

lactic acid USP *pH adjusting agent*

LactiCare lotion OTC *emollient; moisturizer* [lactic acid]

LactiCare-HC lotion ℞ *topical corticosteroidal anti-inflammatory* [hydrocortisone] 1%, 2.5%

Lactinex granules, chewable tablets OTC *dietary supplement; fever blister treatment; not generally regarded as safe and effective as an antidiarrheal* [Lactobacillus acidophilus; Lactobacillus bulgaricus]

Lactinol lotion ℞ *emollient; moisturizer* [lactic acid] 10%

Lactinol-E cream ℞ *emollient; moisturizer* [lactic acid; vitamin E] 10%• 116.67 IU/g

lactitol INN, BAN

Lactobacillus acidophilus natural bacteria [see: acidophilus]

Lactobacillus bulgaricus dietary supplement; not generally regarded as safe and effective as an antidiarrheal

lactobin *investigational (orphan) for AIDS-related diarrhea*

lactobionic acid, calcium salt, dihydrate [see: calcium lactobionate]

Lactocal-F film-coated tablets ℞ *vitamin/mineral/calcium/iron supplement* [multiple vitamins & minerals; calcium; iron; folic acid] ±•200•65•1 mg

lactoflavin [see: riboflavin]

Lactofree liquid, powder OTC *hypoallergenic infant formula* [milk-based formula, lactose free]

β-lactone [see: propiolactone]

γ-lactone D-glucofuranuronic acid [see: glucurolactone]

lactose NF *tablet and capsule diluent; dietary supplement*

Lactrase capsules OTC *digestive aid for lactose intolerance* [lactase enzyme] 250 mg

Lactuca sativa medicinal herb [see: lettuce]

Lactuca virosa medicinal herb [see: wild lettuce]

lactulose USAN, USP, INN, BAN *laxative*

ladakamycin [now: azacitidine]

Lady Esther cream OTC *moisturizer; emollient* [mineral oil]

lady's mantle (Alchemilla xanthochlora; A. vulgaris) plant *medicinal herb for diarrhea and other digestive disorders; also used as an astringent, anti-inflammatory agent, menstrual cycle regulator, and muscle relaxant*

lady's slipper (Cypripedium pubescens) root *medicinal herb for chorea, hysteria, insomnia, nervousness, and restlessness*

laidlomycin INN *veterinary growth stimulant* [also: laidlomycin propionate potassium]

laidlomycin propionate potassium USAN *veterinary growth stimulant* [also: laidlomycin]

Laki-Lorand factor [see: factor XIII]

lamb mint *medicinal herb* [see: peppermint; spearmint]

Lambda ℞ *investigational (Phase III) treatment for renal failure*

lamb's quarter *medicinal herb* [see: birthroot]

Lamictal tablets, chewable/dispersible tablets ℞ *phenyltriazine anticonvulsant; adjunctive treatment for Lennox-Gastaut syndrome (orphan)* [lamotrigine] 25, 100, 150, 200 mg; 5, 25 mg

lamifiban USAN, INN *glycoprotein (GP) IIb/IIIa receptor inhibitor; antiplatelet/ antithrombotic agent for unstable angina*

Laminaria digitata; L. japonica medicinal herb [see: kelp]

Lamisil cream (became OTC and name changed to Lamisil AT in 1999)

Lamisil spray ℞ *topical allylamine antifungal* [terbinafine HCl] 1%

Lamisil tablets ℞ *systemic antifungal for onychomycosis* [terbinafine HCl] 250 mg

Lamisil AT cream OTC *topical allylamine antifungal* [terbinafine HCl] 1%

Lamisil DermGel gel ℞ *topical allylamine antifungal* [terbinafine HCl] 1%

Lamium album medicinal herb [see: blind nettle]

lamivudine USAN, INN, BAN *nucleoside reverse transcriptase inhibitor antiviral for HIV and hepatitis B*

lamotrigine USAN, INN, BAN *phenyltriazine anticonvulsant; adjunctive treatment for Lennox-Gastaut syndrome (orphan)*

Lampit (available only from the Centers for Disease Control) ℞ *investigational anti-infective for Chagas disease* [nifurtimox]

Lamprene capsules ℞ *bactericidal; tuberculostatic; leprostatic (orphan)* [clofazimine] 50 mg

lamtidine INN, BAN

Lanabiotic ointment OTC *topical antibiotic; anesthetic* [polymyxin B sulfate; neomycin sulfate; bacitracin; lidocaine] 10 000 U•3.5 mg•500 U•40 mg per g

Lanacane spray, cream OTC *topical local anesthetic; antiseptic* [benzocaine; benzethonium chloride] 20%•0.1%; 6%•0.1%

Lanacaps (dosage form) *timed-release capsules*

Lanacort 5 cream, ointment OTC *topical corticosteroidal anti-inflammatory* [hydrocortisone acetate] 0.5%

Lanacort 10 cream OTC *topical corticosteroidal anti-inflammatory* [hydrocortisone acetate] 1%

Lanacort 10 ointment (discontinued 1997) OTC *topical corticosteroidal anti-inflammatory* [hydrocortisone acetate] 1%

Lanaphilic cream OTC *moisturizer; emollient; keratolytic* [urea] 20%

Lanaphilic OTC *ointment base*

Lanaphilic with Urea OTC *ointment base* [urea] 10%

Lanatabs (dosage form) *sustained-release tablets*

lanatoside NF, INN, BAN

Laniazid syrup (discontinued 1998) ℞ *tuberculostatic* [isoniazid] 50 mg/5 mL

Laniazid tablets ℞ *tuberculostatic* [isoniazid] 50 mg

Laniazid C.T. tablets ℞ *tuberculostatic* [isoniazid] 300 mg

lanolin USP *ointment base; water-in-oil emulsion; emollient/protectant* ② Lanoline

lanolin, anhydrous USP *absorbent ointment base*

lanolin alcohols *ointment base ingredient*

Lanolor cream OTC *moisturizer; emollient*

Lanophyllin elixir ℞ *antiasthmatic; bronchodilator* [theophylline] 80 mg/15 mL

Lanorinal tablets, capsules ℞ *analgesic; sedative* [aspirin; caffeine; butalbital] 325•40•50 mg

lanoteplase USAN *investigational (Phase III) thrombolytic and tissue plasminogen activator (tPA)*

Lanoxicaps capsules ℞ *cardiac glycoside to increase cardiac output; antiarrhythmic* [digoxin] 0.05, 0.1, 0.2 mg

Lanoxin tablets, pediatric elixir, IV or IM injection ℞ *cardiac glycoside to increase cardiac output; antiarrhythmic* [digoxin] 0.125, 0.25 mg; 0.05 mg/mL; 0.1, 0.25 mg/mL

lanreotide acetate USAN *antineoplastic*

lansoprazole USAN, INN, BAN *proton pump inhibitor for gastric and duodenal ulcers other gastroesophageal disorders*

lanthanum *element (La)*

Lapacho colorado; L. morado *medicinal herb* [see: pau d'arco]

lapirium chloride INN *surfactant* [also: lapyrium chloride]

LAPOCA (L-asparaginase, Oncovin, cytarabine, Adriamycin) *chemotherapy protocol*

laprafylline INN

lapyrium chloride USAN *surfactant* [also: lapirium chloride]

laramycin [see: zorbamycin]

larch (*Larix americana; L. europaea*) bark, resin, young shoots, and needles *medicinal herb used as an anthelmintic, diuretic, laxative, and vulnerary*

Largon IV or IM injection ℞ *sedative; analgesic adjunct* [propiomazine HCl] 20 mg/mL

Lariam tablets ℞ *antimalarial for acute chloroquine-resistant malaria (orphan)* [mefloquine HCl] 250 mg

Larix americana; L. europaea medicinal herb [see: larch]

Larodopa capsules ℞ *dopamine precursor; antiparkinsonian* [levodopa] 100, 250, 500 mg

Larodopa tablets ℞ *dopamine precursor; antiparkinsonian* [levodopa] 100, 250, 500 mg

laroxyl [see: amitriptyline]

Larrea divaricata; L. glutinosa; L. tridentata medicinal herb [see: chaparral]

lasalocid USAN, INN, BAN *coccidiostat for poultry*

Lasan cream, ointment ℞ *topical antipsoriatic* [anthralin] 0.1%, 0.2%, 0.4%; 0.4%

Lasan HP-1 cream ℞ *topical antipsoriatic* [anthralin] 1%

Lasix tablets, oral solution, IM or IV injection ℞ *antihypertensive; loop diuretic* [furosemide] 20, 40, 80 mg; 10 mg/mL; 10 mg/mL ⑨ Esidrix; Lidex

Lassar's paste [betanaphthol (q.v.) + zinc oxide (q.v.)]

latamoxef INN, BAN *anti-infective* [also: moxalactam disodium]

latamoxef disodium [see: moxalactam disodium]

latanoprost USAN, INN *prostaglandin agonist for glaucoma and ocular hypertension*

latex agglutination test *in vitro diagnostic aid*

laudexium methylsulfate [see: laudexium metilsulfate; laudexium methylsulphate]

laudexium methylsulphate BAN [also: laudexium metilsulfate]

laudexium metilsulfate INN [also: laudexium methylsulphate]

lauralkonium chloride INN

laurel *(Laurus nobilis)* leaves and fruit medicinal herb used as an aromatic, astringent, carminative, and stomachic

laurel, mountain; rose laurel; sheep laurel medicinal herb [see: mountain laurel]

laurel, red; swamp laurel medicinal herb [see: magnolia]

laurel, spurge; spurge olive medicinal herb [see: mezereon]

laureth 4 USAN *surfactant*

laureth 9 USAN *spermaticide; surfactant*

laureth 10S USAN *spermaticide*

lauril INN *combining name for radicals or groups*

laurilsulfate INN *combining name for radicals or groups* [also: sodium lauryl sulfate]

laurixamine INN

laurocapram USAN, INN *excipient*

laurocapram & methotrexate *investigational (orphan) for topical treatment of Mycosis fungoides*

lauroguadine INN

laurolinium acetate INN, BAN

lauromacrogol 400 INN

Laurus nobilis medicinal herb [see: laurel]

Laurus persea medicinal herb [see: avocado]

lauryl isoquinolinium bromide USAN *anti-infective*

lavender (Lavandula spp.) flowers, leaves, and oil medicinal herb for acne, bile flow stimulation, diabetes, edema, flatulence, hyperactivity, insomnia, intestinal spasms, migraine headache, and stimulating menstrual flow

lavender oil NF

lavoltidine INN *antiulcerative; histamine H_2-receptor blocker* [also: lavoltidine succinate; loxtidine]

lavoltidine succinate USAN *antiulcerative; histamine H_2-receptor blocker* [also: lavoltidine; loxtidine]

Lavoptik Eye Wash ophthalmic solution OTC *extraocular irrigating solution* [sodium chloride (balanced saline solution)]

lawrencium element (Lr)

Lawsonia inermis medicinal herb [see: henna]

Lax Pills tablets (discontinued 1998) OTC *stimulant laxative* [yellow phenolphthalein] 90 mg

Laxative Pills tablets (discontinued 1998) OTC *stimulant laxative* [yellow phenolphthalein] 90 mg

laxatives *a class of agents that promote evacuation of the bowels or have a mild purgative effect* [see also: cathartics; purgatives]

lazabemide USAN, INN *antiparkinsonian*

lazaroids *a class of potent antioxidants that can protect against oxygen radical–mediated lipid peroxidation and progressive neuronal degeneration following brain or spinal trauma, subarachnoid hemorrhage, or stroke* [also called: 21-aminosteroids]

Lazer Creme OTC *moisturizer; emollient* [vitamins A and E] 3333.3•116.67 U/g

Lazer Formalyde solution ℞ *for hyperhidrosis and bromhidrosis* [formaldehyde] 10%

LazerSporin-C ear drops ℞ *topical corticosteroidal anti-inflammatory; antibiotic* [hydrocortisone; neomycin sulfate; polymyxin B sulfate] 1%•5 mg•10 000 U per mL

LC-65 solution OTC *cleaning solution for hard, soft, or rigid gas permeable contact lenses*

L-Caine injection (discontinued 1995) ℞ *injectable local anesthetic* [lidocaine HCl] 1%

LCD (liquor carbonis detergens) [see: coal tar]

LCR (leurocristine) [see: vincristine]

LCx *Neisseria gonorrhoeae* **Assay** reagent kit for professional use *in vitro diagnostic aid for Neisseria gonorrhoeae*

LDI-200 *investigational (Phase III) apoptosis inducer for myelodysplastic syndrome*

LDP-02 *investigational (Phase II) agent for inflammatory bowel disease*

lead *element (Pb)*

lecimibide USAN *hypocholesterolemic; antihyperlipidemic*

lecithin NF *emulsifier; surfactant; natural phospholipid mixture of various phosphatidylcholines used as an antihypercholesterolemic and cognition enhancer for Alzheimer's and other dementias* 420, 1200 mg oral

lecithol *natural remedy* [see: lecithin]

LED (liposome-encapsulated doxorubicin) [see: doxorubicin HCl, liposome-encapsulated]

Ledercillin VK tablets, powder for oral solution (discontinued 1997) ℞ *natural penicillin antibiotic* [penicillin V potassium] 250, 500 mg; 250 mg/5 mL

Lederject (trademarked delivery system) *prefilled disposable syringe*

Lederplex capsules (discontinued 1995) OTC *vitamin supplement* [multiple B vitamins]

ledoxantrone trihydrochloride USAN *antineoplastic; topoisomerase II inhibitor* [previously: sedoxantrone trihydrochloride]

Ledum groenlandicum; L. latifolium; L. palustre *medicinal herb* [see: Labrador tea]

leeches (Hirudo medicinalis) *natural adjunct to postsurgical wound management*

leek (Allium porrum) *bulb, lower stem, and leaves medicinal herb used as an appetite stimulant, decongestant, and diuretic*

lefetamine INN

leflunomide INN *anti-inflammatory for rheumatoid arthritis; investigational (orphan) for malignant glioma, ovarian cancer, and prevention of rejection of organ transplants; investigational (Phase II) for prostate and non-small cell lung cancers; investigational (Phase III) for first relapse glioblastoma multiforme*

Legalon *orphan status withdrawn 1997* [disodium silibinin dihemisuccinate]

Legatrin tablets (discontinued 1995) OTC *prevention and treatment of nocturnal leg cramps* [quinine sulfate] 162.5 mg

Legatrin PM caplets OTC *prevention and treatment of nocturnal leg cramps* [diphenhydramine HCl; acetaminophen] 50•500 mg

legs, red *medicinal herb* [see: bistort]

leiopyrrole INN

lemidosul INN

lemon *(Citrus limon)* fruit and peel *medicinal herb used as an astringent, refrigerant, and source of vitamin C*

lemon, ground; wild lemon *medicinal herb* [see: mandrake]

lemon balm *(Melissa officinalis)* plant *medicinal herb used as an antispasmodic and sedative; also used for Graves' disease and cold sores*

lemon oil NF

lemon verbena *(Aloysiatriphylla* **spp.)** leaves and flowers *medicinal herb for fever, flatulence, gastrointestinal spasms and other disorders, and sedation*

lemon walnut *medicinal herb* [see: butternut]

lemongrass *(Andropogon citratus; Cymbopogon citratus)* leaves *medicinal herb for colds, cough, fever, gastrointestinal spasm and other disorders, nervousness, pain, and rheumatism; also used as an antiemetic*

lenampicillin INN

lenercept USAN *tumor necrosis factor (TNF) receptor antagonist for septic shock, multiple sclerosis, inflammatory bowel disease, and rheumatoid arthritis*

leniquinsin USAN, INN *antihypertensive*

lenitzol [see: amitriptyline]

lenograstim USAN, INN, BAN *immunomodulator; antineutropenic; hematopoietic stimulant*

lenperone USAN, INN *antipsychotic*

Lens Clear solution (discontinued 1995) OTC *surfactant cleaning solution for soft contact lenses*

Lens Drops solution OTC *rewetting solution for hard or soft contact lenses*

Lens Fresh solution (discontinued 1995) OTC *rewetting solution for hard or soft contact lenses*

Lens Lubricant solution OTC *rewetting solution for hard or soft contact lenses*

Lens Plus Daily Cleaner solution OTC *surfactant cleaning solution for soft contact lenses*

Lens Plus Oxysept products [see: Oxysept]

Lens Plus Rewetting Drops OTC *rewetting solution for soft contact lenses*

Lens Plus Sterile Saline aerosol solution OTC *rinsing/storage solution for soft contact lenses* [sodium chloride (saline solution)]

Lensept solutions (discontinued 1995) OTC *two-step chemical disinfecting system for soft contact lenses* [hydrogen peroxide based] 3%

Lente Iletin I subcu injection (discontinued 1999) OTC *antidiabetic* [insulin zinc (beef-pork)] 100 U/mL

Lente Iletin II subcu injection OTC *antidiabetic* [insulin zinc (pork)] 100 U/mL

Lente Insulin subcu injection (discontinued 1997) OTC *antidiabetic* [insulin zinc (beef)] 100 U/mL

Lente L subcu injection OTC *antidiabetic* [insulin zinc (pork)] 100 U/mL

lentin [see: carbachol]

lentinan JAN *investigational (Phase II/III) immunomodulator for HIV and AIDS*

Lentinula edodes *medicinal herb* [see: shiitake mushrooms]

Leontodon taraxacum *medicinal herb* [see: dandelion]

Leonurus cardiaca *medicinal herb* [see: motherwort]

leopard's bane *medicinal herb* [see: arnica]

Lepidium meyenii *medicinal herb* [see: maca]

lepirudin *anticoagulant for heparin-induced thrombocytopenia (orphan)*

leprosatics *a class of drugs effective against leprosy*

leptacline INN

leptandra; purple leptandra *medicinal herb* [see: Culver's root]

lercanidipine *investigational calcium channel blocker*

lergotrile USAN, INN *prolactin enzyme inhibitor*

lergotrile mesylate USAN *prolactin enzyme inhibitor*

Lescol capsules ℞ *HMG-CoA reductase inhibitor for hypercholesterolemia, hypertriglyceridemia, and atherosclerosis* [fluvastatin sodium] 20, 40 mg

lesopitron INN *investigational anxiolytic*
lesser centaury *medicinal herb* [see: centaury]
leteprinim potassium USAN *investigational (Phase II) nerve growth factor for Alzheimer's disease, spinal cord injury, and stroke*
letimide INN *analgesic* [also: letimide HCl]
letimide HCl USAN *analgesic* [also: letimide]
letosteine INN
letrazuril INN *investigational treatment for AIDS-related cryptosporidial diarrhea*
letrozole USAN, INN *hormone antagonist antineoplastic/aromatase inhibitor for advanced breast cancer in postmenopausal women*
lettuce (Lactuca sativa) *juice and leaves medicinal herb used as an anodyne, antispasmodic, expectorant, and sedative (for herbal medical use, common garden lettuce is harvested after it has gone to seed, and a milky juice is extracted)*
Leucanthemum parthenium *medicinal herb* [see: feverfew]
leucarsone [see: carbarsone]
leucine (L-leucine) USAN, USP, INN, JAN *essential amino acid; symbols: Leu, L*
leucine & isoleucine & valine *investigational (orphan) for hyperphenylalaninemia*
leucinocaine INN
leucocianidol INN
Leucomax (commercially available in 36 foreign countries) Ṛ *antineutropenic; hematopoietic stimulant; investigational (Phase II/III) cytokine for AIDS; orphan status withdrawn 1996* [molgramostim]
leucomycin [see: kitasamycin; spiramycin]
Leucotropin Ṛ *investigational (Phase III) antineoplastic* [regramostim]
L-leucovorin *chemotherapy "rescue" agent (orphan)*
leucovorin calcium USP *antianemic; folate replenisher; antidote to folic acid*

antagonist; chemotherapy "rescue" agent (orphan) [also: calcium folinate] 5, 15, 25 mg oral; 3 mg/mL injection; 50, 100, 350 mg/vial injection
leucovorin & fluorouracil *antineoplastic for metastatic colorectal cancer (orphan)*
leucovorin & methotrexate *antineoplastic for osteosarcoma (orphan)*
LeukArrest Ṛ *investigational (Phase III) treatment for acute ischemic stroke*
Leukeran *tablets* Ṛ *nitrogen mustard-type alkylating antineoplastic for multiple leukemias, lymphomas, and neoplasms* [chlorambucil] 2 mg
Leukine *IV infusion* Ṛ *myeloid reconstitution after autologous bone marrow transplant (orphan); investigational (Phase III) for malignant melanoma; investigational (Phase II) cytokine for AIDS* [sargramostim] 250, 500 µg
leukocyte interferon [now: interferon alfa-n3]
leukocyte protease inhibitor [see: secretory leukocyte protease inhibitor]
leukocyte typing serum USP *in vitro blood test*
leukopoietin [see: sargramostim]
LeukoScan *investigational diagnostic aid for infectious lesions* [technetium Tc 99m sulesomab]
leukotriene receptor antagonists (LTRAs); leukotriene receptor inhibitors *a class of antiasthmatics that inhibit bronchoconstriction when used prophylactically (will not reverse bronchospasm)*
leupeptin *investigational (orphan) aid to microsurgical peripheral nerve repair*
leuprolide acetate USAN *hormonal antineoplastic for various cancers; LHRH agonist for central precocious puberty (orphan)* [also: leuprorelin] 5 mg/mL injection
leuprorelin INN, BAN *antineoplastic; LHRH agonist* [also: leuprolide acetate]
leurocristine (LCR) [see: vincristine]
leurocristine sulfate [see: vincristine sulfate]

Leustatin IV infusion ℞ *antineoplastic for hairy-cell leukemia (orphan); investigational (orphan) for chronic lymphocytic leukemia, multiple sclerosis, and non-Hodgkin's lymphoma* [cladribine] 1 mg/mL

LeuTech ℞ *investigational (Phase III) radiolabeled infection imaging agent for equivocal appendicitis*

leutetium texaphyrin *investigational light-activated agent for dissolving arterial plaque*

Leutrol (name changed to Zyflo upon marketing release in 1997)

Leuvectin ℞ *investigational (Phase I/II) gene-based therapy for advanced metastatic renal cell carcinoma*

levacetylmethadol INN *narcotic analgesic* [also: levomethadyl acetate]

levalbuterol *sympathomimetic bronchodilator; single-isomer albuterol*

levalbuterol HCl USAN *sympathomimetic bronchodilator; single-isomer albuterol*

levalbuterol sulfate USAN *sympathomimetic bronchodilator; single-isomer albuterol*

levallorphan INN, BAN [also: levallorphan tartrate] ② *levorphanol*

levallorphan tartrate USP [also: levallorphan]

levamfetamine INN *anorectic* [also: levamfetamine succinate; levamphetamine]

levamfetamine succinate USAN *anorectic* [also: levamfetamine; levamphetamine]

levamisole INN, BAN *biological response modifier; antineoplastic; veterinary anthelmintic* [also: levamisole HCl]

levamisole HCl USAN, USP *biological response modifier; antineoplastic; veterinary anthelmintic* [also: levamisole]

levamphetamine BAN *anorectic* [also: levamfetamine succinate; levamfetamine]

levant berry (Anamirta cocculus; A. paniculata) leaves and berries *medicinal herb for epilepsy, lice, malaria, morphine poisoning, and worms; not generally regarded as safe and effective for ingestion or topical application on abraded skin*

Levaquin film-coated tablets, IV infusion ℞ *fluoroquinolone antibiotic* [levofloxacin] 250, 500 mg

levarterenol [see: norepinephrine bitartrate]

levarterenol bitartrate [now: norepinephrine bitartrate]

Levatol tablets ℞ *antihypertensive; β-blocker* [penbutolol sulfate] 20 mg

Levbid extended-release tablets ℞ *GI antispasmodic; anticholinergic* [hyoscyamine sulfate] 0.375 mg

levcromakalim USAN, INN, BAN *antiasthmatic; antihypertensive*

levcycloserine USAN, INN *enzyme inhibitor*

levdobutamine INN *cardiotonic* [also: levdobutamine lactobionate]

levdobutamine lactobionate USAN *cardiotonic* [also: levdobutamine]

levdropropizine INN

levemopamil INN *investigational treatment for stroke*

levetiracetam INN *investigational (NDA filed) anticonvulsant*

levisoprenaline INN

Levisticum officinale *medicinal herb* [see: lovage]

Levlen tablets ℞ *monophasic oral contraceptive; emergency "morning after" contraceptive* [levonorgestrel; ethinyl estradiol] 0.15 mg•30 μg

Levlite 21; Levlite 28 tablets (21 active tablets with or without 7 inert "counters") ℞ *ultra low-dose oral contraceptive* [ethinyl estradiol; levonorgestrel] 0.02•0.1 mg

levlofexidine INN

levobetaxolol INN *antiadrenergic (β-receptor)* [also: levobetaxolol HCl]

levobetaxolol HCl USAN *antiadrenergic (β-receptor)* [also: levobetaxolol]

levobunolol INN, BAN *antiadrenergic (β-blocker); topical antiglaucoma agent* [also: levobunolol HCl]

levobunolol HCl USAN, USP *antiadrenergic (β-blocker); topical antiglau-*

coma agent [also: levobunolol]
0.25%, 0.5% eye drops

levobupivacaine HCl USAN *investigational (NDA filed) long-acting local anesthetic*

levocabastine INN, BAN *antihistamine* [also: levocabastine HCl]

levocabastine HCl USAN *antihistamine* [also: levocabastine]

levocarbinoxamine tartrate [see: rotoxamine tartrate]

levocarnitine USAN, USP, INN *dietary amino acid for primary and secondary genetic carnitine deficiency (orphan); investigational (orphan) for end-stage renal disease and pediatric cardiomyopathy* 250 mg oral

levodopa USAN, USP, INN, BAN, JAN *antiparkinsonian; dopamine precursor* ⊘ methyldopa

levodopa & carbidopa *antiparkinsonian* 100•10, 100•25, 250•25 mg oral

Levo-Dromoran tablets, subcu or IV injection ℞ *narcotic analgesic* [levorphanol tartrate] 2 mg; 2 mg/mL

levofacetoperane INN

levofenfluramine INN

levofloxacin USAN, INN, JAN *fluoroquinolone antibiotic*

levofuraltadone USAN, INN *antibacterial; antiprotozoal*

levoglutamide INN *nonessential amino acid*

levoleucovorin calcium USAN *antidote to folic acid antagonists*

levomenol INN

levomepate [see: atromepine]

levomepromazine INN *analgesic* [also: methotrimeprazine]

levomethadone INN

levomethadyl acetate USAN *narcotic analgesic* [also: levacetylmethadol]

levomethadyl acetate HCl USAN *narcotic analgesic for management of opiate addiction (orphan)*

levomethorphan INN, BAN

levometiomeprazine INN

levomoprolol INN

levomoramide INN, BAN

levonantradol INN, BAN *analgesic* [also: levonantradol HCl]

levonantradol HCl USAN *analgesic* [also: levonantradol]

levonordefrin USP *adrenergic; vasoconstrictor* [also: corbadrine]

levonorgestrel USAN, USP, INN, BAN *progestin; contraceptive implant*

Levophed IV infusion ℞ *vasopressor for acute hypotensive shock* [norepinephrine bitartrate] 1 mg/mL

levophenacylmorphan INN, BAN

Levoprome IM injection ℞ *central analgesic; CNS depressant* [methotrimeprazine HCl] 20 mg/mL

levopropicillin INN *antibacterial* [also: levopropylcillin potassium]

levopropicillin potassium [see: levopropylcillin potassium]

levopropoxyphene INN, BAN *antitussive* [also: levopropoxyphene napsylate]

levopropoxyphene napsylate USAN *antitussive* [also: levopropoxyphene]

levopropylcillin potassium USAN *antibacterial* [also: levopropicillin]

levopropylhexedrine INN

levoprotiline INN

Levora tablets (21 or 28) ℞ *monophasic oral contraceptive* [levonorgestrel; ethinyl estradiol] 0.15•0.03 mg

levorin INN

levormeloxifene *investigational (Phase III) partial estrogen receptor agonist for osteoporosis (clinical trials discontinued 1998)*

levorphanol INN, BAN *narcotic analgesic* [also: levorphanol tartrate] ⊘ levallorphan

levorphanol tartrate USP *narcotic analgesic* [also: levorphanol]

levosimendan USAN *investigational cardiotonic and vasodilator for congestive heart failure*

Levo-T tablets ℞ *thyroid hormone* [levothyroxine sodium] 25, 50, 75, 100, 125, 150, 200, 300 μg

Levothroid tablets, powder for injection ℞ *thyroid hormone* [levothyroxine sodium] 25, 50, 75, 88, 100, 112,

125, 137, 150, 175, 200, 300 μg; 200, 500 μg

Levothroid ⒼⓂ (U.S. product: Synthroid) tablets ℞ *thyroid hormone* [levothyroxine sodium] 25, 50, 75, 100, 112, 125, 150, 175, 200, 300 μg

levothyroxine sodium (T₄) USP, INN *thyroid hormone* [also: thyroxine] 0.1, 0.15, 0.2, 0.3 mg oral; 200, 500 μg/ vial injection ⊡ liothyronine

levothyroxine sodium & tiratricol *investigational (orphan) to suppress thyroid-stimulating hormone (TSH) in thyroid cancer*

Levovist ⒼⓂ powder for IV injection ℞ *ultrasound contrast medium for echocardiography* [galactose]

levoxadrol INN *local anesthetic; smooth muscle relaxant* [also: levoxadrol HCl]

levoxadrol HCl USAN *local anesthetic; smooth muscle relaxant* [also: levoxadrol]

Levoxyl tablets ℞ *thyroid hormone* [levothyroxine sodium] 25, 50, 75, 88, 100, 112, 125, 137, 150, 175, 200, 300 μg

Levsin tablets, drops, IV, subcu or IM injection, elixir ℞ *GI antispasmodic; anticholinergic* [hyoscyamine sulfate] 0.125 mg; 0.125 mg/mL; 0.5 mg/mL; 0.125 mg/5 mL

Levsin PB drops ℞ *GI antispasmodic; anticholinergic; sedative* [hyoscyamine sulfate; phenobarbital; alcohol 5%] 0.125•15 mg/mL

Levsin with Phenobarbital tablets ℞ *GI antispasmodic; anticholinergic; sedative* [hyoscyamine sulfate; phenobarbital] 0.125•15 mg

Levsinex Timecaps (timed-release capsules) ℞ *GI antispasmodic; anticholinergic* [hyoscyamine sulfate] 0.375 mg

Levsin-PB drops ℞ *GI antispasmodic; anticholinergic; sedative* [hyoscyamine sulfate; phenobarbital; alcohol 5%] 0.125•15 mg/mL

Levsin/SL sublingual tablets (also may be chewed or swallowed) ℞ *GI antispasmodic; anticholinergic* [hyoscyamine sulfate] 0.125 mg

Levulan ℞ *investigational (NDA filed) photosensitizer for photodynamic therapy of precancerous actinic keratoses of the face and scalp* [aminolevulinic acid HCl]

levulose BAN *nutrient; caloric replacement* [also: fructose]

LEX-032 *investigational (Phase II) serine protease inhibitor for treatment of reperfusion injury*

lexipafant USAN *platelet activating factor (PAF) antagonist; investigational (Phase III) treatment for acute pancreatitis*

lexithromycin USAN, INN *antibacterial*

lexofenac INN

Lexxel film-coated combination-release tablets ℞ *antihypertensive; angiotensin-converting enzyme (ACE) inhibitor; calcium channel blocker* [enalapril maleate (immediate release); felodipine (extended release)] 5•5, 5•2.5 mg

LHRF (luteinizing hormone-releasing factor) acetate hydrate [see: gonadorelin acetate]

LHRF diacetate tetrahydrate [now: gonadorelin acetate]

LHRF dihydrochloride [now: gonadorelin HCl]

LHRF HCl [see: gonadorelin HCl]

liarozole INN, BAN *antipsoriatic; aromatase inhibitor* [also: liarozole fumarate]

liarozole fumarate USAN *antipsoriatic; aromatase inhibitor* [also: liarozole]

liarozole HCl USAN *antineoplastic for prostate cancer; aromatase inhibitor*

Liatris scariosa; L. spicata; L. squarrosa *medicinal herb* [see: blazing star]

libecillide INN

libenzapril USAN, INN *angiotensin-converting enzyme (ACE) inhibitor*

Librax capsules ℞ *GI anticholinergic; anxiolytic* [clidinium bromide; chlordiazepoxide HCl] 2.5•5 mg

Libritabs film-coated tablets ℞ *benzodiazepine anxiolytic* [chlordiazepoxide] 10, 25 mg

Librium capsules, powder for injection ℞ *benzodiazepine anxiolytic; sometimes abused as a street drug* [chlordiazepoxide HCl] 5, 10, 25 mg; 100 mg

Lice-Enz foam shampoo OTC *pediculi-cide for lice* [pyrethrins; piperonyl butoxide] 0.3%•3%

Licoplex DS IM injection (discontinued 1995) ℞ *hematinic* [ferrous gluconate; multiple B vitamins; procaine HCl] 3 mg/mL• ± •2%

licorice (Glycyrrhiza glabra; G. pallidiflora; G. uralensis) root *medicinal herb for Addison's disease, blood cleansing, colds, cough, drug withdrawal, female disorders, hoarseness, hypoglycemia, lung disorders, sore throat, and stomach ulcers; also used as an expectorant and to increase energy*

licostinel USAN *investigational (Phase I) NMDA receptor antagonist for stroke*

licryfilcon A USAN *hydrophilic contact lens material*

licryfilcon B USAN *hydrophilic contact lens material*

Lid Wipes-SPF solution, pads OTC *eyelid cleansing wipes for blepharitis or contact lenses*

Lidakol cream ℞ *investigational (NDA filed) topical oral antiviral lipase inhibitor for herpes simplex* [n-docosanol] 10%

Lida-Mantle-HC cream ℞ *local anesthetic; topical corticosteroidal antiinflammatory* [lidocaine; hydrocortisone acetate] 3%•0.5%

lidamidine INN *antiperistaltic* [also: lidamidine HCl]

lidamidine HCl USAN *antiperistaltic* [also: lidamidine]

Lidex cream, gel, ointment, topical solution ℞ *topical corticosteroidal anti-inflammatory* [fluocinonide] 0.05% ⍰ Lasix; Lidox; Wydase

Lidex-E cream ℞ *topical corticosteroidal anti-inflammatory; emollient* [fluocinonide] 0.05%

lidimycin INN *antifungal* [also: lydimycin]

lidocaine USP, INN *topical local anesthetic; investigational (orphan) transdermal delivery for post-herpetic neuralgia* [also: lignocaine]

lidocaine benzyl benzoate [see: denatonium benzoate]

lidocaine HCl USP *local anesthetic; antiarrhythmic* [also: lignocaine HCl] 2%, 4%, 5% topical; 1%, 1.5%, 2% injection; 4%, 10%, 20% IV admixture

Lidoderm transdermal patch ℞ *topical anesthetic for post-herpetic neuralgia (orphan)* [lidocaine] 5%

lidofenin USAN, INN *hepatic function test*

lidofilcon A USAN *hydrophilic contact lens material*

lidofilcon B USAN *hydrophilic contact lens material*

lidoflazine USAN, INN, BAN *coronary vasodilator*

Lidoject-1; Lidoject-2 injection ℞ *injectable local anesthetic* [lidocaine HCl] 1%; 2%

LidoPen auto-injector (automatic IM injection device) ℞ *emergency injection for cardiac arrhythmias* [lidocaine HCl] 10%

Lidox capsules (discontinued 1995) ℞ *GI anticholinergic; anxiolytic* [clidinium bromide; chlordiazepoxide HCl] 2.5•5 mg ⍰ Lidex

lifarizine USAN, INN, BAN *platelet aggregation inhibitor*

life everlasting *medicinal herb* [see: everlasting]

life root (Senecio aureus; S. jacoboea; S. vulgaris) *medicinal herb for childbirth pain, diaphoresis, edema, fever, and stimulation of labor and menses; not generally regarded as safe and effective for ingestion because of hepatotoxicity*

life-of-man *medicinal herb* [see: spikenard]

lifibrate USAN, INN *antihyperlipoproteinemic*

lifibrol USAN, INN *antihyperlipidemic*

light mineral oil [see: mineral oil, light]

lignocaine BAN *topical local anesthetic* [also: lidocaine]

lignocaine HCl BAN *local anesthetic; antiarrhythmic* [also: lidocaine HCl]

lignosulfonic acid, sodium salt [see: polignate sodium]

lilopristone INN

lily, conval; May lily *medicinal herb* [see: lily of the valley]

lily, ground *medicinal herb* [see: birth-root]

lily, white pond; sweet water lily; sweet-scented pond lily; sweet-scented water lily; white water lily; toad lily *medicinal herb* [see: white pond lily]

lily of the valley *(Convallaria majalis)* flower, leaves, and rhizome *medicinal herb for arrhythmias, edema, epilepsy, and heart disorders*

limaprost INN

limarsol [see: acetarsone]

Limbitrol DS 10-25 tablets ℞ *antidepressant; anxiolytic* [chlordiazepoxide; amitriptyline HCl] 10•25 mg

lime USP *pharmaceutic necessity*

lime, sulfurated (calcium polysulfide, calcium thiosulfate) USP *wet dressing/soak for cystic acne and seborrhea*

lime tree *medicinal herb* [see: linden tree]

linarotene USAN, INN *antikeratinizing agent*

Lincocin capsules, IV or IM injection ℞ *lincosamide antibiotic* [lincomycin HCl] 500 mg; 300 mg/mL ⊞ Cleocin; Indocin

Lincocin pediatric capsules (discontinued 1998) ℞ *lincosamide antibiotic* [lincomycin HCl] 250 mg ⊞ Cleocin; Indocin

lincomycin USAN, INN, BAN *lincosamide antibiotic*

lincomycin HCl USP *lincosamide antibiotic* 300 mg/mL injection

Lincorex IV or IM injection ℞ *lincosamide antibiotic* [lincomycin HCl] 300 mg/mL

lincosamides *a class of antimicrobial antibiotics with potentially serious side effects, to which bacterial resistance has been shown*

lindane USAN, USP, INN, BAN *pediculicide for lice; scabicide* 1% topical

linden tree *(Tilia americana; T. cordata; T. europaea; T. platyphyllos)* flowers *medicinal herb for diaphoresis,*

diarrhea, headache, hypertension, indigestion, nasal congestion, nervousness, skin moisturizer, stomach disorders, and throat irritation

linezolid USAN *investigational (Phase II) antibiotic against gram-positive bacteria*

Linguets (trademarked form) *buccal tablets*

linogliride USAN, INN *antidiabetic*

linogliride fumarate USAN *antidiabetic*

linolexamide [see: clinolamide]

Linomide ℞ *investigational (Phase II) immunomodulator for HIV; investigational for bone marrow transplant for leukemia; clinical trials for MS discontinued 1997; orphan status withdrawn 1998* [roquinimex]

linopiridine USAN, INN *cognition enhancer for Alzheimer's disease*

linseed *medicinal herb* [see: flaxseed]

linsidomine INN

lint bells *medicinal herb* [see: flaxseed]

lintopride INN

Linum usitatissimum *medicinal herb* [see: flaxseed]

lion's ear; lion's tail *medicinal herb* [see: motherwort]

lion's tooth *medicinal herb* [see: dandelion]

Lioresal intrathecal injection ℞ *skeletal muscle relaxant for intractable spasticity due to spinal cord injury or disease (orphan); investigational (orphan) for trigeminal neuralgia* [baclofen] 10 mg/20 mL (500 μg/mL), 10 mg/5 mL (2000 μg/mL)

Lioresal tablets ℞ *skeletal muscle relaxant* [baclofen] 10, 20 mg

liothyronine INN, BAN *radioactive agent* [also: liothyronine I 125] ⊞ levothyroxine

liothyronine I 125 USAN *radioactive agent* [also: liothyronine]

liothyronine I 131 USAN *radioactive agent*

liothyronine sodium (T₃) USP, BAN *thyroid hormone; treatment of myxedema coma or precoma (orphan)* 25 μg oral

liotrix USAN, USP *thyroid hormone* ⊞ Klotrix

Lip Medex ointment OTC *topical anti-pruritic/counterirritant; mild local anesthetic* [camphor; phenol] 1%•0.54%

lipancreatin [see: pancrelipase]

lipase *digestive enzyme* [24 IU/mg in pancrelipase; 2 IU/mg in pancreatin]

lipase of pancreas [see: pancrelipase]

lipase triacylglycerol [see: pancrelipase]

Lipisorb powder OTC *enteral nutritional therapy* [lactose-free formula]

Lipitor film-coated tablets ℞ *HMG-CoA reductase inhibitor for hypercholesterolemia, dysbetalipoproteinemia, and hypertriglyceridemia* [atorvastatin calcium] 10, 20, 40 mg

Lipoflavonoid capsules OTC *dietary lipotropic with vitamin supplementation* [choline; inositol; multiple B vitamins; vitamin C; lemon bioflavonoids] 111.3•111.3•±•100•100 mg

Lipogen capsules, caplets OTC *dietary lipotropic with vitamin supplementation* [choline; inositol; multiple vitamins] 111•111•± mg

α-lipoic acid; lipoicin *natural antioxidant* [see: alpha lipoic acid]

Lipomul liquid OTC *dietary fat supplement* [corn oil] 10 g/15 mL

Lipo-Nicin/100 tablets (discontinued 1996) ℞ *peripheral vasodilator; antihyperlipidemic* [niacin; niacinamide; multiple vitamins] 100•75•± mg

Lipo-Nicin/300 timed-release capsules (discontinued 1996) ℞ *peripheral vasodilator; antihyperlipidemic* [niacin; multiple vitamins] 300•± mg

Liponol capsules OTC *dietary lipotropic with vitamin supplementation* [choline; inositol; methionine; multiple B vitamins] 115•83•110•± mg

lipoprotein OspA, recombinant *active immunizing agent against Lyme disease*

liposomal gentamicin [see: gentamicin liposome]

liposome-encapsulated doxorubicin HCl (LED) [see: doxorubicin HCl, liposome-encapsulated]

liposome-encapsulated recombinant interleukin-2 [see: interleukin-2, liposome-encapsulated recombinant]

liposome-encapsulated T4 endonuclease V [see: T4 endonuclease V, liposome encapsulated]

Liposyn II 10%; Liposyn III 10% IV infusion (discontinued 1996) ℞ *nutritional therapy* [fat emulsion]

Liposyn II 20%; Liposyn III 20% IV infusion ℞ *nutritional therapy* [fat emulsion]

Lipotriad caplets OTC *dietary lipotropic with vitamin supplementation* [choline; inositol; multiple vitamins] 111•?•± mg

lipotropics *a class of oral nutritional supplements*

Lipovite capsules (discontinued 1995) OTC *vitamin supplement* [multiple B vitamins] ±

Liquaemin Sodium IV or deep subcu injection (discontinued 1997) ℞ *anticoagulant* [heparin sodium] 1000, 5000, 10 000, 20 000, 40 000 U/mL

liquefied phenol [see: phenol, liquefied]

Liquibid; Liquibid-1200 sustained-release tablet ℞ *expectorant* [guaifenesin] 600 mg; 1200 mg

Liquibid-D sustained-release tablets ℞ *decongestant; expectorant* [phenylephrine HCl; guaifenesin] 40•600 mg

Liqui-Char oral liquid OTC *adsorbent antidote for poisoning* [activated charcoal] 12.5 g/60 mL, 15 g/75 mL, 25 g/120 mL, 30 g/120 mL, 50 g/240 mL

Liqui-Coat HD concentrated oral suspension ℞ *radiopaque contrast medium for gastrointestinal imaging* [barium sulfate] 210%

Liquid Caps (dosage form) *soft liquid-filled capsules*

liquid glucose [see: glucose, liquid]

Liquid Lather body wash (discontinued 1995) OTC *bath emollient*

liquid petrolatum [see: mineral oil]

Liquid Pred syrup ℞ *corticosteroid; anti-inflammatory* [prednisone; alcohol 5%] 5 mg/5 mL

Liquid Tabs (dosage form) *liquid-filled tablets*

Liquidambar orientalis; L. styraciflua *medicinal herb* [see: storax]

Liqui-Doss emulsion OTC *emollient laxative* [mineral oil]

Liquifilm Tears; Liquifilm Forte eye drops OTC *ophthalmic moisturizer/lubricant* [polyvinyl alcohol] 1.4%; 3%

Liquifilm Wetting solution OTC *wetting solution for hard contact lenses*

Liqui-Gels (trademarked dosage form) *soft liquid-filled gelatin capsules*

Liqui-Histine DM syrup ℞ *antitussive; decongestant; antihistamine* [dextromethorphan hydrobromide; phenylpropanolamine HCl; brompheniramine maleate] 10•12.5•2 mg/5 mL

Liqui-Histine-D elixir ℞ *decongestant; antihistamine* [phenylpropanolamine HCl; phenyltoloxamine citrate; pyrilamine maleate; pheniramine maleate] 12.5•4•4•4 mg/5 mL

Liquimat lotion OTC *antibacterial and exfoliant for acne* [sulfur] 4%

Liquipake oral/rectal suspension (discontinued 1999) ℞ *radiopaque contrast medium for gastrointestinal imaging* [barium sulfate] 100%

Liquiprin elixir (discontinued 1997) OTC *analgesic; antipyretic* [acetaminophen] 160 mg/5 mL

Liquiprin Drops for Children OTC *analgesic; antipyretic* [acetaminophen] 80 mg/1.66 mL

Liquitab (trademarked dosage form) *chewable tablet*

LiquiVent ℞ *investigational (Phase III) blood substitute; investigational (Phase III) treatment for pediatric acute respiratory distress syndrome (ARDS); investigational (Phase II) agent for adults with acute lung injury or ARDS* [perflubron]

liquor carbonis detergens (LCD) [see: coal tar]

liroldine INN

lisadimate USAN, INN *sunscreen*

lisinopril USAN, INN, BAN *antihypertensive; angiotensin-converting enzyme (ACE) inhibitor*

lisofylline (LSF) USAN *acetyltransferase inhibitor; investigational (Phase III) immunomodulator and cytokine inhibi-*
tor for RBC replenishment following bone marrow transplants; investigational agent for prevention of GI tract damage during chemotherapy; investigational (Phase II/III) for ARDS

Listerex Scrub lotion (discontinued 1995) OTC *topical keratolytic for acne* [salicylic acid] 2%

Listerine; Cool-Mint Listerine; FreshBurst Listerine mouthwash/gargle OTC *topical oral antiseptic; analgesic* [thymol; eucalyptol; methyl salicylate; menthol; alcohol 22%–26%] 0.06%•0.09%•0.06%•0.04%

Listermint Arctic Mint mouthwash/gargle OTC

Listermint with Fluoride oral rinse (discontinued 1995) OTC *topical dental caries preventative* [sodium fluoride] 0.02%

lisuride INN [also: lysuride]

Lithane ⓒ (U.S. product: Eskalith) capsules ℞ *antipsychotic for manic episodes* [lithium carbonate] 150, 300 mg

lithium *element (Li)*

lithium benzoate NF

lithium carbonate USAN, USP *antimanic; immunity booster in chemotherapy and AIDS* 150, 300, 600 mg oral

lithium citrate USP *antimanic; immunity booster in chemotherapy and AIDS* 300 mg/5 mL oral

lithium hydroxide USP *antimanic*

lithium hydroxide monohydrate [see: lithium hydroxide]

lithium salicylate NF

Lithobid slow-release tablets ℞ *antipsychotic for manic episodes* [lithium carbonate] 300 mg

litholytics *a class of agents that dissolve stones or calculi* [see also: antilithics]

Lithonate capsules ℞ *antipsychotic for manic episodes* [lithium carbonate] 300 mg

Lithostat tablets ℞ *adjunctive therapy in chronic urea-splitting urinary tract infections* [acetohydroxamic acid] 250 mg

Lithotabs film-coated tablets ℞ *antipsychotic for manic episodes* [lithium carbonate] 300 mg

litracen INN
liver, desiccated; liver extracts *source of vitamin B$_{12}$*
Liver Combo No. 5 IM injection ℞ *antianemic; vitamin supplement* [liver extracts; vitamin B$_{12}$; folic acid] 10 µg•100 µg•0.4 mg per mL
liver derivative complex *claimed to be an anti-inflammatory for various dermatological conditions*
liver lily *medicinal herb* [see: blue flag]
liverleaf; liverwort *medicinal herb* [see: hepatica]
lividomycin INN
Livitamin capsules (discontinued 1995) OTC *hematinic* [ferrous fumarate; liver, desiccated; multiple vitamins] 33•150• ± mg
Livitamin chewable tablets (discontinued 1995) OTC *hematinic* [ferrous fumarate; multiple B vitamins; vitamin C] 16.4• ± •100 mg
Livitamin liquid (discontinued 1995) OTC *hematinic* [peptonized iron; liver fraction 1; multiple B vitamins] 35.5•500• ± mg/15 mL
Livitamin with Intrinsic Factor capsules (discontinued 1995) ℞ *hematinic* [ferrous fumarate; multiple B vitamins; ascorbic acid; liver, desiccated; intrinsic factor concentrate] 33 mg• ± •100 mg•150 mg•0.33 U
Livitrinsic-f capsules ℞ *hematinic* [ferrous fumarate; cyanocobalamin; ascorbic acid; intrinsic factor concentrate; folic acid] 110 mg•15 µg• 75 mg•240 mg•0.5 mg
Livostin eye drop suspension ℞ *topical antihistamine for allergic conjunctivitis* [levocabastine HCl] 0.05%
Livostin ⓒ nasal spray ℞ *antihistamine for seasonal allergic rhinitis* [levocabastine HCl] 0.05%
lixazinone sulfate USAN *cardiotonic; phosphodiesterase inhibitor*
LJP-394 *investigational (Phase II/III) immunosuppressant for lupus*
LKV Infant Drops powder + liquid OTC *vitamin supplement* [multiple vitamins; biotin] ± •75 µg/0.6 mL

LLD factor [see: cyanocobalamin]
10% LMD IV injection ℞ *plasma volume expander for shock due to hemorrhage, burns, or surgery* [dextran 40] 10%
LMD (low molecular weight dextran) [see: dextran 40]
LMF (Leukeran, methotrexate, fluorouracil) *chemotherapy protocol*
LMWD (low molecular weight dextran) [see: dextran 40]
Lobac capsules ℞ *skeletal muscle relaxant; analgesic* [salicylamide; phenyltoloxamine; acetaminophen] 200• 20•300 mg
Lobana Body lotion OTC *moisturizer; emollient*
Lobana Body Shampoo; Lobana Liquid Lather liquid OTC *soap-free therapeutic skin cleanser* [chloroxylenol]
Lobana Derm-Ade cream OTC *moisturizer; emollient* [vitamins A, D, and E]
Lobana Peri-Garde ointment OTC *moisturizer; emollient; antiseptic* [vitamins A, D, and E; chloroxylenol]
lobelia (*Lobelia inflata*) plant (tincture) *medicinal herb for arthritis, asthma, bronchitis, hay fever, colds, cough, ear infections, epilepsy, fever, food poisoning, lockjaw, nervousness, pain, pneumonia, preventing miscarriage, whooping cough, and worms*
lobeline INN *nicotine withdrawal aid* [also: lobeline HCl]
lobeline HCl JAN *nicotine withdrawal aid* [also: lobeline]
lobeline sulfate *investigational (Phase III) nicotine withdrawal aid; clinical trials discontinued 1997*
lobendazole USAN, INN *veterinary anthelmintic*
lobenzarit INN *antirheumatic* [also: lobenzarit sodium]
lobenzarit sodium USAN *antirheumatic* [also: lobenzarit]
lobucavir USAN, INN *antiviral; investigational (Phase III) for AIDS-related asymptomatic cytomegalovirus (clinical trials discontinued 1999)*
lobuprofen INN

LoCholest; LoCholest Light powder for oral suspension ℞ *cholesterol-lowering antihyperlipidemic; also used for biliary obstruction* [cholestyramine resin] 4 g/dose

locicortolone dicibate INN

locicortone [see: locicortolone dicibate]

Locoid cream, ointment, solution ℞ *topical corticosteroidal anti-inflammatory* [hydrocortisone butyrate] 0.1%

locust plant *medicinal herb* [see: senna]

lodaxaprine INN

lodazecar INN

lodelaben USAN, INN *antiarthritic; emphysema therapy adjunct*

lodenosine USAN *investigational reverse transcriptase antiviral for HIV*

Lodine film-coated tablets, capsules ℞ *nonsteroidal anti-inflammatory drug (NSAID); analgesic; antiarthritic* [etodolac] 200, 300, 400, 500 mg

Lodine XL extended-release film-coated tablets ℞ *once-daily nonsteroidal anti-inflammatory drug (NSAID); analgesic; antiarthritic* [etodolac] 400, 500, 600 mg

lodinixil INN

lodiperone INN

Lodosyn tablets ℞ *decarboxylase inhibitor; antiparkinsonian adjunct (used with levodopa; no effect when given alone)* [carbidopa] 25 mg

lodoxamide INN, BAN *antiallergic; antiasthmatic* [also: lodoxamide ethyl]

lodoxamide ethyl USAN *antiallergic; antiasthmatic* [also: lodoxamide]

lodoxamide trometamol BAN *antiallergic; antiasthmatic* [also: lodoxamide tromethamine]

lodoxamide tromethamine USAN *antiasthmatic; antiallergic for vernal keratoconjunctivitis (orphan)* [also: lodoxamide trometamol]

Lodrane LD sustained-release capsules ℞ *decongestant; antihistamine* [pseudoephedrine HCl; brompheniramine maleate] 60•6 mg

Loestrin 21 1/20; Loestrin 21 1.5/30 tablets ℞ *monophasic oral contraceptive* [norethindrone acetate; ethinyl estradiol] 1 mg•20 μg; 1.5 mg•30 μg

Loestrin Fe 1/20; Loestrin Fe 1.5/30 tablets ℞ *monophasic oral contraceptive; iron supplement* [norethindrone acetate; ethinyl estradiol; ferrous fumarate] 1 mg•20 μg•75 mg; 1.5 mg•30 μg•75 mg

lofemizole INN *anti-inflammatory; analgesic; antipyretic* [also: lofemizole HCl]

lofemizole HCl USAN *anti-inflammatory; analgesic; antipyretic* [also: lofemizole]

Lofenalac powder OTC *special diet for infants with phenylketonuria*

lofendazam INN, BAN

lofentanil INN, BAN *narcotic analgesic* [also: lofentanil oxalate]

lofentanil oxalate USAN *narcotic analgesic* [also: lofentanil]

lofepramine INN, BAN *antidepressant* [also: lofepramine HCl]

lofepramine HCl USAN *antidepressant* [also: lofepramine]

lofexidine INN, BAN *antihypertensive* [also: lofexidine HCl]

lofexidine HCl USAN *antihypertensive* [also: lofexidine]

loflucarban INN

LoFrin ℞ *5-lipoxygenase inhibitor* [fenleuton]

Logen tablets ℞ *antidiarrheal* [diphenoxylate HCl; atropine sulfate] 2.5•0.025 mg

LOMAC (leucovorin, Oncovin, methotrexate, Adriamycin, cyclophosphamide) *chemotherapy protocol*

Lomanate liquid ℞ *antidiarrheal* [diphenoxylate HCl; atropine sulfate] 2.5•0.025 mg/5 mL

lombazole INN, BAN

lomefloxacin USAN, INN, BAN *antibacterial*

lomefloxacin HCl USAN *broad-spectrum fluoroquinolone antibiotic*

lomefloxacin mesylate USAN *antibacterial*

lometraline INN *antipsychotic; antiparkinsonian* [also: lometraline HCl]

lometraline HCl USAN *antipsychotic; antiparkinsonian* [also: lometraline]

lometrexol INN *antineoplastic* [also: lometrexol sodium]

lometrexol sodium USAN *antineoplastic* [also: lometrexol]

lomevactone INN

lomifylline INN

lomofungin USAN *antifungal*

Lomotil tablets, liquid ℞ *antidiarrheal* [diphenoxylate HCl; atropine sulfate] 2.5•0.025 mg; 2.5•0.025 mg/5 mL

lomustine USAN, INN, BAN *nitrosourea-type alkylating antineoplastic for brain tumors and Hodgkin's disease*

Lonalac powder OTC *enteral nutritional therapy* [milk-based formula]

lonapalene USAN *antipsoriatic*

lonaprofen INN

lonazolac INN

lonidamine INN

Loniten tablets ℞ *antihypertensive; vasodilator* [minoxidil] 2.5, 10 mg ⊞ clonidine

Lonox tablets ℞ *antidiarrheal* [diphenoxylate HCl; atropine sulfate] 2.5•0.025 mg ⊞ Lovenox

loop diuretics *a class of diuretic agents that inhibit the reabsorption of sodium and chloride*

Lo/Ovral tablets ℞ *monophasic oral contraceptive; emergency "morning after" contraceptive* [norgestrel; ethinyl estradiol] 0.3 mg•30 μg

loperamide INN, BAN *antiperistaltic; antidiarrheal* [also: loperamide HCl]

loperamide HCl USAN, USP, JAN *antiperistaltic; antidiarrheal* [also: loperamide] 2 mg oral; 1 mg/5 mL oral

loperamide oxide INN, BAN *antiperistaltic; antidiarrheal*

Lophophora williamsii a *flowering Mexican cactus whose heads (mescal buttons) are used to produce mescaline, a hallucinogenic street drug*

Lopid film-coated tablets ℞ *antihyperlipidemic for hypertriglyceridemia and coronary heart disease* [gemfibrozil] 600 mg (300 mg capsules available in Canada)

lopinavir USAN *investigational (Phase II) antiviral protease inhibitor for HIV*

lopirazepam INN

loprazolam INN, BAN

lopremone [now: protirelin]

Lopressor tablets, IV injection ℞ *antianginal; antihypertensive; β-blocker* [metoprolol tartrate] 50, 100 mg; 1 mg/mL

Lopressor HCT 50/25; Lopressor HCT 100/25; Lopressor HCT 100/50 tablets ℞ *antihypertensive; β-blocker; diuretic* [metoprolol tartrate; hydrochlorothiazide] 50•25 mg; 100•25 mg; 100•50 mg

loprodiol INN

Loprox cream, lotion ℞ *topical antifungal* [ciclopirox olamine] 1%

Lorabid Pulvules (capsules), powder for oral suspension ℞ *carbacephem antibiotic* [loracarbef] 200, 400 mg; 100, 200 mg/5 mL

loracarbef USAN, INN *carbacephem antibiotic*

lorajmine INN *antiarrhythmic* [also: lorajmine HCl]

lorajmine HCl USAN *antiarrhythmic* [also: lorajmine]

lorapride INN

loratadine USAN, INN, BAN *second-generation piperidine antihistamine*

lorazepam USAN, USP, INN, BAN *benzodiazepine anxiolytic; minor tranquilizer* 0.5, 1, 2 mg oral; 2 mg/mL oral; 2, 4 mg/mL injection

lorbamate USAN, INN *muscle relaxant*

lorcainide INN, BAN *antiarrhythmic* [also: lorcainide HCl]

lorcainide HCl USAN *antiarrhythmic* [also: lorcainide]

Lorcet tablets (discontinued 1997) ℞ *narcotic analgesic* [hydrocodone bitartrate; acetaminophen] 5•500 mg

Lorcet Plus; Lorcet 10/650 tablets ℞ *narcotic analgesic* [hydrocodone bitartrate; acetaminophen] 7.5•650 mg; 10•650 mg

Lorcet-HD capsules ℞ *narcotic analgesic* [hydrocodone bitartrate; acetaminophen] 5•500 mg ⊞ Fioricet

lorcinadol USAN, INN, BAN *analgesic*

loreclezole USAN, INN, BAN *antiepileptic*

Lorelco tablets (discontinued 1996) ℞ *antihyperlipidemic to reduce serum cholesterol* [probucol] 250, 500 mg

Lorenzo's oil (erucic acid and oleic acid) *natural treatment for childhood adrenoleukodystrophy and adrenomyeloneuropathy in adults*

lorglumide INN

lormetazepam USAN, INN, BAN *sedative; hypnotic*

lornoxicam USAN, INN, BAN *analgesic; anti-inflammatory*

Lorothidol (available only from the Centers for Disease Control) ℞ *investigational anti-infective for paragonimiasis and fascioliasis* [bithionol]

Loroxide lotion OTC *topical keratolytic for acne* [benzoyl peroxide] 5.5%

lorpiprazole INN

Lortab elixir ℞ *narcotic analgesic* [hydrocodone bitartrate; acetaminophen] 2.5•167 mg/5 mL

Lortab 2.5/500; Lortab 5/500; Lortab 7.5/500; Lortab 10/500 tablets ℞ *narcotic analgesic* [hydrocodone bitartrate; acetaminophen] 2.5•500 mg; 5•500 mg; 7.5•500 mg; 10•500 mg

Lortab ASA tablets ℞ *narcotic analgesic* [hydrocodone bitartrate; aspirin] 5•500 mg

lortalamine USAN, INN *antidepressant*

lorzafone USAN, INN *minor tranquilizer*

losartan INN *antihypertensive; angiotensin II receptor antagonist* [also: losartan potassium]

losartan potassium USAN *antihypertensive; angiotensin II receptor antagonist* [also: losartan]

Losec ⓒᴬᴺ (U.S. product: Prilosec) delayed-release tablets ℞ *proton pump inhibitor for gastric and duodenal ulcers and other gastroesophageal disorders* [omeprazole] 10, 20 mg

losigamone INN

losindole INN

losmiprofen INN

losoxantrone INN *antineoplastic* [also: losoxantrone HCl]

losoxantrone HCl USAN *antineoplastic* [also: losoxantrone]

losulazine INN *antihypertensive* [also: losulazine HCl]

losulazine HCl USAN *antihypertensive* [also: losulazine]

Lotemax eye drop suspension ℞ *corticosteroidal anti-inflammatory* [loteprednol etabonate] 0.5%

Lotensin tablets ℞ *antihypertensive; angiotensin-converting enzyme (ACE) inhibitor* [benazepril HCl] 5, 10, 20, 40 mg

Lotensin HCT 5/6.25; Lotensin HCT 10/12.5; Lotensin HCT 20/12.5; Lotensin HCT 20/25 tablets ℞ *antihypertensive; angiotensin-converting enzyme (ACE) inhibitor; diuretic* [benazepril HCl; hydrochlorothiazide] 5•6.25 mg; 10•12.5 mg; 20•12.5 mg; 20•25 mg

loteprednol INN *corticosteroidal anti-inflammatory* [also: loteprednol etabonate]

loteprednol etabonate USAN *ophthalmic corticosteroidal anti-inflammatory* [also: loteprednol]

lotifazole INN

lotrafiban HCl USAN *platelet aggregation inhibitor; GP IIb/IIIa receptor antagonist*

Lotrel capsules ℞ *antihypertensive; angiotensin-converting enzyme (ACE) inhibitor; calcium channel blocker* [amlodipine besylate; benazepril HCl] 2.5•10, 5•10, 5•20 mg

lotrifen INN

Lotrimin cream, solution, lotion ℞ *topical antifungal* [clotrimazole] 1% ⑦ Otrivin

Lotrimin AF cream, solution, lotion OTC *topical antifungal* [clotrimazole] 1%

Lotrimin AF powder, spray powder, spray liquid OTC *topical antifungal* [miconazole nitrate] 2%

Lotrisone cream ℞ *topical corticosteroidal anti-inflammatory; antifungal*

[betamethasone dipropionate; clotrimazole] 0.05%•1%

lotucaine INN

lousewort *medicinal herb* [see: betony; feverweed]

lovage *(Angelica levisticum; Levisticum officinale)* leaves and roots *medicinal herb for bad breath, boils, edema, flatulence, and sore throat; also used topically as a skin emollient*

lovastatin USAN, INN, BAN HMG-CoA *reductase inhibitor for hypercholesterolemia and atherosclerosis*

Lovenox deep subcu injection in prefilled syringes ℞ *anticoagulant/antithrombotic for prevention of deep vein thrombosis (DVT) following knee, hip, or abdominal surgery, unstable angina, and myocardial infarction* [enoxaparin sodium] 30 mg/0.3 mL, 40 mg/0.4 mL, 60 mg/0.6 mL, 80 mg/0.8 mL, 100 mg/mL ⓥ Lonox

loviride USAN, INN *investigational nonnucleoside reverse transcriptase inhibitor (NNRTI) antiviral for HIV*

low molecular weight dextran (LMD; LMWD) [see: dextran 40]

low molecular weight heparins *a class of anticoagulants used for the prophylaxis or treatment of thromboembolic complications of surgery and ischemic complications of unstable angina or myocardial infarction*

low osmolar contrast media (LOCM) *a class of newer radiopaque agents that have a low osmolar concentration of iodine (the contrast agent), which corresponds to a lower incidence of adverse reactions* [also called: nonionic contrast media]

Lowila Cake bar OTC *soap-free therapeutic skin cleanser*

Lowsium Plus oral suspension OTC *antacid; antiflatulent* [magaldrate; simethicone] 540•40 mg/5 mL

loxanast INN

Loxapac ⓐ (U.S. product: Loxitane) capsules ℞ *conventional (typical) antipsychotic* [loxapine] 5, 10, 25, 50 mg

Loxapac ⓐ (U.S. product: Loxitane) oral concentrate, IM injection ℞ *conventional (typical) antipsychotic* [loxapine HCl] 25 mg/mL; 50 mg/mL

loxapine USAN, INN, BAN *minor tranquilizer; dibenzoxazepine antipsychotic*

loxapine HCl *minor tranquilizer; dibenzoxazepine antipsychotic*

loxapine succinate USAN *minor tranquilizer; dibenzoxazepine antipsychotic* 5, 10, 25, 50 mg oral

loxiglumide INN

Loxitane capsules ℞ *conventional (typical) antipsychotic* [loxapine succinate] 5, 10, 25, 50 mg ⓥ doxepin

Loxitane C oral concentrate ℞ *conventional (typical) antipsychotic* [loxapine HCl] 25 mg/mL

Loxitane IM injection ℞ *conventional (typical) antipsychotic* [loxapine HCl] 50 mg/mL

loxoprofen INN

loxoribine USAN, INN *immunostimulant; vaccine adjuvant; orphan status withdrawn 1996*

loxotidine [now: lavoltidine succinate]

loxtidine BAN *antiulcerative; histamine H2-receptor blocker* [also: lavoltidine succinate; lavoltidine]

lozilurea INN

Lozi-Tabs (trademarked form) *lozenges*

Lozol film-coated tablets ℞ *antihypertensive; diuretic* [indapamide] 1.25, 2.5 mg

LP-2307 *investigational (Phase I/II) melanoma vaccine*

L-PAM (L-phenylalanine mustard) [see: melphalan]

LR (lactated Ringer's) solution [see: Ringer's injection, lactated]

LSD (lysergic acid diethylamide) *hallucinogenic street drug associated with disorders of sensory and temporal perception, depersonalization, and ataxia* [medically known as lysergide]

LSF (lisofylline) [q.v.]

LTRAs (leukotriene receptor antagonists) *a class of antiasthmatics*

lubeluzole USAN, INN *investigational neural protective for ischemic stroke*

LubraSol Bath Oil OTC *bath emollient*

Lubricating Gel (name changed to WHF Lubricating Gel in 1998)

Lubricating Jelly OTC *vaginal lubricant* [glycerin; propylene glycol]

Lubriderm cream, lotion OTC *moisturizer; emollient*

Lubriderm Bath Oil OTC *bath emollient*

Lubrin vaginal inserts OTC *lubricant for sexual intercourse* [glycerin; caprylic triglyceride]

LubriTears eye drops OTC *ophthalmic moisturizer/lubricant* [hydroxypropyl methylcellulose] 0.3%

LubriTears ophthalmic ointment OTC *ocular moisturizer/lubricant* [white petrolatum; mineral oil; lanolin]

lucanthone INN, BAN *antischistosomal* [also: lucanthone HCl]

lucanthone HCl USAN, USP *antischistosomal* [also: lucanthone]

lucartamide INN

lucensomycin [see: lucimycin]

Lucilia caesar natural treatment [see: maggots]

lucimycin INN

Ludiomil coated tablets ℞ *tetracyclic antidepressant* [maprotiline HCl] 25, 50, 75 mg

lufironil USAN, INN *collagen inhibitor*

lufuradom INN

Lufyllin tablets, elixir, IM injection ℞ *antiasthmatic; bronchodilator* [dyphylline] 200 mg; 100 mg/15 mL; 250 mg/mL

Lufyllin 400 tablets ℞ *antiasthmatic; bronchodilator* [dyphylline] 400 mg

Lufyllin-EPG tablets, elixir ℞ *antiasthmatic; bronchodilator; decongestant; expectorant; sedative* [dyphylline; ephedrine HCl; guaifenesin; phenobarbital] 100•16•200•16 mg; 150•24•300•24 mg/15 mL

Lufyllin-GG tablets, elixir ℞ *antiasthmatic; bronchodilator; expectorant* [dyphylline; guaifenesin] 200•200 mg; 100•100 mg/15 mL

Lugol solution ℞ *thyroid-blocking therapy; topical antimicrobial* [iodine; potassium iodide] 5%•10%

Luminal Sodium IV or IM injection ℞ *long-acting barbiturate sedative, hypnotic, and anticonvulsant; also abused as a street drug* [phenobarbital sodium] 130 mg/mL ② Tuinal

lung surfactant, synthetic [see: colfosceril palmitate]

lungwort *(Pulmonaria officinalis)* flowering plant *medicinal herb used as an astringent, demulcent, emollient, expectorant, and pectoral*

2,6-lupetidine [see: nanofin]

lupitidine INN *veterinary antagonist to histamine H_2 receptors* [also: lupitidine HCl]

lupitidine HCl USAN *veterinary antagonist to histamine H_2 receptors* [also: lupitidine]

Lupron; Lupron Pediatric subcu injection (daily) ℞ *hormonal antineoplastic for prostatic cancer and central precocious puberty (orphan)* [leuprolide acetate] 5 mg/mL ② Mepron; Napron

Lupron Depot microspheres for IM injection (monthly) ℞ *hormonal antineoplastic for prostatic cancer, endometriosis, and uterine fibroids* [leuprolide acetate] 3.75, 7.5 mg ② Mepron; Napron

Lupron Depot–3 month; Lupron Depot–4 month microspheres for IM injection ℞ *hormonal antineoplastic for prostatic cancer* [leuprolide acetate] 11.5, 22.5 mg; 30 mg ② Mepron; Napron

Lupron Depot-Ped microspheres for IM injection (monthly) ℞ *hormonal antineoplastic for central precocious puberty (orphan)* [leuprolide acetate] 7.5, 11.25, 15 mg ② Mepron; Napron

luprostiol INN, BAN

Luride Lozi-Tabs (chewable tablets), drops, gel ℞ *dental caries preventative* [sodium fluoride] 0.25, 1.1, 2.2 mg; 1.1 mg/mL; 1.2%

Luride SF Lozi-Tabs (lozenges) ℞ *topical dental caries preventative* [sodium fluoride] 2.2 mg

Lurline PMS tablets OTC *analgesic; antipyretic; diuretic; vitamin* [acetaminophen; pamabrom; pyridoxine] 500•25•50 mg

lurosetron mesylate USAN *antiemetic*

lurtotecan dihydrochloride USAN *antineoplastic; topoisomerase I inhibitor*

Lustra cream ℞ *hyperpigmentation bleaching agent* [hydroquinone (in a base containing glycolic acid and vitamins C and E)] 4%

luteinizing hormone-releasing factor acetate hydrate [see: gonadorelin acetate]

luteinizing hormone-releasing factor diacetate tetrahydrate [now: gonadorelin acetate]

luteinizing hormone-releasing factor dihydrochloride [now: gonadorelin HCl]

luteinizing hormone-releasing factor HCl [see: gonadorelin HCl]

lutetium *element (Lu)*

lutetium texaphyrin *investigational for the photodynamic treatment of cancer; investigational photosensitizer for ophthalmology indications including age-related macular degeneration*

Lu-Tex ℞ *investigational for the photodynamic treatment of cancer; investigational photosensitizer for ophthalmology indications including age-related macular degeneration* [lutetium texaphyrin]

lutrelin INN *luteinizing hormone-releasing hormone (LHRH) agonist* [also: lutrelin acetate]

lutrelin acetate USAN *luteinizing hormone-releasing hormone (LHRH) agonist* [also: lutrelin]

Lutrepulse powder for continuous ambulatory infusion ℞ *gonadotropin-releasing hormone for hypothalamic amenorrhea (orphan)* [gonadorelin acetate] 0.8, 3.2 mg

Luvox film-coated tablets ℞ *selective serotonin reuptake inhibitor (SSRI) for obsessive-compulsive disorder (OCD); investigational (Phase III) for depression and panic disorder* [fluvoxamine maleate] 25, 50, 100 mg

luxabendazole INN, BAN

Luxiq foam ℞ *topical corticosteroidal anti-inflammatory for scalp dermatoses* [betamethasone valerate] 0.12%

L-VAM (leuprolide acetate, vinblastine, Adriamycin, mitomycin) *chemotherapy protocol*

LY-315535 *investigational (Phase I) for functional bowel disorders*

lyapolate sodium USAN *anticoagulant* [also: sodium apolate]

lycetamine USAN *topical antimicrobial*

lycine HCl [see: betaine HCl]

lycopene *natural substance found in high concentration in ripe tomatoes; a member of the carotene family; used as an antineoplastic and antioxidant*

Lycopodium clavatum *medicinal herb* [see: club moss]

Lycopus virginicus *medicinal herb* [see: bugleweed]

lydimycin USAN *antifungal* [also: lidimycin]

Lyme borreliosis vaccine [see: lipoprotein OspA, recombinant]

lymecycline INN, BAN

LYMErix IM injection ℞ *active immunizing agent against Lyme disease* [lipoprotein OspA, recombinant] 30 μg/0.5 mL

Lymphazurin 1% subcu injection ℞ *radiopaque contrast medium for lymphography* [isosulfan blue] 10 mg/mL (1%)

LymphoCide ℞ *investigational (orphan) for non-Hodgkin's lymphoma* [monoclonal antibody CD22 antigen on B-cells, radiolabeled]

lymphocyte immune globulin, antithymocyte *passive immunizing agent; investigational (orphan) to prevent allograft rejection in organ and bone marrow transplants*

lymphogranuloma venereum antigen USP

lymphoma antibody, humanized *investigational*

LymphoScan ℞ *investigational (Phase III, orphan) for diagnostic aid for non-Hodgkin's B-cell lymphoma, AIDS-related lymphomas, and other acute* *and chronic B-cell leukemias* [technetium Tc 99m bectumomab]

lynestrenol USAN, INN *progestin* [also: lynoestrenol]

lynoestrenol BAN *progestin* [also: lynestrenol]

Lyo-Ject (trademarked delivery system) *prefilled dual-chambered syringe with lyophilized powder and diluent*

Lyphocin powder for IV or IM injection (discontinued 1998) ℞ *tricyclic glycopeptide antibiotic* [vancomycin HCl] 0.5, 1, 5 g

Lypholized Vitamin B Complex & Vitamin C with B$_{12}$ injection ℞ *parenteral vitamin therapy* [multiple B vitamins; vitamin C] ± •50 mg/mL

Lypholyte; Lypholyte II IV admixture ℞ *intravenous electrolyte therapy* [combined electrolyte solution]

lypressin USAN, USP, INN, BAN *posterior pituitary hormone; antidiuretic; vasoconstrictor*

lysergic acid diethylamide (LSD) *street drug* [see: LSD; lysergide]

lysergide INN, BAN, DCF

lysine (L-lysine) USAN, INN *essential amino acid; symbols: Lys, K; natural*

remedy for the prophylaxis and treatment of recurrent oral and genital herpes simplex outbreaks; inhibits HSV replication 312, 500, 1000 mg oral

lysine acetate USP *amino acid*

DL-lysine acetylsalicylate [see: aspirin DL-lysine]

lysine HCl USAN, USP *amino acid*

L-lysine monoacetate [see: lysine acetate]

L-lysine monohydrochloride [see: lysine HCl]

8-L-lysine vasopressin [see: lypressin]

Lysodase ℞ *investigational (orphan) chronic enzyme replacement therapy for Gaucher's disease* [PEG-glucocerebrosidase]

Lysodren tablets ℞ *antibiotic antineoplastic for inoperable adrenal cortical carcinoma and Cushing syndrome* [mitotane] 500 mg

lysostaphin USAN *antibacterial enzyme; investigational agent for methicillin-resistant Staphylococcus aureus (MRSA) endocarditis*

LysPro [see: Humalog]

lysuride BAN [also: lisuride]

M

M-CSF (macrophage colony-stimulating factor) [now: cilmostim]

M-2 protocol (vincristine, carmustine, cyclophosphamide, melphalan, prednisone) *chemotherapy protocol*

MAA (macroaggregated albumin) [see: albumin, aggregated]

Maalox chewable tablets, oral suspension OTC *antacid* [aluminum hydroxide; magnesium hydroxide] 200•200, 350•350 mg; 225•200 mg/5 mL ⑬ Marax

Maalox, Extra Strength oral suspension OTC *antacid; antiflatulent* [aluminum hydroxide; magnesium

hydroxide; simethicone] 500•450•40 mg/5 mL

Maalox Antacid caplets OTC *antacid* [calcium carbonate] 1 g

Maalox Anti-Diarrheal caplets OTC *antidiarrheal* [loperamide HCl] 2 mg

Maalox Anti-Gas chewable tablets OTC *antiflatulent* [simethicone] 80 mg

Maalox Daily Fiber Therapy powder OTC *bulk laxative* [psyllium hydrophilic mucilloid] 3.4 g/dose

Maalox H2 Acid Controller ⓐ (U.S. product: Pepcid AC) film-coated tablets OTC *histamine H$_2$ antagonist for heartburn and acid indigestion* [famotidine] 10 mg

Maalox HRF (Heartburn Relief Formula) liquid OTC *antacid* [aluminum hydroxide; magnesium carbonate] 140•175 mg/5 mL

Maalox Plus chewable tablets, oral suspension OTC *antacid; antiflatulent* [aluminum hydroxide; magnesium hydroxide; simethicone] 200•200•25 mg; 500•450•40 mg/5 mL

Maalox Therapeutic Concentrate oral suspension OTC *antacid* [aluminum hydroxide; magnesium hydroxide] 600•300 mg/5 mL

MAb; MAB (monoclonal antibody)

MABOP (Mustargen, Adriamycin, bleomycin, Oncovin, prednisone) *chemotherapy protocol*

MabThera (European name for U.S. product Rituxan)

mabuterol INN

MAC (methotrexate, actinomycin D, chlorambucil) *chemotherapy protocol*

MAC; MAC III (methotrexate, actinomycin D, cyclophosphamide) *chemotherapy protocol*

MAC (mitomycin, Adriamycin, cyclophosphamide) *chemotherapy protocol*

maca *(Lepidium meyenii)* root *medicinal herb used as an adaptogen, aphrodisiac in males, fertility aid in females, and to relieve stress*

MACC (methotrexate, Adriamycin, cyclophosphamide, CCNU) *chemotherapy protocol*

mace *(Myristica fragrans)* dried nutmeg aril (the fleshy network surrounding the seed) *medicinal herb* [see: nutmeg]

MACHO (methotrexate, asparaginase, cyclophosphamide, hydroxydaunomycin, Oncovin) *chemotherapy protocol*

MACOP-B (methotrexate, Adriamycin, cyclophosphamide, Oncovin, prednisone, bleomycin) *chemotherapy protocol*

Macritonin injection, intranasal ℞ *investigational (Phase III) oral treatment for osteoporosis* [calcitonin (salmon)]

macroaggregated albumin (MAA) [see: albumin, aggregated]

macroaggregated iodinated (^{131}I) human albumin [see: macrosalb (^{131}I)]

Macrobid capsules ℞ *urinary antibiotic* [nitrofurantoin (macrocrystals); nitrofurantoin monohydrate] 25•75 mg

Macrodantin capsules ℞ *urinary antibiotic* [nitrofurantoin (macrocrystals)] 25, 50, 100 mg

Macrodex IV infusion ℞ *plasma volume expander for shock due to hemorrhage, burns, or surgery* [dextran 70] 6%

macrogol 4000 INN, BAN [also: polyethylene glycol 4000]

macrogol ester 2000 INN *surfactant* [also: polyoxyl 40 stearate]

macrogol ester 400 INN *surfactant* [also: polyoxyl 8 stearate]

macrolides *a class of antibiotics that are bacteriostatic or bactericidal, depending on drug concentration*

macrophage colony-stimulating factor (M-CSF) [now: cilmostim]

macrophage-targeted β-glucocerebrosidase [now: alglucerase]

macrosalb (^{131}I) INN, BAN

macrosalb (^{99m}Tc) INN, BAN [also: technetium (^{99m}Tc) labeled macroaggregated human ...]

Macroscint ℞ *investigational inflammation and infection imaging aid* [indium In 111 IGIV pentetate]

Macrotys actaeoides *medicinal herb* [see: black cohosh]

Macrulin *investigational (Phase I) oral agent for type 2 diabetes* [insulin]

Macstim ℞ *hematopoietic; macrophage colony-stimulating factor; investigational antineoplastic for various cancers; investigational antihyperlipidemic* [cilmostim]

MAD (MeCCNU, Adriamycin) *chemotherapy protocol*

mad-dog weed; mad weed *medicinal herb* [see: skullcap]

MADDOC (mechlorethamine, Adriamycin, dacarbazine, DDP, Oncovin, cyclophosphamide) *chemotherapy protocol*

madnep; madness *medicinal herb* [see: masterwort]

maduramicin USAN, INN *anticoccidal*

mafenide USAN, INN, BAN *bacteriostatic; adjunct to burn therapy*

mafenide acetate USP *broad-spectrum bacteriostatic to prevent meshed autograft loss on second- and third-degree burns (orphan)*

mafenide HCl

mafilcon A USAN *hydrophilic contact lens material*

mafoprazine INN

mafosfamide INN

Mag-200 tablets OTC *magnesium supplement* [magnesium oxide] 400 mg

magaldrate USAN, USP, INN *antacid* 540 mg/5 mL oral

Magaldrate Plus oral suspension OTC *antacid; antiflatulent* [magaldrate; simethicone] 540•40/5 mL

Magalox Plus chewable tablets OTC *antacid; antiflatulent* [aluminum hydroxide; magnesium hydroxide; simethicone] 200•200•25 mg

Magan tablets ℞ *analgesic; antirheumatic* [magnesium salicylate] 545 mg

Mag-Cal tablets OTC *dietary supplement* [calcium carbonate; vitamin D; multiple minerals] 416.7 mg•66.7 IU• ±

Mag-Cal Mega tablets OTC *mineral supplement* [magnesium; calcium] 800•400 mg

Mag-G tablets OTC *magnesium supplement* [magnesium gluconate] 500 mg

maggots (Lucilia caesar; Phaenicia sericata; Pharmia regina) *natural treatment for debriding necrotic tissue in abscesses, burns, cellulitis, gangrene, osteomyelitis, and ulcers*

Magnacal ready-to-use liquid OTC *enteral nutritional therapy* [lactose-free formula]

Magnalox liquid OTC *antacid* [aluminum hydroxide; magnesium hydroxide] 225•220 mg/5 mL

Magnaprin; Magnaprin Arthritis Strength Captabs film-coated tablets OTC *analgesic; antipyretic; antiinflammatory; antirheumatic* [aspirin (buffered with aluminum hydroxide, magnesium hydroxide, and calcium carbonate)] 325 mg

magnesia, milk of USP *antacid; laxative* [also: magnesium hydroxide] 400 mg/5 mL oral

magnesia magma [now: magnesia, milk of]

magnesium *element (Mg)*

magnesium aluminosilicate hydrate [see: almasilate]

magnesium aluminum silicate NF *suspending agent*

magnesium amino acid chelate *dietary magnesium supplement*

magnesium aspartate [see: potassium aspartate & magnesium aspartate]

magnesium carbonate USP *antacid; dietary magnesium supplement*

magnesium carbonate hydrate [see: magnesium carbonate]

magnesium chloride USP *electrolyte replenisher* 1.97 mEq/mL (20%) injection

magnesium chloride hexahydrate [see: magnesium chloride]

magnesium citrate USP *saline laxative*

magnesium clofibrate INN

magnesium D-gluconate dihydrate [see: magnesium gluconate]

magnesium D-gluconate hydrate [see: magnesium gluconate]

magnesium gluconate USP *magnesium replenisher*

magnesium glycinate USAN

magnesium hydroxide USP *antacid; saline laxative* [also: magnesia, milk of]

magnesium hydroxycarbonate *antiurolithic*

magnesium oxide USP *antacid; sorbent* 400, 500 mg oral

magnesium phosphate USP *antacid*

magnesium phosphate pentahydrate [see: magnesium phosphate]

magnesium salicylate USP *analgesic; antipyretic; anti-inflammatory; antirheumatic*

magnesium salicylate tetrahydrate [see: magnesium salicylate]

magnesium silicate NF *tablet excipient*

magnesium silicate hydrate [see: magnesium trisilicate]

magnesium stearate NF *tablet and capsule lubricant*

magnesium sulfate USP, JAN *anticonvulsant; saline laxative; electrolyte replenisher* 0.8, 1, 4 mEq/mL (10%, 12.5%, 50%) injection

magnesium sulfate heptahydrate [see: magnesium sulfate]

magnesium trisilicate USP *antacid*

Magnevist IV injection, prefilled syringes ℞ *MRI contrast medium* [gadopentetate dimeglumine] 469 mg/mL

magnolia (Magnolia glauca) bark *medicinal herb used as an antiperiodic, aromatic, astringent, diaphoretic, febrifuge, stimulant, and tonic*

Magnox oral suspension OTC *antacid* [aluminum hydroxide; magnesium hydroxide] 225•200 mg/5 mL

Magonate tablets, liquid OTC *magnesium supplement* [magnesium gluconate] 500 mg; 54 mg/5 mL

Mag-Ox 400 tablets OTC *antacid; magnesium supplement* [magnesium oxide] 400 mg

Magsal tablets ℞ *analgesic; antipyretic; anti-inflammatory; antihistamine* [magnesium salicylate; phenyltoloxamine citrate] 600•25 mg

Mag-Tab SR sustained-release caplets OTC *magnesium supplement* [magnesium lactate] 7 mEq (84 mg)

Magtrate tablets OTC *magnesium supplement* [magnesium gluconate] 500 mg

mahogany birch; mountain mahogany *medicinal herb* [see: birch]

Mahonia aquifolium *medicinal herb* [see: Oregon grape]

ma-huang *medicinal herb* [see: ephedra]

MAID (mesna [rescue], Adriamycin, ifosfamide, dacarbazine) *chemotherapy protocol*

maitake mushrooms (Grifola frondosa) cap and stem *medicinal herb for cancer, diabetes, hypercholesterolemia, hypertension, obesity, and stimulation of the immune system*

maitansine INN *antineoplastic* [also: maytansine]

Maitec injection ℞ *investigational (orphan) for disseminated Mycobacterium avium-intracellulare infection* [gentamicin sulfate, liposomal]

Majorana hortensis *medicinal herb* [see: marjoram]

Major-Con chewable tablets OTC *antiflatulent* [simethicone] 80 mg

Major-gesic tablets OTC *antihistamine; analgesic* [phenyltoloxamine citrate; acetaminophen] 30•325 mg

MAK 195 F *investigational therapy for graft vs. host disease* [monoclonal antibodies]

malaleuca *medicinal herb* [see: tea tree oil]

Malarone ⓐ film-coated tablets ℞ *antimalarial* [atovaquone; proguanil HCl (chloroguanide HCl)] 250•100 mg

Malatal tablets (discontinued 1997) ℞ *GI antispasmodic; anticholinergic; sedative* [atropine sulfate; scopolamine hydrobromide; hyoscyamine hydrobromide; phenobarbital] 0.0194•0.0065•0.1037•16.2 mg

malathion USP, BAN *pediculicide*

maletamer INN *antiperistaltic* [also: malethamer]

malethamer USAN *antiperistaltic* [also: maletamer]

maleylsulfathiazole INN

malic acid NF *acidifying agent*

malidone [see: aloxidone]

Mallamint chewable tablets OTC *antacid* [calcium carbonate] 420 mg

Mallazine eye drops OTC *topical ophthalmic decongestant and vasoconstrictor* [tetrahydrozoline HCl] 0.05%

Mallisol ointment (discontinued 1999) OTC *broad-spectrum antimicrobial* [povidone-iodine]

mallow *(Malva rotundifolia; M. sylvestris)* plant *medicinal herb used as an astringent, demulcent, emollient, and expectorant*

mallow, marsh *(Althaea officinalis) medicinal herb* [see: marsh mallow]

malonal [see: barbital]

malotilate USAN, INN *liver disorder treatment*

Malpighia glabra; M. punicifolia medicinal herb [see: acerola]

Maltsupex liquid OTC *bulk laxative* [nondiastatic barley malt extract] 16 g/tbsp.

Maltsupex powder OTC *bulk laxative* [nondiastatic barley malt extract] 8 g/tbsp.

Maltsupex tablets OTC *bulk laxative* [nondiastatic barley malt extract] 750 mg

Malva rotundifolia; M. sylvestris medicinal herb [see: mallow]

Mammol ointment OTC *emollient for nipples of nursing mothers* [bismuth subnitrate] 40%

*m***-AMSA (acridinylamine methanesulphon anisidide)** [see: amsacrine]

Mandameth enteric-coated tablets ℞ *urinary antibiotic* [methenamine mandelate] 0.5, 1 g

Mandelamine film-coated tablets (discontinued 1995) ℞ *urinary antibiotic* [methenamine mandelate] 0.5, 1 g

mandelic acid NF

Mandol powder for IV or IM injection ℞ *cephalosporin antibiotic* [cefamandole nafate] 1 g ⊡ nadolol

mandrake *(Mandragora officinarium; Podophyllum peltatum)* root and resin *medicinal herb for cancer, condylomata, constipation, fever, indigestion, liver disorders, lower bowel disorders, warts, and worms; not generally regarded as safe and effective for children or pregnant women*

Manerex ⊛ film-coated tablets ℞ *antidepressant; MAO inhibitor* [moclobemide] 100, 150 mg

mangafodipir trisodium USAN *paramagnetic contrast agent for MRI of the liver*

manganese *element (Mn)*

manganese chloride USP *dietary manganese supplement* 0.1 mg/mL injection

manganese chloride tetrahydrate [see: manganese chloride]

manganese gluconate (manganese D-gluconate) USP *dietary manganese supplement*

manganese glycerophosphate NF

manganese hypophosphite NF

manganese phosphinate [see: manganese hypophosphite]

manganese sulfate USP *dietary manganese supplement* 0.1 mg/mL injection

manganese sulfate monohydrate [see: manganese sulfate]

mangofodipir trisodium *MRI contrast medium for liver imaging*

manidipine 6300 INN

manna sugar [see: mannitol]

mannite [see: mannitol]

mannitol (D-mannitol) USP *renal function test aid; antihypertensive; osmotic diuretic; urologic irrigant* 10%, 15%, 20%, 25% injection

mannitol hexanitrate INN

mannityl nitrate [see: mannitol hexanitrate]

mannomustine INN, BAN

mannosulfan INN

manozodil INN

Mantadil cream (discontinued 1997) ℞ *topical corticosteroidal anti-inflammatory; antihistamine* [hydrocortisone acetate; chlorcyclizine HCl] 0.5%•2%

Mantoux test [see: tuberculin]

MAO inhibitors (monoamine oxidase inhibitors) [q.v.]

Maolate tablets ℞ *skeletal muscle relaxant* [chlorphenesin carbamate] 400 mg

Maox tablets (name changed to Maox 420 in 1995)

Maox 420 tablets OTC *antacid* [magnesium oxide] 420 mg

MAP (mitomycin, Adriamycin, Platinol) *chemotherapy protocol*

Mapap tablets OTC *analgesic; antipyretic* [acetaminophen] 325, 500 mg

Mapap, Children's liquid OTC *analgesic; antipyretic* [acetaminophen] 160 mg/5 mL

Mapap Cold Formula tablets OTC *antitussive; decongestant; antihistamine; analgesic* [dextromethorphan hydrobromide; pseudoephedrine HCl; chlorpheniramine maleate; acetaminophen] 15•30•2•325 mg

Mapap Infant Drops OTC *analgesic; antipyretic* [acetaminophen] 100 mg/mL

maple lungwort *medicinal herb* [see: lungwort]

maprotiline USAN, INN *tetracyclic antidepressant*

maprotiline HCl USP *tetracyclic antidepressant* 25, 50, 75 mg oral

Maranox tablets OTC *analgesic; antipyretic* [acetaminophen] 325 mg

Marax tablets ℞ *antiasthmatic; bronchodilator; decongestant* [theophylline; ephedrine sulfate] 130•25 mg ⊡ Atarax; Maalox

Marax-DF pediatric syrup ℞ *antiasthmatic; bronchodilator; decongestant; antihistamine* [theophylline; ephedrine sulfate; hydroxyzine HCl] 97.5•18.75•7.5 mg/15 mL

Marbec tablets (discontinued 1995) OTC *dietary supplement* [multiple B vitamins; vitamin C; brewer's yeast] ±•300•120 mg

Marblen tablets, liquid OTC *antacid* [calcium carbonate; magnesium carbonate] 520•400 mg; 540•400 mg/5 mL

Marcaine HCl injection ℞ *injectable local anesthetic* [bupivacaine HCl] 0.25%, 0.5%, 0.75%

Marcaine HCl injection ℞ *injectable local anesthetic* [bupivacaine HCl; epinephrine bitartrate] 0.25%•1:200 000, 0.5%•1:200 000, 0.75%•1:200 000 ⊡ Narcan

Marcaine Spinal injection ℞ *injectable local anesthetic* [bupivacaine HCl] 0.75%

Marcaine with Epinephrine injection (discontinued 1996) ℞ *injectable local anesthetic* [bupivacaine HCl; epinephrine] 0.5%•1:200 000

Marcillin capsules ℞ *aminopenicillin antibiotic* [ampicillin] 500 mg

Marcillin powder for oral suspension (discontinued 1998) ℞ *aminopenicillin antibiotic* [ampicillin] 250 mg/100 mL

Marcof Expectorant syrup ℞ *narcotic antitussive; expectorant* [hydrocodone bitartrate; potassium guaiacolsulfonate] 5•300 mg/5 mL

mare's tail *medicinal herb* [see: fleabane; horseweed]

Marezine tablets OTC *antiemetic; anticholinergic; antihistamine; motion sickness preventative* [cyclizine HCl] 50 mg

Margesic capsules ℞ *analgesic; anti-inflammatory; sedative* [acetaminophen; caffeine; butalbital] 325•40•50 mg

Margesic H capsules ℞ *narcotic analgesic* [hydrocodone bitartrate; acetaminophen] 5•500 mg

Margesic No. 3 tablets (discontinued 1996) ℞ *narcotic analgesic* [codeine phosphate; acetaminophen] 30•650 mg

maridomycin INN

marigold (Calendula officinalis) florets *medicinal herb for bruises, cuts, dysmenorrhea, eye infections, fever, and skin diseases; not generally regarded as safe and effective*

marijuana; marihuana (Cannabis sativa) euphoric/hallucinogenic street drug made from the dried leaves and flowering tops of the cannabis plant; *medicinal herb for asthma, analgesia, leprosy, and loss of appetite; investigational for HIV*

marimastat USAN *investigational (Phase III) antineoplastic; matrix metalloproteinase (MMP) inhibitor*

Marine Lipid Concentrate softgels OTC *dietary supplement* [omega-3 fatty acids] 1200 mg

Marinol soft gelatin capsules ℞ *antiemetic for chemotherapy; appetite stim-*

ulant for AIDS patients (orphan) [dronabinol] 2.5, 5, 10 mg

mariptiline INN

marjoram *(Majorana hortensis; Origanum vulgare)* plant *medicinal herb for abdominal cramps, colic, headache, indigestion, respiratory problems, and violent cough*

Marlin Salt System tablets OTC *rinsing/storage solution for soft contact lenses* [sodium chloride (normal saline solution)] 250 mg

Marlin Salt System II tablets OTC *rinsing/storage solution for soft contact lenses* [sodium chloride (normal saline solution)] 250 mg

Marmine IV or IM injection ℞ *antinauseant; antiemetic; antivertigo; motion sickness preventative* [dimenhydrinate] 50 mg/mL

Marmine tablets OTC *antinauseant; antiemetic; antivertigo; motion sickness preventative* [dimenhydrinate] 50 mg

Marnal tablets, capsules (discontinued 1998) ℞ *analgesic; sedative* [aspirin; caffeine; butalbital] 325•40•50 mg

Marnatal-F film-coated tablets ℞ *vitamin/mineral/calcium/iron supplement* [multiple vitamins & minerals; calcium; iron; folic acid] ≛•250•60•1 mg

Marogen ℞ *investigational substitute for blood transfusion; investigational (orphan) for anemia of end-stage renal disease* [epoetin beta]

maroxepin INN

Marplan tablets ℞ *antidepressant; monoamine oxidase (MAO) inhibitor* [isocarboxazid] 10 mg

Marpres tablets ℞ *antihypertensive; vasodilator; diuretic* [hydrochlorothiazide; reserpine; hydralazine HCl] 15•0.1•25 mg

Marrubium vulgare *medicinal herb* [see: horehound]

marsh clover; marsh trefoil *medicinal herb* [see: buckbean]

marsh mallow *(Althaea officinalis)* root *medicinal herb for asthma, boils, bronchial infections, cough, emphy-* sema, infected wounds, kidney disorders, lung congestion, sore throat, and urinary bleeding

MART-1 adenoviral gene therapy *investigational (orphan) for metastatic malignant melanoma*

Marten-Tab caplets ℞ *analgesic; sedative* [acetaminophen; butalbital] 325•50 mg

Marthritic tablets ℞ *analgesic; antipyretic; anti-inflammatory; antirheumatic* [salsalate] 750 mg

masoprocol USAN, INN *antineoplastic for actinic keratoses (AK)*

Massé Breast cream OTC *moisturizer and emollient for nipples of nursing women*

Massengill Baking Soda Freshness solution OTC *vaginal cleanser and deodorizer; acidity modifier* [sodium bicarbonate]

Massengill Disposable Douche solution OTC *antiseptic/germicidal; vaginal cleanser and deodorizer; acidity modifier* [cetylpyridinium chloride; lactic acid; sodium lactate]

Massengill Disposable Douche; Massengill Vinegar & Water Extra Mild solution OTC *vaginal cleanser and deodorizer; acidity modifier* [vinegar (acetic acid)]

Massengill Douche powder OTC *astringent; analgesic; counterirritant; vaginal cleanser and deodorizer* [ammonium alum; phenol; methyl salicylate; menthol; thymol]

Massengill Douche solution concentrate OTC *vaginal cleanser and deodorizer; acidity modifier* [lactic acid; sodium lactate; sodium bicarbonate]

Massengill Feminine Cleansing Wash liquid OTC *for external perivaginal cleansing*

Massengill Medicated towelettes OTC *topical corticosteroidal anti-inflammatory* [hydrocortisone] 0.5%

Massengill Medicated Douche with Cepticin; Massengill Medicated Disposable Douche with Cepticin solution OTC *antiseptic/germici-*

dal; *vaginal cleanser and deodorizer* [povidone-iodine] 12%; 10%

Massengill Unscented solution (discontinued 1995) OTC *vaginal cleanser and deodorizer; acidity modifier* [lactic acid]

Massengill Vinegar & Water Extra Cleansing with Puraclean solution OTC *antiseptic/germicidal; vaginal cleanser and deodorizer; acidity modifier* [cetylpyridinium chloride; vinegar (acetic acid)]

masterwort (Heracleum lanatum) root and seed *medicinal herb used as an antispasmodic, carminative, and stimulant*

maté *medicinal herb* [see: yerba maté]

Materna tablets (discontinued 1997) ℞ *vitamin/mineral/calcium/iron supplement* [multiple vitamins & minerals; calcium; iron; folic acid; biotin] ± • 250•60•1•0.03 mg

Matricaria chamomilla medicinal herb [see: chamomile]

matrix metalloproteinase (MMP) inhibitors *a class of investigational (Phase III) antineoplastics and investigational (orphan) agents to treat corneal ulcers*

Matulane capsules ℞ *antineoplastic for Hodgkin's disease; investigational for lymphoma, brain and lung cancer* [procarbazine HCl] 50 mg

Mavik ⒶⓃ capsules ℞ *antihypertensive; angiotensin-converting enzyme (ACE) inhibitor* [trandolapril] 0.5, 1, 2 mg

Mavik tablets ℞ *antihypertensive; angiotensin-converting enzyme (ACE) inhibitor* [trandolapril] 1, 2, 4 mg

maxacalcitol *investigational vitamin D_3 analog for the topical treatment of psoriasis*

Maxair Autohaler (breath-activated metered-dose inhaler) ℞ *sympathomimetic bronchodilator* [pirbuterol acetate] 0.2 mg/dose

Maxalt tablets ℞ *vascular serotonin 5-HT_1 receptor agonist for migraine headache* [rizatriptan benzoate] 5, 10 mg

Maxalt-MLT orally disintegrating tablets ℞ *vascular serotonin 5-HT_1 receptor agonist for migraine headache* [rizatriptan benzoate] 5, 10 mg

Maxamine ℞ *investigational (Phase III) treatment for malignant melanoma and acute myelogenous leukemia; investigational (Phase I) adjunct to interferon alfa-2b for chronic hepatitis C* [aldesleukin]

Maxaquin; Maxaquin-3 film-coated tablets ℞ *broad-spectrum fluoroquinolone antibiotic* [lomefloxacin HCl] 400 mg

Max-Caro capsules (discontinued 1996) OTC *vitamin A precursor* [beta carotene] 15 mg (25 000 IU)

MaxEPA soft capsules OTC *dietary supplement* [omega-3 fatty acids; multiple vitamins & minerals] 1000• ± mg

Maxibolin *an anabolic steroid abused as a street drug* [see: ethylestrenol]

Maxicam ℞ *investigational (NDA filed) nonsteroidal anti-inflammatory drug (NSAID); antiarthritic; analgesic; antipyretic* [isoxicam]

Maxidex Drop-Tainers (eye drop suspension) ℞ *topical ophthalmic corticosteroidal anti-inflammatory* [dexamethasone] 0.1%

Maxidex ophthalmic ointment (discontinued 1998) ℞ *topical ophthalmic corticosteroidal anti-inflammatory* [dexamethasone] 0.05%

Maxiflor cream, ointment ℞ *topical corticosteroidal anti-inflammatory* [diflorasone diacetate] 0.05%

Maxilube jelly OTC *vaginal lubricant*

Maximum Blue Label; Maximum Green Label tablets OTC *vitamin/ mineral supplement* [multiple vitamins & minerals; folic acid; biotin] ± •130•50 μg

Maximum Red Label tablets OTC *vitamin/mineral/iron supplement* [multiple vitamins & minerals; iron; folic acid; biotin] ± •3.3 mg•0.13 mg•50 μg

"Maximum Strength" products [see under product name]

Maxipime powder for IV or IM injection ℞ *cephalosporin antibiotic* [cefepime HCl] 0.5, 1, 2 g

Maxitrol eye drop suspension, ophthalmic ointment ℞ *topical ophthalmic corticosteroidal anti-inflammatory; antibiotic* [dexamethasone; neomycin sulfate; polymyxin B sulfate] 0.1%•0.35%•10 000 U/mL; 0.1%•0.35%•10 000 U/g

Maxivate ointment, cream, lotion ℞ *topical corticosteroidal anti-inflammatory* [betamethasone dipropionate] 0.05%

Maxi-Vite tablets OTC *vitamin/mineral/calcium/iron supplement* [multiple vitamins & minerals; calcium; iron; folic acid; biotin] ±•53.5•1.5•0.4•0.001 mg

Maxolon tablets ℞ *antidopaminergic; antiemetic for chemotherapy; peristaltic* [metoclopramide HCl] 10 mg

Maxovite sustained-release tablets OTC *vitamin/mineral supplement* [multiple vitamins & minerals; folic acid; biotin] ±•330•11.7 μg

Maxzide tablets ℞ *antihypertensive; diuretic* [triamterene; hydrochlorothiazide] 37.5•25, 75•50 mg ② Microzide

May apple *medicinal herb* [see: mandrake]

May bells; May lily *medicinal herb* [see: lily of the valley]

May bush; May tree *medicinal herb* [see: hawthorn]

May lily *medicinal herb* [see: lily of the valley]

maytansine USAN *antineoplastic* [also: maitansine]

May-Vita elixir ℞ *vitamin supplement* [multiple B vitamins; folic acid] ±•0.1 mg

Mazanor tablets ℞ *anorexiant; CNS stimulant* [mazindol] 1 mg

mazapertine succinate USAN *antipsychotic; dopamine receptor antagonist*

mazaticol INN

MAZE (m-AMSA, azacitidine, etoposide) *chemotherapy protocol*

mazindol USAN, USP, INN, BAN *anorexiant; CNS stimulant; investigational (orphan) treatment for Duchenne muscular dystrophy* ② mebendazole

mazipredone INN

MB (methylene blue) [q.v.]

m-BACOD; M-BACOD (methotrexate, bleomycin, Adriamycin, cyclophosphamide, Oncovin, dexamethasone) *chemotherapy protocol* "m" is 200 mg/m²; "M" is 3 g/m²

M-BACOS (methotrexate, bleomycin, Adriamycin, cyclophosphamide, Oncovin, Solu-Medrol) *chemotherapy protocol*

MBC (methotrexate, bleomycin, cisplatin) *chemotherapy protocol*

MBD (methotrexate, bleomycin, DDP) *chemotherapy protocol*

MBR (methylene blue, reduced) [see: methylene blue]

MC (mitoxantrone, cytarabine) *chemotherapy protocol*

M-Caps capsules ℞ *urinary acidifier to control ammonia production* [racemethionine] 200 mg

MCBP (melphalan, cyclophosphamide, BCNU, prednisone) *chemotherapy protocol*

MCH (microfibrillar collagen hemostat) [q.v.]

MCP (melphalan, cyclophosphamide, prednisone) *chemotherapy protocol*

M-CSF (macrophage colony-stimulating factor) [now: cilmostim]

MCT oil OTC *dietary fat supplement* [medium chain triglycerides from coconut oil]

MCT (medium chain triglycerides) [q.v.]

MCV (methotrexate, cisplatin, vinblastine) *chemotherapy protocol*

MD-60; MD-76 injection (discontinued 1999) ℞ *radiopaque contrast medium* [diatrizoate meglumine; diatrizoate sodium (48.7% total iodine)] 52%•8% (29.3%); 66%•10% (37%)

MD-76 R injection ℞ *radiopaque contrast medium* [diatrizoate meglumine;

diatrizoate sodium (48.7% total iodine)] 660•100 mg/mL (370 mg/mL)

MDA (methylenedioxyamphetamine) [see: MDMA, MDEA]

mda-7 *investigational tumor suppressor gene for cancer therapy*

MDEA (3,4-methylenedioxyethamphetamine) *a hallucinogenic amphetamine derivative closely related to MDMA, abused as a street drug, which causes dependence* [also see: amphetamines; MDMA]

MD-Gastroview oral solution ℞ *radiopaque contrast medium for gastrointestinal imaging* [diatrizoate meglumine; diatrizoate sodium (48.29% total iodine)] 660•100 mg/mL (367 mg/mL)

MDMA (3,4-methylenedioxymethamphetamine) *widely abused hallucinogenic street drug that is chemically related to amphetamines and mescaline and causes dependence* [see also: amphetamines; mescaline; MDEA]

MDP (methylene diphosphonate) [now: medronate disodium]

MDX-210 *investigational (Phase II) HER-2 receptor antibody for prostate cancer*

MDX-240 *investigational (Phase II) treatment for AIDS*

MDX-RA *investigational (Phase III) immunotoxin for the prevention of secondary cataracts (clinical trials discontinued 1998)*

MEA (mercaptoethylamine) [see: mercaptamine]

meadow cabbage *medicinal herb* [see: skunk cabbage]

meadow sorrel *medicinal herb* [see: sorrel]

meadowsweet (Filipendula ulmaria) plant *medicinal herb used for ulcers and upper respiratory problems; also used as an astringent, diaphoretic, and diuretic*

mealberry *medicinal herb* [see: uva ursi]

mealy starwort *medicinal herb* [see: star grass]

measles, mumps & rubella virus vaccine, live USP *active immunizing agent for measles (rubeola), mumps and rubella*

measles immune globulin USP

measles & rubella virus vaccine, live USP *active immunizing agent for measles (rubeola) and rubella*

measles virus vaccine, live USP *active immunizing agent for measles (rubeola)*

Mebadin (available only from the Centers for Disease Control) ℞ *investigational anti-infective for amebiasis and amebic dysentery* [dehydroemetine]

meballymal [see: secobarbital]

mebamoxine [see: benmoxin]

mebanazine INN, BAN

Mebaral tablets ℞ *long-acting barbiturate sedative, hypnotic and anticonvulsant* [mephobarbital] 32, 50, 100 mg ⑫ Medrol

mebendazole USAN, USP, INN *anthelmintic for trichuriasis, enterobiasis, ascariasis, and uncinariasis* 100 mg oral ⑫ mazindol

mebenoside INN

mebeverine INN *smooth muscle relaxant* [also: mebeverine HCl]

mebeverine HCl USAN *smooth muscle relaxant* [also: mebeverine]

mebezonium iodide INN, BAN

mebhydrolin INN, BAN

mebiquine INN

mebolazine INN

mebrofenin USAN, INN *hepatobiliary function test*

mebrophenhydramine HCl [see: embramine HCl]

mebubarbital [see: pentobarbital]

mebumal [see: pentobarbital]

mebutamate USAN, INN *antihypertensive*

mebutizide INN

mecamylamine INN *antihypertensive* [also: mecamylamine HCl]

mecamylamine HCl USP *antihypertensive* [also: mecamylamine]

mecamylamine HCl & nicotine *investigational (Phase III) transdermal patch for smoking cessation*

mecarbinate INN

mecarbine [see: mecarbinate]

mecasermin INN, BAN *investigational (NDA filed, orphan) for amyotrophic lateral sclerosis, growth hormone insufficiency, and post-poliomyelitis syndrome* [previously known as insulin-like growth factor 1 (IGF-1)]

MeCCNU (methyl chloroethyl-cyclohexyl-nitrosourea) [see: semustine]

mecetronium ethylsulfate USAN *antiseptic* [also: mecetronium etilsulfate]

mecetronium etilsulfate INN *antiseptic* [also: mecetronium ethylsulfate]

mechlorethamine HCl USP *nitrogen mustard-type alkylating antineoplastic* [also: chlormethine; mustine; nitrogen mustard N-oxide HCl]

meciadanol INN

mecillinam INN, BAN *antibacterial* [also: amdinocillin]

mecinarone INN

Meclan cream ℞ *topical antibiotic for acne* [meclocycline sulfosalicylate] 1% ② Meclomen; Mezlin

meclizine HCl USP *antiemetic; antihistamine; anticholinergic; motion sickness relief* [also: meclozine] 12.5, 25, 50 mg oral ② mescaline

meclocycline USAN, INN, BAN *topical antibiotic*

meclocycline sulfosalicylate USAN, USP *topical antibiotic*

meclofenamate sodium USAN, USP *analgesic; antiarthritic; nonsteroidal anti-inflammatory drug (NSAID)* 50, 100 mg oral

meclofenamic acid USAN, INN *nonsteroidal anti-inflammatory drug (NSAID)*

meclofenoxate INN, BAN

Meclomen capsules (discontinued 1996) ℞ *nonsteroidal anti-inflammatory drug (NSAID); antiarthritic; analgesic* [meclofenamate sodium] 50, 100 mg ② Meclan

meclonazepam INN

mecloqualone USAN, INN *sedative; hypnotic*

mecloralurea INN

meclorisone INN, BAN *topical anti-inflammatory* [also: meclorisone dibutyrate]

meclorisone dibutyrate USAN *topical anti-inflammatory* [also: meclorisone]

mecloxamine INN

meclozine INN, BAN *antiemetic; antihistamine; anticholinergic; motion sickness relief* [also: meclizine HCl] ② mescaline

mecobalamin USAN, INN *vitamin; hematopoietic*

mecrilate INN *tissue adhesive* [also: mecrylate]

mecrylate USAN *tissue adhesive* [also: mecrilate]

MECY (methotrexate, cyclophosphamide) *chemotherapy protocol*

mecysteine INN

Med Timolol ⓒ (U.S. product: Timoptic) eye drops ℞ *topical antiglaucoma agent (β-blocker)* [timolol maleate] 0.25%, 0.5%

Meda Cap capsules OTC *analgesic; antipyretic* [acetaminophen] 500 mg

Meda Tab tablets OTC *analgesic; antipyretic* [acetaminophen] 325 mg

Medacote lotion OTC *topical antihistamine; astringent; antipruritic* [pyrilamine maleate; zinc oxide] 1% • ②

Medadyne liquid OTC *topical oral anesthetic; antiseptic; astringent* [benzocaine; methylbenzethonium chloride; tannic acid; camphor; menthol]

Medadyne throat spray OTC *topical anesthetic; oral antiseptic* [lidocaine; cetalkonium chloride]

Medalone 40; Medalone 80 [see: depMedalone 40; depMedalone 80]

Medamint throat lozenges OTC *topical oral anesthetic* [benzocaine]

medazepam INN *minor tranquilizer* [also: medazepam HCl]

medazepam HCl USAN *minor tranquilizer* [also: medazepam]

medazomide INN

medazonamide [see: medazomide]

Medebar Plus rectal suspension ℞ *radiopaque contrast medium for gastrointestinal imaging* [barium sulfate] 100%

Medescan oral suspension ℞ *radiopaque contrast medium for gastrointestinal imaging* [barium sulfate] 2.3%

medetomidine INN, BAN *veterinary analgesic; veterinary sedative* [also: medetomidine HCl]

medetomidine HCl USAN *veterinary analgesic; veterinary sedative* [also: medetomidine]

medibazine INN

Medicago sativa medicinal herb [see: alfalfa]

medical air [see: air, medical]

Medicated Acne Cleanser OTC *topical acne treatment* [colloidal sulfur; resorcinol] 4%•2%

medicinal zinc peroxide [see: zinc peroxide, medicinal]

Medicone anorectal ointment OTC *topical local anesthetic* [benzocaine] 20%

Medicone rectal suppositories OTC *topical vasoconstrictor for hemorrhoids* [phenylephrine HCl] 0.25%

Medi-Flu caplets, liquid (discontinued 1995) OTC *antitussive; decongestant; antihistamine; analgesic* [dextromethorphan hydrobromide; pseudoephedrine HCl; chlorpheniramine maleate; acetaminophen] 15•30•2•500 mg; 5•10•0.67•167 mg/5 mL

medifoxamine INN

Medigesic capsules ℞ *analgesic; sedative* [acetaminophen; caffeine; butalbital] 325•40•50 mg

Medihaler-Epi inhalation aerosol (discontinued 1996) OTC *bronchodilator for bronchial asthma* [epinephrine bitartrate] 0.3 mg/dose

Medihaler-Iso inhalation aerosol ℞ *sympathomimetic bronchodilator* [isoproterenol sulfate] 80 μg/dose

Medilax chewable tablets (discontinued 1998) OTC *stimulant laxative* [phenolphthalein] 120 mg

medinal [see: barbital sodium]

Medipain 5 capsules (discontinued 1997) ℞ *narcotic analgesic* [hydrocodone bitartrate; acetaminophen] 5•500 mg

Mediplast plaster OTC *topical keratolytic* [salicylic acid] 40%

Mediplex Tabules (tablets) OTC *vitamin/mineral supplement* [multiple vitamins & minerals] ≛

Medipren tablets, caplets (discontinued 1996) OTC *nonsteroidal anti-inflammatory drug (NSAID); antiarthritic; analgesic* [ibuprofen] 200 mg

Medi-Quik aerosol (discontinued 1995) OTC *topical local anesthetic; antiseptic* [lidocaine HCl; benzalkonium chloride]

Medi-Quik ointment OTC *topical antibiotic* [polymyxin B sulfate; neomycin; bacitracin] 5000 U•3.5 mg•400 U per g

Medi-Quik spray OTC *topical local anesthetic; antiseptic* [lidocaine; benzalkonium chloride] 2%•0.13%

medium chain triglycerides (MCT) *dietary lipid supplement*

medorinone USAN, INN *cardiotonic*

medorubicin INN

Medotar ointment OTC *topical antipsoriatic; antiseborrheic; astringent; antiseptic* [coal tar; zinc oxide] 1%• ≛

Medralone 40; Medralone 80 intralesional, soft tissue, and IM injection ℞ *corticosteroid; anti-inflammatory; immunosuppressant* [methylprednisolone acetate] 40 mg/mL; 80 mg/mL

medrogestone USAN, INN, BAN *progestin*

Medrol tablets, Dosepak (unit of use package) ℞ *corticosteroid; anti-inflammatory; immunosuppressant* [methylprednisolone] 2, 4, 8, 16, 24, 32 mg ⊘ Mebaral

medronate disodium USAN *pharmaceutic aid*

medronic acid USAN, INN, BAN *pharmaceutic aid*

medroxalol USAN, INN, BAN *antihypertensive*

medroxalol HCl USAN *antihypertensive*

medroxiprogesterone acetate [see: medroxyprogesterone acetate]

medroxyprogesterone INN, BAN *progestin for secondary amenorrhea or abnormal uterine bleeding; hormonal* *antineoplastic* [also: medroxyprogesterone acetate]

medroxyprogesterone acetate USP *progestin for secondary amenorrhea, abnormal uterine bleeding, and endometrial hyperplasia; hormonal antineoplastic* [also: medroxyprogesterone] 2.5, 5, 10 mg oral

MED·Rx controlled-release tablets (14-day, 56-tablet regimen) ℞ *decongestant; expectorant* [pseudoephedrine HCl + guaifenesin (blue tablets); guaifenesin (white tablets)] 60•600 mg; 600 mg

MED·Rx DM controlled-release tablets (14-day, 56-tablet regimen) ℞ *decongestant; expectorant; antitussive* [pseudoephedrine HCl + guaifenesin (blue tablets); dextromethorphan hydrobromide + guaifenesin (green tablets)] 60•600 mg; 30•600 mg

medrylamine INN

medrysone USAN, USP, INN *ophthalmic corticosteroidal anti-inflammatory*

mefeclorazine INN

mefenamic acid USAN, USP, INN, BAN *analgesic; nonsteroidal anti-inflammatory drug (NSAID)*

mefenidil USAN, INN *cerebral vasodilator*

mefenidil fumarate USAN *cerebral vasodilator*

mefenidramium metilsulfate INN

mefenorex INN *anorectic* [also: mefenorex HCl]

mefenorex HCl USAN *anorectic* [also: mefenorex]

mefeserpine INN

mefexamide USAN, INN *CNS stimulant*

mefloquine USAN, INN, BAN *antimalarial*

mefloquine HCl USAN *antimalarial for acute chloroquine-resistant malaria (orphan)*

Mefoxin powder or frozen premix for IV or IM injection ℞ *cephamycin antibiotic* [cefoxitin sodium] 1, 2, 10 g

mefruside USAN, INN *diuretic*

Mega B with C tablets (discontinued 1995) OTC *vitamin supplement* [multiple B vitamins; vitamin C; folic acid; biotin] ±•500 mg•400 μg•100 μg

Mega VM-80 tablets OTC *geriatric vitamin/mineral supplement* [multiple vitamins & minerals; folic acid; biotin] ±•400•80 μg

Mega-B tablets OTC *vitamin supplement* [multiple B vitamins; folic acid; biotin] ±•100•100 μg

Megace oral suspension ℞ *treatment for AIDS-related anorexia and cachexia (orphan)* [megestrol acetate] 40 mg/mL

Megace tablets ℞ *hormonal antineoplastic for advanced carcinoma of the breast or endometrium* [megestrol acetate] 20, 40 mg

Megadose tablets (discontinued 1995) OTC *geriatric vitamin/mineral supplement* [multiple vitamins & minerals; folic acid; biotin] ±•400•80 μg

Megagen ℞ *investigational (orphan) adjunct to hematopoietic stem cell transplantation* [megakaryocyte growth and development factor, pegylated, recombinant human]

megakaryocyte growth and development factor, pegylated, recombinant human *investigational (orphan) adjunct to hematopoietic stem cell transplantation*

megallate INN *combining name for radicals or groups*

megalomicin INN *antibacterial* [also: megalomicin potassium phosphate]

megalomicin potassium phosphate USAN *antibacterial* [also: megalomicin]

Megaton elixir ℞ *vitamin/mineral supplement* [multiple B vitamins & minerals; folic acid] ±•0.1 mg

megestrol INN, BAN *hormonal antineoplastic for breast or endometrial cancer* [also: megestrol acetate]

megestrol acetate USAN, USP *hormonal antineoplastic for breast or endometrial cancer; therapy for AIDS-related anorexia and cachexia (orphan)* [also: megestrol] 20, 40 mg oral

meglitinide INN

meglucycline INN

meglumine USP, INN *radiopaque contrast medium*

meglumine diatrizoate BAN *oral/ parenteral radiopaque contrast medium (46.67% iodine)* [also: diatrizoate meglumine]

meglumine iocarmate BAN *radiopaque contrast medium* [also: iocarmate meglumine]

meglumine iothalamate BAN *parenteral radiopaque contrast medium (47% iodine)* [also: iothalamate meglumine]

meglumine ioxaglate BAN *radiopaque contrast medium* [also: ioxaglate meglumine]

meglutol USAN, INN *antihyperlipoproteinemic*

mel B [see: melarsoprol]

mel W [see: melarsonyl potassium]

Melacine ℞ *investigational (NDA filed, orphan) theraccine for invasive stage III-IV melanoma; investigational (Phase III) for early-stage melanoma* [melanoma vaccine]

meladrazine INN, BAN

melafocon A USAN *hydrophobic contact lens material*

Melaleuca alternifolia medicinal herb [see: tea tree oil]

Melanex solution ℞ *hyperpigmentation bleaching agent* [hydroquinone] 3%

melanoma vaccine *investigational (NDA filed, orphan) therapeutic vaccine for invasive stage III-IV melanoma; investigational (Phase III) for early-stage melanoma*

melarsonyl potassium INN, BAN

melarsoprol INN, BAN, DCF *investigational anti-infective for trypanosomiasis*

melatonin *natural sleep aid; investigational (orphan) for circadian rhythm sleep disorders in blind people with no light perception*

melengestrol INN *antineoplastic; progestin* [also: melengestrol acetate]

melengestrol acetate USAN *antineoplastic; progestin* [also: melengestrol]

meletimide INN

melfalan [see: melphalan]

Melfiat-105 Unicelles (sustained-release capsules) ℞ *anorexiant; CNS stimulant* [phendimetrazine tartrate] 105 mg

Melia azedarach medicinal herb [see: pride of China]

melilot *(Melilotus alba; M. officinalis)* flowering plant *medicinal herb used as an antispasmodic, diuretic, emollient, expectorant, and vulnerary*

Melimmune *investigational (orphan) for non-Hodgkin's B-cell lymphoma* [indium In 111 murine MAb (2B8-MXDTPA); yttrium Y 90 murine MAB (2B8-MXDTPA)]

melinamide INN

Melissa officinalis medicinal herb [see: lemon balm]

melitracen INN *antidepressant* [also: melitracen HCl]

melitracen HCl USAN *antidepressant* [also: melitracen]

melizame USAN, INN *sweetener*

Mellaril tablets, oral concentrate ℞ *conventional (typical) antipsychotic* [thioridazine HCl] 10, 15, 25, 50, 100, 150, 200 mg; 30, 100 mg/mL ⊉ Aldoril; Elavil; Eldepryl; Enovil; Equanil; Moderil

Mellaril-S oral suspension ℞ *conventional (typical) antipsychotic* [thioridazine HCl] 25, 100 mg/5 mL (10 mg/5 mL available in Canada)

meloxicam USAN, INN, BAN *investigational (NDA filed) COX-2 inhibitor for rheumatoid arthritis and osteoarthritis*

Melpaque HP cream ℞ *hyperpigmentation bleaching agent; sunscreen* [hydroquinone in a sunblock base] 4%

melperone INN, BAN

melphalan (MPL) USAN, USP, INN, BAN, JAN *nitrogen mustard-type alkylating antineoplastic for multiple myeloma (orphan) and ovarian cancer; investigational (orphan) for metastatic melanoma*

Melquin HP cream ℞ *hyperpigmentation bleaching agent* [hydroquinone] 4%

memantine INN *investigational (Phase II/III) NMDA antagonist for chronic pain of peripheral diabetic neuropathy; investigational (Phase III) cognition adjuvant for Alzheimer's disease and AIDS dementia*

Memorette (trademarked packaging form) *patient compliance package*

memotine INN *antiviral* [also: memotine HCl]

memotine HCl USAN *antiviral* [also: memotine]

menabitan INN *analgesic* [also: menabitan HCl]

menabitan HCl USAN *analgesic* [also: menabitan]

menadiol BAN *vitamin K₄; prothrombogenic* [also: menadiol sodium diphosphate]

menadiol sodium diphosphate USP *vitamin K₄; prothrombogenic* [also: menadiol]

menadiol sodium sulfate INN

menadione USP *vitamin K₃; prothrombogenic*

menadione sodium bisulfite USP, INN

Menadol tablets OTC *nonsteroidal antiinflammatory drug (NSAID); antiarthritic; analgesic* [ibuprofen] 200 mg

menaphthene [see: menadione]

menaphthone [see: menadione]

menaphthone sodium bisulfite [see: menadione sodium bisulfite]

menaquinone *vitamin K₂; prothrombogenic*

menatetrenone INN

menbutone INN, BAN

mendelevium *element (Md)*

Menest film-coated tablets ℞ *estrogen replacement therapy for postmenopausal disorders; palliative therapy for inoperable prostatic and breast cancer* [esterified estrogens] 0.3, 0.625, 1.25, 2.5 mg

menfegol INN

menglytate INN

menichlopholan [see: niclofolan]

Meni-D capsules ℞ *anticholinergic; antivertigo agent; motion sickness preventative* [meclizine HCl] 25 mg

meningococcal polysaccharide vaccine, group A USP *active bacterin for meningitis (Neisseria meningitidis)*

meningococcal polysaccharide vaccine, group C USP *active bacterin for meningitis (Neisseria meningitidis)*

meningococcal polysaccharide vaccine, group W-135 *active bacterin for meningitis (Neisseria meningitidis)*

meningococcal polysaccharide vaccine, group Y *active bacterin for meningitis (Neisseria meningitidis)*

Menispermum cocculus; M. lacunosum medicinal herb [see: levant berry]

menitrazepam INN

menoctone USAN, INN *antimalarial*

menogaril USAN, INN *antibiotic antineoplastic*

Menogen; Menogen H.S. tablets ℞ *estrogen/androgen for menopausal vasomotor symptoms* [esterified estrogens; methyltestosterone] 1.25•2.5 mg; 0.625•1.25 mg

Menomune-A/C/Y/W-135 powder for subcu injection ℞ *meningitis vaccine* [meningococcal polysaccharide vaccine, groups A, C, Y, and W-135] 200 μg/0.5 mL

Menoplex tablets OTC *analgesic; antipyretic; antihistamine* [acetaminophen; phenyltoloxamine citrate] 325•30 mg

Menorest transdermal patch ℞ *investigational estrogen replacement therapy to increase bone mineral density and prevent osteoporosis in postmenopausal women* [estradiol]

menotropins USAN, USP *gonadotropin; gonad-stimulating principle for the induction of ovulation in women and the stimulation of spermatogenesis in men*

menotropins & human luteinizing hormone (hLH), recombinant *investigational for chronic anovulation due to hypogonadotropic hypogonadism; orphan status withdrawn 1998*

Menrium 5-2; Menrium 5-4; Menrium 10-4 tablets (discontinued 1997) ℞ *estrogen replacement therapy for postmenopausal disorders; anxiolytic* [chlordiazepoxide; esterified estrogens] 5•0.2 mg; 5•0.4 mg; 10•0.4 mg

Mentane ℞ *investigational (NDA filed) cholinesterase inhibitor for Alzheimer's disease; (approval denied by the FDA)* [velnacrine]

Mentax cream ℞ *topical benzylamine antifungal* [butenafine HCl] 1%

Mentha piperita medicinal herb [see: peppermint]

Mentha pulegium medicinal herb [see: pennyroyal]

Mentha spicata medicinal herb [see: spearmint]

menthol USP *topical analgesic and antipruritic; counterirritant; mild local anesthetic*

MenthoRub vaporizing ointment OTC *topical analgesic; counterirritant* [menthol; camphor; eucalyptus oil; oil of turpentine] 2.6% • 4.73% • 2 • 2

Menyanthes trifoliata medicinal herb [see: buckbean]

meobentine INN *antiarrhythmic* [also: meobentine sulfate]

meobentine sulfate USAN *antiarrhythmic* [also: meobentine]

mepacrine INN *anthelmintic; antimalarial* [also: quinacrine HCl]

mepacrine HCl [see: quinacrine HCl]

meparfynol [see: methylpentynol]

mepartricin USAN, INN *antifungal; antiprotozoal*

mepazine acetate [see: pecazine]

mepenzolate bromide USP, INN *peptic ulcer adjunct*

mepenzolate methylbromide [see: mepenzolate bromide]

mepenzolone bromide [see: mepenzolate bromide]

Mepergan injection ℞ *narcotic analgesic; sedative* [meperidine HCl; promethazine HCl] 25 • 25 mg/mL

Mepergan Fortis capsules ℞ *narcotic analgesic; sedative* [meperidine HCl; promethazine HCl] 50 • 25 mg

meperidine HCl USP *narcotic analgesic; also abused as a street drug* [also: pethidine] 50, 100 mg oral; 50 mg/5 mL oral; 10, 25, 50, 75, 100 mg/mL injection ② meprobamate

Mephaquin ℞ *antimalarial for acute chloroquine-resistant malaria (orphan)* [mefloquine HCl]

mephenesin NF, INN

mephenhydramine [see: moxastine]

mephenoxalone INN

mephentermine INN *adrenergic; vasoconstrictor; vasopressor for hypotensive shock* [also: mephentermine sulfate]

mephentermine sulfate USP *adrenergic; vasoconstrictor; vasopressor for hypotensive shock* [also: mephentermine]

mephenytoin USAN, USP, INN *hydantoin anticonvulsant* [also: methoin] ② Mephyton; Mesantoin

mephobarbital USP, JAN *anticonvulsant; sedative* [also: methylphenobarbital; methylphenobarbitone]

Mephyton tablets ℞ *coagulant; correct anticoagulant-induced prothrombin deficiency; vitamin K supplement* [phytonadione] 5 mg ② mephenytoin; methadone

mepicycline [see: pipacycline]

MEPIG (mucoid exopolysaccharide *Pseudomonas* **[hyper]-immune globulin)** [q.v.]

mepindolol INN, BAN

mepiperphenidol bromide

mepiprazole INN, BAN

mepirizole [see: epirizole]

mepiroxol INN

mepitiostane INN

mepivacaine INN *local anesthetic* [also: mepivacaine HCl]

mepivacaine HCl USP *local anesthetic* [also: mepivacaine] 1%, 2% injection

mepixanox INN

mepramidil INN

meprednisone USAN, USP, INN

meprobamate USP, INN, BAN, JAN *sedative; hypnotic; anxiolytic; minor tranquilizer; also abused as a street drug* 200, 400 mg oral ② meperidine

Meprogesic Q tablets (discontinued 1995) ℞ *analgesic; antipyretic; antiinflammatory; anxiolytic* [aspirin; meprobamate] 325 • 200 mg

Mepron film-coated tablets (discontinued 1995) ℞ *antiprotozoal for AIDS-related Pneumocystis carinii pneumonia (PCP)* [atovaquone] 250 mg ② Lupron; Napron

Mepron oral suspension ℞ *antiprotozoal for Pneumocystis carinii pneumo-*

nia (orphan); investigational (orphan) for Toxoplasma gondii encephalitis [atovaquone] 750 mg/5 mL ☑ Lupron; Napron

meproscillarin INN, BAN

Meprospan sustained-release capsules (discontinued 1997) ℞ anxiolytic [meprobamate] 200, 400 mg ☑ Naprosyn

meprothixol BAN [also: meprotixol]

meprotixol INN [also: meprothixol]

meprylcaine INN local anesthetic [also: meprylcaine HCl]

meprylcaine HCl USP local anesthetic [also: meprylcaine]

meptazinol INN, BAN analgesic [also: meptazinol HCl]

meptazinol HCl USAN analgesic [also: meptazinol]

mepyramine INN, BAN antihistamine [also: pyrilamine maleate]

mepyramine maleate [see: pyrilamine maleate]

mepyrium [see: amprolium]

mepyrrotazine [see: dimelazine]

mequidox USAN, INN antibacterial

mequinol INN

mequitamium iodide INN

mequitazine INN, BAN

mequitazium iodide [see: mequitamium iodide]

meragidone sodium

meralein sodium USAN, INN topical anti-infective

meralluride NF, INN

merbaphen USP

merbromin NF, INN general antiseptic

mercaptamine INN antiurolithic [also: cysteamine]

mercaptoarsenical [see: arsthinol]

mercaptoarsenol [see: arsthinol]

mercaptoethylamine (MEA) [see: mercaptamine]

mercaptomerin (MT6) INN [also: mercaptomerin sodium]

mercaptomerin sodium USP [also: mercaptomerin]

mercaptopurine (6-MP) USP, INN antimetabolite antineoplastic

mercuderamide INN

mercufenol chloride USAN topical anti-infective

mercumatilin sodium INN

mercuric oxide, yellow NF ophthalmic antiseptic (FDA ruled it "not safe and effective" in 1992)

mercuric salicylate NF

mercuric succinimide NF

mercurobutol INN

Mercurochrome solution OTC antiseptic [merbromin] 2%

mercurophylline NF, INN

mercurous chloride [see: calomel]

mercury element (Hg)

mercury, ammoniated USP topical anti-infective; antipsoriatic

mercury amide chloride [see: mercury, ammoniated]

mercury oleate NF

merethoxylline procaine

mergocriptine INN

Meridia capsules ℞ anorexiant for the treatment of obesity [sibutramine HCl] 5, 10, 15 mg

merisoprol acetate Hg 197 USAN radioactive agent

merisoprol acetate Hg 203 USAN radioactive agent

merisoprol Hg 197 USAN renal function test; radioactive agent

Meritene powder OTC enteral nutritional therapy [milk-based formula]

meropenem USAN, INN, BAN broad-spectrum carbapenem antibiotic for intra-abdominal infections and bacterial meningitis

Merrem powder for IV infusion ℞ broad-spectrum carbapenem antibiotic for intra-abdominal infections and bacterial meningitis [meropenem] 500, 1000 mg

mersalyl INN

mersalyl sodium [see: mersalyl]

Mersol solution, tincture OTC antiseptic; antibacterial; antifungal [thimerosal] 1:1000

mertiatide INN

Meruvax II powder for subcu injection ℞ rubella vaccine [rubella virus vaccine, live] 0.5 mL

mesabolone INN

mesalamine USAN *anti-inflammatory; treatment of ulcerative colitis and proctitis* [also: mesalazine]

mesalazine INN, BAN *anti-inflammatory; treatment of ulcerative colitis and proctitis* [also: mesalamine]

Mesantoin tablets ℞ *hydantoin anticonvulsant* [mephenytoin] 100 mg ② mephenytoin; Mestinon; Metatensin

mescaline *hallucinogenic street drug derived from the flowering heads (mescal buttons) of a Mexican cactus* ② meclizine

Mescolor film-coated, sustained-release tablets ℞ *decongestant; antihistamine; anticholinergic* [pseudoephedrine HCl; chlorpheniramine maleate; methscopolamine nitrate] 120•8•2.5 mg

meseclazone USAN, INN *anti-inflammatory*

mesifilcon A USAN *hydrophilic contact lens material*

mesilate INN *combining name for radicals or groups* [also: mesylate]

mesna USAN, INN, BAN *urotoxic antidote for hemorrhagic cystitis (orphan); investigational (orphan) for cyclophosphamide-induced urotoxicity*

Mesnex IV injection ℞ *urotoxic antidote for hemorrhagic cystitis (orphan); investigational (orphan) for cyclophosphamide-induced urotoxicity* [mesna] 100 mg/mL

mesocarb INN

meso-inositol [see: inositol]

meso-NDGA (nordihydroguaiaretic acid) [see: masoprocol]

meso-nordihydroguaiaretic acid (NDGA) [see: masoprocol]

mesoridazine USAN, INN *phenothiazine antipsychotic*

mesoridazine besylate USP *phenothiazine antipsychotic*

mespiperone C 11 USAN *radiopharmaceutical imaging aid for PET scans of the brain (produced at bedside for immediate administration)*

mespirenone INN

mestanolone INN, BAN

mestenediol [see: methandriol]

mesterolone USAN, INN, BAN *androgen; also abused as a street drug*

Mestinon tablets, Timespan (sustained-release tablets), syrup, IM or IV injection ℞ *cholinergic/anticholinesterase muscle stimulant; muscle relaxant reversal* [pyridostigmine bromide] 60 mg; 180 mg; 60 mg/5 mL; 5 mg/mL ② Mesantoin; Metatensin

mestranol USAN, USP, INN *estrogen*

mesudipine INN

mesulergine INN

mesulfamide INN

mesulfen INN [also: mesulphen]

mesulphen BAN [also: mesulfen]

mesuprine INN *vasodilator; smooth muscle relaxant* [also: mesuprine HCl]

mesuprine HCl USAN *vasodilator; smooth muscle relaxant* [also: mesuprine]

mesuximide INN *anticonvulsant* [also: methsuximide]

mesylate USAN, USP, BAN *combining name for radicals or groups* [also: mesilate]

metabromsalan USAN, INN *disinfectant*

metabutethamine HCl NF

metabutoxycaine HCl NF

metacetamol INN, BAN

metaclazepam INN

metacycline INN *antibacterial* [also: methacycline]

metaglycodol INN

metahexamide INN

metahexanamide [see: metahexamide]

Metahydrin tablets ℞ *diuretic; antihypertensive* [trichlormethiazide] 4 mg ② Metandren

metalkonium chloride INN

metallibure INN *anterior pituitary activator for swine* [also: methallibure]

metalol HCl USAN *antiadrenergic (β-receptor)*

metamelfalan INN

metamfazone INN [also: methamphazone]

metamfepramone INN [also: dimepropion]

metamfetamine INN *CNS stimulant; widely abused as a street drug* [also: methamphetamine HCl]

metamizole sodium INN *analgesic; antipyretic* [also: dipyrone]

metampicillin INN

Metamucil effervescent powder OTC *bulk laxative; antacid* [psyllium hydrophilic mucilloid; sodium bicarbonate; potassium bicarbonate] 3.4•2•2 g/packet

Metamucil powder, wafers OTC *bulk laxative* [psyllium hydrophilic mucilloid] 3.4 g/tsp.; 1.7 g

metandienone INN [also: methandrostenolone; methandienone]

metanixin INN

metaoxedrine chloride [see: phenylephrine HCl]

metaphosphoric acid, potassium salt [see: potassium metaphosphate]

metaphosphoric acid, trisodium salt [see: sodium trimetaphosphate]

metaphyllin [see: aminophylline]

metapramine INN

Metaprel syrup (discontinued 1999) ℞ *sympathomimetic bronchodilator* [metaproterenol sulfate] 10 mg/5 mL

Metaprel tablets, inhalation aerosol powder, solution for inhalation (discontinued 1996) ℞ *sympathomimetic bronchodilator* [metaproterenol sulfate] 10, 20 mg; 0.65 mg/dose; 0.4%, 0.6%, 5%

metaproterenol polistirex USAN *sympathomimetic bronchodilator* [also: orciprenaline] ② metoprolol

metaproterenol sulfate USAN, USP *sympathomimetic bronchodilator* 10, 20 mg oral; 10 mg/5 mL oral; 0.4%, 0.6%, 5% inhalation

metaradrine bitartrate [see: metaraminol bitartrate]

metaraminol INN *adrenergic; vasopressor for acute hypotensive shock, anaphylaxis, or traumatic shock* [also: metaraminol bitartrate]

metaraminol bitartrate USP *adrenergic; vasopressor for acute hypotensive*

shock, anaphylaxis, or traumatic shock [also: metaraminol]

Metaret injection ℞ *investigational (NDA filed, orphan) growth factor antagonist for prostate cancer* [suramin hexasodium] 600 mg

Metastat ℞ *investigational agent for inhibition of cancer invasion and metastases*

Metastron IV injection ℞ *analgesic for metastatic bone pain* [strontium chloride Sr 89] 10.9–22.6 mg/mL (4 mCi)

Metatensin #2; Metatensin #4 tablets ℞ *antihypertensive* [trichlormethiazide; reserpine] 2•0.1 mg; 4•0.1 mg ② Mesantoin; Mestinon

metaterol INN

metaxalone USAN, INN, BAN *skeletal muscle relaxant* ② metolazone

metazamide INN

metazepium iodide [see: buzepide metiodide]

metazide INN

metazocine INN, BAN

metbufen INN

metcaraphen HCl

metembonate INN *combining name for radicals or groups*

meteneprost USAN, INN *oxytocic; prostaglandin*

metenolone INN *anabolic steroid; also abused as a street drug* [also: methenolone acetate; methenolone; metenolone acetate]

metenolone acetate JAN *anabolic steroid; also abused as a street drug* [also: methenolone acetate; metenolone; methenolone]

metenolone enanthate JAN *anabolic steroid; also abused as a street drug* [also: methenolone enanthate]

Metered Solution Inhaler (MSI) *investigational (Phase I/II) pulmonary delivery device for asthma*

metergoline INN, BAN

metergotamine INN

metescufylline INN

metesculetol INN

metesind glucuronate USAN *specific thymidylate synthase (TS) inhibitor antineoplastic* ⑫ medicine

metethoheptazine INN

metetoin INN *anticonvulsant* [also: methetoin]

metformin USAN, INN, BAN *biguanide antidiabetic* [also: metformin HCl]

metformin HCl USAN, JAN *biguanide antidiabetic* [also: metformin]

methacholine bromide NF

methacholine chloride USP, INN *cholinergic; bronchoconstrictor for pulmonary challenge tests*

methacrylic acid copolymer NF *tablet-coating agent*

methacycline USAN *antibacterial* [also: metacycline]

methacycline HCl USP *gram-negative and gram-positive bacteriostatic; antirickettsial*

methadol [see: dimepheptanol]

methadone INN *narcotic analgesic; narcotic addiction detoxicant; often abused as a street drug* [also: methadone HCl] ⑫ Mephyton

methadone HCl USP *narcotic analgesic; narcotic addiction detoxicant; often abused as a street drug* [also: methadone] 5, 10, 40 mg oral; 5, 10 mg/5 mL oral; 10 mg/mL oral

methadonium chloride [see: methadone HCl]

Methadose tablets, oral concentrate, powder ℞ *narcotic analgesic; narcotic addiction detoxicant; often abused as a street drug* [methadone HCl] 5, 10, 40 mg; 10 mg/mL; 50, 100, 500, 1000 g

methadyl acetate USAN *narcotic analgesic* [also: acetylmethadol]

methafilcon B USAN *hydrophilic contact lens material*

Methagual OTC *counterirritant* [methyl salicylate; guaiacol] 8%•2%

Methalgen cream OTC *topical analgesic; counterirritant* [methyl salicylate; menthol; camphor; mustard oil]

methallenestril INN

methallenestrol [see: methallenestril]

methallibure USAN *anterior pituitary activator for swine* [also: metallibure]

methalthiazide USAN *diuretic; antihypertensive*

methamoctol

methamphazone BAN [also: metamfazone]

methamphetamine HCl USP *CNS stimulant; widely abused as a street drug* [also: metamfetamine]

methampyrone [now: dipyrone]

methanabol [see: methandriol]

methandienone BAN [also: methandrostenolone; metandienone]

methandriol

methandrostenolone USP *steroid; discontinued for human use, but the veterinary product is still available and sometimes abused as a street drug* [also: metandienone; methandienone]

methaniazide INN

methanol [see: methyl alcohol]

methantheline bromide USP *peptic ulcer adjunct* [also: methanthelinium bromide]

methanthelinium bromide INN, BAN *anticholinergic* [also: methantheline bromide]

methaphenilene INN, BAN [also: methaphenilene HCl]

methaphenilene HCl NF [also: methaphenilene]

methapyrilene INN [also: methapyrilene fumarate]

methapyrilene fumarate USP [also: methapyrilene]

methapyrilene HCl USP

methaqualone USAN, USP, INN, BAN *hypnotic; sedative; widely abused as a street drug, which leads to dependence*

methaqualone HCl USP

metharbital USP, INN, JAN *anticonvulsant* [also: metharbitone]

metharbitone BAN *anticonvulsant* [also: metharbital]

methastyridone INN

Methatropic capsules OTC *dietary lipotropic with vitamin supplementation* [choline; inositol; methionine; multiple B vitamins] 115•83•110•≛ mg

methazolamide USP, INN *carbonic anhydrase inhibitor for glaucoma* 25, 50 mg oral

Methblue 65 tablets ℞ *urinary antiinfective and antiseptic; antidote to cyanide poisoning* [methylene blue] 65 mg

methcathinone *a highly addictive manufactured street drug similar to cathinone, with amphetamine-like effects* [see also: cathinone; *Catha edulis*]

methdilazine USP, INN *phenothiazine antihistamine; antipruritic*

methdilazine HCl USP *phenothiazine antihistamine; antipruritic*

methenamine USP, INN *urinary antibiotic* ⧄ methionine

methenamine hippurate USAN, USP *urinary antibiotic* [also: hexamine hippurate]

methenamine mandelate USP *urinary antibiotic* 0.5, 1 g oral; 0.5 g/5 mL oral

methenamine sulfosalicylate *topical antipsoriatic*

methenolone BAN *anabolic steroid; also abused as a street drug* [also: methenolone acetate; metenolone; metenolone acetate]

methenolone acetate USAN *anabolic steroid; also abused as a street drug* [also: metenolone; methenolone; metenolone acetate]

methenolone enanthate USAN *anabolic steroid; also abused as a street drug* [also: metenolone enanthate]

metheptazine INN

Methergine coated tablets, IV or IM injection ℞ *oxytocic for induction of labor, control of postpartum uterine atony, and postpartum hemorrhage* [methylergonovine maleate] 0.2 mg; 0.2 mg/mL

methestrol INN

methetharimide [see: bemegride]

methetoin USAN *anticonvulsant* [also: metetoin]

methicillin sodium USAN, USP *penicillinase-resistant penicillin antibiotic* [also: meticillin]

methimazole USP *thyroid inhibitor* [also: thiamazole]

methindizate BAN [also: metindizate]

methiodal sodium USP, INN

methiomeprazine INN

methiomeprazine HCl [see: methiomeprazine]

methionine (DL-methionine) NF, JAN *urinary acidifier* [also: racemethionine] 500 mg oral

methionine (L-methionine) USAN, USP, INN, JAN *essential amino acid; symbols: Met, M; investigational (orphan) for AIDS myelopathy* ⧄ methenamine

methionine-enkephalin *investigational (Phase I) immunomodulator for AIDS*

methionyl neurotropic factor, brain-derived, recombinant *investigational (orphan) for amyotrophic lateral sclerosis*

methionyl stem cell factor, recombinant human *investigational (orphan) for progressive bone marrow failure*

methionyl stem cell factor, recombinant human & filgrastim *investigational adjunct to myelosuppressive or myeloablative therapy; orphan status withdrawn 1998*

methiothepin [see: metitepine]

methisazone USAN *antiviral* [also: metisazone]

methisoprinol [now: inosine pranobex]

methitural INN

methixene HCl USAN *smooth muscle relaxant* [also: metixene] ⧄ methoxsalen

methocamphone methylsulfate [see: trimethidinium methosulfate]

methocarbamol USP, INN, BAN, JAN *skeletal muscle relaxant* 500, 750 mg oral; 100 mg/mL injection

methocidin INN

methohexital USP, INN *barbiturate general anesthetic* [also: methohexitone]

methohexital sodium USP *barbiturate general anesthetic*

methohexitone BAN *barbiturate general anesthetic* [also: methohexital]

methoin BAN *anticonvulsant* [also: mephenytoin]

methonaphthone [see: menbutone]

methophedrine [see: methoxyphedrine]
methophenazine [see: metofenazate]
methopholine USAN analgesic [also: metofoline]
methoprene INN
methopromazine INN
methopromazine maleate [see: methopromazine]
methopyrimazole [see: epirizole]
d-methorphan [see: dextromethorphan]
d-methorphan hydrobromide [see: dextromethorphan hydrobromide]
methoserpidine INN, BAN
methotrexate (MTX) USAN, USP, INN, BAN, JAN antimetabolite antineoplastic; antirheumatic; systemic antipsoriatic; investigational (orphan) for juvenile rheumatoid arthritis 2.5 mg oral; 1 g injection
methotrexate & laurocapram investigational (orphan) for topical treatment of Mycosis fungoides
methotrexate & leucovorin antineoplastic for osteosarcoma (orphan)
Methotrexate LPF Sodium preservative-free injection (discontinued 1994) ℞ antimetabolite antineoplastic for leukemia; systemic antipsoriatic; antirheumatic [methotrexate sodium] 1 g
methotrexate sodium USP antirheumatic; systemic antipsoriatic; antimetabolite antineoplastic for osteogenic sarcoma (orphan) 2.5 mg oral; 20, 1000 mg/vial injection; 2.5, 25 mg/mL injection
methotrimeprazine USAN, USP central analgesic; CNS depressant [also: levomepromazine]
methoxamine INN adrenergic; vasoconstrictor; vasopressor for hypotensive shock during surgery [also: methoxamine HCl]
methoxamine HCl USP adrenergic; vasoconstrictor; vasopressor for hypotensive shock during surgery [also: methoxamine]
methoxiflurane [see: methoxyflurane]
methoxsalen (8-methoxsalen) USP repigmentation agent for vitiligo; antipsoriatic; palliative treatment for cuta-

neous T-cell lymphoma (CTCL); investigational (orphan) for diffuse systemic sclerosis and cardiac allografts ☒ methixene
methoxy polyethylene glycol [see: polyethylene glycol monomethyl ether]
8-methoxycarbonyloctyl oligosaccharides investigational (Phase III) E. coli neutralizer for traveler's diarrhea and hemolytic uremic syndrome (HUS)
methoxyfenoserpin [see: mefeserpine]
methoxyflurane USAN, USP, INN, BAN inhalation general anesthetic
methoxyphedrine INN
p-methoxyphenacyl [see: anisatil]
methoxyphenamine INN [also: methoxyphenamine HCl]
methoxyphenamine HCl USP [also: methoxyphenamine]
4-methoxyphenol [see: mequinol]
o-methoxyphenyl salicylate acetate [see: guacetisal]
methoxypromazine maleate [see: methopromazine]
8-methoxypsoralen (8-MOP) [see: methoxsalen]
5-methoxyresorcinol [see: flamenol]
methphenoxydiol [see: guaifenesin]
methscopolamine bromide USP GI antispasmodic; peptic ulcer adjunct [also: hyoscine methobromide]
methscopolamine nitrate anticholinergic
methsuximide USP, BAN anticonvulsant [also: mesuximide]
methyclothiazide USAN, USP, INN diuretic; antihypertensive 2.5, 5 mg oral
methydromorphine [see: methyldihydromorphine]
methyl alcohol NF solvent
methyl benzoquate BAN coccidiostat for poultry [also: nequinate]
methyl cresol [see: cresol]
methyl cysteine [see: mecysteine]
methyl p-hydroxybenzoate [see: methylparaben]
methyl isobutyl ketone NF alcohol denaturant
methyl nicotinate USAN

methyl palmoxirate USAN *antidiabetic*

methyl phthalate [see: dimethyl phthalate]

methyl salicylate NF *flavoring agent; counterirritant; topical anesthetic*

methyl sulfoxide [see: dimethyl sulfoxide]

methyl violet [see: gentian violet]

l-**methylaminoethanolcatechol** [see: epinephrine]

methylaminopterin [see: methotrexate]

methylandrostenediol [see: methandriol]

methylatropine nitrate USAN *anticholinergic* [also: atropine methonitrate]

methylbenactyzium bromide INN

methylbenzethonium chloride USP, INN *topical anti-infective/antiseptic*

α-**methylbenzylhydrazine** [see: mebanazine]

methylcarbamate of salicylanilide [see: anilamate]

methyl-CCNU (chloroethyl-cyclohexyl-nitrosourea) [see: semustine]

methylcellulose USP, INN *ophthalmic moisturizer; suspending and viscosity-increasing agent*

methylcellulose, propylene glycol ether of [see: hydroxypropyl methylcellulose]

methylchromone INN, BAN

methyldesorphine INN, BAN

methyldigoxin [see: metildigoxin]

methyldihydromorphine INN

methyldihydromorphinone HCl [see: metopon]

methyldinitrobenzamide [see: dinitolmide]

methyldioxatrine [see: meletimide]

N-**methyldiphenethylamine** [see: demelverine]

α-**methyl-DL-thyroxine ethyl ester** [see: etiroxate]

methyldopa USAN, USP, INN, BAN, JAN *centrally acting antiadrenergic antihypertensive* 125, 250, 500 mg oral ⊡ levodopa

α-**methyldopa** [now: methyldopa]

methyldopate BAN *centrally acting antiadrenergic antihypertensive* [also: methyldopate HCl]

methyldopate HCl USAN, USP *centrally acting antiadrenergic antihypertensive* [also: methyldopate] 50 mg/mL injection

6-methylenandrosta-1,4-diene-3,17-dione *orphan status withdrawn 1996*

methylene blue (MB) USP *antimethemoglobinemic; GU antiseptic; antidote to cyanide poisoning; diagnostic aid for gastric secretions* [also: methylthioninium chloride] 65 mg oral; 10 mg/mL injection

methylene chloride NF *solvent*

methylene diphosphonate (MDP) [now: medronate disodium]

methylenedioxyamphetamine (MDA) [see: MDMA, MDEA]

3,4-methylenedioxyethamphetamine (MDEA) [q.v.]

3,4-methylenedioxymethamphetamine (MDMA) [q.v.]

6-methyleneoxytetracycline (MOTC) [see: methacycline]

methylenprednisolone [see: prednylidene]

methylergometrine INN *oxytocic* [also: methylergonovine maleate]

methylergometrine maleate [see: methylergonovine maleate]

methylergonovine maleate USP *oxytocic for induction of labor* [also: methylergometrine]

methylergonovinium bimaleate [see: methylergonovine maleate]

methylergotamine [see: metergotamine]

methylestrenolone [see: normethandrone]

methyl-GAG (methylglyoxal-*bis*-guanylhydrazone) [see: mitoguazone]

methylglyoxal-*bis*-guanylhydrazone (methyl-GAG; MGBG) [see: mitoguazone]

1-methylhexylamine [see: tuaminoheptane]

l-methylhexylamine sulfate [see: tuaminoheptane sulfate]

N-methylhydrazine [see: procarbazine]

Methylin tablets ℞ *CNS stimulant for attention deficit hyperactivity disorders (ADHD) and narcolepsy* [methylphenidate HCl] 5, 10, 20 mg

methylmorphine [see: codeine]

methylnaltrexone *investigational treatment for chronic opioid-induced constipation; orphan status withdrawn 1998*

methyl-nitro-imidazole [see: carnidazole]

methylnortestosterone [see: normethandrone]

methylparaben USAN, NF *antifungal agent; preservative*

methylparaben sodium USAN, NF *antimicrobial preservative*

methylparafynol [see: meparfynol]

methylpentynol INN, BAN

methylperidol [see: moperone]

(+)-methylphenethylamine [see: dextroamphetamine]

(–)-methylphenethylamine [see: levamphetamine]

methylphenethylamine HCl [see: amphetamine HCl]

methylphenethylamine phosphate [see: amphetamine phosphate]

(–)-methylphenethylamine succinate [see: levamfetamine succinate]

methylphenethylamine sulfate [see: amphetamine sulfate]

(+)-methylphenethylamine sulfate [see: dextroamphetamine sulfate]

methylphenidate INN, BAN *CNS stimulant for attention deficit hyperactivity disorder (ADHD) and narcolepsy; also abused as a street drug* [also: methylphenidate HCl]

d-methylphenidate HCl (d-MPH) *investigational (Phase III) stimulant for attention deficit hyperactivity disorder*

methylphenidate HCl (MPH) USP, JAN *CNS stimulant for attention deficit hyperactivity disorder (ADHD) and narcolepsy; also abused as a street drug* [also: methylphenidate] 5, 10, 20 mg oral

methylphenobarbital INN *anticonvulsant; sedative* [also: mephobarbital; methylphenobarbitone]

methylphenobarbitone BAN *anticonvulsant; sedative* [also: mephobarbital; methylphenobarbital]

d-methylphenylamine sulfate [see: dextroamphetamine sulfate]

methylphytyl napthoquinone [see: phytonadione]

methylprednisolone USP, INN, BAN, JAN *corticosteroid; anti-inflammatory; immunosuppressant* 4, 16 mg oral

methylprednisolone aceponate INN

methylprednisolone acetate USP, JAN *corticosteroid; anti-inflammatory; immunosuppressant* 20, 40, 80 mg/mL injection

methylprednisolone hemisuccinate USP *corticosteroid; anti-inflammatory*

methylprednisolone sodium phosphate USAN *corticosteroid; anti-inflammatory* 40, 125, 500, 1000 mg/ vial injection

methylprednisolone sodium succinate USP, JAN *corticosteroid; anti-inflammatory; immunosuppressant*

methylprednisolone suleptanate USAN, INN *corticosteroid; anti-inflammatory*

methylpromazine

4-methylpyrazole (4-MP) [see: fomepizole]

methylrosaniline chloride [now: gentian violet]

methylrosanilinium chloride INN *topical anti-infective* [also: gentian violet]

methylscopolamine bromide [see: methscopolamine bromide]

methylsulfate USP *combining name for radicals or groups* [also: metilsulfate]

methyltestosterone USP, INN, BAN *oral androgen; hormonal antineoplastic for female breast cancer; also abused as a street drug* 10, 25 mg oral

methyltheobromine [see: caffeine]

methylthionine chloride [see: methylene blue]

methylthionine HCl [see: methylene blue]

methylthioninium chloride INN *anti-methemoglobinemic; antidote to cyanide poisoning* [also: methylene blue]

methylthiouracil USP, INN

methyltrienolone [see: metribolone]

methynodiol diacetate USAN *progestin* [also: metynodiol]

methyprylon USP, INN *sedative; hypnotic* [also: methprylone]

methyprylone BAN *sedative* [also: methyprylon]

methyridene BAN [also: metyridine]

methysergide USAN, INN, BAN *migraine-specific vasoconstrictor and peripheral serotonin antagonist for the prophylaxis of vascular headaches*

methysergide maleate USP *migraine-specific vasoconstrictor and peripheral serotonin antagonist for the prophylaxis of vascular headaches*

metiamide USAN, INN *antagonist to histamine H_2 receptors*

metiapine USAN, INN *antipsychotic*

metiazinic acid INN

metibride INN

meticillin INN *penicillinase-resistant penicillin antibiotic* [also: methicillin sodium]

meticillin sodium *penicillinase-resistant penicillin antibiotic* [see: methicillin sodium]

Meticorten tablets ℞ *corticosteroid; anti-inflammatory; immunosuppressant* [prednisone] 1 mg

meticrane INN

metildigoxin INN

metilsulfate INN *combining name for radicals or groups* [also: methylsulfate]

Metimyd eye drop suspension, ophthalmic ointment ℞ *topical ophthalmic corticosteroidal anti-inflammatory; antibiotic* [prednisolone acetate; sulfacetamide sodium] 0.5% • 10%

metindizate INN [also: methindizate]

metioprim USAN, INN, BAN *antibacterial*

metioxate INN

metipirox INN

metipranolol USAN, INN, BAN *topical antiglaucoma agent (β-blocker)*

metipranolol HCl *topical antiglaucoma agent (β-blocker)*

metiprenaline INN

metirosine INN *antihypertensive* [also: metyrosine]

metisazone INN *antiviral* [also: methisazone]

metitepine INN

metixene INN *smooth muscle relaxant* [also: methixene HCl]

metixene HCl [see: methixene HCl]

metizoline INN *adrenergic; vasoconstrictor* [also: metizoline HCl]

metizoline HCl USAN *adrenergic; vasoconstrictor* [also: metizoline]

metkefamide INN *analgesic* [also: metkephamid acetate]

metkefamide acetate [see: metkephamid acetate]

metkephamid acetate USAN *analgesic* [also: metkefamide]

metochalcone INN

metocinium iodide INN

metoclopramide INN, BAN, JAN *antiemetic for chemotherapy; GI stimulant; antidopaminergic; radiosensitizer* [also: metoclopramide HCl]

metoclopramide HCl USAN, USP, JAN *antiemetic for chemotherapy; GI stimulant; antidopaminergic; radiosensitizer* [also: metoclopramide] 5, 10 mg oral; 5, 10 mg/5 mL oral; 10 mg/mL oral; 5 mg/mL injection

metoclopramide monohydrochloride monohydrate [see: metoclopramide HCl]

metocurine iodide USAN, USP *neuromuscular blocker; muscle relaxant* 2 mg/mL injection

metofenazate INN

metofoline INN *analgesic* [also: methopholine]

metogest USAN, INN *hormone*

metolazone USAN, INN *antihypertensive; diuretic* ⑨ metaxalone

metomidate INN, BAN

metopimazine USAN, INN *antiemetic*

Metopirone softgels ℞ *diagnostic aid for pituitary function* [metyrapone] 250 mg ⑨ metyrapone

metopon INN
metopon HCl [see: metopon]
metoprine USAN *antineoplastic*
metoprolol USAN, INN, BAN *antihypertensive; antiadrenergic (β-receptor)* ② metaproterenol
metoprolol fumarate USAN *antihypertensive; antiadrenergic (β-receptor)*
metoprolol succinate USAN *antianginal; antihypertensive; antiadrenergic (β-receptor)*
metoprolol tartrate USAN, USP *antihypertensive; antiadrenergic (β-receptor)* 50, 100 mg oral; 1 mg/mL injection
metoquizine USAN, INN *anticholinergic*
metoserpate INN *veterinary sedative* [also: metoserpate HCl]
metoserpate HCl USAN *veterinary sedative* [also: metoserpate]
metostilenol INN
metoxepin INN
metoxiestrol [see: moxestrol]
metrafazoline INN
metralindole INN
metrazifone INN
metrenperone USAN, INN, BAN *veterinary myopathic*
Metric 21 tablets (discontinued 1995) ℞ *antibiotic; antiprotozoal; amebicide* [metronidazole]
metrifonate INN *veterinary anthelmintic; investigational (NDA filed) acetylcholinesterase inhibitor for Alzheimer's dementia* [also: trichlorfon; metriphonate]
metrifudil INN
metriphonate BAN *veterinary anthelmintic* [also: trichlorfon; metrifonate]
metrizamide USAN, INN *parenteral radiopaque contrast medium (48.25% iodine)*
metrizoate sodium USAN *radiopaque contrast medium* [also: sodium metrizoate]
Metro I.V. ready-to-use injection ℞ *antibiotic; antiprotozoal; amebicide* [metronidazole] 500 mg/100 mL
MetroCream ℞ *topical antibiotic for rosacea* [metronidazole] 0.75%

Metrodin powder for IM injection (discontinued 1997) ℞ *ovulation stimulant in polycystic ovary disease (orphan)* [urofollitropin] 0.83, 1.66 mg/ampule
MetroGel; MetroLotion ℞ *antibacterial for rosacea (orphan); investigational (orphan) for decubitus ulcers and perioral dermatitis* [metronidazole] 0.75%
MetroGel Vaginal gel ℞ *antibacterial for bacterial vaginosis* [metronidazole] 0.75%
metronidazole USAN, USP, INN, BAN *antibiotic; antiprotozoal/amebicide; acne rosacea treatment (orphan); investigational (orphan) for decubitus ulcers and perioral dermatitis* 250, 500 mg oral; 500 mg/100 mL injection
metronidazole benzoate *antiprotozoal (Trichomonas)*
metronidazole HCl USAN *antibiotic; antiprotozoal; amebicide*
metronidazole phosphate USAN *antibacterial; antiprotozoal*
MET-Rx food bar, powder for drink OTC *enteral nutritional therapy* 100 g; 72 g
Metubine Iodide IV injection ℞ *neuromuscular blocker; anesthesia adjunct* [metocurine iodide] 2 mg/mL
metuclazepam [see: metaclazepam]
meturedepa USAN, INN *antineoplastic*
metynodiol INN *progestin* [also: methynodiol diacetate]
metynodiol diacetate [see: methynodiol diacetate]
metyrapone USAN, USP, INN *diagnostic aid for pituitary function* ② Metopirone; metyrosine
metyrapone tartrate USAN *pituitary function test*
metyridine INN [also: methyridene]
metyrosine USAN, USP *antihypertensive; pheochromocytomic agent* ② metyrapone
Mevacor tablets ℞ *HMG-CoA reductase inhibitor for hypercholesterolemia and atherosclerosis* [lovastatin] 10, 20, 40 mg
mevastatin INN
mevinolin [now: lovastatin]

mexafylline INN

mexazolam INN

mexenone INN, BAN

mexiletine INN, BAN *antiarrhythmic* [also: mexiletine HCl]

mexiletine HCl USAN, USP *antiarrhythmic* [also: mexiletine] 150, 200, 250 mg oral

mexiprostil INN

Mexitil capsules ℞ *antiarrhythmic* [mexiletine HCl] 150, 200, 250 mg

mexoprofen INN

Mexoryl SX *investigational UVA sunscreen* [ecamsule]

mexrenoate potassium USAN, INN *aldosterone antagonist*

Mexsana Medicated powder OTC *topical diaper rash treatment* [kaolin; zinc oxide; eucalyptus oil; camphor; corn starch]

mezacopride INN

mezepine INN

mezereon *(Daphne mezereum)* bark *medicinal herb used as a cathartic, diuretic, emetic, and rubefacient; eating the berries can be fatal, and people have been poisoned by eating birds that ate the berries*

mezilamine INN

Mezlin powder for IV or IM injection ℞ *extended-spectrum penicillin antibiotic* [mezlocillin sodium] 1, 2, 3, 4, 20 g ☒ Meclan

mezlocillin USAN, INN *extended-spectrum penicillin antibiotic*

mezlocillin sodium USP *extended-spectrum penicillin antibiotic*

MF (methotrexate [with leucovorin rescue], fluorouracil) *chemotherapy protocol*

MF (mitomycin, fluorouracil) *chemotherapy protocol*

MFP (melphalan, fluorouracil, medroxyprogesterone acetate) *chemotherapy protocol*

MG Cold Sore Formula solution OTC *topical oral anesthetic; antipruritic/counterirritant* [lidocaine; menthol] ≟•1%

MG217 Dual Treatment lotion OTC *topical antipsoriatic; antiseborrheic* [coal tar solution] 5%

MG217 Medicated conditioner OTC *topical antipsoriatic; antiseborrheic* [coal tar solution] 2%

MG217 Medicated ointment OTC *topical antipsoriatic; antiseborrheic; antifungal; keratolytic* [coal tar solution; colloidal sulfur; salicylic acid] 2%•1.1%•1.5%

MG217 Medicated shampoo OTC *topical antipsoriatic; antiseborrheic; antifungal; keratolytic* [coal tar solution; salicylic acid] 5%•2%

MG400 shampoo OTC *antiseborrheic; keratolytic* [salicylic acid; sulfur] 3%•5%

MGA (melengestrol acetate) [q.v.]

MGBG (methylglyoxal-*bis*-guanylhydrazone) [see: mitoguazone]

MGI-114 *investigational (Phase II) antineoplastic for hormone-refractory prostate and ovarian cancers*

MGW (magnesium sulfate + glycerin + water) enema [q.v.]

Miacalcin nasal spray ℞ *calcium regulator for postmenopausal osteoporosis (only)* [calcitonin (salmon)] 200 IU/0.09 mL dose

Miacalcin subcu or IM injection ℞ *calcium regulator for hypercalcemia, Paget's disease, and postmenopausal osteoporosis* [calcitonin (salmon)] 200 IU/mL

Mi-Acid gelcaps OTC *antacid* [calcium carbonate; magnesium carbonate] 311•232 mg

Mi-Acid; Mi-Acid II liquid OTC *antacid; antiflatulent* [aluminum hydroxide; magnesium hydroxide; simethicone] 200•200•20 mg/5 mL; 400•400•40 mg/5 mL

mianserin INN, BAN *serotonin inhibitor; antihistamine* [also: mianserin HCl]

mianserin HCl USAN, JAN *serotonin inhibitor; antihistamine* [also: mianserin]

mibefradil INN *vasodilator and calcium channel blocker for hypertension and* *chronic stable angina* [also: mibefradil dihydrochloride]

mibefradil dihydrochloride USAN *vasodilator and calcium channel blocker for hypertension and chronic stable angina* [also: mibefradil]

M^{131}IBG [now: iobenguane sulfate I 131]

MIBG-I-123 [see: iobenguane sulfate I 123]

mibolerone USAN, INN *anabolic; androgen*

Micanol Ⓒ (U.S. product: Lasan HP-1) cream OTC *topical antipsoriatic* [anthralin] 1%, 3%

Micardis tablets ℞ *long-acting antihypertensive; angiotensin II receptor antagonist* [telmisartan] 40, 80 mg

Micatin cream, powder, aerosol powder, liquid spray OTC *topical antifungal* [miconazole nitrate] 2%

MICE (mesna [rescue], ifosfamide, carboplatin, etoposide) *chemotherapy protocol* [also: ICE]

micinicate INN

Miconal cream ℞ *topical antipsoriatic* [anthralin] 1%

miconazole USP, INN, BAN, JAN *fungicidal*

miconazole nitrate USAN, USP, JAN *antifungal* 2% topical

Micrainin tablets ℞ *analgesic; antipyretic; anti-inflammatory; anxiolytic* [aspirin; meprobamate] 325•200 mg

MICRhoGAM IM injection ℞ *obstetric Rh factor immunity suppressant* [Rh$_0$(D) immune globulin] 50 μg ② microgram

microbubble contrast agent *investigational (orphan) neurosonographic diagnostic aid for intracranial tumors*

Microcaps (trademarked dosage form) *fast-melting tablets*

microcrystalline cellulose [see: cellulose, microcrystalline]

microcrystalline wax [see: wax, microcrystalline]

microfibrillar collagen hemostat (MCH) *topical local hemostatic*

Micro-K; Micro-K 10 Extencaps (controlled-release capsules) ℞ *potassium supplement* [potassium chloride] 600 mg (8 mEq); 750 mg (10 mEq)

Micro-K LS extended-release powder ℞ *potassium supplement* [potassium chloride] 20 mEq/packet

Microlipid emulsion OTC *dietary fat supplement* [safflower oil] 50%

Micronase tablets ℞ *sulfonylurea antidiabetic* [glyburide] 1.25, 2.5, 5 mg

microNefrin solution for inhalation OTC *sympathomimetic bronchodilator for bronchial asthma and COPD* [racepinephrine HCl] 2.25%

micronized aluminum *astringent*

Micronized Glyburide tablets ℞ *sulfonylurea antidiabetic* [glyburide] 1.5, 3 mg

micronomicin INN

Micronor tablets ℞ *oral contraceptive (progestin only)* [norethindrone] 0.35 mg

Microstix-3 reagent strips for professional use *in vitro diagnostic aid for nitrate, uropathogens, or bacteria in the urine*

MicroTrak Chlamydia trachomatis slide test for professional use *in vitro diagnostic aid for Chlamydia trachomatis*

MicroTrak HSV 1/HSV 2 Culture Identification/Typing Test culture test for professional use *in vitro diagnostic aid for herpes simplex virus in tissue cultures*

MicroTrak HSV 1/HSV 2 Direct Specimen Identification/Typing Test slide test for professional use *in vitro diagnostic aid for herpes simplex virus in external lesions*

MicroTrak Neisseria gonorrhoeae Culture Confirmation Test reagent kit for professional use *in vitro diagnostic aid for Neisseria gonorrhoeae*

Microzide capsules ℞ *once-daily antihypertensive; thiazide diuretic* [hydrochlorothiazide] 12.5 mg ② Maxzide

mictine [see: aminometradine]

midaflur USAN, INN *sedative*

midaglizole INN

midalcipran [see: milnacipran]

midamaline INN

Midamine (name changed to ProAmatine upon release in 1996)

Midamor tablets ℞ *antihypertensive; potassium-sparing diuretic* [amiloride HCl] 5 mg

midazogrel INN

midazolam INN, BAN, JAN *short-acting benzodiazepine general anesthetic* [also: midazolam HCl]

midazolam HCl USAN *short-acting benzodiazepine general anesthetic* [also: midazolam]

midazolam maleate USAN *intravenous anesthetic*

Midchlor capsules ℞ *vasoconstrictor; sedative; analgesic (for migraine)* [isometheptene mucate; dichloralphenazone; acetaminophen] 65•100•325 mg

midecamycin INN

midodrine INN, BAN *antihypotensive; vasoconstrictor; vasopressor for orthostatic hypotension (OH)* [also: midodrine HCl]

midodrine HCl USAN, JAN *antihypotensive; vasoconstrictor; vasopressor for orthostatic hypotension (orphan)* [also: midodrine]

Midol; Midol for Cramps caplets (discontinued 1995) OTC *analgesic; antipyretic; anti-inflammatory; muscle relaxant* [aspirin; caffeine; cinnamedrine HCl] 545•32.4•14.9 mg; 500•32.4•14.9 mg

Midol, Teen caplets OTC *analgesic; anti-inflammatory; diuretic* [acetaminophen; pamabrom] 400•25 mg

Midol 200 tablets (discontinued 1996) OTC *nonsteroidal anti-inflammatory drug (NSAID); antiarthritic; analgesic* [ibuprofen] 200 mg

Midol IB tablets OTC *nonsteroidal anti-inflammatory drug (NSAID); antiarthritic; analgesic* [ibuprofen] 200 mg

Midol Multi-Symptom Formula caplets OTC *analgesic; anti-inflammatory; antihistaminic sleep aid* [acetaminophen; pyrilamine maleate] 325•12.5 mg

Midol Multi-Symptom Menstrual caplets OTC *analgesic; anti-inflammatory; antihistaminic sleep aid* [acetaminophen; caffeine; pyrilamine maleate] 500•60•15 mg

Midol PM caplets OTC *analgesic; antipyretic; antihistaminic sleep aid* [acetaminophen; diphenhydramine] 500•25 mg

Midol PMS caplets, gelcaps OTC *analgesic; anti-inflammatory; diuretic; antihistaminic sleep aid* [acetaminophen; pamabrom; pyrilamine maleate] 500•25•15 mg

Midrin capsules ℞ *vasoconstrictor; sedative; analgesic (for migraine)* [isometheptene mucate; dichloralphenazone; acetaminophen] 65•100•325 mg ② Mydfrin

Midstream Pregnancy Test kit for home use OTC *in vitro diagnostic aid for urine pregnancy test*

MIFA (mitomycin, fluorouracil, Adriamycin) *chemotherapy protocol*

mifarmonab [see: imciromab pentetate]

Mifegyne (available in France, Sweden, and the U.K.) ℞ *abortifacient; investigational glucocorticosteroid antagonist for Cushing syndrome* [mifepristone]

mifentidine INN

mifepristone INN, BAN *progesterone antagonist; abortifacient; investigational (Phase III) for unresectable meningioma*

mifobate USAN, INN *antiatherosclerotic*

miglitol USAN, INN, BAN *antidiabetic agent for type 2 diabetes; α-glucosidase inhibitor that delays the digestion of dietary carbohydrates*

mignonette, Jamaica *medicinal herb* [see: henna (*Lawsonia*)]

Migranal nasal spray ℞ *rapid-acting antimigraine agent* [dihydroergotamine mesylate] 0.05 mg/spray

Migratine capsules ℞ *vasoconstrictor; sedative; analgesic (for migraine)* [isometheptene mucate; dichloralphenazone; acetaminophen] 65•100•325 mg

Miguard ℞ *investigational (NDA filed) 5-HT_{1B/1D} agonist for acute treatment of migraine* [frovatriptan succinate]

mikamycin INN, BAN

MiKasome ℞ *investigational (Phase II) liposomal formulation of the antibiotic amikacin for complicated urinary tract infections* [amikacin]

milacemide INN *anticonvulsant; antidepressant* [also: milacemide HCl]

milacemide HCl USAN *anticonvulsant; antidepressant* [also: milacemide]

milameline HCl USAN *partial muscarinic agonist for Alzheimer's disease*

mild silver protein [see: silver protein, mild]

milenperone USAN, INN, BAN *antipsychotic*

Miles Nervine caplets OTC *antihistaminic sleep aid* [diphenhydramine HCl] 25 mg

milfoil *medicinal herb* [see: yarrow]

milipertine USAN, INN *antipsychotic*

milk ipecac *medicinal herb* [see: birthroot; dogbane]

milk of bismuth [see: bismuth, milk of]

milk of magnesia [see: magnesia, milk of]

Milk of Magnesia-Cascara, Concentrated oral suspension OTC *antacid; laxative* [milk of magnesia; aromatic cascara fluidextract; alcohol 7%] 30•5 mL/15 mL

milk thistle *(Silybum marianum)* seeds *medicinal herb for Amanita mushroom poisoning, bronchitis, gallbladder disorders, hemorrhage, liver damage, peritonitis, spleen disorders, stomach disorders, and varicose veins*

Milkinol emulsion OTC *emollient laxative* [mineral oil]

milkweed *(Asclepias syriaca)* roots *medicinal herb used as a diuretic, emetic, purgative, and tonic*

milnacipran INN *investigational antidepressant*

milodistim USAN *antineutropenic; hematopoietic stimulant; granulocyte mac-rophage colony-stimulating factor (GM-CSF) + interleukin 3*

Milontin Kapseals (capsules) ℞ *anticonvulsant* [phensuximide] 500 mg ② Dilantin; Miltown; Mylanta

Milophene tablets (discontinued 1997) ℞ *ovulation stimulant* [clomiphene citrate] 50 mg

miloxacin INN

milrinone USAN, INN, BAN *cardiotonic*

milrinone lactate *vasodilator for congestive heart failure*

miltefosine INN

Miltown; Miltown-600 tablets ℞ *anxiolytic; also abused as a street drug* [meprobamate] 200, 400 mg; 600 mg ② Milontin

milverine INN

MIM D2A21 *investigational for sexually transmitted diseases*

mimbane INN *analgesic* [also: mimbane HCl]

mimbane HCl USAN *analgesic* [also: mimbane]

minalrestat USAN *aldose reductase inhibitor for diabetic neuropathy and other long-term diabetic complications*

minaprine USAN, INN, BAN *psychotropic*

minaprine HCl USAN *antidepressant*

minaxolone USAN, INN *anesthetic*

mindodilol INN

mindolic acid [see: clometacin]

mindoperone INN

MINE (mesna [rescue], ifosfamide, Novantrone, etoposide) *chemotherapy protocol*

MINE-ESHAP (alternating cycles of MINE and ESHAP) *chemotherapy protocol*

minepentate INN, BAN

Mineral Ice [see: Therapeutic Mineral Ice]

mineral oil USP *emollient/protectant; laxative; solvent*

mineral oil, light NF *tablet and capsule lubricant; vehicle*

mineralocorticoids *a class of adrenal cortical steroids that are used for partial replacement therapy in adrenocortical insufficiency*

Minesse ℞ *investigational low-dose oral contraceptive in a 24-day regimen* [ethinyl estradiol; gestodene]

Mini Thin Asthma Relief tablets OTC *decongestant; expectorant* [ephedrine HCl; guaifenesin] 25•100, 25•200 mg

Mini Thin Pseudo tablets OTC *nasal decongestant* [pseudoephedrine HCl] 60 mg

mini-BEAM (BCNU, etoposide, ara-C, melphalan) *chemotherapy protocol*

mini-COAP (cyclophosphamide, Oncovin, ara-C, prednisone) *chemotherapy protocol*

Minidyne solution OTC *broad-spectrum antimicrobial* [povidone-iodine] 10%

Mini-Gamulin Rh IM injection ℞ *obstetric Rh factor immunity suppressant* [Rh₀(D) immune globulin] 50 μg

Miniguard disposable pads *adhesive foam pad to seal urethral opening for stress urinary incontinence in women*

Min-I-Mix (delivery system) *dual-chambered prefilled syringe*

Minipress capsules ℞ *antihypertensive; α-blocker* [prazosin HCl] 1, 2, 5 mg

Minitran transdermal patch ℞ *antianginal; vasodilator* [nitroglycerin] 9, 18, 36, 54 mg

Minit-Rub OTC *topical analgesic; counterirritant* [methyl salicylate; menthol; camphor] 15%•3.5%•2.3%

Minizide 1; Minizide 2; Minizide 5 capsules ℞ *antihypertensive; α-blocker; diuretic* [prazosin HCl; polythiazide] 1•0.5 mg; 2•0.5 mg; 5•0.5 mg

Minocin pellet-filled capsules, oral suspension, powder for IV injection ℞ *tetracycline antibiotic; orphan status withdrawn 1996* [minocycline HCl] 50, 100 mg; 50 mg/5 mL; 100 mg ⊡ Indocin; Mithracin; niacin

minocromil USAN, INN, BAN *prophylactic antiallergic*

minocycline USAN, INN, BAN *gram-negative and gram-positive bacteriostatic; antirickettsial*

minocycline HCl USP *antibacterial; orphan status withdrawn 1996* 50, 100 mg oral

minoxidil USAN, USP, INN, BAN *antihypertensive; peripheral vasodilator; hair growth stimulant* 2.5, 10 mg oral

Minoxidil for Men topical solution OTC *hair growth stimulant* [minoxidil; alcohol 60%] 2%

mint; lamb mint; mackerel mint; Our Lady's mint *medicinal herb* [see: spearmint]

mint, brandy; lamb mint *medicinal herb* [see: peppermint]

mint, mountain *medicinal herb* [see: marjoram; Oswego tea]

mint, squaw *medicinal herb* [see: pennyroyal]

Mintezol chewable tablets, oral suspension ℞ *anthelmintic for strongyloidiasis (threadworm), larva migrans, and trichinosis* [thiabendazole] 500 mg; 500 mg/5 mL

Mintox chewable tablets, oral suspension OTC *antacid* [aluminum hydroxide; magnesium hydroxide] 200•200 mg; 225•200 mg/5 mL

Mintox Plus liquid OTC *antacid; antiflatulent* [aluminum hydroxide; magnesium hydroxide; simethicone] 500•450•40 mg/5 mL

Minute-Gel ℞ *topical dental caries preventative* [acidulated phosphate fluoride] 1.23%

Miochol solution (discontinued 1996) ℞ *direct-acting miotic for ophthalmic surgery* [acetylcholine chloride] 1:100

Miochol-E solution ℞ *direct-acting miotic for ophthalmic surgery* [acetylcholine chloride] 1:100

mioflazine INN, BAN *coronary vasodilator* [also: mioflazine HCl]

mioflazine HCl USAN *coronary vasodilator* [also: mioflazine]

Miostat solution ℞ *direct-acting miotic for ophthalmic surgery* [carbachol] 0.01%

miotics *a class of drugs that cause the pupil of the eye to contract*

mipafilcon A USAN *hydrophilic contact lens material*

mipimazole INN

Miradon tablets ℞ *indandione-derivative anticoagulant* [anisindione] 50 mg

MiraFlow solution OTC *cleaning solution for hard or soft contact lenses*

MiraLax powder for oral solution ℞ *osmotic laxative* [polyethylene glycol 3350] 17 g/dose

Miraluma ℞ *investigational radioactive imaging aid for mammography* [technetium Tc 99m sestamibi]

Mirapex tablets ℞ *dopamine agonist; antiparkinsonian* [pramipexole dihydrochloride] 0.125, 0.25, 1, 1.5 mg

MiraSept Step 2 solution OTC *rinsing/ storage solution for soft contact lenses* [sodium chloride (preserved saline solution)]

MiraSept System solutions OTC *two-step chemical disinfecting system for soft contact lenses* [hydrogen peroxide based] 3%

Mircette tablets ℞ *triphasic oral contraceptive: 21 days, 2 days, 5 days* [Phase 1: ethinyl estradiol + desogestrel; Phase 2: placebo; Phase 3: ethinyl estradiol] 20•150 μg; ⁕; 10 μg

Mireze ⓐ eye drops ℞ *topical antiallergic for seasonal allergic conjunctivitis* [nedocromil sodium] 2%

mirfentanil INN *analgesic* [also: mirfentanil HCl]

mirfentanil HCl USAN *analgesic* [also: mirfentanil]

mirincamycin INN *antibacterial; antimalarial* [also: mirincamycin HCl]

mirincamycin HCl USAN *antibacterial; antimalarial* [also: mirincamycin]

mirisetron maleate USAN *anxiolytic*

miristalkonium chloride INN

miroprofen INN

mirosamicin INN

mirtazapine USAN, INN *tetracyclic antidepressant; 5-HT$_{1A}$ agonist*

misonidazole USAN, INN *antiprotozoal (Trichomonas)*

misoprostol USAN, INN, BAN *prevention of NSAID-induced gastric ulcers*

Mission Prenatal; Mission Prenatal F.A.; Mission Prenatal H.P. tab-

lets OTC *vitamin/iron supplement* [multiple vitamins; ferrous gluconate; folic acid] ⁕•30•0.4 mg; ⁕• 30•0.8 mg; ⁕•30•0.8 mg

Mission Prenatal Rx tablets ℞ *vitamin/calcium/iron supplement* [multiple vitamins; calcium; iron; folic acid] ⁕•175•29.5•1 mg

Mission Surgical Supplement tablets OTC *vitamin/iron supplement* [multiple vitamins; ferrous gluconate] ⁕•27 mg

mistletoe (Phoradendron flavescens; P. serotinum; P. tomentosum; Viscum album) plant *medicinal herb for cancer, chorea, epilepsy, hypertension, internal hemorrhages, menstrual disorders, nervousness, poor circulation, and spleen disorders; not generally regarded as safe and effective for ingestion as it is highly toxic*

Mistometer (trademarked form) *metered-dose inhalation aerosol*

Mitchella repens *medicinal herb* [see: squaw vine]

Mithracin powder for IV infusion ℞ *antibiotic antineoplastic for testicular cancer* [plicamycin] 2.5 mg ⊉ Minocin

mithramycin [now: plicamycin] ⊉ mitomycin

mitindomide USAN, INN *antineoplastic*

mitobronitol INN, BAN

mitocarcin USAN, INN *antineoplastic*

mitoclomine INN, BAN

mitocromin USAN *antineoplastic*

mitoflaxone INN

mitogillin USAN, INN *antineoplastic*

mitoguazone INN *investigational antineoplastic for multiple myeloma and head, esophagus, and prostate cancer; investigational (orphan) for non-Hodgkin's lymphoma*

mitolactol INN *investigational (orphan) antineoplastic for brain tumors and recurrent or metastatic cervical squamous cell carcinoma*

mitomalcin USAN, INN *antineoplastic*

mitomycin USAN, USP, INN, BAN *antibiotic antineoplastic; investigational (orphan) for refractory glaucoma and* *glaucoma surgery* ☑ mithramycin; Mutamycin

mitomycin C (MTC) [see: mitomycin]

mitonafide INN

mitopodozide INN, BAN

mitoquidone INN, BAN

mitosper USAN, INN *antineoplastic*

mitotane USAN, USP, INN *antibiotic antineoplastic; adrenal cytotoxic agent*

mitotenamine INN, BAN

mitotic inhibitors *a class of antineoplastics that inhibit cell division (mitosis)*

mitoxantrone INN *antibiotic antineoplastic* [also: mitoxantrone HCl; mitozantrone]

mitoxantrone HCl USAN *antibiotic antineoplastic for prostate cancer and acute myelogenous (nonlymphocytic) leukemia (orphan)* [also: mitoxantrone; mitozantrone]

mitozantrone BAN *antineoplastic* [also: mitoxantrone HCl; mitoxantrone]

mitozolomide INN, BAN

Mitran capsules ℞ *benzodiazepine anxiolytic* [chlordiazepoxide HCl] 10 mg

Mitrolan chewable tablets OTC *bulk laxative; antidiarrheal* [calcium polycarbophil] 500 mg

mitronal [see: cinnarizine]

MIV (mitoxantrone, ifosfamide, VePesid) *chemotherapy protocol*

Mivacron IV infusion ℞ *muscle relaxant; adjunct to anesthesia* [mivacurium chloride] 0.5, 2 mg/mL

mivacurium chloride USAN, INN, BAN *neuromuscular blocking agent*

mivobulin isethionate USAN *antineoplastic; mitotic inhibitor; tubulin binder*

mixed respiratory vaccine (MRV) *active bacterin for respiratory tract infections*

mixed tocopherols [see: vitamin E]

mixidine USAN, INN *coronary vasodilator*

Mix-O-Vial (trademarked packaging form) *two-compartment vial*

mizoribine INN

MK-869 *investigational (Phase III) antiemetic for chemotherapy-induced emesis*

MKC-442 *investigational non-nucleoside reverse transcriptase inhibitor*

(NNRTI) for treatment of HIV infection and AIDS

M-KYA capsules (discontinued 1996) OTC *prevention and treatment of nocturnal leg cramps* [quinine sulfate] 64.8 mg

MM (mercaptopurine, methotrexate) *chemotherapy protocol*

MMOPP (methotrexate, mechlorethamine, Oncovin, procarbazine, prednisone) *chemotherapy protocol*

MMP (matrix metalloproteinase) inhibitors [q.v.]

MMR (measles, mumps & rubella vaccines) [q.v.]

M-M-R II powder for subcu injection ℞ *measles, mumps and rubella vaccine* [measles, mumps, and rubella virus vaccine, live] 0.5 mL

MOB (mechlorethamine, Oncovin, bleomycin) *chemotherapy protocol*

MOB-III (mitomycin, Oncovin, bleomycin, cisplatin) *chemotherapy protocol*

Moban tablets, oral concentrate ℞ *conventional (typical) antipsychotic* [molindone HCl] 5, 10, 25, 50, 100 mg; 20 mg/mL ☑ Mobidin; Modane

mobecarb INN

mobenzoxamine INN

Mobic ℞ *investigational (NDA filed) once-daily COX-2 inhibitor for rheumatoid arthritis and osteoarthritis* [meloxicam]

Mobidin tablets ℞ *analgesic; antipyretic; anti-inflammatory; antirheumatic* [magnesium salicylate] 600 mg ☑ Moban

Mobigesic tablets OTC *analgesic; antipyretic; anti-inflammatory; antihistamine* [magnesium salicylate; phenyltoloxamine citrate] 325•30 mg

Mobist ℞ *investigational neuroprotectant*

Mobisyl Creme OTC *topical analgesic* [trolamine salicylate] 10%

moccasin snake antivenin [see: antivenin (Crotalidae) polyvalent]

mocimycin INN

mociprazine INN

mock pennyroyal *medicinal herb* [see: pennyroyal]

moclobemide USAN, INN, BAN *antidepressant; MAO inhibitor*

moctamide INN

Moctanin biliary infusion ℞ *anticholelithogenic for dissolution of cholesterol gallstones (orphan)* [monoctanoin]

modafinil USAN, INN *analeptic for excessive daytime sleepiness of narcolepsy (orphan)*

modaline INN *antidepressant* [also: modaline sulfate]

modaline sulfate USAN *antidepressant* [also: modaline]

Modane tablets (discontinued 1998) OTC *stimulant laxative* [white phenolphthalein] 130 mg ☒ Moban; Mudrane

Modane Bulk liquid OTC *bulk laxative* [psyllium hydrophilic mucilloid] 50%

Modane Plus tablets OTC *stimulant laxative; stool softener* [white phenolphthalein; docusate sodium] 65•100 mg

Modane Soft capsules OTC *stool softener* [docusate sodium] 100 mg

modecainide USAN, INN *antiarrhythmic*

Modecate ⒸⒶⓃ (U.S. product: Prolixin Decanoate) subcu or IM injection ℞ *conventional (typical) antipsychotic* [fluphenazine decanoate] 25, 100 mg/mL

Moderil tablets (discontinued 1995) ℞ *antihypertensive* [rescinnamine] 0.25, 0.5 mg ☒ Mellaril

Modicon tablets ℞ *monophasic oral contraceptive* [norethindrone; ethinyl estradiol] 0.5 mg•35 μg ☒ Mylicon

modified bovine lung surfactant extract [see: beractant]

modified Burow solution [see: aluminum acetate solution]

modified cellulose gum [now: croscarmellose sodium]

modified Shohl solution (sodium citrate & citric acid) *urinary alkalinizer; compounding agent*

Modiodal (foreign name for U.S. product Provigil)

Moditen Enanthate ⒸⒶⓃ (U.S. product: Prolixin Enanthate) subcu or IM injection ℞ *conventional (typical)*

antipsychotic [fluphenazine enanthate] 25 mg/mL

Moditen HCl ⒸⒶⓃ (U.S. product: Prolixin) tablets ℞ *conventional (typical) antipsychotic* [fluphenazine HCl] 10 mg

Modivid ℞ *investigational cephalosporin antibiotic* [cefodizime]

Modrastane capsules (discontinued 1995) ℞ *adrenal steroid inhibitor; antisteroidal antineoplastic for Cushing syndrome* [trilostane] 30, 60 mg

Modual powder OTC *carbohydrate caloric supplement* [glucose polymers]

Moduretic tablets ℞ *antihypertensive; diuretic* [amiloride HCl; hydrochlorothiazide] 5•50 mg

moexipril INN, BAN *antihypertensive; angiotensin-converting enzyme (ACE) inhibitor*

moexipril HCl USAN *antihypertensive; angiotensin-converting enzyme (ACE) inhibitor*

moexiprilat INN

MOF (MeCCNU, Oncovin, fluorouracil) *chemotherapy protocol*

mofebutazone INN

mofedione [see: oxazidione]

mofegiline INN *antiparkinsonian* [also: mofegiline HCl]

mofegiline HCl USAN *antiparkinsonian* [also: mofegiline]

mofetil USAN, INN *combining name for radicals or groups*

mofloverine INN

mofoxime INN

MOF-STREP; MOF-Strep (MeCCNU, Oncovin, fluorouracil, streptozocin) *chemotherapy protocol*

Mogadon ℞ *investigational benzodiazepine tranquilizer; anxiolytic; anticonvulsant; hypnotic* [nitrazepam]

moguisteine INN

Moist Again vaginal gel OTC *lubricant* [glycerin; aloe vera]

Moi-Stir oral spray, Swabsticks OTC *saliva substitute* ☒ moisture

Moisture Drops eye drops OTC *ophthalmic moisturizer/lubricant* [hydroxypropyl methylcellulose] 0.5%

Moisture Eyes eye drops OTC *ocular moisturizer/lubricant* [propylene glycol] 0.95%

Moisturel lotion (discontinued 1997) OTC *moisturizer; emollient* [dimethicone] 3%

molecusol & carbamazepine *orphan status withdrawn 1996*

molfarnate INN

molgramostim USAN, INN, BAN *antineutropenic; hematopoietic stimulant; investigational (Phase II/III) cytokine to AIDS; orphan status withdrawn 1996*

molinazone USAN, INN *analgesic*

molindone INN *dihydroindolone antipsychotic* [also: molindone HCl]

molindone HCl USAN *dihydroindolone antipsychotic* [also: molindone]

Mol-Iron tablets (discontinued 1998) OTC *hematinic* [ferrous sulfate (source of iron)] 195 mg (39 mg)

Mol-Iron with Vitamin C tablets (discontinued 1998) OTC *hematinic* [iron (from ferrous sulfate); ascorbic acid] 39•75 mg

Mollifene Ear Wax Removing Formula drops OTC *agent to emulsify and disperse ear wax* [carbamide peroxide] 6.5%

molracetam INN

molsidomine USAN, INN *antianginal; coronary vasodilator*

molybdenum *element (Mo)*

Molypen IV injection ℞ *intravenous nutritional therapy* [ammonium molybdate tetrahydrate] 25 μg/mL

Momentum caplets OTC *analgesic; antipyretic; anti-inflammatory; antihistamine* [aspirin; phenyltoloxamine citrate] 500•15 mg

Momentum Muscular Backache Formula caplets OTC *analgesic; antipyretic; anti-inflammatory* [magnesium salicylate] 580 mg

mometasone INN, BAN *topical corticosteroidal anti-inflammatory* [also: mometasone furoate]

mometasone furoate USAN *topical corticosteroidal anti-inflammatory;*

investigational (NDA filed) inhalation powder for asthma [also: mometasone]

Momordica charantia *medicinal herb* [see: bitter melon]

MOMP (mechlorethamine, Oncovin, methotrexate, prednisone) *chemotherapy protocol*

Monafed sustained-release tablets ℞ *expectorant* [guaifenesin] 600 mg

Monafed DM tablets ℞ *antitussive; expectorant* [dextromethorphan hydrobromide; guaifenesin] 30•600 mg

monalazone disodium INN

monalium hydrate [see: magaldrate]

Monarda didyma *medicinal herb* [see: Oswego tea]

Monarda fistulosa *medicinal herb* [see: wild bergamot]

Monarda punctata *medicinal herb* [see: horsemint]

monascus yeast (*Monascus purpureus*) *natural remedy for gastric disorders, indigestion, lowering cholesterol, and poor circulation*

monatepil INN *antianginal; antihypertensive* [also: monatepil maleate]

monatepil maleate USAN *antianginal; antihypertensive* [also: monatepil]

monensin USAN, INN *antiprotozoal; antibacterial; antifungal*

Monistat 3 vaginal suppositories + cream OTC *antifungal* [miconazole nitrate] 200 mg; 2%

Monistat 7 vaginal suppositories, vaginal cream OTC *antifungal* [miconazole nitrate] 100 mg; 2%

Monistat 7 Combination Pack vaginal suppositories + cream OTC *antifungal* [miconazole nitrate] 100 mg; 2%

Monistat Dual-Pak vaginal suppositories + cream ℞ *antifungal* [miconazole nitrate] 200 mg; 2%

Monistat i.v. intrathecal or IV injection (discontinued 1999) ℞ *systemic antifungal* [miconazole] 10 mg/mL

Monistat-Derm cream ℞ *topical antifungal* [miconazole nitrate] 2%

mono- & di-acetylated monoglycerides NF *plasticizer*

mono- & di-glycerides NF *emulsifying agent*

monoamine oxidase inhibitors (MAOIs) *a class of antidepressants that increase CNS monoamine neurotransmitters (epinephrine, norepinephrine, and serotonin)*

monobactams *a class of bactericidal antibiotics effective against gram-negative aerobic pathogens*

monobasic potassium phosphate [see: potassium phosphate, monobasic]

monobasic sodium phosphate [see: sodium phosphate, monobasic]

monobenzone USP, INN *depigmenting agent for vitiligo*

monobenzyl ether of hydroquinone [see: monobenzone]

monobromated camphor [see: camphor, monobromated]

monocalcium phosphate [see: calcium phosphate, dibasic]

Monocaps tablets OTC *vitamin/mineral/iron supplement* [multiple vitamins & minerals; ferrous fumerate; folic acid; biotin] ± • 14 mg • 0.1 mg • 15 μg ② Monoclate; Monoket

Monocete liquid (discontinued 1995) ℞ *cauterant; keratolytic* [monochloroacetic acid] 80% ② Monocid

Mono-Chlor liquid ℞ *cauterant; keratolytic* [monochloroacetic acid] 80%

monochloroacetic acid *strong keratolytic/cauterant*

monochlorothymol [see: chlorothymol]

monochlorphenamide [see: clofenamide]

Monocid powder for IV or IM injection ℞ *cephalosporin antibiotic* [cefonicid sodium] 1, 10 g ② Monocete

Monoclate powder for IV injection (discontinued 1996) ℞ *antihemophilic to correct coagulation deficiency* [antihemophilic factor VIII:C, heat treated] ± ② Monocaps; Monoket

Monoclate P powder for IV injection ℞ *antihemophilic to correct coagulation deficiency* [antihemophilic factor VIII:C] ± ② Monocaps; Monoket

monoclonal antibody 17-1A *orphan status withdrawn 1997* [now: edrecolomab]

monoclonal antibody 5A8 to CD4 *investigational (orphan) for post-exposure prophylaxis to occupational HIV exposure*

monoclonal antibody 5c8, recombinant humanized *investigational (orphan) for systemic lupus erythematosus (SLE) and immune thrombocytopenic purpura*

monoclonal antibody 7E3 [see: abciximab]

monoclonal antibody anti-idiotype melanoma assorted antigen, murine *orphan status withdrawn 1997*

monoclonal antibody B43.13 *investigational (orphan) for epithelial ovarian cancer*

monoclonal antibody E5 [now: edobacomab]

monoclonal antibody PM-81 *investigational (orphan) for acute myelogenous leukemia*

monoclonal antibody PM-81 & AML-2-23 *investigational (orphan) for bone marrow transplant for acute myelogenous leukemia*

monoclonal antibody r24 *investigational treatment for Hodgkin's disease*

monoclonal antibody to B-cell lymphoma, murine or human *orphan status withdrawn 1996*

monoclonal antibody to CD22 antigen on B-cells, radiolabeled *investigational (orphan) for non-Hodgkin's lymphoma*

monoclonal antibody to CEA, humanized *investigational (orphan) antineoplastic for pancreatic and small cell lung cancer*

monoclonal antibody to cytomegalovirus, human *investigational (orphan) prophylaxis for CMV retinitis and CMV disease in solid organ transplants*

monoclonal antibody to hepatitis B virus, human *investigational (orphan) hepatitis B prophylaxis for liver transplant*

monoclonal antibody to lupus nephritis *investigational (orphan) for immunization against lupus nephritis*

monoclonal antiendotoxin antibody XMMEN-OE5 *orphan status withdrawn 1994; clinical trials discontinued 1997* [now: edobacomab]

monoclonal factor IX [see: factor IX complex]

monoctanoin USAN, BAN *anticholelithogenic for dissolution of cholesterol gallstones (orphan)*

monoctanoin component A
monoctanoin component B
monoctanoin component C
monoctanoin component D

Mono-Diff reagent kit for professional use *in vitro diagnostic aid for mononucleosis*

Monodox capsules ℞ *antibiotic* [doxycycline] 50, 100 mg

Mono-Drop (trademarked delivery system) *prefilled eye drop dispenser*

monoethanolamine NF *surfactant*

monoethanolamine oleate INN *sclerosing agent* [also: ethanolamine oleate]

Mono-Gesic film-coated tablets ℞ *analgesic; antipyretic; anti-inflammatory; antirheumatic* [salsalate] 750 mg

Monoket tablets ℞ *antianginal; vasodilator* [isosorbide mononitrate] 10, 20 mg ② Monocete

Mono-Latex reagent kit for professional use *in vitro diagnostic aid for mononucleosis*

monolaurin *investigational (Phase III, orphan) for nonbullous congenital ichthyosiform erythroderma*

monometacrine INN

Mononine powder for IV infusion ℞ *antihemophilic for factor IX deficiency (hemophilia B; Christmas disease) (orphan)* [coagulation factor IX complex] 100 IU/mL

monooctanoin [see: monoctanoin]

monophenylbutazone [see: mofebutazone]

monophosphoryl lipid A (MPL-A) *investigational (Phase I) vaccine for AIDS*

monophosphothiamine INN

Mono-Plus reagent kit for professional use *in vitro diagnostic aid for mononucleosis*

monopotassium 4-aminosalicylate [see: aminosalicylate potassium]

monopotassium carbonate [see: potassium bicarbonate]

monopotassium D-gluconate [see: potassium gluconate]

monopotassium monosodium tartrate tetrahydrate [see: potassium sodium tartrate]

monopotassium phosphate [see: potassium phosphate, monobasic]

Monopril tablets ℞ *antihypertensive; angiotensin-converting enzyme (ACE) inhibitor* [fosinopril sodium] 10, 20, 40 mg

monosodium p-aminohippurate [see: aminohippurate sodium]

monosodium 4-aminosalicylate dihydrate [see: aminosalicylate sodium]

monosodium carbonate [see: sodium bicarbonate]

monosodium D-gluconate [see: sodium gluconate]

monosodium D-thyroxine hydrate [see: dextrothyroxine sodium]

monosodium glutamate NF *flavoring agent; perfume*

monosodium L-ascorbate [see: sodium ascorbate]

monosodium L-thyroxine hydrate [see: levothyroxine sodium]

monosodium phosphate dihydrate [see: sodium phosphate, monobasic]

monosodium phosphate monohydrate [see: sodium phosphate, monobasic]

monosodium salicylate [see: sodium salicylate]

monosodium sulfite [see: sodium bisulfite]

Monospot slide test for professional use *in vitro diagnostic aid for mononucleosis*

monostearin [see: glyceryl monostearate]

Monosticon Dri-Dot slide test for professional use *in vitro diagnostic aid for mononucleosis*

monosulfiram BAN [also: sulfiram]

Mono-Sure slide test for professional use *in vitro diagnostic aid for mononucleosis*

Mono-Test slide test for professional use *in vitro diagnostic aid for mononucleosis*

monothioglycerol NF *preservative*

Monotropa uniflora medicinal herb [see: fit root]

Mono-Vacc Test (O.T.) single-use intradermal puncture test device ℞ *tuberculosis skin test* [old tuberculin] 5 U

monoxerutin INN

montelukast sodium USAN *antiasthmatic; leukotriene receptor inhibitor*

monteplase INN

montirelin INN

montmorillonite (redmond clay) *natural remedy for bug bites and stings and other skin problems*

Monuril (foreign name for U.S. product Monurol)

Monurol granules for oral solution ℞ *broad-spectrum bactericidal antibiotic for urinary tract infections* [fosfomycin tromethamine] 3 g per packet

moose elm *medicinal herb* [see: slippery elm]

8-MOP capsules ℞ *systemic psoralens for repigmentation of idiopathic vitiligo; used to increase tolerance to sunlight and enhance pigmentation* [methoxsalen] 10 mg

MOP (mechlorethamine, Oncovin, prednisone) *chemotherapy protocol*

MOP (mechlorethamine, Oncovin, procarbazine) *chemotherapy protocol*

8-MOP (8-methoxypsoralen) [see: methoxsalen]

MOP-BAP (mechlorethamine, Oncovin, procarbazine, bleomycin, Adriamycin, prednisone) *chemotherapy protocol*

moperone INN

mopidamol INN

mopidralazine INN

MOPP (mechlorethamine, Oncovin, procarbazine, prednisone) *chemotherapy protocol*

MOPP (mustine HCl, Oncovin, procarbazine, prednisone) *chemotherapy protocol*

MOPP/ABV (mechlorethamine, Oncovin, procarbazine, prednisone, Adriamycin, bleomycin, vinblastine) *chemotherapy protocol*

MOPP/ABVD (alternating cycles of MOPP and ABVD) *chemotherapy protocol*

MOPP-BLEO; MOPP-Bleo (mechlorethamine, Oncovin, procarbazine, prednisone, bleomycin) *chemotherapy protocol*

MOPPHDB (mechlorethamine, Oncovin, procarbazine, prednisone, high-dose bleomycin) *chemotherapy protocol*

MOPPLDB (mechlorethamine, Oncovin, procarbazine, prednisone, low-dose bleomycin) *chemotherapy protocol*

MOPr (mechlorethamine, Oncovin, procarbazine) *chemotherapy protocol*

moprolol INN

moquizone INN

moracizine INN, BAN *antiarrhythmic* [also: moricizine]

morantel INN *anthelmintic* [also: morantel tartrate]

morantel tartrate USAN *anthelmintic* [also: morantel]

Moranyl (available only from the Centers for Disease Control) ℞ *antiparasitic for African trypanosomiasis and onchocerciasis* [suramin sodium]

morazone INN, BAN

morclofone INN

More-Dophilus powder OTC *dietary supplement; fever blister treatment; not generally regarded as safe and effective as an antidiarrheal* [Lactobacillus acidophilus] 4 billion U/g

morforex INN

moricizine USAN *antiarrhythmic* [also: moracizine]

moricizine HCl *antiarrhythmic*

morinamide INN

Morinda citrifolia *medicinal herb* [see: noni]

Mormon tea *medicinal herb* [see: ephedra]

morniflumate USAN, INN *anti-inflammatory*

morning glory *(Ipomoea violacea)* seeds *contain lysergic acid amide, chemically similar to LSD, which produce hallucinations when ingested as a street drug* [see also: LSD]

morocromen INN

moroxydine INN, BAN

morphazinamide [see: morinamide]

morpheridine INN, BAN

MorphiDex ℞ *investigational (NDA filed) agent for the relief of moderate to severe cancer pain* [morphine sulfate; dextromethorphan]

morphine BAN *narcotic analgesic; widely abused as a street drug, which leads to dependence* [also: morphine sulfate]

morphine dinicotinate ester [see: nicomorphine]

morphine HCl USP *narcotic analgesic preferred in Germany and Great Britain; widely abused as a street drug, which leads to dependence*

morphine sulfate (MS) USP *narcotic analgesic preferred in the U.S.; intraspinal microinfusion for intractable chronic pain (orphan); widely abused as a street drug, which leads to dependence* [also: morphine] 10, 15, 30 mg oral; 10, 20 mg/5 mL oral; 0.5, 1, 2, 4, 5, 10, 15, 25, 50 mg/mL injection; 5, 10, 20, 30 mg rectal

4-morpholinecarboximidoylguanidine [see: moroxydine]

2-morpholinoethylrutin [see: ethoxazorutoside]

3-morpholinosydnoneimine [see: linsidomine]

morpholinyl succinimide [see: morsuximide]

morpholinylethyl morphine [see: pholcodine]

morrhuate sodium USP *sclerosing agent* [also: sodium morrhuate] 50 mg/mL injection

morsuximide INN

morsydomine [see: molsidomine]

mortification root *medicinal herb* [see: marsh mallow]

Morton Salt Substitute; Morton Seasoned Salt Substitute OTC *salt substitute* [potassium chloride] 64 mEq/5 g; 56 mEq/5 g

Morus nigra; M. rubra *medicinal herb* [see: mulberry]

Moschus moschiferus *natural remedy* [see: deer musk]

Mosco liquid OTC *topical keratolytic* [salicylic acid in flexible collodion] 17.6%

mosquito plant *medicinal herb* [see: pennyroyal]

motapizone INN

MOTC (methyleneoxytetracycline) [see: methacycline]

mother of thyme *medicinal herb* [see: thyme]

motherwort *(Leonurus cardiaca)* flowering tops and leaves *medicinal herb used as an antispasmodic, astringent, calmative, cardiac, emmenagogue, hepatic, laxative, nervine, and stomachic*

Motilium ⓒ film-coated tablets ℞ *antiemetic for diabetic gastroparesis and chronic gastritis (investigational (NDA filed) in the USA)* [domperidone maleate] 10 mg

Motofen tablets ℞ *antidiarrheal* [difenoxin HCl; atropine sulfate] 1 • 0.025 mg

motrazepam INN

motretinide USAN, INN *keratolytic*

Motrin tablets, chewable tablets, oral suspension ℞ *nonsteroidal anti-inflammatory drug (NSAID); antiarthritic; analgesic* [ibuprofen] 300, 400, 600, 800 mg; 50, 100 mg; 100 mg/5 mL

Motrin, Children's drops OTC *nonsteroidal anti-inflammatory drug (NSAID); analgesic; antipyretic* [ibuprofen] 40 mg/mL

Motrin, Children's oral suspension OTC *nonsteroidal anti-inflammatory drug (NSAID); analgesic; antipyretic* [ibuprofen] 100 mg/5 mL

Motrin, Junior film-coated caplets, chewable tablets OTC *nonsteroidal anti-inflammatory drug (NSAID); antiarthritic; analgesic* [ibuprofen] 100 mg

Motrin IB caplets, tablets, gelcaps OTC *nonsteroidal anti-inflammatory drug (NSAID); antiarthritic; analgesic* [ibuprofen] 200 mg

Motrin IB Sinus caplets OTC *decongestant; analgesic* [pseudoephedrine HCl; ibuprofen] 30•200 mg

mountain ash *(Sorbus americana; S. aucuparia)* fruit *medicinal herb used as an aperient, astringent, and diuretic*

mountain balm *medicinal herb* [see: yerba santa]

mountain box; mountain cranberry *medicinal herb* [see: uva ursi]

mountain laurel *(Kalmia latifolia)* leaves *medicinal herb used as an astringent and sedative*

mountain mahogany *medicinal herb* [see: birch]

mountain mint *medicinal herb* [see: marjoram; Oswego tea]

mountain snuff; mountain tobacco *medicinal herb* [see: arnica]

mountain sorrel *medicinal herb* [see: wood sorrel]

mountain strawberry *medicinal herb* [see: strawberry]

mountain sumach *medicinal herb* [see: sumach]

mountain sweet *medicinal herb* [see: New Jersey tea]

mountain tea *medicinal herb* [see: wintergreen]

mouse ear *(Hieracium pilosella)* plant *medicinal herb used as an astringent, cholagogue, and diuretic*

MouthKote oral spray OTC *saliva substitute*

MouthKote F/R oral rinse (discontinued 1997) OTC *topical dental caries preventative* [sodium fluoride] 0.04%

MouthKote O/R mouthwash OTC *anesthetic and antimicrobial throat irrigation* [benzyl alcohol; menthol]

MouthKote O/R oral solution OTC *topical antihistamine* [diphenhydramine] 1.25%

MouthKote P/R oral solution, ointment OTC *topical antihistamine* [diphenhydramine HCl] 1.25%; 25%

mouthroot *medicinal herb* [see: gold thread]

moveltipril INN

moxadolen INN

moxalactam disodium USAN, USP *bactericidal antibiotic* [also: latamoxef]

moxantrazole [now: teloxantrone HCl]

moxaprindine INN

moxastine INN

moxaverine INN, BAN

moxazocine USAN, INN *analgesic; antitussive*

moxestrol INN

moxicoumone INN

moxidectin USAN, INN *veterinary antiparasitic*

moxifloxacin HCl USAN *fluoroquinolone antibiotic*

moxilubant maleate USAN *leukotriene B₄ receptor antagonist for rheumatoid arthritis and psoriasis*

moxipraquine INN, BAN

moxiraprine INN

moxisylyte INN [also: thymoxamine]

moxnidazole USAN, INN *antiprotozoal (Trichomonas)*

moxonidine INN *investigational antihypertensive*

MP (melphalan, prednisone) *chemotherapy protocol*

MP-351 *investigational 2-5A antisense drug for A and B strains of respiratory syncytial virus*

4-MP (4-methylpyrazole) [see: fomepizole]

6-MP (6-mercaptopurine) [see: mercaptopurine]

MPF [see: Mucoprotective Factor]

m-PFL (methotrexate, Platinol, fluorouracil, leucovorin [rescue]) *chemotherapy protocol*

MPH (methylphenidate HCl) [q.v.]

MPIF-1 (myeloid progenitor inhibitory factor 1) [q.v.]

MPL (melphalan) [q.v.]

MPL + PRED (melphalan, prednisone) *chemotherapy protocol*

MPL-A (monophosphoryl lipid A) [q.v.]

M-Prednisol-40; M-Prednisol-80 intralesional, soft tissue, and IM injection ℞ *corticosteroid; antiinflammatory; immunosuppressant* [methylprednisolone acetate] 40 mg/mL; 80 mg/mL

MRV subcu injection ℞ *active respiratory bacteria immunizing agent* [mixed respiratory vaccine]

MRV (mixed respiratory vaccine) [q.v.]

M-R-Vax II powder for subcu injection ℞ *measles and rubella vaccine* [measles and rubella virus vaccine, live] 0.5 mL

MS (magnesium salicylate) [q.v.]

MS (morphine sulfate) [q.v.]

MS Contin controlled-release tablets ℞ *narcotic analgesic; preoperative sedative and anxiolytic* [morphine sulfate] 15, 30, 60, 100, 200 mg

MS-325 *investigational (Phase II) injectable MRI contrast medium for multiple cardiovascular indications*

MSI (Metered Solution Inhaler) [q.v.]

MSIR tablets, capsules, oral solution, oral concentrate ℞ *narcotic analgesic; preoperative sedative and anxiolytic* [morphine sulfate] 15, 30 mg; 15, 30 mg; 10, 20 mg/5 mL; 20 mg/mL

MS/L; MS/L Concentrate oral liquid (discontinued 1999) ℞ *narcotic analgesic; preoperative sedative and anxiolytic; also abused as a street drug* [morphine sulfate] 10 mg/5 mL; 100 mg/5 mL

MS/S suppositories (discontinued 1998) ℞ *narcotic analgesic; preoperative sedative and anxiolytic* [morphine sulfate] 5, 10, 20, 30 mg

MSTA (Mumps Skin Test Antigen) intradermal injection ℞ *diagnostic aid to assess immune system competency (not effective in testing immunity to mumps virus)* [mumps skin test antigen] 0.1 mL (4 U/0.1 mL)

MT6 (mercaptomerin) [q.v.]

MTC (mitomycin C) [see: mitomycin]

M.T.E.-4; M.T.E.-5; M.T.E.-6; M.T.E.-7; M.T.E.-4 Concentrated; M.T.E.-5 Concentrated; M.T.E.-6 Concentrated IV injection ℞ *intravenous nutritional therapy* [multiple trace elements (metals)]

mTHPC [see: temoporfin]

MTX (methotrexate) [q.v.]

MTX + MP (methotrexate, mercaptopurine) *chemotherapy protocol*

MTX + MP + CTX (methotrexate, mercaptopurine, cyclophosphamide) *chemotherapy protocol*

MTXCP-PDAdr (methotrexate [with leucovorin rescue], cisplatin, doxorubicin) *chemotherapy protocol*

MUC-1 *investigational cancer vaccine*

Muco-Fen-DM timed-release tablets ℞ *antitussive; expectorant* [dextromethorphan hydrobromide; guaifenesin] 30•600 mg

Muco-Fen-LA timed-release tablets ℞ *expectorant* [guaifenesin] 600 mg

mucoid exopolysaccharide *Pseudomonas* hyperimmune globulin (MEPIG) *investigational (orphan) for pulmonary infections of cystic fibrosis*

mucolytics *a class of respiratory inhalant drugs that destroy or inhibit mucin*

Mucomyst solution for nebulization or intratracheal instillation ℞ *mucolytic; investigational (orphan) for severe acetaminophen overdose* [acetylcysteine sodium] 10%, 20%

Mucomyst 10 IV ℞ *mucolytic; investigational (orphan) for severe acetaminophen overdose* [acetylcysteine]

Mucoplex tablets (discontinued 1995) OTC *dietary supplement* [vitamins B_2 and B_{12}; liver fraction] 1.5 mg•5 μg•750 mg

Mucoprotective Factor (MPF) (trademarked ingredient) *aromatic flavored syrup* [eriodictyon]

Mucosil-10; Mucosil-20 solution for nebulization or intratracheal instillation ℞ *mucolytic* [acetylcysteine sodium] 10%; 20%

Mudrane tablets ℞ *antiasthmatic; bronchodilator; decongestant; expectorant; sedative* [aminophylline; ephedrine HCl; potassium iodide; phenobarbital] 111•16•195•8 mg ⬚ Modane

Mudrane GG elixir (discontinued 1995) ℞ *antiasthmatic; decongestant; expectorant; sedative* [theophylline; ephedrine HCl; guaifenesin; phenobarbital] 4•0.8•5.2•0.5 mg/mL

Mudrane GG tablets ℞ *antiasthmatic; decongestant; expectorant; sedative* [theophylline; ephedrine HCl; guaifenesin; phenobarbital] 111•16•100•8 mg

Mudrane GG-2 tablets ℞ *antiasthmatic; bronchodilator; expectorant* [theophylline; guaifenesin] 111•100 mg

Mudrane-2 tablets (discontinued 1995) ℞ *antiasthmatic; expectorant* [aminophylline; potassium iodide] 111•195 mg

mugwort (Artemisia vulgaris) root and plant *medicinal herb used as a diaphoretic, emmenagogue, and laxative*

mulberry (Morus nigra; M. rubra) bark *medicinal herb used as an anthelmintic and cathartic*

mullein (Verbascum nigrum; V. phlomoides; V. thapsiforme; V. thapsus) plant *medicinal herb for asthma, bleeding in bowel and lungs, bronchitis, bruises, cough, croup, diarrhea, earache, gout, hemorrhoids, insomnia, lymphatic system, nervousness, pain, pleurisy, sinus congestion, and tuberculosis*

MulTE-Pak-4; MulTE-Pak-5 IV injection ℞ *intravenous nutritional therapy* [multiple trace elements (metals)] ±

Multi 75 timed-release tablets OTC *vitamin/mineral supplement* [multiple vitamins & minerals; folic acid; biotin] ±•0.4•⅖ mg

Multi Vit with Iron drops OTC *vitamin/iron supplement* [multiple vitamins; iron] ±•10 mg/mL

Multi Vitamin Concentrate injection ℞ *parenteral vitamin supplement* [multiple vitamins] ±

Multibret-500 Hematinic timed-release tablets (discontinued 1995) ℞ *hematinic* [ferrous sulfate; multiple B vitamins; sodium ascorbate] 105•±•500 mg

Multibret-Folic-500 timed-release tablets (discontinued 1995) ℞ *hematinic* [ferrous sulfate; multiple B vitamins; sodium ascorbate; folic acid] 105•±•500•0.8 mg

Multi-Day tablets OTC *vitamin supplement* [multiple vitamins; folic acid] ±•0.4 mg

Multi-Day Plus Iron tablets OTC *vitamin/iron supplement* [multiple vitamins; iron; folic acid] ±•18•0.4 mg

Multi-Day Plus Minerals tablets OTC *vitamin/mineral/iron supplement* [multiple vitamins & minerals; iron; folic acid; biotin] ±•18 mg•0.4 mg•30 μg

Multi-Day with Calcium and Extra Iron tablets OTC *vitamin/calcium/iron supplement* [multiple vitamins; calcium; iron; folic acid] ±•⅖•27•0.4 mg

MultiKine injection ℞ *investigational (Phase III) antineoplastic for prostate cancer; investigational for cancer of the oral cavity* [leukocyte; interleukin]

Multilex; Multilex-T & M tablets OTC *vitamin/mineral/iron supplement* [multiple vitamins & minerals; iron] ±•15 mg

Multilyte-20; Multilyte-40 IV admixture ℞ *intravenous electrolyte therapy* [combined electrolyte solution]

Multi-Mineral tablets OTC *mineral supplement* [multiple minerals]

Multiple Trace Element; Multiple Trace Element Concentrated; Multiple Trace Element Neonatal; Multiple Trace Element Pedi-

atric IV injection ℞ *intravenous nutritional therapy* [multiple trace elements (metals)]

Multiple Trace Element with Selenium; Multiple Trace Element with Selenium Concentrated IV injection ℞ *intravenous nutritional therapy* [multiple trace elements (metals)]

Multistix; Multistix 2; Multistix 7; Multistix 8 SG; Multistix 9; Multistix 9 SG; Multistix 10 SG; Multistix SG reagent strips *in vitro diagnostic aid for multiple urine products*

Multitest CMI single-use intradermal skin test device ℞ *skin test for multiple allergen sensitivity* [skin test antigens (seven different); glycerin (one for test control)]

Multitrace-5 Concentrate IV injection ℞ *intravenous nutritional therapy* [multiple trace elements (metals)] ±

multivitamin infusion, neonatal formula investigational (orphan) total parenteral nutrition for very low birthweight infants

Multi-Vitamin Mineral with Beta-Carotene tablets OTC *vitamin/mineral/iron supplement* [multiple vitamins & minerals; ferrous fumarate; folic acid; biotin] ±•27•0.4•0.45 mg

Multivitamin with Fluoride drops ℞ *pediatric vitamin supplement and dental caries preventative* [multiple vitamins; fluoride] ±•0.25, ±•0.5 mg/mL

Multivitamins capsules OTC *vitamin supplement* [multiple vitamins] ±

Mulvidren-F Softabs (chewable tablets) ℞ *pediatric vitamin supplement and dental caries preventative* [multiple vitamins; fluoride] ±•1 mg

mumps skin test antigen (MSTA) USP *diagnostic aid to assess immune system competency*

mumps vaccine [see: mumps virus vaccine, inactivated]

mumps virus vaccine, inactivated NF

mumps virus vaccine, live USP *active immunizing agent for mumps*

Mumpsvax powder for subcu injection ℞ *mumps vaccine* [mumps virus vaccine, live] 0.5 mL

mupirocin USAN, INN, BAN *topical antibacterial antibiotic*

mupirocin calcium USAN *topical antibacterial antibiotic*

muplestim USAN *progenitor cell stimulator for neutropenia and thrombocytopenia*

murabutide INN

Murine eye drops OTC *ophthalmic moisturizer/lubricant* [polyvinyl alcohol] 0.5%

Murine Ear Drops OTC *agent to emulsify and disperse ear wax* [carbamide peroxide; alcohol] 6.5%•6.3%

murine MAb [see: muromonab-CD3]

Murine Plus eye drops OTC *topical ophthalmic decongestant and vasoconstrictor* [tetrahydrozoline HCl] 0.05%

Muro 128 eye drops, ophthalmic ointment OTC *corneal edema-reducing agent* [sodium chloride (hypertonic saline solution)] 2%, 5%; 5%

murocainide INN

Murocel eye drops OTC *ophthalmic moisturizer/lubricant* [methylcellulose] 1%

Murocoll-2 eye drops ℞ *cycloplegic; mydriatic* [scopolamine hydrobromide; phenylephrine HCl] 0.3%•10%

murodermin INN

muromonab-CD3 USAN, INN *monoclonal antibody immunosuppressive for renal, hepatic, and cardiac transplants*

Muroptic-5 eye drops OTC *corneal edema-reducing agent* [sodium chloride (hypertonic saline solution)] 5%

Muro's Opcon eye drops (discontinued 1995) ℞ *topical ophthalmic decongestant and vasoconstrictor* [naphazoline HCl] 0.1%

muscarinic agonists *a class of investigational analgesics*

MuscleRub ointment OTC *topical analgesic; counterirritant* [methyl salicylate; menthol] 15%•10%

Muse single-use intraurethral suppository ℞ *vasodilator for erectile dysfunction* [alprostadil] 125, 150, 500, 1000 μg

musk *natural remedy* [see: deer musk]
Mus-Lax capsules (discontinued 1996) ℞ *skeletal muscle relaxant; analgesic* [chlorzoxazone; acetaminophen] 250•300 mg
mustaral oil [see: allyl isothiocyanate]
mustard *(Brassica alba; Sinapis alba)* seeds and oil *medicinal herb for indigestion and liver and lung disorders; also used as an appetizer, diuretic, emetic, and soak for aching feet, arthritis, and rheumatism*
mustard oil [see: allyl isothiocyanate]
Mustargen powder for IV or intracavitary injection ℞ *nitrogen mustard-type alkylating antineoplastic for multiple myelomas, lymphomas and leukemias, and breast, lung, and ovarian cancers* [mechlorethamine HCl] 10 mg
Musterole Deep Strength Rub OTC *topical analgesic; counterirritant* [methyl salicylate; methyl nicotinate; menthol] 30%•0.5%•3%
Musterole Extra Strength OTC *topical analgesic; counterirritant* [camphor; menthol] 5%•3%
mustine BAN *nitrogen mustard-type alkylating antineoplastic* [also: mechlorethamine HCl; chlormethine; nitrogen mustard N-oxide HCl]
mustine HCl [see: mechlorethamine HCl]
Mutamycin powder for IV injection ℞ *antibiotic antineoplastic for stomach, pancreatic, breast, colon, head, neck, and lung cancers* [mitomycin] 5, 20, 40 mg ⑫ mitomycin
muzolimine USAN, INN *diuretic; antihypertensive*
MV (mitomycin, vinblastine) *chemotherapy protocol*
MV (mitoxantrone, VePesid) *chemotherapy protocol*
MVAC; M-VAC (methotrexate, vinblastine, Adriamycin, cisplatin) *chemotherapy protocol*
M-Vax ℞ *investigational (Phase III, orphan) theraccine for postsurgical stage III malignant melanoma*

M.V.C. 9+3 injection (discontinued 1995) ℞ *parenteral vitamin supplement* [multiple vitamins; folic acid; biotin] ±•0.4 mg•60 μg per 5 mL
M.V.C. 9+4 Pediatric powder for injection ℞ *vitamin therapy* [multiple vitamins; folic acid; biotin]
MVF (mitoxantrone, vincristine, fluorouracil) *chemotherapy protocol*
M.V.I. Neonatal IV infusion ℞ *investigational (orphan) total parenteral nutrition for very low birthweight infants* [multiple vitamins]
M.V.I. Pediatric injection ℞ *parenteral vitamin supplement* [multiple vitamins; folic acid; biotin] ±•140•20 μg/5 mL
M.V.I.-12 injection ℞ *parenteral vitamin supplement* [multiple vitamins; folic acid; biotin] ±•400•60 μg/5 mL
M.V.M. capsules OTC *vitamin/mineral/iron supplement* [multiple vitamins & minerals; iron; folic acid; biotin] ±•3.6 mg•0.08 mg•160 μg
MVP (mitomycin, vinblastine, Platinol) *chemotherapy protocol*
MVPP (mechlorethamine, vinblastine, procarbazine, prednisone) *chemotherapy protocol*
MVT (mitoxantrone, VePesid, thiotepa) *chemotherapy protocol*
MVVPP (mechlorethamine, vincristine, vinblastine, procarbazine, prednisone) *chemotherapy protocol*
MX-6 *investigational (Phase III) treatment for cervical intraepithelial neoplasia (CIN)*
Myadec tablets OTC *vitamin/mineral/iron supplement* [multiple vitamins & minerals; iron; folic acid; biotin] ±•18 mg•0.4 mg•30 μg
Myambutol film-coated tablets ℞ *tuberculostatic* [ethambutol HCl] 100, 400 mg ⑫ Nembutal
Myapap drops (discontinued 1997) ℞ *analgesic; antipyretic* [acetaminophen] 100 mg/mL
Mycelex cream, solution ℞ *topical antifungal* [clotrimazole] 1%

Mycelex troches ℞ *antifungal; oral candidiasis prophylaxis or treatment* [clotrimazole] 10 mg

Mycelex OTC cream, solution OTC *topical antifungal* [clotrimazole] 1%

Mycelex Twin Pack vaginal tablets + cream ℞ *antifungal* [clotrimazole] 500 mg; 1%

Mycelex-7 vaginal cream, vaginal tablets, combination pack (cream + vaginal suppositories) OTC *antifungal* [clotrimazole] 1%; 100 mg

Mycelex-G vaginal tablets ℞ *antifungal* [clotrimazole] 500 mg

Mycifradin Sulfate oral solution ℞ *aminoglycoside antibiotic* [neomycin sulfate] 125 mg/5 mL

Myciguent ointment, cream OTC *topical antibiotic* [neomycin sulfate] 3.5 mg/g

Mycinette throat spray OTC *topical anesthetic; oral antiseptic; astringent* [phenol; alum] 1.4%•0.3%

Mycinettes lozenges OTC *topical oral anesthetic* [benzocaine] 15 mg

Myci-Spray nasal spray OTC *nasal decongestant; antihistamine* [phenylephrine HCl; pyrilamine maleate] 0.25%•0.15%

Mycitracin Plus ointment OTC *topical antibiotic; local anesthetic* [polymyxin B sulfate; neomycin sulfate; bacitracin; lidocaine] 5000 U•3.5 mg•500 U•40 mg per g

Mycitracin Triple Antibiotic ointment OTC *topical antibiotic* [polymyxin B sulfate; neomycin sulfate; bacitracin] 5000 U•3.5 mg•500 U per g

Mycobacterium avium sensitin RS-10 *investigational (orphan) diagnostic aid for Mycobacterium avium infection in immunocompromised patients*

Myco-Biotic II cream ℞ *topical corticosteroidal anti-inflammatory; antifungal* [triamcinolone acetonide; neomycin sulfate; nystatin] 0.1%•0.5%•100 000 U per g

Mycobutin capsules ℞ *antiviral/antibacterial for prevention of Mycobacterium avium complex (MAC) in* advanced HIV patients (orphan) [rifabutin] 150 mg

Mycocide NS solution OTC *topical antiseptic* [benzalkonium chloride] ⒉

Mycogen II cream, ointment ℞ *topical corticosteroidal anti-inflammatory; antifungal* [triamcinolone acetonide; nystatin] 0.1%•100 000 U per g

Mycolog-II cream, ointment ℞ *topical corticosteroidal anti-inflammatory; antifungal* [triamcinolone acetonide; nystatin] 0.1%•100 000 U per g

Myconel cream ℞ *topical corticosteroidal anti-inflammatory; antifungal* [triamcinolone acetonide; nystatin] 0.1%•100 000 U per g

mycophenolate mofetil USAN *immunosuppressant for allogenic kidney and heart transplants; purine biosynthesis inhibitor*

mycophenolate mofetil HCl USAN *immunosuppressant for allogenic kidney and heart transplants; purine biosynthesis inhibitor*

mycophenolic acid USAN, INN *antineoplastic*

Mycostatin cream, ointment, powder, vaginal tablets ℞ *topical antifungal* [nystatin] 100 000 U/g; 100 000 U/g; 100 000 U/g; 100 000 U

Mycostatin film-coated tablets ℞ *systemic antifungal* [nystatin] 500 000 U

Mycostatin oral suspension, Pastilles (troches) ℞ *antifungal; oral candidiasis treatment* [nystatin] 100 000 U/mL; 200 000 U

Myco-Triacet II cream, ointment ℞ *topical corticosteroidal anti-inflammatory; antifungal* [triamcinolone acetonide; nystatin] 0.1%•100 000 U per g

mydeton [see: tolperisone]

Mydfrin 2.5% eye drops ℞ *topical ophthalmic decongestant and vasoconstrictor; mydriatic* [phenylephrine HCl] 2.5% ⓓ Midrin; Myfedrine

Mydriacyl Drop-Tainers (eye drops) ℞ *cycloplegic; mydriatic* [tropicamide] 0.5%, 1%

mydriatics *a class of drugs that cause the pupil of the eye to dilate*

myelin *investigational (orphan) for multiple sclerosis*

myeloid progenitor inhibitory factor 1 (MPIF-1) *investigational prophylactic for chemotherapy side effects*

myelosan [see: busulfan]

myfadol INN

Mygel; Mygel II oral suspension OTC *antacid; antiflatulent* [aluminum hydroxide; magnesium hydroxide; simethicone] 200•200•20 mg/5 mL; 400•400•40 mg/5 mL

Myidyl syrup (discontinued 1997) ℞ *antihistamine* [triprolidine HCl] 1.25 mg/5 mL

Mykinac cream ℞ *topical antifungal* [nystatin]

Mykrox tablets ℞ *antihypertensive; diuretic* [metolazone] 0.5 mg

Mylagen gelcaps OTC *antacid* [calcium carbonate; magnesium carbonate] 311•232 mg

Mylagen; Mylagen II liquid OTC *antacid; antiflatulent* [aluminum hydroxide; magnesium hydroxide; simethicone] 200•200•20 mg/5 mL; 400•400•40 mg/5 mL

Mylanta chewable tablets, liquid OTC *antacid; antiflatulent* [aluminum hydroxide; magnesium hydroxide; simethicone] 200•200•20, 400•400•40 mg; 200•200•20, 400•400•40 mg/5 mL ⊠ Dilantin; Milontin

Mylanta gelcaps OTC *antacid* [calcium carbonate; magnesium carbonate] 311•232 mg

Mylanta lozenges OTC *antacid* [calcium carbonate] 600 mg

Mylanta, Children's oral liquid, chewable tablets OTC *antacid* [calcium carbonate] 400 mg/5 mL; 400 mg

Mylanta AR ("acid reducer") tablets OTC *histamine H_2 antagonist for heartburn and acid indigestion* [famotidine] 10 mg

Mylanta Gas chewable tablets OTC *antiflatulent* [simethicone] 40, 80, 125 mg

Mylanta Natural Fiber Supplement powder OTC *bulk laxative* [psyllium hydrophilic mucilloid] 3.4 g/tsp.

Myleran tablets ℞ *alkylating antineoplastic for chronic myelogenous leukemia (CML)* [busulfan] 2 mg ⊠ Mylicon

Mylicon drops OTC *antiflatulent* [simethicone] 40 mg/0.6 mL ⊠ Modicon; Myleran

Myloral ℞ *investigational (Phase III) oral treatment for multiple sclerosis* [bovine myelin]

Myminic Expectorant liquid OTC *decongestant; expectorant* [phenylpropanolamine HCl; guaifenesin; alcohol 5%] 12.5•100 mg/5 mL

Myminicol liquid OTC *antitussive; decongestant; antihistamine* [dextromethorphan hydrobromide; phenylpropanolamine HCl; chlorpheniramine maleate] 10•12.5•2 mg/5 mL

Mynatal capsules ℞ *vitamin/mineral/calcium/iron supplement* [multiple vitamins & minerals; calcium; iron; folic acid; biotin] ≛•300•65•1•0.03 mg

Mynatal FC caplets ℞ *vitamin/mineral/calcium/iron supplement* [multiple vitamins & minerals; calcium; iron; folic acid; biotin] ≛•250•60•1•0.03 mg

Mynatal P.N. captabs ℞ *vitamin/calcium/iron supplement* [multiple vitamins; calcium; iron; folic acid] ≛•125•60•1 mg

Mynatal P.N. Forte caplets ℞ *vitamin/mineral/calcium/iron supplement* [multiple vitamins & minerals; calcium; iron; folic acid] ≛•250•60•1 mg

Mynatal Rx caplets ℞ *vitamin/mineral/calcium/iron supplement* [multiple vitamins & minerals; calcium; iron; folic acid; biotin] ≛•200•60•1•0.03 mg

Mynate 90 Plus delayed-release caplets ℞ *vitamin/calcium/iron supplement* [multiple vitamins; calcium; iron; folic acid] ≛•250•90•1 mg

Myochrysine IM injection (discontinued 1996) ℞ *antirheumatic* [gold sodium thiomalate] 25, 50 mg/mL

Myocide NS solution OTC *topical antiseptic* [benzalkonium chloride] ≛

Myoflex Creme OTC *topical analgesic* [trolamine salicylate] 10%

Myolin IV or IM injection ℞ *skeletal muscle relaxant* [orphenadrine citrate] 30 mg/mL

Myoscint (commercially available in Europe) ℞ *investigational (orphan) imaging agent for cardiac necrosis and myocarditis* [imciromab pentetate]

Myotonachol tablets ℞ *cholinergic urinary stimulant for postsurgical and postpartum urinary retention* [bethanechol chloride] 10, 25 mg

Myotrophin injection ℞ *investigational (NDA filed, orphan) for amyotrophic lateral sclerosis, growth hormone insufficiency, and post-poliomyelitis syndrome* [mecasermin]

Myphetane DC Cough syrup ℞ *narcotic antitussive; decongestant; antihistamine* [codeine phosphate; phenylpropanolamine HCl; brompheniramine maleate; alcohol 1.2%] 10•12.5•2 mg/5 mL

Myphetane DX Cough syrup ℞ *antitussive; decongestant; antihistamine* [dextromethorphan hydrobromide; pseudoephedrine HCl; brompheniramine maleate; alcohol 1%] 10•30•2 mg/5 mL

myralact INN, BAN

Myrica cerifera medicinal herb [see: bayberry]

myricodine [see: myrophine]

Myristica fragrans medicinal herb [see: nutmeg; mace]

myristica oil [see: nutmeg oil]

myristyl alcohol NF *stiffening agent*

myristyltrimethylammonium bromide *antiseborrheic*

myrophine INN, BAN

Myroxylon balsamum; M. pereirae medicinal herb [see: Peruvian balsam]

myrrh (*Commiphora abssynica; C. molmol; C. myrrha*) seeds *medicinal herb for bad breath, bronchitis, cancer, constipation, hay fever, hemorrhoids, leprosy, lung diseases, mouth and skin sores, sore throat, syphilis, and stimu-*

lating menses; also used as an antiseptic and astringent

myrtecaine INN

Myrtilli fructus medicinal herb [see: bilberry]

myrtle *medicinal herb* [see: periwinkle]

myrtle, bog *medicinal herb* [see: buckbean]

myrtle, wax *medicinal herb* [see: bayberry]

myrtle flag; grass myrtle; sweet myrtle *medicinal herb* [see: calamus]

Mysoline tablets, oral suspension ℞ *anticonvulsant for grand mal, psychomotor, or focal epileptic seizures* [primidone] 50, 250 mg; 250 mg/5 mL

myspamol [see: proquamezine]

Mytelase caplets ℞ *anticholinesterase muscle stimulant; myasthenia gravis treatment* [ambenonium chloride] 10 mg

Mytrex cream, ointment ℞ *topical corticosteroidal anti-inflammatory; antifungal* [triamcinolone acetonide; nystatin] 0.1%•100 000 U/g

Mytussin syrup OTC *expectorant* [guaifenesin; alcohol 3.5%] 100 mg/5 mL

Mytussin AC Cough syrup ℞ *narcotic antitussive; expectorant* [codeine phosphate; guaifenesin; alcohol 3.5%] 10•100 mg/5 mL

Mytussin DAC syrup ℞ *narcotic antitussive; decongestant; expectorant* [codeine phosphate; pseudoephedrine HCl; guaifenesin; alcohol 1.7%] 10•30•100 mg/5 mL

Mytussin DM liquid OTC *antitussive; expectorant* [dextromethorphan hydrobromide; guaifenesin; alcohol 1.6%] 10•100 mg/5 mL

myuizone [see: thioacetazone; thiacetazone]

My-Vitalife capsules OTC *vitamin/mineral/calcium/iron supplement* [multiple vitamins & minerals; calcium; iron; folic acid; biotin] ±•130•27•0.4•0.03 mg

MZM tablets ℞ *carbonic anhydrase inhibitor for glaucoma* [methazolamide] 25, 50 mg

MZM (methazolamide) [q.v.]
M-Zole 3 Combination Pack vaginal suppositories + cream OTC *antifungal* [miconazole nitrate] 200 mg; 2%

M-Zole 7 Dual Pack vaginal suppositories + cream OTC *antifungal* [miconazole nitrate] 100 mg; 2%

N-0923 *investigational (Phase II) dopamine agonist in a transdermal patch for Parkinson's disease*
N₂ (nitrogen) [q.v.]
N-3 polyunsaturated fatty acids [see: doconexent; icosapent; omega-3 marine triglycerides]
²²**Na** [see: sodium chloride Na 22]
nabazenil USAN, INN *anticonvulsant*
Nabi-HB IM injection ℞ *immunizing agent following exposure to hepatitis B surface antigen* [hepatitis B immune globulin] 5%
nabilone USAN, INN, BAN *minor tranquilizer*
nabitan INN *analgesic* [also: nabitan HCl]
nabitan HCl USAN *analgesic* [also: nabitan]
naboctate INN *antiglaucoma agent; antinauseant* [also: naboctate HCl]
naboctate HCl USAN *antiglaucoma agent; antinauseant* [also: naboctate]
nabumetone USAN, INN, BAN *antiarthritic; nonsteroidal anti-inflammatory drug (NSAID)*
nabutan HCl [now: nabitan HCl]
NAC (nitrogen mustard, Adriamycin, CCNU) *chemotherapy protocol*
nacartocin INN
NaCl (sodium chloride) [q.v.]
NAD (nicotinamide-adenine dinucleotide) [see: nadide]
nadide USAN, INN *antagonist to alcohol and narcotics*
nadisan [see: carbutamide]
nadolol USAN, USP, INN, BAN *antianginal; antihypertensive; antiadrenergic (β-receptor)* 20, 40, 80, 120, 160 mg oral ⑨ Nandol

nadoxolol INN
nadroparin calcium INN, BAN *anticoagulant; low molecular weight heparin*
naepaine HCl NF
nafamostat INN *anticoagulant; antifibrinolytic* [also: nafamostat mesylate; nafamostat mesilate]
nafamostat mesilate JAN *anticoagulant; antifibrinolytic* [also: nafamostat mesylate; nafamostat]
nafamostat mesylate USAN *anticoagulant; antifibrinolytic* [also: nafamostat; nafamostat mesilate]
nafarelin INN, BAN *luteinizing hormone-releasing hormone (LHRH) agonist* [also: nafarelin acetate]
nafarelin acetate USAN *luteinizing hormone-releasing hormone (LHRH) agonist for central precocious puberty (orphan) and endometriosis* [also: nafarelin]
Nafazair eye drops ℞ *topical ophthalmic decongestant and vasoconstrictor* [naphazoline HCl] 0.1%
Nafazair A eye drops (discontinued 1995) ℞ *topical ophthalmic decongestant and antihistamine* [naphazoline HCl; pheniramine maleate] 0.025%•0.3%
nafazatrom INN, BAN
nafcaproic acid INN
Nafcil powder for IV or IM injection (discontinued 1998) ℞ *penicillinase-resistant penicillin antibiotic* [nafcillin sodium] 0.5, 1, 2, 10 g
nafcillin INN *penicillinase-resistant penicillin antibiotic* [also: nafcillin sodium]
nafcillin sodium USAN, USP *penicillinase-resistant penicillin antibiotic* [also: nafcillin]

nafenodone INN
nafenopin USAN, INN *antihyperlipoproteinemic*
nafetolol INN
nafimidone INN *anticonvulsant* [also:
nafimidone HCl]
nafimidone HCl USAN *anticonvulsant*
[also: nafimidone]
nafiverine INN
naflocort USAN, INN *topical adrenocortical steroid*
nafomine INN *muscle relaxant* [also:
nafomine malate]
nafomine malate USAN *muscle relaxant* [also: nafomine]
nafoxadol INN
nafoxidine HCl USAN, INN *antiestrogen*
nafronyl oxalate USAN *vasodilator*
[also: naftidrofuryl]
naftalofos USAN, INN *veterinary anthelmintic*
naftazone INN, BAN
naftidrofuryl INN *vasodilator* [also:
nafronyl oxalate]
naftifine INN, BAN *broad-spectrum antifungal* [also: naftifine HCl]
naftifine HCl USAN *broad-spectrum
antifungal* [also: naftifine]
Naftin cream, gel ℞ *topical antifungal*
[naftifine HCl] 1%
naftopidil INN
naftoxate INN
naftypramide INN *antibacterial*
Naganol (available only from the
Centers for Disease Control) ℞ *antiparasitic for African trypanosomiasis
and onchocerciasis* [suramin sodium]
naganol [see: suramin sodium]
nagrestipen USAN *stem cell inhibitory
protein*
nalazosulfamide [see: salazosulfamide]
nalbuphine INN, BAN *narcotic agonist-
antagonist analgesic; narcotic antagonist* [also: nalbuphine HCl]
nalbuphine HCl USAN *narcotic agonist-antagonist analgesic; narcotic
antagonist* [also: nalbuphine] 10, 20
mg/mL injection
Naldec Pediatric syrup ℞ *decongestant; antihistamine* [phenylpropanol-

amine HCl; phenylephrine HCl;
phenyltoloxamine citrate; chlorpheniramine maleate]
Naldecon sustained-release tablets,
syrup, pediatric syrup, pediatric
drops ℞ *decongestant; antihistamine*
[phenylpropanolamine HCl; phenylephrine HCl; chlorpheniramine
maleate; phenyltoloxamine citrate]
40•10•5•15 mg; 20•5•2.5•7.5
mg/5 mL; 5•1.25•0.5•2 mg/5 mL;
5•1.25•0.5•2 mg/mL 🔊 Nalfon
Naldecon CX Adult liquid ℞ *narcotic
antitussive; decongestant; expectorant*
[codeine phosphate; phenylpropanolamine HCl; guaifenesin] 10•
12.5•200 mg/5 mL
Naldecon DX children's syrup, pediatric drops OTC *pediatric antitussive,
decongestant, and expectorant* [dex-
tromethorphan hydrobromide;
phenylpropanolamine HCl; guaifen-
esin] 5•6.25•100 mg/5 mL; 5•
6.25•50 mg/mL
Naldecon DX Adult liquid OTC *antitussive; decongestant; expectorant*
[dextromethorphan hydrobromide;
phenylpropanolamine HCl; guaifen-
esin] 10•12.5•200 mg/5 mL
Naldecon EX children's syrup, pediatric drops OTC *pediatric decongestant
and expectorant* [phenylpropanol-
amine HCl; guaifenesin] 6.25•100
mg/5 mL; 6.25•50 mg/mL
Naldecon Senior DX liquid OTC *antitussive; expectorant* [dextromethor-
phan hydrobromide; guaifenesin]
10•200 mg/5 mL
Naldecon Senior EX liquid OTC *expectorant* [guaifenesin] 200 mg/5 mL
Naldegesic tablets OTC *decongestant;
analgesic* [pseudoephedrine HCl;
acetaminophen]
Naldelate syrup, pediatric syrup ℞
decongestant; antihistamine [phenylpro-
panolamine HCl; phenylephrine
HCl; chlorpheniramine maleate;
phenyltoloxamine citrate] 20•5•2.5•
7.5 mg/5 mL; 5•1.25•0.5•2 mg/5 mL

Naldelate DX Adult liquid OTC *antitussive; decongestant; expectorant* [dextromethorphan hydrobromide; phenylpropanolamine HCl; guaifenesin] 10•12.5•200 mg/5 mL

Nalfon Pulvules (capsules) ℞ *nonsteroidal anti-inflammatory drug (NSAID); antiarthritic; analgesic* [fenoprofen calcium] 200, 300 mg ⑨ Naldecon

Nalgest sustained-release tablets, syrup, pediatric syrup, pediatric drops ℞ *decongestant; antihistamine* [phenylpropanolamine HCl; phenylephrine HCl; chlorpheniramine maleate; phenyltoloxamine citrate] 40•10•5•15 mg; 20•5•2.5•7.5 mg/5 mL; 5•1.25•0.5•2 mg/5 mL; 5•1.25•0.5•2 mg/mL

nalidixane [see: nalidixic acid]

nalidixate sodium USAN *antibacterial*

nalidixic acid USAN, USP, INN *urinary antibiotic*

Nallpen powder for IV or IM injection ℞ *penicillinase-resistant penicillin antibiotic* [nafcillin sodium] 0.5, 1, 2, 10 g

nalmefene USAN, INN, BAN *narcotic antagonist*

nalmefene HCl *narcotic antagonist*

nalmetrene [now: nalmefene]

nalmexone INN *analgesic; narcotic antagonist* [also: nalmexone HCl]

nalmexone HCl USAN *analgesic; narcotic antagonist* [also: nalmexone]

nalorphine INN [also: nalorphine HCl]

nalorphine HCl USP [also: nalorphine]

naloxiphane tartrate [see: levallorphan tartrate]

naloxone INN, BAN *narcotic antagonist* [also: naloxone HCl]

naloxone HCl USAN, USP, JAN *narcotic antagonist* [also: naloxone] 0.02, 0.4 mg/mL injection

naloxone HCl & buprenorphine HCl *investigational (orphan) for opiate addictions*

naloxone HCl & pentazocine *narcotic agonist-antagonist analgesic* 0.5• 50 mg oral

naltrexone USAN, INN, BAN *narcotic antagonist*

naltrexone HCl *opiate blockage and maintenance in formerly opiate-dependent individuals (orphan)*

naminterol INN

[¹³N]ammonia [see: ammonia N 13]

namoxyrate USAN, INN *analgesic*

namuron [see: cyclobarbitone]

nanafrocin INN

nandrolone BAN *anabolic* [also: nandrolone cyclotate]

nandrolone cyclotate USAN *anabolic* [also: nandrolone]

nandrolone decanoate USAN, USP *androgen/anabolic steroid for anemia of renal insufficiency; sometimes abused as a street drug* 50, 100, 200 mg/mL injection (in oil)

nandrolone phenpropionate USP *androgen/anabolic steroid for metastatic breast cancer in women; sometimes abused as a street drug* 25, 50 mg/mL injection (in oil)

naniopine [see: nanofin]

nanofin INN

nanterinone INN, BAN

nantradol INN *analgesic* [also: nantradol HCl]

nantradol HCl USAN *analgesic* [also: nantradol]

NAPA (N-acetyl-*p*-aminophenol) [see: acetaminophen]

NAPA (N-acetyl-procainamide) [q.v.]

napactadine INN *antidepressant* [also: napactadine HCl]

napactadine HCl USAN *antidepressant* [also: napactadine]

napadisilate INN *combining name for radicals or groups* [also: napadisylate]

napadisylate BAN *combining name for radicals or groups* [also: napadisilate]

napamezole INN *antidepressant* [also: napamezole HCl]

napamezole HCl USAN *antidepressant* [also: napamezole]

Napamide capsules ℞ *antiarrhythmic* [disopyramide phosphate]

Naphazole-A eye drops (discontinued 1995) ℞ *topical ophthalmic deconges-*

tant and antihistamine [naphazoline HCl; pheniramine maleate] 0.025%•0.3%

naphazoline INN, BAN *topical ophthalmic decongestant and vasoconstrictor; nasal decongestant* [also: naphazoline HCl; naphazoline nitrate]

naphazoline HCl USP *topical ophthalmic decongestant and vasoconstrictor; nasal decongestant* [also: naphazoline; naphazoline nitrate] 0.1% eye drops

naphazoline HCl & antazoline phosphate *topical ocular decongestant and antihistamine* 0.05%•0.5%

naphazoline HCl & pheniramine maleate *topical ocular decongestant and antihistamine* 0.025%•0.3% eye drops

naphazoline nitrate JAN *topical ocular vasoconstrictor; nasal decongestant* [also: naphazoline HCl; naphazoline]

Naphazoline Plus eye drops OTC *topical ophthalmic decongestant and antihistamine* [naphazoline HCl; pheniramine maleate] 0.025%•0.3%

Naphcon eye drops OTC *topical ophthalmic decongestant and vasoconstrictor* [naphazoline HCl] 0.012%

Naphcon Forte Drop-Tainers (eye drops) ℞ *topical ophthalmic decongestant and vasoconstrictor* [naphazoline HCl] 0.1%

Naphcon-A Drop-Tainers (eye drops) OTC *topical ophthalmic decongestant and antihistamine* [naphazoline HCl; pheniramine maleate] 0.025%•0.3%

Naphoptic-A eye drops ℞ *topical ophthalmic decongestant and antihistamine* [naphazoline HCl; pheniramine maleate] 0.025%•0.3%

2-naphthol [see: betanaphthol]

naphthonone INN

naphthypramide [see: naftypramide]

Naphuride (available only from the Centers for Disease Control) ℞ *antiparasitic for African trypanosomiasis and onchocerciasis* [suramin sodium]

napirimus INN

napitane mesylate USAN *antidepressant; α-adrenergic blocker; norepinephrine uptake antagonist*

Naprelan controlled-release tablets ℞ *once-daily nonsteroidal anti-inflammatory drug (NSAID); antiarthritic; analgesic* [naproxen (from naproxen sodium)] 375 (412.5), 500 (550) mg

naprodoxime INN

Napron X tablets ℞ *nonsteroidal anti-inflammatory drug (NSAID); antiarthritic; analgesic* [naproxen] 500 mg ⊠ Lupron; Mepron

Naprosyn tablets, oral suspension ℞ *nonsteroidal anti-inflammatory drug (NSAID); antiarthritic; analgesic* [naproxen] 250, 375, 500 mg; 125 mg/5 mL ⊠ Meprospan; Natacyn

Naprosyn EC [see: EC-Naprosyn]

naproxen USAN, USP, INN, BAN, JAN *analgesic; antiarthritic; nonsteroidal anti-inflammatory drug (NSAID); antipyretic* 250, 375, 500 mg oral; 125 mg/5 mL oral

naproxen sodium USAN, USP *analgesic; antiarthritic; nonsteroidal anti-inflammatory drug (NSAID); antipyretic* 220, 250, 500 mg oral

naproxol USAN, INN *anti-inflammatory; analgesic; antipyretic*

napsagatran USAN, INN *antithrombotic*

napsilate INN *combining name for radicals or groups* [also: napsylate]

napsylate USAN, BAN *combining name for radicals or groups* [also: napsilate]

Naqua tablets ℞ *diuretic; antihypertensive* [trichlormethiazide] 2, 4 mg

naranol INN *antipsychotic* [also: naranol HCl]

naranol HCl USAN *antipsychotic* [also: naranol]

narasin USAN, INN, BAN *coccidiostat; veterinary growth stimulant*

naratriptan INN, BAN *vascular serotonin 5-HT$_1$ receptor agonist for migraine headache* [also: naratriptan HCl]

naratriptan HCl USAN *vascular serotonin 5-HT$_1$ receptor agonist for migraine headache* [also: naratriptan]

Narcan IV, IM, or subcu injection, neonatal injection ℞ *narcotic antagonist for opiate dependence or overdose; hypo-*

tension treatment [naloxone HCl] 0.4, 1 mg/mL; 0.02 mg/mL ⑨ Marcaine

narcotic agonist-antagonists *a class of opioid or morphine-like analgesics with lower abuse potential than pure narcotic agonist analgesics*

narcotic agonists; narcotics *a class of opioid or morphine-like analgesics that relieve pain and induce sleep*

narcotine [see: noscapine]

narcotine HCl [see: noscapine HCl]

nard *medicinal herb* [see: spikenard]

Nardil sugar-coated tablets ℞ *antipsychotic; monoamine oxidase inhibitor (MAOI) for treatment-resistant atypical depression* [phenelzine sulfate] 15 mg ⑨ Norinyl

Naropin injection ℞ *long-acting local anesthetic* [ropivacaine HCl] 2, 5, 7.5, 10 mg/mL

narrow dock *medicinal herb* [see: yellow dock]

Nasabid prolonged-action capsules ℞ *decongestant; expectorant* [pseudoephedrine HCl; guaifenesin] 90•250 mg

Nasabid SR long-acting tablets ℞ *decongestant; expectorant* [pseudoephedrine HCl; guaifenesin] 90•500 mg

Nasacort nasal spray ℞ *corticosteroidal anti-inflammatory for seasonal or perennial rhinitis* [triamcinolone acetonide] 55 µg/spray

Nasacort AQ metered-dose aerosol ℞ *corticosteroidal anti-inflammatory for seasonal or perennial rhinitis* [triamcinolone acetonide] 55 µg/spray

Nasahist B subcu or IM injection (discontinued 1997) ℞ *antihistamine; anaphylaxis* [brompheniramine maleate] 10 mg/mL

NāSal nasal spray, nose drops OTC *nasal moisturizer* [sodium chloride (saline solution)] 0.65%

Nasal Decongestant spray OTC *nasal decongestant* [oxymetazoline HCl] 0.05%

Nasal Jelly ointment OTC *nasal moisturizer* [phenol; camphor; menthol; eucalyptus oil; oil of lavender]

Nasal Moist nasal spray OTC *nasal moisturizer* [sodium chloride (saline solution)] 0.65%

Nasal Relief nasal spray OTC *nasal decongestant* [oxymetazoline HCl] 0.05%

NasalCrom; Children's NasalCrom nasal spray OTC *anti-inflammatory/ mast cell stabilizer for the prophylaxis of allergic rhinitis* [cromolyn sodium] 4% (5.2 mg/dose)

NasalCrom A nasal spray + tablets OTC *anti-inflammatory/mast cell stabilizer for the prophylaxis of allergic rhinitis; antihistamine* [cromolyn sodium; chlorpheniramine maleate] 4% (5.2 mg/dose); 4 mg

NasalCrom CA nasal spray + tablets OTC *anti-inflammatory/mast cell stabilizer for the prophylaxis of allergic rhinitis; decongestant; analgesic* [cromolyn sodium; pseudoephedrine HCl; acetaminophen] 4% (5.2 mg/dose); 30 mg•500 mg

Nasalide nasal spray ℞ *corticosteroidal anti-inflammatory for seasonal or perennial rhinitis* [flunisolide] 25 µg/dose

Nasarel metered dose nasal spray ℞ *corticosteroidal anti-inflammatory for seasonal or perennial rhinitis* [flunisolide] 25 µg/dose

Nasatab LA long-acting film-coated tablets ℞ *decongestant; expectorant* [pseudoephedrine HCl; guaifenesin] 120•500 mg

Nascobal nasal gel in metered-dose applicator ℞ *maintenance administration following intramuscular vitamin B_{12} therapy* [cyanocobalamin] 500 µg/0.1 mL dose

Nashville rabbit antithymocyte serum [see: lymphocyte immune globulin, antithymocyte]

Nashville Rabbit Antithymocyte Serum ℞ *investigational (orphan) passive immunizing agent to prevent allograft rejection in organ and bone*

marrow transplants [lymphocyte immune globulin, antithymocyte (rabbit)]

Nasonex nasal spray ℞ *corticosteroid for the prophylaxis and treatment of seasonal and perennial allergic rhinitis* [mometasone furoate] 50 μg/spray

Nasturtium officinale *medicinal herb* [see: watercress]

Natabec Rx Kapseals (capsules) (discontinued 1995) ℞ *vitamin/calcium/ iron supplement* [multiple vitamins; calcium; iron; folic acid] ±•240• 30•1 mg

Natacyn eye drop suspension ℞ *ophthalmic antifungal agent* [natamycin] 5% ② Naprosyn

Natafort Filmseal (film-coated tablets) (discontinued 1995) ℞ *vitamin/calcium/iron supplement* [multiple vitamins; calcium; iron; folic acid] ±• 350•65•1 mg

NatalCare Plus film-coated tablets ℞ *vitamin/mineral/calcium/iron supplement* [multiple vitamins & minerals; calcium; iron; folic acid] ±•200• 27•1 mg

Natalins tablets OTC *vitamin/calcium/ iron supplement* [multiple vitamins; calcium; iron; folic acid] ±•200• 30•0.5 mg

Natalins Rx tablets ℞ *vitamin/calcium/ iron supplement* [multiple vitamins; calcium; iron; folic acid; biotin] ±• 200•60•1•0.03 mg

natamycin USAN, USP, INN, BAN *ophthalmic fungicidal antibiotic* [also: pimaricin]

Natarex Prenatal tablets ℞ *vitamin/ calcium/iron supplement* [multiple vitamins; calcium; iron; folic acid; biotin] ±•200•60•1•0.03 mg

Natrecor ℞ *investigational (NDA filed) brain natriuretic peptide (BNP) for acute congestive heart failure* [nesiritide]

natural killer cell stimulatory factor [see: edodekin alfa]

Natural Vegetable powder OTC *bulk laxative* [psyllium hydrophilic mucilloid] 3.4 g/tsp.

Naturalyte oral solution OTC *electrolyte replacement* [sodium, potassium, and chloride electrolytes] 240 mL, 1 L

Nature's Bounty 1 timed-release tablets (discontinued 1995) OTC *vitamin/mineral/calcium/iron supplement* [multiple vitamins & minerals; calcium; iron; folic acid; biotin] ±• 50•10•0.4•0.05 mg

Nature's Remedy tablets OTC *laxative* [cascara sagrada] 150 mg

Nature's Tears eye drops OTC *ophthalmic moisturizer/lubricant* [hydroxypropyl methylcellulose] 0.4%

Naturetin tablets ℞ *antihypertensive; diuretic* [bendroflumethiazide] 5, 10 mg

Naturvus *hydrophilic contact lens material* [hefilcon B]

Naus-A-Way solution (discontinued 1997) OTC *antinauseant; antiemetic* [phosphorated carbohydrate solution (fructose, dextrose, and orthophosphoric acid)]

Nausea Relief solution OTC *antinauseant; antiemetic* [phosphorated carbohydrate solution (dextrose, fructose, and phosphoric acid)] 1.87 g•1.87 g•21.5 mg

Nausetrol solution OTC *antinauseant; antiemetic* [phosphorated carbohydrate solution (fructose, dextrose, and orthophosphoric acid)]

Navane capsules ℞ *conventional (typical) antipsychotic* [thiothixene] 1, 2, 5, 10, 20 mg

Navane IM solution (discontinued 1997) ℞ *conventional (typical) antipsychotic* [thiothixene HCl] 2 mg/mL

Navane oral concentrate ℞ *conventional (typical) antipsychotic* [thiothixene HCl] 5 mg/mL

Navane powder for IM injection (discontinued 1998) ℞ *conventional (typical) antipsychotic* [thiothixene HCl] 5 mg/mL

Navelbine IV injection ℞ *antineoplastic for Hodgkin's disease and lung, breast and ovarian cancer* [vinorelbine tartrate] 10 mg/mL

naxagolide INN *antiparkinsonian; dopamine agonist* [also: naxagolide HCl]

naxagolide HCl USAN *antiparkinsonian; dopamine agonist* [also: naxagolide]

naxaprostene INN

9-NC (9-nitro-20-(S)-camptothecin) [q.v.]

ND Clear sustained-release capsules ℞ *decongestant; antihistamine* [pseudoephedrine HCl; chlorpheniramine maleate] 120•8 mg

ND Stat subcu or IM injection (discontinued 1997) ℞ *antihistamine for anaphylaxis* [brompheniramine maleate] 10 mg/mL

ND-Gesic tablets OTC *decongestant; antihistamine; analgesic* [phenylephrine HCl; chlorpheniramine maleate; pyrilamine maleate; acetaminophen] 5•2•12.5•300 mg

NE-1530 *investigational (Phase I) agent for the prevention of otitis media*

nealbarbital INN [also: nealbarbitone]

nealbarbitone BAN [also: nealbarbital]

nebacumab USAN, INN, BAN *antiendotoxin monoclonal antibody; investigational (orphan) for gram-negative bacteremia in endotoxin shock*

Nebcin IV or IM injection, pediatric injection, powder for injection ℞ *aminoglycoside antibiotic* [tobramycin sulfate] 10, 40 mg/mL; 10 mg/mL; 1.2 g

nebidrazine INN

nebivolol USAN, INN *antihypertensive (β-blocker)*

nebracetam INN

nebramycin USAN, INN *antibacterial*

nebramycin factor 6 [see: tobramycin]

NebuPent inhalation aerosol ℞ *antiprotozoal; treatment and prophylaxis of Pneumocystis carinii pneumonia (orphan)* [pentamidine isethionate] 300 mg

Necon 0.5/35-21; Necon 0.5/35-28 tablets ℞ *monophasic oral contraceptive* [norethindrone; ethinyl estradiol] 0.5 mg•35 μg

Necon 1/35-21; Necon 1/35-28 tablets ℞ *monophasic oral contraceptive* [norethindrone; ethinyl estradiol] 1 mg•35 μg

Necon 1/50-21; Necon 1/50-28 tablets ℞ *monophasic oral contraceptive* [norethindrone; mestranol] 1 mg•50 μg

Necon 10/11-21; Necon 10/11-28 tablets ℞ *biphasic oral contraceptive* [norethindrone; ethinyl estradiol] Phase 1: 0.5 mg•35 μg; Phase 2: 1 mg•35 μg

nedocromil USAN, INN, BAN *antiinflammatory; prophylactic antiallergic*

nedocromil calcium USAN *antiinflammatory; prophylactic antiallergic*

nedocromil sodium USAN *antiinflammatory; prophylactic antiallergic; antiasthmatic*

N.E.E. 1/35 tablets ℞ *monophasic oral contraceptive* [norethindrone; ethinyl estradiol] 1 mg•35 μg

neem tree (Azadirachta indica) fruit, leaves, root, and oil *medicinal herb for contraception, diabetes, heart disease, malaria, skin diseases, ulcers, and worms; also used as a pesticide and insect repellent; not generally regarded as safe and effective for infants as it may cause death*

nefazodone INN *antidepressant; serotonin and norepinephrine uptake inhibitor* [also: nefazodone HCl]

nefazodone HCl USAN *antidepressant; serotonin and norepinephrine uptake inhibitor* [also: nefazodone]

neflumozide INN *antipsychotic* [also: neflumozide HCl]

neflumozide HCl USAN *antipsychotic* [also: neflumozide]

nefocon A USAN *hydrophobic contact lens material*

nefopam INN *analgesic* [also: nefopam HCl]

nefopam HCl USAN *analgesic* [also: nefopam]

nefrolan [see: clorexolone]

NegGram caplets, oral suspension ℞ *urinary antibiotic* [nalidixic acid] 250, 500, 1000 mg; 250 mg/5 mL

neldazosin INN

nelezaprine INN *muscle relaxant* [also: nelezaprine maleate]

nelezaprine maleate USAN *muscle relaxant* [also: nelezaprine]

nelfilcon A USAN *hydrophilic contact lens material*

nelfinavir mesylate USAN *antiretroviral HIV-1 protease inhibitor*

Nelova 1/35E; Nelova 0.5/35E tablets ℞ *monophasic oral contraceptive* [norethindrone; ethinyl estradiol] 1 mg●35 μg; 0.5 mg●35 μg

Nelova 1/50M tablets ℞ *monophasic oral contraceptive* [norethindrone; mestranol] 1 mg●50 μg

Nelova 10/11 tablets ℞ *biphasic oral contraceptive* [norethindrone; ethinyl estradiol] Phase 1: 0.5 mg●35 μg; Phase 2: 1 mg●35 μg

nelzarabine USAN *antineoplastic for T-cell and B-cell lymphomas*

nemadectin USAN, INN *veterinary antiparasitic*

nemazoline INN *nasal decongestant* [also: nemazoline HCl]

nemazoline HCl USAN *nasal decongestant* [also: nemazoline]

Nembutal elixir ℞ *sedative; hypnotic; also abused as a street drug* [pentobarbital] 20 mg/5 mL ② Myambutal

Nembutal Sodium capsules, IV or IM injection, suppositories ℞ *sedative; hypnotic; also abused as a street drug* [pentobarbital sodium] 50, 100 mg; 50 mg/mL; 30, 60, 120, 200 mg

neoarsphenamine NF, INN

Neocaf ℞ *investigational (orphan) for apnea of prematurity* [caffeine]

Neo-Calglucon syrup OTC *calcium supplement* [calcium glubionate] 1.8 g/5 mL

neocarzinostatin [now: zinostatin]

Neo-Castaderm liquid (discontinued 1995) OTC *topical antifungal; astringent; antiseptic* [resorcinol; boric acid; acetone; sodium bisulfite; phenol; alcohol]

Neocate One + ready-to-use liquid OTC *pediatric enteral nutritional therapy* [lactose-free formula] 237 mL

Neocera (trademarked ingredient) *suppository base* [polyethylent glycol 400, 1450, and 8000; polysorbate 60]

neocid [see: chlorophenothane]

neocinchophen NF, INN

NeoCitran DM Coughs & Colds ⒸⒶⓃ powder for oral solution OTC *antitussive; decongestant; antihistamine* [dextromethorphan hydrobromide; phenylephrine HCl; pheniramine maleate] 30●10●20 mg/dose

Neo-Cortef ointment (discontinued 1997) ℞ *topical corticosteroidal anti-inflammatory; antibiotic* [hydrocortisone; neomycin sulfate] 0.5%●0.5%, 1%●0.5%

Neo-Cultol jelly OTC *emollient laxative* [mineral oil]

NeoDecadron cream (discontinued 1998) ℞ *topical corticosteroidal anti-inflammatory; antibiotic* [dexamethasone sodium phosphate; neomycin sulfate] 0.1%●0.5%

NeoDecadron Ocumeter (eye drops), ophthalmic ointment ℞ *topical ophthalmic corticosteroidal anti-inflammatory; antibiotic* [dexamethasone sodium phosphate; neomycin sulfate] 0.1%●0.35%; 0.05%●0.35%

Neo-Dexair eye drops ℞ *topical ophthalmic corticosteroidal anti-inflammatory; antibiotic* [dexamethasone sodium phosphate; neomycin sulfate] 0.1%●0.35%

Neo-Dexameth eye drops ℞ *topical ophthalmic corticosteroidal anti-inflammatory; antibiotic* [dexamethasone sodium phosphate; neomycin sulfate] 0.1%●0.35%

Neo-Diaral capsules OTC *antidiarrheal* [loperamide] 2 mg

Neo-Durabolic IM injection ℞ *anabolic steroid for anemia of renal insufficiency* [nandrolone decanoate] 50, 200 mg/mL

neodymium *element (Nd)*

Neo-fradin oral solution ℞ *aminoglycoside antibiotic* [neomycin sulfate] 125 mg/5 mL

Neoloid oil OTC *stimulant laxative* [castor oil] 36.4%

Neomac ointment OTC *topical antibiotic* [polymyxin B sulfate; neomycin sulfate; bacitracin]

Neomark ℞ *investigational (NDA filed, orphan) radiosensitizer for breast and brain tumors* [broxuridine]

neo-mercazole [see: carbimazole]

Neomixin ointment OTC *topical antibiotic* [polymyxin B sulfate; neomycin sulfate; bacitracin zinc] 5000 U•3.5 mg•400 U per g ② neomycin

neomycin INN, BAN *antibacterial* [also: neomycin palmitate] ② Neomixin

neomycin B [see: framycetin]

neomycin palmitate USAN *antibacterial* [also: neomycin]

neomycin sulfate USP *aminoglycoside antibiotic* 500 mg oral; 3.5 mg/g topical

neomycin undecenoate [see: neomycin undecylenate]

neomycin undecylenate USAN *antibacterial; antifungal*

neon *element (Ne)*

Neopap suppositories OTC *analgesic; antipyretic* [acetaminophen] 125 mg

neopenyl [see: clemizole penicillin]

neoquate [see: nequinate]

Neoral soft gels for microemulsion, oral solution for microemulsion ℞ *immunosuppressant for allogenic kidney, liver, and heart transplants, rheumatoid arthritis, and psoriasis* [cyclosporine; alcohol 9.5%] 25, 100 mg; 100 mg/mL

NeoRespin timed-release capsules OTC *bronchodilator for bronchial asthma and bronchospasm* [ephedrine HCl]

Neosar powder for IV injection ℞ *nitrogen mustard-type alkylating antineoplastic for multiple leukemias, lymphomas, blastomas, sarcomas and organ cancers* [cyclophosphamide] 100 mg

Neosporin cream OTC *topical antibiotic* [polymyxin B sulfate; neomycin sulfate] 10 000 U•3.5 mg per g

Neosporin Drop Dose (eye drops) ℞ *topical ophthalmic antibiotic* [polymyxin B sulfate; neomycin sulfate; gramicidin] 10 000 U•1.75 mg• 0.025 mg per mL

Neosporin ointment OTC *topical antibiotic* [polymyxin B sulfate; neomycin sulfate; bacitracin] 5000 U•3.5 mg• 400 U, 10 000 U•3.5 mg•500 U /g

Neosporin ophthalmic ointment ℞ *ophthalmic antibiotic* [polymyxin B sulfate; neomycin sulfate; bacitracin zinc] 10 000 U•3.5 mg•400 U per g

Neosporin G.U. Irrigant solution ℞ *bactericidal* [neomycin sulfate; polymyxin B sulfate] 40 mg•200 000 U per mL

Neosporin Plus cream OTC *topical antibiotic; anesthetic* [polymyxin B sulfate; neomycin; lidocaine] 10 000 U•3.5 mg•40 mg per g

Neosporin Plus ointment OTC *topical antibiotic; anesthetic* [polymyxin B sulfate; bacitracin zinc; neomycin; lidocaine] 10 000 U•500 U•3.5 mg•40 mg per g

neostigmine BAN *cholinergic/anticholinesterase muscle stimulant* [also: neostigmine bromide]

neostigmine bromide USP, INN, BAN *cholinergic/anticholinesterase muscle stimulant* [also: neostigmine] 15 mg oral

neostigmine methylsulfate USP *cholinergic/anticholinesterase muscle stimulant; urinary stimulant* 1:1000 (1 mg/mL), 1:2000 (0.5 mg/mL) injection

Neostrata AHA for Age Spots and Skin Lightening gel (discontinued 1997) OTC *hyperpigmentation bleaching agent; sunscreen* [hydroquinone; glycolic acid] 2%•10%

Neo-Synalar cream (discontinued 1995) ℞ *topical corticosteroidal anti-inflammatory; antibacterial* [fluocinolone acetonide; neomycin sulfate] 0.025%•0.5%

Neo-Synephrine eye drops, viscous solution ℞ *topical ophthalmic decongestant and vasoconstrictor; mydriatic* [phenylephrine HCl] 2.5%, 10%; 10%

Neo-Synephrine nasal spray, nose drops OTC *nasal decongestant* [phenylephrine HCl] 0.25%, 0.5%, 1%; 0.125%, 0.25%, 0.5%, 1%

Neo-Synephrine 12 Hour nasal spray OTC *nasal decongestant* [oxymetazoline HCl] 0.05%

Neo-Synephrine IV, IM, or subcu injection ℞ *vasopressor for hypotensive or cardiac shock* [phenylephrine HCl] 1% (10 mg/mL)

Neo-Tabs tablets ℞ *aminoglycoside antibiotic* [neomycin sulfate] 500 mg

Neotal ophthalmic ointment (discontinued 1995) ℞ *topical ophthalmic antibiotic* [polymyxin B sulfate; neomycin sulfate; bacitracin zinc] 5000 U•5 mg•400 U per g

NeoTect kit for injection preparation ℞ *radiopharmaceutical imaging agent for lung cancer; investigational (NDA filed) for malignant melanoma and neuroendocrine disorders* [depreotide]

Neothylline tablets (discontinued 1996) ℞ *antiasthmatic; bronchodilator* [dyphylline] 200, 400 mg

Neothylline-GG tablets (discontinued 1995) ℞ *antiasthmatic; bronchodilator; expectorant* [dyphylline; guaifenesin] 200•200 mg

Neotrace-4 IV injection ℞ *intravenous nutritional therapy* [multiple trace elements (metals)]

Neotricin HC ophthalmic ointment ℞ *topical ophthalmic corticosteroidal anti-inflammatory; antibiotic* [hydrocortisone acetate; neomycin sulfate; bacitracin zinc; polymyxin B sulfate] 1%•3.5%•400 U/g•10 000 U/g

Neotrofin ℞ *investigational (Phase II) nerve growth factor for Alzheimer's disease, spinal cord injuries, and stroke* [leteprinim potassium]

Neovastat ℞ *investigational (Phase III) antineoplastic/angiogenesis inhibitor for lung, prostate, and breast cancers* [AE-941 (code name—generic name not yet assigned)] ② Novastan

nepafenac USAN *topical ophthalmic anti-inflammatory and analgesic*

Nepeta cataria medicinal herb [see: catnip]

Nephlex Rx tablets ℞ *vitamin supplement* [multiple B vitamins; ascorbic acid; folic acid; biotin] ±•60•1•0.3 mg

NephrAmine 5.4% IV infusion ℞ *nutritional therapy for renal failure* [multiple essential amino acids; electrolytes]

nephritics *a class of agents that affect the kidney (a term used in folk medicine)*

Nephro-Calci tablets OTC *calcium supplement* [calcium carbonate] 1.5 g

Nephrocaps capsules ℞ *vitamin supplement* [multiple B vitamins; vitamin C; folic acid; biotin] ±•100 mg•1 mg•150 μg

Nephro-Derm cream (discontinued 1996) OTC *topical analgesic; moisturizer; emollient; antipruritic; counterirritant* [camphor; menthol]

Nephro-Fer tablets OTC *hematinic* [ferrous fumarate (source of iron)] 350 mg (115 mg)

Nephro-Fer Rx film-coated tablets ℞ *hematinic* [ferrous fumarate; folic acid] 106.9•1 mg

Nephron solution for inhalation OTC *sympathomimetic bronchodilator* [racepinephrine HCl] 2.25%

Nephron FA tablets (name changed to Nephplex Rx in 1995; reintroduced with a different formulation in 1996—see below)

Nephron FA tablets ℞ *hematinic* [ferrous fumarate; multiple B vitamins; ascorbic acid; folic acid; biotin; docusate sodium] 66.6•±•40•1•0.3•75 mg

Nephro-Vite Rx film-coated tablets ℞ *vitamin supplement* [multiple B vitamins; vitamin C; folic acid; biotin] ±•60 mg•1 mg•300 μg

Nephro-Vite Rx + Fe film-coated tablets ℞ *hematinic* [ferrous fumarate; multiple B vitamins; ascorbic acid; folic acid; biotin] 100•±•60•1•0.3 mg

Nephro-Vite Vitamin B Complex and C Supplement tablets OTC *vitamin supplement* [multiple B vita-

mins; vitamin C; folic acid; biotin]
± •60•0.8•0.3 mg

Nephrox oral suspension OTC *antacid; laxative* [aluminum hydroxide; mineral oil 10%] 320 mg/5 mL

Nepro oral liquid OTC *enteral nutritional therapy for acute or chronic renal failure* [lactose-free formula] 240 mL

neptamustine INN *antineoplastic* [also: pentamustine]

Neptazane tablets ℞ *carbonic anhydrase inhibitor for glaucoma* [methazolamide] 25, 50 mg

neptunium *element (Np)*

nequinate USAN, INN *coccidiostat for poultry* [also: methyl benzoquate]

neraminol INN

nerbacadol INN

nerelimomab USAN *monoclonal antibody; investigational (Phase III) cytokine modulator for septic shock*

neridronic acid INN

Nerium indicum; N. oleander medicinal herb [see: oleander]

nerve growth factor (NGF) *investigational agent for chemotherapy-induced peripheral neuropathy*

nervines *a class of agents that have a calming or soothing effect on the nerves (a term used in folk medicine)*

Nervocaine 1% injection ℞ *injectable local anesthetic* [lidocaine HCl] 1%

Nervocaine 2% injection (discontinued 1995) ℞ *injectable local anesthetic* [lidocaine HCl] 2%

Nesacaine; Nesacaine MPF injection ℞ *injectable local anesthetic* [chloroprocaine HCl] 1%, 2%; 2%, 3%

nesapidil INN

nesiritide *investigational (NDA filed) brain natriuretic peptide (BNP) for acute congestive heart failure*

nesosteine INN

Nestabs tablets OTC *vitamin/calcium/iron supplement* [multiple vitamins; calcium; ferrous fumarate; folic acid]
± •200•36•0.8 mg

Nestabs FA tablets ℞ *vitamin/calcium/iron supplement* [multiple vitamins;

calcium; ferrous fumarate; folic acid]
± •200•36•1 mg

Nestrex tablets OTC *vitamin supplement* [pyridoxine HCl] 25 mg

nethalide [see: pronetalol]

netilmicin INN, BAN *aminoglycoside antibiotic* [also: netilmicin sulfate]

netilmicin sulfate USAN, USP *aminoglycoside antibiotic* [also: netilmicin]

netobimin USAN, INN, BAN *veterinary anthelmintic*

netrafilcon A USAN *hydrophilic contact lens material*

Netromicina (Mexican name for U.S. product Netromycin)

Netromycin IV or IM injection ℞ *aminoglycoside antibiotic* [netilmicin sulfate] 100 mg/mL

nettle *(Urtica dioica; U. urens)* leaves and root *medicinal herb for blood cleansing, bronchitis, diarrhea, edema, hypertension, internal and external bleeding, and rheumatism; also being investigated for hay fever and urinary tract irrigation*

nettle, hemp; bee nettle; dog nettle; hemp dead nettle *medicinal herb* [see: hemp nettle]

nettle flowers; dead nettle; stingless nettle; white nettle *medicinal herb* [see: blind nettle]

Neumega subcu injection ℞ *platelet growth factor for prevention of thrombocytopenia following chemotherapy or radiation (orphan)* [oprelvekin] 5 mg

Neupogen IV or subcu injection ℞ *hematopoietic stimulant for severe chronic neutropenia and myelodysplastic syndrome (orphan); investigational (Phase III, orphan) cytokine for CMV retinitis of AIDS* [filgrastim] 300 µg/mL

Neuprex ℞ *investigational (Phase III, orphan) agent for gram-negative sepsis, hemorrhagic shock, and meningococcemia; investigational agent for lung infection in cystic fibrosis* [bactericidal and permeability-increasing (BPI) protein, recombinant]

neural dopaminergic cells (or precursors), porcine fetal *investiga-*

tional (orphan) intracerebral implant for stage 4 and 5 Parkinson's disease

neural gabaergic cells (or precursors), porcine fetal investigational (orphan) intracerebral implant for Huntington's disease

Neuralgon (name changed to Lioresal upon marketing release in 1996)

Neuramate tablets ℞ anxiolytic [meprobamate] 400 mg

NeuRecover-DA; NeuRecover-LT; NeuRecover-SA capsules OTC dietary supplement [multiple vitamins & minerals; multiple amino acids; folic acid] ≛●0.067 mg; ≛●0.03 mg; ≛● 0.067 mg

Neurelan investigational (orphan) for multiple sclerosis and spinal cord injury [fampridine]

Neurobloc ℞ investigational (Phase III, orphan) treatment for cervical dystonia [botulinum toxin, type B]

NeuroCell-HD ℞ investigational (orphan) intracerebral implant for patients with Huntington's disease [neural gabaergic cells, porcine fetal]

NeuroCell-PD ℞ investigational (Phase I, orphan) intracerebral implant for patients with advanced Parkinson's disease [neural dopaminergic cells, porcine fetal]

Neurodep injection ℞ parenteral vitamin therapy [multiple B vitamins; vitamin C] ≛●50 mg/mL

Neurodep-Caps capsules OTC vitamin supplement [vitamins B_1, B_6, and B_{12}] 125●125●1 mg

Neurolite injection ℞ imaging aid for SPECT brain scans [technetium Tc 99m bicisate]

Neurontin capsules ℞ anticonvulsant; investigational (orphan) for amyotrophic lateral sclerosis [gabapentin] 100, 300, 400 mg

neurosin [see: calcium glycerophosphate]

NeuroSlim capsules OTC dietary supplement [multiple vitamins & minerals; multiple amino acids; folic acid; biotin] ≛●0.066●0.05 mg

neurotrophic growth factor [see: methionyl neurotrophic factor]

neurotrophin-1 investigational (orphan) for motor neuron disease and amyotrophic lateral sclerosis

neustab [see: thioacetazone; thiacetazone]

Neut IV or subcu injection ℞ pH buffer for metabolic acidosis; urinary alkalinizer [sodium bicarbonate] 4% (0.48 mEq/mL)

neutral acriflavine [see: acriflavine]

neutral insulin INN, BAN, JAN antidiabetic [also: insulin, neutral]

Neutralase investigational (Phase III) agent for the reversal of heparin-induced anticoagulation for bypass surgery [heparinase 1]

neutramycin USAN, INN antibacterial

Neutra-Phos powder OTC phosphorus supplement [monobasic sodium phosphate; monobasic potassium phosphate; dibasic sodium phosphate; dibasic potassium phosphate] 250 mg/packet (P)

Neutra-Phos-K powder OTC phosphorus supplement [monobasic potassium phosphate; dibasic potassium phosphate] 250 mg/packet (P)

NeuTrexin powder for IV injection ℞ antiprotozoal for AIDS-related Pneumocystis carinii pneumonia (orphan); investigational (orphan) antineoplastic for multiple cancers [trimetrexate glucuronate] 25 mg

neutroflavine [see: acriflavine]

Neutrogena Acne Mask OTC topical keratolytic cleansing mask for acne [benzoyl peroxide] 5%

Neutrogena Antiseptic Cleanser for Acne-Prone Skin liquid OTC topical cleanser for acne [benzethonium chloride]

Neutrogena Body lotion, oil OTC moisturizer; emollient

Neutrogena Drying gel OTC topical astringent and antiseptic for acne [hamamelis water; isopropyl alcohol]

Neutrogena Moisture lotion OTC moisturizer; emollient

Neutrogena Non-Drying Cleansing
lotion OTC *soap-free therapeutic skin cleanser*

Neutrogena Norwegian Formula Hand cream OTC *moisturizer; emollient*

Neutrogena Oil-Free Acne Wash liquid OTC *topical keratolytic cleanser for acne* [salicylic acid] 2%

Neutrogena Soap; Neutrogena Cleansing for Acne-Prone Skin; Neutrogena Baby Cleansing Formula Soap; Neutrogena Dry Skin Soap; Neutrogena Oily Skin Soap bar OTC *therapeutic skin cleanser*

Neutrogena T/Derm oil OTC *topical antipsoriatic; antiseborrheic* [coal tar] 5%

Neutrogena T/Gel shampoo, conditioner OTC *antiseborrheic; antipsoriatic; antipruritic; antibacterial* [coal tar] 2%; 1.5%

Neutrogena T/Sal shampoo OTC *antiseborrheic; antipsoriatic; antipruritic; antibacterial* [salicylic acid; coal tar] 2%•2%

nevirapine USAN, INN *antiviral nonnucleoside reverse transcriptase inhibitor (NNRTI) for HIV-1*

New Decongest Pediatric syrup, drops (name changed to Tri-Phen-Mine in 1995)

New Jersey tea (*Ceanothus americanus*) root bark *medicinal herb used as an astringent, expectorant, and sedative*

New Zealand green-lipped mussel (*Perna canaliculus*) freeze-dried body or gonads *natural treatment for osteoarthritis and rheumatoid arthritis*

new-estranol 1 [see: diethylstilbestrol]

new-oestranol 1 [see: diethylstilbestrol]

new-oestranol 11 [see: diethylstilbestrol dipropionate]

NewPaks (trademarked delivery form) *ready-to-use closed system containers*

New-Skin liquid, spray OTC *skin protectant; antiseptic* [hydroxyquinoline]

nexeridine INN *analgesic* [also: nexeridine HCl]

nexeridine HCl USAN *analgesic* [also: nexeridine]

NFL (Novantrone, fluorouracil, leucovorin [rescue]) *chemotherapy protocol*

NG-29 *investigational (orphan) diagnostic aid for pituitary release of growth hormone*

NGF (nerve growth factor) [q.v.]

N-Graft ℞ *investigational (orphan) intracerebral implant for patients with advanced Parkinson's disease (for co-implantation with fetal neural cells)* [Sertoli cells, porcine]

N.G.T. cream ℞ *topical corticosteroidal anti-inflammatory; antifungal* [triamcinolone acetonide; nystatin] 0.1%•100 000 U per g

Nia-Bid sustained-action capsules OTC *vitamin supplement* [niacin] 400 mg

Niacels timed-release capsules (discontinued 1997) OTC *vitamin supplement* [niacin] 400 mg

niacin USP *vitamin B_3; peripheral vasodilator; antihyperlipidemic* [also: nicotinic acid] 25, 50, 100, 125, 250, 500 mg oral; 100 mg/mL injection ② Minocin

niacinamide USP *vitamin B_3; enzyme cofactor* [also: nicotinamide] 50, 100, 125, 250, 500 mg oral

niacinamide hydroiodide *expectorant*

Niacor immediate-release tablets ℞ *antihyperlipidemic; peripheral vasodilator* [niacin] 500 mg

nialamide NF, INN

niaprazine INN

Niaspan extended-release tablets, 21-day starter pack (7 tablets of each strength) ℞ *peripheral vasodilator; antihyperlipidemic; vitamin B_3* [niacin] 375, 500, 750, 1000 mg

nibroxane USAN, INN *topical antimicrobial*

Nicabate (European name for U.S. product Nicoderm)

nicafenine INN

nicainoprol INN

nicametate INN, BAN

nicaraven INN

nicarbazin BAN

nicardipine INN, BAN *vasodilator; calcium channel blocker* [also: nicardipine HCl]

nicardipine HCl USAN *antianginal; antihypertensive; vasodilator; calcium channel blocker* [also: nicardipine] 20, 30 mg oral

NicCheck I reagent strips *in vitro diagnostic aid for urine nicotine, used to determine the smoking status of the subject*

NicCheck II reagent strips *investigational in vitro diagnostic aid for urine nicotine, used to determine exposure to passive cigarette smoke*

N'Ice throat spray OTC *topical analgesic; counterirritant; mild local anesthetic* [menthol] 0.12%

N'Ice; N'Ice 'n Clear lozenges OTC *topical oral analgesic; counterirritant; mild local anesthetic* [menthol] 5 mg

N'Ice Vitamin C Drops (lozenges) OTC *vitamin supplement* [ascorbic acid; menthol; sorbitol] 60 mg

NicErase-SL ℞ *investigational (Phase III) treatment for nicotine withdrawal; clinical trials discontinued 1997* [lobeline sulfate]

nicergoline USAN, INN *vasodilator*

niceritrol INN, BAN

nicethamide BAN [also: nikethamide]

niceverine INN

nickel *element (Ni)*

Niclocide chewable tablets (discontinued 1995) ℞ *anthelmintic for cestodiasis (tapeworm)* [niclosamide] 500 mg

niclofolan INN, BAN

niclosamide USAN, INN *anthelmintic for cestodiasis (tapeworm)*

Nico-400 timed-release capsules OTC *vitamin supplement* [niacin] 400 mg

Nicobid Tempules (timed-release capsules) OTC *niacin therapy; antihyperlipidemic* [niacin] 125, 250, 500 mg ② Nitro-Bid

nicoboxil INN

nicoclonate INN

nicocodine INN, BAN

nicocortonide INN

Nicoderm transdermal patch ℞ *smoking deterrent; nicotine withdrawal aid* [nicotine] 36, 78, 114 mg

Nicoderm CQ transdermal patch OTC *smoking deterrent; nicotine withdrawal aid* [nicotine] 7, 14, 21 mg/day

nicodicodine INN, BAN

nicoduozide (isoniazid + nicothiazone)

nicofibrate INN

nicofuranose INN

nicofurate INN

nicogrelate INN

Nicolar tablets ℞ *niacin therapy; antihyperlipidemic* [niacin] 500 mg

nicomol INN

nicomorphine INN, BAN

nicopholine INN

nicorandil USAN, INN *coronary vasodilator*

Nicorette chewing pieces OTC *smoking deterrent; nicotine withdrawal aid* [nicotine polacrilex] 2 mg

Nicorette DS chewing pieces (discontinued 1997) ℞ *smoking deterrent; nicotine withdrawal aid* [nicotine polacrilex] 4 mg

nicothiazone INN

nicotinaldehyde thiosemicarbazone [see: nicothiazone]

nicotinamide INN, BAN, JAN *vitamin B_3; enzyme cofactor* [also: niacinamide]

nicotinamide-adenine dinucleotide (NAD) [now: nadide]

nicotine *a very poisonous alkaloid used as an insecticide and external parasiticide; the principal drug in tobacco* [also see: tobacco]

nicotine & mecamylamine HCl *investigational (Phase III) transdermal patch for smoking cessation*

nicotine OT *investigational (Phase II) oral transmucosal form for smoking cessation*

nicotine polacrilex USAN *smoking deterrent; nicotine withdrawal aid* 2, 4 mg oral

nicotine resin complex [see: nicotine polacrilex]

Nicotinex elixir OTC *vitamin supplement* [niacin] 50 mg/5 mL
nicotinic acid INN, BAN, JAN *vitamin B₃; vasodilator; antihyperlipidemic* [also: niacin]
nicotinic acid amide [see: niacinamide]
nicotinic acid 1-oxide [see: oxiniacic acid]
nicotinohydroxamic acid [see: nicoxamat]
6-nicotinoyl dihydrocodeine [see: nicodicodine]
6-nicotinoylcodeine [see: nicocodine]
4-nicotinoylmorpholine [see: nicopholine]
nicotinyl alcohol USAN, BAN *peripheral vasodilator*
nicotinyl tartrate
Nicotrol oral inhaler Ṟ *smoking deterrent; nicotine withdrawal aid* [nicotine] 4 mg
Nicotrol transdermal patch OTC *smoking deterrent; nicotine withdrawal aid* [nicotine] 15 mg
Nicotrol transdermal patch Ṟ *smoking deterrent; nicotine withdrawal aid* [nicotine] 8.3, 16.6, 24.9 mg
Nicotrol NS nasal spray Ṟ *smoking deterrent; nicotine withdrawal aid* [nicotine] 0.5 mg/spray
nicotylamide [see: niacinamide]
nicoumalone BAN [also: acenocoumarol]
Nico-Vert capsules (discontinued 1995) Ṟ *anticholinergic; antiemetic; antivertigo agent; motion sickness preventative* [meclizine HCl] 30, 50 mg
nicoxamat INN
nictiazem INN
nictindole INN
Nidagel ⓐ (U.S. product: MetroGel Vaginal) vaginal gel Ṟ *antibacterial for bacterial vaginosis* [metronidazole] 0.75%
nidroxyzone INN
Nidryl elixir (discontinued 1996) OTC *antihistamine; antitussive* [diphenhydramine HCl] 12.5 mg/5 mL
nifedipine USAN, USP, INN, BAN *antianginal; antihypertensive; coronary*

vasodilator; calcium channel blocker; investigational (orphan) for interstitial cystitis 10, 20 mg oral
nifenalol INN
nifenazone INN, BAN
Niferex tablets, elixir OTC *hematinic* [polysaccharide-iron complex] 50 mg; 100 mg/5 mL
Niferex Forte elixir (discontinued 1996) Ṟ *hematinic* [polysaccharide-iron complex; cyanocobalamin; folic acid] 300 mg•75 μg•3 mg per 15 mL
Niferex with Vitamin C chewable tablets (discontinued 1998) OTC *hematinic* [polysaccharide-iron complex; ascorbic acid; sodium ascorbate] 50•100•169 mg
Niferex-150 capsules OTC *hematinic* [polysaccharide-iron complex] 150 mg
Niferex-150 Forte capsules Ṟ *hematinic* [polysaccharide-iron complex; cyanocobalamin; folic acid] 150 mg•25 μg•1 mg
Niferex-PN film-coated tablets Ṟ *prenatal vitamin/iron supplement* [polysaccharide-iron complex; multiple vitamins & minerals; folic acid] 60• ± •1 mg
Niferex-PN Forte film-coated tablets Ṟ *prenatal vitamin/mineral/calcium/iron supplement* [multiple vitamins & minerals; calcium; polysaccharide-iron complex; folic acid] ± •250• 60•1 mg
niflumic acid INN
nifluridide USAN *ectoparasiticide*
nifungin USAN, INN
nifuradene USAN, INN *antibacterial*
nifuralazine [see: furalazine]
nifuraldezone USAN, INN *antibacterial*
nifuralide INN
nifuramizone [see: nifurethazone]
nifuratel USAN, INN *antibacterial; antifungal; antiprotozoal (Trichomonas)*
nifuratrone USAN, INN *antibacterial*
nifurazolidone [see: furazolidone]
nifurdazil USAN, INN *antibacterial*
nifurethazone INN
nifurfoline INN
nifurhydrazone [see: nihydrazone]

nifurimide USAN, INN *antibacterial*
nifurizone INN
nifurmazole INN
nifurmerone USAN, INN *antifungal*
nifuroquine INN
nifuroxazide INN
nifuroxime NF, INN
nifurpipone (NP) INN
nifurpirinol USAN, INN *antibacterial*
nifurprazine INN
nifurquinazol USAN, INN *antibacterial*
nifursemizone USAN, INN *antiprotozoal for poultry (Histomonas)*
nifursol USAN, INN *antiprotozoal for poultry (Histomonas)*
nifurthiazole USAN, INN *antibacterial*
nifurthiline [see: thiofuradene]
nifurtimox INN, BAN *investigational anti-infective for Chagas disease (available only from Centers for Disease Control and Prevention)*
nifurtoinol INN
nifurvidine INN
nifurzide INN
Night Time Cold/Flu Relief oral liquid OTC *antitussive; decongestant; antihistamine; analgesic* [dextromethorphan hydrobromide; pseudoephedrine HCl; doxylamine succinate; acetaminophen; alcohol 10%] 30•60•12.5•1000 mg/30 mL
nightshade; nightshade vine *medicinal herb* [see: bittersweet nightshade]
nightshade, American *medicinal herb* [see: pokeweed]
nightshade, deadly *medicinal herb* [see: belladonna]
nightshade, fetid; stinking nightshade *medicinal herb* [see: henbane]
nightshade, three-leaved *medicinal herb* [see: birthroot]
Night-Time Effervescent Cold tablets for oral solution OTC *decongestant; antihistamine; analgesic; antipyretic* [phenylpropanolamine HCl; diphenhydramine citrate; aspirin] 15•38.33•325 mg
Nighttime Sleep Aid tablets OTC *antihistaminic sleep aid* [diphenhydramine HCl] 50 mg

niguldipine INN
nihydrazone INN
nikethamide NF, INN [also: nicethamide]
Nilandron tablets ℞ *antiandrogen antineoplastic adjunct to surgical or chemical castration for metastatic prostate cancer* [nilutamide] 50 mg
nileprost INN
nilestriol INN *estrogen* [also: nylestriol]
nilprazole INN
Nilstat cream, ointment ℞ *topical antifungal* [nystatin] 100 000 U/g ⑨ Nitrostat; nystatin
Nilstat film-coated tablets ℞ *systemic antifungal* [nystatin] 500 000 U
Nilstat oral suspension, powder for oral suspension ℞ *antifungal; oral candidiasis treatment* [nystatin] 100 000 U/mL; 150 million, 500 million, 1 billion, 2 billion U
niludipine INN
nilutamide USAN, INN, BAN *antiandrogen antineoplastic adjunct to surgical or chemical castration for metastatic prostate cancer*
nilvadipine USAN, INN, JAN *calcium channel antagonist*
nimazone USAN, INN *anti-inflammatory*
Nimbex IV infusion ℞ *nondepolarizing neuromuscular blocking agent for anesthesia* [cisatracurium besylate] 2, 10 mg/mL
Nimbus; Nimbus Quick Strip test kit for home use OTC *in vitro diagnostic aid for urine pregnancy test* [monoclonal antibody-based enzyme immunoassay]
Nimbus Plus test kit for professional use *in vitro diagnostic aid for urine pregnancy test*
nimesulide INN, BAN
nimetazepam INN
nimidane USAN, INN *veterinary acaricide*
nimodipine USAN, INN, BAN *vasodilator; calcium channel blocker; investigational Alzheimer's treatment*
nimorazole INN, BAN
Nimotop soft liquid-filled capsules ℞ *calcium channel blocker for subarach-*

noid hemorrhage; investigational Alzheimer's treatment [nimodipine] 30 mg

nimustine INN

niobium *element (Nb)*

niometacin INN

Nion B Plus C caplets OTC *vitamin supplement* [multiple B vitamins; vitamin C] ≛ • 300 mg

Nipent powder for IV injection ℞ *antibiotic antineoplastic for hairy cell leukemia (orphan); investigational (orphan) for chronic lymphocytic leukemia and cutaneous T-cell lymphoma* [pentostatin] 10 mg

niperotidine INN

nipradilol INN

niprofazone INN

niridazole USAN, INN *antischistosomal*

nisbuterol INN *bronchodilator* [also: nisbuterol mesylate]

nisbuterol mesylate USAN *bronchodilator* [also: nisbuterol]

nisin *investigational agent for severe colonic bacterial infections*

nisobamate USAN, INN *minor tranquilizer*

nisoldipine USAN, INN, BAN, JAN *coronary vasodilator; calcium channel blocker for hypertension*

nisoxetine USAN, INN *antidepressant*

nisterime INN *androgen* [also: nisterime acetate]

nisterime acetate USAN *androgen* [also: nisterime]

nitarsone USAN, INN *antiprotozoal (Histomonas)*

nitazoxanide (NTZ) INN *investigational (NDA filed, orphan) anti-infective for AIDS-related cryptosporidial diarrhea (NDA withdrawn 1998)*

Nite Time Cold Formula liquid OTC *antitussive; decongestant; antihistamine; analgesic* [dextromethorphan hydrobromide; pseudoephedrine HCl; doxylamine succinate; acetaminophen; alcohol 25%] 5 • 10 • 1.25 • 167 mg/5 mL

nithiamide USAN *veterinary antibacterial* [also: aminitrozole; acinitrazole]

nitracrine INN

nitrafudam INN *antidepressant* [also: nitrafudam HCl]

nitrafudam HCl USAN *antidepressant* [also: nitrafudam]

nitralamine HCl USAN *antifungal*

nitramisole INN *anthelmintic* [also: nitramisole HCl]

nitramisole HCl USAN *anthelmintic* [also: nitramisole]

nitraquazone INN

nitrates *a class of antianginal agents that cause the relaxation of vascular smooth muscles*

nitratophenylmercury [see: phenylmercuric nitrate]

nitrazepam USAN, INN, BAN, JAN *anticonvulsant; hypnotic*

Nitrazine paper for professional use *in vitro diagnostic aid for urine pH determination*

nitre, sweet spirit of [see: ethyl nitrite]

nitrefazole INN, BAN

Nitrek transdermal patch ℞ *antianginal; vasodilator* [nitroglycerin] 22.4, 44.8, 67.2 mg (0.2, 0.4, 0.6 mg/hr.)

nitrendipine USAN, INN, BAN, JAN *antihypertensive; calcium channel blocker*

nitric acid NF *acidifying agent*

nitric oxide *investigational (orphan) for neonatal persistent pulmonary hypertension and acute adult respiratory distress syndrome; investigational to prevent reperfusion injury following lung transplants*

nitricholine perchlorate INN

9-nitro-20-(S)-camptothecin (9-NC) *investigational (orphan) for pancreatic cancer*

***p*-nitrobenzenearsonic acid** [see: nitarsone]

Nitro-Bid ointment ℞ *antianginal; vasodilator* [nitroglycerin] 2% (15 mg/inch) ⓦ Nicobid

Nitro-Bid Plateau Caps (controlled-release capsules) (discontinued 1996) ℞ *antianginal; vasodilator* [nitroglycerin] 2.5, 6.5, 9 mg ⓦ Nicobid

Nitro-Bid IV infusion ℞ *antianginal; vasodilator; perioperative antihypertensive; for congestive heart failure*

with myocardial infarction [nitroglycerin] 5 mg/mL

9-nitrocamptothecin *investigational (Phase III) antineoplastic for pancreatic cancer*

Nitrocine Timecaps (timed-release capsules) (discontinued 1996) ℞ *antianginal; vasodilator* [nitroglycerin] 2.5, 6.5, 9 mg

Nitrocine transdermal patch (discontinued 1995) ℞ *antianginal; vasodilator* [nitroglycerin] 187.5 mg

nitroclofene INN

nitrocycline USAN, INN *antibacterial*

nitrodan USAN, INN *anthelmintic*

Nitro-Derm transdermal patch ℞ *antianginal; vasodilator* [nitroglycerin] 160 mg

Nitrodisc transdermal patch ℞ *antianginal; vasodilator* [nitroglycerin] 16, 24, 32 mg

Nitro-Dur transdermal patch ℞ *antianginal; vasodilator* [nitroglycerin] 20, 40, 60, 80, 120, 160 mg

nitroethanolamine [see: aminoethyl nitrate]

nitrofuradoxadone [see: furmethoxadone]

nitrofural INN *broad-spectrum bactericidal; adjunct to burn treatment* [also: nitrofurazone]

nitrofurantoin USP, INN *urinary antibiotic* 50, 100 mg oral

nitrofurantoin sodium *urinary antibiotic*

nitrofurazone USP, BAN *broad-spectrum bactericidal; adjunct to burn treatment and skin grafting* [also: nitrofural] 0.2% topical

nitrofurmethone [see: furaltadone]

nitrofuroxizone [see: nidroxyzone]

Nitrogard transmucosal extended-release tablets ℞ *antianginal; vasodilator* [nitroglycerin] 1, 2, 3 mg

nitrogen (N$_2$) NF *air displacement agent; element (N)*

nitrogen monoxide [see: nitrous oxide]

nitrogen mustard N-oxide HCl JAN *alkylating antineoplastic* [also: mechlorethamine HCl; chlormethine; mustine]

nitrogen mustards *a class of alkylating antineoplastics*

nitrogen oxide (N$_2$O) [see: nitrous oxide]

nitroglycerin USP *coronary vasodilator; antianginal; antihypertensive* [also: glyceryl trinitrate] 2.5, 6.5, 9 mg oral; 5 mg/mL injection; 16–187.5 mg transdermal; 2% topical ☑ Nitroglyn

Nitroglyn extended-release capsules ℞ *antianginal; vasodilator* [nitroglycerin] 2.5, 6.5, 9, 13 mg ☑ nitroglycerin

nitrohydroxyquinoline [see: nitroxoline]

Nitrol ointment, Appli-Kit (ointment & adhesive dosage covers) ℞ *antianginal; vasodilator* [nitroglycerin] 2% (15 mg/inch)

Nitrolan liquid OTC *enteral nutritional therapy* [lactose-free formula]

Nitrolingual Pumpspray ⊛ CFC-free sublingual aerosol ℞ *antianginal; vasodilator* [nitroglycerin] 0.4 mg/spray

nitromannitol [see: mannitol hexanitrate]

nitromersol USP *topical anti-infective*

nitromide USAN *coccidiostat for poultry; antibacterial*

nitromifene INN

nitromifene citrate USAN *antiestrogen*

Nitrong sustained-release tablets ℞ *antianginal; vasodilator* [nitroglycerin] 2.6, 6.5, 9 mg

Nitropress powder for IV injection, flip-top vials ℞ *vasodilator for hypertensive emergency* [sodium nitroprusside] 50 mg/dose

nitroprusside sodium [see: sodium nitroprusside]

NitroQuick sublingual tablets ℞ *antianginal; vasodilator* [nitroglycerin] 0.3, 0.4, 0.6 mg

nitroscanate USAN, INN *veterinary anthelmintic*

nitrosoureas *a class of alkylating antineoplastics*

Nitrostat sublingual tablets ℞ *antianginal; vasodilator* [nitroglycerin] 0.3, 0.4, 0.6 mg

nitrosulfathiazole INN [also: para-nitrosulfathiazole]

Nitro-Time extended-release capsules R antianginal; vasodilator [nitroglycerin] 2.5, 6.5, 9 mg

nitrous acid, sodium salt [see: sodium nitrite]

nitrous oxide (N₂O) USP a weak inhalation general anesthetic; sometimes abused as a street drug to create a dreamy or floating sensation

nitroxinil INN

nitroxoline INN, BAN

nivacortol INN corticosteroid; anti-inflammatory [also: nivazol]

nivadipine [see: nilvadipine]

nivaquine [see: chloroquine phosphate]

nivazol USAN corticosteroid; anti-inflammatory [also: nivacortol]

Nivea After Tan; Nivea Moisturizing; Nivea Moisturizing Extra Enriched lotion OTC moisturizer; emollient

Nivea Moisturizing; Nivea Skin oil OTC moisturizer; emollient

Nivea Moisturizing Creme Soap bar OTC therapeutic skin cleanser

Nivea Ultra Moisturizing Creme OTC moisturizer; emollient

nivimedone sodium USAN antiallergic

nixylic acid INN

nizatidine USAN, USP, INN, BAN, JAN histamine H₂ antagonist for gastric and duodenal ulcers

nizofenone INN

Nizoral cream, shampoo R topical antifungal [ketoconazole] 2%

Nizoral tablets R systemic antifungal; orphan status withdrawn 1996 [ketoconazole] 200 mg

Nizoral A-D shampoo OTC topical antifungal for dandruff [ketoconazole] 1%

NMP-22 investigational (NDA filed) bladder cancer test kit

N-Multistix; N-Multistix SG reagent strips in vitro diagnostic aid for multiple urine products

NNRTIs (non-nucleoside reverse transcriptase inhibitors) [q.v.]

no more burn; no more ouchies spray (discontinued 1995) OTC topical local anesthetic; antiseptic [lidocaine HCl; benzethonium chloride] 2.3%•0.13%

no more germies soap (discontinued 1995) OTC antiseptic; disinfectant [triclosan] 0.25%

no more germies towelettes (discontinued 1995) OTC antiseptic wipes [benzalkonium chloride]

no more itchies spray (discontinued 1995) OTC topical corticosteroidal anti-inflammatory [hydrocortisone] 1%

No Pain-HP roll-on OTC topical analgesic [capsaicin] 0.075%

nobelium element (No)

noberastine USAN, INN, BAN antihistamine

noble yarrow medicinal herb [see: yarrow]

nocloprost INN

nocodazole USAN, INN antineoplastic

nodding wakerobin medicinal herb [see: birthroot]

NōDōz tablets, chewable tablets OTC CNS stimulant; analeptic [caffeine] 200 mg; 100 mg

nofecainide INN

nofetumomab merpentan monoclonal antibody imaging agent for small cell lung cancer

nogalamycin USAN, INN antineoplastic

No-Hist capsules R nasal decongestant [phenylephrine HCl; phenylpropanolamine HCl; pseudoephedrine HCl] 5•40•40 mg

Nolahist tablets OTC antihistamine [phenindamine tartrate] 25 mg

Nolamine timed-release tablets R decongestant; antihistamine [phenylpropanolamine HCl; chlorpheniramine maleate; phenindamine tartrate] 50•4•24 mg

nolinium bromide USAN, INN antisecretory; antiulcerative

Nolvadex tablets R antiestrogen antineoplastic for advanced postmenopausal breast cancer; breast cancer prevention *for high-risk patients* [tamoxifen citrate] 10, 20 mg

nomegestrol INN

nomelidine INN

nomifensine INN *antidepressant* [also: nomifensine maleate]

nomifensine maleate USAN *antidepressant* [also: nomifensine]

nonabine INN, BAN

nonabsorbable surgical suture [see: suture, nonabsorbable surgical]

nonachlazine [now: azaclorzine HCl]

nonanedioic acid [see: azelaic acid]

nonaperone INN

nonapyrimine INN

nonathymulin INN

nondestearinated cod liver oil [see: cod liver oil, nondestearinated]

noni *(Morinda citrifolia)* berries *medicinal herb for arthritis, bacterial infections, diabetes, drug addiction, headache, hypertension, liver and skin disorders, pain, and slowing aging; also used as an antioxidant*

nonionic contrast media *a class of newer radiopaque agents that, in general, have a low osmolar concentration of iodine (the contrast agent), which corresponds to a lower incidence of adverse reactions* [also called: low osmolar contrast media (LOCM)]

nonivamide INN

non-nucleoside reverse transcriptase inhibitors (NNRTIs) *a class of antivirals that inhibit HIV replication* [reverse transcriptase is also known as DNA polymerase]

nonoxinol 4 INN *surfactant* [also: nonoxynol 4]

nonoxinol 9 INN *wetting and solubilizing agent; spermaticide* [also: nonoxynol 9]

nonoxinol 15 INN *surfactant* [also: nonoxynol 15]

nonoxinol 30 INN *surfactant* [also: nonoxynol 30]

nonoxynol 4 USAN *surfactant* [also: nonoxinol 4]

nonoxynol 9 USAN, USP *wetting and solubilizing agent; spermicide* [also: nonoxinol 9]

nonoxynol 10 NF *surfactant*

nonoxynol 15 USAN *surfactant* [also: nonoxinol 15]

nonoxynol 30 USAN *surfactant* [also: nonoxinol 30]

nonsteroidal anti-inflammatory drugs (NSAIDs) *a class of anti-inflammatory drugs that have analgesic and antipyretic effects*

nonylphenoxypolyethoxyethanol [see: nonoxynol 4, 9, 15, & 30]

Nootropil ℞ *cognition adjuvant; investigational (orphan) for myoclonus* [piracetam]

nopal *plant medicinal herb for cleansing the lymphatic system, diabetes, digestion, obesity, neutralizing toxins, and preventing arteriosclerosis*

noracymethadol INN *analgesic* [also: noracymethadol HCl]

noracymethadol HCl USAN *analgesic* [also: noracymethadol]

noradrenaline bitartrate [see: norepinephrine bitartrate]

noramidopyrine methanesulfonate sodium [see: dipyrone]

norandrostenolone phenylpropionate [see: nandrolone phenpropionate]

norastemizole *investigational (Phase III) third generation, nonsedating antihistamine for allergy*

norbolethone USAN *anabolic* [also: norboletone]

norboletone INN *anabolic* [also: norbolethone]

norbudrine INN [also: norbutrine]

norbutrine BAN [also: norbudrine]

Norcet capsules (discontinued 1995) ℞ *narcotic analgesic* [hydrocodone bitartrate; acetaminophen] 5•500 mg

norclostebol INN

Norco tablets ℞ *narcotic analgesic* [hydrocodone bitartrate; acetaminophen] 10•325 mg

norcodeine INN, BAN

Norcuron powder for IV injection ℞ *nondepolarizing neuromuscular blocker; adjunct to anesthesia* [vecuronium bromide] 10, 20 mg/vial

norcycline [see: sancycline]

nordazepam INN

nordefrin HCl NF

Nordette tablets ℞ *monophasic oral contraceptive; emergency "morning after" contraceptive* [levonorgestrel; ethinyl estradiol] 0.15 mg•30 μg

nordinone INN

Norditropin powder for subcu injection ℞ *growth hormone for adults or children with congenital or endogenous growth hormone deficiency, children with Turner syndrome or renal-induced growth failure, or AIDS-wasting syndrome (orphan)* [somatropin] 4, 8 mg (12, 24 IU) per vial

Norel capsules ℞ *decongestant; expectorant* [phenylephrine HCl; phenylpropanolamine HCl; guaifenesin] 5•45•200 mg

Norel Plus capsules ℞ *decongestant; antihistamine; analgesic* [phenylpropanolamine HCl; chlorpheniramine maleate; phenyltoloxamine dihydrogen citrate; acetaminophen] 25•4•25•325 mg

norephedrine HCl [see: phenylpropanolamine HCl]

norepinephrine INN *adrenergic; vasoconstrictor; vasopressor for shock* [also: norepinephrine bitartrate]

norepinephrine bitartrate USAN, USP *adrenergic; vasoconstrictor; vasopressor for acute hypotensive shock* [also: norepinephrine]

norethandrolone NF, INN

Norethin 1/35E tablets ℞ *monophasic oral contraceptive* [norethindrone; ethinyl estradiol] 1 mg•35 μg

Norethin 1/50M tablets ℞ *monophasic oral contraceptive* [norethindrone; mestranol] 1 mg•50 μg

norethindrone USP *progestin for amenorrhea, abnormal uterine bleeding, and endometriosis* [also: norethisterone]

norethindrone acetate USP *progestin for amenorrhea, abnormal uterine bleeding, and endometriosis*

norethisterone INN, BAN, JAN *progestin* [also: norethindrone]

norethynodrel USAN, USP *progestin* [also: noretynodrel]

noretynodrel INN *progestin* [also: norethynodrel]

noreximide INN

norfenefrine INN

Norflex sustained-release tablets, IV or IM injection ℞ *skeletal muscle relaxant* [orphenadrine citrate] 100 mg; 30 mg/mL

norfloxacin USAN, USP, INN, BAN, JAN *broad-spectrum bactericidal antibiotic*

norfloxacin succinil INN

norflurane USAN, INN *inhalation anesthetic*

Norforms powder (discontinued 1998) OTC *absorbs vaginal moisture; astringent* [cornstarch; zinc oxide]

Norforms vaginal suppositories OTC *feminine deodorant* [polyethylene glycol]

Norgesic; Norgesic Forte tablets ℞ *skeletal muscle relaxant; analgesic* [orphenadrine citrate; aspirin; caffeine] 25•385•30 mg; 50•770•60 mg

norgesterone INN

norgestimate USAN, INN, BAN *progestin*

norgestomet USAN, INN *progestin*

norgestrel USAN, USP, INN *progestin*

d-norgestrel *(incorrect enantiomer designation)* [now: levonorgestrel]

D-norgestrel [see: levonorgestrel]

norgestrienone INN

Norinyl 1 + 35 tablets ℞ *monophasic oral contraceptive* [norethindrone; ethinyl estradiol] 1 mg•35 μg ② Nardil

Norinyl 1 + 50 tablets ℞ *monophasic oral contraceptive* [norethindrone; mestranol] 1 mg•50 μg

Norisodrine Aerotrol (inhalation aerosol) ℞ *bronchodilator* [isoproterenol HCl]

Norisodrine with Calcium Iodide syrup ℞ *bronchodilator; expectorant* [isoproterenol sulfate; calcium iodide; alcohol 6%] 3•150 mg

Noritate cream ℞ *antibacterial for inflammatory lesions and acne rosacea* [metronidazole (in an emollient base)] 1%

Norlac Rx tablets (discontinued 1995) ℞ *vitamin/mineral/calcium/iron supplement* [multiple vitamins & minerals; calcium; iron; folic acid] ± •200•60•1 mg

norletimol INN

norleusactide INN [also: pentacosactride]

norlevorphanol INN, BAN

norlupinanes *a class of antibiotics* [also called: quinolizidines]

Norlutate tablets (discontinued 1995) ℞ *progestin for amenorrhea, abnormal uterine bleeding, or endometriosis* [norethindrone acetate] 5 mg ② Norlutin

Norlutin tablets (discontinued 1995) ℞ *progestin for amenorrhea, abnormal uterine bleeding, or endometriosis* [norethindrone] 5 mg ② Norlutate

½ normal saline (½ NS; 0.45% sodium chloride) *electrolyte replacement*

normal saline (NS; 0.9% sodium chloride) *electrolyte replacement* [also: saline solution]

normal serum albumin [see: albumin, human]

normethadone INN, BAN

normethandrolone [see: normethandrone]

normethandrone

normethisterone [see: normethandrone]

Normiflo deep subcu injection in prefilled syringes ℞ *low molecular weight heparin-type anticoagulant for the prevention of deep vein thrombosis (DVT) following knee replacement surgery* [ardeparin sodium] 5000, 10 000 U/0.5 mL

Normix ℞ *investigational (orphan) antibacterial for hepatic encephalopathy* [rifaximin]

Normodyne film-coated tablets, IV infusion ℞ *antihypertensive; α- and β-blocker* [labetalol HCl] 100, 200, 300 mg; 5 mg/mL

normorphine INN, BAN

Normosang ℞ *investigational (orphan) for acute symptomatic porphyria and myelodysplastic syndrome* [heme arginate]

Normosol-M and 5% Dextrose; Normosol-R and 5% Dextrose IV infusion ℞ *intravenous nutritional/ electrolyte therapy* [combined electrolyte solution; dextrose]

Normosol-R; Normosol-R pH 7.4 IV infusion ℞ *intravenous electrolyte therapy* [combined electrolyte solution]

Noroxin film-coated tablets ℞ *broadspectrum fluoroquinolone antibiotic* [norfloxacin] 400 mg

Norpace capsules ℞ *antiarrhythmic* [disopyramide phosphate] 100, 150 mg

Norpace CR controlled-release capsules ℞ *antiarrhythmic* [disopyramide phosphate] 100, 500 mg

norpipanone INN, BAN

Norplant implantable Silastic capsules ℞ *implant contraceptive system* [levonorgestrel] 36 mg

Norpramin film-coated tablets ℞ *tricyclic antidepressant* [desipramine HCl] 10, 25, 50, 75, 100, 150 mg ② imipramine

norpseudoephedrine [see: cathine]

Nor-Q.D. tablets ℞ *oral contraceptive (progestin only)* [norethindrone] 0.35 mg

nortestosterone phenylpropionate [see: nandrolone phenpropionate]

Nor-Tet capsules ℞ *broad-spectrum antibiotic* [tetracycline HCl] 250, 500 mg

nortetrazepam INN

nortriptyline HCl USAN, USP, INN *tricyclic antidepressant* [10, 25, 50, 75 mg oral] ② amitriptyline

Norvasc tablets ℞ *antianginal; antihypertensive; calcium channel blocker* [amlodipine] 2.5, 5, 10 mg

norvinisterone INN

norvinodrel [see: norgesterone]

Norvir soft capsules, oral solution ℞ *antiviral protease inhibitor for HIV* [ritonavir] 100 mg; 80 mg/mL

Norway pine; Norway spruce *medicinal herb* [see: spruce]

Norwich tablets OTC *analgesic; antipyretic; anti-inflammatory; antirheumatic* [aspirin] 325, 500 mg

Norzine IM injection, suppositories, tablets ℞ *antiemetic* [thiethylperazine maleate] 5 mg/mL; 10 mg; 10 mg

NoSalt; NoSalt Seasoned (discontinued 1997) OTC *salt substitute* [potassium chloride] 64 mEq/5 g; 34 mEq/5 g

nosantine INN, BAN

noscapine USP, INN *antitussive*

noscapine HCl NF

nosebleed *medicinal herb* [see: yarrow]

nosiheptide USAN, INN *veterinary growth stimulant*

Nōstril; Children's Nōstril nasal spray OTC *nasal decongestant* [phenylephrine HCl] 0.5%; 0.25%

Nōstrilla nasal spray OTC *nasal decongestant* [oxymetazoline HCl] 0.05%

notensil maleate [see: acepromazine]

Novacet lotion ℞ *topical acne treatment* [sulfacetamide sodium; sulfur] 10%•5%

Nova-Dec tablets OTC *vitamin/mineral/iron supplement* [multiple vitamins & minerals; iron; folic acid; biotin] ±• 30 mg•0.4 mg•30 µg

Novafed timed-release capsules (discontinued 1996) ℞ *nasal decongestant* [pseudoephedrine HCl] 120 mg

Novafed A sustained-release capsules ℞ *decongestant; antihistamine* [pseudoephedrine HCl; chlorpheniramine maleate] 120•8 mg

Novagest Expectorant with Codeine liquid ℞ *narcotic antitussive; decongestant; expectorant* [codeine phosphate; pseudoephedrine HCl; guaifenesin; alcohol 1.4%] 10•30•100 mg/5 mL

Novahistine elixir (discontinued 1997) OTC *decongestant; antihistamine* [phenylephrine HCl; chlorpheniramine maleate] 5•2 mg/5 mL

Novahistine DH liquid (discontinued 1997) ℞ *narcotic antitussive; decongestant; antihistamine* [codeine phosphate; pseudoephedrine HCl; chlor-

pheniramine maleate; alcohol 5%] 10•30•2 mg/5 mL

Novahistine DMX liquid (discontinued 1997) OTC *antitussive; decongestant; expectorant* [dextromethorphan hydrobromide; pseudoephedrine HCl; guaifenesin; alcohol 10%] 10• 30•100 mg/5 mL

Novahistine Expectorant liquid (discontinued 1997) ℞ *narcotic antitussive; decongestant; expectorant* [codeine phosphate; pseudoephedrine HCl; guaifenesin; alcohol 7.5%] 10•30•100 mg/5 mL

novamidon [see: aminopyrine]

Novamine; Novamine 15% IV infusion ℞ *total parenteral nutrition; peripheral parenteral nutrition* [multiple essential and nonessential amino acids]

Novantrone IV injection ℞ *antibiotic antineoplastic for prostate cancer or acute myelogenous (nonlymphocytic) leukemia (orphan)* [mitoxantrone HCl] 2 mg/mL

Novapren ℞ *investigational (Phase I) antiviral for HIV*

NovaSource Renal ⦿ oral liquid OTC *nutritional therapy for renal failure* [multiple vitamins & minerals] 237 mL

Novastan ℞ *investigational (NDA filed) thrombin inhibitor for heparin-induced thrombocytopenia (HIT) and thrombosis (NDA disapproved in 1998); investigational (Phase II) for myocardial infarction* [argatroban] ⑨ Neovastat; Ovastat

novel (atypical) antipsychotics *a class of agents with a high affinity to the serotonin receptors and varying degrees of affinity to other neurotransmitter receptors; "atypical" due to the low incidence of extrapyramidal side effects (EPS)* [compare to: conventional (typical) antipsychotics]

novobiocin INN, BAN *bacteriostatic antibiotic* [also: novobiocin calcium]

novobiocin calcium USP *bacteriostatic antibiotic* [also: novobiocin]

novobiocin sodium USP *bacteriostatic antibiotic*

Novocain injection ℞ *injectable local anesthetic* [procaine HCl] 1%, 2%, 10%

Novo-Cyproterone 🄬 tablets ℞ *antiandrogen antineoplastic for advanced prostatic carcinoma* [cyproterone acetate] 50 mg

Novo-Domperidone 🄬 film-coated tablets ℞ *antiemetic for diabetic gastroparesis and chronic gastritis* [domperidone maleate] 10 mg

Novo-Gemfibrozil 🄬 (U.S. product: Lopid) tablets ℞ *antihyperlipidemic for hypertriglyceridemia and coronary heart disease* [gemfibrozil] 600 mg

Novolin 70/30 subcu injection OTC *antidiabetic* [isophane human insulin (rDNA); human insulin (rDNA)] 100 U/mL

Novolin 70/30 PenFill NovoPen cartridge OTC *antidiabetic* [isophane human insulin (rDNA); human insulin (rDNA)] 150 U/1.5 mL

Novolin 70/30 Prefilled syringes OTC *antidiabetic* [isophane human insulin (rDNA); human insulin (rDNA)] 150 U/1.5 mL

Novolin 85/15 PenFill NovoPen cartridge OTC *investigational (NDA filed) antidiabetic* [isophane human insulin (rDNA); human insulin (rDNA)]

Novolin ge 30/70 🄬 (U.S. product: Novolin 70/30) vials for subcu injection, prefilled cartridges OTC *antidiabetic* [insulin; isophane insulin] 100 U/mL; 1.5, 3 mL

Novolin ge 50/50 🄬 (U.S. product: Novolin 50/50) prefilled cartridges OTC *antidiabetic* [insulin; isophane insulin] 300 U/3 mL

Novolin ge Lente 🄬 (U.S. product: Novolin L) vials for subcu injection, prefilled cartridges OTC *antidiabetic* [insulin zinc] 100 U/mL; 3 mL

Novolin ge NPH 🄬 (U.S. product: Novolin N) vials for subcu injection, prefilled cartridges OTC *antidiabetic* [isophane insulin] 100 U/mL; 1.5, 3 mL

Novolin ge Toronto 🄬 (U.S. product: Novolin R) vials for subcu injection, prefilled cartridges OTC *antidiabetic* [insulin] 100 U/mL; 1.5, 3 mL

Novolin ge Ultralente 🄬 (U.S. product: Humulin U Ultralente) vials for subcu injection, prefilled cartridges OTC *antidiabetic* [insulin zinc] 100 U/mL; 1.5 mL

Novolin L subcu injection OTC *antidiabetic* [human insulin zinc (rDNA)] 100 U/mL

Novolin N subcu injection OTC *antidiabetic* [isophane human insulin (rDNA)] 100 U/mL

Novolin N PenFill NovoPen cartridge OTC *antidiabetic* [isophane human insulin (rDNA)] 150 U/1.5 mL

Novolin N Prefilled syringes OTC *antidiabetic* [isophane human insulin (rDNA)] 150 U/1.5 mL

Novolin R subcu injection OTC *antidiabetic* [human insulin (rDNA)] 100 U/mL

Novolin R PenFill NovoPen cartridges OTC *antidiabetic* [human insulin (rDNA)] 150 U/1.5 mL

Novolin R Prefilled syringes OTC *antidiabetic* [human insulin (rDNA)] 150 U/1.5 mL

NovoNorm (European name for U.S. product Prandin)

Novopaque oral/rectal suspension ℞ *radiopaque contrast medium for gastrointestinal imaging* [barium sulfate] 60%

NovoPen 1.5 prefilled reusable syringe *uses Novolin PenFill cartridges and NovoFine 30-gauge disposable needles* [insulin (several types available)] 1–40 U/injection

NovoRapid ℞ *investigational (NDA filed) rapid-acting insulin analog* [insulin aspart]

NovoSeven powder for IV injection ℞ *coagulant for hemophilia A and B (orphan); investigational (orphan) for von Willebrand's disease* [factor VIIa, recombinant] 1.2, 4.8 mg/vial

Novo-Terazosin 🄬 (U.S. product: Hytrin) tablets ℞ *antihypertensive*

(α-blocker); treatment for benign prostatic hyperplasia (BPH) [terazosin HCl] 1, 2, 5, 10 mg

Novo-Timol ⓐ (U.S. product: Timoptic) eye drops ℞ topical antiglaucoma agent (β-blocker) [timolol maleate] 0.25%, 0.5%

NOVP (Novantrone, Oncovin, vinblastine, prednisone) chemotherapy protocol

noxiptiline INN [also: noxiptyline]

noxiptyline BAN [also: noxiptiline]

noxythiolin BAN [also: noxytiolin]

noxytiolin INN [also: noxythiolin]

NP (nifurpipone) [q.v.]

NP-27 solution, powder, spray powder, cream (discontinued 1998) OTC topical antifungal [tolnaftate] 1%

NPH (neutral protamine Hagedorn) insulin [see: insulin, isophane]

NPH Iletin I subcu injection (discontinued 1999) OTC antidiabetic [isophane insulin (beef-pork)] 100 U/mL

NPH Iletin II subcu injection OTC antidiabetic [isophane insulin (pork)] 100 U/mL

NPH Insulin subcu injection (discontinued 1997) OTC antidiabetic [isophane insulin (beef)] 100 U/mL

NPH-N subcu injection OTC antidiabetic [isophane insulin (pork)] 100 U/mL

NS (normal saline) [q.v.]

NS-2710 investigational (Phase II) anxiolytic

NSAIDs (nonsteroidal anti-inflammatory drugs) [q.v.]

NTBC investigational (orphan) for tyrosinemia type I

NTS transdermal patches ℞ antianginal; vasodilator [nitroglycerin]

NTZ (nitazoxanide) [q.v.]

NTZ Long Acting nasal spray, nose drops OTC nasal decongestant [oxymetazoline HCl] 0.05%

Nubain IV, subcu or IM injection ℞ narcotic agonist-antagonist analgesic [nalbuphine HCl] 10, 20 mg/mL

nuclomedone INN

nuclotixene INN

Nucofed capsules, syrup ℞ narcotic antitussive; decongestant [codeine phosphate; pseudoephedrine HCl] 20•60 mg; 20•60 mg/5 mL

Nucofed Expectorant; Nucofed Pediatric Expectorant syrup ℞ narcotic antitussive; decongestant; expectorant [codeine phosphate; pseudoephedrine HCl; guaifenesin; alcohol 12.5%•6%] 20•60•200 mg/5 mL; 10•30•100 mg/5 mL

Nucotuss Expectorant; Nucotuss Pediatric Expectorant liquid narcotic antitussive; decongestant; expectorant [codeine phosphate; pseudoephedrine HCl; guaifenesin; alcohol 12.5%•6%] 20•60•200 mg/5 mL; 10•30•100 mg/5 mL

nufenoxole USAN, INN antiperistaltic

Nu-Iron elixir OTC hematinic [polysaccharide-iron complex] 100 mg/5 mL

Nu-Iron 150 capsules OTC hematinic [polysaccharide-iron complex] 150 mg

Nu-Iron Plus elixir ℞ hematinic [polysaccharide-iron complex; cyanocobalamin; folic acid] 300 mg•75 µg•3 mg per 15 mL

Nu-Iron V film-coated tablets ℞ vitamin/iron supplement [polysaccharide-iron complex; multiple vitamins; folic acid] 60• ± •1 mg

Nu-knit (trademarked form) oxidized cellulose hemostatic pad

Nulicaine injection (discontinued 1995) ℞ injectable local anesthetic [lidocaine HCl] 1%, 2%

Nullo tablets (discontinued 1996) OTC vulnerary; fecal and urinary odor control [chlorophyllin copper complex] 33.3 mg

NuLytely powder for oral solution ℞ pre-procedure bowel evacuant [polyethylene glycol-electrolyte solution] 105 g/L

Numorphan IV, IM, or subcu injection, suppositories ℞ narcotic analgesic; preoperative support of anesthesia; investigational (orphan) for intractable pain in narcotic-tolerant patients [oxymorphone HCl] 1, 1.5 mg/mL; 5 mg

Numzident gel OTC *topical oral anesthetic* [benzocaine] 10%

Numzit Teething gel OTC *topical oral anesthetic* [benzocaine] 7.5%

Numzit Teething lotion OTC *topical oral anesthetic* [benzocaine; alcohol 12.1%] 0.2%

Nupercainal ointment, cream OTC *topical local anesthetic* [dibucaine] 1%; 0.5%

Nupercainal rectal suppositories OTC *emollient; astringent* [cocoa butter; zinc oxide] 2.1•0.25 g

Nuprin tablets, caplets OTC *nonsteroidal anti-inflammatory drug (NSAID); antiarthritic; analgesic* [ibuprofen] 200 mg

Nuprin Backache caplets OTC *analgesic; antipyretic; anti-inflammatory* [magnesium salicylate] 580 mg

Nu-Prochlor ⓒᴬᴺ (U.S. product: Compazine) film-coated tablets ℞ *conventional (typical) antipsychotic; antiemetic* [prochlorperazine bimaleate] 5, 10 mg

Nuquin HP cream, gel ℞ *hyperpigmentation bleaching agent; sunscreen* [hydroquinone; dioxybenzone] 4%•30 mg

Nuromax IV injection ℞ *nondepolarizing neuromuscular blocker; adjunct to anesthesia* [doxacurium chloride] 1 mg/mL

Nursette (trademarked form) *prefilled disposable bottle*

Nursoy liquid, powder (discontinued 1996) OTC *hypoallergenic infant food* [soy protein formula]

Nu-Salt OTC *salt substitute* [potassium chloride] 68 mEq/5 g

nut, oil *medicinal herb* [see: butternut]

Nu-Tears eye drops OTC *ophthalmic moisturizer/lubricant* [polyvinyl alcohol] 1.4%

Nu-Tears II eye drops OTC *ophthalmic moisturizer/lubricant* [polyvinyl alcohol; polyethylene glycol 400] 1%•1%

Nu-Timolol ⓒᴬᴺ (U.S. product: Timoptic) eye drops ℞ *topical antiglaucoma agent (β-blocker)* [timolol maleate] 0.25%, 0.5%

nutmeg *(Myristica fragrans)* seed and aril *medicinal herb for diarrhea, flatulence, inducing expectoration, insomnia, mouth sores, rheumatism, salivary stimulation, and stimulating menstruation*

nutmeg oil NF

Nutracort cream ℞ *topical corticosteroidal anti-inflammatory* [hydrocortisone] 1%

Nutracort lotion (discontinued 1997) ℞ *topical corticosteroidal anti-inflammatory* [hydrocortisone] 1%

Nutraderm cream, lotion OTC *moisturizer; emollient*

Nutraderm OTC *lotion base*

Nutraderm Bath Oil OTC *bath emollient*

Nutraloric powder OTC *enteral nutritional therapy* [milk-based formula]

Nutramigen liquid, powder OTC *hypoallergenic infant food* [enzymatically hydrolyzed protein formula]

Nutra-Plex liquid (discontinued 1995) OTC *vitamin/mineral supplement* [multiple B vitamins & minerals; alcohol 13.5%]

Nutraplus cream, lotion OTC *moisturizer; emollient; keratolytic* [urea] 10%

Nutra-Soothe bath oil OTC *bath emollient* [colloidal oatmeal; light mineral oil]

Nutren 1.0 liquid OTC *enteral nutritional therapy* [lactose-free formula]

Nutren 1.5 liquid OTC *enteral nutritional therapy* [lactose-free formula]

Nutren 2.0 ready-to-use liquid OTC *enteral nutritional therapy* [lactose-free formula]

Nutricon tablets OTC *vitamin/mineral/calcium/iron supplement* [multiple vitamins & minerals; calcium; iron; folic acid; biotin] ±•200•20•0.4•0.15 mg

Nutrilan ready-to-use liquid OTC *enteral nutritional therapy* [lactose-free formula]

Nutrilyte; Nutrilyte II IV admixture ℞ *intravenous electrolyte therapy* [combined electrolyte solution]

Nutrineal Peritoneal Dialysis Solution with 1.1% Amino Acid ℞

investigational (orphan) nutritional supplement for continuous ambulatory peritoneal dialysis patients

Nutropin powder for subcu injection ℞ *growth hormone for adults or children with congenital or endogenous growth hormone deficiency, children with Turner syndrome or renal-induced growth failure, or AIDS-wasting syndrome (orphan)* [somatropin] 5, 10 mg (13, 26 IU) per vial

Nutropin AQ subcu injection ℞ *growth hormone for congenital or renal-induced growth failure and Turner syndrome (orphan); investigational (orphan) for severe burns* [somatropin] 10 mg (30 IU) per vial

Nutropin Depot sustained-release injection ℞ *investigational delivery form* [somatropin]

Nutrox capsules OTC *dietary supplement* [multiple vitamins & minerals; multiple amino acids] ±

Nuvance ℞ *investigational (Phase II) treatment for allergy, asthma, transplant rejection, and infectious diseases* [interleukin-4 receptor]

nuvenzepine INN

nyctal [see: carbromal]

nydrane [see: benzchlorpropamid]

Nydrazid IM injection ℞ *tuberculostatic* [isoniazid] 100 mg/mL

nylestriol USAN *estrogen* [also: nilestriol]

nylidrin HCl USP *peripheral vasodilator* [also: buphenine]

Nymphaea odorata medicinal herb [see: white pond lilly]

Nyotran ℞ *investigational (NDA filed) systemic antifungal for Aspergillus fumigatus infections* [nystatin liposomal]

NyQuil Allergy/Head Cold, Children's liquid (discontinued 1995) OTC *pediatric decongestant and antihistamine* [pseudoephedrine HCl; chlorpheniramine maleate] 10•0.67 mg/5 mL

NyQuil Hot Therapy powder for oral solution OTC *antitussive; decongestant; antihistamine; analgesic* [dextromethorphan hydrobromide; pseudoephedrine HCl; doxylamine succinate;

acetaminophen] 30•60•12.5•1000 mg/packet

NyQuil LiquiCaps (liquid-filled capsules) OTC *antitussive; decongestant; antihistamine; analgesic* [dextromethorphan hydrobromide; pseudoephedrine HCl; doxylamine succinate; acetaminophen] 10•30•6.25•250 mg

NyQuil Multisymptom Cold Flu Relief; NyQuilNighttime Cold/ Flu Medicine liquid OTC *antitussive; decongestant; antihistamine; analgesic* [dextromethorphan hydrobromide; pseudoephedrine HCl; doxylamine succinate; acetaminophen; alcohol 10%•25%] 5•10•2.1•167 mg/5 mL; 5•10•1.25•167 mg/5 mL

NyQuil Nighttime Cough/Cold, Children's liquid OTC *pediatric antitussive, decongestant, and antihistamine* [dextromethorphan hydrobromide; pseudoephedrine HCl; chlorpheniramine maleate] 5•10•0.67 mg/5 mL

nystatin USP, INN, BAN, JAN *polyene antifungal* 100 000, 500 000 U/mL oral; 100 000 mg vaginal; 100 000 U/g topical ② Nilstat; Nitrostat

Nystatin-LF (liposomal formulation) IV injection ℞ *investigational (NDA filed) systemic therapy for fungal infections; investigational (Phase II) antiviral for HIV* [nystatin]

Nystex cream, ointment ℞ *topical antifungal* [nystatin] 100 000 U/g

Nystex oral suspension ℞ *antifungal; oral candidiasis treatment* [nystatin] 100 000 U/mL

Nytcold Medicine liquid OTC *antitussive; decongestant; antihistamine; analgesic* [dextromethorphan hydrobromide; pseudoephedrine HCl; doxylamine succinate; acetaminophen; alcohol 25%] 5•10•1.25•167 mg/5 mL

Nytol tablets OTC *antihistaminic sleep aid* [diphenhydramine HCl] 25, 50 mg

NZGLM (New Zealand green-lipped mussel) [q.v.]

O$_2$ (oxygen) [q.v.]
oak *medicinal herb* [see: white oak]
OAP (Oncovin, ara-C, prednisone) *chemotherapy protocol*
oatmeal, colloidal *demulcent*
oats (Avena sativa) *grain and straw medicinal herb for dry itchy skin, hyperlipidemia, indigestion, insomnia, nervousness, opium addiction, reducing the desire to smoke, and strengthening the heart*
Obalan tablets (discontinued 1996) ℞ *anorexiant; CNS stimulant* [phendimetrazine tartrate] 35 mg
obecalp *placebo (spelled backward)*
Obenix capsules ℞ *anorexiant; CNS stimulant* [phentermine HCl] 37.5 mg
Obephen capsules (discontinued 1997) ℞ *anorexiant; CNS stimulant* [phentermine HCl] 30 mg
obidoxime chloride USAN, INN *cholinesterase reactivator*
Oby-Cap capsules (discontinued 1998) ℞ *anorexiant; CNS stimulant* [phentermine HCl] 30 mg
O-Cal f.a. tablets ℞ *vitamin/mineral/calcium/iron supplement and dental caries preventative* [multiple vitamins & minerals; calcium; iron; folic acid; sodium fluoride] ≛•200•66•1•1.1 mg
ocaperidone USAN, INN, BAN *antipsychotic*
Occlusal-HP liquid OTC *topical keratolytic* [salicylic acid in polyacrylic vehicle] 17%
Occucoat ophthalmic solution ℞ *ophthalmic surgical aid* [hydroxypropyl methylcellulose] 2%
Ocean Mist nasal spray OTC *nasal moisturizer* [sodium chloride (saline solution)] 0.65%
ocfentanil INN *narcotic analgesic* [also: ocfentanil HCl]
ocfentanil HCl USAN *narcotic analgesic* [also: ocfentanil]
ociltide INN
Ocimum basilicum *medicinal herb* [see: basil]

ocinaplon USAN *anxiolytic*
OCL oral solution ℞ *pre-procedure bowel evacuant* [polyethylene glycol-electrolyte solution]
ocrase INN
ocrilate INN *tissue adhesive* [also: ocrylate]
ocrylate USAN *tissue adhesive* [also: ocrilate]
octabenzone USAN, INN *ultraviolet screen*
octacaine INN
octacosactrin BAN [also: tosactide]
octacosanol (wheat germ oil) *natural supplement for increasing muscle endurance*
octadecafluorodecehydronaphthalene [see: perflunafene]
octadecanoic acid, calcium salt [see: calcium stearate]
octadecanoic acid, sodium salt [see: sodium stearate]
octadecanoic acid, zinc salt [see: zinc stearate]
1-octadecanol [see: stearyl alcohol]
9-octadecenylamine hydrofluoride [see: dectaflur]
octafonium chloride INN
Octamide PFS IV or IM injection ℞ *antiemetic for chemotherapy; GI stimulant; peristaltic* [metoclopramide HCl] 5 mg/mL
octamoxin INN
octamylamine INN
octanoic acid USAN, INN *antifungal*
octapinol INN
octastine INN
octatropine methylbromide INN, BAN *anticholinergic; peptic ulcer adjunct* [also: anisotropine methylbromide]
octatropone bromide [see: anisotropine methylbromide]
octaverine INN, BAN
octazamide USAN, INN *analgesic*
octenidine INN, BAN *topical anti-infective* [also: octenidine HCl]
octenidine HCl USAN *topical anti-infective* [also: octenidine]

octenidine saccharin USAN *dental plaque inhibitor*

Octicare ear drops, ear drop suspension ℞ *topical corticosteroidal anti-inflammatory; antibiotic* [hydrocortisone; neomycin sulfate; polymyxin B sulfate] 1%•5 mg•10 000 U per mL

octicizer USAN *plasticizer*

octil INN *combining name for radicals or groups*

octimibate INN

octisamyl [see: octamylamine]

Octocaine HCl injection ℞ *injectable local anesthetic* [lidocaine HCl; epinephrine] 2%•1:50 000, 2%•1:100 000

octoclothepine [see: clorotepine]

octocrilene INN *ultraviolet screen* [also: octocrylene]

octocrylene USAN *ultraviolet screen* [also: octocrilene]

octodecactide [see: codactide]

octodrine USAN, INN *adrenergic; vasoconstrictor; local anesthetic*

octopamine INN

octotiamine INN

octoxinol INN *surfactant/wetting agent* [also: octoxynol 9]

octoxynol 9 USAN, NF *surfactant/wetting agent; spermicide* [also: octoxinol]

OctreoScan powder for injection ℞ *radiopaque contrast medium* [oxidronate sodium] 2 mg

OctreoScan 111 ℞ *investigational radioactive imaging agent for SPECT scans of neuroendocrine tumors* [indium In 111 pentetreotide]

octreotide USAN, INN, BAN *gastric antisecretory*

octreotide acetate USAN *gastric antisecretory for acromegaly and severe diarrhea due to VIPomas and other tumors (orphan)*

octreotide pamoate USAN *antineoplastic*

octriptyline INN *antidepressant* [also: octriptyline phosphate]

octriptyline phosphate USAN *antidepressant* [also: octriptyline]

octrizole USAN, INN *ultraviolet screen*

S-**octyl thiobenzoate** [see: tioctilate]

octyl-2-cyanoacrylate [see: ocrylate]

octyldodecanol NF *oleaginous vehicle*

OcuCaps caplets OTC *vitamin/mineral supplement* [vitamins A, C, and E; multiple minerals] 5000 IU•400 mg•182 mg• ≜

Ocu-Carpine eye drops (discontinued 1995) ℞ *topical antiglaucoma agent; direct-acting miotic* [pilocarpine HCl] 0.5%, 1%, 2%, 3%, 4%, 6%

OcuClear eye drops OTC *topical ophthalmic decongestant and vasoconstrictor* [oxymetazoline HCl] 0.025%

OcuClenz solution, pads (discontinued 1996) OTC *eyelid cleanser for blepharitis or contact lenses*

OcuCoat prefilled syringe OTC *ophthalmic surgical aid* [hydroxypropyl methylcellulose] 2%

OcuCoat; OcuCoat PF eye drops OTC *ophthalmic moisturizer/lubricant* [hydroxypropyl methylcellulose] 0.8%

Ocudose (trademarked delivery device) *single-use eye drop dispenser*

Ocufen eye drops ℞ *topical ophthalmic nonsteroidal anti-inflammatory drug (NSAID); intraoperative miosis inhibitor* [flurbiprofen sodium] 0.03%

ocufilcon A USAN *hydrophilic contact lens material*

ocufilcon B USAN *hydrophilic contact lens material*

ocufilcon C USAN *hydrophilic contact lens material*

ocufilcon D USAN *hydrophilic contact lens material*

Ocuflox eye drops ℞ *topical ophthalmic quinolone antibiotic for corneal ulcers (orphan)* [ofloxacin] 3 mg/mL

Ocumeter (trademarked delivery device) *prefilled eye drop dispenser*

Ocupress eye drops ℞ *topical antiglaucoma agent (β-blocker)* [carteolol HCl] 1%

Ocusert Pilo-20; Ocusert Pilo-40 continuous-release ocular wafer ℞ *topical antiglaucoma agent; direct-acting miotic* [pilocarpine] 20 μg/hr.; 40 μg/hr.

OCuSOFT solution, pads OTC *eyelid cleanser for blepharitis or contact lenses*

OCuSoft VMS film-coated tablets OTC *vitamin/mineral supplement* [vitamins A, C, and E; multiple minerals] 5000 IU•60 mg•30 mg• ±

Ocusulf-10 eye drops ℞ *topical ophthalmic antibiotic* [sulfacetamide sodium] 10%

Ocutears ⊛ eye drops OTC *ophthalmic moisturizer/lubricant* [hydroxypropyl methylcellulose] 0.5%

Ocutricin eye drops (discontinued 1995) ℞ *topical ophthalmic antibiotic* [polymyxin B sulfate; neomycin sulfate; gramicidin] 10 000 U•1.75 mg•0.025 mg per mL

Ocutricin ophthalmic ointment ℞ *topical ophthalmic antibiotic* [polymyxin B sulfate; neomycin sulfate; bacitracin zinc] 10 000 U•3.5 mg•400 U per g

Ocuvite film-coated tablets OTC *vitamin/mineral supplement* [vitamins A, C, and E; multiple minerals] 5000 IU•60 mg•30 IU• ±

Ocuvite Extra tablets OTC *vitamin/mineral supplement* [vitamins A, C, and E; multiple minerals] 6000 IU•200 mg•50 IU• ±

OCuZIN tablets OTC *vitamin/mineral supplement* [vitamins A, C, and E; zinc; copper; selenium]

Odor Free ArthriCare [see: ArthriCare, Odor Free]

Oenothera biennis medicinal herb [see: evening primrose]

OEP (oil of evening primrose) [see: evening primrose]

Oesto-Mins powder OTC *vitamin/mineral supplement* [vitamins C and D; calcium; magnesium; potassium] 500 mg•100 IU•250 mg•250 mg•45 mg per 4.5 g

oestradiol BAN *estrogen replacement therapy for postmenopausal disorders; palliative therapy for prostatic and breast cancers* [also: estradiol]

oestradiol benzoate BAN [also: estradiol benzoate]

oestradiol valerate BAN *estrogen* [also: estradiol valerate]

oestriol succinate BAN *estrogen* [also: estriol; estriol succinate]

oestrogenine [see: diethylstilbestrol]

oestromenin [see: diethylstilbestrol]

oestrone BAN *estrogen replacement therapy for postmenopausal disorders; palliative therapy for prostatic and breast cancers* [also: estrone]

Off-Ezy Corn & Callus Remover kit (liquid + cushion pads) OTC *topical keratolytic* [salicylic acid in a collodion-like vehicle] 17%

Off-Ezy Wart Remover liquid OTC *topical keratolytic* [salicylic acid in a collodion-like vehicle] 17%

ofloxacin USAN, INN, BAN, JAN *broad-spectrum quinolone bactericidal antibiotic; topical corneal ulcer treatment (orphan)*

ofornine USAN, INN *antihypertensive*

oftasceine INN

Ogen tablets ℞ *estrogen replacement therapy for postmenopausal disorders* [estrone (from estropipate)] 0.625 (0.75), 1.25 (1.5), 2.5 (3) mg

Ogen vaginal cream ℞ *estrogen replacement for postmenopausal atrophic vaginitis* [estropipate] 1.5 mg/g

OGT-918 investigational (orphan) *glucosidase inhibitor for Gaucher's disease and Fabry's disease*

oidiomycin *diagnostic aid for cell-mediated immunity; extract of the Oidiomycetes fungus family*

oil nut medicinal herb [see: butternut]

oil of evening primrose (OEP) [see: evening primrose]

oil of mustard [see: allyl isothiocyanate]

Oil of Olay Foaming Face Wash liquid OTC *topical cleanser for acne*

oil ricini [see: castor oil]

Oilatum Soap bar OTC *therapeutic skin cleanser*

ointment, hydrophilic USP *ointment base; oil-in-water emulsion*

ointment, white USP *oleaginous ointment base*

ointment, yellow USP *ointment base*

OK-B7 *investigational monoclonal antibody used for the treatment of lymphoma*

olaflur USAN, INN, BAN *dental caries prophylactic*

olamine USAN, INN *combining name for radicals or groups*

olanzapine USAN, INN *thienobenzodiazepine antipsychotic*

olaquindox INN, BAN

old man's beard *medicinal herb* [see: fringe tree; woodbine]

old tuberculin (OT) [see: tuberculin]

Olea europaea medicinal herb [see: olive]

oleander (Nerium indicum; N. oleander) *plant medicinal herb for asthma, cancer, corns, epilepsy, and heart disease; not generally regarded as safe and effective in any form as it is extremely toxic*

oleandomycin INN [also: oleandomycin phosphate]

oleandomycin, triacetate ester [see: troleandomycin]

oleandomycin phosphate NF [also: oleandomycin]

oleic acid NF *emulsion adjunct*

oleic acid I 125 USAN *radioactive agent*

oleic acid I 131 USAN *radioactive agent*

oleovitamin A [now: vitamin A]

oleovitamin A & D USP *source of vitamins A and D*

oleovitamin D, synthetic [now: ergocalciferol]

olethytan 20 [see: polysorbate 80]

oletimol INN

oleum caryophylii [see: clove oil]

oleum gossypii seminis [see: cottonseed oil]

oleum maydis [see: corn oil]

oleum ricini [see: castor oil]

oleyl alcohol NF *emulsifying agent; emollient*

oligomycin D [see: rutamycin]

olive (Olea europaea) leaves, bark, and fruit *medicinal herb used as an antiseptic, astringent, cholagogue, demulcent, emollient, febrifuge, hypoglycemic, laxative, and tranquilizer*

olive, spurge; spurge laurel *medicinal herb* [see: mezereon]

olive oil NF *pharmaceutic aid*

olivomycin INN

olmidine INN

olopatadine INN *antiallergic; antiasthmatic*

olopatadine HCl USAN *antiallergic; antiasthmatic; ophthalmic antihistamine*

olpimedone INN

olsalazine INN, BAN *GI anti-inflammatory* [also: olsalazine sodium]

olsalazine sodium USAN *GI anti-inflammatory; treatment of ulcerative colitis* [also: olsalazine]

oltipraz INN

Olux foam ℞ *investigational (Phase III) topical corticosteroidal anti-inflammatory for scalp dermatoses* [clobetasol]

olvanil USAN, INN *analgesic*

OM 401 *investigational (orphan) for sickle cell disease*

OMAD (Oncovin, methotrexate/ citrovorum factor, Adriamycin, dactinomycin) *chemotherapy protocol*

omega-3 fatty acids [see: doconexent; icosapent; omega-3 marine triglycerides]

omega-3 fatty acids with all double bonds in the cis configuration *investigational (orphan) preventative for organ graft rejection*

omega-3 marine triglycerides BAN [12% doconexent (q.v.) + 18% icosapent (q.v.)]

omeprazole USAN, INN, BAN, JAN *proton pump inhibitor for gastric and duodenal ulcers and other gastroesophageal disorders*

omeprazole sodium USAN *gastric antisecretory*

omidoline INN

Omnicef capsules, oral suspension ℞ *cephalosporin antibiotic* [cefdinir] 300 mg; 125 mg/5 mL

Omniferon ℞ *investigational (Phase I) for genital herpes, multiple sclerosis, and AIDS* [interferon alfa]

OmniHIB powder for IM injection, prefilled syringes ℞ *Haemophilus influenzae type b (HIB) vaccine*

[Hemophilus b conjugate vaccine; tetanus toxoid] 10•24 μg/0.5 mL

OMNIhist L.A. long-acting tablets ℞ *decongestant; antihistamine; anticholinergic* [phenylephrine HCl; chlorpheniramine maleate; methscopolamine nitrate] 20•8•2.5 mg

Omnipaque injection ℞ *radiopaque contrast medium* [iohexol (46.36% iodine)] 302, 388, 453, 518, 647, 755 mg/mL (140, 180, 210, 240, 300, 350 mg/mL)

Omnipen capsules, powder for oral suspension ℞ *aminopenicillin antibiotic* [ampicillin] 250, 500 mg; 125, 250 mg/5 mL ⊡ Unipen

Omnipen-N powder for IV or IM injection ℞ *aminopenicillin antibiotic* [ampicillin sodium] 125, 250, 500 mg, 1, 2, 10 g

Omniscan IV injection ℞ *MRI contrast medium* [gadodiamide] 287 mg/mL

omoconazole INN *antifungal*

omoconazole nitrate USAN *antifungal*

omonasteine INN

OMS Concentrate drops ℞ *narcotic analgesic* [morphine sulfate] 20 mg/mL

onapristone INN *investigational antineoplastic for hormone-dependent cancers*

Oncaspar IV or IM injection ℞ *antineoplastic for acute lymphocytic leukemia (orphan) and acute lymphoblastic leukemia* [pegaspargase] 750 IU/mL

Oncet capsules ℞ *narcotic antitussive; analgesic* [hydrocodone bitartrate; acetaminophen] 5•500 mg

Oncocine-HspE7 ℞ *investigational (Phase I) agent for cervical cancer*

Oncolym ℞ *investigational (Phase III, orphan) treatment for non-Hodgkin's B-cell lymphoma* [iodine I 131 Lym-1 MAb]

Oncolysin B ℞ *investigational (Phase III) antineoplastic for B-cell lymphoma, leukemia, AIDS lymphoma, and myeloma; clinical trials discontinued 1997* [anti-B4-blocked ricin MAb]

Onconase ℞ *investigational (Phase III) treatment for pancreatic, breast, colo-* rectal, prostate, and small cell lung cancers [p30 protein]

OncoRad OV103 ℞ *investigational (orphan) antineoplastic for ovarian cancer* [CYT-103-Y-90 (code name —generic name not yet assigned)]

OncoScint CR/OV ℞ *radiodiagnostic imaging aid for ovarian (orphan) and colorectal cancer* [indium In 111 satumomab pendetide]

Oncostate ℞ *investigational (orphan) for renal cell carcinoma* [coumarin]

Onco-TCS *investigational (Phase II) antineoplastic for advanced non-Hodgkin's lymphoma* [vincristine liposomal]

OncoTICE ⊛ (U.S. product: Tice BCG) powder for intravesical instillation ℞ *antineoplastic for urinary bladder cancer* [BCG vaccine, Tice strain] 50 mg

OncoTrac imaging kit ℞ *investigational (orphan) for diagnostic imaging agent for metastasis of malignant melanoma* [technetium Tc 99m antimelanoma murine MAb]

OncoVax-CL ℞ *investigational (Phase I/II) therapeutic vaccine for colorectal cancer*

OncoVax-P ℞ *investigational (Phase II) therapeutic vaccine for prostate cancer*

Oncovin IV injection, Hyporets (prefilled syringes) ℞ *antineoplastic for lung and breast cancers, various leukemias, lymphomas, and sarcomas* [vincristine sulfate] 1 mg/mL ⊡ Ancobon

Oncovite tablets OTC *vitamin supplement* [multiple vitamins] ±

ondansetron INN, BAN $5-HT_3$ *antiemetic for chemotherapy; antischizophrenic; anxiolytic* [also: ondansetron HCl]

ondansetron HCl USAN $5-HT_3$ *antiemetic for chemotherapy; antischizophrenic; anxiolytic* [also: ondansetron]

Ondrox sustained-release tablets OTC *vitamin/mineral/calcium/iron supplement* [multiple vitamins & minerals; multiple amino acids; calcium; iron; folic acid; biotin] ±•25•3•0.67•0.005 mg

1+1·F Creme ℞ *topical corticosteroidal anti-inflammatory; antifungal; antibacterial; local anesthetic* [hydrocortisone; clioquinol; pramoxine] 1%•3%•1%

1% HC ointment ℞ *topical corticosteroidal anti-inflammatory* [hydrocortisone] 1%

One Step Midstream Pregnancy Test stick for home use (discontinued 1998) OTC *in vitro diagnostic aid for urine pregnancy test*

One Touch reagent strips for home use OTC *in vitro diagnostic aid for blood glucose*

15AU81 *investigational (orphan) for primary pulmonary hypertension*

One·A·Day 55 Plus tablets OTC *geriatric vitamin/mineral supplement* [multiple vitamins & minerals; folic acid; biotin] ±•400•30 µg

One·A·Day Essential tablets OTC *vitamin supplement* [multiple vitamins; folic acid] ±•0.4 mg

One·A·Day Extras Antioxidant softgel capsules OTC *vitamin/mineral supplement* [vitamins A, C, and E; multiple minerals] 5000 IU•250 mg•200 IU•±

One·A·Day Extras Vitamin C tablets OTC *vitamin supplement* [vitamin C] 500 mg

One·A·Day Extras Vitamin E soft gel capsules OTC *vitamin supplement* [vitamin E] 400 IU

One·A·Day Maximum Formula tablets OTC *vitamin/mineral/iron supplement* [multiple vitamins & minerals; iron; folic acid; biotin] ±•18 mg•0.4 mg•30 µg

One·A·Day Men's Vitamins tablets OTC *vitamin supplement* [multiple vitamins; folic acid] ±•0.4 mg

One·A·Day Women's Formula tablets OTC *vitamin/calcium/iron supplement* [multiple vitamins; calcium; iron; folic acid] ±•450•27•0.4 mg

1-alpha-D2 *investigational (Phase III) for secondary hyperparathyroidism in hemodialysis patients*

One·Tablet·Daily OTC *vitamin supplement* [multiple vitamins; folic acid] ±•0.4 mg

One·Tablet·Daily with Iron OTC *vitamin/iron supplement* [multiple vitamins; iron; folic acid] ±•18•0.4 mg

One·Tablet·Daily with Minerals OTC *vitamin/mineral/iron supplement* [multiple vitamins & minerals; iron; folic acid; biotin] ±•18 mg•0.4 mg•30 µg

onion (Allium cepa) bulb *medicinal herb used as an anthelmintic, antiseptic, antispasmodic, carminative, diuretic, expectorant, and stomachic*

Onkolox ℞ *investigational (orphan) for renal cell carcinoma* [coumarin]

Ontak frozen solution for IV injection ℞ *antineoplastic for recurrent or persistent cutaneous T-cell lymphoma (orphan)* [denileukin diftitox] 150 µg/mL

ontazolast USAN *antiasthmatic; leukotriene biosynthesis inhibitor*

ontianil INN

Ony·Clear solution ℞ *topical antifungal* [miconazole nitrate] 2%

Ony·Clear Nail (name changed to Ony·Clear in 1996)

ONYX·015 *investigational (Phase II) adenovirus E1B, in combination with cisplatin and 5-FU, for recurrent head and neck cancer*

OP·1 (osteogenic protein·1) [q.v.]

OPA (Oncovin, prednisone, Adriamycin) *chemotherapy protocol*

OPAL (Oncovin, prednisone, L-asparaginase) *chemotherapy protocol*

OPC·14117 *investigational vitamin E-like antioxidant for cognitive impairment and HIV-related nerve damage*

Opcon·A eye drops OTC *topical ophthalmic decongestant, antihistamine, and lubricant* [naphazoline HCl; pheniramine maleate; hydroxypropyl methylcellulose] 0.027%•0.315%•0.5%

OPEN (Oncovin, prednisone, etoposide, Novantrone) *chemotherapy protocol*

Operand solution, prep pads, swab sticks, surgical scrub, perineal wash concentrate, aerosol, Iofoam skin cleanser, ointment OTC *broad-spectrum antimicrobial* [povidone-iodine] 1%; 1%; 1%; 7.5%; 1%; 0.5%; 1%; 1%

Operand Douche concentrate OTC *antiseptic/germicidal; vaginal cleanser and deodorizer* [povidone-iodine]

Ophthaine eye drops (discontinued 1997) ℞ *topical ophthalmic anesthetic* [proparacaine HCl] 0.5%

Ophthalgan eye drops ℞ *corneal edema-reducing and clearing agent* [glycerin]

Ophthetic eye drops ℞ *topical ophthalmic anesthetic* [proparacaine HCl] 0.5%

Ophthifluor antecubital venous injection ℞ *ophthalmic diagnostic agent* [fluorescein sodium] 10%

Ophthocort ophthalmic ointment (discontinued 1996) ℞ *topical ophthalmic corticosteroidal anti-inflammatory; antibiotic* [hydrocortisone acetate; chloramphenicol; polymyxin B sulfate] 0.5%•1%•10 000 U/g ⚕

Ophthochlor

opiniazide INN

opipramol INN *antidepressant; antipsychotic* [also: opipramol HCl]

opipramol HCl USAN *antidepressant; antipsychotic* [also: opipramol]

opium USP *narcotic analgesic; widely abused as a street drug, which is highly addictive* 10% oral

opium, powdered USP *narcotic analgesic*

Oplopanax horridus medicinal herb [see: devil's club]

OPP (Oncovin, procarbazine, prednisone) *chemotherapy protocol*

OPPA (Oncovin, prednisone, procarbazine, Adriamycin) *chemotherapy protocol*

oprelvekin USAN *platelet growth factor for prevention of thrombocytopenia following chemotherapy or radiation (orphan)* [also: interleukin 11, recombinant human]

Opticare PMS tablets OTC *vitamin/mineral supplement; digestive enzymes* [multiple vitamins & minerals; iron; folic acid; biotin; amylase; protease; lipase] ±•2.5 mg•0.033 mg•10.4 μg•2500 U•2500 U•200 U

Opti-Clean solution OTC *cleaning solution for hard, soft, or rigid gas permeable contact lenses*

Opti-Clean II solution OTC *cleaning solution for hard or soft contact lenses*

Opti-Clean II Especially for Sensitive Eyes solution OTC *cleaning solution for rigid gas permeable contact lenses*

Opticrom 4% eye drops ℞ *topical ophthalmic antiallergic for vernal keratoconjunctivitis (orphan)* [cromolyn sodium]

Opticyl eye drops ℞ *cycloplegic; mydriatic* [tropicamide] 0.5%, 1%

Opti-Free solution OTC *chemical disinfecting solution for soft contact lenses* [note: one of four different products with the same name]

Opti-Free solution OTC *rewetting solution for soft contact lenses* [note: one of four different products with the same name]

Opti-Free solution OTC *surfactant cleaning solution for soft contact lenses* [note: one of four different products with the same name]

Opti-Free tablets OTC *enzymatic cleaner for soft contact lenses* [pork pancreatin; note: one of four different products with the same name]

Optigene ophthalmic solution OTC *extraocular irrigating solution* [sterile isotonic solution]

Optigene 3 eye drops OTC *topical ophthalmic decongestant and vasoconstrictor* [tetrahydrozoline HCl] 0.05%

Optilets-500 Filmtabs (film-coated tablets) OTC *vitamin supplement* [multiple vitamins] ±

Optilets-M-500 Filmtabs (film-coated tablets) OTC *vitamin/mineral/iron supplement* [multiple vitamins & minerals; iron] ±•20 mg

Optimark ℞ *investigational (NDA filed) MRI contrast agent*

Optimental liquid OTC *enteral nutritional therapy* 237 mL

Optimine tablets ℞ *antihistamine* [azatadine maleate] 1 mg

Optimmune ℞ *investigational (orphan) for severe keratoconjunctivitis sicca in Sjögren syndrome* [cyclosporine]

Optimoist oral spray OTC *saliva substitute*

Optimox Prenatal tablets OTC *vitamin/mineral/calcium/iron supplement* [multiple vitamins & minerals; calcium; iron; folic acid] ≜•100•5•0.133 mg

Optimyd eye drops (discontinued 1995) ℞ *topical ophthalmic corticosteroidal anti-inflammatory; antibiotic* [prednisolone sodium phosphate; sulfacetamide sodium] 0.5%•10%

Opti-One solution OTC *rewetting solution for soft contact lenses*

Opti-One Multi-Purpose solution OTC *chemical disinfecting solution for soft contact lenses*

OptiPranolol eye drops ℞ *topical antiglaucoma agent (β-blocker)* [metipranolol HCl] 0.3%

Optiray 160; Optiray 240; Optiray 300; Optiray 320; Optiray 350 injection ℞ *radiopaque contrast medium* [ioversol (47.3% iodine)] 339 mg/mL (160 mg/mL); 509 mg/mL (240 mg/mL); 636 mg/mL (300 mg/mL); 678 mg/mL (320 mg/mL); 741 mg/mL (350 mg/mL)

Opti-Soft Especially for Sensitive Eyes solution OTC *rinsing/storage solution for soft contact lenses* [sodium chloride (preserved saline solution)]

Optison injectable suspension *ultrasound contrast medium for cardiac imaging; investigational (Phase III) diagnostic aid for infertility due to obstructed fallopian tubes* [human albumin (sonicated with octafluoropropane)] 3 mL

Opti-Tears solution OTC *rewetting solution for hard or soft contact lenses*

Optivite P.M.T. tablets OTC *geriatric vitamin/mineral supplement* [multiple vitamins & minerals; folic acid; biotin] ≜•30•≜ μg

Opti-Zyme Enzymatic Cleaner Especially for Sensitive Eyes tablets OTC *enzymatic cleaner for soft or rigid gas permeable contact lenses* [pork pancreatin]

Optro ℞ *investigational agent for chronic anemia* [human hemoglobin, recombinant]

OPV (oral poliovirus vaccine) [see: poliovirus vaccine, live oral]

ORA5 liquid OTC *oral anti-infective* [copper sulfate; iodine; potassium iodide] ≜•≜•≜

Orabase gel OTC *mucous membrane anesthetic* [benzocaine] 15%

Orabase Baby gel OTC *topical oral anesthetic* [benzocaine] 7.5%

Orabase HCA oral paste ℞ *topical corticosteroidal anti-inflammatory* [hydrocortisone acetate] 0.5%

Orabase Lip Healer cream OTC *topical oral anesthetic; antipruritic/counterirritant; vulnerary* [benzocaine; menthol; allantoin] 5%•0.5%•1.5%

Orabase-B oral paste OTC *topical oral anesthetic* [benzocaine] 20% ⊡ Orinase

Orabase-Plain oral paste OTC *relief from minor oral irritations* [plasticized hydrocarbon gel]

Oracit solution ℞ *urinary alkalinizing agent* [sodium citrate; citric acid] 490•640 mg/5 mL

Oradex-C lozenges (discontinued 1995) OTC *topical anesthetic; counterirritant* [dyclonine HCl] 3 mg

Oragrafin Calcium granules for oral suspension (discontinued 1999) ℞ *radiopaque contrast medium for cholecystography* [ipodate calcium (61.7% iodine)] 3 g/packet

Oragrafin Sodium capsules ℞ *radiopaque contrast medium for cholecystography* [ipodate sodium (61.4% iodine)] 500 mg (307 mg)

Orajel liquid OTC *topical oral anesthetic* [benzocaine; alcohol 44.2%] 20%

Orajel; Orajel Brace-aid; Orajel/d; Denture Orajel; Baby Orajel; Baby Orajel Nighttime Formula gel OTC *topical oral anesthetic* [benzocaine] 20%; 20%; 10%; 10%; 7.5%; 10%

Orajel Mouth-Aid liquid, gel OTC *mucous membrane anesthetic* [benzocaine] 20%

Orajel Perioseptic liquid OTC *topical oral anti-inflammatory and anti-infective for braces* [carbamide peroxide] 15%

Orajel Tooth & Gum Cleanser, Baby gel OTC *removes plaque-like film* [poloxamer 407; simethicone] 2%•0.12%

Oralease ℞ *investigational (Phase III) analgesic for pain due to oral ulcers*

Oralet (trademarked dosage form) *oral lozenge/lollipop*

Oralgen; Oralin ⒸⒶⓃ ℞ *investigational (Phase II/III) oral insulin formulation*

Oralone Dental paste ℞ *topical corticosteroidal anti-inflammatory* [triamcinolone acetonide] 0.1%

Oramide tablets ℞ *sulfonylurea antidiabetic* [tolbutamide]

Oraminic II subcu or IM injection (discontinued 1997) ℞ *antihistamine for anaphylaxis* [brompheniramine maleate] 10 mg/mL

Oramorph SR sustained-release tablets ℞ *narcotic analgesic* [morphine sulfate] 15, 30, 60, 100 mg

orange flower oil NF *flavoring agent; perfume*

orange flower water NF

orange oil NF

orange peel tincture, sweet NF

orange root *medicinal herb* [see: goldenseal]

orange spirit, compound NF

orange swallow wort *medicinal herb* [see: pleurisy root]

orange syrup NF

Orap tablets ℞ *antidyskinetic for Tourette syndrome* [pimozide] 2 mg (4 mg available in Canada)

Oraphen-PD elixir OTC *analgesic; antipyretic* [acetaminophen] 120 mg/5 mL

orarsan [see: acetarsone] Ⓓ Oracin; Orasone

Orasept liquid OTC *oral astringent; antiseptic* [tannic acid; methylbenzethonium chloride; alcohol 53.31%] 12.16%•1.53%

Orasept throat spray OTC *topical oral anesthetic; antiseptic* [benzocaine; methylbenzethonium chloride] 0.996%•1.037%

Orasol liquid OTC *topical oral anesthetic; antipruritic/counterirritant; antiseptic* [benzocaine; phenol; alcohol 70%] 6.3%•0.5%

Orasone tablets ℞ *corticosteroid; anti-inflammatory; immunosuppressant* [prednisone] 1, 5, 10, 20, 50 mg Ⓓ Oracin; orarsan

OraSure reagent kit for home use OTC *in vitro diagnostic aid for HIV antibodies*

OraSure HIV-1 reagent kit for professional use ℞ *in vitro diagnostic aid for HIV antibodies using oral mucosal transudate* [single-sample, three-test kit: two ELISA assays + Western Blot assay]

Oratect gel (discontinued 1995) OTC *topical oral anesthetic* [benzocaine; alcohol 65.8%] 15%

orazamide INN

Orazinc capsules, tablets OTC *zinc supplement* [zinc sulfate] 220 mg; 110 mg

orbofiban acetate USAN *platelet aggregation inhibitor; fibrinogen receptor antagonist*

orbutopril INN

orchanet *medicinal herb* [see: henna (Alkanna)]

orciprenaline INN, BAN *bronchodilator* [also: metaproterenol polistirex]

orciprenaline polistirex [see: metaproterenol polistirex]

orconazole INN *antifungal* [also: orconazole nitrate]

orconazole nitrate USAN *antifungal* [also: orconazole]

Ordrine AT extended-release capsules ℞ *antitussive; decongestant* [caramiphen edisylate; phenylpropanolamine HCl] 40•75 mg

Ordrine S.R. sustained-release capsules ℞ *decongestant; antihistamine* [phenylpropanolamine HCl; chlorpheniramine maleate]

oregano *medicinal herb* [see: marjoram]

Oregon grape *(Mahonia aquifolium)* rhizome and root *medicinal herb for acne, blood disorders, eczema, jaundice, liver disorders, promoting digestion, psoriasis, and staphylococcal infections*

orestrate INN

orestrol [see: diethylstilbestrol dipropionate]

Oretic tablets ℞ *antihypertensive; diuretic* [hydrochlorothiazide] 25, 50 mg ⊡ Oreton

Oreton Methyl tablets, buccal tablets ℞ *androgen for male hypogonadism, impotence and breast cancer* [methyltestosterone] 10 mg ⊡ Oretic

Orexin chewable tablets OTC *vitamin supplement* [vitamins B_1, B_6, and B_{12}] 8.1 mg•4.1 mg•25 µg

Organidin NR tablets, oral liquid ℞ *expectorant* [guaifenesin] 200 mg; 100 mg/5 mL

organoclay [see: bentoquatam]

Orgaran subcu injection ℞ *anticoagulant/antithrombotic for prevention of deep vein thrombosis (DVT) following hip replacement surgery* [danaparoid sodium] 750 anti-Xa IU/0.6 mL

orgotein USAN, INN, BAN *anti-inflammatory; antirheumatic; investigational (orphan) for amyotrophic lateral sclerosis and to prevent donor organ reperfusion injury* [previously known as superoxide dismutase (SOD)]

orgotein, recombinant human *investigational (orphan) for bronchopulmonary dysplasia of premature neonates*

orienticine A; orienticine D [see: orientiparcin]

orientiparcin INN [a mixture of orienticine A and orienticine D]

Origanum vulgare medicinal herb [see: marjoram]

Orimune oral suspension ℞ *poliomyelitis vaccine* [poliovirus vaccine, live oral trivalent] 0.5 mL

Orinase tablets ℞ *sulfonylurea antidiabetic* [tolbutamide] 500 mg ⊡ Orabase; Ornade; Ornex; Tolinase

Orinase Diagnostic powder for IV injection ℞ *in vivo diagnostic aid for pancreas function and diabetes* [tolbutamide sodium] 1 g

Orlaam IV injection ℞ *narcotic analgesic for management of opiate addiction (orphan)* [levomethadyl acetate HCl] 10 mg/mL

orlipastat [see: orlistat]

orlistat USAN, INN *lipase inhibitor to suppress the absorption of dietary fats, leading to weight loss*

ormaplatin USAN *antineoplastic*

Ormazine IV or IM injection (discontinued 1998) ℞ *conventional (typical) antipsychotic* [chlorpromazine HCl] 25 mg/mL

ormetroprim USAN, INN *antibacterial*

Ornade Spansules (sustained-release capsules) ℞ *decongestant; antihistamine* [phenylpropanolamine HCl; chlorpheniramine maleate] 75•12 mg ⊡ Orinase; Ornex

Ornex caplets (name changed to Ornex No Drowsiness in 1995)

Ornex No Drowsiness caplets OTC *decongestant; analgesic; antipyretic* [pseudoephedrine HCl; acetaminophen] 30•325 mg ⊡ Orex; Orinase; Ornade

Ornex Severe Cold No Drowsiness caplets (discontinued 1995) OTC *antitussive; decongestant; analgesic* [dextromethorphan hydrobromide; pseudoephedrine HCl; acetaminophen] 15•30•500 mg ⊡ Orex; Orinase; Ornade

ornidazole USAN, INN *anti-infective*

Ornidyl IV injection concentrate ℞ *antiprotozoal for Trypanosoma brucei gambiense (sleeping sickness) infection (orphan)* [eflornithine HCl] 200 mg/mL

ornipressin INN

ornithine (L-ornithine) INN

ornithine vasopressin [see: ornipressin]

ornoprostil INN

orotic acid INN

orotirelin INN

orpanoxin USAN, INN *anti-inflammatory*

orphenadine citrate [see: orphenadrine citrate]

orphenadrine INN, BAN *skeletal muscle relaxant; antihistamine* [also: orphenadrine citrate]

orphenadrine citrate USP *skeletal muscle relaxant; antihistamine* [also: orphenadrine] 100 mg oral; 30 mg/mL injection

orphenadrine HCl *anticholinergic; antiparkinsonian*

Orphengesic; Orphengesic Forte tablets (discontinued 1996) ℞ *skeletal muscle relaxant; analgesic; CNS stimulant* [orphenadrine citrate; aspirin; caffeine] 25•385•30 mg; 50•770•60 mg

orpressin [see: ornipressin]

orris root *(Iris florentina) medicinal herb used as a diuretic and stomachic*

ortetamine INN

orthesin [see: benzocaine]

Ortho Dienestrol vaginal cream ℞ *estrogen replacement for postmenopausal atrophic vaginitis* [dienestrol] 0.01%

Ortho Tri-Cyclen tablets, Dialpak (tablet dispenser) ℞ *triphasic oral contraceptive; treatment for acne vulgaris in females* [norgestimate; ethinyl estradiol] Phase 1: 0.18 mg•35 μg; Phase 2: 0.215 mg•35 μg; Phase 3: 0.25 mg•35 μg

Ortho-Cept tablets ℞ *monophasic oral contraceptive* [desogestrel; ethinyl estradiol] 0.15 mg•30 μg

Orthoclone OKT3 IV injection ℞ *immunosuppressant for renal, cardiac, and hepatic transplants* [muromonab-CD3] 5 mg/5 mL ② Ortho-Creme

orthocresol NF

Ortho-Cyclen tablets, Dialpak (tablet dispenser) ℞ *monophasic oral contraceptive* [norgestimate; ethinyl estradiol] 0.25 mg•35 μg

Ortho-Est tablets ℞ *estrogen replacement therapy for postmenopausal disorders* [estrone (from estropipate)] 0.625 (0.75), 1.25 (1.5) mg

Ortho-Gynol vaginal gel OTC *spermicidal contraceptive (for use with a diaphragm)* [octoxynol 9] 1%

Ortholinum ℞ *investigational (orphan) for spasmodic torticollis* [botulinum toxin, type F]

Ortho-Novum 1/35 tablets ℞ *monophasic oral contraceptive* [norethindrone; ethinyl estradiol] 1 mg•35 μg

Ortho-Novum 1/50 tablets ℞ *monophasic oral contraceptive* [norethindrone; mestranol] 1 mg•50 μg

Ortho-Novum 7/7/7 tablets ℞ *triphasic oral contraceptive* [norethindrone; ethinyl estradiol] Phase 1: 0.5 mg•35 μg; Phase 2: 0.75 mg•35 μg; Phase 3: 1 mg•35 μg

Ortho-Novum 10/11 tablets ℞ *biphasic oral contraceptive* [norethindrone; ethinyl estradiol] Phase 1: 0.5 mg•35 μg; Phase 2: 1 mg•35 μg

orthotolidine

Orthovisc (European name for U.S. product Hyalgan)

Orthoxicol Cough syrup OTC *antitussive; decongestant; antihistamine* [dextromethorphan hydrobromide; phenylpropanolamine HCl; chlorpheniramine maleate; alcohol 8%] 6.7•8.3•1.3 mg/5 mL

Orudis capsules ℞ *nonsteroidal anti-inflammatory drug (NSAID); antiarthritic; analgesic* [ketoprofen] 25, 50, 75 mg

Orudis KT tablets OTC *nonsteroidal anti-inflammatory drug (NSAID); analgesic; antiarthritic* [ketoprofen] 12.5 mg

Oruvail sustained-release pellets in capsules ℞ *once-daily nonsteroidal anti-inflammatory drug (NSAID); antiarthritic; analgesic* [ketoprofen] 100, 150, 200 mg

oryzanol A, B, and C *medicinal herb* [see: rice bran oil]

Orzel ℞ *investigational (NDA filed) oral therapy for colorectal cancer*

osalmid INN

osarsal [see: acetarsone]

Os-Cal 250+D; Os-Cal 500+D film-coated tablets OTC *dietary supplement* [calcium carbonate; vitamin D] 250 mg•125 IU; 500 mg•125 IU

Os-Cal 500 tablets, chewable tablets OTC *calcium supplement* [calcium carbonate] 1.25 g

Os-Cal Fortified tablets OTC *vitamin/ calcium/iron supplement* [multiple vitamins; calcium carbonate; iron] ≛•250•5 mg

Os-Cal Fortified Multivitamin & Minerals tablets OTC *vitamin/mineral/calcium/iron supplement* [multiple vitamins & minerals; calcium carbonate; iron] ≛•250•5 mg

Os-Cal Plus tablets (discontinued 1995) OTC *vitamin/calcium/iron supplement* [multiple vitamins; calcium carbonate; iron] ≛•250•16.6 mg

osmadizone INN

Osmitrol IV infusion ℞ *antihypertensive; osmotic diuretic* [mannitol] 5%, 10%, 15%, 20%

osmium *element (Os)*

Osmoglyn solution ℞ *osmotic diuretic* [glycerin] 50%

Osmolite; Osmolite HN liquid OTC *enteral nutritional therapy* [lactose-free formula]

Osmorhiza longistylis medicinal herb [see: sweet cicely]

osmotic diuretics *a class of diuretics that increase excretion of sodium and chloride and decrease tubular absorption of water*

Osmovist injection (discontinued 1995) ℞ *radiopaque contrast medium* [iotrolan]

Osmunda cinnamomea; O. regalis medicinal herb [see: buckhorn brake]

OspA [see: lipoprotein OspA, recombinant]

Ossigel ℞ *investigational (Phase I) agent to accelerate healing of bone fractures* [ersofermin; hyaluronate sodium]

OST-577 *investigational human anti-hepatitis B antibody*

Ostac ⓐ capsules, IV infusion ℞ *bisphosphonate bone resorption inhibitor for hypercalcemia of malignancy and osteolysis due to bone metastasis of*

malignant tumors [clodronate disodium] 400 mg; 30 mg/mL

Ostavir ℞ *investigational (Phase II) anti-hepatitis B monoclonal antibody* [tuvirumab]

Osteocalcin subcu or IM injection ℞ *calcium regulator for hypercalcemia, Paget's disease, and postmenopausal osteoporosis* [calcitonin (salmon)] 200 IU/mL

Osteo-D ℞ *calcium regulator; investigational (orphan) for familial hypophosphatemic rickets* [secalciferol]

Osteo-F slow-release tablets ℞ *investigational treatment for postmenopausal osteoporosis* [sodium fluoride]

osteogenic protein-1 (OP-1) *investigational that enhances motor function following stroke*

Osteomark ℞ *investigational enzyme-linked immunoassay for monitoring bone resorption; investigational agent for primary hyperparathyroidism and metastatic bone tumors* [monoclonal antibodies]

OsteoMax effervescent powder for oral solution OTC *dietary supplement* [calcium citrate; vitamin D; magnesium] 500 mg•200 IU•200 mg

Osteo-Mins powder OTC *dietary supplement* [multiple minerals; vitamins C and D] ≛•500 mg•100 IU

Ostiderm lotion OTC *for hyperhidrosis and bromhidrosis* [aluminum sulfate; zinc oxide] 14.5•≛ mg/g

Ostiderm roll-on OTC *for hyperhidrosis and bromhidrosis* [aluminum chlorohydrate; camphor; alcohol] ≛•≛•≛

ostreogrycin INN, BAN

osvarsan [see: acetarsone]

Oswego tea (*Monarda didyma*) leaves and flowers *medicinal herb used as a calmative, rubefacient, and stimulant*

OT (old tuberculin) [see: tuberculin]

Otic Domeboro ear drops ℞ *antibacterial; antifungal* [acetic acid; aluminum acetate] 2%•≛

Otic Tridesilon ear drops (discontinued 1995) ℞ *topical corticosteroidal anti-inflammatory; antibacterial; anti-*

fungal [desonide; acetic acid]
0.05%•2%

Otic-Care ear drops, otic suspension
℞ *topical corticosteroidal anti-inflammatory; antibiotic* [hydrocortisone; neomycin sulfate; polymyxin B sulfate] 1%•5 mg•10 000 U per mL

otilonium bromide INN, BAN

Oti-Med ear drops ℞ *topical corticosteroidal anti-inflammatory; antibacterial; topical local anesthetic* [hydrocortisone; chloroxylenol; pramoxine HCl] 10•1•10 mg/mL

otimerate sodium INN

OtiTricin otic suspension ℞ *topical corticosteroidal anti-inflammatory; antibiotic* [hydrocortisone; neomycin sulfate; polymyxin B sulfate] 1%•5 mg•10 000 U per mL

Otobiotic Otic ear drops ℞ *topical corticosteroidal anti-inflammatory; antibiotic* [hydrocortisone; polymyxin B sulfate] 0.5%•10 000 U per mL ⊡ Urobiotic

Otocain ear drops ℞ *topical local anesthetic* [benzocaine] 20%

Otocalm ear drops ℞ *topical local anesthetic; analgesic* [benzocaine; antipyrine] 1.4%•5.4%

Otocort ear drops, otic suspension ℞ *topical corticosteroidal anti-inflammatory; antibiotic* [hydrocortisone; neomycin sulfate; polymyxin B sulfate] 1%•5 mg•10 000 U per mL

Otomar-HC ear drops ℞ *topical corticosteroidal anti-inflammatory; local anesthetic; antibacterial* [hydrocortisone; pramoxine HCl; chloroxylenol] 10•10•1 mg/mL

Otomycet-HC ear drops ℞ *topical corticosteroidal anti-inflammatory; antibacterial; antifungal* [hydrocortisone; acetic acid] 1%•2%

Otomycin-HPN Otic ear drops ℞ *topical corticosteroidal anti-inflammatory; antibiotic* [hydrocortisone; neomycin sulfate; polymyxin B sulfate] 1%•5 mg•10 000 U per mL

Otosporin ear drops ℞ *topical corticosteroidal anti-inflammatory; antibiotic* [hydrocortisone; neomycin sulfate; polymyxin B sulfate] 1%•5 mg•10 000 U per mL

Otrivin nasal spray, nose drops, pediatric drops OTC *nasal decongestant* [xylometazoline HCl] 0.1%; 0.1%; 0.05% ⊡ Lotrimin

ouabain USP

Our Lady's mint *medicinal herb* [see: spearmint]

Outgro solution OTC *pain relief for ingrown toenails* [tannic acid; chlorobutanol; isopropyl alcohol 83%] 25%•5%

ovandrotone albumin INN, BAN

OvaRex ℞ *investigational (Phase II, orphan) therapeutic vaccine for epithelial ovarian cancer* [monoclonal antibody B43.13] ⊡ O-Vax

Ovastat ℞ *investigational (orphan) for ovarian cancer* [treosulfan] ⊡ Novastan

O-Vax ℞ *investigational (Phase III) therapeutic vaccine for ovarian cancer* ⊡ Ovarex

Ovcon-35; Ovcon-50 tablets ℞ *monophasic oral contraceptive* [norethindrone; ethinyl estradiol] 1 mg•35 μg; 1 mg•50 μg

Ovide lotion ℞ *pediculicide* [malathion; isopropyl alcohol 78%] 0.5%

ovine corticotropin-releasing hormone [see: corticorelin ovine triflutate]

Ovoid (trademarked dosage form) *sugar-coated tablet*

Ovral tablets ℞ *monophasic oral contraceptive; emergency "morning after" contraceptive* [norgestrel; ethinyl estradiol] 0.5 mg•50 μg

Ovrette tablets ℞ *oral contraceptive (progestin only)* [norgestrel] 0.075 mg

OvuGen test kit OTC *in vitro diagnostic aid to predict ovulation time*

OvuKIT Self-Test kit for home use OTC *in vitro diagnostic aid to predict ovulation time*

OvuQuick Self-Test kit for home use OTC *in vitro diagnostic aid to predict ovulation time*

[^{15}O]water [see: water O 15]

ox bile extract [see: bile salts]
oxabolone cipionate INN
oxabrexine INN
22-oxacalcitriol [see: maxacalcitol]
oxaceprol INN
oxacillin INN *penicillinase-resistant penicillin antibiotic* [also: oxacillin sodium]
oxacillin sodium USAN, USP *penicillinase-resistant penicillin antibiotic* [also: oxacillin] 250, 500 mg oral; 250 mg/5 mL oral; 0.25, 0.5, 1, 2, 4, 10 g injection
oxadimedine INN
oxadimedine HCl [see: oxadimedine]
oxadoddy *medicinal herb* [see: Culver's root]
oxaflozane INN
oxaflumazine INN
oxafuradene [see: nifuradene]
oxagrelate USAN, INN *platelet antiaggregatory agent*
oxalinast INN
oxaliplatin USAN, INN *investigational (orphan) alkylating antineoplastic for ovarian and colorectal cancers*
Oxalis acetosella *medicinal herb* [see: wood sorrel]
oxamarin INN *hemostatic* [also: oxamarin HCl]
oxamarin HCl USAN *hemostatic* [also: oxamarin]
oxametacin INN
oxamisole INN *immunoregulator* [also: oxamisole HCl]
oxamisole HCl USAN *immunoregulator* [also: oxamisole]
oxamniquine USAN, USP, INN *antischistosomal; anthelmintic for schistosomiasis (flukes)*
oxamphetamine hydrobromide [see: hydroxyamphetamine hydrobromide]
oxamycin [see: cycloserine]
oxanamide INN
Oxandrin tablets ℞ *anabolic steroid for weight gain; investigational (orphan) for muscular dystrophy, AIDS-wasting syndrome, and alcoholic hepatitis; also abused as a street drug* [oxandrolone] 2.5 mg

oxandrolone USAN, USP, INN, BAN, JAN *anabolic steroid for weight gain; investigational (orphan) for muscular dystrophy, AIDS-wasting syndrome, and alcoholic hepatitis; also abused as a street drug*
oxantel INN *anthelmintic* [also: oxantel pamoate]
oxantel pamoate USAN *anthelmintic* [also: oxantel]
oxantrazole HCl [see: piroxantrone HCl]
oxapadol INN
oxapium iodide INN
oxaprazine
oxapropanium iodide INN
oxaprotiline INN *antidepressant* [also: oxaprotiline HCl]
oxaprotiline HCl USAN *antidepressant* [also: oxaprotiline]
oxaprozin USAN, INN, BAN *nonsteroidal anti-inflammatory drug (NSAID) for rheumatoid arthritis and osteoarthritis*
oxarbazole USAN, INN *antiasthmatic*
oxarutine [see: ethoxazorutoside]
oxatomide USAN, INN *antiallergic; antiasthmatic*
oxazafone INN
oxazepam USAN, USP, INN *benzodiazepine anxiolytic; minor tranquilizer; alcohol withdrawal therapy* 10, 15, 30 mg oral
oxazidione INN
oxazolam INN
oxazolidin [see: oxyphenbutazone]
oxazolidinediones *a class of anticonvulsants*
oxazorone INN
oxcarbazepine INN *antiepileptic*
oxdralazine INN
oxeladin INN, BAN
oxendolone USAN, INN *antiandrogen for benign prostatic hypertrophy*
oxepinac INN
oxerutins BAN
oxetacaine INN *topical anesthetic* [also: oxethazaine]
oxetacillin INN
2-oxetanone [see: propiolactone]

446 oxethazaine

oxethazaine USAN, BAN *topical anesthetic* [also: oxetacaine]

oxetorone INN *migraine-specific analgesic* [also: oxetorone fumarate]

oxetorone fumarate USAN *migraine-specific analgesic* [also: oxetorone]

Oxeze ⓐ Turbuhaler (dry powder in a metered-dose inhaler) ℞ *twice-daily bronchodilator for asthma* [formoterol fumarate] 6, 12 μg/dose

oxfenamide [see: oxiramide]

oxfendazole USAN, INN *anthelmintic*

oxfenicine USAN, INN, BAN *vasodilator*

oxibendazole USAN, INN *anthelmintic*

oxibetaine INN

oxibuprocaine chloride [see: benoxinate HCl]

oxichlorochine sulfate [see: hydroxychloroquine sulfate]

oxicinchophen [see: oxycinchophen]

oxiconazole INN, BAN *broad-spectrum topical antifungal* [also: oxiconazole nitrate]

oxiconazole nitrate USAN *broad-spectrum topical antifungal* [also: oxiconazole]

oxicone [see: oxycodone]

oxidized cellulose [see: cellulose, oxidized]

oxidized cholic acid [see: dehydrocholic acid]

oxidized regenerated cellulose [see: cellulose, oxidized regenerated]

oxidopamine USAN, INN *ophthalmic adrenergic*

oxidronate sodium *parenteral radiopaque contrast medium*

oxidronic acid USAN, INN, BAN *calcium regulator*

oxifenamate [see: hydroxyphenamate]

oxifentorex INN

Oxi-Freeda tablets OTC *dietary supplement* [multiple vitamins & minerals; multiple amino acids]

oxifungin INN *antifungal* [also: oxifungin HCl]

oxifungin HCl USAN *antifungal* [also: oxifungin]

oxilorphan USAN, INN *narcotic antagonist*

oximetazoline HCl [see: oxymetazoline HCl]

oximetholone [see: oxymetholone]

oximonam USAN, INN *antibacterial*

oximonam sodium USAN *antibacterial*

oxindanac INN

oxiniacic acid INN

oxiperomide USAN, INN *antipsychotic*

oxipertine [see: oxypertine]

oxipethidine [see: hydroxypethidine]

oxiphenbutazone [see: oxyphenbutazone]

oxiphencyclimine chloride [see: oxyphencyclimine HCl]

Oxipor VHC lotion OTC *topical antipsoriatic; antiseborrheic; keratolytic* [coal tar solution; alcohol 79%] 25%

oxiprocaine [see: hydroxyprocaine]

oxiprogesterone caproate [see: hydroxyprogesterone caproate]

oxipurinol INN *xanthine oxidase inhibitor* [also: oxypurinol]

oxiracetam INN, BAN *investigational treatment for Alzheimer's disease*

oxiramide USAN, INN *antiarrhythmic*

oxisopred INN

Oxistat cream, lotion ℞ *broad-spectrum topical antifungal* [oxiconazole nitrate] 1%

oxistilbamidine isethionate [see: hydroxystilbamidine isethionate]

oxisuran USAN, INN *antineoplastic*

oxitefonium bromide INN

oxitetracaine [see: hydroxytetracaine]

oxitetracycline [see: oxytetracycline]

oxitriptan INN

oxitriptyline INN

oxitropium bromide INN, BAN

Oxizole ⓐ (U.S. product: Oxistat) cream, lotion ℞ *broad-spectrum topical antifungal* [oxiconazole nitrate] 1%

oxmetidine INN, BAN *antagonist to histamine H_2 receptors* [also: oxmetidine HCl]

oxmetidine HCl USAN *antagonist to histamine H_2 receptors* [also: oxmetidine]

oxmetidine mesylate USAN *antagonist to histamine H_2 receptors*

oxodipine INN

oxogestone INN *progestin* [also: oxogestone phenpropionate]

oxogestone phenpropionate USAN *progestin* [also: oxogestone]

oxoglurate INN *combining name for radicals or groups*

oxolamine INN

oxolinic acid USAN, INN *antibacterial*

oxomemazine INN

oxonazine INN

4-oxopentanoic acid, calcium salt [see: calcium levulinate]

oxophenarsine INN [also: oxophenarsine HCl]

oxophenarsine HCl USP [also: oxophenarsine]

5-oxoproline [see: pidolic acid]

oxoprostol INN, BAN

oxothiazolidine carboxylate (L-2-oxothiazolidine-4-carboxylic acid) *investigational (Phase II) immunomodulator for AIDS; investigational (orphan) for adult respiratory distress syndrome and amyotrophic lateral sclerosis (ARDS trials discontinued 1998)*

oxozepam [see: oxazepam]

oxpentifylline BAN *peripheral vasodilator; hemorheologic agent* [also: pentoxifylline]

oxpheneridine INN

oxprenoate potassium INN

oxprenolol INN *coronary vasodilator* [also: oxprenolol HCl]

oxprenolol HCl USAN, USP *coronary vasodilator* [also: oxprenolol]

OxSODrol ℞ *investigational (Phase III) anti-inflammatory and antirheumatic; investigational (Phase II) for the prevention of bronchopulmonary dysplasia* [orgotein (previously known as superoxide dismutase, or SOD)]

Oxsoralen lotion ℞ *topical psoralens for repigmentation of idiopathic vitiligo* [methoxsalen] 1%

Oxsoralen-Ultra capsules ℞ *systemic psoralens for the treatment of severe recalcitrant psoriasis* [methoxsalen] 10 mg

oxtriphylline USP *bronchodilator* [also: choline theophyllinate] 100, 200 mg oral; 50, 100 mg/5 mL oral

Oxy 5 Advanced Formula for Sensitive Skin gel (name changed to Advanced Formula Oxy 5 for Sensitive Skin in 1995)

Oxy 5 for Sensitive Skin, Advanced Formula; Oxy for Sensitive Skin, Advanced Formula gel OTC *topical keratolytic for acne* [benzoyl peroxide] 5%; 2.5%

Oxy 5 Tinted lotion OTC *topical keratolytic for acne* [benzoyl peroxide] 5%

Oxy 10 Advanced Formula gel OTC *topical keratolytic for acne* [benzoyl peroxide] 10%

Oxy 10 Wash liquid OTC *topical keratolytic for acne* [benzoyl peroxide] 10%

Oxy Medicated Cleanser & Pads OTC *topical keratolytic cleanser for acne* [salicylic acid; alcohol] 0.5%•22%, 0.5%•40%, 2%•50%

Oxy Medicated Soap bar OTC *medicated cleanser for acne* [triclosan] 1%

Oxy Night Watch; Oxy Night Watch for Sensitive Skin lotion OTC *topical keratolytic for acne* [salicylic acid] 2%; 1%

Oxy ResiDon't Medicated Face Wash liquid (discontinued 1997) OTC *medicated cleanser for acne* [triclosan] 0.6%

oxybenzone USAN, USP, INN *ultraviolet screen*

oxybuprocaine INN, BAN *topical anesthetic* [also: benoxinate HCl; oxybuprocaine HCl]

oxybuprocaine HCl JAN *topical anesthetic* [also: benoxinate HCl; oxybuprocaine]

oxybutynin INN, BAN *anticholinergic; urinary antispasmodic* [also: oxybutynin chloride]

oxybutynin chloride USAN, USP *anticholinergic; urinary antispasmodic for urge urinary incontinence and frequency* [also: oxybutynin] 5 mg oral; 5 mg/5 mL oral

Oxycel pads, pledgets, strips ℞ *topical local hemostat for surgery* [cellulose, oxidized]

oxychlorosene USAN *topical anti-infective*

oxychlorosene sodium USAN *topical anti-infective*

oxycinchophen INN, BAN

oxyclipine INN *anticholinergic* [also: propenzolate HCl]

oxyclipine HCl [see: propenzolate HCl]

oxyclozanide INN, BAN

oxycodone USAN, INN, BAN *narcotic analgesic; also abused as a street drug*

oxycodone HCl USAN, USP *narcotic analgesic; also abused as a street drug*

oxycodone terephthalate USP *narcotic analgesic; also abused as a street drug*

OxyContin controlled-release tablets ℞ *narcotic analgesic* [oxycodone HCl] 10, 20, 40, 80 mg

Oxydess II tablets ℞ *CNS stimulant; amphetamine* [dextroamphetamine sulfate] 10 mg

oxydimethylquinazine [see: antipyrine]

oxydipentonium chloride INN

oxyethyltheophylline [see: etofylline]

OxyFast oral drops ℞ *narcotic analgesic* [oxycodone HCl] 20 mg/mL

oxyfedrine INN, BAN

oxyfenamate INN *minor tranquilizer* [also: hydroxyphenamate]

oxyfilcon A USAN *hydrophilic contact lens material*

oxygen (O$_2$) USP *medicinal gas; element (O)*

oxygen, polymeric *investigational (orphan) for sickle cell anemia*

oxygen 93 percent USP *medicinal gas*

Oxygent emulsion ℞ *investigational (Phase III) blood substitute* [perflubron]

OxyIR immediate-release capsules ℞ *narcotic analgesic* [oxycodone HCl] 5 mg

oxymesterone INN, BAN

oxymetazoline INN, BAN *topical ocular vasoconstrictor; nasal decongestant* [also: oxymetazoline HCl] ⊠ oxymetholone

oxymetazoline HCl USAN, USP *topical ocular vasoconstrictor; nasal decongestant* [also: oxymetazoline] 0.05% nasal

oxymetholone USAN, USP, INN, BAN *androgen; anabolic steroid; also abused as a street drug* ⊠ oxymetazoline; oxymorphone

oxymethylene urea [see: polynoxylin]

oxymorphone INN, BAN *narcotic analgesic* [also: oxymorphone HCl] ⊠ oxymetholone

oxymorphone HCl USP *narcotic analgesic; investigational (orphan) for intractable pain in narcotic-tolerant patients* [also: oxymorphone]

oxypendyl INN

oxypertine USAN, INN *antidepressant*

oxyphenbutazone USP, INN *anti-inflammatory; antirheumatic; antipyretic; analgesic*

oxyphencyclimine INN *anticholinergic* [also: oxyphencyclimine HCl]

oxyphencyclimine HCl USP *peptic ulcer adjunct* [also: oxyphencyclimine]

oxyphenhydrazine [see: carsalam]

oxyphenisatin BAN *laxative* [also: oxyphenisatin acetate; oxyphenisatine]

oxyphenisatin acetate USAN *laxative* [also: oxyphenisatine; oxyphenisatin]

oxyphenisatine INN *laxative* [also: oxyphenisatin acetate; oxyphenisatin]

oxyphenonium bromide

oxyphylline [see: etofylline]

oxypurinol USAN *xanthine oxidase inhibitor* [also: oxipurinol]

oxypyrronium bromide INN

oxyquinoline USAN *disinfectant/antiseptic*

oxyquinoline benzoate [see: benzoxiquine]

oxyquinoline sulfate USAN, NF *complexing agent*

oxyridazine INN

Oxysept solution + tablets OTC *two-step chemical disinfecting system for soft contact lenses* [hydrogen peroxide-based] 3%

Oxysept 2 solution OTC *rinsing/storage solution for soft contact lenses* [sodium chloride (saline solution)]

oxysonium iodide INN

oxytetracycline USP, INN *bacteriostatic antibiotic; antirickettsial*

oxytetracycline calcium USP *antibacterial*

oxytetracycline HCl USP *bacteriostatic antibiotic; antirickettsial* 250 mg oral

oxytocics *a class of agents that promote rapid labor and childbirth*

oxytocics *a class of posterior pituitary hormones that stimulate contraction of the myometrium (uterine muscle)*

oxytocin USP, INN *posterior pituitary hormone; oxytocic for induction of labor* 10 U/mL injection

Oxyzal Wet Dressing liquid OTC *antiseptic dressing for minor infections* [oxyquinoline sulfate; benzalkonium chloride]

Oysco 500 chewable tablets OTC *calcium supplement* [calcium carbonate] 1.25 g

Oyst-Cal 500 film-coated tablets OTC *calcium supplement* [calcium carbonate] 1.25 g

Oyst-Cal-D film-coated tablets OTC *dietary supplement* [calcium carbonate; vitamin D] 250 mg•125 IU

Oyster Calcium tablets OTC *dietary supplement* [calcium carbonate; vitamins A and D] 375 mg•800 IU•200 IU

Oyster Calcium 500 + D tablets OTC *dietary supplement* [calcium carbonate; vitamin D] 500 mg•125 IU

Oyster Calcium with Vitamin D tablets OTC *dietary supplement* [calcium carbonate; vitamin D] 250 mg•125 IU

Oyster Shell Calcium with Vitamin D tablets OTC *calcium supplement* [calcium carbonate; vitamin D] 250 mg•125 IU

Oyster Shell Calcium-500 tablets OTC *calcium supplement* [calcium carbonate] 1.25 g

Oystercal 500 tablets OTC *calcium supplement* [calcium carbonate] 1.25 g

Oystercal-D 250 tablets OTC *dietary supplement* [calcium carbonate; vitamin D] 250 mg•125 IU

oz; gamma-oz *medicinal herb* [see: rice bran oil]

ozagrel INN *investigational antiasthmatic* [also: ozagrel sodium]

ozagrel sodium JAN *investigational antiasthmatic* [also: ozagrel]

ozolinone USAN, INN *diuretic*

P & S liquid OTC *antimicrobial hair dressing* [phenol]

P & S shampoo OTC *antiseborrheic; keratolytic* [salicylic acid] 2%

P & S Plus gel OTC *topical antipsoriatic; antiseborrheic; keratolytic* [coal tar solution; salicylic acid] 8%•2%

p30 protein *investigational (Phase III) adjunct to chemotherapy for pancreatic, breast, colorectal, prostate, and small cell lung cancers*

³²**P** [see: chromic phosphate P 32]

³²**P** [see: polymetaphosphate P 32]

³²**P** [see: sodium phosphate P 32]

P-53 *investigational (Phase II) antipsoriatic*

p53 adenoviral gene *investigational (Phase II) gene therapy for cancer* [also: adenoviral p53 gene]

P-54 *investigational (Phase II) COX-2 inhibitor for osteoarthritis*

P₁E₁; P₂E₁; P₄E₁; P₆E₁ Drop-Tainers (eye drops) ℞ *topical antiglaucoma agent* [pilocarpine HCl; epinephrine bitartrate] 1%•1%; 2%•1%; 4%•1%; 6%•1%

P₃E₁ Drop-Tainers (eye drops) (discontinued 1998) ℞ *topical antiglaucoma agent* [pilocarpine HCl; epinephrine bitartrate] 3%•1%

P-414 *investigational (Phase II) oral heparin for deep vein thrombosis*

P-748 *investigational (Phase II) imaging agent for pulmonary emboli*

PAB (para-aminobenzoate) [see: aminobenzoic acid]

PABA (para-aminobenzoic acid) [now: aminobenzoic acid]

PABA sodium [see: aminobenzoate sodium]

Pabalate enteric-coated tablets OTC *analgesic; antipyretic; anti-inflammatory* [sodium salicylate; aminobenzoate sodium] 300•300 mg

Pabalate-SF enteric-coated tablets (discontinued 1995) ℞ *analgesic; antipyretic; anti-inflammatory* [potassium salicylate; aminobenzoate potassium] 300•300 mg

PAB-Esc-C (Platinol, Adriamycin, bleomycin, escalating doses of cyclophosphamide) *chemotherapy protocol*

pabestrol D [see: diethylstilbestrol dipropionate]

P-A-C tablets (discontinued 1995) OTC *analgesic; antipyretic; anti-inflammatory* [aspirin; caffeine] 400•32 mg

PAC; PAC-I (Platinol, Adriamycin, cyclophosphamide) *chemotherapy protocol*

PACE (Platinol, Adriamycin, cyclophosphamide, etoposide) *chemotherapy protocol*

Pacerone tablets ℞ *antiarrhythmic for acute ventricular tachycardia and fibrillation (orphan)* [amiodarone HCl] 200 mg

Pacis ⒸⒶⓃ powder for intravesical instillation ℞ *antineoplastic for urinary bladder cancer* [BCG vaccine, Montreal strain] 120 mg

Packer's Pine Tar shampoo, soap OTC *antiseborrheic; antipsoriatic; antipruritic; antibacterial* [pine tar]

paclitaxel USAN, INN, BAN *antineoplastic for AIDS-related Kaposi sarcoma (orphan), and breast and ovarian cancers*

pacrinolol INN

padimate INN *ultraviolet screen* [also: padimate A]

padimate A USAN *ultraviolet screen* [also: padimate]

padimate O USAN *ultraviolet screen*

Paeonia officinalis medicinal herb [see: peony]

PAF-AH (platelet-activating factor acetylhydrolase) [see: platelet-activating factor acetylhydrolast, recombinant]

pafenolol INN

Pagoclone ℞ *investigational (Phase II) treatment for panic disorders*

pagoclone USAN *anxiolytic*

PAH (para-aminohippurate) [see: aminohippuric acid]

PAHA (para-aminohippuric acid) [see: aminohippuric acid]

Pain Bust-R II cream OTC *topical analgesic; counterirritant* [methyl salicylate; menthol] 17%•12%

Pain Doctor cream OTC *topical analgesic; topical anesthetic; antipruritic* [capsaicin; methyl salicylate; menthol] 0.025%•25%•10%

Pain Gel Plus OTC *topical analgesic; counterirritant* [menthol] 4%

Pain Reliever tablets OTC *analgesic; antipyretic; anti-inflammatory* [acetaminophen; aspirin; caffeine] 250•250•65 mg

paint, Indian medicinal herb [see: bloodroot]

paint, yellow Indian medicinal herb [see: goldenseal]

paint root, red medicinal herb [see: bloodroot]

Pain-X gel OTC *topical analgesic; counterirritant* [capsaicin; menthol; camphor] 0.05%•5%•4%

PALA disodium [see: sparfosate sodium]

palatrigine INN, BAN

paldimycin USAN, INN *antibacterial*

paldimycin A [see: paldimycin]

paldimycin B [see: paldimycin]

pale gentian medicinal herb [see: gentian]

palestrol [see: diethylstilbestrol]

palinavir USAN *antiviral; HIV-1 protease inhibitor*

palinum [see: cyclobarbitone]

palivizumab *monoclonal antibody for prophylaxis of respiratory syncytial virus (RSV) in infants*

palladium *element (Pd)*

palm, dwarf; dwarf palmetto; pan palm *medicinal herb* [see: saw palmetto]

palmidrol INN

Palmitate-A 5000 tablets OTC *vitamin supplement* [vitamin A] 5000 IU

palmoxirate sodium USAN *antidiabetic* [also: palmoxiric acid]

palmoxiric acid INN *antidiabetic* [also: palmoxirate sodium]

palonosetron HCl USAN *antiemetic; antinauseant; 5-HT$_3$ antagonist*

PALS coated tablets OTC *systemic deodorant for ostomy, breath, and body odors* [chlorophyllin copper complex] 100 mg

PAM; L-PAM (phenylalanine mustard) [see: melphalan]

2-PAM (2-pyridine aldoxime methylchloride) [see: pralidoxime chloride]

pamabrom USAN *nonprescription diuretic*

pamaqueside USAN *hypocholesterolemic; cholesterol absorption inhibitor; antiatherosclerotic*

pamaquine naphthoate NF

pamatolol INN *antiadrenergic (β-receptor)* [also: pamatolol sulfate]

pamatolol sulfate USAN *antiadrenergic (β-receptor)* [also: pamatolol]

Pamelor capsules, oral solution ℞ *tricyclic antidepressant* [nortriptyline HCl] 10, 25, 50, 75 mg; 10 mg/5 mL ⃞ Dymelor

pamidronate disodium USAN *bisphosphonate bone resorption inhibitor for Paget's disease, hypercalcemia of malignancy, breast cancer, and multiple myeloma*

pamidronic acid INN, BAN

Pamine tablets ℞ *GI antispasmodic; anticholinergic; peptic ulcer treatment* [methscopolamine bromide] 2.5 mg

Pamisyl ℞ *investigational (orphan) for ulcerative colitis* [aminosalicylic acid]

pamoate USAN, USP *combining name for radicals or groups* [also: embonate]

Pamprin, Multi-Symptom caplets, tablets OTC *analgesic; antipyretic; diuretic; antihistaminic sleep aid* [acetaminophen; pamabrom; pyrilamine maleate] 500•25•15 mg

Pamprin, Nighttime powder OTC *antihistaminic sleep aid; analgesic* [diphenhydramine HCl; acetaminophen] 50•650 mg

Pamprin Maximum Pain Relief caplets OTC *analgesic; antipyretic; diuretic* [acetaminophen; magnesium salicylate; pamabrom] 250•250•25 mg

Pan C-500 tablets OTC *dietary supplement* [vitamin C; citrus bioflavonoids & hesperidin] 1000•250 mg

Panacet 5/500 tablets ℞ *narcotic analgesic* [hydrocodone bitartrate; acetaminophen] 5•500 mg

panadiplon USAN, INN *anxiolytic*

Panadol tablets, caplets OTC *analgesic; antipyretic* [acetaminophen] 500 mg

Panadol, Children's chewable tablets, liquid OTC *analgesic; antipyretic* [acetaminophen] 80 mg; 160 mg/5 mL

Panadol, Infants' drops OTC *analgesic; antipyretic* [acetaminophen] 100 mg/mL

Panadol, Junior caplets OTC *analgesic; antipyretic* [acetaminophen] 160 mg

Panafil ointment ℞ *topical enzyme for wound debridement; vulnerary; wound deodorant* [papain; urea; chlorophyllin copper complex] 10%•10%•0.5%

Panafil White ointment ℞ *topical enzyme for wound debridement; vulnerary* [papain; urea] 10%•10%

Panalgesic cream OTC *topical analgesic; counterirritant* [methyl salicylate; menthol] 35%•4%

Panalgesic Gold liniment OTC *topical analgesic; counterirritant; antiseptic*

[methyl salicylate; camphor; menthol; alcohol 22%] 55%•3.1%•1.25%

Panasal 5/500 tablets ℞ *narcotic analgesic* [hydrocodone bitartrate; aspirin] 5•500 mg

Panasol-S tablets ℞ *corticosteroid; anti-inflammatory; immunosuppressant* [prednisone] 1 mg ② Panscol

Panavir ℞ *investigational (Phase II) antiviral for HIV and AIDS* [probucol]

Panax ginseng; P. shin-seng (**Korean ginseng**) *medicinal herb* [see: ginseng]

Panax horridum medicinal herb [see: devil's club]

Panax pseudoginseng (**Chikusetsu ginseng; Himalayan ginseng; Sanchi ginseng; Zhuzishen**) *medicinal herb* [see: ginseng]

Panax quinquefolia (**American ginseng**) *medicinal herb* [see: ginseng]

Panax spp. medicinal herb [see: ginseng]

Panax trifolius (**dwarf ginseng**) *medicinal herb* [see: ginseng]

Pancof-HC oral liquid ℞ *narcotic antitussive; decongestant; antihistamine* [hydrocodone bitartrate; pseudoephedrine HCl; chlorpheniramine maleate; alcohol 5%] 2.5•15•2 mg/5 mL

pancopride USAN, INN *antiemetic; anxiolytic; peristaltic stimulant*

Pancrease; Pancrease MT 4; Pancrease MT 10; Pancrease MT 16; Pancrease MT 20 capsules containing enteric-coated microtablets ℞ *digestive enzymes* [lipase; protease; amylase] 4.5•25•20; 4.5•12•12; 10•30•30; 16•48•48; 20•44•56 thousand USP units

pancreatin USP *digestive enzyme*

Pancreatin, 4X; Pancreatin, 8X tablets OTC *digestive enzymes* [pancreatin; lipase; protease; amylase] 2400 mg•12 000 U•60 000 U•60 000 U; 7200 mg•22 500 U•180 000 U•180 000 U

Pancrecarb MS-8 delayed-release capsules ℞ *digestive enzymes for exocrine pancreatic insufficiency in cystic fibrosis and chronic pancreatitis* [lipase; protease; amylase] 8•45•40 thousand USP units

pancrelipase USAN, USP *digestive enzyme*

Pancrezyme 4X tablets OTC *digestive enzymes* [pancreatin; lipase; protease; amylase] 2400 mg•12 000 U•60 000 U•60 000 U

pancuronium bromide USAN, INN *nondepolarizing neuromuscular blocker; muscle relaxant; adjunct to anesthesia* 1, 2 mg/mL injection

Pandel cream ℞ *topical corticosteroidal anti-inflammatory* [hydrocortisone probutate] 0.1%

Panex; Panex 500 tablets (discontinued 1997) OTC *analgesic; antipyretic* [acetaminophen] 325 mg; 500 mg

Panhematin powder for IV injection ℞ *enzyme inhibitor for acute intermittent porphyria (AIP), porphyria variegata, and hereditary coproporphyria (orphan)* [hemin] 7 mg/mL

Pan-HER ℞ *investigational (Phase I) treatment for breast, ovarian, stomach, and lung cancer*

panidazole INN, BAN

Panitone-500 tablets OTC *analgesic; antipyretic* [acetaminophen] 500 mg

Panmist JR long-acting tablets ℞ *decongestant; expectorant* [pseudoephedrine HCl; guaifenesin] 45•600 mg

Panmycin capsules ℞ *broad-spectrum antibiotic* [tetracycline HCl] 250 mg

Pannaz tablets ℞ *decongestant; antihistamine; anticholinergic* [phenylpropanolamine HCl; chlorpheniramine maleate; methscopolamine bromide] 75•6•2.5 mg

panomifene INN

Panorex ℞ *antineoplastic adjunct (orphan status withdrawn 1997)* [edrecolomab] ② Panarex

Panoxyl cleansing bar ℞ *topical keratolytic for acne* [benzoyl peroxide] 5%, 10% ② Benoxyl

Panoxyl AQ 2½; Panoxyl 5; Panoxyl AQ 5; Panoxyl 10; Panoxyl AQ 10 gel ℞ *topical keratolytic for*

acne [benzoyl peroxide] 2.5%; 5%; 5%; 10%; 10%

Panretin capsules ℞ *investigational (Phase III, orphan) treatment for Kaposi sarcoma, psoriasis, myelodysplastic syndrome (MDS), and acute promyelocytic leukemia (APL); investigational (Phase I/II) for HIV* [alitretinoin]

Panretin gel ℞ *topical treatment for cutaneous lesions of AIDS-related Kaposi sarcoma (orphan)* [alitretinoin] 0.1%

Panscol lotion, ointment OTC *topical keratolytic* [salicylic acid] 3% ☑ Panasol

pansy *(Viola tricolor)* plant *medicinal herb used as an anodyne, demulcent, diaphoretic, diuretic, expectorant, laxative, and vulnerary*

pantenicate INN

panthenol USAN, USP, INN *B complex vitamin*

D-**panthenol** [see: dexpanthenol]

Panthoderm cream OTC *antipruritic; vulnerary; emollient* [dexpanthenol] 2%

pantoprazole USAN, INN, BAN *proton pump inhibitor for gastric and duodenal ulcers*

pantothenic acid BAN *vitamin B_5; enzyme cofactor* [also: calcium pantothenate]

DL-**pantothenic acid** [see: calcium pantothenate, racemic]

pantothenol [see: dexpanthenol]

pantothenyl alcohol [see: panthenol]

D-**pantothenyl alcohol** [see: dexpanthenol]

Pantozol ℞ *investigational proton pump inhibitor for gastroesophageal reflux disease (GERD)* [pantoprazole]

panuramine INN, BAN

Papadeine #3 tablets ℞ *narcotic analgesic* [codeine phosphate; acetaminophen]

papain USP *topical proteolytic enzyme for necrotic tissue debridement*

papaverine BAN *peripheral vasodilator; smooth muscle relaxant; orphan status withdrawn 1996* [also: papaverine HCl]

papaverine HCl USP *peripheral vasodilator; smooth muscle relaxant for cere-*

bral, myocardial, and peripheral ischemias [also: papaverine] 150 mg oral; 30 mg/mL

papaveroline INN, BAN

papaya *(Carica papaya)* leaves, fruit, juice, and seeds *medicinal herb for aiding digestion, gas, insect bites, and intestinal worms*

Papaya Enzyme chewable tablets OTC *digestive enzymes* [papain; amylase] 60•60 mg

Papirine ℞ *investigational antiviral*

Paplex Ultra solution ℞ *topical keratolytic* [salicylic acid in flexible collodion] 26%

papoose root *medicinal herb* [see: blue cohosh]

Par Glycerol elixir ℞ *expectorant* [iodinated glycerol] 60 mg/5 mL

para-aminobenzoate (PAB) [see: aminobenzoic acid]

Para-Aminobenzoic Acid tablets, powder OTC *"possibly effective" for scleroderma and other skin diseases, and Peyronie's disease* [aminobenzoic acid] 100, 500 mg; 120 g

para-aminobenzoic acid (PABA) [now: aminobenzoic acid]

para-aminohippurate (PAH) [see: aminohippuric acid]

para-aminohippurate sodium [see: aminohippurate sodium]

para-aminohippuric acid (PAHA) [see: aminohippuric acid]

para-aminosalicylate (PAS) [see: aminosalicylic acid]

para-aminosalicylic acid (PASA) [see: aminosalicylic acid]

Parabolan *brand name for trenbolone hexahydrobenzylcarbonate, a European veterinary anabolic steroid abused as a street drug*

parabromdylamine maleate [see: brompheniramine maleate]

paracetaldehyde [see: paraldehyde]

paracetamol INN, BAN *analgesic; antipyretic* [also: acetaminophen]

parachlorometaxylenol (PCMX) *topical antiseptic; broad-spectrum antibacterial*

parachlorophenol (PCP) USP *topical antibacterial*

parachlorophenol, camphorated USP *topical dental anti-infective*

paracodin [see: dihydrocodeine]

paraffin NF *stiffening agent*

paraffin, liquid [see: mineral oil]

paraffin, synthetic NF *stiffening agent*

Paraflex caplets ℞ *skeletal muscle relaxant* [chlorzoxazone] 250 mg

paraflutizide INN

Parafon Forte DSC caplets ℞ *skeletal muscle relaxant* [chlorzoxazone] 500 mg ⑦ Pantopon

paraformaldehyde USP

Paraguay tea *medicinal herb* [see: yerba maté]

Para-Hist HD liquid ℞ *narcotic antitussive; decongestant; antihistamine* [hydrocodone bitartrate; phenylephrine HCl; chlorpheniramine maleate] 1.67•5•2 mg/5 mL

parahydrecin [now: isomerol]

Paral oral liquid, rectal liquid ℞ *sedative; hypnotic* [paraldehyde]

paraldehyde USP *hypnotic; sedative; anticonvulsant* 1 g/mL oral or rectal

paramethadione USP, INN, BAN *anticonvulsant* ⑦ paramethasone

paramethasone INN *corticosteroid; anti-inflammatory* [also: paramethasone acetate] ⑦ paramethadione

paramethasone acetate USAN, USP *corticosteroid; anti-inflammatory* [also: paramethasone]

para-nitrosulfathiazole NF [also: nitrosulfathiazole]

paranyline HCl USAN *anti-inflammatory* [also: renytoline]

parapenzolate bromide USAN, INN *anticholinergic*

Paraplatin powder for IV injection ℞ *alkylating antineoplastic for ovarian and other cancers* [carboplatin] 50, 150, 450 mg

parapropamol INN

pararosaniline embonate INN *antischistosomal* [also: pararosaniline pamoate]

pararosaniline pamoate USAN *antischistosomal* [also: pararosaniline embonate]

parasympathomimetics *a class of agents that produce effects similar to those of the parasympathetic nervous system* [also called: cholinergic agonists]

Parathar powder for IV injection ℞ *in vivo diagnostic aid for parathyroid-induced hypocalcemia* (orphan) [teriparatide acetate] 200 U

parathesin [see: benzocaine]

parathiazine INN

parathyroid USP *hormone*

parathyroid hormone (1-34), biosynthetic human [see: teriparatide]

parathyroid hormone (1-84), recombinant human *investigational (Phase III) agent to increase bone mineral content and density in postmenopausal osteoporosis*

paraxazone INN

parbendazole USAN, INN *anthelmintic*

parconazole INN *antifungal* [also: parconazole HCl]

parconazole HCl USAN *antifungal* [also: parconazole]

Paredrine eye drops ℞ *mydriatic* [hydroxyamphetamine hydrobromide] 1%

paregoric (PG) USP (a preparation of opium, anise oil, benzoic acid, camphor, alcohol, and glycerin) *antiperistaltic; narcotic analgesic; sometimes abused as a street drug* 2 mg/5 mL oral

Paremyd eye drops ℞ *mydriatic; weak cycloplegic* [hydroxyamphetamine hydrobromide; tropicamide] 1%• 0.25%

parenabol [see: boldenone undecylenate]

Parepectolin concentrated liquid OTC *GI adsorbent; antidiarrheal* [attapulgite] 600 mg/15 mL

pareptide INN *antiparkinsonian* [also: pareptide sulfate]

pareptide sulfate USAN *antiparkinsonian* [also: pareptide]

parethoxycaine INN

parethoxycaine HCl [see: parethoxycaine]

Par-F tablets ℞ vitamin/mineral/calcium/iron supplement [multiple vitamins & minerals; calcium; iron; folic acid] ± • 250 • 60 • 1 mg

pargeverine INN

pargolol INN

pargyline INN antihypertensive [also: pargyline HCl]

pargyline HCl USAN, USP antihypertensive [also: pargyline]

Parhist SR sustained-release capsules (discontinued 1995) ℞ decongestant; antihistamine [phenylpropanolamine HCl; chlorpheniramine maleate] 75 • 12 mg

paricalcitol synthetic vitamin D analog for hyperparathyroidism secondary to chronic renal failure

paridocaine INN

Parlodel SnapTabs (scored tablets), capsules ℞ dopamine agonist; antiparkinsonian; lactation preventative; treats acromegaly, infertility, and hypogonadism [bromocriptine mesylate] 2.5 mg; 5 mg

Par-Natal Plus 1 Improved tablets ℞ vitamin/calcium/iron supplement [multiple vitamins; calcium; iron; folic acid] ± • 200 • 65 • 1 mg

Parnate film-coated tablets ℞ monoamine oxidase inhibitor (MAOI) for reactive depression (a major depressive episode without melancholia) [tranylcypromine sulfate] 10 mg

parodilol INN

parodyne [see: antipyrine]

paroleine [see: mineral oil]

paromomycin INN, BAN aminoglycoside antibiotic; amebicide [also: paromomycin sulfate]

Paromomycin ℞ investigational (orphan) for tuberculosis, Mycobacterium avium complex, and visceral leishmaniasis [aminosidine]

paromomycin sulfate USP aminoglycoside antibiotic; amebicide [also: paromomycin]

paroxetine USAN, INN, BAN selective serotonin reuptake inhibitor (SSRI) for depression, obsessive-compulsive disorder, and panic disorder

paroxetine HCl selective serotonin reuptake inhibitor (SSRI) for depression, obsessive-compulsive disorder, panic disorder, and social phobia

paroxyl [see: acetarsone]

paroxypropione INN

parpanit HCl [see: caramiphen HCl]

parsalmide INN

Parsidol tablets (discontinued 1997) ℞ anticholinergic; antiparkinsonian [ethopropazine HCl] 10, 50 mg

parsley (Petroselinum sativum) leaves and root medicinal herb for amenorrhea, bladder infections, blood building and cleansing, body lice, colic, dysmenorrhea, flatulence, gallstones, inducing abortion, jaundice, nephritis, prostate disorders, and urinary retention

parsley fern medicinal herb [see: tansy]

parsnip, cow; wooly parsnip medicinal herb [see: masterwort]

Partapp TD timed-release tablets (discontinued 1995) ℞ decongestant; antihistamine [phenylpropanolamine HCl; phenylephrine HCl; brompheniramine maleate] 15 • 15 • 12 mg

Parthenocissus quinquefolia medicinal herb [see: American ivy]

partricin USAN, INN antifungal; antiprotozoal

partridge berry medicinal herb [see: squaw vine; wintergreen]

Partuss LA long-acting tablets ℞ decongestant; expectorant [phenylpropanolamine HCl; guaifenesin] 75 • 400 mg

parvaquone INN, BAN ge

Parvlex tablets OTC hematinic [ferrous fumarate; multiple B vitamins & minerals; vitamin C; folic acid] 100 • ± • 50 • 0.1 mg

PAS (para-aminosalicylate) [see: aminosalicylic acid]

PASA (para-aminosalicylic acid) [see: aminosalicylic acid]

Paser granules ℞ tuberculostatic (orphan) [aminosalicylic acid] 4 g/packet

pasiniazid INN

pasque flower *(Anemone patens)* plant *medicinal herb used as a diaphoretic, diuretic, and rubefacient; not generally regarded as safe and effective due to toxicity*

passion flower *(Passiflora incarnata)* plant *medicinal herb for asthma, bronchitis, eye infections, fever, inflamed hemorrhoids, insomnia, menopause, nervousness, pain related to neurasthenia, and attention deficit disorders, nervousness, and excitability in children*

Pastilles (dosage form) *troches*

Patanol Drop-Tainer (eye drops) ℞ *topical ophthalmic antihistamine for allergic conjunctivitis* [olopatadine HCl] 0.1%

PATCO (prednisone, ara-C, thioguanine, cyclophosphamide, Oncovin) *chemotherapy protocol*

Pathilon film-coated tablets ℞ *peptic ulcer treatment adjunct* [tridihexethyl chloride] 25 mg ⊡ Pathocil

Pathocil capsules, powder for oral suspension ℞ *penicillinase-resistant penicillin antibiotic* [dicloxacillin sodium] 250, 500 mg; 62.5 mg/5 mL ⊡ Bactocill; Pathilon; Placidyl

patience, garden *medicinal herb* [see: yellow dock]

patience dock *medicinal herb* [see: bistort]

pau d'arco *(Lapacho colorado; L. morado)* inner bark *medicinal herb for boils, blood cleansing, cancer, Candida albicans infections, chlorosis, diabetes, leukemia, pain, skin wounds, and syphilis*

Paullinia cupana; P. sorbilis *medicinal herb* [see: guarana]

paulomycin USAN, INN *antibacterial*

Pausinystalia johimbe *medicinal herb* [see: yohimbe]

pauson *medicinal herb* [see: bloodroot]

Pavabid Plateau Caps (controlled-release capsules) ℞ *peripheral vasodilator; smooth muscle relaxant for cerebral, myocardial, and peripheral ischemias* [papaverine HCl] 150 mg ⊡ Pavased

Pavabid HP capsulets (tablets) (discontinued 1995) ℞ *peripheral vasodilator; smooth muscle relaxant for cerebral, myocardial, and peripheral ischemias* [papaverine HCl] 300 mg

Pavagen TD timed-release capsules ℞ *peripheral vasodilator; smooth muscle relaxant for cerebral, myocardial, and peripheral ischemias* [papaverine HCl] 150 mg

Pavarine Spancaps (timed-release capsules) (discontinued 1997) ℞ *peripheral vasodilator; smooth muscle relaxant for cerebral, myocardial, and peripheral ischemias* [papaverine HCl] 150 mg

Pavased timed-release capsules (discontinued 1996) ℞ *peripheral vasodilator; smooth muscle relaxant for cerebral, myocardial, and peripheral ischemias* [papaverine HCl] 150 mg

Pavatine timed-release capsules (discontinued 1997) ℞ *peripheral vasodilator; smooth muscle relaxant for cerebral, myocardial, and peripheral ischemias* [papaverine HCl] 150 mg ⊡ Pavatym

PAVe (procarbazine, Alkeran, Velban) *chemotherapy protocol*

Paverolan Lanacaps (timed-release capsules) (discontinued 1997) ℞ *peripheral vasodilator; smooth muscle relaxant for cerebral, myocardial, and peripheral ischemias* [papaverine HCl] 150 mg ⊡ Pavulon

Pavulon IM injection ℞ *nondepolarizing neuromuscular blocker; adjunct to anesthesia* [pancuronium bromide] 1, 2 mg/mL ⊡ Paverolan

pawpaw *(Asimina triloba)* fruit *medicinal herb used as an antimicrobial and antineoplastic*

paxamate INN

Paxarel tablets ℞ *anxiolytic; sedative* [acecarbromal] 250 mg

Paxene ℞ *antineoplastic for AIDS-related Kaposi sarcoma (orphan), and breast and ovarian cancers* [paclitaxel]

Paxil film-coated tablets, oral suspension ℞ *selective serotonin reuptake inhibitor (SSRI) for depression, obses-*

*sive-compulsive disorder (OCD), panic
disorder, and social phobia* [paroxetine
HCl] 10, 20, 30, 40 mg; 10 mg/5 mL

Paxil CR film-coated controlled-
release tablets ℞ *selective serotonin
reuptake inhibitor (SSRI) for depression* [paroxetine HCl] 12.5, 25 mg

Paxipam tablets (discontinued 1995)
℞ *anxiolytic* [halazepam] 20, 40 mg

pazelliptine INN

pazinaclone USAN *anxiolytic*

Pazo Hemorrhoid ointment OTC *temporary relief of hemorrhoidal symptoms; topical vasoconstrictor; counterirritant; astringent* [ephedrine sulfate;
camphor; zinc oxide] 0.2%•2%•5%

Pazo Hemorrhoid suppositories OTC
*temporary relief of hemorrhoidal symp-
toms; topical vasoconstrictor; astringent*
[ephedrine sulfate; zinc oxide] 3.8•
96.5 mg

pazoxide USAN, INN *antihypertensive*

**PBV (Platinol, bleomycin, vinblas-
tine)** *chemotherapy protocol*

PBZ elixir (discontinued 1997) ℞
antihistamine [tripelennamine HCl]
37.5 mg/5 mL

PBZ tablets ℞ *antihistamine* [tripelen-
namine HCl] 25, 50 mg

PBZ (pyribenzamine) [see: tripelen-
namine]

PBZ-SR extended-release tablets ℞
antihistamine [tripelennamine HCl]
100 mg

PC (paclitaxel, carboplatin) *chemotherapy protocol*

PC (phosphatidylcholine) [see: leci-
thin]

PCE Dispertabs (delayed-release tablets) ℞ *macrolide antibiotic* [erythro-
mycin] 333, 500 mg

**PCE (Platinol, cyclophosphamide,
etoposide)** *chemotherapy protocol*

**PCE (polymer-coated erythromy-
cin)** [see: erythromycin]

PCMX (parachlorometaxylenol)
[q.v.]

PCOs (procyanidolic oligomers) [q.v.]

PCP (parachlorophenol) [q.v.]

PCP (phenylcyclohexyl piperidine)
*a powerful veterinary analgesic/anes-
thetic widely abused as a hallucinogenic
street drug* [medically known as
phencyclidine HCl]

**PCV (procarbazine, CCNU, vin-
cristine)** *chemotherapy protocol*

**PDE III (phosphodiesterase III)
inhibitors** *a class of platelet aggregation inhibitors*

PDGA (pteroyldiglutamic acid)

PDLA (phosphinicodilactic acid)
[see: foscolic acid]

PDP Liquid Protein OTC *dietary supplement* [hydrolyzed protein; L-tryp-
tophan] 15•⁴ g/30 mL

PE (phenylephrine) [q.v.]

PE (polyethylene) [q.v.]

pea, ground squirrel *medicinal herb*
[see: twin leaf]

pea, turkey; wild turkey pea *medicinal herb* [see: turkey corn]

peach (*Prunus persica*) bark and
leaves *medicinal herb for bladder disorders, chest congestion, chronic bronchitis, nausea, and water retention*

peanut oil NF *solvent*

**PEB (Platinol, etoposide, bleomy-
cin)** *chemotherapy protocol*

pecazine INN, BAN

pecazine acetate [see: pecazine]

pecilocin INN, BAN

pecocycline INN

pectin USP *suspending agent; protectant;
GI adsorbent*

pectorals *a class of agents that relieve
disorders of the respiratory tract, such
as expectorants*

Pedameth capsules, liquid ℞ *urinary
acidifier to control ammonia production*
[racemethionine] 200 mg; 75 mg/5 mL

PediaCare Allergy Formula liquid
OTC *antihistamine* [chlorpheniramine
maleate] 1 mg/5 mL

PediaCare Cold-Allergy chewable
tablets OTC *pediatric decongestant and
antihistamine* [pseudoephedrine HCl;
chlorpheniramine maleate] 15•1 mg

PediaCare Cough-Cold Formula
chewable tablets, liquid OTC *pediatric*

antitussive, decongestant, and antihistamine [dextromethorphan hydrobromide; pseudoephedrine HCl; chlorpheniramine maleate] 5•15•1 mg; 5•15•1 mg/5 mL

PediaCare Fever Drops suspension OTC *pediatric analgesic and antipyretic* [ibuprofen] 50 mg/1.25 mL

PediaCare Fever Liquid suspension OTC *pediatric analgesic and antipyretic* [ibuprofen] 100 mg/5 mL

PediaCare Infant's Decongestant drops OTC *nasal decongestant* [pseudoephedrine HCl] 7.5 mg/0.8 mL

PediaCare NightRest Cough-Cold liquid OTC *pediatric antitussive, decongestant, and antihistamine* [dextromethorphan hydrobromide; pseudoephedrine HCl; chlorpheniramine maleate] 7.5•15•1 mg/5 mL

Pediacof syrup ℞ *pediatric narcotic antitussive, decongestant, antihistamine, and expectorant* [codeine phosphate; phenylephrine HCl; chlorpheniramine maleate; potassium iodide; alcohol 5%] 5•2.5•0.75•75 mg/5 mL

Pediacon DX children's syrup, pediatric drops OTC *pediatric antitussive, decongestant, and expectorant* [dextromethorphan hydrobromide; phenylpropanolamine HCl; guaifenesin] 5•6.25•100 mg/5 mL; 5•6.25•50 mg/mL

Pediacon EX pediatric drops OTC *pediatric decongestant and expectorant* [phenylpropanolamine HCl; guaifenesin] 6.25•50 mg/mL

Pediaflor drops ℞ *dental caries preventative* [sodium fluoride] 1.1 mg/mL

Pedialyte oral solution, freezer pops OTC *electrolyte replacement* [sodium, potassium, and chloride electrolytes]

Pediamist low-pressure nasal spray OTC *nasal moisturizer for children* [sodium chloride (saline solution)]

PediaPatch transdermal patch (name changed to Trans-Ver-Sal Pedia-Patch in 1995)

Pediapred oral solution ℞ *corticosteroid; anti-inflammatory* [prednisolone sodium phosphate] 5 mg/5 mL

PediaSure ready-to-use liquid OTC *total or supplementary infant feeding*

Pediatric Electrolyte oral solution OTC *electrolyte replacement* [dextrose; multiple electrolytes] 1 L

Pediazole oral suspension ℞ *antibiotic* [erythromycin ethylsuccinate; sulfisoxazole acetyl] 200•600 mg/5 mL

Pedi-Bath Salts OTC *bath emollient*

Pedi-Boro Soak Paks powder packets OTC *astringent wet dressing (modified Burow solution)* [aluminum sulfate; calcium acetate]

Pedi-Cort V Creme ℞ *topical corticosteroidal anti-inflammatory; antifungal; antibacterial* [hydrocortisone; clioquinol] 1%•3%

pediculocides *a class of agents effective against head and pubic lice*

Pedi-Dri powder ℞ *topical antifungal* [nystatin] 100 000 U/g

Pediotic ear drop suspension ℞ *topical corticosteroidal anti-inflammatory; antibiotic* [hydrocortisone; neomycin sulfate; polymyxin B sulfate] 1%•5 mg•10 000 U per mL

Pedi-Pro foot powder OTC *topical antifungal; anhidrotic* [zinc undecylenate; aluminum chlorohydrate; menthol; chloroxylenol]

Pedituss Cough syrup ℞ *pediatric narcotic antitussive, decongestant, antihistamine, and expectorant* [codeine phosphate; phenylephrine HCl; chlorpheniramine maleate; potassium iodide] 5•2.5•0.75•75 mg/5 mL

Pedi-Vit-A Creme OTC *moisturizer; emollient* [vitamin A] 100 000 U/30 g

Pedotic otic suspension ℞ *topical corticosteroidal anti-inflammatory; antibiotic* [hydrocortisone; neomycin sulfate; polymyxin B sulfate] 1%•5 mg•10 000 U per mL

PedTE-Pak-4 IV injection ℞ *intravenous nutritional therapy* [multiple trace elements (metals)] ≛

Pedtrace-4 IV injection ℞ *intravenous nutritional therapy* [multiple trace elements (metals)]

PedvaxHIB powder for IM injection
℞ *Haemophilus influenzae type b
(HIB) vaccine* [Hemophilus b conju-
gate vaccine]

PeeWee's Children's Vitamins
chewable tablets (discontinued
1995) OTC *vitamin/iron supplement*
[multiple vitamins; iron; folic acid]
≐•15•0.3 mg

pefloxacin USAN, INN, BAN *antibacterial*

pefloxacin mesylate USAN *antibacterial*

PEG (polyethylene glycol) [q.v.]

**PEG-ADA (polyethylene glycol-
adenosine deaminase)** [see:
pegademase bovine]

pegademase INN *adenosine deaminase
(ADA) replacement* [also: pegademase bovine]

pegademase bovine USAN *adenosine
deaminase (ADA) replacement for
severe combined immunodeficiency disease (orphan)* [also: pegademase]

**PEG-adenosine deaminase (PEG-
ADA)** [see: pegademase bovine]

Peganone tablets ℞ *hydantoin anticonvulsant* [ethotoin] 250, 500 mg

PEG-L-asparaginase [see: pegaspargase]

pegaspargase (PEG-L-asparaginase)
USAN, INN *antineoplastic for acute
lymphocytic leukemia (orphan) and
acute lymphoblastic leukemia*

pegasys *investigational (orphan) for
renal call carcinoma*

PEG-camptothecin *investigational pro-
drug form of camptothecin, a hormonal
antineoplastic topoisomerase I inhibitor*

**PEG-ES (polyethylene glycol-elec-
trolyte solution)** [q.v.]

PEG-glucocerebrosidase *investigational (orphan) chronic enzyme replacement therapy for Gaucher's disease*

PEG-hemoglobin *investigational blood
replacement*

PEG-interleukin-2 *investigational
(Phase II) cytokine for AIDS; investigational (orphan) for primary immunod-
eficiencies associated with T-cell defects*

PEG-Intron A *long-acting formulation
of Intron A; investigational (Phase III)
for hepatitis C, malignant melanoma,*

and chronic myelogenous leukemia
[interferon alfa-2b in a polyethylene
glycol carrier]

peglicol 5 oleate USAN *emulsifying agent*

pegorgotein USAN, INN *free-radical scavenger; investigational to prevent irreversible brain damage after head trauma*

pegoterate USAN, INN *suspending agent*

pegoxol 7 stearate USAN *emulsifying
agent*

**PEG-SOD (polyethylene glycol-
superoxide dismutase)** [see: pegor-
gotein]

**PEG-uricase (polyethylene glycol-
urate oxidase)** *investigational*

**pegylated megakaryocyte growth
factor** [see: megakaryocyte growth
and development factor, pegylated,
recombinant human]

Pelamine tablets (discontinued 1997)
℞ *antihistamine* [tripelennamine
HCl] 50 mg

pelanserin INN *antihypertensive; vasodilator; serotonin adrenergic blocker*
[also: pelanserin HCl]

pelanserin HCl USAN *antihypertensive;
vasodilator; serotonin adrenergic
blocker* [also: pelanserin]

peldesine USAN *purine nucleoside phosphorylase inhibitor for psoriasis; investigational (orphan) for cutaneous T-cell
lymphoma; investigational (Phase III)
for HIV*

peliomycin USAN, INN *antineoplastic*

pellants *a class of agents that purify or
cleanse the system, particularly the blood*
[also called: depurants; depuratives]

pelretin USAN, INN *antikeratinizing agent*

pelrinone INN *cardiotonic* [also: pelrinone HCl]

pelrinone HCl USAN *cardiotonic* [also:
pelrinone]

pemedolac USAN, INN *analgesic*

pemerid INN *antitussive* [also: pemerid
nitrate]

pemerid nitrate USAN *antitussive* [also:
pemerid]

pemetrexed disodium USAN *antineoplastic; thymidylate synthase inhibitor;
dihydrofolate reductase inhibitor; glyci-*

namide ribonucleotide formyl transferase inhibitor

pemirolast INN *antiallergic; mediator
release inhibitor* [also: pemirolast
potassium]

pemirolast potassium USAN *antiallergic; mediator release inhibitor* [also:
pemirolast]

pemoline USAN, INN, BAN, JAN *CNS
stimulant for attention deficit hyperactivity disorders (ADHD) and narcolepsy* 37.5, 75 mg oral

pempidine INN, BAN

penamecillin USAN, INN, BAN *antibacterial*

penbutolol INN, BAN *antiadrenergic (β-
receptor)* [also: penbutolol sulfate]

penbutolol sulfate USAN *antiadrenergic (β-receptor)* [also: penbutolol]

penciclovir USAN, INN, BAN *topical
antiviral for herpes*

pendecamaine INN, BAN

pendiomide [see: azamethonium bro-
mide]

Penecare cream, lotion OTC *moisturizer; emollient* [lactic acid] ℥

Penecort cream, solution ℞ *topical
corticosteroidal anti-inflammatory*
[hydrocortisone] 1%

penems *a class of broad-spectrum antibiotics*

Penetrex film-coated tablets ℞ *broad-
spectrum fluoroquinolone antibiotic*
[enoxacin] 200, 400 mg

PenFill (trademarked form) *insulin
injector refill cartridge*

penfluridol USAN, INN *antipsychotic*

penflutizide INN

pengitoxin INN

penicillamine USAN, USP, INN *metal
chelating agent; antirheumatic* ℥ penicillin

penicillin aluminum

**penicillin benzathine phenoxy-
methyl** [now: penicillin V benza-
thine]

penicillin calcium USP

penicillin G benzathine USP *natural
penicillin antibiotic* [also: benzathine

benzylpenicillin; benzathine penicillin; benzylpenicillin benzathine]

penicillin G hydrabamine *natural
penicillin antibiotic*

penicillin G potassium USP *natural
penicillin antibiotic* [also: benzylpenicillin potassium] 1, 2, 3, 5, 10, 20
million U injection

penicillin G procaine USP *natural
penicillin antibiotic* [also: procaine
penicillin]

penicillin G redox [see: redox-penicillin G]

penicillin G sodium USP *natural penicillin antibiotic* [also: benzylpenicillin
sodium] 5 million U injection

**penicillin hydrabamine phenoxy-
methyl** [now: penicillin V hydraba-
mine]

penicillin N [see: adicillin]

penicillin O [see: almecillin]

penicillin O chloroprocaine

penicillin O potassium

penicillin O sodium

penicillin phenoxymethyl [now:
penicillin V]

penicillin potassium G [see: penicillin G potassium]

penicillin potassium phenoxymethyl
[now: penicillin V potassium]

penicillin V USAN, USP *natural penicillin antibiotic* [also: phenoxymethyl-
penicillin]

penicillin V benzathine USAN, USP
natural penicillin antibiotic

penicillin V hydrabamine USAN, USP
natural penicillin antibiotic

penicillin V potassium USAN, USP
natural penicillin antibiotic

Penicillin VK tablets, oral solution ℞
natural penicillin antibiotic [penicillin
V potassium] 250, 500 mg; 125, 250
mg/5 mL

penicillin-152 potassium [see: phenethicillin potassium] ℥ penicillamine; Polycillin

penicillinase INN, BAN

penicillinase-resistant penicillins *a
subclass of penicillins (q.v.)*

penicillinphenyrazine [see: phenyracillin]

penicillins *a class of bactericidal antibiotics, divided into natural, penicillinase-resistant, aminopenicillin, and extended-spectrum penicillins, and effective against both gram-positive and gram-negative bacteria*

penidural [see: benzathine penicillin]

penimepicycline INN

penimocycline INN

penirolol INN

Pen-Kera cream OTC *moisturizer; emollient*

penmesterol INN

Pennsaid ℞ *investigational (NDA filed) topical NSAID for rheumatoid arthritis and osteoarthritis pain* [diclofenac potassium]

pennyroyal (*Hedeoma pulegeoides; Mentha pulegium*) plant *medicinal herb for childbirth pain, colds, colic, fever, gas, inducing abortion and menstruation, mouth sores, respiratory illnesses, and venomous bites; also used as an insect repellent; not generally regarded as safe and effective for ingestion as it is toxic*

penoctonium bromide INN

penprostene INN

penta tea *medicinal herb* [see: jiaogulan]

pentabamate USAN, INN *minor tranquilizer*

Pentacarinat IV or IM injection ℞ *antiprotozoal; treatment and prophylaxis of Pneumocystis carinii pneumonia (orphan)* [pentamidine isethionate] 300 mg

Pentacef powder for IV or IM injection ℞ *cephalosporin antibiotic* [ceftazidime]

pentacosactride BAN [also: norleusactide]

pentacynium chloride INN

pentacyone chloride [see: pentacynium chloride]

pentaerithritol tetranicotinate [see: niceritrol]

pentaerithrityl tetranitrate INN *vasodilator* [also: pentaerythritol tetranitrate]

pentaerythritol tetranitrate (PETN) USP *coronary vasodilator; antianginal* [also: pentaerithrityl tetranitrate]

pentaerythritol trinitrate [see: pentrinitrol]

pentafilcon A USAN *hydrophilic contact lens material*

pentafluranol INN, BAN

pentafuside *investigational (Phase II) antiviral fusion inhibitor for HIV*

pentagastrin USAN, INN, JAN *gastric secretion indicator*

pentagestrone INN

pentalamide INN, BAN

pentalyte USAN, USP, NF *electrolyte combination*

Pentam 300 IV or IM injection ℞ *antiprotozoal; treatment and prophylaxis of Pneumocystis carinii pneumonia (orphan)* [pentamidine isethionate] 300 mg

pentamethazene [see: azamethonium bromide]

pentamethonium bromide INN, BAN

pentamethylenetetrazol [see: pentylenetetrazol]

pentamidine INN, BAN

pentamidine isethionate *antiprotozoal; treatment and prophylaxis of Pneumocystis carinii pneumonia (orphan)* 300 mg injection

pentamin [see: azamethonium bromide]

pentamorphone USAN, INN *narcotic analgesic*

pentamoxane INN

pentamoxane HCl [see: pentamoxane]

pentamustine USAN *antineoplastic* [also: neptamustine]

pentanedial [see: glutaral]

pentanitrol [see: pentaerythritol tetranitrate]

pentaphonate

pentapiperide INN

pentapiperium methylsulfate USAN *anticholinergic* [also: pentapiperium metilsulfate]

pentapiperium metilsulfate INN *anticholinergic* [also: pentapiperium methylsulfate]

pentaquine INN [also: pentaquine phosphate]

pentaquine phosphate USP [also: pentaquine]

Pentasa controlled-release capsules ℞ *for ulcerative colitis, proctosigmoiditis, and proctitis; investigational for Crohn's disease* [mesalamine] 250 mg

pentasodium colistinmethanesulfonate [see: colistimethate sodium]

Pentaspan ℞ *leukapheresis adjunct to improve leukocyte yield (orphan)* [pentastarch]

pentastarch USAN, BAN *leukapheresis adjunct; red cell sedimenting agent; centrifugal leukocyte harvesting aid (orphan)*

pentavalent gas gangrene antitoxin

Pentazine injection (discontinued 1997) ℞ *antihistamine; sedative; antiemetic; motion sickness relief* [promethazine HCl] 50 mg/mL ② Phenazine

Pentazine VC with Codeine liquid ℞ *narcotic antitussive; antihistamine* [codeine phosphate; promethazine HCl] 10•6.25 mg/5 mL

pentazocine USAN, USP, INN, BAN *narcotic agonist-antagonist analgesic; also abused as a street drug*

pentazocine HCl USAN, USP *narcotic agonist-antagonist analgesic; also abused as a street drug*

pentazocine lactate USAN, USP *analgesic*

pentazocine & naloxone HCl *narcotic agonist-antagonist analgesic; also abused as a street drug* 50•0.5 mg oral

pentetate calcium trisodium USAN *plutonium chelating agent* [also: calcium trisodium pentetate]

pentetate calcium trisodium Yb 169 USAN *radioactive agent*

pentetate disodium [see: pentetic acid, sodium salts]

pentetate indium disodium In 111 USAN *diagnostic aid; radioactive agent*

pentetate monosodium [see: pentetic acid, sodium salts]

pentetate pentasodium [see: pentetic acid, sodium salts]

pentetate tetrasodium [see: pentetic acid, sodium salts]

pentetate trisodium [see: pentetic acid, sodium salts]

pentetate trisodium calcium [see: pentetate calcium trisodium]

pentethylcyclanone [see: cyclexanone]

pentetic acid USAN, BAN *diagnostic aid*

pentetic acid, sodium salts *diagnostic aid*

pentetrazol INN [also: pentylenetetrazol]

penthanil diethylenetriamine pentaacetic acid (DTPA) [see: pentetic acid]

penthienate bromide NF

Penthrane liquid for vaporization ℞ *inhalation general anesthetic* [methoxyflurane]

penthrichloral INN, BAN

pentiapine INN *antipsychotic* [also: pentiapine maleate]

pentiapine maleate USAN *antipsychotic* [also: pentiapine]

penticide [see: chlorophenothane]

pentifylline INN, BAN

pentigetide USAN, INN *antiallergic*

pentisomicin USAN, INN *anti-infective*

pentisomide INN

pentizidone INN *antibacterial* [also: pentizidone sodium]

pentizidone sodium USAN *antibacterial* [also: pentizidone]

pentobarbital USP, INN *sedative; hypnotic; also abused as a street drug* [also: pentobarbitone; pentobarbital calcium] ② phenobarbital

pentobarbital calcium JAN *sedative; hypnotic; also abused as a street drug* [also: pentobarbital; pentobarbitone]

pentobarbital sodium USP, JAN *sedative; hypnotic; also abused as a street drug* [also: pentobarbitone sodium] 100 mg oral; 50 mg/mL injection

pentobarbitone BAN *sedative; hypnotic; also abused as a street drug* [also: pentobarbital]

pentobarbitone sodium BAN *sedative; hypnotic; also abused as a street drug* [also: pentobarbital sodium]

Pentolair eye drops ℞ *mydriatic; cycloplegic* [cyclopentolate HCl] 1%

pentolinium tartrate NF [also: pentolonium tartrate]

pentolonium tartrate INN [also: pentolinium tartrate]

pentolonum bitartrate [see: pentolinium tartrate]

pentomone USAN, INN *prostate growth inhibitor*

pentopril USAN, INN *angiotensin-converting enzyme (ACE) inhibitor*

pentorex INN

pentosalen BAN

pentosan polysulfate sodium USAN, INN *urinary tract anti-inflammatory and analgesic for interstitial cystitis (orphan)* [also: pentosan polysulphate sodium]

pentosan polysulphate sodium BAN *urinary tract anti-inflammatory and analgesic* [also: pentosan polysulfate sodium]

Pentostam (available only from the Centers for Disease Control) ℞ *investigational anti-infective for leishmaniasis* [sodium stibogluconate]

pentostatin USAN, INN *potentiator; antibiotic antineoplastic for hairy cell leukemia (orphan); investigational (orphan) for chronic lymphocytic leukemia and cutaneous T-cell lymphoma*

Pentothal powder for IV injection ℞ *barbiturate general anesthetic* [thiopental sodium] 2%, 2.5% (20, 25 mg/mL) ② pentrinitrol

Pentothal rectal suspension (discontinued 1997) ℞ *barbiturate general anesthetic* [thiopental sodium] 400 mg/g ② pentrinitrol;

pentoxifylline USAN, INN *peripheral vasodilator; hemorheologic agent* [also: oxpentifylline] 400 mg oral

pentoxiverine citrate [see: carbetapentane citrate]

pentoxyverine INN [also: carbetapentane citrate]

pentoxyverine citrate [see: carbetapentane citrate]

Pentrax; Pentrax Gold shampoo OTC *antiseborrheic; antipsoriatic; antipruritic; antibacterial* [coal tar] 4.3%; 4%

pentrinitrol USAN, INN *coronary vasodilator* ② Pentothal

tert-**pentyl alcohol** [see: amylene hydrate]

Pentylan tablets (discontinued 1995) ℞ *antianginal; vasodilator* [pentaerythritol tetranitrate] 10, 20 mg

6-pentyl-*m*-cresol [see: amylmetacresol]

pentylenetetrazol NF [also: pentetrazol]

pentymal [see: amobarbital]

Pen-V tablets (discontinued 1998) ℞ *natural penicillin antibiotic* [penicillin V potassium] 250, 500 mg

Pen-Vee K tablets, powder for oral solution ℞ *natural penicillin antibiotic* [penicillin V potassium] 250, 500 mg; 125, 250 mg/5 mL

peony (*Paeonia officinalis*) root (other parts are poisonous) *medicinal herb used as an antispasmodic, diuretic, and sedative*

Pepcid film-coated tablets, powder for oral suspension, IV injection, pre-loaded syringes for IV ℞ *histamine H_2 antagonist for gastric and duodenal ulcers* [famotidine] 20, 40 mg; 40 mg/5 mL; 10 mg/mL; 20 mg

Pepcid AC ("acid controller") tablets, chewable tablets OTC *histamine H_2 antagonist for heartburn and acid indigestion* [famotidine] 10 mg

Pepcid RPD rapidly disintegrating tablets ℞ *histamine H_2 antagonist for gastric and duodenal ulcers* [famotidine] 20, 40 mg

pepleomycin [see: peplomycin sulfate]

peplomycin INN *antineoplastic* [also: peplomycin sulfate]

peplomycin sulfate USAN *antineoplastic* [also: peplomycin]

pepper, African red; American red pepper; bird pepper; cayenne pepper; chili pepper; cockspur pepper; garden pepper; red pepper; Spanish pepper *medicinal herb* [see: cayenne]

pepper, Jamaica *medicinal herb* [see: allspice]

pepper, java; tailed pepper *medicinal herb* [see: cubeb]

pepper, water *medicinal herb* [see: knotweed]

pepper, wild *medicinal herb* [see: mezereon]

pepperidge bush *medicinal herb* [see: barberry]

peppermint NF *flavoring agent; perfume*

peppermint *(Mentha piperita)* leaves *medicinal herb for appetite stimulation, colds, colic, indigestion, fever, gas and heartburn, headache, shock, sore throat, and toothache*

peppermint oil NF *flavoring agent*

peppermint spirit USP *flavoring agent; perfume*

peppermint water NF *flavored vehicle*

pepsin *digestive aid*

pepstatin USAN, INN *pepsin enzyme inhibitor*

Peptamen ready-to-use liquid OTC *enteral nutritional therapy for GI impairment*

Peptavlon subcu injection ℞ *in vivo diagnostic aid for gastrointestinal function* [pentagastrin] 250 μg/mL

Pepto Diarrhea Control oral solution OTC *antidiarrheal* [loperamide HCl] 1 mg/5 mL

Pepto-Bismol chewable tablets, caplets, liquid OTC *antidiarrheal; antinauseant* [bismuth subsalicylate] 262 mg; 262 mg; 262, 524 mg/15 mL

peraclopone INN

peradoxime INN

perafensine INN

peralopride INN

peraquinsin INN

perastine INN

peratizole INN, BAN

perbufylline INN

Perchloracap capsules ℞ *radioimaging adjunct* [potassium perchlorate] 200 mg

Percocet tablets ℞ *narcotic analgesic* [oxycodone HCl; acetaminophen] 5•325 mg

Percodan; Percodan-Demi tablets ℞ *narcotic analgesic; also abused as a street drug* [oxycodone HCl; oxycodone terephthalate; aspirin] 4.5•0.38•325 mg; 2.25•0.19•325 mg ② Decadron

Percogesic tablets OTC *antihistamine; analgesic* [phenyltoloxamine citrate; acetaminophen] 30•325 mg

Percolone tablets ℞ *narcotic analgesic* [oxycodone HCl] 5 mg

Perdiem granules OTC *stimulant/bulk laxative* [psyllium husks; senna extract] 3.25•0.74 g/tsp. ② Pyridium

Perdiem Fiber granules OTC *bulk laxative* [psyllium] 4.03 g/tsp.

Perfectoderm gel OTC *topical keratolytic for acne* [benzoyl peroxide] 5%

perfilcon A USAN *hydrophilic contact lens material*

perflenapent USAN *ultrasound contrast medium*

perflisopent USAN *ultrasound contrast medium*

perfluamine INN, BAN

perflubron USAN, INN *blood substitute; oral MRI contrast medium; investigational (Phase III) agent for pediatric acute respiratory distress syndrome (ARDS)*

perflunafene INN, BAN

perfluorochemical (PFC) emulsion (discontinued 1995) *synthetic blood oxygen carrier for PTCA*

perflutren *investigational (NDA filed) ultrasound contrast medium*

perfomedil INN

perfosfamide USAN *antineoplastic; orphan status withdrawn 1996*

Pergamid ℞ *investigational antineoplastic; orphan status withdrawn 1996* [perfosfamide]

pergolide INN, BAN *dopamine agonist; antiparkinsonian* [also: pergolide mesylate]

pergolide mesylate USAN *dopamine agonist; antiparkinsonian; investigational (orphan) for Tourette syndrome* [also: pergolide]

Pergonal powder for IM injection ℞ *ovulation stimulant for women; spermatogenesis stimulant for men* [menotropins] 75, 150 IU/ampule

perhexiline INN *coronary vasodilator* [also: perhexiline maleate]

perhexiline maleate USAN *coronary vasodilator* [also: perhexiline]

Periactin tablets, syrup ℞ *antihistamine* [cyproheptadine HCl] 4 mg; 2 mg/5 mL ② Taractan

periciazine INN *phenothiazine antipsychotic* [also: pericyazine]

Peri-Colace capsules, syrup OTC *stimulant laxative; stool softener* [casanthranol; docusate sodium] 30•100 mg; 30•60 mg/15 mL

pericyazine BAN *phenothiazine antipsychotic* [also: periciazine]

Peridex mouth rinse ℞ *antimicrobial; gingivitis treatment; investigational (orphan) for oral mucositis in bone marrow transplant patients* [chlorhexidine gluconate; alcohol 11.6%] 0.12%

Peridin-C tablets OTC *vitamin supplement* [ascorbic acid; hesperidin complex; hesperidin methyl chalcone bioflavonoids] 200•150•50 mg

Peri-Dos softgels OTC *stimulant laxative; stool softener* [casanthranol; docusate sodium] 30•100 mg

perilla (Perilla frutescens) plant *medicinal herb for asthma, inducing sweating, nausea, gastrointestinal spasms, and sunstroke*

perillyl alcohol (POH) *investigational (Phase II) monoterpene antineoplastic*

perimetazine INN

perindopril USAN, INN, BAN *antihypertensive; angiotensin-converting enzyme (ACE) inhibitor*

perindopril erbumine USAN *antihypertensive; angiotensin-converting enzyme (ACE) inhibitor*

perindoprilat INN, BAN

PerioChip biodegradable polymer implant ℞ *antimicrobial adjunct to scaling and root planing procedures in periodontitis* [chlorhexidine gluconate] 2.5 mg

PerioGard mouth rinse ℞ *antimicrobial; gingivitis treatment* [chlorhexidine gluconate; alcohol 11.6%] 0.12%

Periostat capsules ℞ *collagenase inhibitor for periodontal disease* [doxycycline hyclate] 20 mg

peripheral vasodilators *a class of cardiovascular drugs that cause dilation of the blood vessels*

Periploca sylvestris *medicinal herb* [see: gymnema]

perisoxal INN

Peritrate tablets (discontinued 1995) ℞ *antianginal; vasodilator* [pentaerythritol tetranitrate] 10, 20, 40 mg

Peritrate SA sustained-action tablets (discontinued 1995) ℞ *antianginal; vasodilator* [pentaerythritol tetranitrate] 80 mg

periwinkle (Catharanthus roseus) plant *medicinal herb for cancer, diabetes, diarrhea, insect stings, nervousness, ocular inflammation, and ulcers; not generally regarded as safe and effective for ingestion because of toxicity*

perlapine USAN, INN *hypnotic*

Perles (dosage form) *soft gelatin capsule*

permanganic acid, potassium salt [see: potassium permanganate]

Permapen Isoject (unit dose syringe) ℞ *natural penicillin antibiotic* [penicillin G benzathine] 1200 thousand U

Permax tablets ℞ *dopamine agonist; antiparkinsonian; investigational (orphan) for Tourette syndrome* [pergolide mesylate] 0.05, 0.25, 1 mg

permethrin USAN, INN, BAN *ectoparasiticide*

Permitil tablets, oral concentrate ℞ *conventional (typical) antipsychotic* [fluphenazine HCl] 2.5, 5, 10 mg; 5 mg/mL

Perna canaliculus *natural remedy* [see: New Zealand green-lipped mussel]

Pernox Scrub; Pernox Lathering Lotion OTC *abrasive cleanser for acne* [sulfur; salicylic acid]

peroxide, dibenzoyl [see: benzoyl peroxide]

Peroxin A 5; Peroxin A 10 gel ℞ *topical keratolytic for acne* [benzoyl peroxide] 5%; 10%

Peroxyl mouth rinse, oral gel OTC *cleansing of oral wounds* [hydrogen peroxide] 1.5%

perphenazine USP, INN *phenothiazine antipsychotic; antiemetic; intractable hiccough relief* 2, 4, 8, 16 mg oral

Persa-Gel; Persa-Gel W 5%; Persa-Gel W 10% gel ℞ *topical keratolytic for acne* [benzoyl peroxide] 5%, 10%; 5%; 10%

Persantine sugar-coated tablets ℞ *platelet aggregation inhibitor* [dipyridamole] 25, 50, 75 mg ⊡ Pertofrane

Persantine IV injection ℞ *diagnostic aid for coronary artery function* [dipyridamole] 10 mg

Persea americana; P. gratissima medicinal herb [see: avocado]

Persian bark; Persian berries *medicinal herb* [see: buckthorn]

Persian walnut *medicinal herb* [see: English walnut]

persic oil NF *vehicle*

persilic acid INN

Pertofrane capsules (discontinued 1996) ℞ *tricyclic antidepressant* [desipramine HCl] 25, 50 mg ⊡ Persantine

Pertropin capsules OTC *dietary lipotropic agent* [linolenic acid; multiple essential fatty acids] 7 mins.

Pertussin CS; Pertussin ES syrup OTC *antitussive* [dextromethorphan hydrobromide] 3.5 mg/5 mL; 15 mg/5 mL

pertussis immune globulin USP *passive immunizing agent*

pertussis immune human globulin [now: pertussis immune globulin]

pertussis vaccine USP *active immunizing agent*

pertussis vaccine adsorbed USP *active immunizing agent*

Peruvian balsam NF *topical local protectant; rubefacient*

Peruvian balsam *(Myroxylon balsamum; M. pereirae)* oil *medicinal herb for edema, expelling worms,* hemostasis, topical infections, and wound healing

Peruvian bark; yellow Peruvian bark *medicinal herb* [see: quinine]

Peruvian ginseng *medicinal herb* [see: maca]

Petasites hybridus medicinal herb [see: butterbur]

pethidine INN, BAN *narcotic analgesic; also abused as a street drug* [also: meperidine HCl]

pethidine HCl [see: meperidine HCl]

PETN (pentaerythritol tetranitrate) [q.v.]

petrichloral INN

petrolatum USP *ointment base; emollient/ protectant* [also: yellow petrolatum]

petrolatum, hydrophilic USP *absorbent ointment base; topical protectant*

petrolatum, liquid [see: mineral oil]

petrolatum, liquid emulsion [see: mineral oil emulsion]

petrolatum, white USP, JAN *oleaginous ointment base; topical protectant*

petrolatum gauze [see: gauze, petrolatum]

petroleum benzin [see: benzin, petroleum]

petroleum distillate inhalants *vapors from butane, toluene, acetone, benzene, gasoline, etc. which produce psychoactive effects, abused as street drugs* [see also: nitrous oxide; volatile nitrites]

petroleum jelly [see: petrolatum]

Petroselinum sativum medicinal herb [see: parsley]

Peumus boldus medicinal herb [see: boldo]

pexantel INN

pexiganan acetate *investigational (NDA filed) broad-spectrum topical antibiotic for impetigo and diabetic foot ulcers*

PFA (phosphonoformic acid) [see: foscarnet sodium]

Pfaffia paniculata medicinal herb [see: suma]

PFC (perfluorochemical) emulsion [q.v.]

Pfeiffer's Allergy tablets (discontinued 1997) OTC *antihistamine* [chlorpheniramine maleate] 4 mg

Pfeiffer's Cold Sore lotion OTC *topical oral anesthetic; analgesic; counterirritant* [gum benzoin; camphor; menthol; eucalyptol; alcohol 85%] 7% • ? • ? • ?

Pfizerpen powder for injection ℞ *natural penicillin antibiotic* [penicillin G potassium] 1, 5, 20 million U

Pfizerpen-AS IM injection (discontinued 1997) ℞ *bactericidal antibiotic* [penicillin G procaine] 300 000 U/mL

PFL (Platinol, fluorouracil, leucovorin [rescue]) *chemotherapy protocol*

PFT (L-phenylalanine mustard, fluorouracil, tamoxifen) *chemotherapy protocol*

PG (paregoric) [q.v.]

PG (prostaglandin) [q.v.]

PGA (pteroylglutamic acid) [see: folic acid]

PGE$_1$ (prostaglandin E$_1$) [now: alprostadil]

PGE$_2$ (prostaglandin E$_2$) [now: dinoprostone]

PGF$_{2\alpha}$ (prostaglandin F$_{2\alpha}$) [see: dinoprost]

PGF$_{2\alpha}$ (prostaglandin F$_{2\alpha}$) THAM [see: dinoprost tromethamine]

PGG glucan *investigational (Phase III) immunotherapeutic to prevent postsurgical infections following non-colorectal GI surgery (clinical trials discontinued 1999)*

PGI$_2$ (prostaglandin I$_2$) [now: epoprostenol]

PGX (prostaglandin X) [now: epoprostenol]

Phaenicia sericata natural treatment [see: maggots]

Phanacōl Cough syrup (discontinued 1995) OTC *decongestant; antitussive; expectorant; analgesic; antipyretic* [phenylpropanolamine HCl; dextromethorphan hydrobromide; guaifenesin; acetaminophen] 25 • 10 • 100 • 325 mg/5 mL

Phanadex Cough syrup OTC *antitussive; decongestant; antihistamine;*

expectorant [dextromethorphan hydrobromide; phenylpropanolamine HCl; pyrilamine maleate; guaifenesin] 15 • 25 • 40 • 100 mg/5 mL

Phanatuss Cough syrup OTC *antitussive; expectorant* [dextromethorphan hydrobromide; guaifenesin] 10 • 85 mg/5 mL

phanchinone [see: phanquinone; phanquone]

phanquinone INN [also: phanquone]

phanquone BAN [also: phanquinone]

pharmaceutical glaze [see: glaze, pharmaceutical]

Pharmaflur; Pharmaflur df; Pharmaflur 1.1 chewable tablets ℞ *dental caries preventative* [sodium fluoride] 2.2 mg; 2.2 mg; 1.1 mg

Pharmalgen subcu or IM injection ℞ *venom sensitivity testing (subcu); venom desensitization therapy (IM)* [extracts of honeybee, yellow jacket, yellow hornet, white-faced hornet, mixed vespid, and wasp venom]

Pharmia regina natural treatment [see: maggots]

Pharmorubicin PFS; Pharmorubicin RDF ⓒ injection ℞ *antibiotic antineoplastic* [epirubicin HCl] 2 mg/mL; 10, 20, 50, 150 mg

Phazyme tablets, drops OTC *antiflatulent* [simethicone] 60 mg; 40 mg/0.6 mL ⓓ Pherazine

Phazyme ⓒ oral liquid OTC *antiflatulent* [simethicone] 125 mg/5 mL

Phazyme 95 tablets OTC *antiflatulent* [simethicone] 95 mg

Phazyme 125 softgels OTC *antiflatulent* [simethicone] 125 mg

phebutazine [see: febuverine]

phebutyrazine [see: febuverine]

phemfilcon A USAN *hydrophilic contact lens material*

phenacaine INN [also: phenacaine HCl]

phenacaine HCl USP [also: phenacaine]

phenacemide USP, INN, BAN *anticonvulsant*

phenacetin USP, INN (*withdrawn from market*) ⓓ phenazocine

phenacon [see: fenaclon]

phenactropinium chloride INN, BAN

phenacyl 4-morpholineacetate [see: mobecarb]

N-phenacylhomatropinium chloride [see: phenactropinium chloride]

phenacylpivalate [see: pibecarb]

Phenadex Children's Cough/Cold syrup (discontinued 1998) OTC *pediatric antitussive, decongestant, and expectorant* [dextromethorphan hydrobromide; phenylpropanolamine HCl; guaifenesin; alcohol 5%] 5•6.25•100 mg/5 mL

Phenadex Pediatric Cough/Cold drops (discontinued 1998) OTC *pediatric antitussive, decongestant, and expectorant* [dextromethorphan hydrobromide; phenylpropanolamine HCl; guaifenesin] 5•6.25•50 mg/mL

Phenadex Senior liquid (discontinued 1998) OTC *antitussive; expectorant* [dextromethorphan hydrobromide; guaifenesin] 10•200 mg/5 mL

phenadoxone INN, BAN

phenaglycodol INN

Phenahist-TR sustained-release tablets ℞ *decongestant; antihistamine; anticholinergic* [phenylpropanolamine HCl; phenylephrine HCl; chlorpheniramine maleate; hyoscyamine sulfate; atropine sulfate; scopolamine hydrobromide] 50•25•8•0.19•0.04•0.01 mg

phenamazoline INN

phenamazoline HCl [see: phenamazoline]

Phenameth tablets (discontinued 1997) ℞ *antihistamine; sedative; antiemetic; motion sickness relief* [promethazine HCl] 25 mg

Phenameth DM syrup ℞ *antitussive; antihistamine* [dextromethorphan hydrobromide; promethazine HCl; alcohol] 15•6.25 mg/5 mL

phenampromide INN

Phenapap Sinus Headache & Congestion tablets OTC *decongestant; antihistamine; analgesic* [pseudoephedrine HCl; chlorpheniramine maleate; acetaminophen] 30•2•325 mg

Phenaphen with Codeine No. 3 & No. 4 capsules ℞ *narcotic analgesic* [codeine phosphate; acetaminophen] 30•325 mg; 60•325 mg

Phenaphen-650 with Codeine tablets (discontinued 1995) ℞ *narcotic analgesic* [codeine phosphate; acetaminophen] 30•650 mg

phenaphthazine

phenarbutal [see: phetharbital]

phenarsone sulfoxylate INN

Phenaseptic mouthwash/gargle (discontinued 1995) OTC *topical antipruritic/counterirritant; mild local anesthetic* [phenol] 1.4%

Phenate timed-release tablets ℞ *decongestant; antihistamine; analgesic* [phenylpropanolamine HCl; chlorpheniramine maleate; acetaminophen] 40•4•325 mg

Phenazine 25 injection (discontinued 1996) ℞ *antihistamine; sedative; antiemetic; motion sickness relief* [promethazine HCl] 25 mg/mL ② Pentazine; phenelzine; Phenoxine; Pherazine

Phenazine 50 injection (discontinued 1997) ℞ *antihistamine; sedative; antiemetic; motion sickness relief* [promethazine HCl] 50 mg/mL ② Pentazine; phenelzine; Phenoxine; Pherazine

Phenazo ⊛ (U.S. product: Pyridium) tablets ℞ *urinary analgesic* [phenazopyridine HCl] 100, 200 mg

phenazocine INN ② phenacetin

phenazocine hydrobromide [see: phenazocine]

Phenazodine tablets (discontinued 1996) ℞ *urinary analgesic* [phenazopyridine HCl] 100, 200 mg

phenazone INN, BAN *analgesic* [also: antipyrine]

phenazopyridine INN, BAN *urinary tract analgesic* [also: phenazopyridine HCl]

phenazopyridine HCl USAN, USP *urinary tract analgesic* [also: phenazopyridine] 100, 200 mg oral

phenbenicillin BAN [also: fenbenicillin]

phenbutazone sodium glycerate USAN *anti-inflammatory*

phenbutrazate BAN [also: fenbutrazate]

phencarbamide USAN *anticholinergic* [also: fencarbamide]

Phenchlor S.H.A. sustained-release tablets ℞ *decongestant; antihistamine; anticholinergic* [phenylpropanolamine HCl; phenylephrine HCl; chlorpheniramine maleate; hyoscyamine sulfate; atropine sulfate; scopolamine hydrobromide] 50•25•8•0.19•0.04•0.01 mg

phencyclidine INN *anesthetic* [also: phencyclidine HCl]

phencyclidine HCl USAN *anesthetic* [also: phencyclidine]

phendimetrazine INN *anorexiant* [also: phendimetrazine tartrate]

phendimetrazine tartrate USP *anorexiant; CNS stimulant* [also: phendimetrazine] 35, 105 mg oral

Phendryl; Phendryl Children's Allergy Medicine elixir (discontinued 1997) OTC *antihistamine* [diphenhydramine HCl] 12.5 mg/5 mL

phenelzine INN, BAN *antidepressant; MAO inhibitor* [also: phenelzine sulfate] ☒ Phenazine; Phenylzin

phenelzine sulfate USP *antidepressant; MAO inhibitor* [also: phenelzine]

phenemal [see: phenobarbital]

Phenerbel-S tablets ℞ *GI anticholinergic; sedative; analgesic* [belladonna alkaloids; phenobarbital; ergotamine tartrate] 0.2•40•0.6 mg

Phenergan tablets, suppositories, injection ℞ *antihistamine; sedative; antiemetic; motion sickness relief* [promethazine HCl] 12.5, 25, 50 mg; 12.5, 25, 50 mg; 25, 50 mg/mL ☒ Phenaphen; Theragran

Phenergan Fortis syrup ℞ *antihistamine; sedative; antiemetic; motion sickness relief* [promethazine HCl; alcohol 1.5%] 25 mg/5 mL

Phenergan Plain syrup ℞ *antihistamine; sedative; antiemetic; motion sickness relief* [promethazine HCl] 6.25 mg/5 mL

Phenergan VC syrup ℞ *decongestant; antihistamine* [phenylephrine HCl; promethazine HCl; alcohol 7%] 5•6.25 mg/5 mL

Phenergan VC with Codeine syrup ℞ *narcotic antitussive; decongestant; antihistamine* [codeine phosphate; phenylephrine HCl; promethazine HCl; alcohol 7%] 10•5•6.25 mg/5 mL

Phenergan with Codeine syrup ℞ *narcotic antitussive; antihistamine* [codeine phosphate; promethazine HCl; alcohol 7%] 10•6.25 mg/5 mL

Phenergan with Dextromethorphan syrup ℞ *antitussive; antihistamine* [dextromethorphan hydrobromide; promethazine HCl; alcohol 7%] 15•6.25 mg/5 mL

pheneridine INN

phenethanol [see: phenylethyl alcohol]

phenethazine [see: fenethazine]

phenethicillin potassium USAN [also: pheneticillin]

phenethyl alcohol BAN *antimicrobial agent* [also: phenylethyl alcohol]

N-phenethylanthranilic acid [see: enfenamic acid]

phenethylazocine bromide [see: phenazocine hydrobromide]

phenethylhydrazine sulfate [see: phenelzine sulfate]

pheneticillin INN [also: phenethicillin potassium]

pheneticillin potassium [see: phenethicillin potassium]

Phenetron tablets, syrup (discontinued 1997) ℞ *antihistamine; antitussive* [chlorpheniramine maleate] 4 mg; 2 mg/5 mL

phenetsal [see: acetaminosalol]

pheneturide INN, BAN [also: acetylpheneturide]

Phenex-1 powder OTC *formula for infants with phenylketonuria*

Phenex-2 powder OTC *enteral nutritional therapy for phenylketonuria (PKU)*

phenformin INN, BAN *biguanide hypoglycemic agent* [also: phenformin HCl]

phenformin HCl USP *hypoglycemic agent (removed from market by FDA in 1977, now available as an investigational drug)* [also: phenformin]

phenglutarimide INN, BAN
Phenhist DH with Codeine liquid ℞ narcotic antitussive; decongestant; antihistamine [codeine phosphate; pseudoephedrine HCl; chlorpheniramine maleate; alcohol 5%] 10•30•2 mg/5 mL
Phenhist Expectorant liquid ℞ narcotic antitussive; decongestant; expectorant [codeine phosphate; pseudoephedrine HCl; guaifenesin; alcohol 7.5%] 10•30•100 mg/5 mL
phenicarbazide INN
phenidiemal [see: phetharbital]
phenindamine INN piperidine antihistamine [also: phenindamine tartrate]
phenindamine tartrate USAN piperidine antihistamine [also: phenindamine]
phenindione USP, INN anticoagulant
pheniodol sodium INN [also: iodoalphionic acid]
pheniprazine INN, BAN
pheniprazine HCl [see: pheniprazine]
pheniramine INN [also: pheniramine maleate]
pheniramine maleate USAN antihistamine [also: pheniramine]
pheniramine maleate & naphazoline HCl topical ocular antihistamine and decongestant 0.3%•0.025% eye drops
phenisonone hydrobromide
phenmetraline HCl [see: phenmetrazine HCl]
phenmetrazine INN, BAN anorexiant; CNS stimulant; also abused as a street drug [also: phenmetrazine HCl]
phenmetrazine HCl USP anorexiant; CNS stimulant; also abused as a street drug [also: phenmetrazine]
phenobamate [see: febarbamate]
phenobarbital USP, INN, JAN anticonvulsant; hypnotic; sedative; also abused as a street drug [also: phenobarbitone] 15, 30, 60, 100 mg oral; 15, 20 mg/5 mL oral ② pentobarbital
phenobarbital sodium USP, INN, JAN anticonvulsant; hypnotic; sedative; also abused as a street drug 30, 60, 65, 130 mg/mL injection

phenobarbitone BAN anticonvulsant; hypnotic; sedative; also abused as a street drug [also: phenobarbital]
phenobutiodil INN
phenododecinium bromide [see: domiphen bromide]
Phenoject-50 injection (discontinued 1997) ℞ antihistamine; motion sickness relief; sleep aid; antiemetic; sedative [promethazine HCl] 50 mg/mL
phenol USP topical antiseptic/antipruritic; local anesthetic; preservative
phenol, liquefied USP topical antipruritic
phenol, sodium salt [see: phenolate sodium]
phenol red [see: phenolsulfonphthalein]
phenolate sodium USAN disinfectant
Phenolated Calamine lotion OTC topical poison ivy treatment [calamine; zinc oxide; phenol] 8%•8%•1%
Phenolax wafers OTC stimulant laxative [phenolphthalein] 64.8 mg
phenolphthalein USP, INN stimulant laxative [banned in all OTC laxatives in 1999]
phenolphthalein, white [see: phenolphthalein]
phenolphthalein, yellow USP stimulant laxative banned in all OTC laxatives in 1999
phenolsulfonphthalein USP
phenolsulphonate sodium USP
phenomorphan INN, BAN
phenomycilline [see: penicillin V]
phenoperidine INN, BAN
phenopryldiasulfone sodium [see: solasulfone]
Phenoptic eye drops ℞ topical ophthalmic decongestant and vasoconstrictor; mydriatic [phenylephrine HCl] 2.5%
phenosulfophthalein [see: phenolsulfonphthalein]
phenothiazine NF, INN antipsychotic
phenothiazines a class of dopamine receptor antagonists with antipsychotic, hypotensive, antiemetic, antispasmodic, and antihistaminic activity
phenothrin INN, BAN
phenoxazoline HCl [see: fenoxazoline HCl]

Phenoxine tablets OTC *diet aid* [phenylpropanolamine HCl] 25 mg ②
Phenazine
phenoxybenzamine INN *antihypertensive* [also: phenoxybenzamine HCl]
phenoxybenzamine HCl USP *antihypertensive; pheochromocytomic agent* [also: phenoxybenzamine]
phenoxymethylpenicillin INN *natural penicillin antibiotic* [also: penicillin V]
phenoxypropazine BAN [also: fenoxypropazine]
phenoxypropylpenicillin [see: propicillin]
phenozolone [see: fenozolone]
phenprobamate INN, BAN
phenprocoumon USAN, USP, INN *anticoagulant*
phenprocumone [see: phenprocoumon]
phenpromethadrine [see: phenpromethamine]
phenpromethamine INN
phenpropamine citrate [see: alverine citrate]
phensuximide USP, INN, BAN *anticonvulsant*
phentermine USAN, INN *anorexiant; CNS stimulant; an adrenergic isomer of amphetamine* ② phentolamine
phentermine HCl USP *anorexiant; CNS stimulant; the water-soluble form of phentermine for oral administration* 8, 15, 18.75, 30, 37.5 mg oral
phenthiazine [see: phenothiazine]
phentolamine INN, BAN *antihypertensive; pheochromocytomic agent* [also: phentolamine HCl] ② phentermine; Ventolin
phentolamine HCl USP *antihypertensive; pheochromocytomic agent* [also: phentolamine]
phentolamine mesilate INN, JAN *antiadrenergic; antihypertensive; pheochromocytomic agent* [also: phentolamine mesylate]
phentolamine mesylate USP *antihypertensive; α-adrenergic blocker; pheochromocytomic agent; investigational (Phase III) oral treatment for*

erectile dysfunction [also: phentolamine mesilate] 5 mg injection
phentolamine methanesulfonate [now: phentolamine mesylate]
Phentrol tablets (discontinued 1996) ℞ *anorexiant; CNS stimulant* [phentermine HCl] 8 mg
Phentrol 2; Phentrol 4; Phentrol 5 capsules ℞ *anorexiant; CNS stimulant* [phentermine HCl] 30 mg
phentydrone
Phenurone tablets (discontinued 1997) ℞ *anticonvulsant* [phenacemide] 500 mg
phenyl aminosalicylate USAN, BAN *antibacterial; tuberculostatic* [also: fenamisal]
phenyl salicylate NF *analgesic; not generally regarded as safe and effective as an antidiarrheal*
phenylalanine (L-phenylalanine) USAN, USP, INN *essential amino acid; symbols: Phe, F*
phenylalanine ammonia-lyase *investigational (orphan) for hyperphenylalaninemia*
phenylalanine mustard (PAM) [see: melphalan]
L-phenylalanine mustard (L-PAM) [see: melphalan]
Phenylase *investigational (orphan) for hyperphenylalaninemia* [phenylalanine ammonia-lyase]
phenylazo diamino pyridine HCl [see: phenazopyridine HCl]
phenylbenzyl atropine [see: xenytropium bromide]
phenylbutazone USP, INN *antirheumatic; anti-inflammatory; antipyretic; analgesic*
phenylbutylpiperadines *a class of dopamine receptor antagonists with conventional (typical) antipsychotic activity* [also called: butyrophenones]
phenylbutyrate sodium [see: sodium phenylbutyrate]
2-phenylbutyrylurea [see: phenetiride; acetylpheneturide]
phenylcarbinol [see: benzyl alcohol]

phenylcinchoninic acid [now: cinchophen]

α-phenyl-p-cresol carbamate [see: diphenan]

phenylcyclohexyl piperidine (PCP) [see: PCP; phencyclidine HCl]

2-phenylcyclopentylamine HCl [see: cypenamine HCl]

phenyldimazone [see: normethadone]

Phenyldrine timed-release tablets OTC diet aid [phenylpropanolamine HCl] 75 mg

phenylephrine (PE) INN, BAN nasal decongestant; ocular vasoconstrictor; vasopressor for hypotensive or cardiac shock [also: phenylephrine HCl]

phenylephrine bitartrate bronchodilator; vasoconstrictor

phenylephrine HCl USP nasal decongestant; ocular vasoconstrictor; vasopressor for hypotensive or cardiac shock [also: phenylephrine] 0.25%, 0.5%, 1% nose drops or spray; 2.5%, 10% eye drops; 1% injection

phenylephrine tannate nasal decongestant

phenylephrine tannate, chlorpheniramine tannate, and pyrilamine tannate decongestant; antihistamine 25•8•25 mg oral

phenylethanol [see: phenylethyl alcohol]

phenylethyl alcohol USP antimicrobial agent; preservative [also: phenethyl alcohol]

phenylethylmalonylurea [see: phenobarbital]

Phenylfenesin L.A. extended-action tablets ℞ decongestant; expectorant [phenylpropanolamine HCl; guaifenesin] 75•400 mg

Phenylfenesin L.A. long-acting tablets ℞ decongestant; expectorant [phenylpropanolamine HCl; guaifenesin] 75•400 mg

Phenyl-Free liquid OTC special diet for infants with phenylketonuria (PKU)

Phenylgesic tablets OTC antihistamine; analgesic [phenyltoloxamine citrate; acetaminophen] 30•325 mg

phenylindanedione [see: phenindione]

phenylmercuric acetate NF antimicrobial agent; preservative

phenylmercuric borate INN

phenylmercuric chloride NF

phenylmercuric nitrate NF antimicrobial agent; preservative; topical antiseptic

phenylone [see: antipyrine]

phenylpropanolamine (PPA) INN, BAN vasoconstrictor; nasal decongestant; nonprescription diet aid [also: phenylpropanolamine HCl]

phenylpropanolamine HCl USP vasoconstrictor; nasal decongestant; nonprescription diet aid [also: phenylpropanolamine] 25, 50, 75 mg oral

phenylpropanolamine polistirex USAN adrenergic; vasoconstrictor

1-phenylsemicarbazide [see: phenicarbazide]

phenylthilone [see: phenythilone]

phenyltoloxamine INN antihistamine

phenyltoloxamine citrate antihistamine

phenyltriazines a class of anticonvulsants

phenyracillin INN

phenyramidol HCl USAN analgesic; skeletal muscle relaxant [also: fenyramidol]

phenythilone INN

phenytoin USAN, USP, INN, BAN hydantoin anticonvulsant 125 mg/5 mL oral

phenytoin redox [see: redox-phenytoin]

phenytoin sodium USP hydantoin anticonvulsant 100 mg oral; 50 mg/mL injection

Pherazine DM syrup ℞ antitussive; antihistamine [dextromethorphan hydrobromide; promethazine HCl; alcohol 7%] 15•6.25 mg/5 mL

Pherazine VC syrup (name changed to Promethazine VC Plain in 1995)

Pherazine VC with Codeine syrup ℞ narcotic antitussive; decongestant; antihistamine [codeine phosphate; phenylephrine HCl; promethazine HCl; alcohol 7%] 10•5•6.25 mg/5 mL

Pherazine with Codeine syrup ℞ narcotic antitussive; antihistamine [codeine phosphate; promethazine HCl; alcohol 7%] 10•6.25 mg/5 mL

phetharbital INN

phezathion [see: fezatione]

Phicon cream OTC *topical anesthetic; emollient* [pramoxine HCl; vitamins A and E] 0.5%•7500 IU•2000 IU

Phicon F cream OTC *topical anesthetic; antifungal* [pramoxine HCl; undecylenic acid] 0.05%•8%

Phillips' Chewable tablets OTC *antacid* [magnesium hydroxide] 311 mg

Phillips' Laxative gelcaps (discontinued 1998) OTC *stimulant laxative; stool softener* [phenolphthalein; docusate sodium] 90•83 mg

Phillips' LaxCaps capsules OTC *stimulant laxative; stool softener* [phenolphthalein; docusate sodium] 90•83 mg

Phillips' Milk of Magnesia; Concentrated Phillips' Milk of Magnesia liquid OTC *antacid; laxative* [magnesium hydroxide] 400 mg/5 mL; 800 mg/5 mL

pHisoDerm; pHisoDerm for Baby liquid OTC *soap-free therapeutic skin cleanser*

pHisoDerm Cleansing Bar OTC *therapeutic skin cleanser*

pHisoHex liquid Ŗ *bacteriostatic skin cleanser* [hexachlorophene] 3% ▨ Fostex

phloropropiophenone [see: flopropione]

pholcodine INN

pholedrine INN, BAN

pholescutol [see: folescutol]

Phoradendron flavescens; P. serotinum; P. tomentosum medicinal herb [see: mistletoe]

PhosChol softgels, liquid concentrate OTC *neurotransmitter; lipotropic* [phosphatidylcholine] 565, 900 mg; 3 g/5 mL

phoscolic acid [see: foscolic acid]

Phos-Flur oral rinse Ŗ *topical dental caries preventative* [acidulated phosphate fluoride] 0.44 mg/mL

PhosLo tablets Ŗ *buffering agent for hyperphosphatemia in end-stage renal disease (orphan)* [calcium acetate] 667 mg

phosphate salt of tricyclic nucleoside [now: triciribine phosphate]

phosphatidylcholine (PC) [see: lecithin]

phosphatidylglycerol *investigational (orphan) for neonatal respiratory distress syndrome*

phosphinic acid [see: hypophosphorous acid]

2,2'-phosphinicodilactic acid (PDLA) [see: foscolic acid]

Phosphocol P 32 suspension for intracavitary instillation, interstitial injection Ŗ *radiopharmaceutical antineoplastic* [chromic phosphate P 32] 10, 15 mCi

phosphocysteamine *investigational (orphan) for cystinosis*

phosphodiesterase III (PDE III) inhibitors *a class of platelet aggregation inhibitors*

Phospholine Iodide powder for eye drops Ŗ *topical antiglaucoma agent; irreversible cholinesterase inhibitor miotic* [echothiophate iodide] 0.03%, 0.06%, 0.125%, 0.25%

phosphonoformic acid (PFA) [see: foscarnet sodium]

phosphorated carbohydrate solution (hyperosmolar solution with phosphoric acid) *antinauseant; antiemetic*

phosphoric acid NF *solvent; acidifying agent*

phosphoric acid, aluminum salt [see: aluminum phosphate gel]

phosphoric acid, calcium salt [see: calcium phosphate, dibasic]

phosphoric acid, chromium salt [see: chromic phosphate Cr 51 & P 32]

phosphoric acid, diammonium salt [see: ammonium phosphate]

phosphoric acid, dipotassium salt [see: potassium phosphate, dibasic]

phosphoric acid, disodium salt heptahydrate [see: sodium phosphate, dibasic]

phosphoric acid, disodium salt hydrate [see: sodium phosphate, dibasic]

phosphoric acid, magnesium salt [see: magnesium phosphate]

phosphoric acid, monopotassium salt [see: potassium phosphate, monobasic]

phosphoric acid, monosodium salt dihydrate [see: sodium phosphate, monobasic]

phosphoric acid, monosodium salt monohydrate [see: sodium phosphate, monobasic]

phosphorofluoridic acid, disodium salt [see: sodium monofluorophosphate]

phosphorus *element (P)*

Phospho-Soda [see: Fleet Phospho-Soda]

phosphothiamine [see: monophosphothiamine]

Photofrin powder for IV injection ℞ *laser light–activated antineoplastic for photodynamic therapy of esophageal (orphan) and non-small cell lung cancers; investigational (orphan) for bladder cancer* [porfimer sodium] 75 mg

PhotoPoint ℞ *investigational (Phase I/II) photosensitizer for age-related macular degeneration (AMD)* [tin etiopurpurin dichloride]

phoxim INN, BAN

Phrenilin tablets ℞ *analgesic; sedative* [acetaminophen; butalbital] 325•50 mg

Phrenilin Forte capsules ℞ *analgesic; sedative* [acetaminophen; butalbital] 650•50 mg

PHRT (procarbazine, hydroxyurea, radiotherapy) *chemotherapy protocol*

phthalofyne USAN *veterinary anthelmintic* [also: ftalofyne]

phthalylsulfacetamide NF

phthalylsulfamethizole INN

phthalylsulfathiazole USP, INN

phylcardin [see: aminophylline]

phyllindon [see: aminophylline]

Phyllocontin controlled-release tablets ℞ *antiasthmatic; bronchodilator* [aminophylline] 225 mg

phylloquinone [see: phytonadione]

Phylorinol liquid OTC *topical antipruritic/counterirritant; mild local anesthetic; antiseptic; astringent; oral deodorant* [phenol; boric acid; strong iodine solution; chlorophyllin copper complex] 0.6%•?•?•?

Phylorinol mouthwash/gargle OTC *topical antipruritic/counterirritant; mild local anesthetic* [phenol] 0.6%

physic root *medicinal herb* [see: Culver's root]

physiological irrigating solution *for general irrigating, washing and rinsing; not for injection*

Physiolyte liquid ℞ *sterile irrigant* [physiological irrigating solution]

PhysioSol liquid ℞ *sterile irrigant* [physiological irrigating solution]

physostigmine USP, BAN *reversible cholinesterase inhibitor miotic for glaucoma; investigational (NDA filed) for Alzheimer's disease* ② pyridostigmine; Prostigmin

physostigmine salicylate USP *cholinergic to reverse anticholinergic overdose; investigational (orphan) for Friedreich's and other inherited ataxias*

physostigmine sulfate USP *ophthalmic cholinergic for glaucoma; miotic*

phytate persodium USAN *pharmaceutic aid*

phytate sodium USAN *calcium-chelating agent*

phytic acid [see: fytic acid]

Phytolacca americana; P. decandra; P. rigida *medicinal herb* [see: pokeweed]

phytomenadione INN, BAN *vitamin K₁; prothrombogenic* [also: phytonadione]

phytonadiol sodium diphosphate INN

phytonadione USP, JAN *vitamin K₁; prothrombogenic* [also: phytomenadione] 2 mg/mL injection

PIA (Platinol, ifosfamide, Adriamycin) *chemotherapy protocol*

pibecarb INN

piberaline INN

picafibrate INN
picartamide INN
Picea excelsa; P. mariana medicinal herb [see: spruce tree]
picenadol INN analgesic [also: picenadol HCl]
picenadol HCl USAN analgesic [also: picenadol]
picilorex INN
pick purse; pickpocket medicinal herb [see: shepherd's purse]
piclamilast USAN phosphodiesterase type IV inhibitor for asthma
piclonidine INN
piclopastine INN
picloxydine INN, BAN
picobenzide INN
picodralazine INN
picolamine INN
piconol INN
picoperine INN
picoprazole INN
picotrin INN keratolytic [also: picotrin diolamine]
picotrin diolamine USAN keratolytic [also: picotrin]
Picrasma excelsa medicinal herb [see: quassia]
picric acid [see: trinitrophenol]
picrotoxin NF
picumast INN, BAN
picumeterol INN, BAN bronchodilator [also: picumeterol fumarate]
picumeterol fumarate USAN bronchodilator [also: picumeterol]
pidolacetamol INN
pidolic acid INN
pifarnine USAN, INN gastric antiulcerative
pifenate INN, BAN
pifexole INN
piflutixol INN
pifoxime INN
pigeonberry medicinal herb [see: pokeweed]
piketoprofen INN
Pilagan eye drops Ŗ topical antiglaucoma agent; direct-acting miotic [pilocarpine nitrate] 1%, 2%, 4%
pildralazine INN

pilewort *(Erechtites hieracifolia)* plant medicinal herb used as an astringent and emetic
Pilocar eye drops Ŗ topical antiglaucoma agent; direct-acting miotic [pilocarpine HCl] 0.5%, 1%, 2%, 3%, 4%, 6%
pilocarpine USP, BAN antiglaucoma agent; ophthalmic cholinergic
pilocarpine HCl USP ophthalmic cholinergic; antiglaucoma; miotic; treatment of xerostomia and keratoconjunctivitis sicca due to radiotherapy or Sjögren syndrome (orphan); also for dry mouth 0.5%, 1%, 2%, 4%, 6%, 8% eye drops
pilocarpine nitrate USP ophthalmic cholinergic; antiglaucoma; miotic
Pilopine HS ophthalmic gel Ŗ topical antiglaucoma agent; direct-acting miotic [pilocarpine HCl] 4%
Piloptic-½; Piloptic-1; Piloptic-2; Piloptic-3; Piloptic-4; Piloptic-6 eye drops Ŗ topical antiglaucoma agent; direct-acting miotic [pilocarpine HCl] 0.5%; 1%; 2%; 3%; 4%; 6%
Pilopto-Carpine eye drops Ŗ topical antiglaucoma agent; direct-acting miotic [pilocarpine HCl] 4%
Pilostat eye drops Ŗ topical antiglaucoma agent; direct-acting miotic [pilocarpine HCl] 0.5%, 1%, 2%, 3%, 4%, 6%
Pilpak (trademarked packaging form) patient compliance package
Pima syrup Ŗ expectorant [potassium iodide] 325 mg/5 mL
pimagedine HCl USAN advanced glycosylation inhibitor for type 1 diabetes; investigational (Phase III) for diabetics in end-stage renal disease
pimaricin JAN ophthalmic antibacterial/antifungal antibiotic [also: natamycin]
pimeclone INN
pimefylline INN
pimelautide INN
Pimenta dioica; P. officinalis medicinal herb [see: allspice]
pimetacin INN
pimethixene INN
pimetine INN antihyperlipoproteinemic [also: pimetine HCl]

pimetine HCl USAN *antihyperlipoproteinemic* [also: pimetine]

pimetixene [see: pimethixene]

pimetremide INN

pimeverine [see: pimetremide]

piminodine INN [also: piminodine esylate]

piminodine esylate NF [also: piminodine]

piminodine ethanesulfonate [see: piminodine esylate]

pimobendan USAN, INN *cardiotonic*

pimonidazole INN, BAN

pimozide USAN, USP, INN, BAN, JAN *antidyskinetic for Tourette syndrome; diphenylbutylpiperidine antipsychotic; neuroleptic*

pimpernel; small pimpernel *medicinal herb* [see: burnet]

pimpernel, blue *medicinal herb* [see: skullcap]

pimpernel, water *medicinal herb* [see: brooklime]

Pimpinella anisum medicinal herb [see: anise]

Pimpinella magna; P. saxifrage medicinal herb [see: burnet]

pinacidil USAN, INN *antihypertensive*

pinadoline USAN, INN *analgesic*

pinafide INN

pinaverium bromide INN *GI antispasmodic*

pinazepam INN

pincainide INN

Pindac (approved but not currently being marketed) ℞ *antihypertensive* [pinacidil]

pindolol USAN, USP, INN, BAN *antianginal; antihypertensive; vasodilator; antiadrenergic (β-receptor)* 5, 10 mg oral

pine, Norway *medicinal herb* [see: spruce]

pine, prince's *medicinal herb* [see: pipsissewa]

pine bark extract *natural free radical scavenger for inflammatory collagen disease and peripheral vascular disease; contains 80%–85% procyanidolic oligomers (PCOs)*

pine needle oil NF

pine tar USP

pineapple *(Ananas comosus) fruit medicinal herb for constipation, jaundice, soft tissue inflammation, and topical wound debridement*

Pink Bismuth liquid OTC *antidiarrheal; antinauseant* [bismuth subsalicylate] 130, 262 mg/15 mL

pinolcaine INN

pinoxepin INN *antipsychotic* [also: pinoxepin HCl]

pinoxepin HCl USAN *antipsychotic* [also: pinoxepin]

Pin-Rid soft gel capsules, liquid OTC *anthelmintic for ascariasis (roundworm) and enterobiasis (pinworm)* [pyrantel pamoate] 180 mg; 50 mg/mL

Pinus palustris natural remedy [see: turpentine]

Pinus strobus medicinal herb [see: white pine]

Pin-X liquid OTC *anthelmintic for ascariasis (roundworm) and enterobiasis (pinworm)* [pyrantel pamoate] 50 mg/mL

pioglitazone INN *thiazolidinedione antidiabetic; increases cellular response to insulin without increasing insulin secretion* [also: pioglitazone HCl]

pioglitazone HCl USAN *thiazolidinedione antidiabetic; increases cellular response to insulin without increasing insulin secretion* [also: pioglitazone]

pipacycline INN

pipamazine INN

pipamperone USAN, INN *antipsychotic*

pipaneperone [see: pipamperone]

pipazetate INN *antitussive* [also: pipazethate]

pipazethate USAN *antitussive* [also: pipazetate]

pipe plant; Dutchman's pipe; Indian pipe *medicinal herb* [see: fit root]

pipebuzone INN

pipecuronium bromide USAN, INN, BAN *muscle relaxant; nondepolarizing neuromuscular blocker; adjunct to anesthesia*

pipemidic acid INN

pipenzolate bromide INN

pipenzolate methylbromide [see: pipenzolate bromide]

pipenzolone bromide [see: pipenzolate bromide]

pipequaline INN

Piper cubeba medicinal herb [see: cubeb]

Piper methysticum medicinal herb [see: kava kava]

piperacetazine USAN, USP, INN *antipsychotic* ② piperazine

piperacillin INN, BAN *extended-spectrum penicillin antibiotic* [also: piperacillin sodium]

piperacillin sodium USAN, USP, JAN *extended-spectrum penicillin antibiotic* [also: piperacillin]

piperamide INN *anthelmintic* [also: piperamide maleate]

piperamide maleate USAN *anthelmintic* [also: piperamide]

piperamine [see: bamipine]

piperazine USP *anthelmintic for enterobiasis (pinworm) and ascariasis (roundworm)* ② piperacetazine

piperazine calcium edetate INN *anthelmintic* [also: piperazine edetate calcium]

piperazine citrate USP *anthelmintic* 250 mg oral; 500 mg/mL oral

piperazine citrate hydrate [see: piperazine citrate]

piperazine edetate calcium USAN *anthelmintic* [also: piperazine calcium edetate]

piperazine estrone sulfate [now: estropipate]

piperazine hexahydrate [see: piperazine citrate]

piperazine phosphate

piperazine phosphate monohydrate [see: piperazine phosphate]

piperazine theophylline ethanoate [see: acefylline piperazine]

piperidine phosphate

piperidines *a class of antihistamines*

piperidolate INN [also: piperidolate HCl]

piperidolate HCl USP [also: piperidolate]

piperilate [see: pipethanate]

piperine USP

piperocaine INN [also: piperocaine HCl]

piperocaine HCl USP [also: piperocaine]

piperonyl butoxide *pediculicide for lice*

piperoxan INN

piperphenidol HCl

piperylone INN

pipethanate INN

pipobroman USAN, USP, INN *alkylating antineoplastic*

pipoctanone INN

pipofezine INN

piposulfan USAN, INN *antineoplastic*

pipotiazine INN *phenothiazine antipsychotic* [also: pipotiazine palmitate]

pipotiazine palmitate USAN *phenothiazine antipsychotic* [also: pipotiazine]

pipoxizine INN

pipoxolan INN *muscle relaxant* [also: pipoxolan HCl]

pipoxolan HCl USAN *muscle relaxant* [also: pipoxolan]

Pipracil powder for IV or IM injection ℞ *extended-spectrum penicillin antibiotic* [piperacillin sodium] 2, 3, 4, 40 g

pipradimadol INN

pipradrol INN [also: pipradrol HCl]

pipradrol HCl NF [also: pipradrol]

pipramadol INN

pipratecol INN

piprinhydrinate INN, BAN

piprocurarium iodide INN

piprofurol INN

piprozolin USAN, INN *choleretic*

pipsissewa (Chimaphila umbellata) plant *medicinal herb used as an astringent, diaphoretic, and diuretic*

piquindone INN *antipsychotic* [also: piquindone HCl]

piquindone HCl USAN *antipsychotic* [also: piquindone]

piquizil INN *bronchodilator* [also: piquizil HCl]

piquizil HCl USAN *bronchodilator* [also: piquizil]

piracetam USAN, INN, BAN *cognition adjuvant; investigational (orphan) for myoclonus* ② piroxicam

pirandamine INN *antidepressant* [also: pirandamine HCl]

pirandamine HCl USAN *antidepressant*
[also: pirandamine]
pirarubicin INN
piraxelate INN
pirazmonam INN *antimicrobial* [also:
pirazmonam sodium]
pirazmonam sodium USAN *antimicrobial* [also: pirazmonam]
pirazofurin INN *antineoplastic* [also:
pyrazofurin]
pirazolac USAN, INN, BAN *antirheumatic*
pirbenicillin INN *antibacterial* [also:
pirbenicillin sodium]
pirbenicillin sodium USAN *antibacterial* [also: pirbenicillin]
pirbuterol INN *sympathomimetic bronchodilator* [also: pirbuterol acetate]
pirbuterol acetate USAN *sympathomimetic bronchodilator* [also: pirbuterol]
pirbuterol HCl USAN *bronchodilator*
pirdonium bromide INN
pirenoxine INN
pirenperone USAN, INN, BAN *tranquilizer*
pirenzepine INN, BAN *treatment for
peptic ulcers* [also: pirenzepine HCl]
pirenzepine HCl USAN, JAN *treatment
for peptic ulcers* [also: pirenzepine]
pirepolol INN
piretanide USAN, INN *diuretic*
pirfenidone USAN, INN *analgesic; anti-
inflammatory; antipyretic*
piribedil INN
piribenzyl methylsulfate [see: bevonium metilsulfate]
piridicillin INN *antibacterial* [also: piridicillin sodium]
piridicillin sodium USAN *antibacterial*
[also: piridicillin]
piridocaine INN
piridocaine HCl [see: piridocaine]
piridoxilate INN, BAN
piridronate sodium USAN *calcium regulator*
piridronic acid INN
pirifibrate INN
pirinidazole INN
pirinitramide [see: piritramide]
pirinixic acid INN
pirinixil INN
piriprost USAN *antiasthmatic*

piriprost potassium USAN *antiasthmatic*
piriqualone INN
pirisudanol INN
piritramide INN, BAN
piritrexim INN *antiproliferative agent*
[also: piritrexim isethionate]
piritrexim isethionate USAN *antiproliferative; orphan status withdrawn
1996* [also: piritrexim]
pirlimycin HCl USAN *antibacterial*
pirlindole INN
pirmagrel USAN, INN *thromboxane synthetase inhibitor*
pirmenol INN *antiarrhythmic* [also: pirmenol HCl]
pirmenol HCl USAN *antiarrhythmic*
[also: pirmenol]
pirnabin INN *antiglaucoma agent* [also:
pirnabine]
pirnabine USAN *antiglaucoma agent*
[also: pirnabin]
piroctone USAN, INN *antiseborrheic*
piroctone olamine USAN *antiseborrheic*
pirodavir USAN, INN, BAN *antiviral*
pirogliride INN *antidiabetic* [also: pirogliride tartrate]
pirogliride tartrate USAN *antidiabetic*
[also: pirogliride]
piroheptine INN
pirolate USAN, INN *antiasthmatic*
pirolazamide USAN, INN *antiarrhythmic*
piromidic acid INN
piroxantrone INN *antineoplastic* [also:
piroxantrone HCl]
piroxantrone HCl USAN *antineoplastic*
[also: piroxantrone]
piroxicam USAN, USP, INN, BAN, JAN
*antiarthritic; nonsteroidal anti-inflam-
matory drug (NSAID); analgesic; antiarthritic 10, 20 mg oral ⊡ piracetam*
piroxicam beta-cyclodextrin [see:
piroxicam betadex]
piroxicam betadex USAN *investigational analgesic, anti-inflammatory,
and antirheumatic*
piroxicam cinnamate USAN *anti-
inflammatory*
piroxicam olamine USAN *analgesic;
anti-inflammatory*
piroxicillin INN

piroximone USAN, INN, BAN *cardiotonic*

pirozadil INN

pirprofen USAN, INN, BAN *anti-inflammatory*

pirquinozol USAN, INN *antiallergic*

pirralkonium bromide INN

pirroksan [now: proroxan HCl]

pirsidomine USAN, INN *vasodilator*

pirtenidine INN

pistachio *medicinal herb* [see: witch hazel]

pitch tree, Canada; hemlock pitch tree *medicinal herb* [see: hemlock]

pitcher plant (*Sarracenia purpurea*) root *medicinal herb used as an astringent, diuretic, and stimulant*

pitenodil INN

Pitocin IV, IM injection ℞ *oxytocic for induction of labor, postpartum bleeding, and incomplete abortion* [oxytocin] 10 U/mL ⊉ Pitressin

pitofenone INN

Pitressin Synthetic IM or subcu injection ℞ *pituitary antidiuretic hormone for diabetes insipidus or prevention of abdominal distention* [vasopressin] 20 U/mL ⊉ Pitocin

Pitrex ⒸⒶⓃ (U.S. product: Tinactin) cream OTC *topical antifungal* [tolnaftate] 1%

pituitary, anterior

pituitary, posterior USP *antidiuretic hormone*

pituxate INN

pivalate USAN, INN, BAN *combining name for radicals or groups*

pivampicillin INN *aminopenicillin antibiotic* [also: pivampicillin HCl]

pivampicillin HCl USAN *aminopenicillin antibiotic* [also: pivampicillin]

pivampicillin pamoate USAN *antibacterial*

pivampicillin probenate USAN *antibacterial*

Pivanex ℞ *investigational (Phase II) small-molecule antineoplastic for stage III and IV non-small cell lung cancer*

pivenfrine INN

pivmecillinam INN, BAN *aminopenicillin antibiotic* [also: amdinocillin pivoxil; pivmecillinam HCl]

pivmecillinam HCl JAN *aminopenicillin antibiotic* [also: amdinocillin pivoxil; pivmecillinam]

pivopril USAN *antihypertensive*

pivoxazepam INN

pivoxetil USAN, INN *combining name for radicals or groups*

pivoxil USAN, INN *combining name for radicals or groups*

pivsulbactam BAN *β-lactamase inhibitor; penicillin/cephalosporin synergist* [also: sulbactam pivoxil]

pix pini [see: pine tar]

Pixykine ℞ *investigational second-generation colony stimulating factor for neutropenia and thrombocytopenia* [milodistim]

pizotifen INN, BAN *anabolic; antidepressant; serotonin inhibitor (migraine specific)* [also: pizotyline]

pizotyline USAN *anabolic; antidepressant; serotonin inhibitor (migraine specific)* [also: pizotifen]

placebo *no medicinal value* [also: obecalp]

Placidyl capsules ℞ *hypnotic* [ethchlorvynol] 200, 500, 750 mg ⊉ Pathocil

plafibride INN

plague vaccine USP *active bacterin for plague (Yersinia pestis)* $1.8–2.2 \times 10^8$ bacilli/mL IM injection

Plan B tablets ℞ *emergency "morning after" oral contraceptive (progestin only)* [levonorgestrel] 0.75 mg

planadalin [see: carbromal]

Plantago lanceolata; P. major **and other species** *medicinal herb* [see: plantain]

Plantago ovata **(psyllium)** *medicinal herb* [see: plantain]

plantago seed USP *laxative*

plantain (*Plantago lanceolata; P. major* and other species) leaves and seeds *medicinal herb for bed-wetting, bladder infections, blood poisoning, constipation, diarrhea, diverticulitis, edema, hyperlipidemia, kidney* *disorders, neuralgia, snake bites, sores, and topical inflammation*

Plaquase powder for injection ℞ *investigational (orphan) for Peyronie's disease* [collagenase]

Plaquenil Sulfate tablets ℞ *antimalarial; antirheumatic* [hydroxychloroquine sulfate] 200 mg

Plasbumin-5; Plasbumin-25 IV infusion ℞ *blood volume expander for shock, burns, and hypoproteinemia* [human albumin] 5%; 25%

plasma, antihemophilic human USP

plasma concentrate factor IX [see: factor IX complex]

plasma expanders *a class of therapeutic blood modifiers used to increase the volume of circulating blood* [also called: blood volume expanders]

plasma protein fraction USP *blood volume supporter*

plasma protein fraction, human [now: plasma protein fraction]

plasma protein fractions *a class of therapeutic blood modifiers used to regulate the volume of circulating blood*

plasma thromboplastin component (PTC) [see: factor IX]

Plasma-Lyte A pH 7.4; Plasma-Lyte R; Plasma-Lyte 56; Plasma-Lyte 148 IV infusion ℞ *intravenous electrolyte therapy* [combined electrolyte solution]

Plasma-Lyte M (R; 56; 148) and 5% Dextrose IV infusion ℞ *intravenous nutritional/electrolyte therapy* [combined electrolyte solution; dextrose]

Plasmanate IV infusion ℞ *blood volume expander for shock due to burns, trauma and surgery* [plasma protein fraction] 5%

Plasma-Plex IV infusion ℞ *blood volume expander for shock due to burns, trauma and surgery* [plasma protein fraction] 5%

Plasmatein IV infusion ℞ *blood volume expander for shock due to burns, trauma and surgery* [plasma protein fraction] 5%

plasmin BAN [also: fibrinolysin, human]

Plateau Cap (trademarked dosage form) *controlled-release capsule*

platelet cofactor II [see: factor IX]

platelet concentrate USP *platelet replenisher*

platelet factor 4, recombinant (rPF4) *investigational antineoplastic for various cancers and heparin neutralizer*

platelet-activating factor acetylhydrolase, recombinant (rPAF-AH) *investigational (Phase II) for asthma; investigational (Phase II) for endoscopic retrograde cholangiopancreatography (ERCP)*

Platinol powder for IV injection (discontinued 1997) ℞ *alkylating antineoplastic for testicular, ovarian, bladder, lung, head, neck, and esophageal cancers* [cisplatin] 10, 50 mg

Platinol-AQ IV injection ℞ *alkylating antineoplastic for metastatic testicular tumors, metastatic ovarian tumors, and advanced bladder cancer* [cisplatin] 1 mg/mL

platinum *element (Pt)*

cis-**platinum** [now: cisplatin]

cis-**platinum II** [now: cisplatin]

platinum diamminodichloride [see: cisplatin]

plaunotol INN

plauracin USAN, INN *veterinary growth stimulant*

Plavix coated tablets ℞ *platelet aggregation inhibitor for stroke, myocardial infarction, and peripheral artery disease* [clopidogrel bisulfate] 75 mg

Plax, Advanced Formula mouthwash/gargle OTC [sodium pyrophosphate]

pleconaril USAN *investigational (Phase II) viral replication inhibitor for treatment of asthmatics with common cold*

Plegine tablets ℞ *anorexiant; CNS stimulant* [phendimetrazine tartrate] 35 mg

Plegisol solution ℞ *cardioplegic solution* [calcium chloride; magnesium chloride; potassium chloride; sodium chloride] 17.6•325.3•119.3•643 mg/100 mL

Plendil extended-release tablets ℞ *antihypertensive; calcium channel blocker* [felodipine] 2.5, 5, 10 mg

Pletal tablets ℞ *vasodilator and platelet aggregation inhibitor for intermittent claudication* [cilostazol] 50, 100 mg

pleurisy root *(Asclepias tuberosa) medicinal herb for asthma, bronchitis, dysentery, emphysema, fever, pleurisy, and pneumonia*

pleuromulin INN

Pliagel solution OTC *surfactant cleaning solution for soft contact lenses*

plicamycin USAN, USP, INN *antibiotic antineoplastic*

plomestane USAN *antineoplastic; aromatase inhibitor*

plum *(Prunus americana; P. domestica; P. spinosa)* fruit and bark *medicinal herb used as an anthelmintic, astringent, and laxative*

plutonium *element (Pu)*

PMB 200; PMB 400 tablets (discontinued 1998) ℞ *estrogen replacement therapy for postmenopausal disorders; anxiolytic* [conjugated estrogens; meprobamate] 0.45•200 mg; 0.45•400 mg

PMEA *investigational (Phase I/II) antiviral nucleoside analog for HIV and various herpesvirus types* [also: GS 393]

PMMA (polymethylmethacrylate) [q.v.]

PMPA *investigational (Phase I/II) treatment for HIV*

PMS-Bethanechol Chloride Ⓒ (U.S. product: Duvoid) tablets ℞ *cholinergic urinary stimulant for postsurgical and postpartum urinary retention* [bethanechol chloride] 10, 25, 50 mg

PMS-Dicitrate Ⓒ (U.S. product: Bicitra) oral solution ℞ *urinary alkalinizing agent* [sodium citrate; citric acid] 500•334 mg/5 mL

PMS-Fluphenazine Ⓒ (U.S. product: Prolixin) tablets, elixir ℞ *conventional (typical) antipsychotic* [fluphenazine decanoate] 1, 2, 5 mg; 2.5 mg/5 mL

PMS-Fluphenazine Ⓒ (U.S. product: Prolixin Decanoate) subcu or IM injection ℞ *conventional (typical) antipsychotic* [fluphenazine decanoate] 25 mg/mL

PMS-Haloperidol; PMS-Haloperidol LA Ⓒ (U.S. product: Haldol) IM injection ℞ *conventional (typical) antipsychotic; antidyskinetic for Tourette syndrome* [haloperidol lactate] 2 mg/mL

PMS-Lithium Carbonate Ⓒ (U.S. product: Eskalith) capsules ℞ *antipsychotic for manic episodes* [lithium carbonate] 150, 300, 600 mg

PMS-Lithium Citrate Ⓒ syrup ℞ *antipsychotic for manic episodes* [lithium citrate] 300 mg/5 mL

P-MVAC (Platinol, methotrexate, vinblastine, Adriamycin, carboplatin) *chemotherapy protocol*

Pneumo 23 Ⓒ subcu or IM injection ℞ *pneumonia vaccine* [pneumococcal polysaccharide vaccine] 0.5 mL

pneumococcal polysaccharide vaccine *active bacterin for pneumococcal pneumonia (23 types)*

pneumococcal vaccine, polyvalent *active bacterin for pneumococcal pneumonia (23 types)*

Pneumomist sustained-release tablets ℞ *expectorant* [guaifenesin] 600 mg

Pneumopent for inhalation ℞ *investigational (orphan) prophylaxis of Pneumocystis carinii pneumonia* [pentamidine isethionate]

Pneumotussin HC syrup ℞ *narcotic antitussive; expectorant* [hydrocodone bitartrate; guaifenesin] 5•100 mg/5 mL

Pneumovax 23 subcu or IM injection ℞ *pneumonia vaccine* [pneumococcal vaccine, polyvalent] 0.5 mL

Pnu-Imune 23 subcu or IM injection ℞ *pneumonia vaccine* [pneumococcal vaccine, polyvalent] 0.5 mL

pobilukast edamine USAN *antiasthmatic*

POC (procarbazine, Oncovin, CCNU) *chemotherapy protocol*

POCA (prednisone, Oncovin, cytarabine, Adriamycin) *chemotherapy protocol*

POCC (procarbazine, Oncovin, cyclophosphamide, CCNU) *chemotherapy protocol*

Pockethaler (trademarked delivery device) *nasal inhalation aerosol*

pod pepper *medicinal herb* [see: cayenne]

podilfen INN

Podocon-25 liquid ℞ *topical keratolytic for genital warts* [podophyllum resin] 25%

podofilox USAN *topical antimitotic for genital warts* [also: podophyllotoxin]

Podofin liquid ℞ *topical keratolytic for genital warts* [podophyllum resin] 25% ⊡ podophyllin

podophyllin [see: podophyllum resin] ⊡ Podofin

podophyllotoxin BAN *topical antimitotic* [also: podofilox]

podophyllotoxins *a class of mitotic-inhibiting antineoplastics derived from podophyllotoxin*

podophyllum USP *caustic; cytotoxic agent for genital warts*

Podophyllum peltatum medicinal herb [see: mandrake]

podophyllum resin USP *caustic; cytotoxic agent for genital warts*

POH (perillyl alcohol) [q.v.]

poinsettia (Euphorbia pulcherrima; E. poinsettia; Poinsettia pulcherrima) *plant and sap medicinal herb for fever, pain relief, stimulating lactation, toothache, and warts; also used as an antibacterial and depilatory*

Point-Two oral rinse ℞ *topical dental caries preventative* [sodium fluoride; alcohol 6%] 0.2%

poison, dog *medicinal herb* [see: dog poison]

Poison Antidote Kit OTC *emergency treatment for various poisons* [syrup of ipecac; charcoal suspension] 30•60 mL

poison ash *medicinal herb* [see: fringe tree]

poison flag *medicinal herb* [see: blue flag]

poison hemlock (Conium maculatum) *plant medicinal herb that has been used for analgesia and sedation and as a method of execution; it is extremely poisonous*

poison ivy extract, alum precipitated USAN *ivy poisoning counteractant*

poison oak (Tocicodendron diversilobum) extract *medicinal herb used in homeopathic remedies for osteoarthritis*

poison oak extract USAN *antiallergic*

Poison Oak-N-Ivy Armor lotion OTC *topical poison ivy protectant*

poke root (Phytolacca decandra) *medicinal herb* [see: pokeweed]

pokeweed (Phytolacca americana; P. decandra; P. rigida) *root and young shoots medicinal herb for arthritis, blood cleansing, bowel evacuation, dysmenorrhea, mucous membrane inflammation and discharge, mumps, pain, rheumatism, ringworm, scabies, syphilis, and tonsillitis; not generally regarded as safe and effective*

polacrilin USAN, INN *pharmaceutic aid*

polacrilin potassium USAN, NF *tablet disintegrant*

Poladex timed-release tablets (discontinued 1997) ℞ *antihistamine* [dexchlorpheniramine maleate] 4, 6 mg

Polaramine tablets, Repetabs (repeat-action tablets), syrup ℞ *antihistamine* [dexchlorpheniramine maleate] 2 mg; 4, 6 mg; 2 mg/5 mL

Polaramine Expectorant liquid ℞ *decongestant; antihistamine; expectorant* [pseudoephedrine sulfate; dexchlorpheniramine maleate; guaifenesin; alcohol 7.2%] 20•2•100 mg/5 mL

poldine methylsulfate USAN, USP *anticholinergic* [also: poldine metilsulfate]

poldine metilsulfate INN *anticholinergic* [also: poldine methylsulfate]

polecat weed *medicinal herb* [see: skunk cabbage]

policapram USAN, INN *tablet binder*

policresulen INN

polidexide sulfate INN

polidocanol

polifeprosan INN *pharmaceutic aid; implantable, biodegradable drug carrier* [also: polifeprosan 20]

polifeprosan 20 USAN *pharmaceutic aid; implantable, biodegradable drug carrier* [also: polifeprosan]

poligeenan USAN, INN *dispersing agent*

poliglecaprone 25 USAN *absorbable surgical suture material*

poliglecaprone 90 USAN *absorbable surgical suture coating*

poliglusam USAN *antihemorrhagic*

polignate sodium USAN *pepsin enzyme inhibitor*

polihexanide INN [also: polyhexanide]

poliomyelitis vaccine [now: poliovirus vaccine, inactivated]

poliovirus vaccine, enhanced inactivated (eIPV) *active immunizing agent for poliomyelitis*

poliovirus vaccine, inactivated (IPV) USP *active immunizing agent for poliomyelitis*

poliovirus vaccine, live oral (OPV) USP *active immunizing agent for poliomyelitis*

polipropene 25 USAN *tablet excipient*

polisaponin INN

politef INN *prosthetic aid* [also: polytef]

polixetonium chloride USAN, INN *preservative*

Polocaine injection ℞ *injectable local anesthetic* [mepivacaine HCl] 1%, 2%, 3%

Polocaine injection ℞ *injectable local anesthetic* [mepivacaine HCl; levonordefrin] 2%•1:20 000

Polocaine MPF injection ℞ *injectable local anesthetic* [mepivacaine HCl] 1%, 1.5%, 2%

polonium *element (Po)*

poloxalene USAN, INN, BAN *surfactant*

poloxamer USAN, NF, INN, BAN *ointment and suppository base; tablet binder*

poloxamer 124 USAN *surfactant; emulsifier; solubilizer; stabilizer*

poloxamer 188 USAN *surfactant; emulsifier; solubilizer; investigational (Phase III, orphan) for sickle cell crisis; investigational (orphan) for severe burns and vasospasm following cerebral aneurysm repair*

poloxamer 237 USAN *surfactant; emulsifier; solubilizer; stabilizer*

poloxamer 331 *investigational (orphan) for toxoplasmosis of AIDS*

poloxamer 338 USAN *surfactant; emulsifier; solubilizer; stabilizer*

poloxamer 407 USAN *surfactant; emulsifier; solubilizer; stabilizer*

poly I: poly C12U *investigational (Phase III, orphan) antiviral/immunomodulator for AIDS, renal cell carcinoma, metastatic melanoma, and chronic fatigue syndrome*

polyamine resin [see: polyamine-methylene resin]

polyamine-methylene resin

polyanhydroglucose [see: dextran]

polyanhydroglucuronic acid [see: dextran]

polybenzarsol INN

polybutester USAN *surgical suture material*

polybutilate USAN *surgical suture coating*

polycarbokane [see: polycarbophil]

polycarbophil USP, INN, BAN *bulk laxative*

Polycillin capsules, powder for oral suspension, pediatric drops (discontinued 1998) ℞ *aminopenicillin antibiotic* [ampicillin] 250, 500 mg; 125, 250, 500 mg/5 mL; 100 mg/mL ② penicillin

Polycillin-N powder for IV or IM injection (discontinued 1998) ℞ *aminopenicillin antibiotic* [ampicillin sodium] 0.125, 0.25, 0.5, 1, 2, 10 g

Polycillin-PRB powder for oral suspension (discontinued 1998) ℞ *antibiotic for Neisseria gonorrhoeae* [ampicillin; probenecid] 3.5•1 g

Polycitra syrup ℞ *urinary alkalinizing agent* [potassium citrate; sodium citrate; citric acid] 550•500•334 mg/5 mL

Polycitra-K oral solution, crystals for oral solution ℞ *urinary alkalizing agent* [potassium citrate; citric acid] 1100•334 mg/5 mL; 3300•1002 mg/packet

Polycitra-LC solution ℞ *urinary alkalizing agent* [potassium citrate; sodium citrate; citric acid] 550•500•334 mg/5 mL

Polycose liquid, powder OTC *carbohydrate caloric supplement* [glucose polymers]

polydextrose USAN *food additive*

polydimethylsiloxane *surgical aid (retinal tamponade) for retinal detachment*

Polydine ointment, scrub, solution OTC *broad-spectrum antimicrobial* [povidone-iodine]

polydioxanone USAN *absorbable surgical suture material*

polyelectrolyte 211 [see: sodium alginate]

polyenes *a class of antifungals produced by a species of Streptomyces that damage fungal cell membranes*

polyestradiol phosphate INN, BAN *antineoplastic; estrogen*

polyetadene INN *antacid* [also: polyethadene]

polyethadene USAN *antacid* [also: polyetadene]

polyethylene excipient NF *stiffening agent*

polyethylene glycol (PEG) NF *ophthalmic moisturizer; ointment and suppository base; solvent*

polyethylene glycol *n* (*n* refers to the molecular weight: 300, 400, 1000, etc.)

polyethylene glycol *n* **dioleate** (*n* refers to the molecular weight: 300, 400, 1000, etc.)

polyethylene glycol 8 monostearate [see: polyoxyl 8 stearate]

polyethylene glycol 1000 monocetyl ether [see: cetomacrogol 1000]

polyethylene glycol 1540 NF

polyethylene glycol 4000 USP [also: macrogol 4000]

polyethylene glycol 6000 USP

polyethylene glycol monoleyl ether [see: polyoxyl 10 oleyl ether]

polyethylene glycol monomethyl ether NF *excipient*

polyethylene glycol monostearate [see: polyoxyl 40 & 50 stearate]

polyethylene glycol-electrolyte solution (PEG-ES) *pre-procedure bowel evacuant* [contains PEG 3350]

polyethylene glycol-superoxide dismutase (PEG-SOD) [see: pegorgotein]

polyethylene oxide NF *suspending and viscosity agent; tablet binder*

polyferose USAN *hematinic*

Polygala senega medicinal herb [see: senega]

Polygam powder for IV infusion ℞ *passive immunizing agent for HIV* [immune globulin] 50 mg/mL

Polygam S/D freeze-dried powder for IV infusion ℞ *passive immunizing agent for HIV, idiopathic thrombocytopenic purpura (ITP), and B-cell chronic lymphocytic leukemia* [immune globulin, solvent/detergent treated] 50 mg/mL

polygeline INN, BAN

polyglactin 370 USAN *absorbable surgical suture coating*

polyglactin 910 USAN *absorbable surgical suture material*

polyglycolic acid USAN, INN *surgical suture material*

polyglyconate USAN, BAN *absorbable surgical suture material*

Polygonatum multiflorum; P. odoratum medicinal herb [see: Solomon's seal]

Polygonum aviculare; P. hydropiper; P. persicaria; P. punctatum medicinal herb [see: knotweed]

Polygonum bistorta medicinal herb [see: bistort]

Polygonum multiflorum medicinal herb [see: fo-ti; ho-shou-wu]

PolyHeme ℞ *investigational (Phase III) blood substitute* [human hemoglobin cross-linked with glutaral]

polyhexanide BAN [also: polihexanide]

Poly-Histine elixir ℞ *antihistamine* [pheniramine maleate; pyrilamine maleate; phenyltoloxamine citrate] 4•4•4 mg/5 mL

Poly-Histine CS syrup ℞ *narcotic antitussive; decongestant; antihistamine* [codeine phosphate; phenylpropanolamine HCl; brompheniramine maleate] 10•12.5•2 mg/5 mL

Poly-Histine DM syrup ℞ *antitussive; decongestant; antihistamine* [dextromethorphan hydrobromide; phenylpropanolamine HCl; brompheniramine maleate] 10•12.5•2 mg/5 mL

Poly-Histine-D sustained-release capsules, elixir ℞ *decongestant; antihistamine* [phenylpropanolamine HCl; phenyltoloxamine citrate; pyrilamine maleate; pheniramine maleate] 50• 16•16•16 mg; 12.5•4•4•4 mg/5 mL

Poly-Histine-D Ped Caps sustained-release capsules ℞ *pediatric decongestant and antihistamine* [phenylpropanolamine HCl; phenyltoloxamine citrate; pyrilamine maleate; pheniramine maleate] 25•8•8•8 mg

poly-ICLC *investigational (orphan) for primary brain tumors*

polyloxyl 8 stearate USAN *surfactant*

polymacon USAN *hydrophilic contact lens material*

polymanoacetate [now: acemannan]

polymeric oxygen [see: oxygen, polymeric]

polymetaphosphate P 32 USAN *radioactive agent*

polymethyl methacrylate (PMMA) *rigid hydrophobic polymer used for hard contact lenses*

polymixin E [see: colistin sulfate]

polymonine

Polymox capsules, powder for oral suspension, pediatric drops (discontinued 1998) ℞ *aminopenicillin antibiotic* [amoxicillin] 250, 500 mg; 125, 250 mg/5 mL; 50 mg/mL

polymyxin BAN *bactericidal antibiotic* [also: polymyxin B sulfate; polymyxin B]

polymyxin B INN *bactericidal antibiotic* [also: polymyxin B sulfate; polymyxin]

polymyxin B sulfate USP *bactericidal antibiotic* [also: polymyxin B; polymyxin] 500 000 U/vial eye drops or injection

polymyxin B$_1$ [see: polymyxin B]

polymyxin B$_2$ [see: polymyxin B]

polymyxin B$_3$ [see: polymyxin B]

polymyxin E [see: colistin sulfate]

polynoxylin INN, BAN

polyoxyethylene 20 sorbitan monolaurate [see: polysorbate 20]

polyoxyethylene 20 sorbitan monooleate [see: polysorbate 80]

polyoxyethylene 20 sorbitan monopalmitate [see: polysorbate 40]

polyoxyethylene 20 sorbitan monostearate [see: polysorbate 60]

polyoxyethylene 20 sorbitan trioleate [see: polysorbate 85]

polyoxyethylene 20 sorbitan tristearate [see: polysorbate 65]

polyoxyethylene 50 stearate [now: polyoxyl 50 stearate]

polyoxyethylene glycol 1000 monocetyl ether [see: cetomacrogol 1000]

polyoxyethylene nonyl phenol *surfactant/wetting agent*

polyoxyl 10 oleyl ether NF *surfactant*

polyoxyl 20 cetostearyl ether NF *surfactant*

polyoxyl 35 castor oil NF *emulsifying agent; surfactant*

polyoxyl 40 hydrogenated castor oil NF *emulsifying agent; surfactant*

polyoxyl 40 stearate USAN, NF *surfactant*

polyoxyl 50 stearate NF *surfactant; emulsifying agent*

polyoxypropylene 15 stearyl ether USAN *solvent*

polyphosphoric acid, sodium salt [see: sodium polyphosphate]

Polypodium vulgare medicinal herb [see: female fern]

Poly-Pred eye drop suspension ℞ *topical ophthalmic corticosteroidal anti-inflammatory; antibiotic* [prednisolone acetate; neomycin sulfate; polymyxin B sulfate] 0.5%•0.35%•10 000 U per mL

polypropylene glycol NF

polyribonucleotide [see: poly I: poly C12U]

polysaccharide-iron complex *hematinic* 150 mg oral

Polysorb Hydrate cream OTC *moisturizer; emollient*

polysorbate 20 USAN, NF, INN *surfactant/wetting agent*

polysorbate 40 USAN, NF, INN *surfactant*

polysorbate 60 USAN, NF, INN *surfactant*

polysorbate 65 USAN, INN *surfactant*

polysorbate 80 USAN, NF, INN *surfactant/wetting agent; viscosity-increasing agent*

polysorbate 85 USAN, INN *surfactant*

Polysporin ointment, powder OTC *topical antibiotic* [polymyxin B sulfate; bacitracin zinc] 10 000•500 U/g

Polysporin ophthalmic ointment OTC *topical ophthalmic antibiotic* [polymyxin B sulfate; bacitracin zinc] 10 000•500 U/g

Polytabs-F chewable tablets ℞ *pediatric vitamin supplement and dental caries preventative* [multiple vitamins; fluoride; folic acid] ± •1•0.3 mg

Polytar shampoo, soap OTC *antiseborrheic; antipsoriatic; antipruritic; antibacterial* [coal tar, pine tar, and juniper tar solution] 2.5%; 1%

Polytar Bath oil OTC *antipsoriatic; antiseborrheic; antipruritic; emollient* [coal tar, pine tar, and juniper tar solution] 25%

polytef USAN *prosthetic aid* [also: politef]

polytetrafluoroethylene (PTFE) [see: polytef]

polythiazide USAN, USP, INN *diuretic; antihypertensive*

Polytrim eye drops ℞ *topical ophthalmic antibiotic* [polymyxin B sulfate; trimethoprim] 10 000 U•1 mg per mL

polyurethane foam USAN *internal bone splint*

polyvalent Crotaline antivenin [see: antivenin (Crotalidae) polyvalent]

polyvalent gas gangrene antitoxin [see: gas gangrene antitoxin, pentavalent]

polyvidone INN *dispersing, suspending and viscosity-increasing agent* [also: povidone]

Poly-Vi-Flor chewable tablets ℞ *pediatric vitamin supplement and dental caries preventative* [multiple vitamins; sodium fluoride; folic acid] ± •0.25• 0.3, ± •0.5•0.3, ± •1•0.3 mg

Poly-Vi-Flor drops ℞ *pediatric vitamin supplement and dental caries preventative* [multiple vitamins; sodium fluoride] ± •0.25, ± •0.5 mg/mL

Poly-Vi-Flor with Iron chewable tablets ℞ *pediatric vitamin/iron supplement and dental caries preventative* [multiple vitamins & minerals; sodium fluoride; iron; folic acid] ± • 0.25•12•0.3, ± •0.5•12•0.3, ± •1• 12•0.3 mg

Poly-Vi-Flor with Iron drops ℞ *pediatric vitamin/iron supplement and dental caries preventative* [multiple vitamins & minerals; sodium fluoride; iron] ± •0.25•10, ± •0.5•10 mg/mL

polyvinyl acetate phthalate NF *coating agent*

polyvinyl alcohol (PVA) USP *ophthalmic moisturizer; viscosity-increasing agent*

polyvinyl chloride, radiopaque *oral radiopaque contrast medium for severe constipation*

polyvinylpyrrolidone [now: povidone]

Poly-Vi-Sol chewable tablets OTC *vitamin supplement* [multiple vitamins; folic acid] ± •0.3 mg

Poly-Vi-Sol drops OTC *vitamin supplement* [multiple vitamins] ±

Poly-Vi-Sol with Iron chewable tablets OTC *vitamin/iron supplement* [multiple vitamins; iron; folic acid] ± •12•0.3 mg

Poly-Vi-Sol with Iron drops OTC *vitamin/iron supplement* [multiple vitamins; iron] ± •10 mg/mL

Poly-Vitamin drops OTC *vitamin supplement* [multiple vitamins] ±

Polyvitamin Fluoride chewable tablets ℞ *pediatric vitamin supplement and dental caries preventative* [multiple vitamins; fluoride; folic acid] ± • 0.5•0.3, ± •1•0.3 mg

Polyvitamin Fluoride drops ℞ *pediatric vitamin supplement and dental caries preventative* [multiple vitamins; fluoride] ± •0.25, ± •0.5 mg/mL

Polyvitamin Fluoride with Iron chewable tablets ℞ *pediatric vitamin/iron supplement and dental caries preventative* [multiple vitamins & minerals; fluoride; iron; folic acid] ± •1• 12•0.3 mg

Poly-Vitamin with Iron drops OTC *vitamin/iron supplement* [multiple vitamins; iron] ± • 10 mg/mL

Polyvitamin with Iron and Fluoride drops ℞ *pediatric vitamin/iron supplement and dental caries preventative* [multiple vitamins; iron; fluoride] ± •10•0.25 mg/mL

Polyvitamins with Fluoride and Iron chewable tablets ℞ *pediatric vitamin/iron supplement and dental caries preventative* [multiple vitamins; fluoride; iron; folic acid] ± •0.5•12•0.3 mg

pomegranate (*Punica granatum***)** seeds and fruit rind *medicinal herb used as an anthelmintic and astringent*

POMP (prednisone, Oncovin, methotrexate, Purinethol) *chemotherapy protocol*

ponalrestat USAN, INN, BAN *aldose reductase inhibitor*

Pondimin tablets (discontinued 1997) ℞ *anorexiant; CNS depressant* [fenfluramine HCl] 20 mg

ponfibrate INN

Ponstel capsules ℞ *nonsteroidal antiinflammatory drug (NSAID); analgesic; for primary dysmenorrhea* [mefenamic acid] 250 mg ⊡ Pronestyl

Pontocaine cream OTC *topical local anesthetic* [tetracaine HCl] 1%

Pontocaine ointment OTC *topical local anesthetic* [tetracaine; menthol] 0.5%•0.5%

Pontocaine HCl Mono-Drop (eye drops) ℞ *topical ophthalmic anesthetic* [tetracaine HCl] 0.5%

Pontocaine HCl ophthalmic ointment (discontinued 1995) ℞ *topical ophthalmic anesthetic* [tetracaine HCl] 0.5%

Pontocaine HCl solution ℞ *nose/throat anesthetic to abolish laryngeal and esophageal reflex* [tetracaine HCl; chlorobutanol] 2%•0.4%

Pontocaine HCl spinal injection, powder for reconstitution ℞ *injectable local anesthetic* [tetracaine HCl] 0.2%, 0.3%, 1%

poplar (*Populus tremuloides***)** bark and buds *medicinal herb used as an antiperiodic, balsamic, febrifuge, and stomachic*

poplar, balsam *medicinal herb* [see: balm of Gilead]

poplar, black *medicinal herb* [see: black poplar]

Po-Pon-S sugar-coated tablets OTC *vitamin/mineral supplement* [multiple vitamins & minerals] ±

Populus balsamifera; P. candicans *medicinal herb* [see: balm of Gilead]

Populus nigra; P. tremula *medicinal herb* [see: black poplar]

Populus tremuloides *medicinal herb* [see: poplar]

poractant alfa BAN *porcine lung extract containing 90% phospholipids*

Porcelana cream OTC *hyperpigmentation bleaching agent* [hydroquinone] 2%

Porcelana with Sunscreen cream OTC *hyperpigmentation bleaching agent; sunscreen* [hydroquinone; padimate O] 2%•2.5%

porcine islet preparation, encapsulated *investigational (orphan) antidiabetic for type 1 patients on immunosuppression*

porfimer sodium USAN, INN *laser light–activated antineoplastic for photodynamic therapy (PDT) of esophageal (orphan) and non-small cell lung cancers; investigational (orphan) for bladder cancer*

porfiromycin USAN, INN, BAN *antibacterial; investigational (Phase III, orphan) antineoplastic for head, neck, and cervical cancers*

Porites spp. *natural material* [see: coral]

porofocon A USAN *hydrophobic contact lens material*

porofocon B USAN *hydrophobic contact lens material*

Portagen powder OTC *enteral nutritional therapy* [lactose-free formula]

porton asparaginase [see: Erwinia L-asparaginase]

posatirelin INN

posedrine [see: benzchlorpropamid]

Posicor tablets (discontinued 1998) ℞ *vasodilator and calcium channel blocker for hypertension and chronic stable angina* [mibefradil dihydrochloride] 50, 100 mg ② Proscar

poskine INN, BAN

posterior pituitary [see: pituitary, posterior]

Posture tablets OTC *calcium supplement* [calcium phosphate, tribasic] 1565.2 mg

Posture-D film-coated tablets OTC *dietary supplement* [calcium phosphate, tribasic; vitamin D] 600 mg•125 IU

Potaba tablets, capsules, Envules (powder for reconstitution), powder ℞ "possibly effective" for scleroderma and other skin diseases, and Peyronie's disease [aminobenzoate potassium] 500 mg; 500 mg; 2 g; 100 g, 1 lb.

Potable Aqua tablets OTC *emergency disinfectant for drinking water* [tetraglycine hydroperiodide (source of iodine)] 16.7% (6.68%)

Potasalan liquid ℞ *potassium supplement* [potassium chloride; alcohol 4%] 20 mEq/15 mL

potash, sulfurated USP *source of sulfides*

potassic saline, lactated NF

potassium *element (K)*

potassium acetate USP *electrolyte replenisher* 2, 4 mEq/mL injection

potassium acid phosphate *urinary acidifier*

potassium alpha-phenoxyethyl penicillin [see: phenethicillin potassium]

potassium alum [see: alum, potassium]

potassium aminobenzoate [see: aminobenzoate potassium]

potassium aspartate [see: L-aspartate potassium]

potassium aspartate & magnesium aspartate USAN *nutrient*

potassium benzoate NF *preservative*

potassium benzyl penicillin [see: penicillin G potassium]

potassium bicarbonate USP *pH buffer; electrolyte replacement*

potassium bitartrate USAN

potassium borate *pH buffer*

potassium canrenoate JAN *aldosterone antagonist* [also: canrenoate potassium; canrenoic acid]

potassium carbonate USP *alkalizing agent*

potassium chloride (KCl) USP *electrolyte replenisher* 600, 750 mg oral; 20, 40 mEq/15 mL oral; 20 mEq/pkt oral; 2, 10, 20, 30, 40, 60, 90 mEq/mL injection

potassium chloride K 42 USAN *radioactive agent*

potassium citrate USP *electrolyte replacement; urinary alkalizer for nephrolithiasis and hypocitruria prevention* (orphan)

potassium clavulanate & amoxicillin [see: amoxicillin]

potassium clavulanate & ticarcillin [see: ticarcillin disodium]

potassium dichloroisocyanurate [see: troclosene potassium]

potassium glucaldrate USAN, INN *antacid*

potassium gluconate USP *electrolyte replenisher* 500, 595 mg oral; 20 mEq/15 mL oral

potassium guaiacolsulfonate USP *expectorant* [also: sulfogaiacol]

potassium hydroxide (KOH) NF *alkalizing agent*

potassium hydroxymethoxybenzenesulfonate hemihydrate [see: potassium guaiacolsulfonate]

potassium iodide USP *antifungal; expectorant; iodine supplement; thyroid agent* 1 g/mL oral

potassium mercuric iodide NF

potassium metabisulfite NF *antioxidant*

potassium metaphosphate NF *buffering agent*

potassium nitrate *tooth desensitizer*

potassium nitrazepate INN

potassium para-aminobenzoate (PAB) [see: aminobenzoate potassium]

potassium penicillin G [see: penicillin G potassium]

potassium perchlorate *radioimaging adjunct*

potassium permanganate USP *topical anti-infective*

potassium phosphate, dibasic USP *calcium regulator; phosphorus replacement; pH buffer*

potassium phosphate, monobasic NF *pH buffer; phosphorus replacement*

potassium sodium tartrate USP *laxative*

potassium sorbate NF *antimicrobial agent*

potassium tetraborate *pH buffer*

potassium thiocyanate NF

potassium-sparing diuretics *a class of diuretic agents that interfere with sodium reabsorption, thus decreasing potassium secretion*

potato, wild; wild sweet potato vine *medicinal herb* [see: wild jalap]

Potentilla anserina; P. canadensis; P. reptans medicinal herb [see: cinquefoil]

Potentilla tormentilla medicinal herb [see: tormentil]

Povidine *ointment, scrub, solution* OTC *broad-spectrum antimicrobial* [povidone-iodine] 10%, 5%, 10%

povidone USAN, USP *dispersing, suspending and viscosity-increasing agent* [also: polyvidone]

povidone I 125 USAN *radioactive agent*

povidone I 131 USAN *radioactive agent*

povidone-iodine USP, BAN *broad-spectrum antimicrobial* 10% topical

powdered cellulose [see: cellulose, powdered]

powdered ipecac [see: ipecac, powdered]

powdered opium [see: opium, powdered]

PowderJect (trademarked device) ℞ *investigational device for the needleless injection of drugs in powder form*

PowerMate *tablets* OTC *vitamin/mineral supplement* [multiple vitamins & minerals] ±

PowerVites *tablets* OTC *vitamin/mineral supplement* [multiple vitamins & minerals; folic acid; biotin] ± • 150 • 25 μg

PPA (phenylpropanolamine) [q.v.]

PPD (purified protein derivative [of tuberculin]) [see: tuberculin]

PPG-15 stearyl ether [now: polyoxypropylene 15 stearyl ether]

PPI-002 *orphan status withdrawn 1996*

PPRT-321 *investigational (Phase II) saw palmetto derivative for benign prostatic hyperplasia*

PR-122 (redox-phenytoin) *orphan status withdrawn 1996*

PR-225 (redox-acyclovir) *orphan status withdrawn 1996*

PR-239 (redox penicillin G) *orphan status withdrawn 1996*

PR-320 (molecusol & carbamazepine) *orphan status withdrawn 1996*

practolol USAN, INN *antiadrenergic (β-receptor)*

prajmalium bitartrate INN, BAN

pralidoxime chloride USAN, USP *cholinesterase reactivator for organophosphate poisoning and anticholinesterase overdose* 600 mg injection ⊠ pyridoxine; pramoxine

pralidoxime iodide USAN, INN *cholinesterase reactivator* ⊠ pyridoxine; pramoxine

pralidoxime mesylate USAN *cholinesterase reactivator* ⊠ pyridoxine; pramoxine

pralmorelin dihydrochloride USAN *growth hormone secretagogue*

PrameGel *gel* OTC *topical local anesthetic* [pramoxine HCl; menthol] 1% • 0.5%

Pramet FA *controlled-release Filmtabs (film-coated tablets) (discontinued 1995)* ℞ *prenatal vitamin/calcium/iron supplement* [multiple vitamins; calcium; iron; folic acid] ± •250•60•1 mg

Pramidin nasal spray (commercially available in Italy) ℞ *investigational antiemetic for chemotherapy* [metoclopramide HCl]

Pramilet FA Filmtabs (film-coated tablets) ℞ *prenatal vitamin/mineral/ calcium/iron supplement* [multiple vitamins & minerals; calcium; iron; folic acid] ± •250•40•1 mg

pramipexole USAN, INN *dopamine agonist; antiparkinsonian; investigational for depression and schizophrenia*

pramipexole dihydrochloride USAN *dopamine agonist; antiparkinsonian; investigational for depression and schizophrenia*

pramiracetam INN *cognition adjuvant* [also: pramiracetam HCl]

pramiracetam HCl USAN *cognition adjuvant* [also: pramiracetam]

pramiracetam sulfate USAN *cognition adjuvant; orphan status withdrawn 1996*

pramiverine INN, BAN

pramlintide USAN *investigational (Phase III) antidiabetic for type 1 and type 2 diabetes mellitus*

pramocaine INN *topical anesthetic* [also: pramoxine HCl; pramoxine]

pramocaine HCl [see: pramoxine HCl]

Pramosone cream, lotion, ointment ℞ *topical corticosteroidal anti-inflammatory; local anesthetic* [hydrocortisone acetate; pramoxine] 1%•1%, 2.5%•1%; 2.5%•1%; 2.5%•1% ⓦ pramoxine

pramoxine BAN *topical local anesthetic* [also: pramoxine HCl; pramocaine] ⓦ pralidoxime; Pramosone

Pramoxine HC anorectal aerosol foam ℞ *topical corticosteroidal anti-inflammatory; local anesthetic* [hydrocortisone acetate; pramoxine HCl] 1%•1%

pramoxine HCl USP *topical local anesthetic* [also: pramocaine; pramoxine]

prampine INN, BAN

Prandase ⓒⒶⓃ (U.S. product: Precose) tablets ℞ *alpha-glucosidase inhibitor*

for type 2 diabetes mellitus [acarbose] 50, 100 mg

Prandin tablets ℞ *oral antidiabetic agent that stimulates release of insulin from the pancreas in type 2 diabetes mellitus* [repaglinide] 0.5, 1, 2 mg

pranidipine INN

pranlukast INN, BAN *investigational treatment for asthma*

pranolium chloride USAN, INN *antiarrhythmic*

pranoprofen INN

pranosal INN

praseodymium *element (Pr)*

prasterone INN

Pravachol tablets ℞ *HMG-CoA reductase inhibitor for hyperlipidemia, atherosclerosis, coronary procedures, and recurrent myocardial infarctions* [pravastatin sodium] 10, 20, 40 mg ⓦ Primacor

pravadoline INN *analgesic* [also: pravadoline maleate]

pravadoline maleate USAN *analgesic* [also: pravadoline]

pravastatin INN, BAN *HMG-CoA reductase inhibitor for hyperlipidemia, atherosclerosis, coronary procedures, and recurrent myocardial infarctions* [also: pravastatin sodium]

pravastatin sodium USAN, JAN *HMG-CoA reductase inhibitor for hyperlipidemia, atherosclerosis, coronary procedures, and recurrent myocardial infarctions* [also: pravastatin]

Prax lotion, cream OTC *topical local anesthetic* [pramoxine HCl] 1%

praxadine INN

prazepam USAN, USP, INN *sedative; anxiolytic* 5 mg oral ⓦ prazepine; prazosin

prazepine INN ⓦ prazepam

praziquantel USAN, USP, INN, BAN *anthelmintic for schistosomiasis (flukes)*

prazitone INN, BAN

prazocillin INN

prazosin INN, BAN *antihypertensive; α_1-adrenergic blocker* [also: prazosin HCl] ⓦ prazepam

prazosin HCl USAN, USP, JAN *antihypertensive; α₁-adrenergic blocker* [also: prazosin] 1, 2, 5 mg oral

Pre-Attain liquid OTC *enteral nutritional therapy* [lactose-free formula]

precatory bean *(Abrus precatorius)* plant *medicinal herb for eye inflammation, hastening labor, and stimulating abortion; not generally regarded as safe and effective as it is highly toxic and ingestion may be fatal*

precipitated calcium carbonate JAN *antacid; calcium replenisher* [also: calcium carbonate]

precipitated chalk [see: calcium carbonate]

precipitated sulfur [see: sulfur, precipitated]

Precision High Nitrogen Diet powder OTC *enteral nutritional therapy* [lactose-free formula]

Precision LR Diet powder OTC *enteral nutritional therapy* [lactose-free formula]

preclamol INN

Precose tablets ℞ *alpha-glucosidase inhibitor for type 2 diabetes mellitus* [acarbose] 25, 50, 100 mg

Pred Mild; Pred Forte eye drop suspension ℞ *topical ophthalmic corticosteroidal anti-inflammatory* [prednisolone acetate] 0.12%; 1%

Predaject-50 IM injection (discontinued 1996) ℞ *corticosteroid; anti-inflammatory* [prednisolone acetate] 50 mg/mL

Predalone 50 IM injection ℞ *corticosteroid; anti-inflammatory* [prednisolone acetate] 50 mg/mL

Predcor-50 IM injection ℞ *corticosteroid; anti-inflammatory* [prednisolone acetate] 50 mg/mL

Pred-G eye drop suspension ℞ *topical ophthalmic corticosteroidal anti-inflammatory; antibiotic* [prednisolone acetate; gentamicin sulfate] 1%•0.3%

Pred-G S.O.P. ophthalmic ointment ℞ *ophthalmic topical corticosteroidal anti-inflammatory; antibiotic* [prednisolone acetate; gentamicin sulfate; chlorobutanol] 0.6%•0.3%•0.5%

prednazate USAN, INN *anti-inflammatory*

prednazoline INN

prednicarbate USAN, INN *corticosteroid; anti-inflammatory*

Prednicen-M tablets ℞ *corticosteroid; anti-inflammatory; immunosuppressant* [prednisone] 5 mg

prednimustine USAN, INN *antineoplastic; investigational for malignant non-Hodgkin's lymphomas; orphan status withdrawn 1998*

Prednisol TBA intra-articular, intra-lesional, or soft tissue injection ℞ *corticosteroid; anti-inflammatory* [prednisolone tebutate] 20 mg/mL

prednisolamate INN, BAN

prednisolone USP, INN *corticosteroidal anti-inflammatory* 5 mg oral ⊘ prednisone

prednisolone acetate USP, BAN *corticosteroidal anti-inflammatory* 1% eye drops; 25, 50 mg/mL injection

prednisolone hemisuccinate USP *corticosteroidal anti-inflammatory*

prednisolone sodium phosphate USP *corticosteroidal anti-inflammatory* 0.125%, 1% eye drops

prednisolone sodium succinate USP *corticosteroidal anti-inflammatory*

prednisolone steaglate INN, BAN *corticosteroidal anti-inflammatory*

prednisolone tebutate USP *corticosteroidal anti-inflammatory* 20 mg/mL injection

prednisone USP, INN *corticosteroid; anti-inflammatory; immunosuppressant* 1, 5, 20 mg oral ⊘ prednisolone

prednival USAN *corticosteroid; anti-inflammatory*

prednylidene INN, BAN

prefenamate INN

Prefill (dosage form) *prefilled applicator*

Preflex Daily Cleaner Especially for Sensitive Eyes solution OTC *surfactant cleaning solution for soft contact lenses*

Prefrin Liquifilm eye drops OTC *topical ophthalmic decongestant* [phenylephrine HCl] 0.12%

pregabalin USAN *gabamimetic anticonvulsant*

pregelatinized starch [see: starch, pregelatinized]

Pregestimil powder OTC *hypoallergenic infant food for severe malabsorption disorders* [enzymatically hydrolyzed protein formula]

pregnandiol JAN

pregneninolone [see: ethisterone]

pregnenolone INN *non-hormonal sterol derivative* [also: pregnenolone succinate]

pregnenolone succinate USAN *non-hormonal sterol derivative* [also: pregnenolone]

Pregnosis slide test for home use OTC *in vitro diagnostic aid for urine pregnancy test* [latex agglutination test]

Pregnyl powder for IM injection R *hormone for prepubertal cryptorchidism and hypogonadism; ovulation stimulant* [chorionic gonadotropin] 1000 U/mL

Pre-H Cal tablets (discontinued 1995) R *vitamin/calcium/iron supplement* [multiple vitamins; calcium; iron; folic acid] ±•47.5•51.7•0.5 mg

Prehist sustained-release capsules R *decongestant; antihistamine* [phenylephrine HCl; chlorpheniramine maleate] 20•8 mg

Prehist D sustained-release tablets, sustained-release capsules R *decongestant; antihistamine; anticholinergic* [phenylephrine HCl; chlorpheniramine maleate; methscopolamine nitrate] 20•8•2.5 mg

Prelone syrup R *corticosteroid; anti-inflammatory* [prednisolone; alcohol 5%] 5, 15 mg/5 mL

Prelu-2 timed-release capsules R *anorexiant; CNS stimulant* [phendimetrazine tartrate] 105 mg

premafloxacin USAN, INN *veterinary antibacterial*

Premarin tablets R *estrogen replacement therapy for postmenopausal disorders; palliative therapy for prostatic and breast cancer* [conjugated estrogens] 0.3, 0.625, 0.9, 1.25, 2.5 mg

Premarin vaginal cream R *estrogen replacement for postmenopausal atrophic vaginitis* [conjugated estrogens] 0.625 mg/g

Premarin Intravenous IV or IM injection R *treatment of abnormal uterine bleeding due to hormonal imbalance* [conjugated estrogens] 25 mg

Premarin with Methyltestosterone tablets R *estrogen/androgen for menopausal vasomotor symptoms* [conjugated estrogens; methyltestosterone] 0.625•5, 1.25•10 mg

premazepam INN, BAN

Premphase tablets (28 per package, 14 of each phase) R *hormone replacement therapy for postmenopausal disorders* [Phase 1: conjugated estrogens; Phase 2: conjugated estrogens; medroxyprogesterone acetate] 0.625 mg; 0.625•5 mg

Prempro tablets R *hormone replacement therapy for postmenopausal disorders* [conjugated estrogens; medroxyprogesterone acetate] 0.625•2.5, 0.625•5 mg

Prempro tablets (the single-phase product replaced the two-phase product in 1996) [Phase 1: conjugated estrogens; Phase 2: medroxyprogesterone acetate] 0.625 mg; 2.5 mg

Prēmsyn PMS caplets OTC *analgesic; antipyretic; diuretic; antihistaminic sleep aid* [acetaminophen; pamabrom; pyrilamine maleate] 500•25•15 mg

prenalterol INN, BAN *adrenergic* [also: prenalterol HCl]

prenalterol HCl USAN *adrenergic* [also: prenalterol]

Prenatal H.P. tablets R *vitamin/calcium/iron supplement* [multiple vitamins; calcium; iron; folic acid] ±• 50•30•0.8 mg

Prenatal Maternal tablets R *vitamin/mineral/calcium/iron supplement* [multiple vitamins & minerals; calcium; iron; folic acid; biotin] ±•250•60• 1•0.03 mg

Prenatal MR 90 film-coated delayed-release tablets R *vitamin/calcium/iron*

supplement [multiple vitamins; calcium; iron; folic acid] ± •250•90•1 mg

Prenatal One film-coated tablets (discontinued 1995) ℞ *vitamin/calcium/ iron supplement* [multiple vitamins; calcium; iron; folic acid] ± •200• 65•1 mg

Prenatal Plus; Prenatal Plus Improved tablets ℞ *vitamin/calcium/ iron supplement* [multiple vitamins; calcium; iron; folic acid] ± •200• 65•1 mg

Prenatal Plus Iron tablets ℞ *vitamin/ calcium/iron supplement* [multiple vitamins; calcium; iron; folic acid] ± •200•27•1 mg

Prenatal Plus with Betacarotene tablets ℞ *vitamin/calcium/iron supplement* [multiple vitamins; calcium; iron; folic acid] ± •200•65•1 mg

Prenatal Rx tablets ℞ *vitamin/calcium/ iron supplement* [multiple vitamins; calcium; iron; folic acid] ± •175• 29.5•1 mg

Prenatal Rx with Betacarotene tablets ℞ *vitamin/calcium/iron supplement* [multiple vitamins; calcium; iron; folic acid; biotin] ± •200•60• 1•0.03 mg

Prenatal with Folic Acid tablets OTC *vitamin/calcium/iron supplement* [multiple vitamins; calcium; iron; folic acid] ± •200•60•0.8 mg

Prenatal Z film-coated delayed-release tablets ℞ *vitamin/calcium/iron supplement* [multiple vitamins; calcium; iron; folic acid] ± •300•65•1 mg

Prenatal-1 + Iron tablets ℞ *vitamin/ calcium/iron supplement* [multiple vitamins; calcium; iron; folic acid] ± •200•65•1 mg

Prenatal-S tablets OTC *vitamin/calcium/ iron supplement* [multiple vitamins; calcium; iron; folic acid] ± •200• 60•0.8 mg

Prenate 90; Prenate Ultra film-coated delayed-release tablets ℞ *vitamin/calcium/iron supplement* [multiple vitamins; calcium; iron; folic acid] ± •250•90•1 mg; ± •200•90•1 mg

Prenavite tablets OTC *vitamin/calcium/ iron supplement* [multiple vitamins; calcium; iron; folic acid] ± •200• 60•0.8 mg

prenisteine INN

prenoverine INN

prenoxdiazine INN

prenylamine USAN, INN *coronary vasodilator*

Preparation H anorectal cream, anorectal ointment OTC *temporary relief of hemorrhoidal symptoms* [shark liver oil; phenylephrine HCl] 3%•0.25%

Preparation H cleansing tissues OTC *moisturizer and cleanser for external rectal/vaginal areas* [propylene glycol]

Preparation H rectal suppositories OTC *temporary relief of hemorrhoidal symptoms* [shark liver oil] 3%

Preparation H Cooling Gel ⊛ OTC *temporary relief of hemorrhoidal symptoms* [phenylephrine HCl; hamamelis water] 0.25%•50%

prepared chalk [see: calcium carbonate]

Prepcat oral suspension ℞ *radiopaque contrast medium for gastrointestinal imaging* [barium sulfate] 1.5%

Pre-Pen solution for dermal scratch test ℞ *diagnostic aid for penicillin hypersensitivity* [benzylpenicilloyl polylysine] 0.25 mL

Pre-Pen/MDM solution for dermal scratch test ℞ *investigational (orphan) for penicillin hypersensitivity assessment* [benzylpenicillin]

Prepidil gel ℞ *prostaglandin for cervical ripening at term* [dinoprostone] 0.5 mg

Prepulsid ⊛ (U.S. product: Propulsid) tablets ℞ *treatment for nocturnal heartburn due to gastroesophageal reflux disease (GERD)* [cisapride] 10, 20 mg

Presalin tablets (discontinued 1995) OTC *analgesic; antipyretic; anti-inflammatory; antacid* [acetaminophen; aspirin; salicylamide; aluminum hydroxide] 120•260•120•100 mg

pretamazium iodide INN, BAN

prethcamide

prethrombin [see: prothrombin complex, activated]

pretiadil INN

Pretts Diet-Aid chewable tablets OTC *diet aid* [sodium carboxymethylcellulose; alginic acid; sodium bicarbonate] 100•200•70 mg

Pretty Feet & Hands cream OTC *moisturizer; emollient*

Pretz solution OTC *nasal moisturizer* [sodium chloride (saline solution)] 0.6%

Pretz Irrigating solution OTC *for postoperative irrigation* [sodium chloride (saline solution); glycerin; eriodictyon] 0.75%

Pretz Moisturizing nose drops OTC *nasal moisturizer* [sodium chloride (saline solution); glycerin; eriodictyon] 0.75%

Pretz-D nasal spray OTC *nasal decongestant and moisturizer* [ephedrine sulfate] 0.25%

PretzPak ointment OTC *antimicrobial postoperative nasal pack* [benzyl alcohol; polyethylene glycol; carboxymethylcellulose; urea; allantoin]

Prevacid delayed-release capsules ℞ *proton pump inhibitor for gastric and duodenal ulcers and other gastroesophageal disorders* [lansoprazole] 15, 30 mg

Prevalite powder for oral suspension ℞ *cholesterol-lowering antihyperlipidemic; also used for biliary obstruction* [cholestyramine resin] 4 g/dose

Prevatac ℞ *investigational (Phase II/III) agent to prevent recurrence of prostate cancer* [exisulind]

Preven emergency contraceptive kit (4 film-coated tablets + pregnancy test) ℞ *for "morning after" contraception* [ethinyl estradiol; levonorgestrel] 0.05•0.25 mg ② Preveon

Prevent-X powder for oral solution OTC *dietary supplement* [multiple vitamins & minerals; multiple amino acids] ≛

Preveon ℞ *investigational (Phase III) agent for advanced HIV infection; investigational (Phase III) treatment for chronic hepatitis B virus (HBV) infections* [adefovir dipivoxil] ② Preven

PreviDent gel (for self-application) ℞ *topical dental caries preventative* [sodium fluoride] 1.1%

PreviDent Rinse oral solution ℞ *topical dental caries preventative* [sodium fluoride] 0.2%

Prevpac three-drug daily pack ℞ *triple therapy for H. pylori: an antisecretory and two antibiotics* [lansoprazole; clarithromycin; amoxicillin] 2 × 30 mg; 2 × 500 mg; 4 × 500 mg

PreVue B. *burgdorferi* Antibody Detection Assay reagent kit for professional use *in vitro diagnostic aid for Lyme disease*

prezatide copper acetate USAN, INN *immunomodulator; investigational (Phase II) wound-healing gel for venous leg ulcers*

pribecaine INN

prickly ash (*Xanthoxylum americanum; X. fraxineum*) bark *medicinal herb for fever, mouth sores, poor circulation, ulcers, and wounds*

prickly juniper (*Juniperus oxycedrus*) *medicinal herb* [see: juniper]

prickly pear *medicinal herb* [see: nopal]

pride of China (*Melia azedarach*) root bark and fruit *medicinal herb used as an anthelmintic, astringent, bitter tonic, emetic, emmenagogue, and purgative*

pride weed *medicinal herb* [see: fleabane; horseweed]

pridefine INN *antidepressant* [also: pridefine HCl]

pridefine HCl USAN *antidepressant* [also: pridefine]

prideperone INN

pridinol INN

priest's crown *medicinal herb* [see: dandelion]

prifelone USAN, INN *dermatologic antiinflammatory*

prifinium bromide INN

Priftin film-coated tablets ℞ *antibacterial for tuberculosis (orphan); investiga-*

tional (orphan) for AIDS-related Myco-bacterium avium complex (MAC) [rifa-pentine] 150 mg

prifuroline INN

priliximab USAN, INN *monoclonal anti-body to treat autoimmune lymphoprolif-erative diseases and in organ transplants*

prilocaine USAN, INN, BAN *topical local anesthetic*

prilocaine HCl USAN, USP *topical local anesthetic* [also: propitocaine HCl]

Prilosec delayed-release capsules ℞ *proton pump inhibitor for gastric and duodenal ulcers and other gastroesopha-geal disorders* [omeprazole] 10, 20 mg ⌸ Prozac

primachine phosphate [see: prima-quine phosphate]

Primacor IV infusion ℞ *vasodilator for congestive heart failure* [milrinone lac-tate] 0.2, 1 mg/mL ⌸ Pravachol

Primacor in 5% Dextrose IV infu-sion ℞ *vasodilator for congestive heart failure* [milrinone lactate; dextrose] 200 μg/mL; 5% ⌸ Pravachol

Primaderm-B anorectal ointment (discontinued 1995) OTC *topical anesthetic; astringent* [benzocaine; zinc oxide; cod liver oil]

primaperone INN

primaquine INN *antimalarial* [also: primaquine phosphate]

primaquine phosphate USP *anti-malarial; prevention of malarial relapse* [also: primaquine] 26.3 mg oral

primaquine phosphate & clinda-mycin HCl *investigational (orphan) for AIDS-associated Pneumocystis carinii pneumonia*

Primatene tablets (discontinued 1998) OTC *antiasthmatic; bronchodila-tor; decongestant; sedative* [theophyl-line; ephedrine HCl; phenobarbital] 130•24•7.5 mg

Primatene Dual Action tablets OTC *antiasthmatic; bronchodilator; decon-gestant; expectorant* [theophylline; ephedrine HCl; guaifenesin] 60•12.5•100 mg

Primatene Mist inhalation aerosol OTC *sympathomimetic bronchodilator* [epinephrine] 0.2 mg/dose

Primatene Mist Suspension inhala-tion aerosol (discontinued 1999) OTC *sympathomimetic bronchodilator* [epinephrine bitartrate] 0.3 mg/dose

Primatuss Cough Mixture 4 liquid OTC *antitussive; antihistamine* [dextro-methorphan hydrobromide; chlor-pheniramine maleate; alcohol 10%] 15•2 mg/5 mL

Primatuss Cough Mixture 4D liquid OTC *antitussive; decongestant; expecto-rant* [dextromethorphan hydrobro-mide; pseudoephedrine HCl; guaifene-sin; alcohol 10%] 10•20•67 mg/5 mL

Primaxin I.M. powder for injection ℞ *carbapenem antibiotic* [imipenem; cilas-tatin sodium] 500•500, 750•750 mg

Primaxin I.V. powder for injection ℞ *carbapenem antibiotic* [imipenem; cilas-tatin sodium] 250•250, 500•500 mg

primidolol USAN, INN *antihypertensive; antianginal; antiarrhythmic*

primidone USP, INN, BAN *anticonvul-sant for grand mal, psychomotor, or focal epileptic seizures* 250 mg oral

Primobolan *brand name for metheno-lone acetate, a European anabolic ste-roid abused as a street drug*

Primobolan Depot *brand name for methenolone enanthate, a European anabolic steroid abused as a street drug*

primycin INN

prince's pine *medicinal herb* [see: pip-sissewa]

Principen capsules, powder for oral suspension ℞ *aminopenicillin antibi-otic* [ampicillin] 250, 500 mg; 125, 250 mg/5 mL

Principen with Probenecid capsules ℞ *antibiotic for Neisseria gonorrhoeae* [ampicillin trihydrate; probenecid]

Prinivil tablets ℞ *antihypertensive; angio-tensin-converting enzyme (ACE) inhibi-tor* [lisinopril] 2.5, 5, 10, 20, 40 mg

prinodolol [see: pindolol]

prinomide INN *antirheumatic* [also: pri-nomide tromethamine]

prinomide tromethamine USAN *antirheumatic* [also: prinomide]

prinoxodan USAN, INN *cardiotonic*

Prinzide tablets ℞ *antihypertensive; angiotensin-converting enzyme (ACE) inhibitor; diuretic* [hydrochlorothiazide; lisinopril] 12.5•10 mg

Prinzide 12.5; Prinzide 25 tablets ℞ *antihypertensive; angiotensin-converting enzyme (ACE) inhibitor; diuretic* [hydrochlorothiazide; lisinopril] 12.5•20 mg; 25•20 mg

Priorix (commercially available in Europe) ℞ *investigational vaccine* [measles, mumps, and rubella virus vaccine, live]

Priscoline HCl IV injection ℞ *peripheral vasodilator for neonatal persistent pulmonary hypertension* [tolazoline HCl] 25 mg/mL ⧉ Apresoline

pristinamycin INN, BAN

privet, Egyptian *medicinal herb* [see: henna (*Lawsonia*)]

Privine nasal spray, nose drops OTC *nasal decongestant* [naphazoline HCl] 0.05%

prizidilol INN, BAN *antihypertensive* [also: prizidilol HCl]

prizidilol HCl USAN *antihypertensive* [also: prizidilol]

Pro Skin capsules OTC *vitamin/zinc supplement* [vitamins A, B_5, C, and E; zinc] 6250 IU•10 mg•100 mg•100 IU•10 mg

PRO-2000 gel ℞ *investigational (Phase I) topical microbicide that functions as a chemical barrier to prevent HIV infection and sexually transmitted diseases*

Pro-50 injection (discontinued 1997) ℞ *antihistamine; sedative; antiemetic; motion sickness relief* [promethazine HCl] 50 mg/mL

PRO-542 *investigational (Phase I/II) recombinant fusion protein for HIV and AIDS*

proadifen INN *non-specific synergist* [also: proadifen HCl]

proadifen HCl USAN *non-specific synergist* [also: proadifen]

ProAmatine tablets ℞ *vasopressor for orthostatic hypotension (orphan)* [midodrine HCl] 2.5, 5 mg

proanthocyanidins *natural free radical scavenger found in grape seed extract and pine bark extract* [also: procyanidolic oligomers (PCOs); procyanidins]

Probalan tablets (discontinued 1997) ℞ *uricosuric for gout* [probenecid] 500 mg

Probampacin powder for oral suspension (discontinued 1998) ℞ *antibiotic for Neisseria gonorrhoeae* [ampicillin; probenecid] 3.5•1 g

Pro-Banthīne tablets ℞ *peptic ulcer treatment adjunct; antispasmodic; antisecretory* [propantheline bromide] 7.5, 15 mg

probarbital sodium NF, INN

Probax gel OTC *relief from minor oral irritations* [propolis] 2%

Probec-T tablets OTC *vitamin supplement* [multiple B vitamins; vitamin C] ≟•600 mg

Proben-C tablets (discontinued 1997) ℞ *treatment for frequent, recurrent attacks of gouty arthritis* [probenecid; colchicine] 500•0.5 mg

probenecid USP, INN, BAN *uricosuric for gout* 500 mg oral

probenecid & colchicine *treatment for frequent, recurrent attacks of gouty arthritis*

probicromil calcium USAN *prophylactic antiallergic* [also: ambicromil]

Pro-Bionate capsules, powder OTC *dietary supplement; fever blister treatment; not generally regarded as safe and effective as an antidiarrheal* [Lactobacillus acidophilus] 2 billion U; 2 billion U/g

probucol USAN, USP, INN *antihyperlipidemic; investigational (Phase II) antiviral for HIV and AIDS*

probutate USAN *combining name for radicals or groups* [also: buteprate]

procainamide INN *antiarrhythmic* [also: procainamide HCl]

procainamide HCl USP *antiarrhythmic* [also: procainamide] 250, 375, 500,

750 mg oral; 100, 500 mg/mL injection

procaine INN *local anesthetic* [also: procaine borate] ⊠ Procan

procaine borate NF *local anesthetic* [also: procaine] ⊠ Procan

procaine HCl USP *injectable local anesthetic; sometimes used as a treatment for the overall effects of aging, such as alopecia, arthritis, cerebral atherosclerosis, hypertension, progressive dementia, and sexual dysfunction* 1%, 2% ⊠ Procan

procaine penicillin BAN *bactericidal antibiotic* [also: penicillin G procaine] ⊠ Procan

ProcalAmine IV infusion ℞ *peripheral parenteral nutrition* [multiple essential and nonessential amino acids; electrolytes]

Pro-Cal-Sof capsules OTC *stool softener* [docusate calcium] 240 mg

Procan SR sustained-release tablets (replaced by Procanbid in 1996) ℞ *antiarrhythmic* [procainamide HCl] 250, 500, 750, 1000 mg ⊠ procaine

Procanbid extended-release film-coated tablets ℞ *twice-daily antiarrhythmic* [procainamide HCl] 500, 1000 mg

procarbazine INN *antineoplastic* [also: procarbazine HCl] ⊠ dacarbazine

procarbazine HCl USAN, USP *antineoplastic for Hodgkin's disease* [also: procarbazine]

Procardia capsules ℞ *antianginal; antihypertensive; calcium channel blocker* [nifedipine] 10, 20 mg

Procardia XL film-coated sustained-release tablets ℞ *antianginal; antihypertensive; calcium channel blocker* [nifedipine] 30, 60, 90 mg

procaterol INN, BAN *bronchodilator* [also: procaterol HCl]

procaterol HCl USAN *bronchodilator* [also: procaterol]

prochlorperazine USP, INN *phenothiazine antipsychotic; antiemetic*

prochlorperazine bimaleate *phenothiazine antipsychotic; antiemetic*

prochlorperazine edisylate USP *phenothiazine antipsychotic; antiemetic* 5 mg/mL injection

prochlorperazine ethanedisulfonate [see: prochlorperazine edisylate]

prochlorperazine maleate USP *phenothiazine antipsychotic; antiemetic* 5, 10, 25 mg oral

prochlorperazine mesylate *phenothiazine antipsychotic; antiemetic*

procinolol INN

procinonide USAN, INN *adrenocortical steroid*

proclonol USAN, INN *anthelmintic; antifungal*

procodazole INN

proconvertin [see: factor VII]

Procort cream, spray OTC *topical corticosteroidal anti-inflammatory* [hydrocortisone] 1%

Procrit IV or subcu injection ℞ *stimulates RBC production; for anemia of chronic renal failure, HIV, or chemotherapy (orphan)* [epoetin alfa] 2000, 3000, 4000, 10 000, 20 000 U/mL

Proctocort anorectal cream, suppositories ℞ *topical corticosteroidal anti-inflammatory* [hydrocortisone] 1%; 30 mg

ProctoCream-HC anorectal cream ℞ *topical corticosteroidal anti-inflammatory* [hydrocortisone acetate] 2.5%

ProctoCream-HC anorectal cream ℞ *topical corticosteroidal anti-inflammatory; local anesthetic* [hydrocortisone acetate; pramoxine HCl] 1%•1%

ProctoFoam NS anorectal aerosol foam OTC *topical local anesthetic* [pramoxine HCl] 1%

Proctofoam-HC anorectal aerosol foam ℞ *topical corticosteroidal anti-inflammatory; local anesthetic* [hydrocortisone acetate; pramoxine HCl] 1%•1%

Pro-Cute lotion OTC *moisturizer; emollient*

procyanidolic oligomers (PCOs) *natural free radical scavenger found in grape seed extract and pine bark extract* [also: proanthocyanidins; procyanidins]

ProCycle Gold tablets OTC *vitamin/ mineral/iron supplement* [multiple vitamins & minerals; iron; folic acid; biotin] ± •3•0.067• ± mg

procyclidine HCl USP *anticholinergic; antiparkinsonian; skeletal muscle relaxant* [also: procyclidine]

procymate INN

Procysteine ℞ *investigational (Phase II) immunomodulator for AIDS; investigational (orphan) for amyotrophic lateral sclerosis; investigational (Phase III, orphan) for adult respiratory distress syndrome (ARDS trials discontinued 1998)* [oxothiazolidine carboxylate]

prodeconium bromide INN

Proderm Topical dressing OTC *dressing for decubitus ulcers* [castor oil; peruvian balsam] 650•72.5 mg/0.82 mL

prodilidine INN *analgesic* [also: prodilidine HCl]

prodilidine HCl USAN *analgesic* [also: prodilidine]

prodipine INN

Prodium tablets OTC *urinary analgesic* [phenazopyridine HCl] 95 mg

prodolic acid USAN, INN *anti-inflammatory*

pro-drugs *a class of agents which metabolize into a therapeutic or more potent form in the body*

profadol INN *analgesic* [also: profadol HCl]

profadol HCl USAN *analgesic* [also: profadol]

Profasi powder for IM injection ℞ *hormone for prepubertal cryptorchidism and hypogonadism; ovulation stimulant* [chorionic gonadotropin] 500, 1000 U/mL

Profen II; Profen LA timed-release tablets ℞ *decongestant; expectorant* [phenylpropanolamine HCl; guaifenesin] 37.5•600 mg; 75•600 mg

Profen II DM timed-release tablets ℞ *decongestant; expectorant; antitussive* [phenylpropanolamine HCl; guaifenesin; dextromethorphan hydrobromide] 37.5•600•30 mg

Profenal Drop-Tainers (eye drops) ℞ *ocular nonsteroidal anti-inflammatory drug (NSAID); intraoperative miosis inhibitor* [suprofen] 1%

profenamine INN *antiparkinsonian* [also: ethopropazine HCl; ethopropazine]

profenamine HCl [see: ethopropazine HCl]

profexalone INN

Profiber liquid OTC *enteral nutritional therapy* [lactose-free formula]

Profilate HP IV injection (discontinued 1997) ℞ *antihemophilic to correct coagulation deficiency* [antihemophilic factor VIII:C in heptane]

Profilate OSD IV injection (discontinued 1996) ℞ *antihemophilic to correct coagulation deficiency* [antihemophilic factor VIII:C] ±

Profilnine Heat-Treated IV suspension (discontinued 1995) ℞ *anticoagulant to correct factor IX deficiency (hemophilia B; Christmas disease)* [coagulation factor IX complex, heat treated]

Profilnine SD powder for IV injection ℞ *anticoagulant to correct factor IX deficiency (hemophilia B; Christmas disease)* [coagulation factors II, VII, IX, and X, solvent/detergent treated]

proflavine INN [also: proflavine dihydrochloride]

proflavine dihydrochloride NF [also: proflavine]

proflavine sulfate NF

proflazepam INN

ProFree/GP Weekly Enzymatic Cleaner tablets OTC *enzymatic cleaner for rigid gas permeable contact lenses* [papain]

progabide USAN, INN *anticonvulsant; muscle relaxant*

Pro-gesic liquid (discontinued 1995) OTC *topical analgesic* [trolamine salicylate] 10%

Progestasert IUD ℞ *intrauterine contraceptive* [progesterone] 38 mg

progesterone USP, INN *progestin; intrauterine contraceptive; investigational* (*orphan*) *for in vitro fertilization and embryo transfer* 50 mg/mL injection

progestins *a class of sex hormones that cause a sloughing of the endometrial lining, also used as a hormonal antineoplastic*

proglumetacin INN

proglumide USAN, INN, BAN, JAN *anticholinergic*

Proglycem capsules, oral suspension ℞ *emergency antihypertensive; vasodilator; glucose-elevating agent* [diazoxide] 50 mg; 50 mg/mL

Prograf capsules ℞ *liver and kidney transplant rejection preventative; investigational preventative for other transplant rejection* [tacrolimus] 1, 5 mg

Prograf IV infusion ℞ *liver transplant rejection preventative* [tacrolimus] 5 mg/mL

proguanil INN, BAN, DCF *antimalarial; dihydrofolate reductase inhibitor* [also: chloroguanide HCl]

proguanil HCl [see: chloroguanide HCl]

ProHance injection ℞ *MRI contrast media for brain and spine imaging* [gadoteridol] 279.3 mg/mL

proheptazine INN

ProHIBiT IM injection ℞ *Haemophilus influenzae type b (HIB) vaccine* [Hemophilus b conjugate vaccine] 0.5 mL

proinsulin human USAN *antidiabetic*

Prolastin inhalation aerosol ℞ *investigational (Phase II) delivery form* [alpha$_1$-proteinase inhibitor]

Prolastin IV injection ℞ *chronic replacement therapy for hereditary alpha$_1$-proteinase inhibitor deficiency, which leads to progressive panacinar emphysema (orphan)* [alpha$_1$-proteinase inhibitor] 20 mg/mL

ProLease (trademarked delivery system) *sustained-release injection*

Proleukin powder for IV infusion ℞ *antineoplastic for metastatic melanoma and renal cell carcinoma (orphan); investigational (Phase II, orphan) agent for immunodeficiency diseases; investigational (Phase III, orphan) for acute*

myelogenous leukemia (AML) [aldesleukin] 18 million IU/mL

proligestone INN

proline (L-proline) USAN, USP, INN *nonessential amino acid; symbols: Pro, P* ⒫ Prolene

prolintane INN *antidepressant* [also: prolintane HCl]

prolintane HCl USAN *antidepressant* [also: prolintane]

Prolixin tablets, elixir, oral concentrate, IM injection ℞ *conventional (typical) antipsychotic* [fluphenazine HCl] 1, 2.5, 5, 10 mg; 2.5 mg/5 mL; 5 mg/mL; 2.5 mg/mL

Prolixin Decanoate subcu or IM injection, Unimatic (prefilled) syringe ℞ *conventional (typical) antipsychotic* [fluphenazine decanoate] 25 mg/mL

Prolixin Enanthate subcu or IM injection ℞ *conventional (typical) antipsychotic* [fluphenazine enanthate] 25 mg/mL

prolonium iodide INN

Proloprim tablets ℞ *anti-infective; antibacterial* [trimethoprim] 100, 200 mg

ProMACE (prednisone, methotrexate [with leucovorin rescue], Adriamycin, cyclophosphamide, etoposide) *chemotherapy protocol*

ProMACE/cytaBOM (ProMACE [above], cytarabine, bleomycin, Oncovin, mitoxantrone) *chemotherapy protocol*

ProMACE/MOPP (full course of ProMACE, followed by MOPP) *chemotherapy protocol*

ProMaxx-100 extended release ℞ *investigational LH-RH analog for prostate cancer*

promazine INN *phenothiazine antipsychotic* [also: promazine HCl] ⒫ Promethazine

promazine HCl USP *phenothiazine antipsychotic* [also: promazine] 25, 50 mg/mL injection

Promega Pearls (softgels) OTC *dietary supplement* [omega-3 fatty acids; multiple vitamins & minerals] 600• ≛, 1000•≛ mg

promegestone INN
promelase INN
promestriene INN
Prometa syrup (discontinued 1995) ℞ *bronchodilator* [metaproterenol sulfate] 10 mg/5 mL
Prometh syrup (discontinued 1996) ℞ *antihistamine* [promethazine HCl; alcohol]
Prometh VC Plain liquid ℞ *decongestant; antihistamine* [phenylephrine HCl; promethazine HCl] 5•6.25 mg/5 mL
Prometh VC with Codeine syrup ℞ *narcotic antitussive; decongestant; antihistamine* [codeine phosphate; phenylephrine HCl; promethazine HCl; alcohol] 10•5•6.25 mg/5 mL
Prometh with Codeine syrup ℞ *narcotic antitussive; antihistamine* [codeine phosphate; promethazine HCl] 10•6.25 mg/5 mL
Prometh with Dextromethorphan syrup ℞ *antitussive; antihistamine* [dextromethorphan hydrobromide; promethazine HCl; alcohol 7%] 15•6.25 mg/5 mL
Prometh-50 injection (discontinued 1997) ℞ *antihistamine; sedative; antiemetic; motion sickness relief* [promethazine HCl] 50 mg/mL
promethazine INN *phenothiazine antihistamine; antiemetic; antidopaminergic; motion sickness relief* [also: promethazine HCl]
Promethazine DM syrup ℞ *antitussive; antihistamine* [dextromethorphan hydrobromide; promethazine HCl; alcohol] 15•6.25 mg/5 mL
promethazine HCl USP *phenothiazine antihistamine; antiemetic; antidopaminergic; motion sickness relief* [also: promethazine] 25, 50 mg oral; 6.25 mg/5 mL oral; 50 mg suppositories; 25, 50 mg/mL injection
promethazine teoclate INN *phenothiazine antihistamine*
Promethazine VC syrup ℞ *decongestant; antihistamine* [phenylephrine HCl; promethazine HCl] 5•6.25 mg/5 mL
Promethazine VC Plain syrup ℞ *decongestant; antihistamine* [phenylephrine HCl; promethazine HCl; alcohol 7%] 5•6.25 mg/5 mL
Promethazine VC with Codeine syrup ℞ *narcotic antitussive; decongestant; antihistamine* [codeine phosphate; phenylephrine HCl; promethazine HCl; alcohol] 10•5•6.25 mg/5 mL
promethestrol [see: methestrol]
Promethist with Codeine syrup ℞ *narcotic antitussive; decongestant; antihistamine* [codeine phosphate; phenylephrine HCl; promethazine HCl; alcohol] 10•5•6.25 mg/5 mL
promethium *element (Pm)*
Prometrium capsules ℞ *progestin for secondary amenorrhea and to prevent endometrial hyperplasia* [progesterone, micronized] 100 mg
Promine capsules ℞ *antiarrhythmic* [procainamide HCl]
Prominol tablets ℞ *analgesic; antipyretic; sedative* [acetaminophen; butalbital] 650•50 mg
Promit IV injection ℞ *monovalent hapten for prophylaxis of dextran-induced anaphylactic reactions* [dextran 1] 150 mg/mL
ProMod powder OTC *oral protein supplement* [D-whey protein concentrate; soy lecithin]
promolate INN
promoxolane INN
prompt insulin zinc [see: insulin zinc, prompt]
Promycin *investigational (Phase III, orphan) antineoplastic for head, neck, and cervical cancers* [porfiromycin]
Pronemia Hematinic capsules ℞ *hematinic* [ferrous fumarate; cyanocobalamin; ascorbic acid; intrinsic factor concentrate; folic acid] 115 mg•15 μg•150 mg•75 mg•1 mg
Pronestyl capsules, tablets, IV or IM injection ℞ *antiarrhythmic* [procainamide HCl] 250, 375, 500 mg; 250,

375, 500 mg; 100, 500 mg/mL ② Ponstel

Pronestyl-SR sustained-release tablets ℞ *antiarrhythmic* [procainamide HCl] 500 mg

pronetalol INN [also: pronethalol]

pronethalol BAN [also: pronetalol]

Pronto shampoo + creme rinse OTC *pediculicide for lice* [pyrethrins; piperonyl butoxide] 0.33%•4%

Propac powder OTC *oral protein supplement* [whey protein; lactose]

Propacet 100 film-coated tablets ℞ *narcotic analgesic* [propoxyphene napsylate; acetaminophen] 100•650 mg

propacetamol INN

propafenone INN, BAN *antiarrhythmic* [also: propafenone HCl]

propafenone HCl USAN *antiarrhythmic* [also: propafenone]

Propagest tablets OTC *nasal decongestant* [phenylpropanolamine HCl] 25 mg

propamidine INN, BAN, DCF

propamidine isethionate *investigational (orphan) eye drops for Acanthamoeba keratitis*

propaminodiphen [see: pramiverine]

propane NF *aerosol propellant*

1,2-propanediol [see: propylene glycol]

propanidid USAN, INN *intravenous anesthetic*

propanocaine INN

propanoic acid, sodium salt hydrate [see: sodium propionate]

2-propanol [see: isopropyl alcohol]

2-propanone [see: acetone]

propantheline bromide USP, INN GI *antispasmodic; peptic ulcer adjunct* 15 mg oral

PROPApH Acne cream OTC *topical keratolytic for acne* [salicylic acid] 2%

PROPApH Cleansing; PROPApH Cleansing for Sensitive Skin; PROPApH Cleansing Maximum Strength pads OTC *topical keratolytic for acne* [salicylic acid] 0.5%; 0.5%; 2%

PROPApH Cleansing for Normal/ Combination Skin; PROPApH Cleansing for Oily Skin lotion

OTC *topical keratolytic for acne* [salicylic acid] 0.5%

PROPApH Foaming Face Wash liquid ℞ *topical keratolytic cleanser for acne* [salicylic acid] 2%

PROPApH Peel-Off Acne Mask OTC *topical keratolytic for acne* [salicylic acid] 2%

proparacaine HCl USP *topical ophthalmic anesthetic* [also: proxymetacaine] 0.5% eye drops

proparacaine HCl & fluorescein sodium *topical ophthalmic anesthetic; corneal disclosing agent* 0.5%•0.25%

propatyl nitrate USAN *coronary vasodilator* [also: propatylnitrate]

propatylnitrate INN *coronary vasodilator* [also: propatyl nitrate]

propazolamide INN

Propecia film-coated tablets ℞ *androgen hormone inhibitor for androgenic alopecia in men* [finasteride] 1 mg

1-propene homopolymer [see: polipropene 25]

propenidazole INN

propentofylline INN

p-**propenylanisole** [see: anethole]

propenzolate HCl USAN *anticholinergic* [also: oxyclipine]

propericiazine [see: periciazine]

properidine INN, BAN

propetamide INN

propetandrol INN

prophenamine HCl [see: ethopropazine HCl]

Pro-Phree powder OTC *supplement to breast milk* [protein-free formula with vitamins & minerals]

Prophyllin ointment OTC *topical antifungal; vulnerary; wound deodorant* [sodium propionate; chlorophyll derivatives] 5%•0.0125%

propicillin INN, BAN

propikacin USAN, INN *antibacterial*

Propimex-1 powder OTC *formula for infants with propionic or methylmalonicacidemia*

Propimex-2 powder OTC *enteral nutritional therapy for propionic or methylmalonic acidemia*

Propine eye drops ℞ *topical antiglaucoma agent* [dipivefrin HCl] 0.1%

propinetidine INN

propiodal [see: prolonium iodide]

propiolactone (β-propiolactone) USAN, INN *disinfectant*

propiomazine USAN, INN *preanesthetic sedative*

propiomazine HCl USP *sedative; analgesic adjunct*

propionic acid NF *antimicrobial; acidifying agent*

propionyl erythromycin lauryl sulfate [see: erythromycin estolate]

propipocaine INN

propiram INN, BAN *narcotic agonist-antagonist analgesic* [also: propiram fumarate]

propiram fumarate USAN *investigational (Phase III) narcotic agonist-antagonist analgesic* [also: propiram]

propisergide INN

propitocaine HCl JAN *topical local anesthetic* [also: prilocaine HCl]

propiverine INN

propizepine INN

Proplex T IV infusion ℞ *antihemophilic to correct factor VII, VIII (hemophilia A), and IX (hemophilia B; Christmas disease) deficiencies* [coagulation factors II, VII, IX, and X, heat treated] 30 mL

propofol USAN, INN, BAN *rapid-acting general anesthetic* 1% injection

propolis *natural resin collected from the buds of certain trees by bees and used as an antibiotic, anti-inflammatory, antioxidant, antineoplastic, fungicide, immune system stimulant, and vulnerary*

propoxate INN

propoxycaine INN *local anesthetic* [also: propoxycaine HCl]

propoxycaine HCl USP *local anesthetic* [also: propoxycaine]

propoxyphene HCl USAN, USP *narcotic analgesic* [also: dextropropoxyphene HCl] 65 mg oral

propoxyphene napsylate USAN, USP *narcotic analgesic*

propranolol INN, BAN *antianginal; antiarrhythmic; antihypertensive; antiadrenergic (β-receptor); migraine preventative* [also: propranolol HCl]

propranolol HCl USAN, USP *antianginal; antiarrhythmic; antihypertensive; antiadrenergic (β-receptor); migraine preventative* [also: propranolol] 10, 20, 40, 60, 80, 90, 120, 160 mg oral; 4, 8, 80 mg/mL oral; 1 mg/mL injection

Propulsid tablets, oral suspension ℞ *treatment for nocturnal heartburn due to gastroesophageal reflux disease (GERD)* [cisapride] 10, 20 mg; 1 mg/mL

propyl p-aminobenzoate [see: risocaine]

propyl docetrizoate INN, BAN

propyl gallate NF *antioxidant*

propyl p-hydroxybenzoate [see: propylparaben]

propyl p-hydroxybenzoate, sodium salt [see: propylparaben sodium]

N-propylajmalinium tartrate [see: prajmalinum bitartrate]

propylene carbonate NF *gelling agent*

propylene glycol USP *humectant; solvent; suspending and viscosity-increasing agent*

propylene glycol alginate NF *suspending agent; viscosity-increasing agent*

propylene glycol diacetate NF *solvent*

propylene glycol ether of methylcellulose [see: hydroxypropyl methylcellulose]

propylene glycol monostearate NF *emulsifying agent*

propylhexedrine USP, INN, BAN *vasoconstrictor; nasal decongestant*

propyliodone USP, INN *radiopaque contrast medium (56.7% iodine)*

propylorvinol [see: etorphine]

propylparaben USAN, NF *antifungal agent; preservative*

propylparaben sodium USAN, NF *antimicrobial preservative*

2-propylpentanoic acid [see: valproic acid]

propylthiouracil (PTU) USP, INN *thyroid inhibitor*

2-propylvaleramide [see: valpromide]

propylvaleric acid [see: valproic acid]

propyperone INN

propyphenazone INN, BAN

propyromazine bromide INN

proquamezine BAN [also: aminopromazine]

proquazone USAN, INN *anti-inflammatory*

proquinolate USAN, INN *coccidiostat for poultry*

prorenoate potassium USAN, INN *aldosterone antagonist*

Prorex-25; Prorex-50 injection (discontinued 1997) ℞ *antihistamine; sedative; antiemetic; motion sickness relief* [promethazine HCl] 25 mg/mL; 50 mg/mL

proroxan INN *antiadrenergic (α-receptor)* [also: proroxan HCl]

proroxan HCl USAN *antiadrenergic (α-receptor)* [also: proroxan]

Proscar film-coated tablets ℞ *androgen hormone inhibitor for benign prostatic hyperplasia (BPH)* [finasteride] 5 mg ⊇ Posicor

proscillaridin USAN, INN *cardiotonic*

proscillaridin A [see: proscillaridin]

Prosed/DS sugar-coated tablets ℞ *urinary antibiotic; antiseptic; analgesic; antispasmodic* [methenamine; phenyl salicylate; methylene blue; benzoic acid; atropine sulfate; hyoscyamine sulfate] 81.6•36.2•10.8•9•0.06•0.06 mg

ProSobee liquid, powder OTC *hypoallergenic infant food* [soy protein formula]

Pro-Sof Plus capsules OTC *stimulant laxative; stool softener* [casanthranol; docusate sodium] 30•100 mg

ProSol 20% IV infusion ℞ *total parenteral nutrition* [multiple essential and nonessential amino acids] 20 g

ProSom tablets ℞ *sedative; hypnotic* [estazolam] 1, 2 mg

Prosorba Column for dialysis ℞ *treatment for rheumatoid arthritis* [protein A]

prospidium chloride INN

prostacyclin [now: epoprostenol]

prostaglandin agonists *a class of antiglaucoma agents that reduce intraocular*

pressure (IOP) by increasing the outflow of aqueous humor

prostaglandin E₁ (PGE₁) [now: alprostadil]

prostaglandin E₁ alphacyclodextrin *orphan status withdrawn 1996*

prostaglandin E₁ enol ester *investigational (orphan) for advanced chronic critical limb ischemia*

prostaglandin E₂ (PGE₂) [see: dinoprostone]

prostaglandin F₂α (PGF₂α) [see: dinoprost]

prostaglandin I₂ (PGI₂) [now: epoprostenol]

prostaglandin X (PGX) [now: epoprostenol]

prostaglandins *a class of agents that stimulate uterine contractions, used for abortions, cervical ripening, and postpartum hemorrhage*

prostalene USAN, INN *prostaglandin*

Prostaphlin capsules, powder for oral solution, powder for IV or IM injection (discontinued 1998) ℞ *penicillinase-resistant penicillin antibiotic* [oxacillin sodium] 250, 500 mg; 250 mg/5 mL; 0.5, 1, 2, 4, 10 g

ProstaScint ℞ *imaging agent for prostate cancer and its metastases* [capromab pendetide]

ProStep transdermal patch ℞ *smoking deterrent; nicotine withdrawal aid* [nicotine] 15, 30 mg

Prostigmin subcu or IM injection ℞ *cholinergic urinary stimulant for postsurgical urinary retention* [neostigmine methylsulfate] 1:1000 (1 mg/mL), 1:2000 (0.5 mg/mL), 1:4000 (0.25 mg/mL) (1:400 [2.5 mg/mL] available in Canada) ⊇ physostigmine

Prostigmin tablets ℞ *myasthenia gravis treatment; antidote for neuromuscular blockers* [neostigmine bromide] 15 mg

Prostin E2 vaginal suppository ℞ *prostaglandin-type abortifacient* [dinoprostone] 20 mg

Prostin VR Pediatric IV injection ℞ *vasodilator; platelet aggregation inhibitor* [alprostadil] 500 μg/mL

prosulpride INN
prosultiamine INN
protactinium *element (Pa)*
protamine sulfate USP, INN *antidote to heparin overdose* [also: protamine sulphate] 10 mg/mL injection
protamine sulphate BAN *antidote to heparin overdose* [also: protamine sulfate]
protamine zinc insulin (PZI) INN *antidiabetic* [also: insulin, protamine zinc; insulin zinc protamine]
Protar Protein shampoo (discontinued 1998) OTC *antiseborrheic; antipsoriatic; antipruritic; antibacterial* [coal tar] 5%
protargin, mild [see: silver protein, mild]
protease *digestive enzyme* [100 IU/mg in pancrelipase; 25 IU/mg in pancreatin]
protease inhibitors *a class of antivirals that block HIV replication*
ProTec ℞ *investigational immunomodulator* [lisofylline]
ProTech First Aid Stick liquid OTC *topical antiseptic; analgesic* [lidocaine; povidone-iodine] 2.5%•10%
Protectol Medicated powder OTC *topical antifungal* [calcium undecylenate] 15%
Protegra softgels OTC *vitamin/mineral supplement* [multiple vitamins & minerals] ≛
protein A *treatment for rheumatoid arthritis*
protein C concentrate *investigational (orphan) anticoagulant for protein C deficiency*
protein hydrolysate USP *fluid and nutrient replenisher*
α₁-proteinase inhibitor [see: alpha₁-proteinase inhibitor]
Protenate IV infusion ℞ *blood volume expander for shock due to burns, trauma and surgery* [plasma protein fraction] 5%
proterguride INN
Prothazine subcu or IM injection (discontinued 1997) ℞ *antihistamine; sedative; antiemetic; motion sickness relief* [promethazine HCl] 25, 50 mg/mL

Prothazine Plain syrup (discontinued 1997) ℞ *antihistamine; sedative; antiemetic; motion sickness relief* [promethazine HCl] 6.25 mg/5 mL
Prothecan ℞ *investigational hormonal antineoplastic for solid tumors* [PEG-camptothecin]
protheobromine INN
Prothera liquid (discontinued 1995) OTC *soap-free therapeutic skin cleanser*
Prothiaden ℞ *investigational (NDA filed) tricyclic antidepressant* [dothiepin HCl]
prothionamide BAN [also: protionamide]
prothipendyl INN
prothipendyl HCl [see: prothipendyl]
prothixene INN
prothrombin complex, activated BAN
Protilase capsules containing enteric-coated spheres ℞ *digestive enzymes* [lipase; protease; amylase] 4000• 25 000•20 000 U
ProTime test kit for home use OTC *in vitro diagnostic aid for the management of anticoagulation therapy*
protiofate INN
protionamide INN [also: prothionamide]
protirelin USAN, INN, BAN *prothyrotropin; diagnostic aid for thyroid function; investigational (orphan) for infant respiratory distress syndrome of prematurity*
protizinic acid INN
protokylol HCl
proton pump inhibitors *a class of gastric antisecretory agents that inhibit the ATPase "proton pump" within the gastric parietal cell* [also called: ATPase inhibitors; substituted benzimidazoles]
Protopam Chloride IV injection ℞ *antidote for organophosphate poisoning and anticholinesterase overdose* [pralidoxime chloride] 1 g ⊠ Protamine
Protopam Chloride tablets (discontinued 1995) ℞ *antidote for organophosphate and anticholinesterase chemicals* [pralidoxime chloride] 500 mg ⊠ Protamine

Protostat tablets ℞ *antibiotic; antiprotozoal; amebicide* [metronidazole] 250, 500 mg

protoveratrine A

Protovir ℞ *investigational (Phase I) antiviral for AIDS-related cytomegalovirus* [sevirumab]

Protox ℞ *investigational (orphan) for toxoplasmosis of AIDS; investigational (Phase II) for treatment of bacterial and viral infections* [poloxamer 331]

protriptyline INN *tricyclic antidepressant* [also: protriptyline HCl]

protriptyline HCl USAN, USP *tricyclic antidepressant* [also: protriptyline] 5, 10 mg oral

Protropin powder for IM or subcu injection ℞ *growth hormone for congenital growth failure (orphan) or due to chronic renal insufficiency* [somatrem] 5, 10 mg (13, 26 IU) per vial

Protropin II ℞ *growth hormone for adults or children with congenital or endogenous growth hormone deficiency, children with Turner syndrome or renal-induced growth failure, or AIDS-wasting syndrome (orphan); investigational (orphan) for severe burns* [somatropin]

Protuss liquid ℞ *narcotic antitussive; expectorant* [hydrocodone bitartrate; potassium guaiacolsulfonate] 5•300 mg/5 mL

Protuss DM film-coated tablets ℞ *antitussive; decongestant; expectorant* [dextromethorphan hydrobromide; pseudoephedrine HCl; guaifenesin] 30•60•600 mg

Protuss-D liquid ℞ *narcotic antitussive; decongestant; expectorant* [hydrocodone bitartrate; pseudoephedrine HCl; potassium guaiacolsulfonate] 5•30•300 mg/5 mL

prourokinase [see: saruplase]

Provatene soft gel perles (discontinued 1996) OTC *vitamin A precursor* [beta carotene] 15 mg (25 000 IU)

Proventil inhalation aerosol ℞ *sympathomimetic bronchodilator* [albuterol] 90 μg/dose

Proventil tablets, Repetabs (extended-release tablets), syrup, solution for inhalation ℞ *sympathomimetic bronchodilator* [albuterol sulfate] 2, 4 mg; 4 mg; 2 mg/5 mL; 0.083%, 0.5%

Proventil HFA CFC-free inhalation aerosol ℞ *sympathomimetic bronchodilator* [albuterol sulfate] 90 μg/dose

Provera tablets ℞ *progestin for secondary amenorrhea, abnormal uterine bleeding, and endometrial hyperplasia* [medroxyprogesterone acetate] 2.5, 5, 10 mg ⊡ Covera; Provir; Trovert

Provigil tablets ℞ *analeptic for excessive daytime sleepiness of narcolepsy (orphan)* [modafinil] 100, 200 mg

Provir ℞ *investigational (Phase III) treatment for AIDS-related diarrhea* [SP-303 (code name—generic name not yet assigned)] ⊡ Provera; Trovert

Proviron brand name for mesterolone, an androgen abused with anabolic steroid street drugs

provitamin A [see: beta carotene]

Provocholine powder for reconstitution for inhalation ℞ *bronchoconstrictor for in vivo pulmonary function challenge test* [methacholine chloride] 100 mg/5 mL

proxazole USAN, INN *smooth muscle relaxant; analgesic; anti-inflammatory*

proxazole citrate USAN *smooth muscle relaxant; analgesic; anti-inflammatory*

proxetil INN *combining name for radicals or groups*

proxibarbal INN

proxibutene INN

proxicromil USAN, INN *antiallergic*

proxifezone INN

Proxigel OTC *topical oral anti-inflammatory and anti-infective for braces* [carbamide peroxide] 10%

proxorphan INN *analgesic; antitussive* [also: proxorphan tartrate]

proxorphan tartrate USAN *analgesic; antitussive* [also: proxorphan]

Proxy 65 tablets ℞ *narcotic analgesic* [propoxyphene HCl; acetaminophen]

proxymetacaine INN, BAN *topical ophthalmic anesthetic* [also: proparacaine HCl]

proxymetacaine HCl [see: proparacaine HCl]

proxyphylline INN, BAN

Prozac tablets, Pulvules (capsules), oral solution ℞ *selective serotonin reuptake inhibitor (SSRI) for depression, obsessive-compulsive disorder, and bulimia nervosa* [fluoxetine HCl] 10 mg; 10, 20 mg; 20 mg/5 mL ② Prilosec

prozapine INN

Prozine-50 IM injection ℞ *conventional (typical) antipsychotic* [promazine HCl] 50 mg/mL

Prulet tablets OTC *stimulant laxative* [white phenolphthalein] 60 mg

Prunella vulgaris medicinal herb [see: woundwort]

Prunus africana medicinal herb [see: pygeum]

Prunus americana; P. domestica; P. spinosa medicinal herb [see: plum]

Prunus amygdalus medicinal herb [see: almond]

Prunus armeniaca medicinal herb [see: apricot]

Prunus persica medicinal herb [see: peach]

Prunus serotina medicinal herb [see: wild black cherry]

Prunus virginiana medicinal herb [see: wild cherry]

Pryme (name changed to LYMErix upon release in 1999)

PSC-833 *investigational (Phase III) adjunct to chemotherapy for multi–drug-resistant tumors and acute myelogenous leukemia (AML)*

Pseudo liquid OTC *nasal decongestant* [pseudoephedrine HCl] 30 mg/5 mL

Pseudo-Car DM syrup ℞ *antitussive; decongestant; antihistamine* [dextromethorphan hydrobromide; pseudoephedrine HCl; carbinoxamine maleate] 15•60•4 mg/5 mL

Pseudo-Chlor sustained-release capsules ℞ *decongestant; antihistamine*
[pseudoephedrine HCl; chlorpheniramine maleate] 120•8 mg

pseudoephedrine INN, BAN *vasoconstrictor; nasal decongestant* [also: pseudoephedrine HCl]

pseudoephedrine HCl USAN, USP *vasoconstrictor; nasal decongestant* [also: pseudoephedrine] 30, 60 mg oral; 30 mg/5 mL oral

pseudoephedrine HCl & carbinoxamine maleate *decongestant; antihistamine* 60•4 mg/5 mL oral; 25•2 mg/mL oral

pseudoephedrine polistirex USAN *nasal decongestant*

pseudoephedrine sulfate USAN, USP *bronchodilator; nasal decongestant*

pseudoephedrine tannate *bronchodilator; nasal decongestant*

Pseudo-Gest tablets OTC *nasal decongestant* [pseudoephedrine HCl] 30, 60 mg

Pseudo-Gest Plus tablets OTC *decongestant; antihistamine* [pseudoephedrine HCl; chlorpheniramine maleate] 60•4 mg

Pseudomonas aeruginosa **purified extract** *investigational (orphan) agent to increase platelet count in immune thrombocytopenic purpura*

Pseudomonas **immune globulin** [see: mucoid exopolysaccharide *Pseudomonas* hyperimmune globulin]

pseudomonic acid A [see: mupirocin]

Pseudostat ℞ *investigational (Phase II) theraccine for chronic bronchitis*

psilocin *a hallucinogenic street drug closely related to psilocybin*

psilocybin BAN *a hallucinogenic street drug derived from the Psilocybe mexicana mushroom* [also: psilocybine]

psilocybine INN, DCF *a hallucinogenic street drug derived from the Psilocybe mexicana mushroom* [also: psilocybin]

psoralens *a class of oral or topical skin photosensitizing agents used with ultraviolet A light (320–400 nm wavelength) for the treatment of severe recalcitrant psoriasis*

Psor-a-set bar OTC *therapeutic skin cleanser; topical keratolytic* [salicylic acid] 2%

Psorcon cream, ointment ℞ *topical corticosteroidal anti-inflammatory* [diflorasone diacetate] 0.05%

PsoriGel OTC *topical antipsoriatic; antiseborrheic; antiseptic* [coal tar solution; alcohol 33%] 7.5%

Psorion cream (discontinued 1995) ℞ *topical corticosteroidal anti-inflammatory* [betamethasone dipropionate] 0.05%

Psovascar *investigational (Phase I/II) angiogenesis inhibitor for psoriasis*

psyllium *(Plantago ovata) medicinal herb* [see: plantain]

psyllium husk USP *bulk laxative*

psyllium hydrocolloid *bulk laxative*

psyllium hydrophilic mucilloid *bulk laxative*

psyllium seed [see: plantago seed]

PT-14 *investigational peptide analog for erectile dysfunction*

PTC (plasma thromboplastin component) [see: factor IX]

P.T.E.-4; P.T.E.-5 IV injection ℞ *intravenous nutritional therapy* [multiple trace elements (metals)]

pterins *a class of investigational antineoplastics*

pteroyldiglutamic acid (PDGA)

pteroylglutamic acid (PGA) [see: folic acid]

PTFE (polytetrafluoroethylene) [see: polytef]

PTU (propylthiouracil) [q.v.]

ptyalagogues *a class of agents that stimulate the secretion of saliva* [also called: sialagogues]

puccoon, yellow *medicinal herb* [see: goldenseal]

Pueraria lobata; P. thunbergiana medicinal herb [see: kudzu]

puffball *medicinal herb* [see: dandelion]

Pulmicort Turbuhaler (dry powder in a metered-dose inhaler) ℞ *corticosteroidal anti-inflammatory for chronic asthma* [budesonide] 160 μg/dose

Pulmocare ready-to-use liquid OTC *enteral nutritional therapy for pulmonary problems*

Pulmonaria officinalis medicinal herb [see: lungwort]

pulmonary surfactant replacement, porcine *investigational (orphan) for infant respiratory distress syndrome of prematurity*

Pulmozyme solution for nebulization ℞ *reduces respiratory viscoelasticity of sputum in cystic fibrosis (orphan)* [dornase alfa] 1 mg/mL

pulse VAC (vincristine, actinomycin D, cyclophosphamide) *chemotherapy protocol* [also: VAC]

pulse VAC (vincristine, Adriamycin, cyclophosphamide) *chemotherapy protocol* [also: VAC]

PulsePak (trademarked dosage form) *one-week dosage pack*

Pulvule (trademarked dosage form) *bullet-shaped capsule*

pumice USP *dental abrasive*

pumitepa INN

Punctum Plug ℞ *blocks the puncta and canaliculus to eliminate tear loss in keratitis sicca* [silicone plug]

Punica granatum medicinal herb [see: pomegranate]

Puralube ophthalmic ointment OTC *ocular moisturizer/lubricant* [white petrolatum; mineral oil]

Puralube Tears eye drops OTC *ophthalmic moisturizer/lubricant* [polyvinyl alcohol; polyethylene glycol 400] 1%•1%

Puregon Ⓐ (U.S. product: Follistim) subcu or IM injection ℞ *recombinant follicle-stimulating hormone (FSH) for the induction of ovulation and development of multiple follicles for assisted reproductive technology (ART)* [follitropin beta] 50, 100 IU

purgatives *a class of agents that cause vigorous evacuation of the bowels by increasing bulk, stimulating peristaltic action, etc.* [also called: cathartics]

Purge liquid OTC *stimulant laxative* [castor oil] 95%

purified cotton [see: cotton, purified]
purified protein derivative (PPD) of tuberculin [see: tuberculin]
purified rayon [see: rayon, purified]
purified siliceous earth [see: siliceous earth, purified]
purified water [see: water, purified]
H-purin-6-amine [see: adenine]
purine nucleoside phosphorylase *investigational (Phase III) treatment for psoriasis*
Purinethol tablets ℞ *antimetabolite antineoplastic for multiple leukemias* [mercaptopurine] 50 mg
Purinol ⓒ (U.S. product: Zyloprim) tablets ℞ *xanthine oxidase inhibitor for gout and hyperuricemia* [allopurinol] 100, 300 mg
Purlytin *investigational (Phase III) PhotoPoint photodynamic therapy for advanced metastatic breast cancer involving the skin and age-related macular degeneration* [tin ethyl etiopurpurin]
puromycin USAN, INN *antineoplastic; antiprotozoal (Trypanosoma)*
puromycin HCl USAN *antineoplastic; antiprotozoal (Trypanosoma)*
purple angelica *medicinal herb* [see: angelica]
purple boneset *medicinal herb* [see: boneset]
purple cone flower *medicinal herb* [see: echinacea]
purple leptandra *medicinal herb* [see: Culver's root]
Purpose Alpha Hydroxy Moisture lotion, cream OTC *moisturizer; emollient; exfoliant* [glycolic acid] 8%
Purpose Dry Skin cream OTC *moisturizer; emollient*
Purpose Soap bar OTC *therapeutic skin cleanser*
purshiana bark *medicinal herb* [see: cascara sagrada]
purslain, water *medicinal herb* [see: brooklime]
purvain *medicinal herb* [see: blue vervain]
pussywillow *medicinal herb* [see: willow]

PUVA *an acronym for psoralens (P) and ultraviolet A (UVA) light, used as a treatment for severe recalcitrant psoriasis* [see: psoralens; methoxsalen]
PVA (polyvinyl alcohol) [q.v.]
PVB (Platinol, vinblastine, bleomycin) *chemotherapy protocol*
PVC (polyvinyl chloride) [see: polyvinyl chloride, radiopaque]
PVDA (prednisone, vincristine, daunorubicin, asparaginase) *chemotherapy protocol*
PVP; PVP-16 (Platinol, VP-16) *chemotherapy protocol*
P-V-Tussin syrup ℞ *narcotic antitussive; decongestant; antihistamine* [hydrocodone bitartrate; pseudoephedrine HCl; chlorpheniramine maleate; alcohol 5%] 2.5•30•2 mg/5 mL
P-V-Tussin tablets ℞ *narcotic antitussive; antihistamine; expectorant* [hydrocodone bitartrate; phenindamine tartrate; guaifenesin] 5•25•200 mg
Pycnanthemum virginianum *medicinal herb* [see: wild hyssop]
Pycnogenol *natural free radical scavenger; a registered trade name for pine bark extract* [see: pine bark extract]
pygeum (Prunus africana; Pygeum africanum) bark *medicinal herb for prostate gland enlargement and urinary disorders*
Pylori-Check test kit for professional use *in vivo diagnostic aid for H. pylori in the breath*
Pylorid ⓒ (U.S. product: Tritec) film-coated tablets ℞ *histamine H₂ antagonist for duodenal ulcers with H. pylori infection* [ranitidine bismuth citrate] 400 mg
Pyloriset reagent kit for professional use *in vitro diagnostic aid for GI disorders*
pyrabrom USAN *antihistamine*
pyradone [see: aminopyrine]
pyrantel INN *anthelmintic for ascariasis (roundworm) and enterobiasis (pinworm)* [also: pyrantel pamoate]
pyrantel pamoate USAN, USP *anthelmintic for ascariasis (roundworm) and enterobiasis (pinworm)* [also: pyrantel]

pyrantel tartrate USAN *anthelmintic*
pyrathiazine HCl [see: parathiazine]
pyrazinamide (PZA) USP, INN, BAN *bactericidal; primary tuberculostatic* 500 mg oral
pyrazinecarboxamide [see: pyrazinamide]
pyrazofurin USAN *antineoplastic* [also: pirazofurin]
pyrazoline [see: antipyrine]
pyrbenzindole [see: benzindopyrine HCl]
pyrbuterol HCl [see: pirbuterol HCl]
pyrethrins *a class of natural pesticides derived from pyrethrum flowers, especially Chrysanthemum cinerariaefolium and C. coccineum*
Pyrethrum parthenium *medicinal herb* [see: feverfew]
pyribenzamine (PBZ) [see: tripelennamine]
pyricarbate INN
pyridarone INN
Pyridiate; Pyridate No. 2 tablets ℞ *urinary analgesic* [phenazopyridine HCl] 100 mg; 200 mg
4-pyridinamine [see: fampridine]
2-pyridine aldoxime methylchloride (2-PAM) [see: pralidoxime chloride]
3-pyridinecarboxamide [see: niacinamide]
3-pyridinecarboxylic acid [see: niacin]
4-pyridinecarboxylic acid hydrazide [see: isoniazid]
3-pyridinecarboxylic acid methyl ester [see: methyl nicotinate]
3-pyridinemethanol [see: nicotinyl alcohol]
2-pyridinemethanol [see: piconol]
3-pyridinemethanol tartrate [see: nicotinyl tartrate]
Pyridium tablets ℞ *urinary analgesic* [phenazopyridine HCl] 100, 200 mg ⊡ Dyrenium; pyridoxine; pyrithione; pyritidium
Pyridium Plus tablets ℞ *urinary analgesic; antispasmodic; sedative* [phenazopyridine HCl; hyoscyamine

hydrobromide; butabarbital] 150•0.3•15 mg
pyridofylline INN
pyridostigmine bromide USP, INN *cholinergic/anticholinesterase muscle stimulant* ⊡ physostigmine
pyridoxal [see: pyridoxine HCl]
pyridoxamine [see: pyridoxine HCl]
pyridoxine INN *vitamin B_6; enzyme cofactor* [also: pyridoxine HCl] ⊡ pralidoxime; Pyridium
pyridoxine HCl USP *vitamin B_6; enzyme cofactor* [also: pyridoxine] 25, 50, 100 mg oral; 100 mg/mL injection ⊡ pralidoxime; Pyridium
β-pyridylcarbinol [see: nicotinyl alcohol]
pyridylmethanol *me+* [see: nicotinyl alcohol]
9-[3-pyridylmethyl]-9-deazaguanine *investigational for cutaneous T-cell lymphoma; orphan status withdrawn 1998*
pyrilamine maleate USP *anticholinergic; antihistamine; sleep aid* [also: mepyramine]
pyrilamine tannate, phenylephrine tannate, and chlorpheniramine tannate *antihistamine; decongestant* 25•25•8 mg oral
pyrimethamine USP, INN *malaria suppression and transmission control; folic acid antagonist*
pyrimethamine & sulfadiazine *Toxoplasma gondii encephalitis treatment (orphan)*
pyrimidinedione [see: uracil]
pyrimitate INN, BAN
Pyrinex Pediculicide shampoo OTC *pediculicide for lice* [pyrethrins; piperonyl butoxide; deodorized kerosene] 0.2%•2%•0.8%
pyrinoline USAN, INN *antiarrhythmic*
Pyrinyl liquid OTC *pediculicide for lice* [pyrethrins; piperonyl butoxide; deodorized kerosene] 0.2%•2%•0.8%
Pyrinyl II liquid OTC *pediculicide for lice* [pyrethrins; piperonyl butoxide] 0.3%•3%

Pyrinyl Plus shampoo OTC *pediculicide for lice* [pyrethrins; piperonyl butoxide] 0.3%•3%

pyrithen [see: chlorothen citrate]

pyrithione sodium USAN *topical antimicrobial* 🔟 Pyridium

pyrithione zinc USAN, INN, BAN *antibacterial; antifungal; antiseborrheic*

pyrithyldione INN

pyritidium bromide INN 🔟 Pyridium

pyritinol INN, BAN

pyrodifenium bromide [see: prifinium bromide]

pyrogallic acid [see: pyrogallol]

pyrogallol NF

pyrophendane INN

pyrophenindane [see: pyrophendane]

pyrovalerone INN *CNS stimulant* [also: pyrovalerone HCl]

pyrovalerone HCl USAN *CNS stimulant* [also: pyrovalerone]

pyroxamine INN *antihistamine* [also: pyroxamine maleate]

pyroxamine maleate USAN *antihistamine* [also: pyroxamine]

pyroxylin USP, INN *pharmaceutic necessity for collodion*

pyrrobutamine phosphate USP

pyrrocaine USAN, INN *local anesthetic*

pyrrocaine HCl NF

pyrrolifene INN *analgesic* [also: pyrroliphene HCl]

pyrrolifene HCl [see: pyrroliphene HCl]

pyrroliphene HCl USAN *analgesic* [also: pyrrolifene]

pyrrolnitrin USAN, INN *antifungal*

pyrroxane [now: proroxan HCl]

Pyrroxate capsules OTC *decongestant; antihistamine; analgesic* [phenylpropanolamine HCl; chlorpheniramine maleate; acetaminophen] 25•4•650 mg

Pyrus malus medicinal herb [see: apple]

pyrvinium chloride INN

pyrvinium embonate [see: pyrvinium pamoate]

pyrvinium pamoate USP *anthelmintic* [also: viprynium embonate]

pytamine INN

PYtest reagent kit for professional use ℞ *in vitro diagnostic aid for H. pylori in the breath* [carbon C 14 urea] 1 mCi

PZA (pyrazinamide) [q.v.]

PZI (protamine zinc insulin) [q.v.]

QS-21 *investigational (Phase I/II) immune system stimulant for AIDS vaccines*

QTest test stick for home use OTC *in vitro diagnostic aid for urine pregnancy test*

QTest Ovulation test kit for professional use *in vitro diagnostic aid to predict ovulation time*

quadazocine INN, BAN *opioid antagonist* [also: quadazocine mesylate]

quadazocine mesylate USAN *opioid antagonist* [also: quadazocine]

Quadra-Hist extended-release tablets (discontinued 1995) ℞ *decongestant; antihistamine* [phenylpropanolamine HCl; phenylephrine HCl; chlor-pheniramine maleate; phenyltoloxamine citrate] 40•10•5•15 mg

Quadra-Hist Pediatric syrup (discontinued 1995) ℞ *pediatric decongestant and antihistamine* [phenylpropanolamine HCl; phenylephrine HCl; chlorpheniramine maleate; phenyltoloxamine citrate] 5•1.25•0.5•2 mg/5 mL

Quadramet IV injection ℞ *radiopharmaceutical for treatment of bone pain from osteoblastic metastatic tumors* [samarium Sm 153 lexidronam] 1850 MBq/mL (50 mCi/mL)

Quadrinal tablets ℞ *antiasthmatic; bronchodilator; decongestant; expecto-*

rant; sedative [theophylline; ephedrine HCl; potassium iodide; phenobarbital] 65•24•320•24 mg

quadrosilan INN

quaking aspen medicinal herb [see: poplar]

Quantaffirm reagent kit for professional use in vitro diagnostic aid for mononucleosis

Quarzan capsules ℞ anticholinergic; peptic ulcer treatment [clidinium bromide] 2.5, 5 mg ⏃ Questran

quassia (Picrasma excelsa; Quassia amara) bark medicinal herb used as an anthelmintic, antimalarial, appetizer, digestive aid, febrifuge, insecticide, pediculicide, and tonic

quatacaine INN

quaternium-18 bentonite [see: bentoquatam]

quazepam USAN, INN sedative; hypnotic

quazinone USAN, INN cardiotonic

quazodine USAN, INN cardiotonic; bronchodilator

quazolast USAN, INN antiasthmatic; mediator release inhibitor

Queen Anne's lace medicinal herb [see: carrot]

queen of the meadow medicinal herb [see: boneset; meadowsweet]

queen of the meadow (Eupatorium purpureum) leaves medicinal herb for bursitis, gallstones, kidney infections and stones, neuralgias, rheumatism, ringworm, urinary disorders, and water retention

Quelicin IV or IM injection ℞ neuromuscular blocker [succinylcholine chloride] 20, 50, 100 mg/mL

Quelidrine Cough syrup OTC antitussive; decongestant; antihistamine; expectorant [dextromethorphan hydrobromide; ephedrine HCl; phenylephrine HCl; chlorpheniramine maleate; ammonium chloride; ipecac; alcohol 2%] 10 mg•5 mg•5 mg•2 mg•40 mg•0.005 mL per 5 mL

Quercetin tablets OTC dietary supplement [eucalyptus bioflavonoids] 50, 250 mg

Quercus alba medicinal herb [see: white oak]

Questran; Questran Light powder for oral suspension ℞ cholesterol-lowering antihyperlipidemic; also used for biliary obstruction [cholestyramine resin] 4 g/dose

quetiapine fumarate USAN dibenzothiazepine antipsychotic

Quibron; Quibron-300 capsules ℞ antiasthmatic; bronchodilator; expectorant [theophylline; guaifenesin] 150•90 mg; 300•180 mg

Quibron-T Dividose (multiple-scored tablets) ℞ antiasthmatic; bronchodilator [theophylline] 300 mg

Quibron-T/SR sustained-release Dividose (multiple-scored tablets) ℞ antiasthmatic; bronchodilator [theophylline] 300 mg

Quick AC Enema Kit concentrated rectal suspension ℞ radiopaque contrast medium for gastrointestinal imaging [barium sulfate] 150%

Quick Care solutions OTC two-step chemical disinfecting system for soft contact lenses [hydrogen peroxide-based]

Quick Pep tablets OTC CNS stimulant; analeptic [caffeine] 150 mg

Quicklets (trademarked dosage form) quickly dissolving tablets

Quickscreen test kit for home use OTC in vitro diagnostic aid for detection of multiple illicit drugs in the urine

quick-set medicinal herb [see: hawthorn]

QuickVue test cassettes for professional use in vitro diagnostic aid for urine pregnancy test

Quiess IM injection (discontinued 1998) ℞ anxiolytic; antiemetic [hydroxyzine HCl] 50 mg/mL

quifenadine INN

quiflapon sodium USAN leukotriene biosynthesis inhibitor for asthma and inflammatory bowel disease

Quilimmune-M ℞ investigational (Phase II) vaccine against malaria

Quilimmune-P ℞ investigational (Phase II) vaccine against pneumonia in elderly patients

quillaia (*Quillaja saponaria*) bark
medicinal herb for bronchitis and
cough; also used topically for dandruff
and scalp itchiness

quillifoline INN

quilostigmine USAN cholinesterase
inhibitor for Alzheimer's disease

quinacainol INN

quinacillin INN, BAN

quinacrine HCl USP antimalarial; anthelmintic for giardiasis and cestodiasis
(*tapeworm*) [also: mepacrine] ⚕
quinidine

Quinaglute Dura-Tabs (sustained-
release tablets) ℞ antiarrhythmic
[quinidine gluconate] 324 mg

Quinalan sustained-release tablets ℞
antiarrhythmic [quinidine gluconate]
324 mg

quinalbarbitone sodium BAN hypnotic;
sedative [also: secobarbital sodium]

quinaldine blue USAN obstetric diagnostic aid

quinambicide [see: clioquinol]

Quinamm tablets (discontinued
1996) ℞ antimalarial [quinine sul-
fate] 260 mg

quinapril INN, BAN antihypertensive;
angiotensin-converting enzyme (ACE)
inhibitor [also: quinapril HCl]

quinapril HCl USAN antihypertensive;
angiotensin-converting enzyme (ACE)
inhibitor [also: quinapril]

quinaprilat USAN, INN antihypertensive; angiotensin-converting enzyme
(ACE) inhibitor

quinazosin INN antihypertensive [also:
quinazosin HCl]

quinazosin HCl USAN antihypertensive
[also: quinazosin]

quinbolone USAN, INN anabolic

quincarbate INN

quindecamine INN antibacterial [also:
quindecamine acetate]

quindecamine acetate USAN antibacterial [also: quindecamine]

quindonium bromide USAN, INN
antiarrhythmic

quindoxin INN, BAN

quinelorane INN antihypertensive; antiparkinsonian [also: quinelorane HCl]

quinelorane HCl USAN antihypertensive;
antiparkinsonian [also: quinelorane]

quinestradol INN, BAN

quinestrol USAN, USP, INN, BAN estrogen replacement therapy for postmenopausal disorders

quinetalate INN smooth muscle relaxant
[also: quinetolate]

quinethazone USP, INN diuretic; antihypertensive

quinetolate USAN smooth muscle relaxant [also: quinetalate]

quinezamide INN

quinfamide USAN, INN antiamebic

quingestanol INN progestin [also: quingestanol acetate]

quingestanol acetate USAN progestin
[also: quingestanol]

quingestrone USAN, INN progestin

Quinidex Extentabs (extended-release
tablets) ℞ antiarrhythmic [quinidine
sulfate] 300 mg

quinidine NF, BAN antiarrhythmic ⚕
clonidine; quinacrine; Quinatime;
quinine

quinidine gluconate USP antiarrhythmic; antimalarial 324 mg oral; 80
mg/mL injection

quinidine polygalacturonate antiarrhythmic

quinidine sulfate USP antiarrhythmic
300 mg oral

**quinine (*Cinchona calisaya; C. led-
geriana; C. succirubra*)** NF, BAN
bark medicinal herb for cancer, fever,
hemorrhoids, indigestion, inducing
abortion, jaundice, malaria, mouth and
throat diseases, parasites, stimulation of
hair growth, and varicose veins ⚕
quinidine

quinine ascorbate USAN smoking
deterrent

quinine biascorbate [now: quinine
ascorbate]

quinine bisulfate NF

quinine dihydrochloride NF investigational anti-infective for pernicious malaria

quinine ethylcarbonate NF

quinine glycerophosphate NF

quinine HCl NF

quinine hydrobromide NF

quinine hypophosphite NF

quinine monohydrobromide [see: quinine hydrobromide]

quinine monohydrochloride [see: quinine HCl]

quinine monosalicylate [see: quinine salicylate]

quinine phosphate NF

quinine phosphinate [see: quinine hypophosphite]

quinine salicylate NF

quinine sulfate USP *antimalarial; treatment of nocturnal leg cramps* 200, 260, 325 mg oral

quinine sulfate dihydrate [see: quinine sulfate]

quinine tannate USP

quinisocaine INN [also: dimethisoquin HCl; dimethisoquin]

quinocide INN

8-quinolinol [see: oxyquinoline]

8-quinolinol benzoate [see: benzoxiquine]

quinolizidines *a class of antibiotics based on the quinolizidine (norlupinane) structure* [also called: norlupinanes]

quinolones [see: fluoroquinolones]

Quinora tablets R *antiarrhythmic* [quinidine sulfate] 300 mg

quinoxyl [see: chiniofon]

quinpirole INN *antihypertensive* [also: quinpirole HCl]

quinpirole HCl USAN *antihypertensive* [also: quinpirole]

quinprenaline INN *bronchodilator* [also: quinterenol sulfate]

quinprenaline sulfate [see: quinterenol sulfate]

Quin-Release sustained-release tablets R *antiarrhythmic* [quinidine gluconate]

Quinsana Plus powder OTC *topical antifungal* [tolnaftate] 1%

quinsy berry *medicinal herb* [see: currant]

Quintabs tablets OTC *vitamin supplement* [multiple vitamins; folic acid] ± •0.1 mg

Quintabs-M tablets OTC *vitamin/mineral/iron supplement* [multiple vitamins & minerals; iron; folic acid] ± •18•0.4 mg

quinterenol sulfate USAN *bronchodilator* [also: quinprenaline]

quintiofos INN, BAN

3-quinuclidinol benzoate [see: benzoclidine]

quinuclium bromide USAN, INN *antihypertensive*

quinupramine INN

quinupristin USAN, INN *streptogramin antibiotic bacteriostatic to gram-positive infections*

quinupristin & dalfopristin *two streptogramin antibiotics that are synergistically bactericidal to gram-positive infections; investigational (NDA filed) for pneumonia*

quipazine INN *antidepressant; oxytocic* [also: quipazine maleate]

quipazine maleate USAN *antidepressant; oxytocic* [also: quipazine]

Quiphile tablets (discontinued 1996) R *antimalarial* [quinine sulfate] 260 mg

quisultazine INN

quisultidine [see: quisultazine]

Q-Vel soft caplets (discontinued 1996) OTC *prevention and treatment of nocturnal leg cramps* [quinine sulfate] 64.8 mg

r24 antibody [see: monoclonal antibody r24]

R & C shampoo OTC *pediculicide for lice* [pyrethrins; piperonyl butoxide] 0.3%•3%

R & D Calcium Carbonate/600 ℞ *investigational (orphan) for hyperphosphatemia of end-stage renal disease* [calcium carbonate]

R-121919 *investigational (Phase I) agent for anxiety and depression*

RA Lotion OTC *topical acne treatment* [resorcinol; alcohol 43%] 3%

RabAvert IM injection ℞ *rabies vaccine for pre-exposure vaccination or post-exposure prophylaxis* [rabies vaccine, chick embryo cell] 2.5 IU

rabeprazole INN *proton pump inhibitor for gastroesophageal reflux disease and ulcers* [also: rabeprazole sodium]

rabeprazole sodium USAN *investigational (NDA filed) proton pump inhibitor for gastroesophageal reflux disease and ulcers* [also: rabeprazole]

rabies immune globulin (RIG) USP *passive immunizing agent*

rabies vaccine USP *active immunizing agent* Challenge Virus Standard (CVS)

rabies vaccine, adsorbed (RVA) [see: rabies vaccine]

rabies vaccine, HDCV (human diploid cell vaccine) [see: rabies vaccine]

race ginger *medicinal herb* [see: ginger]

racefemine INN

racefenicol INN *antibacterial* [also: racephenicol]

racemethadol [see: dimepheptanol]

racemethionine USAN, USP *urinary acidifier* [also: methionine (the DL- form)]

racemethorphan INN, BAN

racemetirosine INN

racemic amphetamine phosphate

racemic amphetamine sulfate [see: amphetamine sulfate]

racemic calcium pantothenate [see: calcium pantothenate, racemic]

racemoramide INN, BAN

racemorphan INN

racephedrine HCl USAN

racephenicol USAN *antibacterial* [also: racefenicol]

racepinefrine INN *sympathomimetic bronchodilator* [also: racepinephrine]

racepinephrine USP *sympathomimetic bronchodilator* [also: racepinefrine]

racepinephrine HCl USP *sympathomimetic bronchodilator*

raclopride INN, BAN

raclopride C 11 USAN *radiopharmaceutical*

racoonberry *medicinal herb* [see: mandrake]

ractopamine INN *veterinary growth stimulant* [also: ractopamine HCl]

ractopamine HCl USAN *veterinary growth stimulant* [also: ractopamine]

radio-chromated serum albumin [see: albumin, chromated]

radio-iodinated I 125 serum albumin [see: albumin, iodinated]

radio-iodinated I 131 serum albumin [see: albumin, iodinated]

radiomerisoprol ^{197}Hg [see: merisoprol Hg 197]

radioselenomethionine ^{75}Se [see: selenomethionine Se 75]

radiotolpovidone I 131 INN *hypoalbuminemia test; radioactive agent* [also: tolpovidone I 131]

radish (Raphanus sativus) root *medicinal herb used as an antispasmodic, astringent, cholagogue, and diuretic*

radium *element (Ra)*

radon *element (Rn)*

rAd/p53 gene therapy *investigational (Phase I) therapy for cancer*

rafoxanide USAN, INN *anthelmintic*

ragged cup (Silphium perfoliatum) root and gum *medicinal herb used as an antispasmodic, diaphoretic, and stimulant*

ragwort *medicinal herb* [see: life root]

ralitoline USAN, INN *anticonvulsant*

raloxifene INN *antiestrogen; selective estrogen receptor modulator (SERM) for the prevention for postmenopausal osteoporosis* [also: raloxifene HCl]

raloxifene HCl USAN *antiestrogen; selective estrogen receptor modulator (SERM) for the prevention of postmenopausal osteoporosis* [also: raloxifene]

raltitrexed USAN *antimetabolite antineoplastic; investigational (Phase III) thymidylate synthase inhibitor for advanced colorectal cancer*

raluridine USAN *antiviral*

rambufaside [see: meproscillarin]

ramciclane INN

ramifenazone INN

ramipril USAN, INN, BAN *antihypertensive; angiotensin-converting enzyme (ACE) inhibitor*

ramiprilat INN

ramixotidine INN

ramnodigin INN

ramoplanin USAN, INN *investigational (Phase II) antibiotic for vancomycin-resistant Enterococcus faecium (VREF)*

Ramses vaginal jelly OTC *spermicidal contraceptive* [nonoxynol 9] 5%

Ramses Extra premedicated condom OTC *spermicidal/barrier contraceptive* [nonoxynol 9] 15%

ranimustine INN

ranimycin USAN, INN *antibacterial*

ranitidine USAN, INN, BAN *histamine H_2 antagonist for gastric ulcers* 150, 300 mg oral

ranitidine bismuth citrate USAN *histamine H_2 antagonist for gastric ulcers with H. pylori infection* [also: ranitidine bismutrex]

ranitidine bismutrex BAN *histamine H_2 antagonist for gastric ulcers with H. pylori infection* [also: ranitidine bismuth citrate]

ranitidine HCl USP, JAN *histamine H_2 antagonist for gastric ulcers* 15 mg/mL oral

ranolazine INN *antianginal* [also: ranolazine HCl]

ranolazine HCl USAN *investigational (Phase III) antianginal for chronic stable angina* [also: ranolazine]

Ranunculus acris; R. bulbosus; R. scleratus *medicinal herb* [see: buttercup]

rapacuronium bromide USAN *neuromuscular blocker*

Rapamune ℞ *investigational immunosuppressant for organ transplants* [sirolimus]

rapamycin [now: sirolimus]

Raphanus sativus *medicinal herb* [see: radish]

RapidTest Strep test kit for professional use (discontinued 1995) *in vitro diagnostic test for streptococcal antigens in throat swabs*

RapidVue test kit for home use OTC *in vitro diagnostic aid for urine pregnancy test*

Rapimine (name changed to Emadine upon marketing release in 1998)

rasagiline INN

rasagiline mesylate USAN *antiparkinsonian; monoamine oxidase B (MAO-B) inhibitor*

raspberry, ground *medicinal herb* [see: goldenseal]

raspberry, red; wild red raspberry *medicinal herb* [see: red raspberry]

raspberry [syrup] USP

rathyronine INN

rattleroot *medicinal herb* [see: black cohosh]

rattlesnake antivenin [see: antivenin (Crotalidae) polyvalent]

rattlesnake root *medicinal herb* [see: birthroot; black cohosh; senega]

rattleweed *medicinal herb* [see: black cohosh]

Raudixin tablets (discontinued 1995) ℞ *antihypertensive; antipsychotic* [rauwolfia serpentina (whole root)] 50, 100 mg

Rauverid tablets (discontinued 1995) ℞ *antihypertensive; antipsychotic* [rauwolfia serpentina (whole root)] 50 mg

rauwolfia derivatives *all rauwolfia derivatives except reserpine were discontinued 1991–1995*

rauwolfia serpentina USP *antihypertensive; peripheral antiadrenergic; antipsychotic*

Rauzide tablets ℞ *antihypertensive; diuretic* [bendroflumethiazide; rauwolfia serpentina] 4•50 mg

Ravocaine & Novocaine with Levophed injection ℞ *injectable local anesthetic for dental procedures* [propoxycaine HCl; procaine; norepinephrine bitartrate] 7.2•36•0.12 mg/1.8 mL

Ravocaine & Novocaine with Neo-Cobefrin injection (discontinued 1995) ℞ *injectable local anesthetic for dental procedures* [propoxycaine HCl; procaine; levonordefrin] 7.2•36•0.09 mg/1.8 mL

Raxar film-coated tablets; Rax-Pack (10 tablets) ℞ *broad-spectrum fluoroquinolone antibiotic* [grepafloxacin HCl] 200, 400, 600 mg

rayon, purified USAN, USP *surgical aid*

razinodil INN

razobazam INN

razoxane INN, BAN

86Rb [see: rubidium chloride Rb 86]

RBC-CD4 *investigational (Phase I/II) antiviral for HIV*

rBPI (bactericidal and permeability-increasing protein, recombinant) [q.v.]

rCD4 (recombinant soluble human CD4) [see: CD4, recombinant soluble human]

RCF liquid OTC *hypoallergenic infant formula* [soy protein formula, carbohydrate free]

Reabilan; Reabilan HN ready-to-use liquid OTC *enteral nutritional therapy* [lactose-free formula]

Reactine ⓒ (U.S. product: Zyrtec) film-coated tablets, syrup ℞ *once-daily antihistamine* [cetirizine HCl] 5, 10 mg; 5 mg/5 mL

reactrol [see: clemizole HCl]

rebamipide INN

Rebetol capsules ℞ *nucleoside antiviral* [ribavirin] 200 mg

Rebetron capsules + subcu or IM injection ℞ *combination treatment for chronic hepatitis C* [Rebetol (ribavirin capsules); Intron A (interferon alfa-2b injection)] 200 mg•3 million IU

Rebif ⓒ (U.S. product: Avonex) powder for injection, prefilled syringe ℞ *immunomodulator for relapsing remitting multiple sclerosis (orphan) and condyloma acuminata; investigational (orphan) for malignant melanoma, metastatic renal cell carcinoma, T-cell lymphoma, and Kaposi sarcoma* [interferon beta-1a] 3, 12 MIU/vial; 6, 12 MIU/0.5 mL

reboxetine INN *investigational (NDA filed) fast-acting selective norepinephrine reuptake inhibitor for depression*

recainam INN, BAN *antiarrhythmic* [also: recainam HCl]

recainam HCl USAN *antiarrhythmic* [also: recainam]

recainam tosylate USAN *antiarrhythmic*

recanescin [see: deserpidine]

Receptin ℞ *investigational (Phase II) antiviral for AIDS; orphan status withdrawn 1997* [CD4, recombinant soluble human]

reclazepam USAN, INN *sedative*

Reclomide tablets ℞ *antidopaminergic; antiemetic for chemotherapy; peristaltic* [metoclopramide HCl] 10 mg

Recombigen HIV-1 LA Test reagent kit for professional use *in vitro diagnostic aid for HIV-1 antibodies in blood, serum, or plasma* [latex agglutination test]

recombinant alpha₁ antitrypsin [see: alpha₁ antitrypsin, recombinant]

recombinant antihemophilic factor [see: antihemophilic factor, recombinant]

recombinant factor VIIa [see: factor VIIa, recombinant]

recombinant factor VIII [see: antihemophilic factor, recombinant]

recombinant human CD4 immunoglobulin G [CD4 immunoglobulin G, recombinant human]

recombinant human deoxyribonuclease (rhDNase) [see: dornase alfa]

recombinant human erythropoietin
[see: erythropoietin, recombinant
human]

recombinant human growth hormone (rhGH) [see: somatropin]

recombinant human interferon
beta [see: interferon beta, recombinant human]

recombinant human interleukin-1
receptor (rhIL-1R; rhu IL-1R)
[see: interleukin-1 receptor]

recombinant human nerve growth
factor (rhNGF) [see: nerve growth
factor]

recombinant human superoxide
dismutase (SOD) [see: superoxide
dismutase, recombinant human]

recombinant interferon alfa-2a [see:
interferon alfa-2a, recombinant]

recombinant interferon alfa-2b [see:
interferon alfa-2b, recombinant]

recombinant interferon beta [see:
interferon beta, recombinant]

recombinant interleukin-2 [see:
interleukin-2, recombinant]

recombinant methionyl granulocyte CSF [see: methionyl granulocyte CSF, recombinant]

recombinant methionyl human
granulocyte CSF [see: methionyl
human granulocyte CSF, recombi-
nant]

recombinant soluble human CD4
(rCD4) [see: CD4, recombinant soluble human]

recombinant tissue plasminogen
activator (rtPA; rt-PA) [see: alte-
plase]

Recombinate powder for IV injection
℞ antihemophilic to correct coagulation
deficiency [antihemophilic factor VIII,
recombinant] 250, 500, 1000 IU

Recombivax HB adult IM injection,
pediatric/adolescent IM injection,
dialysis formulation ℞ active immunizing agent for hepatitis B and D [hep-
atitis B virus vaccine, recombinant]
10 μg/mL; 5 μg/0.5 mL; 40 μg/mL

Rectacort rectal suppositories ℞ corticosteroidal anti-inflammatory [hydro-
cortisone acetate] 10%

Rectagene rectal suppositories OTC
temporary relief of hemorrhoidal symptoms [live yeast cell derivative; shark
liver oil] 2000 SRF U/oz.

Rectagene II rectal suppositories (discontinued 1997) OTC temporary relief
of hemorrhoidal symptoms [bismuth
subgallate; bismuth resorcin compound; benzyl benzoate; peruvian
balsam; zinc oxide] 2.25%•1.75%•
1.2%•1.8%•11%

Rectagene Medicated Rectal Balm
ointment OTC temporary relief of hemorrhoidal symptoms [shark liver oil;
phenyl mercuric nitrate; live yeast cell
derivative] 3%•1:10 000•66.67 U/g

Rectolax suppositories OTC stimulant
laxative [bisacodyl] 10 mg

red bay; red laurel medicinal herb [see:
magnolia]

red bearberry medicinal herb [see: uva
ursi]

red blood cells [see: blood cells, red]

red bush tea (Aspalathus contaminata; A. linearis; Borbonia pinifolia)
leaves and stems medicinal herb used as
a free radical scavenger; investigational
antineoplastic; investigational for preventing brain damage caused by aging

red clover (Trifolium pratense)
flower medicinal herb for blood cleansing, bronchitis, cancer, clearing toxins,
nervous disorders, and spasms

Red Cross Toothache liquid OTC topical oral analgesic [eugenol] 85%

red currant (Ribes rubrum) medicinal
herb [see: currant]

red elm medicinal herb [see: slippery elm]

red ferric oxide [see: ferric oxide, red]

red ink berries; red ink plant medicinal herb [see: pokeweed]

red laurel; red bay medicinal herb [see:
magnolia]

red legs medicinal herb [see: bistort]

red mulberry (Morus rubra) medicinal herb [see: mulberry]

red oak (*Quercus rubra*) *medicinal herb* [see: white oak]

red paint root *medicinal herb* [see: bloodroot]

red pepper; African red pepper; American red pepper *medicinal herb* [see: cayenne]

red pimpernel (*Anagallis arvensis*) plant *medicinal herb used as a chola-gogue, diaphoretic, diuretic, expectorant, nervine, purgative, and stimulant*

red puccoon *medicinal herb* [see: bloodroot]

red raspberry (*Rubus idaeus; R. strigosus*) leaves *medicinal herb for childbirth afterpains, diarrhea and other bowel disorders, fever, flu, morning sickness, menstrual disorders, mouth sores, nausea, and vomiting*

red root *medicinal herb* [see: bloodroot; danshen; New Jersey tea]

red sarsaparilla *medicinal herb* [see: sarsaparilla]

red veterinarian petrolatum (RVP) [see: petrolatum]

red weed *medicinal herb* [see: pokeweed]

redberry *medicinal herb* [see: ginseng]

Redi Vial (trademarked packaging form) *dual-compartment vial*

Redi Vial (trademarked packaging form) *two-compartment vial*

Rediject (trademarked delivery system) *prefilled disposable syringe*

Redipak (trademarked packaging form) *unit dose or unit-of-issue package*

RediTabs (trademarked dosage form) *rapidly disintegrating tablets*

redmond clay (montmorillonite) *natural remedy for bug bites and stings and other skin problems*

redox-acyclovir *orphan status withdrawn 1996*

redox-penicillin G *orphan status withdrawn 1996*

redox-phenytoin *orphan status withdrawn 1996*

Reducin ℞ *investigational (orphan) for nonoperative management of cutaneous fistulas of the GI tract and bleeding esophageal varices* [somatostatin]

Redutemp tablets OTC *analgesic; antipyretic* [acetaminophen] 500 mg

Redux capsules (discontinued 1997) ℞ *anorexiant and appetite suppressant for long-term dieting* [dexfenfluramine HCl] 15 mg

Reese's Pinworm soft gel capsules, liquid OTC *anthelmintic for ascariasis (roundworm) and enterobiasis (pinworm)* [pyrantel pamoate] 180 mg; 50 mg/mL

ReFacto *investigational (Phase III, orphan) long-term treatment for hemophilia A and for surgical procedures* [factor VIII SQ, recombinant]

Refludan powder for IV injection *anticoagulant for heparin-induced thrombocytopenia (orphan)* [lepirudin] 50 mg

Refresh eye drops OTC *ophthalmic moisturizer/lubricant* [polyvinyl alcohol] 1.4%

Refresh Plus; Refresh Tears eye drops OTC *ophthalmic moisturizer/lubricant* [carboxymethylcellulose] 0.5%

Refresh P.M. ophthalmic ointment OTC *ocular moisturizer/lubricant* [white petrolatum; mineral oil; lanolin]

refrigerants *a class of agents that lower abnormal body heat (a term used in folk medicine)*

Rēgain snack bar OTC *enteral nutritional therapy for impaired renal function* [multiple essential amino acids] ⊠ Rogaine

Regitine IV or IM injection ℞ *antihypertensive for pheochromocytoma; α-blocker* [phentolamine mesylate] 5 mg/mL

Reglan tablets, syrup, IV infusion ℞ *antidopaminergic; antiemetic for chemotherapy; peristaltic* [metoclopramide HCl] 5, 10 mg; 5 mg/5 mL; 5 mg/mL ⊠ Regonol

Regonol IM or IV injection ℞ *cholinergic/anticholinesterase muscle stimulant; muscle relaxant reversal* [pyridostigmine bromide] 5 mg/mL ⊠ Reglan

regramostim USAN, INN *antineutropenic; hematopoietic stimulant; biologic response modifier; bone marrow stimulant*

Regranex gel ℞ *recombinant platelet-derived growth factor B for chronic diabetic foot ulcers* [becaplermin] 0.01%

Regressin ℞ *investigational tumor growth inhibitor and apoptosis inducer for bladder cancer*

Regroton tablets ℞ *antihypertensive; diuretic* [chlorthalidone; reserpine] 50•0.25 mg ⍰ Hygroton

Regulace capsules OTC *stimulant laxative; stool softener* [casanthranol; docusate sodium] 30•100 mg

Regular Iletin I subcu injection (discontinued 1999) OTC *antidiabetic* [insulin (beef-pork)] 100 U/mL

Regular Iletin II subcu injection OTC *antidiabetic* [insulin (pork)] 100 U/mL

Regular Iletin II U-500 (concentrated) subcu or IM injection ℞ *antidiabetic* [insulin (pork)] 500 U/mL

Regular Insulin subcu injection (discontinued 1997) OTC *antidiabetic* [insulin (pork)] 100 U/mL

Regular Purified Pork Insulin subcu injection OTC *antidiabetic* [insulin] 100 U/mL

regulator, female *medicinal herb* [see: life root]

Regulax SS capsules OTC *stool softener* [docusate sodium] 100, 250 mg

Reguloid powder OTC *bulk laxative* [psyllium hydrophilic mucilloid] 3.4 g/tsp.

Regutol tablets (discontinued 1997) OTC *stool softener* [docusate sodium] 100 mg

Rehydralyte oral solution OTC *electrolyte replacement* [sodium, potassium, and chloride electrolytes]

reishi mushrooms body and stem *medicinal herb for AIDS, allergies, fatigue, heart problems, and insomnia*

Rejuva-A ⓒ (U.S. product: Retin-A) cream ℞ *treatment for photodamaged skin* [tretinoin] 0.025%

Relafen film-coated tablets ℞ *antiarthritic; nonsteroidal anti-inflammatory drug (NSAID)* [nabumetone] 500, 750 mg

Relaxadon tablets (discontinued 1995) ℞ *GI antispasmodic; anticholin-*ergic; sedative [atropine sulfate; scopolamine hydrobromide; hyoscyamine hydrobromide; phenobarbital] 0.0194•0.0065•0.1037•16.2 mg

relaxin *investigational (orphan) for progressive systemic sclerosis; investigational (Phase II/III) for scleroderma*

Release-Tabs (dosage form) *timed-release tablets*

Relefact TRH IV injection (name changed to Thyrel-TRH in 1995)

Relenza Rotadisks (powder for oral inhalation, for use with Diskhaler device) *influenza neuraminidase inhibitor for the treatment of acute influenza types A and B* [zanamivir] 5 mg

Relief eye drops OTC *topical ophthalmic decongestant* [phenylephrine HCl] 0.12%

relomycin USAN, INN *antibacterial*

remacemide INN *neuroprotective anticonvulsant* [also: remacemide HCl]

remacemide HCl USAN *neuroprotective anticonvulsant* [also: remacemide]

Remcol Cold capsules (discontinued 1995) OTC *decongestant; antihistamine; analgesic* [phenylpropanolamine HCl; chlorpheniramine maleate; acetaminophen] 25•2•300 mg

Remcol-C capsules (discontinued 1995) OTC *antitussive; antihistamine; analgesic* [dextromethorphan hydrobromide; chlorpheniramine maleate; acetaminophen] 15•2•300 mg

Remeron coated tablets ℞ *tetracyclic antidepressant* [mirtazapine] 15, 30, 45 mg ⍰ Femiron

Remicade powder for IV infusion ℞ *anti-inflammatory; anti-TNFα monoclonal antibody for severe and fistulizing Crohn's disease (orphan); investigational (NDA filed) for rheumatoid arthritis* [infliximab] 100 mg

remifentanil INN, BAN *short-acting narcotic analgesic for general anesthesia* [also: remifentanil HCl]

remifentanil HCl USAN *short-acting narcotic analgesic for general anesthesia* [also: remifentanil]

remikiren INN

Reminyl ℞ *investigational (Phase III) cognition enhancer for Alzheimer's disease* [galantamine]

remiprostol USAN, INN *antiulcerative*

remoxipride USAN, INN, BAN *antipsychotic*

remoxipride HCl USAN *antipsychotic*

Remular-S tablets ℞ *skeletal muscle relaxant* [chlorzoxazone] 250 mg

Remune ℞ *investigational (Phase III) immunostimulant theraccine for HIV* [HIV-1 immunogen, gp120-depleted, inactivated]

Renacidin powder for solution ℞ *bladder and catheter irrigant for apatite or struvite calculi (orphan)* [citric acid; D-gluconic acid lactone; magnesium hydroxycarbonate] 6.602•0.198•3.177 g/100 mL

Renacidin Irrigation solution ℞ *bladder and catheter irrigant for apatite or struvite calculi (orphan)* [citric acid; glucono-delta-lactone; magnesium carbonate]

Renagel capsules ℞ *phosphate-binding polymer for hyperphosphatemia of end-stage renal disease* [sevelamer HCl] 403 mg

RenAmin IV infusion ℞ *nutritional therapy for renal failure* [multiple essential and nonessential amino acids; electrolytes]

renanolone INN

Renese tablets ℞ *diuretic; antihypertensive* [polythiazide] 1, 2, 4 mg

Renese-R tablets ℞ *antihypertensive; diuretic* [polythiazide; reserpine] 2•0.25 mg

rennet, cheese *medicinal herb* [see: bedstraw]

Reno-30 intracavitary instillation ℞ *radiopaque contrast medium for urological imaging* [diatrizoate meglumine (46.67% iodine)] 300 mg/mL (141 mg/mL)

RenoCal-76 injection ℞ *radiopaque contrast medium* [diatrizoate meglumine; diatrizoate sodium (48.7% total iodine)] 660•100 mg/mL (370 mg/mL)

Reno-Dip; Reno-60 injection ℞ *radiopaque contrast medium* [diatrizoate meglumine (46.67% iodine)] 300 mg/mL (141 mg/mL); 600 mg/mL (282 mg/mL)

Renografin-60 injection ℞ *radiopaque contrast medium* [diatrizoate meglumine; diatrizoate sodium (48.75% total iodine)] 520•80 mg/mL (292.5 mg/mL)

Renografin-76 injection (discontinued 1999) ℞ *radiopaque contrast medium* [diatrizoate meglumine; diatrizoate sodium (48.75% total iodine)] 66%•10% (37%)

Reno-M-Dip; Reno-M-30; Reno-M-60 injection (name changed to Reno-Dip, Reno-30, and Reno-60 in 1999)

Renoquid tablets ℞ *broad-spectrum bacteriostatic* [sulfacytine] 250 mg

Renormax tablets (discontinued 1995) ℞ *antihypertensive; ACE inhibitor* [spirapril HCl] 3, 6, 12, 24 mg

Renova cream ℞ *retinoid for photodamage, fine wrinkles, mottled hyperpigmentation, and roughness of facial skin* [tretinoin] 0.05%

Renovist; Renovist II injection (discontinued 1999) ℞ *radiopaque contrast medium* [diatrizoate meglumine; diatrizoate sodium (53.8% total iodine)] 34.3%•35% (37%); 28.5%•29.1% (31%)

Renovue-Dip; Renovue-65 injection (discontinued 1999) ℞ *radiopaque contrast medium* [iodamide meglumine (46% iodine)] 24%; 65%

Rentamine Pediatric oral suspension ℞ *pediatric antitussive, decongestant, and antihistamine* [carbetapentane tannate; phenylephrine tannate; ephedrine tannate; chlorpheniramine tannate] 30•5•5•4 mg/5 mL

rentiapril INN

ReNu solution OTC *rinsing/storage solution for soft contact lenses* [sodium chloride (preserved saline solution)]

ReNu Effervescent Enzymatic Cleaner; ReNu Thermal Enzymatic Cleaner tablets OTC *enzy-*

matic cleaner for soft contact lenses [subtilisin]

ReNu Multi-Purpose solution OTC *chemical disinfecting solution for soft contact lenses*

renytoline INN *anti-inflammatory* [also: paranyline HCl]

renytoline HCl [see: paranyline HCl]

renzapride INN, BAN

ReoPro IV injection ℞ *platelet aggregation inhibitor for acute arterial occlusive disorders (antianginal trials discontinued 1995)* [abciximab] 2 mg/mL

repaglinide *oral antidiabetic agent that stimulates release of insulin from the pancreas in type 2 diabetes mellitus*

Repan tablets, capsules ℞ *analgesic; sedative* [acetaminophen; caffeine; butalbital] 325•40•50 mg ⊡ Riopan

Repan CF tablets ℞ *analgesic; antipyretic; sedative* [acetaminophen; butalbital] 650•50 mg

Repetab (trademarked dosage form) *extended-release tablet*

repirinast USAN, INN *antiallergic; antiasthmatic*

Replens vaginal gel OTC *lubricant* [glycerin; mineral oil]

Replete ready-to-use liquid OTC *enteral nutritional therapy* [lactose-free formula]

rEPO (recombinant erythropoietin) [see: epoetin alfa; epoetin beta]

Reposans-10 capsules ℞ *benzodiazepine anxiolytic* [chlordiazepoxide HCl] 10 mg

repository corticotropin [see: corticotropin, repository]

repromicin USAN, INN *antibacterial*

Repronex powder for IM injection ℞ *ovulation stimulant for women; spermatogenesis stimulant for men* [menotropins] 75, 150 IU/ampule

reproterol INN, BAN *bronchodilator* [also: reproterol HCl]

reproterol HCl USAN *bronchodilator* [also: reproterol]

Requip film-coated tablets ℞ *dopamine agonist; antiparkinsonian; investigational for restless leg syndrome (RLS)* [ropinirole HCl] 0.25, 0.5, 1, 2, 5 mg

Resaid sustained-release capsules ℞ *decongestant; antihistamine* [phenylpropanolamine HCl; chlorpheniramine maleate] 75•12 mg

Rescaps-D S.R. sustained-release capsules ℞ *antitussive; decongestant* [caramiphen edisylate; phenylpropanolamine HCl] 40•75 mg

rescimetol INN

rescinnamine NF, INN, BAN *antihypertensive; rauwolfia derivative*

Rescon liquid OTC *decongestant; antihistamine* [phenylpropanolamine HCl; chlorpheniramine maleate] 12.5•2 mg/5 mL

Rescon sustained-release capsules ℞ *decongestant; antihistamine* [pseudoephedrine HCl; chlorpheniramine maleate] 120•12 mg

Rescon JR controlled-release capsules ℞ *pediatric decongestant and antihistamine* [pseudoephedrine HCl; chlorpheniramine maleate] 60•4 mg

Rescon-DM liquid OTC *antitussive; decongestant; antihistamine* [dextromethorphan hydrobromide; pseudoephedrine HCl; chlorpheniramine maleate] 10•30•2 mg/5 mL

Rescon-ED controlled-release capsules ℞ *decongestant; antihistamine* [pseudoephedrine HCl; chlorpheniramine maleate] 120•8 mg

Rescon-GG liquid OTC *decongestant; expectorant* [phenylephrine HCl; guaifenesin] 5•100 mg/5 mL

Rescriptor tablets ℞ *antiretroviral; non-nucleoside reverse transcriptase inhibitor (NNRTI) for HIV-1* [delavirdine mesylate] 100, 200 mg

Rescue Pak (trademarked dosage form) *unit dose package*

Rescula ℞ *investigational (Phase III) antiglaucoma agent* [isopropyl unoprostone]

Resectisol solution ℞ *genitourinary irrigant* [mannitol] 5 g/100 mL

reserpine USP, INN *antihypertensive; peripheral antiadrenergic; rauwolfia derivative* 0.1, 0.25 mg oral

resibufogenin [see: bufogenin]

Retin-A cream, gel, liquid Ŗ *topical keratolytic for acne* [tretinoin] 0.025%, 0.05%, 0.1% (0.01% available in Canada); 0.025%, 0.1%; 0.05%

Retin-A Micro gel Ŗ *topical keratolytic for acne* [tretinoin] 0.1%

retinal pigmented epithelial cells, human, on collagen microcarriers *investigational (orphan) for stage 3 and 4 Parkinson's disease*

retinamide R-II *investigational (orphan) for myelodysplastic syndrome*

retinoic acid (all-*trans*-retinoic acid) [see: tretinoin]

9-*cis*-retinoic acid [see: alitretinoin]

13-*cis*-retinoic acid [see: isotretinoin]

retinoids *a class of antineoplastics chemically related to vitamin A*

Retinol cream OTC *moisturizer; emollient* [vitamin A] 100 000 IU

retinol INN, BAN *vitamin A_1*

Retinol-A cream OTC *moisturizer; emollient* [vitamin A palmitate] 10 000 IU/g

Retrovector Ŗ *investigational (Phase II) gene therapy for asymptomatic HIV infection* [HIV immunotherapeutic (HIV-IT)]

Retrovir film-coated tablets, capsules, syrup, IV injection Ŗ *nucleoside antiviral for HIV, AIDS, and AIDS-related complex (orphan)* [zidovudine] 300 mg; 100 mg; 50 mg/5 mL; 10 mg/mL

Revasc Ŗ *investigational thrombin inhibitor* [desirudin]

revenast INN

reverse transcriptase (RT) inhibitors *a class of antivirals that inhibit HIV replication* [reverse transcriptase is also known as DNA polymerase]

reversible proton pump inhibitors [see: proton pump inhibitors]

Reversol IV or IM injection Ŗ *myasthenia gravis treatment; antidote to curare overdose* [edrophonium chloride] 10 mg/mL

Revex IV, IM, or subcu injection Ŗ *opioid antagonist for narcotic overdose* [nalmefene] 100 μg/mL, 1 mg/mL

Rēv-Eyes powder for eye drops Ŗ *miotic to reverse iatrogenic mydriasis* [dapiprazole HCl] 0.5%

ReVia tablets Ŗ *narcotic antagonist for opiate dependence or overdose (orphan) and alcoholism* [naltrexone HCl] 50 mg

revospirone INN, BAN

Rexigen Forte sustained-release capsules Ŗ *anorexiant; CNS stimulant* [phendimetrazine tartrate] 105 mg

Rexolate IM injection Ŗ *analgesic; antipyretic; anti-inflammatory; antirheumatic* [sodium thiosalicylate] 50 mg/mL

Rezamid lotion OTC *topical acne treatment* [sulfur; resorcinol; alcohol] 5%•2%•28%

Rezine tablets (discontinued 1995) Ŗ *anxiolytic* [hydroxyzine HCl] 10, 25 ml

Rezipas Ŗ *investigational (orphan) for ulcerative colitis* [aminosalicylic acid]

Rezulin film-coated tablets Ŗ *thiazolidinedione antidiabetic; increases cellular response to insulin without increasing insulin secretion* [troglitazone] 200, 300, 400 mg

R-Frone Ŗ *investigational (orphan) for metastatic renal cell carcinoma, malignant melanoma, and Kaposi sarcoma* [interferon beta-1a, recombinant]

RG 201 *investigational (Phase I) antiinfective for AIDS-related Pneumocystis carinii pneumonia (PCP)*

rGCR (recombinant glucocerebrosidase) [see: glucocerebrosidase, recombinant retroviral vector]

rG-CSF (recombinant granulocyte colony-stimulating factor) [see: lenograstim]

R-Gel OTC *topical analgesic* [capsaicin] 0.025%

R-Gen elixir Ŗ *expectorant* [iodinated glycerol] 60 mg/5 mL

R-gene 10 IV injection Ŗ *diagnostic aid for pituitary (growth hormone) function* [arginine HCl] 10% (950 mOsm/L)

RGG0853, E1A lipid complex *investigational (orphan) for advanced ovarian cancer*

rGM-CSF; rhGM-CSF; rhuGM-CSF (granulocyte-macrophage colony-stimulating factor) [q.v.]

rgp160; rgp160 IIIB; rgp160 MN (recombinant glycoprotein) *investigational (Phase I–III) antiviral (treatment) and vaccine (preventative) for HIV* [also: AIDS vaccine]

$Rh_0(D)$ immune globulin USP *passive immunizing agent; treatment for immune thrombocytopenic purpura (orphan)*

$Rh_0(D)$ immune human globulin [now: $Rh_0(D)$ immune globulin]

Rhamnus cathartica; R. frangula medicinal herb [see: buckthorn]

Rhamnus purshiana medicinal herb [see: cascara sagrada]

(rhATIII) recombinant human antithrombin III) [see: antithrombin III]

rHb1.1 (recombinant human hemoglobin) [see: hemoglobin, recombinant human]

rhDNase (recombinant human deoxyribonuclease) [see: dornase alfa]

Rheaban caplets OTC *antidiarrheal; GI adsorbent* [activated attapulgite] 750 mg

rhenium *element (Re)*

Rheomacrodex IV infusion ℞ *plasma volume expander for shock due to hemorrhage, burns, or surgery* [dextran 40] 10%

RheothRx Copolymer (name changed to Flocor in 1998)

rheotran (45) [see: dextran 45]

Rhesonativ IM injection (discontinued 1995) ℞ *obstetric Rh factor immunity suppressant* [$Rh_0(D)$ immune globulin]

rhetinic acid [see: enoxolone]

Rheum palmatum medicinal herb [see: rhubarb]

Rheumatex slide tests for professional use *in vitro diagnostic aid for rheumatoid factor in the blood* ② Rheumatrex

rheumatism root *medicinal herb* [see: twin leaf; wild yam]

rheumatism weed *medicinal herb* [see: pipsissewa]

Rheumaton slide tests for professional use *in vitro diagnostic aid for rheumatoid factor in serum or synovial fluid*

Rheumatrex Dose Pack (tablets) ℞ *antimetabolite antineoplastic for leukemia; systemic antipsoriatic; antirheumatic; investigational (orphan) for juvenile rheumatoid arthritis* [methotrexate sodium] 2.5 mg ② Rheumatex

rhFSH (recombinant human follicle-stimulating hormone) [see: menotropins]

rhGH (recombinant human growth hormone) [see: somatropin]

rhIGF-1 (recombinant human insulin-like growth factor-1) [now: mecasermin]

rhIL-1R; rhu IL-1R (recombinant human interleukin-1 receptor) [see: interleukin-1 receptor]

rhIL-11 (recombinant human interleukin-11) [see: interleukin-11, recombinant human]

rhIL-12 (recombinant human interleukin-12) [see: interleukin-12]

Rhinall nasal spray, nose drops OTC *nasal decongestant* [phenylephrine HCl] 0.25%

Rhinatate tablets ℞ *decongestant; antihistamine* [phenylephrine tannate; chlorpheniramine tannate; pyrilamine tannate] 25•8•25 mg

Rhinocaps capsules OTC *decongestant; analgesic; antipyretic* [phenylpropanolamine HCl; acetaminophen; aspirin] 20•162•162 mg

Rhinocort nasal inhalation aerosol ℞ *corticosteroidal anti-inflammatory for seasonal or perennial rhinitis* [budesonide] 32 μg/dose

Rhinocort Aqua ⓒ nasal spray ℞ *intranasal steroidal anti-inflammatory* [budesonide] 100 μg/spray

Rhinocort Turbuhaler ⓒ (U.S. product: Pulmicort Turbuhaler) (dry powder in a metered-dose inhaler) ℞ *intranasal steroidal anti-inflammatory* [budesonide] 100 μg/dose

Rhinogesic tablets (discontinued 1995) OTC *decongestant; antihistamine; analgesic* [phenylephrine HCl; chlorpheniramine maleate; acetaminophen; salicylamide] 5•2•150•250 mg

Rhinolar sustained-release capsules (discontinued 1995) ℞ *decongestant; antihistamine; anticholinergic* [phenylpropanolamine HCl; chlorpheniramine maleate; methscopolamine nitrate] 75•8•2.5 mg

Rhinolar-EX; Rhinolar-EX 12 sustained-release capsules ℞ *decongestant; antihistamine* [phenylpropanolamine HCl; chlorpheniramine maleate] 75•8 mg; 75•12 mg

Rhinosyn; Rhinosyn-PD liquid OTC *decongestant; antihistamine* [pseudoephedrine HCl; chlorpheniramine maleate; alcohol] 60•4 mg/5 mL; 30•2 mg/5 mL

Rhinosyn-DM liquid OTC *antitussive; decongestant; antihistamine* [dextromethorphan hydrobromide; pseudoephedrine HCl; chlorpheniramine maleate; alcohol 1.4%] 15•30•2 mg/5 mL

Rhinosyn-DMX syrup OTC *antitussive; expectorant* [dextromethorphan hydrobromide; guaifenesin] 15•100 mg/5 mL

Rhinosyn-X liquid OTC *antitussive; decongestant; expectorant* [dextromethorphan hydrobromide; pseudoephedrine HCl; guaifenesin; alcohol 7.5%] 10•30•100 mg/5 mL

rhNGF (recombinant human nerve growth factor) [see: nerve growth factor]

rhodine [see: aspirin]

rhodium *element (Rh)*

Rho-Fluphenazine Ⓒᴬᴺ (U.S. product: Prolixin Decanoate) subcu or IM injection ℞ *conventional (typical) antipsychotic* [fluphenazine decanoate] 25, 100 mg/mL

RhoGAM IM injection ℞ *obstetric Rh factor immunity suppressant* [Rh₀(D) immune globulin] 300 μg

rhubarb *(Rheum palmatum)* root *medicinal herb for colon and liver disorders*

Rhuli gel OTC *topical poison ivy treatment* [benzyl alcohol; menthol; camphor] 2%•0.3%•0.3%

Rhuli spray OTC *topical poison ivy treatment* [benzocaine; calamine; camphor] 5%•13.8%•0.7%

rhuMab-E25 *investigational (Phase III) monoclonal antibody for allergic asthma*

Rhus glabra medicinal herb [see: sumach]

Rhythmin sustained-release tablets ℞ *antiarrhythmic* [procainamide HCl]

Riba 3.0 SIA reagent kit for professional use *in vitro diagnostic aid for hepatitis C* [strip immunoblot assay (SIA)]

ribaminol USAN, INN *memory adjuvant*

ribavirin USP, INN *antiviral for severe lower respiratory tract infections; investigational (Phase II/III) for HIV; investigational (orphan) for hemorrhagic fever with renal syndrome* [also: tribavirin]

Ribes nigrum; R. rubrum medicinal herb [see: currant]

ribgrass; ribwort *medicinal herb* [see: plantain]

riboflavin USP, INN *vitamin B_2; vitamin G; enzyme cofactor* 25, 50, 100 mg oral

riboflavin 5′-phosphate sodium USP *vitamin*

riboflavine [see: riboflavin]

riboprine USAN, INN *antineoplastic*

ribostamycin INN, BAN

riboxamide [see: tiazofurin]

ricainide [see: indecainide HCl]

rice bran oil (gamma oryzanol) extract *medicinal herb used as a hypolipidemic and to treat gastrointestinal and menopausal symptoms*

richweed *medicinal herb* [see: black cohosh; stone root]

ricin (blocked) conjugated murine MAb (anti-B4) *investigational (orphan) for B-cell lymphoma, leukemia, and treatment of bone marrow in non-T-cell ALL; clinical trials discontinued 1997*

ricin (blocked) conjugated murine MAb (anti-MY9) *investigational (orphan) for myeloid leukemia (including AML), ex vivo treatment of autologous bone marrow in AML, and blast crisis in CML*

ricin (blocked) conjugated murine MAb (CD6) *investigational (orphan) for T-cell leukemias, lymphomas, and other mature T-cell malignancies*

ricin (blocked) conjugated murine MAb (N901) *investigational (orphan) for small cell lung cancer*

RID liquid OTC *pediculicide for lice* [pyrethrins; piperonyl butoxide; petroleum distillate] 0.3%•3•1.2%

Rid-A-Pain gel OTC *topical oral anesthetic* [benzocaine] 10%

Rid-A-Pain with Codeine tablets (discontinued 1995) ℞ *narcotic analgesic* [codeine phosphate; acetaminophen; aspirin; caffeine; salicylamide] 1•97.2•226.8•32.4•32.4 mg

Ridaura capsules ℞ *antirheumatic* [auranofin] 3 mg

ridazolol INN

RIDD (recombinant interleukin-2, dacarbazine, DDP) *chemotherapy protocol*

Ridenol elixir OTC *analgesic; antipyretic* [acetaminophen] 80 mg/5 mL

ridogrel USAN, INN, BAN *thromboxane synthetase inhibitor*

rifabutin USAN, INN *antiviral; antibacterial; for prevention of Mycobacterium avium complex (MAC) in advanced HIV patients (orphan)*

Rifadin capsules, powder for IV injection ℞ *tuberculostatic (orphan)* [rifampin] 150, 300 mg; 600 mg ② Ritalin

rifalazil USAN *investigational (Phase II) rifampin derivative for Mycobacterium avium complex (MAC) and Mycobacterium tuberculosis*

Rifamate capsules ℞ *tuberculostatic* [rifampin; isoniazid] 300•150 mg

rifametane USAN, INN *antibacterial*

rifamexil USAN *antibacterial*

rifamide USAN, INN *antibacterial*

rifampicin INN, BAN, JAN *antibacterial* [also: rifampin]

rifampin USAN, USP *antibacterial; antituberculosis agent (orphan)* [also: rifampicin]

rifampin & isoniazid & pyrazinamide *short-course treatment of tuberculosis (orphan)*

rifamycin INN, BAN

rifamycin diethylamide [see: rifamide]

rifamycin M-14 [see: rifamide]

rifapentine USAN, INN, BAN *antibacterial for tuberculosis (orphan); investigational (orphan) for AIDS-related Mycobacterium avium complex (MAC)*

Rifater tablets ℞ *short-course treatment for tuberculosis (orphan)* [rifampin; isoniazid; pyrazinamide] 120•50•300 mg

rifaxidin [see: rifaximin]

rifaximin USAN, INN *antibacterial; investigational (orphan) for hepatic encephalopathy*

rIFN-A (recombinant interferon alfa) [see: interferon alfa-2a, recombinant]

rIFN-α2 (recombinant interferon alfa-2) [see: interferon alfa-2b, recombinant]

rIFN-B (recombinant interferon beta) [see: interferon beta-1b, recombinant]

r-IFN-beta ℞ *investigational (orphan) for malignant melanoma, metastatic renal cell carcinoma, T-cell lymphoma, and Kaposi sarcoma* [interferon beta, recombinant]

rifomycin [see: rifamycin]

RIG (rabies immune globulin) [q.v.]

RIGScan ℞ *investigational imaging agent*

rilapine INN

rilmazafone INN

rilmenidine INN

rilopirox INN

rilozarone INN

Rilutek film-coated tablets ℞ *amyotrophic lateral sclerosis (ALS) treatment (orphan); investigational (orphan) for Huntington's disease; investiga-*

tional (Phase III) for Parkinson's disease [riluzole] 50 mg

riluzole USAN, INN *amyotrophic lateral sclerosis (ALS) treatment (orphan); investigational (orphan) for Huntington's disease; investigational (Phase III) for Parkinson's disease*

Rimactane capsules ℞ *tuberculostatic* [rifampin] 300 mg

Rimactane/INH Dual Pack (two-product package) (discontinued 1996) ℞ *tuberculostatic* [rifampin (2 capsules); isoniazid (1 tablet)] 300 mg; 300 mg

Rimadyl (approved but not currently being marketed) ℞ *nonsteroidal anti-inflammatory drug (NSAID); analgesic; antipyretic* [carprofen]

rimantadine INN *antiviral* [also: rimantadine HCl]

rimantadine HCl USAN *antiviral* [also: rimantadine]

rimazolium metilsulfate INN

rimcazole INN *antipsychotic* [also: rimcazole HCl]

rimcazole HCl USAN *antipsychotic* [also: rimcazole]

rimexolone USAN, INN, BAN *ophthalmic corticosteroidal anti-inflammatory*

rimiterol INN *bronchodilator* [also: rimiterol hydrobromide]

rimiterol hydrobromide USAN *bronchodilator* [also: rimiterol]

rimoprogin INN

Rimso-50 solution for bladder instillation ℞ *anti-inflammatory for symptomatic relief of interstitial cystitis* [dimethyl sulfoxide (DMSO)] 50%

Rinade B.I.D. sustained-release capsules ℞ *decongestant; antihistamine* [pseudoephedrine HCl; chlorpheniramine maleate] 120•8 mg

Ringer's injection USP *fluid and electrolyte replenisher* [also: compound solution of sodium chloride]

Ringer's injection, lactated USP *fluid and electrolyte replenisher; systemic alkalizer* [also: compound solution of sodium lactate]

Ringer's irrigation USP *irrigation solution*

Ringer's solution [now: Ringer's irrigation]

riodipine INN

Riopan suspension OTC *antacid* [magaldrate] 540 mg/5 mL

Riopan Plus chewable tablets, oral suspension OTC *antacid; antiflatulent* [magaldrate; simethicone] 480•20, 1080•20 mg; 540•40, 1080•40 mg/5 mL

rioprostil USAN, INN *gastric antisecretory*

ripazepam USAN, INN *minor tranquilizer*

ripple grass *medicinal herb* [see: plantain]

risedronate sodium USAN *bisphosphonate bone resorption inhibitor for Paget's disease*

rismorelin porcine USAN *growth stimulant for growth hormone deficiencies*

risocaine USAN, INN *local anesthetic*

risotilide HCl USAN *antiarrhythmic*

Risperdal tablets, oral solution ℞ *novel (atypical) antipsychotic* [risperidone] 0.25, 0.5, 1, 2, 3, 4 mg; 1 mg/mL ② Restoril

risperidone USAN, INN, BAN *benzisoxazole antipsychotic; neuroleptic*

ristianol INN, BAN *immunoregulator* [also: ristianol phosphate]

ristianol phosphate USAN *immunoregulator* [also: ristianol]

ristocetin USP, INN, BAN

Ritalin tablets ℞ *CNS stimulant for attention deficit hyperactivity disorders (ADHD) and narcolepsy; also abused as a street drug* [methylphenidate HCl] 5, 10, 20 mg ② Ismelin; Rifadin

Ritalin-SR sustained-release tablets ℞ *CNS stimulant for attention deficit hyperactivity disorders (ADHD) and narcolepsy* [methylphenidate HCl] 20 mg

ritanserin USAN, INN, BAN *serotonin S₂ antagonist; investigational agent for various psychiatric illnesses and substance abuse* 10 mg oral

ritiometan INN

ritodrine USAN, INN *smooth muscle relaxant*

ritodrine HCl USAN, USP *smooth muscle relaxant; uterine relaxant to arrest* *preterm labor* 0.3, 10, 15 mg/mL injection

ritolukast USAN, INN *antiasthmatic; leukotriene antagonist*

ritonavir USAN, INN *antiviral protease inhibitor for HIV*

ritropirronium bromide INN

ritrosulfan INN

Rituxan IV infusion ℞ *monoclonal antibody for non-Hodgkin's B-cell lymphoma (orphan)* [rituximab] 10 mg/mL

rituximab USAN *monoclonal antibody for non-Hodgkin's B-cell lymphoma (orphan)*

rivastigmine tartrate *investigational (NDA filed) acetylcholinesterase inhibitor for Alzheimer's disease*

rizatriptan benzoate USAN *vascular serotonin 5-HT$_1$ receptor agonist for migraine headache*

rizatriptan sulfate USAN *vascular serotonin 5-HT$_{1B/1D}$ receptor agonist for migraine*

rizolipase INN

RMP-7 (receptor-mediated permeabilizer) *investigational (Phase III) for AIDS; investigational (Phase II) blood-brain barrier permeability-enhancing agent for carrying carboplatin to brain tumors*

RMS suppositories ℞ *narcotic analgesic* [morphine sulfate] 5, 10, 20, 30 mg

rNPA (recombinant novel plasminogen activator) [see: novel plasminogen activator]

Ro 64-0796 *investigational (NDA filed) neuraminidase inhibitor that decreases influenza viral replication and symptom duration*

rob elder *medicinal herb* [see: elderberry]

Robafen AC Cough syrup ℞ *narcotic antitussive; expectorant* [codeine phosphate; guaifenesin; alcohol 3.5%] 10•100 mg/5 mL

Robafen CF liquid OTC *antitussive; decongestant; expectorant* [dextromethorphan hydrobromide; phenylpropanolamine HCl; guaifenesin] 10•12.5•100 mg/5 mL

Robafen DAC syrup ℞ *narcotic antitussive; decongestant; expectorant* [codeine phosphate; pseudoephedrine HCl; guaifenesin; alcohol 1.4%] 10•30•100 mg/5 mL

Robafen DM syrup OTC *antitussive; expectorant* [dextromethorphan hydrobromide; guaifenesin; alcohol 1.4%] 10•100 mg/5 mL

RoBathol Bath Oil OTC *bath emollient*

Robaxin tablets, IV or IM injection ℞ *skeletal muscle relaxant* [methocarbamol] 500, 750 mg; 100 mg/mL

Robaxisal tablets ℞ *skeletal muscle relaxant; analgesic* [methocarbamol; aspirin] 400•325 mg ⊡ Robaxacet

robenidine INN *coccidiostat for poultry* [also: robenidine HCl]

robenidine HCl USAN *coccidiostat for poultry* [also: robenidine]

Robicap (trademarked dosage form) *capsule*

Robicillin VK tablets (discontinued 1998) ℞ *natural penicillin antibiotic* [penicillin V potassium] 250, 500 mg

Robimycin Robitabs (enteric-coated tablets) (discontinued 1998) ℞ *macrolide antibiotic* [erythromycin] 250 mg

Robinul tablets, IV or IM injection ℞ *GI antispasmodic; anticholinergic; peptic ulcer treatment adjunct; antisecretory* [glycopyrrolate] 1 mg; 0.2 mg/5 mL

Robinul Forte tablets ℞ *GI antispasmodic; anticholinergic; peptic ulcer treatment adjunct; antisecretory* [glycopyrrolate] 2 mg

Robitab (trademarked dosage form) *tablet*

Robitet Robicaps (capsules) (discontinued 1997) ℞ *broad-spectrum antibiotic* [tetracycline HCl] 250, 500 mg

Robitussin syrup OTC *expectorant* [guaifenesin; alcohol 3.5%] 100 mg/5 mL

Robitussin A-C syrup ℞ *narcotic antitussive; expectorant* [codeine phosphate; guaifenesin; alcohol 3.5%] 10•100 mg/5 mL

Robitussin Cold & Cough Liqui-Gels (capsules) OTC *antitussive; decongestant; expectorant* [dextromethorphan hydrobromide; pseudoephedrine HCl; guaifenesin] 10•30•200 mg

Robitussin Cough Calmers lozenge OTC *antitussive* [dextromethorphan hydrobromide] 5 mg

Robitussin Cough & Cold; Robitussin Pediatric Cough & Cold liquid OTC *antitussive; decongestant* [dextromethorphan hydrobromide; pseudoephedrine HCl] 15•30 mg/5 mL; 7.5•15 mg/5 mL

Robitussin Cough Drops lozenge OTC *topical analgesic; mild anesthetic* [menthol] 7.4, 10 mg

Robitussin Liquid Center Cough Drops lozenges OTC *topical analgesic; counterirritant; mild local anesthetic* [menthol] 10 mg

Robitussin Night Relief liquid OTC *antitussive; decongestant; antihistamine; analgesic* [dextromethorphan hydrobromide; pseudoephedrine HCl; pyrilamine maleate; acetaminophen] 5•10•8.3•108.3 mg/5 mL

Robitussin Pediatric liquid OTC *antitussive* [dextromethorphan hydrobromide] 7.5 mg/5 mL

Robitussin Severe Congestion Liqui-Gels (capsules) OTC *expectorant; decongestant* [guaifenesin; pseudoephedrine HCl] 200•30 mg

Robitussin-CF liquid OTC *antitussive; decongestant; expectorant* [dextromethorphan hydrobromide; phenylpropanolamine HCl; guaifenesin; alcohol 4.75%] 10•12.5•100 mg/5 mL

Robitussin-DAC syrup ℞ *narcotic antitussive; decongestant; expectorant* [codeine phosphate; pseudoephedrine HCl; guaifenesin; alcohol 1.9%] 10•30•100 mg/5 mL

Robitussin-DM liquid OTC *antitussive; expectorant* [dextromethorphan hydrobromide; guaifenesin] 10•100 mg/5 mL

Robitussin-PE syrup OTC *decongestant; expectorant* [pseudoephedrine HCl; guaifenesin; alcohol 1.4%] 30•100 mg/5 mL

Rocaltrol capsules; oral solution ℞ *vitamin D therapy for hypocalcemia and hypoparathyroidism; decreases severity of psoriatic lesions* [calcitriol] 0.25, 0.5 μg; 1 μg/mL

rocastine INN *antihistamine* [also: rocastine HCl]

rocastine HCl USAN *antihistamine* [also: rocastine]

Rocephin powder or frozen premix for IV or IM injection ℞ *cephalosporin antibiotic* [ceftriaxone sodium] 0.25, 0.5, 1, 2, 10 g

rochelle salt [see: potassium sodium tartrate]

rociverine INN

rock brake; rock polypod *medicinal herb* [see: female fern]

rock elm *medicinal herb* [see: slippery elm]

rock parsley *medicinal herb* [see: parsley]

rock rose (*Helianthemum canadense*) plant *medicinal herb used as an astringent and tonic*

Rocky Mountain grape *medicinal herb* [see: Oregon grape]

Rocky Mountain spotted fever vaccine USP

rocuronium bromide USAN, INN, BAN *neuromuscular blocking agent*

R.O.-Dexsone ⊛ (U.S. product: Decadron Phosphate) eye drops ℞ *topical ophthalmic corticosteroidal anti-inflammatory* [dexamethasone sodium phosphate] 0.1%

rodocaine USAN, INN *local anesthetic*

rodorubicin INN

rofecoxib *COX-2 inhibitor anti-inflammatory and analgesic for osteoarthritis, acute pain, and primary dysmenorrhea*

rofelodine INN

Roferon-A subcu or IM injection, prefilled syringes ℞ *antineoplastic/ antiviral for hairy cell leukemia and Kaposi sarcoma (orphan); hepatitis C treatment; investigational (orphan) for chronic myelogenous leukemia and renal cell carcinoma* [interferon alfa-2a] 3, 6, 9, 36 million IU/mL; 3, 6, 9 million IU

roflurane USAN, INN *inhalation anesthetic*

Rogaine for Men; Rogaine for Women; Rogaine Extra Strength for Men topical solution OTC *hair growth stimulant* [minoxidil] 2%; 2%; 5% ⑨ Rēgain

rogletimide USAN, INN, BAN *antineoplastic; aromatase inhibitor*

rokitamycin INN

Rolaids, Calcium Rich chewable tablets OTC *antacid* [magnesium hydroxide; calcium carbonate] 80•412 mg

Rolatuss Expectorant liquid ℞ *narcotic antitussive; decongestant; antihistamine; expectorant* [codeine phosphate; phenylephrine HCl; chlorpheniramine maleate; ammonium chloride; alcohol 5%] 9.85•5•2•33.3 mg/5 mL

Rolatuss Plain liquid OTC *decongestant; antihistamine* [phenylephrine HCl; chlorpheniramine maleate; alcohol 5%] 5•2 mg/5 mL

Rolatuss with Hydrocodone liquid ℞ *narcotic antitussive; decongestant; antihistamine* [hydrocodone bitartrate; phenylpropanolamine HCl; phenylephrine HCl; pyrilamine maleate; pheniramine maleate] 1.7•3.3•5•3.3•3.3 mg/5 mL

Rolazar ℞ *investigational antineoplastic* [pemetrexed disodium]

roletamide USAN, INN *hypnotic*

rolgamidine USAN, INN, BAN *antidiarrheal*

rolicton [see: amisometradine]

rolicyclidine INN

rolicypram BAN *antidepressant* [also: rolicyprine]

rolicyprine USAN, INN *antidepressant* [also: rolicypram]

rolipram USAN, INN *tranquilizer*

rolitetracycline USAN, USP, INN *antibacterial*

rolitetracycline nitrate USAN *antibacterial*

rolodine USAN, INN *skeletal muscle relaxant*

rolziracetam INN, BAN

Roman camomile *medicinal herb* [see: chamomile]

Roman laurel *medicinal herb* [see: laurel]

romazarit USAN, INN, BAN *anti-inflammatory; antirheumatic*

Romazicon IV injection ℞ *benzodiazepine antagonist to reverse anesthesia or treat overdose* [flumazenil] 0.1 mg/mL

rometin [see: clioquinol]

romifenone INN

romifidine INN

romurtide INN

Romycin topical solution (discontinued 1995) ℞ *topical antibiotic for acne* [erythromycin] 2%

ronactolol INN

Rondamine-DM pediatric drops ℞ *pediatric antitussive, decongestant, and antihistamine* [dextromethorphan hydrobromide; pseudoephedrine HCl; carbinoxamine maleate] 4•25•2 mg/5 mL

Rondec chewable tablets ℞ *decongestant; antihistamine* [pseudoephedrine HCl; brompheniramine maleate] 60•4 mg

Rondec film-coated tablets, syrup, pediatric drops ℞ *decongestant; antihistamine* [pseudoephedrine HCl; carbinoxamine maleate] 60•4 mg; 60•4 mg/5 mL; 25•2 mg/mL

Rondec-DM syrup, pediatric drops ℞ *antitussive; decongestant; antihistamine* [dextromethorphan hydrobromide; pseudoephedrine HCl; carbinoxamine maleate] 15•60•4 mg/5 mL; 4•25•2 mg/mL

Rondec-TR timed-release Filmtabs (film-coated tablets) ℞ *decongestant; antihistamine* [pseudoephedrine HCl; carbinoxamine maleate] 120•8 mg

ronidazole USAN, INN *antiprotozoal*

ronifibrate INN

ronipamil INN

ronnel USAN *systemic insecticide* [also: fenclofos; fenchlorphos]

ropinirole INN, BAN *dopamine agonist; antiparkinsonian* [also: ropinirole HCl]

ropinirole HCl USAN *dopamine agonist; antiparkinsonian* [also: ropinirole]

ropitoin INN *antiarrhythmic* [also: ropitoin HCl]

ropitoin HCl USAN *antiarrhythmic* [also: ropitoin]

ropivacaine INN *long-acting local anesthetic*

ropivacaine HCl *long-acting local anesthetic*

ropizine USAN, INN *anticonvulsant*

roquinimex USAN, INN *investigational (Phase II) immunomodulator for HIV; investigational for bone marrow transplant for leukemia; clinical trials for MS discontinued 1997; orphan status withdrawn 1998*

Rosa acicularis; R. canina; R. rugosa **and other species** *medicinal herb* [see: rose]

rosamicin [now: rosaramicin]

rosamicin butyrate [now: rosaramicin butyrate]

rosamicin propionate [now: rosaramicin propionate]

rosamicin sodium phosphate [now: rosaramicin sodium phosphate]

rosamicin stearate [now: rosaramicin stearate]

rosaprostol INN

rosaramicin USAN, INN *antibacterial*

rosaramicin butyrate USAN *antibacterial*

rosaramicin propionate USAN *antibacterial*

rosaramicin sodium phosphate USAN *antibacterial*

rosaramicin stearate USAN *antibacterial*

rosary pea *medicinal herb* [see: precatory bean]

rose (*Rosa acicularis; R. canina; R. rugosa* and other species) *flowers and hips medicinal herb for blood cleansing, cancer, colds, flu, infections, and sore throat; also used as a diuretic, mild laxative, and source of vitamin C*

rose, sun *medicinal herb* [see: rock rose]

rose bengal *diagnostic aid for corneal injury and pathology* 1.3 mg/strip

rose bengal sodium (^{131}I) INN *hepatic function test; radioactive agent* [also: rose bengal sodium I 131]

rose bengal sodium I 125 USAN *radioactive agent*

rose bengal sodium I 131 USAN, USP *hepatic function test; radioactive agent* [also: rose bengal sodium (^{131}I)]

rose laurel *medicinal herb* [see: mountain laurel]

rose oil NF *perfume*

rose petal aqueous infusion *ocular emollient*

rose water, stronger NF *perfume*

rose water ointment USP *emollient; ointment base*

rosemary (*Rosmarinus officinalis*) leaves *medicinal herb for flatulence, gastrointestinal spasm, halitosis, heart tonic, inducing diaphoresis, migraine headache, promoting menstrual flow, stimulating abortion, and stomach disorders*

Rosets ophthalmic strips OTC *corneal disclosing agent* [rose bengal] 1.3 mg

rosiglitazone maleate USAN *thiazolidinedione antidiabetic; increases cellular response to insulin without increasing insulin secretion*

rosin USP

rosoxacin USAN, INN *antibacterial* [also: acrosoxacin]

rosterolone INN

Rotacaps (trademarked form) *encapsulated powder for inhalation*

Rotadisk (trademarked dosage form) *powder for inhalation* [used in a Diskhaler]

Rotalex test kit for professional use (discontinued 1995) *in vitro diagnostic aid for fecal rotavirus* [latex agglutination test]

rotamicillin INN

Rotamune ℞ *investigational oral rotavirus vaccine*

RotaShield powder for oral liquid ℞ *immunization against gastroenteritis in infants* [rotavirus vaccine, live] 2.5 mL

rotavirus vaccine *live oral immunization against gastroenteritis in infants*

rotoxamine USAN, INN *antihistamine*

rotoxamine tartrate NF

rotraxate INN

round-leaved plantain *medicinal herb* [see: plantain]

Rowasa suppositories, rectal suspension enema ℞ *treatment of active ulcerative colitis, proctosigmoiditis and proctitis* [mesalamine] 500 mg; 4 g/60 mL

roxadimate USAN, INN *sunscreen*

Roxanol suppositories ℞ *narcotic analgesic* [morphine sulfate] 5, 10, 20, 30 mg

Roxanol; Roxanol 100; Roxanol Rescudose; Roxanol T; Roxanol UD oral solution ℞ *narcotic analgesic* [morphine sulfate] 20 mg/mL; 100 mg/5 mL; 10 mg/2.5 mL; 20 mg/mL; 10 mg/2.5 mL, 20 mg/5 mL, 30 mg/1.5 mL

roxarsone USAN, INN *antibacterial*

roxatidine INN, BAN *histamine H_2 antagonist for gastric and duodenal ulcers* [also: roxatidine acetate HCl]

roxatidine acetate HCl USAN *histamine H_2 antagonist for gastric and duodenal ulcers* [also: roxatidine]

roxibolone INN

Roxicet tablets, oral solution ℞ *narcotic analgesic* [oxycodone HCl; acetaminophen] 5•325 mg; 5•325 mg/5 mL

Roxicet 5/500 caplets ℞ *narcotic analgesic* [oxycodone HCl; acetaminophen] 5•500 mg

Roxicodone tablets, oral solution, Intensol (concentrated oral solution) ℞ *narcotic analgesic* [oxycodone HCl] 5 mg; 5 mg/5 mL; 20 mg/mL

roxifiban acetate USAN *antithrombotic; fibrinogen receptor antagonist*

Roxilox capsules ℞ *narcotic analgesic* [oxycodone HCl; acetaminophen] 5•500 mg

Roxin ℞ *investigational (NDA filed) histamine H_2 antagonist for duodenal and gastric ulcers* [roxatidine acetate HCl]

roxindole INN

Roxiprin tablets ℞ *narcotic analgesic* [oxycodone HCl; oxycodone terephthalate; aspirin] 4.5•0.38•325 mg

roxithromycin USAN, INN *antibacterial*

roxolonium metilsulfate INN

roxoperone INN

royal jelly *natural remedy for improving fertility and increasing longevity*

rp24 *investigational antiviral for AIDS* [also: AIDS vaccine]

rPAF-AH (recombinant platelet-activating factor acetylhydrolase) [see: platelet-activating factor acetylhydrolase, recombinant]

rPF4 (recombinant platelet factor 4) [see: platelet factor 4, recombinant]

RPI-4610 *investigational anticancer agent*

r-ProUK ℞ *investigational (Phase III) prourokinase clot-dissolving agent for stroke* [saruplase, recombinant]

R/S lotion OTC *topical acne treatment* [sulfur; resorcinol; alcohol] 5%•2%•28%

RSD-921 *investigational (Phase II) local anesthetic and antiarrhythmic*

RSR-13 *investigational synthetic allosteric modifier of hemoglobin for neuroprotective effect*

RSV-IG (respiratory syncytial virus immune globulin) [q.v.]

RT (reverse transcriptase) inhibitors [q.v.]

R-Tannamine tablets, pediatric oral suspension ℞ *decongestant; antihistamine* [phenylephrine tannate; chlorpheniramine tannate; pyrilamine tannate] 25•8•25 mg; 5•2•12.5 mg/5 mL

R-Tannate tablets, pediatric oral suspension ℞ *decongestant; antihistamine* [phenylephrine tannate; chlorpheniramine tannate; pyrilamine tannate] 25•8•25 mg; 5•2•12.5 mg/5 mL

rtPA; rt-PA (recombinant tissue plasminogen activator) [see: alteplase]

RTX (resiniferatoxin) [q.v.]

Rubacell II test for professional use (discontinued 1995) *in vitro diagnostic aid for rubella virus antibodies in serum or plasma* [passive hemagglutination (PHA) test]

Rubazyme reagent kit for professional use *in vitro diagnostic aid for rubella virus IgG antibodies in serum* [enzyme immunoassay (EIA)]

rubbing alcohol [see: alcohol, rubbing]

rubbing isopropyl alcohol [see: isopropyl alcohol, rubbing]

rubefacients *a class of gentle local irritants that redden the skin by producing active or passive hyperemia*

rubella & mumps virus vaccine, live *active immunizing agent for rubella and mumps*

rubella virus vaccine, live USP *active immunizing agent for rubella*

rubeola vaccine [see: measles virus vaccine, live]

Rubesol-1000 IM or subcu injection (discontinued 1996) ℞ *antianemic; vitamin B$_{12}$ supplement* [cyanocobalamin] 1000 µg/mL

Rubex powder for IV injection ℞ *anthracycline antibiotic antineoplastic* [doxorubicin HCl] 50, 100 mg

rubidium *element (Rb)*

rubidium chloride Rb 82 USAN *radioactive diagnostic aid for cardiac disease*

rubidium chloride Rb 86 USAN *radioactive agent*

Rubramin PC IM or subcu injection ℞ *antianemic; vitamin B$_{12}$ supplement* [cyanocobalamin] 100, 1000 µg/mL

Rubus fructicosus; R. villosus medicinal herb [see: blackberry]

Rubus idaeus; R. strigosus medicinal herb [see: red raspberry]

rue (Ruta bracteosa; R. graveolens; R. montana) *plant medicinal herb for cramps, hypertension, hysteria, muscle strains, neuralgia, nervous disorders, sciatica, stimulation of abortion and menstruation, tendon strains, and trauma*

Rufen film-coated tablets (discontinued 1995) ℞ *nonsteroidal anti-inflammatory drug (NSAID); antiarthritic; analgesic* [ibuprofen] 400, 600, 800 mg

rufloxacin INN

rufocromomycin INN, BAN *antineoplastic* [also: streptonigrin]

Ru-lets 500 film-coated tablets (discontinued 1995) OTC *vitamin/mineral supplement* [multiple vitamins & minerals] ≛

Ru-lets M 500 film-coated tablets OTC *vitamin/mineral supplement* [multiple vitamins & minerals] ≛

RuLox oral suspension OTC *antacid* [aluminum hydroxide; magnesium hydroxide] 225•200 mg/5 mL

RuLox #1; RuLox #2 chewable tablets OTC *antacid* [aluminum hydroxide; magnesium hydroxide] 200•200 mg; 400•400 mg

RuLox Plus chewable tablets, oral suspension OTC *antacid; antiflatulent* [aluminum hydroxide; magnesium hydroxide; simethicone] 200•200•25 mg; 500•450•40 mg/5 mL

rum cherry *medicinal herb* [see: wild black cherry]

Rumex acetosa medicinal herb [see: sorrel]

Rumex crispus medicinal herb [see: yellow dock]

Rumex hymenosepalus medicinal herb [see: canaigre]

Rum-K liquid ℞ *potassium supplement* [potassium chloride] 30 mEq/15 mL

Ruscus aculeatus medicinal herb [see: butcher's broom]

rush, sweet *medicinal herb* [see: calamus]

Ruta bracteosa; R. graveolens; R. montana medicinal herb [see: rue]

rutamycin USAN, INN *antifungal*

ruthenium *element (Ru)*

rutin NF [also: rutoside]

rutoside INN [also: rutin]

Ru-Tuss liquid OTC *decongestant; antihistamine* [phenylephrine HCl; chlorpheniramine maleate; alcohol 5%] 5•2 mg/5 mL

Ru-Tuss sustained-release tablets (discontinued 1995) ℞ *decongestant; antihistamine; anticholinergic* [phenylpropanolamine HCl; phenylephrine HCl; chlorpheniramine maleate; hyoscyamine sulfate; atropine sulfate; scopolamine hydrobromide] 50•25•8•0.19•0.04•0.01 mg

Ru-Tuss II slow-release capsules (discontinued 1995) ℞ *decongestant; antihistamine* [phenylpropanolamine HCl; chlorpheniramine maleate] 75•12 mg

Ru-Tuss DE prolonged-action film-coated tablets ℞ *decongestant; expec-*

torant [pseudoephedrine HCl; guaifenesin] 120•600 mg

Ru-Tuss Expectorant liquid OTC *antitussive; decongestant; expectorant* [dextromethorphan hydrobromide; pseudoephedrine HCl; guaifenesin; alcohol 10%] 10•30•100 mg/5 mL

Ru-Tuss with Hydrocodone liquid ℞ *narcotic antitussive; decongestant; antihistamine* [hydrocodone bitartrate; phenylpropanolamine HCl; phenylephrine HCl; pyrilamine maleate; pheniramine maleate; alcohol 5%] 1.7•3.3•5•3.3•3.3 mg/5 mL

ruvazone INN

Ru-Vert-M film-coated tablets (discontinued 1998) ℞ *anticholinergic; antivertigo agent; motion sickness preventative* [meclizine HCl] 25 mg

RVA (rabies vaccine, adsorbed) [see: rabies vaccine]

RVP (red veterinarian petrolatum) [see: petrolatum]

RxPak; ℞Pak (trademarked form) *prescription package*

Rymed capsules ℞ *decongestant; expectorant* [pseudoephedrine HCl; guaifenesin] 30•250 mg

Rymed liquid OTC *decongestant; expectorant* [pseudoephedrine HCl; guaifenesin; alcohol 1.4%] 30•100 mg/5 mL

Rymed-TR long-acting caplets ℞ *decongestant; expectorant* [phenylpropanolamine HCl; guaifenesin] 75•400 mg

Ryna liquid OTC *decongestant; antihistamine* [pseudoephedrine HCl; chlorpheniramine maleate] 30•2 mg/5 mL

Ryna-C liquid ℞ *narcotic antitussive; decongestant; antihistamine* [codeine phosphate; pseudoephedrine HCl; chlorpheniramine maleate] 10•30•2 mg/5 mL

Ryna-CX liquid ℞ *narcotic antitussive; decongestant; expectorant* [codeine phosphate; pseudoephedrine HCl; guaifenesin] 10•30•100 mg/5 mL

Rynatan pediatric oral suspension ℞ *decongestant; antihistamine* [phenylephrine tannate; chlorpheniramine tannate; pyrilamine tannate] 5•2•12.5 mg/5 mL

Rynatan tablets ℞ *decongestant; antihistamine* [pseudoephedrine sulfate; azatadine maleate] 120•1 mg

Rynatan-S oral suspension ℞ *pediatric decongestant and antihistamine* [phenylephrine tannate; chlorpheniramine tannate; pyrilamine tannate] 5•2•12.5 mg/5 mL

Rynatuss tablets, pediatric suspension ℞ *antitussive; decongestant; antihistamine* [carbetapentane tannate; phenylephrine tannate; ephedrine tannate; chlorpheniramine tannate] 60•10•10•5 mg; 30•5•5•4 mg/5 mL

Rythmol film-coated tablets ℞ *antiarrhythmic* [propafenone HCl] 150, 225, 300 mg

S-2 solution for inhalation OTC *sympathomimetic bronchodilator* [racepinephrine HCl] 2.25%

³⁵**S** [see: sodium sulfate S 35]

SA (salicylic acid) [q.v.]

SA (serum albumin) [see: albumin, human]

Sabatia angularis medicinal herb [see: American centaury]

sabcomeline HCl USAN *muscarinic receptor agonist for Alzheimer's disease*

sabeluzole USAN, INN, BAN *anticonvulsant; antihypoxic*

Sabin vaccine [see: poliovirus vaccine, live oral]

Sabril (commercially available in 40 foreign countries) ℞ *investigational anticonvulsant* [vigabatrin]

S-A-C tablets (discontinued 1995) OTC *analgesic; antipyretic; anti-inflammatory* [acetaminophen; salicylamide; caffeine] 150•230•30 mg

Sacarasa (name changed to Sucraid in 1997)

saccharin NF *flavoring agent*

saccharin calcium USP *non-nutritive sweetener*

saccharin sodium USP *non-nutritive sweetener*

sacred bark *medicinal herb* [see: cascara sagrada]

sacrosidase *enzyme replacement therapy for congenital sucrase-isomaltase deficiency (orphan)*

Saf-Clens spray OTC *wound cleanser*

Safe Tussin 30 liquid OTC *antitussive; expectorant* [dextromethorphan hydrobromide; guaifenesin] 15•100 mg/5 mL

safflower (Carthamus tinctorius) flowers *medicinal herb for delirium, digestive disorders, fever, gout, inducing sweating, jaundice, liver disorders, lowering cholesterol, promoting expectoration, uric acid build-up, and urinary disorders*

safflower oil USP *oleaginous vehicle; essential fatty acid supplement*

saffron (Crocus sativus) flowers *medicinal herb for fever, gout, inducing sweating, measles, rheumatism, scarlet fever, and sedation; also used as an aphrodisiac and expectorant*

saffron, American; bastard saffron *medicinal herb* [see: safflower]

safingol USAN *antipsoriatic; antineoplastic adjunct*

safingol HCl USAN *antipsoriatic; antineoplastic adjunct*

safrole USP

sagackhomi *medicinal herb* [see: uva ursi]

sage (Salvia lavandulaefolia; S. lyrata; S. officinalis) leaves *medicinal herb for cough, diarrhea, dysmenorrhea, fever, gastritis, gum and mouth sores, memory improvement, nausea, nervous disorders, and sore throat*

sailor's tobacco *medicinal herb* [see: mugwort]

St. Benedict thistle *medicinal herb* [see: blessed thistle]

St. James' weed; St. James' wort *medicinal herb* [see: shepherd's purse]

St. John's wort (Hypericum perforatum) plant *medicinal herb for AIDS, antiviral therapy, anxiety, bronchitis, cancer, childbirth afterpains, depression, gastritis, insomnia, and skin disorders*

St. Joseph Adult Chewable Aspirin chewable tablets OTC *analgesic; antipyretic; anti-inflammatory* [aspirin] 81 mg

St. Joseph Anti-Diarrheal for Children liquid OTC *antidiarrheal; GI adsorbent* [attapulgite]

St. Joseph Aspirin-Free Fever Reducer for Children liquid (discontinued 1997) OTC *analgesic; antipyretic* [acetaminophen] 160 mg/5 mL

St. Joseph Aspirin-Free for Children chewable tablets (discontinued 1997) OTC *analgesic; antipyretic* [acetaminophen] 80 mg

St. Joseph Aspirin-Free Infant Drops (discontinued 1997) OTC *analgesic; antipyretic* [acetaminophen] 100 mg/mL

St. Joseph Cold Tablets for Children chewable tablets OTC *pediatric decongestant and analgesic* [phenylpropanolamine HCl; acetaminophen] 3.125•80 mg

St. Joseph Cough Suppressant syrup OTC *antitussive* [dextromethorphan hydrobromide] 7.5 mg/5 mL

St. Josephwort *medicinal herb* [see: basil]

Saizen powder for subcu or IM injection ℞ *growth hormone for adults or children with congenital or endogenous growth hormone deficiency, children with Turner syndrome or renal-induced growth failure, or AIDS-wasting syndrome (orphan)* [somatropin] 5 mg (15 IU) per vial

SalAc liquid OTC *topical keratolytic cleanser for acne* [salicylic acid] 2%

salacetamide INN

salacetin [see: aspirin]

Sal-Acid plaster OTC *topical keratolytic* [salicylic acid in a collodion-like vehicle] 40%

Salactic Film liquid OTC *topical keratolytic* [salicylic acid in a collodion-like vehicle] 17%

salafibrate INN

Salagen film-coated tablets ℞ *treatment of xerostomia and keratoconjunctivitis sicca due to radiotherapy or Sjögren syndrome (orphan); also for dry mouth* [pilocarpine HCl] 5 mg

salantel USAN, INN *veterinary anthelmintic*

Salazide; Salazide-Demi tablets ℞ *antihypertensive* [hydroflumethiazide; reserpine]

salazodine INN

Salazopyrin (European name for U.S. product Azulfidine)

salazosulfadimidine INN [also: salazosulphadimidine]

salazosulfamide INN

salazosulfapyridine JAN *broad-spectrum bacteriostatic; anti-inflammatory for ulcerative colitis; antirheumatic* [also: sulfasalazine; sulphasalazine]

salazosulfathiazole INN

salazosulphadimidine BAN [also: salazosulfadimidine]

salbutamol INN, BAN *sympathomimetic bronchodilator* [also: albuterol]

salbutamol sulfate JAN *sympathomimetic bronchodilator* [also: albuterol sulfate]

salcatonin BAN *synthetic analog of calcitonin (salmon); calcium regulator; investigational osteoporosis treatment* [also: calcitonin salmon (synthesis)]

salcetogen [see: aspirin]

Sal-Clens Acne Cleanser gel OTC *topical keratolytic for acne* [salicylic acid] 2%

salcolex USAN, INN *analgesic; anti-inflammatory; antipyretic*

SalEst test kit for professional use *in vitro diagnostic aid for estriol levels in saliva, used to predict spontaneous preterm labor and delivery*

saletamide INN *analgesic* [also: salethamide maleate]

saletamide maleate [see: salethamide maleate]

salethamide maleate USAN *analgesic* [also: saletamide]

saletin [see: aspirin]

Saleto tablets OTC *analgesic; antipyretic; anti-inflammatory* [acetaminophen; aspirin; salicylamide; caffeine] 115•210•65•16 mg

Saleto CF tablets OTC *antitussive; decongestant; analgesic* [dextromethorphan hydrobromide; phenylpropanolamine; acetaminophen] 10•12.5•325 mg

Saleto-200 tablets OTC *nonsteroidal anti-inflammatory drug (NSAID); antiarthritic; analgesic* [ibuprofen] 200 mg

Saleto-400; Saleto-600; Saleto-800 tablets ℞ *nonsteroidal anti-inflammatory drug (NSAID); antiarthritic; analgesic* [ibuprofen] 400 mg; 600 mg; 800 mg

Saleto-D capsules OTC *decongestant; analgesic; antipyretic* [phenylpropanolamine HCl; acetaminophen; salicylamide; caffeine] 18•240•120•16 mg

Salflex film-coated tablets OTC *analgesic; antipyretic; anti-inflammatory; antirheumatic* [salsalate] 500, 750 mg

salfluverine INN

salicain [now: salicyl alcohol]

salicin USP

salicin willow *medicinal herb* [see: willow]

salicyl alcohol USAN *local anesthetic*

salicylamide USP *analgesic*

salicylanilide NF

salicylate meglumine USAN *antirheumatic; analgesic*

salicylates *a class of drugs that have analgesic, antipyretic, and anti-inflammatory effects*

salicylazosulfapyridine [now: sulfasalazine]

salicylic acid (SA) USP *keratolytic; antiseborrheic; antipsoriatic*

salicylic acid, bimolecular ester [see: salsalate]

salicylic acid acetate [see: aspirin]

Salicylic Acid Acne Treatment bar (discontinued 1995) OTC *medicated cleanser for acne* [salicylic acid] 2%

Salicylic Acid and Sulfur Soap bar OTC *medicated cleanser for acne* [salicylic acid; precipitated sulfur] 3%• 10%

Salicylic Acid Cleansing bar OTC *medicated cleanser for acne* [salicylic acid] 2%

salicylic acid dihydrogen phosphate [see: fosfosal]

salicylsalicylic acid [see: salsalate]

saligenin [now: salicyl alcohol]

saligenol [now: salicyl alcohol]

salinazid INN, BAN

saline, lactated potassic [see: potassic saline, lactated]

saline solution (SS) [also: normal saline]

SalineX nasal mist, nose drops OTC *nasal moisturizer* [sodium chloride (saline solution)] 0.4%

saliniazid [see: salinazid]

salinomycin INN, BAN

Saliva Substitute oral solution OTC *saliva substitute*

Salivart oral spray OTC *saliva substitute*

Salix lozenges OTC *saliva substitute*

Salix alba; S. caprea; S. nigra; S. purpurea medicinal herb [see: willow]

salmaterol [see: salmeterol]

salmefamol INN, BAN

salmeterol USAN, INN, BAN *sympathomimetic bronchodilator*

salmeterol xinafoate USAN *adrenergic; sympathomimetic bronchodilator*

salmisteine INN

salmon calcitonin [see: salcatonin]

Salmonella typhi **vaccine** [see: typhoid vaccine]

Salmonine subcu or IM injection R *calcium regulator for hypercalcemia, Paget's disease, and postmenopausal osteoporosis* [calcitonin (salmon)] 200 IU/mL

salmotin [see: adicillin]

salnacedin USAN *topical anti-inflammatory*

Salocol tablets (discontinued 1995) OTC *analgesic; antipyretic; anti-inflammatory* [acetaminophen; aspirin; salicylamide; caffeine] 115•210•65•16 mg

Salofalk ⒸⒶⓃ (U.S. product: Pentasa) enteric-coated tablets R *for acute ulcerative colitis and the prevention of Crohn's disease relapse following bowel resection* [mesalamine (5-aminosalicylic acid)] 250, 500 mg

Salofalk ⒸⒶⓃ (U.S. product: Rowasa) suppositories, rectal suspension enema R *treatment of distal ulcerative colitis (DUC) and ulcerative proctitis* [mesalamine (5-aminosalicylic acid)] 250, 500 mg; 2, 4 g/58 mL

Sal-Oil-T hair dressing R *antipsoriatic; antiseborrheic; keratolytic* [coal tar; salicylic acid] 10%•6%

salol [see: phenyl salicylate]

Salphenyl capsules (discontinued 1995) OTC *decongestant; antihistamine; analgesic* [phenylephrine HCl; chlorpheniramine maleate; acetaminophen; salicylamide] 10•2• 130•200 mg

Sal-Plant gel OTC *topical keratolytic* [salicylic acid in a collodion-like vehicle] 17%

Salprofen IV injection R *investigational (orphan) for patent ductus arteriosus* [ibuprofen]

salprotoside INN

salsalate USAN, USP, INN, BAN *analgesic; antipyretic; anti-inflammatory; antirheumatic* 500, 750 mg oral

Salsitab film-coated tablets R *analgesic; antipyretic; anti-inflammatory; antirheumatic* [salsalate] 500, 750 mg

Sal-Tropine tablets R *GI anticholinergic and antispasmodic* [atropine sulfate] 0.4 mg

Saluron tablets R *diuretic; antihypertensive* [hydroflumethiazide] 50 mg

Salutensin; Salutensin-Demi tablets R *antihypertensive* [hydroflumethiazide; reserpine] 50•0.125 mg; 25• 0.125 mg ⑦ Diutensen

saluzide [see: opiniazide]

salvarsan [see: arsphenamine]

salverine INN

Salvia lavandulaefolia; S. lyrata; S. officinalis medicinal herb [see: sage]

Salvia miltiorrhiza medicinal herb [see: danshen]

samarium *element (Sm)*

samarium Sm 153 EDTMP (ethylenediaminetetramethylenephosphoric acid) [see: samarium Sm 153 lexidronam]

samarium Sm 153 lexidronam USAN *radiopharmaceutical for treatment of bone pain from osteoblastic metastatic tumors*

Sambucus canadensis; S. ebulus; S. nigra; S. racemosa medicinal herb [see: elder flower; elderberry]

Sanchi ginseng *(Panax pseudoginseng)* medicinal herb [see: ginseng]

sancycline USAN, INN *antibacterial*

sandalwood *(Santalum album)* oil *medicinal herb for headache, stomach ache, and urogenital disorders; also used topically as an antiseptic and astringent*

Sandimmune gel capsules, oral solution, IV injection R *immunosuppressant for allogenic kidney, liver, and heart transplants; investigational for many other uses* [cyclosporine] 25, 50, 100 mg; 100 mg/mL; 50 mg/mL

Sandimmune ophthalmic ointment R *investigational (orphan) for keratoconjunctivitis sicca, keratoplasty graft rejection, and corneal melting syndrome* [cyclosporine] 2%

Sandimmune Neoral ⓒᴬᴺ (U.S. product: Neoral) soft gels for microemulsion, oral solution for microemulsion R *immunosuppressant for allogenic kidney, liver, and heart transplants, rheumatoid arthritis, and psoriasis* [cyclosporine] 25, 50, 100 mg; 100 mg/mL

Sandoglobulin powder for IV infusion R *passive immunizing agent for HIV and idiopathic thrombocytopenic purpura (ITP)* [immune globulin] 1, 3, 6, 12 g

SandoPak (trademarked packaging form) *unit dose blister package*

Sandostatin subcu or IV injection R *gastric antisecretory for acromegaly and severe diarrhea due to VIPomas and other tumors (orphan)* [octreotide acetate] 0.05, 0.1, 0.2, 0.5, 1 mg/mL ⅁ simvastatin; zinostatin

Sandostatin LAR Depot suspension for IM injection R *gastric antisecretory for acromegaly and severe diarrhea due to VIPomas and other tumors (orphan)* [octreotide acetate]

sanfetrinem INN, BAN *antibacterial* [also: sanfetrinem sodium]

sanfetrinem cilexetil USAN *antibacterial*

sanfetrinem sodium USAN *antibacterial* [also: sanfetrinem]

SangCya oral solution R *immunosuppressive to prevent solid organ transplant rejection* [cyclosporine; alcohol 10.5%] 100 mg/mL

Sanguinaria canadensis medicinal herb [see: bloodroot]

sanguinarine chloride [now: sanguinarium chloride]

sanguinarium chloride USAN, INN *antifungal; antimicrobial; anti-inflammatory*

sanicle *(Sanicula europea; S. marilandica)* root *medicinal herb used as an astringent, expectorant, discutient, depurative, nervine, and vulnerary*

Sani-Pak (trademarked packaging form) *sanitary dispensing box*

Sani-Supp suppositories OTC *hyperosmolar laxative* [glycerin]

Sanitube ointment (discontinued 1996) OTC *venereal prophylactic* [calomel; benzoxiquine; trolamine] 30% • ? • ?

Sanorex tablets R *anorexiant; CNS stimulant; investigational (orphan) treatment for Duchenne muscular dystrophy* [mazindol] 1, 2 mg

Sansert tablets R *agent for migraine and vascular headaches* [methysergide maleate] 2 mg

Santalum album medicinal herb [see: sandalwood]

santonin NF

Santyl ointment ℞ *topical enzyme for biochemical debridement* [collagenase] 250 U/g

saperconazole USAN, INN, BAN *antifungal*

Saponaria officinalis medicinal herb [see: soapwort]

saprisartan INN, BAN *antihypertensive; angiotensin II antagonist* [also: saprisartan potassium]

saprisartan potassium USAN *antihypertensive; angiotensin II antagonist* [also: saprisartan]

sapropterin INN

saquinavir INN, BAN *antiviral protease inhibitor for HIV* [also: saquinavir mesylate]

saquinavir mesylate USAN *antiviral protease inhibitor for HIV* [also: saquinavir]

sarafloxacin INN, BAN *anti-infective; DNA gyrase inhibitor* [also: sarafloxacin HCl]

sarafloxacin HCl USAN *anti-infective; DNA gyrase inhibitor* [also: sarafloxacin]

saralasin INN *antihypertensive* [also: saralasin acetate]

saralasin acetate USAN *antihypertensive* [also: saralasin]

Saratoga ointment OTC *astringent; antiseptic; wound protectant* [zinc oxide; boric acid; eucalyptol]

sarcolysin INN

L-sarcolysin [see: melphalan]

Sardo Bath & Shower oil OTC *bath emollient*

Sardoettes towelettes OTC *moisturizer; emollient*

sargramostim USAN, INN, BAN *antineutropenic for bone marrow transplant and graft delay (orphan); investigational (Phase III) for malignant melanoma; investigational (Phase II) cytokine for HIV*

sarmazenil INN

sarmoxicillin USAN, INN *antibacterial*

Sarna Anti-Itch foam, lotion OTC *topical analgesic; counterirritant* [camphor; menthol] 0.5%•0.5%

saroten [see: amitriptyline]

Sarothamnus scoparius medicinal herb [see: broom]

sarpicillin USAN, INN *antibacterial*

Sarracenia purpurea medicinal herb [see: pitcher plant]

sarsaparilla (*Smilax* spp.) root medicinal herb for blood cleansing (binding and expulsion of endotoxins), joint aches including arthritis and rheumatism, hormonal disorders, skin diseases including leprosy and psoriasis, and syphilis

saruplase INN *investigational (Phase III) prourokinase clot-dissolving agent for stroke*

sassafras (*Sassafras albidum; S. officinale*) root and bark medicinal herb for acne, blood cleansing, insect bites and stings, obesity, psoriasis, skin diseases, and water retention; not generally regarded as safe and effective and banned by the FDA as a carcinogen with other serious side effects

sassafras, swamp medicinal herb [see: magnolia]

Sastid cream OTC *topical keratolytic for acne* [precipitated sulfur; salicylic acid]

SAStid Soap bar OTC *medicated cleanser for acne* [precipitated sulfur] 10%

saterinone INN

satinflower medicinal herb [see: chickweed]

satranidazole INN

satumomab INN, BAN *radiodiagnostic monoclonal antibody for ovarian and colorectal carcinoma* [also: indium In 111 satumomab pendetide]

satumomab pendetide [see: indium In 111 satumomab pendetide]

Satureja hortensis medicinal herb [see: summer savory]

Satureja montana; S. obovata medicinal herb [see: winter savory]

savory medicinal herb [see: summer savory; winter savory]

savoxepin INN

saw palmetto (*Serenoa repens; S. serrulata*) berries medicinal herb for benign prostatic hypertrophy and geni-

tourinary, glandular, and reproductive disorders; also used to enlarge breasts, increase sperm production, promote weight gain, and enhance sexual vigor

saxifrage, burnet; European burnet saxifrage; small burnet saxifrage; small saxifrage *medicinal herb* [see: burnet]

saxifrax *medicinal herb* [see: sassafras]

SB-210396 *investigational (Phase III) anti-CD4 antibody for rheumatoid arthritis* [also: IDEC-CE9.1]

SB-217969 *investigational (Phase I/II) anti-CD4 antibody for the treatment of rheumatoid arthritis*

SC (succinylcholine) [see: succinylcholine chlorine]

SC-49483 *investigational pro-drug that prevents the clumping of HIV cells which leads to drug resistance*

SCA proteins (single-chain antigen-binding proteins) *a class of investigational antineoplastics*

Scabene lotion, shampoo (discontinued 1998) ℞ *pediculicide for lice; scabicide* [lindane] 1%

scabicides *a class of agents effective against scabies*

scabwort *medicinal herb* [see: elecampane]

Scadan scalp lotion OTC *antiseptic; antiseborrheic* [myristyltrimethylammonium bromide; stearyl dimethyl benzyl ammonium chloride] 1%•0.1%

Scalpicin liquid OTC *topical antiseborrheic* [salicylic acid] 3%

Scalpicin liquid (discontinued 1999) OTC *topical corticosteroidal anti-inflammatory* [hydrocortisone] 1%

scaly dragon's claw *medicinal herb* [see: coral root]

scammony, wild *medicinal herb* [see: wild jalap]

scandium *element (Sc)*

scarlet bergamot *medicinal herb* [see: Oswego tea]

scarlet berry *medicinal herb* [see: bittersweet nightshade]

scarlet fever streptococcus toxin

scarlet red NF *promotes wound healing*

Scarlet Red Ointment Dressings medication-impregnated gauze ℞ *wound dressing; vulnerary* [scarlet red] 5%

scarlet sumach *medicinal herb* [see: sumach]

SCCS (simethicone-coated cellulose suspension) [see: SonoRx]

sCD4-PE40 [see: alvircept sudotox]

SCF (stem cell factor) [q.v.]

Schamberg lotion OTC *topical analgesic; antiseptic; astringent; antifungal; counterirritant* [zinc oxide; menthol; phenol] 8.25%•0.25%•1.5%

Scheinpharm Tobramycin ⓒ (U.S. product: Nebcin) IV or IM injection ℞ *aminoglycoside antibiotic* [tobramycin sulfate] 10, 40 mg/mL

Schick test [see: diphtheria toxin for Schick test]

Schick test control USP *dermal reactivity indicator*

Schirmer Tear Test ophthalmic strips OTC *diagnostic tear flow test aid*

schizandra (Schisandra arisanensis; S. chinensis; S. rubriflora; S. sphenanthera) berries *medicinal herb for cough, gastrointestinal disorders, increasing energy and mental alertness, nervous disorders, respiratory illnesses, and stress; also used as a liver protectant*

Sclavo PPD Solution intradermal injection (discontinued 1995) ℞ *tuberculosis skin test* [tuberculin purified protein derivative] 5 U/0.1 mL

Sclavo Test-PPD single-use intradermal puncture test device (discontinued 1995) ℞ *tuberculosis skin test* [tuberculin purified protein derivative] 5 U

Scleromate IV injection ℞ *sclerosing agent for varicose veins* [morrhuate sodium] 50 mg/mL

Sclerosol aerosol ℞ *investigational (NDA filed, orphan) treatment for malignant pleural effusion and pneumothorax via intrapleural thoracoscopy administration* [talc, sterile]

scoke *medicinal herb* [see: pokeweed]

Scopace tablets ℞ *GI antispasmodic; anticholinergic; motion sickness preventative* [scopolamine hydrobromide] 0.4 mg

scopafungin USAN *antibacterial; antifungal*

Scope mouthwash OTC *oral antiseptic* [cetylpyridinium chloride]

scopolamine *transdermal motion sickness preventative*

scopolamine hydrobromide USP *GI antispasmodic; anticholinergic; motion sickness preventative; cycloplegic; mydriatic* [also: hyoscine hydrobromide] 0.3, 0.4, 0.86, 1 mg/mL injection

scopolamine methyl nitrate [see: methscopolamine nitrate]

scopolamine methylbromide [see: methscopolamine bromide]

Scott's Emulsion OTC *vitamin supplement* [vitamins A and D] 1250•100 IU/5 mL

Scot-Tussin Allergy liquid OTC *antihistamine* [diphenhydramine HCl] 12.5 mg/5 mL

Scot-Tussin DM liquid OTC *antitussive; antihistamine* [dextromethorphan hydrobromide; chlorpheniramine maleate] 15•2 mg/5 mL

Scot-Tussin DM Cough Chasers lozenges OTC *antitussive* [dextromethorphan hydrobromide] 2.5 mg

Scot-Tussin Expectorant sugar-free liquid OTC *expectorant* [guaifenesin; alcohol 3.5%] 100 mg/5 mL

Scot-Tussin Original 5-Action Cold Formula syrup, sugar-free liquid OTC *decongestant; antihistamine; analgesic* [phenylephrine HCl; pheniramine maleate; sodium citrate; sodium salicylate; caffeine citrate] 4.2•13.3• 83.3•83.3•25 mg

Scot-Tussin Senior Clear liquid OTC *antitussive; expectorant* [dextromethorphan hydrobromide; guaifenesin] 15•200 mg/5 mL

sCR1 (soluble complement receptor 1) *investigational (Phase I/II) complement inhibitor for severe burns,*

adult respiratory distress syndrome, and reperfusion injury [also: TP-10]

Scriptene ℞ *investigational (Phase I) antiviral for AIDS* [zidovudine; didanosine]

scrofula plant *medicinal herb* [see: figwort]

Scrophularia nodosa *medicinal herb* [see: figwort]

scullcap *medicinal herb* [see: skullcap]

scuroforme [see: butyl aminobenzoate]

Scutellaria lateriflora *medicinal herb* [see: skullcap]

SD (streptodornase) [q.v.]

75Se [see: selenomethionine Se 75]

sea girdles *medicinal herb* [see: kelp (*Laminaria*)]

Sea Mist nasal spray OTC *nasal moisturizer* [sodium chloride (saline solution)] 0.65%

Seale's Lotion Modified OTC *topical acne treatment* [sulfur] 6.4%

sealroot; sealwort *medicinal herb* [see: Solomon's seal]

Sea-Omega 30; Sea-Omega 50 softgels OTC *dietary supplement* [omega-3 fatty acids] 1200 mg; 1000 mg

seawrack *medicinal herb* [see: kelp (*Fucus*)]

Seba-Nil Cleansing Mask scrub OTC *abrasive cleanser for acne*

Seba-Nil Oily Skin Cleanser liquid OTC *topical cleanser for acne* [alcohol; acetone]

Sebasorb lotion OTC *topical keratolytic for acne* [salicylic acid; attapulgite] 2%•10%

Sebex shampoo OTC *antiseborrheic; keratolytic* [sulfur; salicylic acid] 2%•2%

Sebex-T shampoo OTC *antiseborrheic; antipsoriatic; keratolytic* [sulfur; salicylic acid; coal tar] 2%•2%•5%

Sebizon lotion ℞ *bacteriostatic; antiseborrheic* [sulfacetamide sodium] 10%

Sebucare hair lotion OTC *antiseborrheic; keratolytic* [salicylic acid; alcohol 61%] 1.8%

Sebulex shampoo (discontinued 1997) OTC *antiseborrheic; keratolytic* [sulfur; salicylic acid] 2%•2%

Sebulex with Conditioners shampoo
OTC *antiseborrheic; keratolytic* [sulfur;
salicylic acid] 2%•2%

Sebulon shampoo (discontinued
1997) OTC *antiseborrheic; antibacterial; antifungal* [pyrithione zinc] 2%

Sebutone cream shampoo, liquid
shampoo (discontinued 1997) OTC
antiseborrheic; antipsoriatic; keratolytic
[coal tar; sulfur; salicylic acid]
0.5%•2%•2%

secalciferol USAN, INN, BAN *calcium
regulator; investigational (orphan) for
familial hypophosphatemic rickets*

secbutabarbital sodium INN *sedative;
hypnotic* [also: butabarbital sodium]

secbutobarbitone BAN *sedative; hypnotic* [also: butabarbital]

seclazone USAN, INN *anti-inflammatory; uricosuric*

secnidazole INN, BAN

secobarbital USP, INN *hypnotic; sedative*

secobarbital sodium USP, JAN *hypnotic; sedative; also abused as a street
drug* [also: quinalbarbitone sodium]
100 mg oral; 50 mg/mL injection

Seconal Sodium Pulvules (capsules) ℞
*sedative; hypnotic; also abused as a street
drug* [secobarbital sodium] 100 mg

secoverine INN

Secran liquid OTC *vitamin supplement*
[vitamins B₁, B₃, and B₁₂; alcohol
17%] 10 mg•10 mg•25 μg per 5 mL

Secran Prenatal tablets (discontinued
1995) ℞ *vitamin/calcium/iron supplement* [multiple vitamins; calcium;
iron; folic acid] ±•250•60•1 mg

secretin INN, BAN *diagnostic aid for
pancreatic function*

Secretin Ferring powder for IV injection ℞ *diagnostic aid for pancreatic
function* [secretin] 10 CU/mL

**secretory leukocyte protease inhib-
itor** *investigational (orphan) for congenital alpha₁-antitrypsin deficiency,
cystic fibrosis, and bronchopulmonary
dysplasia*

Sectral capsules ℞ *antianginal; antihypertensive; antiarrhythmic; β-blocker*
[acebutolol HCl] 200, 400 mg

Secule (trademarked packaging form)
single-dose vial

securinine INN

sedaform [see: chlorobutanol]

Sedapap tablets ℞ *analgesic; sedative*
[acetaminophen; butalbital] 650•50
mg

sedatine [see: antipyrine]

sedatives *a class of soothing agents that
reduce excitement, nervousness, distress,
or irritation* [also called: calmatives]

sedecamycin USAN, INN *veterinary
antibacterial*

sedeval [see: barbital]

sedge, sweet *medicinal herb* [see: cala-
mus]

sedoxantrone trihydrochloride
[now: ledoxantrone trihydrochloride]

seganserin INN, BAN

seglitide INN *antidiabetic* [also: seglitide
acetate]

seglitide acetate USAN *antidiabetic*
[also: seglitide]

SelCID ℞ *investigational (Phase I)
selective cytokine inhibitory drug*

Seldane tablets (discontinued 1998)
℞ *nonsedating antihistamine* [terfena-
dine] 60 mg

Seldane-D sustained-release tablets
(discontinued 1998) ℞ *decongestant;
antihistamine* [pseudoephedrine HCl;
terfenadine] 120•60 mg

Selecor tablets ℞ *investigational (NDA
filed) antihypertensive; antianginal; β-
blocker* [celiprolol HCl]

Select-A-Jet (trademarked delivery
system) *syringe system*

**selective estrogen receptor modula-
tors (SERMs)** *a class of osteoporosis
prevention agents that reduce bone
resorption and decrease overall bone
turnover in postmenopausal women*

**selective serotonin 5-HT₃ (hydroxy-
tryptamine) blockers** *a class of
antiemetic and antinauseant agents
used primarily after emetogenic cancer
chemotherapy* [also called: 5-HT₃
receptor antagonists]

**selective serotonin reuptake inhibi-
tors (SSRIs)** *a class of oral antide-*

pressants that inhibit neuronal uptake of 5-HT (serotonin), a CNS neurotransmitter

selegiline INN, BAN dopaminergic antiparkinsonian; investigational (Phase III) transdermal treatment for depression [also: selegiline HCl]

selegiline HCl USAN dopaminergic antiparkinsonian (orphan) [also: selegiline] 5 mg oral

selenious acid USP dietary selenium supplement 65.4 µg/mL injection

selenium element (Se)

selenium dioxide, monohydrated [see: selenious acid]

selenium sulfide USP antifungal; antiseborrheic 1%, 2.5% topical

selenomethionine (⁷⁵Se) INN pancreas function test; radioactive agent [also: selenomethionine Se 75]

selenomethionine Se 75 USAN, USP pancreas function test; radioactive agent [also: selenomethionine (⁷⁵Se)]

Sele-Pak IV injection ℞ intravenous nutritional therapy [selenious acid] 65.4 µg/mL

Selepen IV injection ℞ intravenous nutritional therapy [selenious acid] 65.4 µg/mL

Selestoject IV, IM injection (discontinued 1996) ℞ corticosteroid; antiinflammatory [betamethasone sodium phosphate] 4 mg/mL

selfotel USAN N-methyl-D-aspartate (NMDA) antagonist for treatment of stroke-induced impairment

Seloken (foreign name for U.S. product Lopressor)

Seloken ZOC (foreign name for U.S. product Toprol XL)

selprazine INN

Selsun lotion/shampoo ℞ antiseborrheic; antifungal [selenium sulfide] 2.5%

Selsun Blue; Selsun Gold for Women lotion/shampoo OTC antiseborrheic [selenium sulfide] 1%

sematilide INN antiarrhythmic [also: sematilide HCl]

sematilide HCl USAN antiarrhythmic [also: sematilide]

semduramicin USAN, INN coccidiostat

semduramicin sodium USAN coccidiostat

Semicid vaginal suppositories OTC spermicidal contraceptive [nonoxynol 9] 100 mg

semisodium valproate BAN anticonvulsant; antipsychotic for manic episodes; migraine prophylaxis [also: divalproex sodium; valproate semisodium]

Semprex-D capsules ℞ decongestant; antihistamine [pseudoephedrine HCl; acrivastine] 60•8 mg

semustine USAN, INN antineoplastic

senecio, golden medicinal herb [see: life root]

Senecio aureus; S. jacobaea; S. vulgaris medicinal herb [see: life root]

senega (*Polygala senega*) root medicinal herb used as an antitussive for asthma, chronic bronchitis, croup, lung congestion, and pneumonia

Senexon tablets OTC stimulant laxative [senna concentrate] 187 mg

Senilezol elixir ℞ vitamin/iron supplement [multiple B vitamins; ferric pyrophosphate] ± •3.3 mg

senna USP stimulant laxative

senna (*Cassia acutifolia; C. angustifolia; C. senna*) leaves medicinal herb for bowel evacuation before gastrointestinal procedures, constipation, edema, and expelling worms

Senna-Gen tablets OTC stimulant laxative [sennosides] 8.6 mg

sennosides USP stimulant laxative

Senokot tablets, granules, suppositories, syrup OTC stimulant laxative [senna concentrate] 187 mg; 326 mg/tsp.; 652 mg; 218 mg/5 mL

Senokot-S tablets OTC stimulant laxative; stool softener [docusate sodium; senna concentrate] 50•187 mg

Senokotxtra tablets OTC stimulant laxative [senna concentrate] 374 mg

Senolax tablets (discontinued 1997) OTC stimulant laxative [senna concentrate] 187 mg

Sensamide ℞ investigational (Phase II/III) radiosensitizer for inoperable *non-small cell lung cancer (NSCLC)* [metoclopramide HCl]

Sensitive Eyes; Sensitive Eyes Plus solution OTC *rinsing/storage solution for soft contact lenses* [sodium chloride (preserved saline solution)]

Sensitive Eyes Daily Cleaner; Sensitive Eyes Saline/Cleaning Solution OTC *surfactant cleaning solution for soft contact lenses*

Sensitive Eyes Drops OTC *rewetting solution for soft contact lenses*

Sensitivity Protection Crest toothpaste OTC *tooth desensitizer; topical dental caries preventative* [potassium nitrate; sodium fluoride]

Sensodyne Cool Gel toothpaste OTC *tooth desensitizer; topical dental caries preventative* [potassium nitrate; sodium fluoride]

Sensodyne Fresh Mint toothpaste OTC *tooth desensitizer; dental caries preventative* [potassium nitrate; sodium monofluorophosphate] ?

Sensodyne-SC toothpaste OTC *tooth desensitizer* [strontium chloride hexahydrate] 10%

SensoGARD gel OTC *topical oral anesthetic* [benzocaine] 20%

Sensorcaine injection ℞ *injectable local anesthetic* [bupivacaine HCl] 0.25%, 0.5%

Sensorcaine injection ℞ *injectable local anesthetic* [bupivacaine HCl; epinephrine] 0.25%•1:200 000; 0.5%•1:200 000

Sensorcaine MPF injection ℞ *injectable local anesthetic* [bupivacaine HCl] 0.25%, 0.5%, 0.75%

Sensorcaine MPF injection ℞ *injectable local anesthetic* [bupivacaine HCl; epinephrine] 0.25%•1:200 000, 0.5%•1:200 000, 0.75%•1:200 000

Sensorcaine MPF Spinal injection ℞ *injectable local anesthetic* [bupivacaine HCl] 0.75%

Sentinel test kit for professional use ℞ *urine test for HIV-1 antibodies* ⌐ fentanyl

sepazonium chloride USAN, INN *topical anti-infective*

seperidol HCl USAN *antipsychotic* [also: clofluperol]

Seprafilm hydrated gel film *to reduce the incidence, extent, and severity of postoperative adhesions* [hyaluronate sodium; carboxymethylcellulose]

seprilose USAN *antirheumatic*

seproxetine HCl USAN *antidepressant*

Septa ointment OTC *topical antibiotic* [polymyxin B sulfate; neomycin sulfate; bacitracin] 5000 U•3.5 mg• 400 U per g ⌐ Cipro; Septra

Septi-Soft solution ℞ *antiseptic; disinfectant* [triclosan] 0.25%

Septisol foam ℞ *bacteriostatic skin cleanser* [hexachlorophene; alcohol 56%] 0.23%

Septisol solution ℞ *antiseptic; disinfectant* [triclosan] 0.25%

septomonab [see: nebacumab]

Septopal polymethyl methacrylate (PMMA) beads on surgical wire ℞ *investigational (orphan) for chronic osteomyelitis* [gentamicin sulfate]

Septra tablets, oral suspension ℞ *anti-infective; antibacterial* [trimethoprim; sulfamethoxazole] 80•400 mg; 40• 200 mg/5 mL ⌐ Cipro; Septa

Septra DS tablets ℞ *anti-infective; antibacterial* [trimethoprim; sulfamethoxazole] 160•800 mg

Septra IV infusion ℞ *anti-infective; antibacterial* [trimethoprim; sulfamethoxazole] 80•400 mg/5 mL

Sequels (trademarked dosage form) *sustained-release capsule or tablet*

sequifenadine INN

seractide INN *adrenocorticotropic hormone* [also: seractide acetate]

seractide acetate USAN *adrenocorticotropic hormone* [also: seractide]

Ser-Ap-Es tablets ℞ *antihypertensive; vasodilator; diuretic* [hydrochlorothiazide; reserpine; hydralazine HCl] 15•0.1•25 mg ⌐ Catapres

seratrodast USAN, INN *anti-inflammatory; antiasthmatic; thromboxane receptor antagonist*

Serax capsules, tablets ℞ *benzodiaze-pine anxiolytic* [oxazepam] 10, 15, 30 mg; 15 mg ② Eurax; Urex; Xerac

serazapine HCl USAN *anxiolytic*

Sereine solution OTC *cleaning solution for hard contact lenses* [note: one of three different products with the same name]

Sereine solution OTC *wetting solution for hard contact lenses* [note: one of three different products with the same name]

Sereine solution OTC *wetting/soaking solution for hard contact lenses* [note: one of three different products with the same name]

Serenoa repens; S. serrulata *medicinal herb* [see: saw palmetto]

Serentil tablets, oral concentrate, IM injection ℞ *conventional (typical) antipsychotic* [mesoridazine besylate] 10, 25, 50, 100 mg; 25 mg/mL; 25 mg/mL ② Surital

Serevent oral metered dose inhaler, Diskus (oral inhalation powder device) ℞ *twice-daily sympathomi-metic bronchodilator for asthma and bronchospasm* [salmeterol xinafoate] 25 μg/dose; 50 μg/dose

serfibrate INN

sergolexole INN *antimigraine* [also: ser-golexole maleate]

sergolexole maleate USAN *antimigraine* [also: sergolexole]

serine (L-serine) USAN, USP, INN *non-essential amino acid; symbols: Ser, S*

L-serine diazoacetate [see: azaserine]

84-L-serineplasminogen activator [see: monteplase]

sermetacin USAN, INN *anti-inflammatory*

sermorelin INN, BAN *growth hormone deficiency diagnosis and treatment* [also: sermorelin acetate]

sermorelin acetate USAN *diagnostic aid for pituitary function; treatment for growth hormone deficiency (orphan), anovulation, and AIDS-related weight loss* [also: sermorelin]

SERMs (selective estrogen receptor modulators) [q.v.]

Seromycin Pulvules (capsules) ℞ *tuberculostatic* [cycloserine] 250 mg

Serophene tablets ℞ *ovulation stimu-lant* [clomiphene citrate] 50 mg

Seroquel tablets ℞ *novel (atypical) antipsychotic* [quetiapine fumarate] 25, 100, 200 mg

Serostim powder for subcu injection ℞ *growth hormone for adults or chil-dren with congenital or endogenous growth hormone deficiency, children with Turner syndrome or renal-induced growth failure, or AIDS-wasting syn-drome (orphan)* [somatropin] 5, 6 mg (15, 18 IU) per vial

serotonin (5-hydroxytryptamine₁; 5-HT₁) [see: selective serotonin reuptake inhibitors; vascular seroto-nin receptor antagonists]

Seroxat (European name for U.S. product Paxil)

Serpalan tablets (discontinued 1995) ℞ *antihypertensive; antipsychotic* [reserpine] 0.1, 0.25 mg

Serpazide tablets ℞ *antihypertensive; vasodilator; diuretic* [hydrochlorothia-zide; reserpine; hydralazine HCl]

serrapeptase INN

Serratia marcescens extract (polyri-bosomes) *investigational (orphan) for primary brain malignancies*

sertaconazole INN

sertindole USAN, INN *antipsychotic; neuroleptic*

Sertoli cells, porcine *investigational (orphan) intracerebral implant for stage 4 and 5 Parkinson's disease (for co-implantation with fetal neural cells)*

sertraline INN, BAN *selective serotonin reuptake inhibitor (SSRI) for depres-sion, obsessive-compulsive disorder, and panic disorder* [also: sertraline HCl]

sertraline HCl USAN *selective serotonin reuptake inhibitor (SSRI) for depres-sion, obsessive-compulsive disorder, and panic disorder* [also: sertraline]

serum albumin (SA) [see: albumin, human]

serum albumin, iodinated (^{125}I) human [see: albumin, iodinated I 125 serum]

serum albumin, iodinated (^{131}I) human [see: albumin, iodinated I 131 serum]

serum fibrinogen (SF) [see: fibrinogen, human]

serum globulin (SG) [see: globulin, immune]

serum gonadotrophin [see: gonadotrophin, serum]

serum gonadotropin [see: gonadotrophin, serum]

serum prothrombin conversion accelerator (SPCA) factor [see: factor VII]

Serutan powder, granules OTC *bulk laxative* [psyllium] 3.4 g/tsp.; 2.5 g/tsp.

Serzone tablets ℞ *antidepressant* [nefazodone HCl] 50, 100, 150, 200, 250 mg

sesame oil NF *solvent; oleaginous vehicle*

Sesame Street Complete chewable tablets OTC *vitamin/mineral/calcium/iron supplement* [multiple vitamins & minerals; calcium; iron; folic acid; biotin] ±•80•10•0.2•0.015 mg

Sesame Street Plus Extra C chewable tablets OTC *vitamin supplement* [multiple vitamins; folic acid] ±•0.2 mg

Sesame Street Plus Iron chewable tablets OTC *vitamin/iron supplement* [multiple vitamins; iron; folic acid] ±•10•0.2 mg

setastine INN

setazindol INN

setiptiline INN

setoperone USAN, INN *antipsychotic*

setwall *medicinal herb* [see: valerian]

Seudotabs tablets OTC *nasal decongestant* [pseudoephedrine HCl] 30 mg

sevelamer HCl USAN *phosphate-binding polymer for hyperphosphatemia of end-stage renal disease*

7 + 3 protocol (cytarabine, daunorubicin) *chemotherapy protocol*

7 + 3 protocol (cytarabine, idarubicin) *chemotherapy protocol*

7 + 3 protocol (cytarabine, mitoxantrone) *chemotherapy protocol*

seven barks *medicinal herb* [see: hydrangea]

7E3 MAb [see: abciximab]

sevirumab USAN, INN *investigational (Phase I) antiviral for AIDS; orphan status withdrawn 1996*

sevitropium mesilate INN

sevoflurane USAN, INN *inhalation general anesthetic*

sevopramide INN

sezolamide HCl USAN *carbonic anhydrase inhibitor*

SF (serum fibrinogen) [see: fibrinogen, human]

SFC lotion OTC *soap-free therapeutic skin cleanser*

sfericase INN

SG (serum globulin) [see: globulin, immune]

SG (soluble gelatin) [see: gelatin]

shamrock, Indian *medicinal herb* [see: birthroot]

shamrock, water *medicinal herb* [see: buckbean]

shark cartilage (derived from *Sphyrna lewini, Squalus acanthias,* **and other species)** *natural remedy for cancer* [also: squalamine]

shark liver oil *emollient/protectant*

shavegrass *medicinal herb* [see: horsetail]

sheep laurel *medicinal herb* [see: mountain laurel]

Sheik Elite premedicated condom OTC *spermicidal/barrier contraceptive* [nonoxynol 9] 8%

shell flower *medicinal herb* [see: turtlebloom]

shellac NF *tablet coating agent*

Shepard's Cream Lotion; Shepard's Skin Cream OTC *moisturizer; emollient*

shepherd's club *medicinal herb* [see: mullein]

shepherd's heart *medicinal herb* [see: shepherd's purse]

shepherd's purse (*Capsella bursa-pastoris***)** plant *medicinal herb for bleeding, ear disease, hypertension, painful menstruation, and urinary bleeding*

shigoka *medicinal herb* [see: Siberian ginseng]

shiitake mushrooms (*Lentinula edodes; Tricholomopsis edodes*) stem and cap *medicinal herb for boosting the immune system, cancer, lowering cholesterol, and viral illnesses*

Shohl solution, modified (sodium citrate & citric acid) *urinary alkalizer; compounding agent*

short chain fatty acids *investigational (orphan) for left-sided ulcerative colitis and chronic radiation proctitis*

short-leaved buchu *medicinal herb* [see: buchu]

Shur-Clens solution OTC *wound cleanser* [poloxamer 188] 20%

Shur-Seal vaginal gel OTC *spermicidal contraceptive (for use with a diaphragm)* [nonoxynol 9] 2%

siagoside INN

sialagogues *a class of agents that stimulate the secretion of saliva* [also called: ptyalagogues]

SIB-1508Y *investigational (Phase II) nicotinic agonist for Parkinson's disease*

Sibelium ℞ *investigational (orphan) vasodilator for alternating hemiplegia* [flunarizine HCl]

Siberian ginseng (*Acanthopanax senticosus; Eleutherococcus senticosus*) root *medicinal herb for age spots, blood diseases, depression, hemorrhage, immune system stimulation, increasing endurance and longevity, normalizing blood pressure, platelet aggregation inhibition, sexual stimulation, and stress* [also see: ginseng]

Siblin granules (discontinued 1997) OTC *bulk laxative* [blond psyllium seed coatings] 2.5 g/tsp.

sibopirdine USAN *cognition enhancer for Alzheimer's disease; nootropic*

sibrafiban USAN *platelet inhibitor; fibrinogen receptor antagonist*

sibutramine INN, BAN *anorexiant for the treatment of obesity; monoamine reuptake inhibitor antidepressant* [also: sibutramine HCl]

sibutramine HCl USAN *anorexiant for the treatment of obesity; monoamine reuptake inhibitor antidepressant* [also: sibutramine]

siccanin INN

Sickledex *test kit for professional use in vitro diagnostic aid for hemoglobin S (sickle cell)*

sicklewort *medicinal herb* [see: woundwort]

side-flowering skullcap *medicinal herb* [see: skullcap]

SigPak (trademarked packaging form) *unit-of-use package*

Sigtab tablets OTC *vitamin supplement* [multiple vitamins; folic acid] ≛•0.4 mg

Sigtab-M tablets OTC *vitamin/mineral/calcium/iron supplement* [multiple vitamins & minerals; calcium; iron; folic acid; biotin] ≛•200•18•0.4•0.045 mg

siguazodan INN, BAN

Silace syrup OTC *stool softener* [docusate sodium] 20 mg/5 mL

Silace-C syrup OTC *stimulant laxative; stool softener* [casanthranol; docusate sodium; alcohol 10%] 30•60 mg/15 mL

SilaClean 20/20 solution (discontinued 1995) OTC *cleaning solution for hard contact lenses*

Siladryl elixir OTC *antihistamine* [diphenhydramine HCl] 12.5 mg/5 mL

Silafed syrup OTC *decongestant; antihistamine* [pseudoephedrine HCl; triprolidine HCl] 30•1.25 mg/5 mL

silafilcon A USAN *hydrophilic contact lens material*

silafocon A USAN *hydrophobic contact lens material*

Silaminic Cold syrup OTC *decongestant; antihistamine* [phenylpropanolamine HCl; chlorpheniramine maleate] 12.5•2 mg/5 mL

Silaminic Expectorant syrup OTC *decongestant; expectorant* [phenylpropanolamine HCl; guaifenesin; alcohol 5%] 12.5•100 mg/5 mL

silandrone USAN, INN *androgen*

Silapap, Children's liquid OTC *analgesic; antipyretic* [acetaminophen] 80 mg/2.5 mL

Silapap, Infant's drops OTC *analgesic; antipyretic* [acetaminophen] 100 mg/mL

Sildec-DM syrup, pediatric drops ℞ *antitussive; decongestant; antihistamine* [dextromethorphan hydrobromide; pseudoephedrine HCl; carbinoxamine maleate] 15•60•4 mg/5 mL; 4•25•2 mg/mL

sildenafil citrate USAN *selective vasodilator for erectile dysfunction*

Sildicon-E pediatric drops OTC *pediatric decongestant and expectorant* [phenylpropanolamine HCl; guaifenesin] 6.25•30 mg/mL

Silfedrine, Children's liquid OTC *nasal decongestant* [pseudoephedrine HCl] 30 mg/5 mL

silibinin INN

silica, dental-type NF *pharmaceutic aid*

silica gel [now: silicon dioxide]

siliceous earth, purified NF *filtering medium*

silicic acid, magnesium salt [see: magnesium trisilicate]

silicon *element (Si)*

silicon dioxide NF *dispersing and suspending agent*

silicon dioxide, colloidal NF *suspending agent; tablet and capsule diluent*

silicone

Silicone No. 2 ointment OTC *skin protectant* [silicone; hydrophobic starch derivative] 10%• ②

silicone oil [see: polydimethylsiloxane]

silicristin INN

silidianin INN

silkweed *medicinal herb* [see: milkweed; pleurisy root]

silky swallow wort; Virginia silk *medicinal herb* [see: milkweed]

silodrate USAN *antacid* [also: simaldrate]

Silphen Cough syrup OTC *antihistamine; antitussive* [diphenhydramine HCl; alcohol 5%] 12.5 mg/5 mL

Silphen DM syrup OTC *antitussive* [dextromethorphan hydrobromide; alcohol 5%] 10 mg/5 mL

Silphium perfoliatum *medicinal herb* [see: ragged cup]

Siltapp with Dextromethorphan HBr Cold & Cough elixir ℞ *antitussive; decongestant; antihistamine* [dextromethorphan hydrobromide; phenylpropanolamine HCl; brompheniramine maleate] 10•12.5•2 mg/5 mL

Sil-Tex liquid ℞ *decongestant; expectorant* [phenylpropanolamine HCl; phenylephrine HCl; guaifenesin; alcohol 5%] 20•5•100 mg/5 mL

Siltussin syrup OTC *expectorant* [guaifenesin; alcohol 3.5%] 100 mg/5 mL

Siltussin DM syrup OTC *antitussive; expectorant* [dextromethorphan hydrobromide; guaifenesin] 10•100 mg/5 mL

Siltussin-CF liquid OTC *antitussive; decongestant; expectorant* [dextromethorphan hydrobromide; phenylpropanolamine HCl; guaifenesin; alcohol 4.75%] 10•12.5•100 mg/5 mL

Silvadene cream ℞ *broad-spectrum bactericidal for adjunctive burn treatment* [silver sulfadiazine] 10 mg/g ② Azulfidine

silver *element (Ag)*

silver nitrate USP *ophthalmic neonatal anti-infective; strong caustic* 1% eye drops; 10%, 25%, 50%, 75% topical

silver nitrate, toughened USP *caustic*

silver protein, mild NF *ophthalmic antiseptic; ophthalmic surgical aid*

silver sulfadiazine (SSD) USAN, USP *broad-spectrum bactericidal; adjunct to burn therapy* [also: sulfadiazine silver]

silverweed; silver cinquefoil *medicinal herb* [see: cinquefoil]

Silybum marianum *medicinal herb* [see: milk thistle]

Simaal Gel; Simaal Gel 2 liquid OTC *antacid; antiflatulent* [aluminum hydroxide; magnesium hydroxide; simethicone] 200•200•20 mg/5 mL; 500•400•40 mg/5 mL

simaldrate INN *antacid* [also: silodrate]

Simdax *investigational cardiotonic and vasodilator for congestive heart failure* [levosimendan]

simethicone USAN, USP *antiflatulent* 80 mg oral; 40 mg/0.6 mL oral

simethicone-coated cellulose suspension (SCCS) [see: SonoRx]

simetride INN

simfibrate INN

Similac Low Iron liquid, powder OTC *total or supplementary infant feeding*

Similac PM 60/40 Low-Iron liquid OTC *formula for infants predisposed to hypocalcemia* [whey formula with lowered mineral levels]

Similac with Iron liquid, powder OTC *total or supplementary infant feeding*

simple syrup [see: syrup]

Simpler's joy *medicinal herb* [see: blue vervain]

Simplet tablets OTC *decongestant; antihistamine; analgesic* [pseudoephedrine HCl; chlorpheniramine maleate; acetaminophen] 60●4●650 mg ② Singlet

Simron soft gelatin capsules (discontinued 1998) OTC *hematinic* [ferrous gluconate (source of iron)] 86 mg (10 mg)

Simron Plus capsules OTC *vitamin/iron supplement* [multiple vitamins; ferrous gluconate; folic acid] ≛●10●0.1 mg

simtrazene USAN, INN *antineoplastic*

Simulect powder for IV infusion *immunosuppressant; IL-2 receptor antagonist for the prevention of acute rejection of renal transplants (orphan)* [basiliximab] 20 mg

simvastatin USAN, INN, BAN *HMG-CoA reductase inhibitor for hyperlipidemia and coronary heart disease* ② Sandostatin; zinostatin

Sinapils tablets OTC *decongestant; antihistamine; analgesic* [phenylpropanolamine HCl; chlorpheniramine maleate; acetaminophen; caffeine] 12.5●2●325●32.5 mg

Sinapis alba *medicinal herb* [see: mustard]

sinapultide USAN *pulmonary surfactant for respiratory distress syndrome*

Sinarest; Sinarest Sinus tablets OTC *decongestant; antihistamine; analgesic* [pseudoephedrine HCl; chlorpheniramine maleate; acetaminophen] 30●2●500 mg; 30●2●325 mg

Sinarest, No Drowsiness tablets OTC *decongestant; analgesic; antipyretic* [pseudoephedrine HCl; acetaminophen] 30●500 mg

Sinarest 12 Hour nasal spray OTC *nasal decongestant* [oxymetazoline HCl] 0.05%

sincalide USAN, INN *choleretic; diagnostic aid for gallbladder function*

Sine-Aid tablets, caplets, gelcaps OTC *decongestant; analgesic; antipyretic* [pseudoephedrine HCl; acetaminophen] 30●500 mg

Sine-Aid IB caplets OTC *decongestant; analgesic* [pseudoephedrine HCl; ibuprofen] 30●200 mg

sinefungin USAN, INN *antifungal*

Sinemet 10/100; Sinemet 25/100; Sinemet 25/250 tablets ℞ *antiparkinsonian; dopamine precursor; decarboxylase inhibitor* [carbidopa; levodopa] 10●100 mg; 25●100 mg; 25●250 mg

Sinemet CR sustained-release tablets ℞ *antiparkinsonian; dopamine precursor; decarboxylase inhibitor* [carbidopa; levodopa] 25●100, 50●200 mg

Sine-Off Allergy/Sinus caplets (name changed to Sine-Off Sinus Medicine in 1995)

Sine-Off No Drowsiness Formula caplets OTC *decongestant; analgesic; antipyretic* [pseudoephedrine HCl; acetaminophen] 30●500 mg

Sine-Off Sinus Medicine caplets OTC *decongestant; antihistamine; analgesic* [pseudoephedrine HCl; chlorpheniramine maleate; acetaminophen] 30●2●500 mg

Sine-Off Sinus Medicine tablets (discontinued 1995) OTC *decongestant; antihistamine; analgesic; antipyretic* [phenylpropanolamine HCl; chlorpheniramine maleate; aspirin] 12.5●2●325 mg

Sinequan capsules, oral concentrate ℞ *tricyclic antidepressant and anxiolytic* [doxepin HCl] 10, 25, 50, 75, 100, 150 mg; 10 mg/mL

Sinex nasal spray OTC *nasal decongestant* [phenylephrine HCl] 0.5%

Sinex 12-Hour nasal spray OTC *nasal decongestant* [oxymetazoline HCl] 0.05%

single-chain antigen-binding proteins (SCA proteins) *a class of investigational antineoplastics*

SingleJect (trademarked dosage form) *prefilled syringe*

Singlet for Adults tablets OTC *decongestant; antihistamine; analgesic* [pseudoephedrine HCl; chlorpheniramine maleate; acetaminophen] 60•4•650 mg ☑ Simplet

Singulair chewable tablets, film-coated tablets ℞ *leukotriene receptor inhibitor for prophylaxis and chronic treatment of asthma* [montelukast sodium] 5 mg; 10 mg

Sinografin intracavitary instillation ℞ *radiopaque contrast medium for gynecological imaging* [diatrizoate meglumine; iodipamide meglumine (47.8% total iodine)] 727•268 mg/mL (380 mg/mL)

sinorphan [now: ecadotril]

sintropium bromide INN

Sinufed Timecelles (sustained-release capsules) ℞ *decongestant; expectorant* [pseudoephedrine HCl; guaifenesin] 60•300 mg

Sinulin tablets OTC *decongestant; antihistamine; analgesic* [phenylpropanolamine HCl; chlorpheniramine maleate; acetaminophen] 25•4•650 mg

Sinumist-SR sustained-release Capsulets (capsule-shaped tablet) ℞ *expectorant* [guaifenesin] 600 mg

Sinupan controlled-release capsules ℞ *decongestant; expectorant* [phenylephrine HCl; guaifenesin] 40•200 mg

Sinus Headache & Congestion tablets OTC *decongestant; antihistamine; analgesic* [pseudoephedrine HCl; chlorpheniramine maleate; acetaminophen] 30•2•500 mg

Sinus Relief tablets OTC *decongestant; analgesic* [pseudoephedrine HCl; acetaminophen] 30•325 mg

Sinusol-B subcu or IM injection (discontinued 1997) ℞ *antihistamine for anaphylaxis* [brompheniramine maleate] 10 mg/mL

SinuStat capsules OTC *decongestant* [pseudoephedrine HCl]

Sinustop Pro capsules OTC *nasal decongestant* [pseudoephedrine HCl] 60 mg

Sinutab Non-Drying liquid capsules OTC *decongestant; expectorant* [pseudoephedrine HCl; guaifenesin] 30•200 mg

Sinutab Sinus Allergy caplets, tablets OTC *decongestant; antihistamine; analgesic* [pseudoephedrine HCl; chlorpheniramine maleate; acetaminophen] 30•2•500 mg

Sinutab Without Drowsiness caplets OTC *decongestant; analgesic; antipyretic* [pseudoephedrine HCl; acetaminophen] 30•500 mg

Sinutab Without Drowsiness tablets OTC *decongestant; analgesic; antipyretic* [pseudoephedrine HCl; acetaminophen] 30•325 mg; 30•500 mg

Sinutrex tablets (discontinued 1995) OTC *decongestant; antihistamine; analgesic* [pseudoephedrine HCl; chlorpheniramine maleate; acetaminophen] 30•2•500 mg

SinuVent long-acting tablets ℞ *decongestant; expectorant* [phenylpropanolamine HCl; guaifenesin] 75•600 mg

Sirdalud (foreign name for U.S. product Zanaflex)

sirolimus USAN *investigational immunosuppressant for organ transplants*

sisomicin USAN, INN *antibacterial* [also: sissomicin]

sisomicin sulfate USAN, USP *antibacterial*

sissomicin BAN *antibacterial* [also: sisomicin]

sitalidone INN

sitofibrate INN

sitogluside USAN, INN *antiprostatic hypertrophy*

sitosterols NF

Sitzmarks capsules ℞ *radiopaque contrast medium for severe constipation* [polyvinyl chloride, radiopaque] 24 rings/capsule

sizofiran INN

SK (streptokinase) [q.v.]

Skeeter Stik liquid OTC *topical local anesthetic; counterirritant* [lidocaine; menthol] 4%•1%

Skelaxin tablets ℞ *skeletal muscle relaxant* [metaxalone] 400 mg

Skelid tablets ℞ *bisphosphonate bone resorption inhibitor for Paget's disease* [tiludronate disodium] 240 mg

SK&F 110679 *orphan status withdrawn 1996*

skin respiratory factor (SRF) *claimed to promote wound healing*

Skin Shield liquid OTC *skin protectant; topical local anesthetic* [dyclonine HCl; benzethonium chloride] 0.75%•0.2%

Skinoren (German name for U.S. product Azelex)

skullcap (Scutellaria lateriflora) plant *medicinal herb for convulsions, epilepsy, fever, hypertension, infertility, insomnia, nervous disorders, rabies, and restlessness*

skunk cabbage (Symplocarpus foetidus) root *medicinal herb used as an antispasmodic, diuretic, emetic, expectorant, pectoral, stimulant, and sudorific*

skunk weed *medicinal herb* [see: skunk cabbage]

SL (sodium lactate) [q.v.]

Sleep-Eze 3 tablets OTC *antihistaminic sleep aid* [diphenhydramine HCl] 25 mg

Sleepinal capsules, soft gels OTC *antihistaminic sleep aid* [diphenhydramine HCl] 50 mg

Sleepwell 2-nite tablets OTC *antihistaminic sleep aid* [diphenhydramine HCl] 25 mg

Slim-Mint gum OTC *decrease taste perception of sweetness* [benzocaine] 6 mg

slippery elm (Ulmus fulva; U. rubra) inner bark *medicinal herb for asthma, blackened or bruised eyes, boils, bronchitis, burns, cold sores, colitis, cough, diaper rash, diarrhea, indigestion, lung disorders, sore throat, and urinary tract inflammation*

slippery root *medicinal herb* [see: comfrey]

Slo-bid Gyrocaps (extended-release capsules) ℞ *antiasthmatic; bronchodilator* [theophylline] 50, 75, 100, 125, 200, 300 mg

Slocaps (trademarked form) *sustained-release capsules*

Slo-Niacin controlled-release tablets OTC *vitamin supplement* [niacin] 250, 500, 750 mg

Slonnon (Japanese name for U.S. investigational product Novastan)

Slo-phyllin tablets, syrup, Gyrocaps (extended-release capsules) ℞ *antiasthmatic; bronchodilator* [theophylline] 100, 200 mg; 80 mg/15 mL; 60, 125, 250 mg

Slo-phyllin GG capsules, syrup ℞ *antiasthmatic; bronchodilator; expectorant* [theophylline; guaifenesin] 150•90 mg; 150•90 mg/15 mL

Slo-Salt-K slow-release tablets OTC *sodium chloride/potassium replacement; dehydration preventative* [sodium chloride; potassium chloride] 410•150 mg

slow channel blockers *a class of coronary vasodilators that inhibit cardiac muscle contraction and slow cardiac electrical conduction velocity* [also called: calcium channel blockers; calcium antagonists]

Slow Fe slow-release tablets OTC *hematinic* [ferrous sulfate, dried (source of iron)] 160 mg (50 mg)

Slow Fe with Folic Acid slow-release tablets OTC *hematinic* [ferrous sulfate; folic acid] 50•0.4 mg

Slow Fluoride slow-release tablets ℞ *investigational agent for postmenopausal osteoporosis* [sodium fluoride]

Slow-K controlled-release tablets ℞ *potassium supplement* [potassium chloride] 600 mg (8 mEq)

Slow-Mag delayed-release enteric-coated tablets OTC *magnesium supplement* [magnesium chloride] 535 mg ⓓ Flomax; Zomig

SLT hair lotion OTC *antiseborrheic; antipsoriatic; keratolytic; antiseptic* [coal tar; salicylic acid; lactic acid; alcohol 65%] 2%•3%•5%

SMA Iron Fortified liquid, powder (discontinued 1996) OTC *total or supplementary infant feeding*

SMA Lo-Iron liquid, powder (discontinued 1996) OTC *total or supplementary infant feeding*

small burnet saxifrage *medicinal herb* [see: burnet]

small pimpernel *medicinal herb* [see: burnet]

small saxifrage *medicinal herb* [see: burnet]

smallpox vaccine USP *active immunizing agent*

SMART anti-CD3 antibody *investigational (Phase I) immunosuppressant*

SMART anti-gpIIb/IIIa monoclonal antibody *investigational cardiovascular antiplatelet agent*

SMART anti-tac; humanized anti-tac [now: dacliximab]

SmartMist (trademarked form) *hand-held inhalation device*

smartweed; water smartweed *medicinal herb* [see: knotweed]

SMF (streptozocin, mitomycin, fluorouracil) *chemotherapy protocol*

Smilax **spp.** *medicinal herb* [see: sarsaparilla]

smooth sumach *medicinal herb* [see: sumach]

SMX; SMZ (sulfamethoxazole) [q.v.]

SMZ-TMP (sulfamethoxazole & trimethoprim) [q.v.]

SN (streptonigrin) [q.v.]

snake bite *medicinal herb* [see: birthroot]

snake head *medicinal herb* [see: turtlebloom]

snake lily *medicinal herb* [see: blue flag]

snake weed *medicinal herb* [see: bistort; plantain]

snakebite antivenin [see: antivenin, Crotalidae & Micrurus fulvius]

snakeroot *medicinal herb* [see: echinacea]

snakeroot, black *medicinal herb* [see: black cohosh; sanicle]

Snaplets-D granules (discontinued 1995) OTC *pediatric decongestant and antihistamine* [phenylpropanolamine HCl; chlorpheniramine maleate] 6.25•1 mg/packet

Snaplets-DM granules OTC *pediatric antitussive and decongestant* [dextromethorphan hydrobromide; phenylpropanolamine HCl] 5•6.25 mg/packet

Snaplets-EX granules OTC *pediatric decongestant and expectorant* [phenylpropanolamine HCl; guaifenesin] 6.25•50 mg/packet

Snaplets-FR granules (discontinued 1997) OTC *analgesic; antipyretic* [acetaminophen] 80 mg/packet

Snaplets-Multi granules OTC *pediatric antitussive, decongestant, and antihistamine* [dextromethorphan hydrobromide; phenylpropanolamine HCl; chlorpheniramine maleate] 5•6.25•1 mg/packet

snapping hazel *medicinal herb* [see: witch hazel]

SnapTab (trademarked dosage form) *scored tablet*

SnET2 [see: tin ethyl etiopurpurin]

Snooze Fast tablets OTC *antihistaminic sleep aid* [diphenhydramine HCl] 50 mg

Sno-Strips ophthalmic strips OTC *diagnostic tear flow test aid*

snout, swine *medicinal herb* [see: dandelion]

snowball, wild *medicinal herb* [see: New Jersey tea]

snowdrop tree; snowflower *medicinal herb* [see: fringe tree]

SNX-482 *investigational selective R-type calcium channel blocker for treatment of brain and neurological disorders*

Soac-Lens solution OTC *wetting/soaking solution for hard contact lenses* soap, green USP *detergent*

soapwort *(Saponaria officinalis)* plant and roots *medicinal herb for acne, boils, eczema, poison ivy rash and psoriasis; also used in skin disinfectants and soaps*

SOD (superoxide dismutase) [see: orgotein]

soda lime NF *carbon dioxide absorbent*

sodium *element (Na)*

sodium acetate USP *dialysis aid; electrolyte replenisher; pH buffer* 2, 4 mEq/mL (16.4%, 32.8%) injection

sodium acetate trihydrate [see: sodium acetate]

sodium acetrizoate INN, BAN [also: acetrizoate sodium]

sodium acetylsalicylate *analgesic*

sodium acid phosphate *urinary acidifier*

sodium acid pyrophosphate *urinary acidifier*

sodium alginate NF *suspending agent*

sodium amidotrizoate INN *oral/rectal/ parenteral radiopaque contrast medium (59.87% iodine)* [also: diatrizoate sodium; sodium diatrizoate]

sodium aminobenzoate [see: aminobenzoate sodium]

sodium amylopectin sulfate [see: sodium amylosulfate]

sodium amylosulfate USAN *enzyme inhibitor*

sodium anoxynaphthonate BAN *blood volume and cardiac output test* [also: anazolene sodium]

sodium antimony gluconate [see: sodium stibogluconate]

sodium antimonylgluconate BAN

sodium apolate INN, BAN *anticoagulant* [also: lyapolate sodium]

sodium arsenate, exsiccated NF

sodium arsenate As 74 USAN *radioactive agent*

sodium ascorbate USP, INN *vitamin C; antiscorbutic* 500 mg oral; 1800 mg/½ tsp. oral; 222, 500 mg/mL injection

sodium aurothiomalate INN *antirheumatic* [also: gold sodium thiomalate]

sodium aurotiosulfate INN [also: gold sodium thiosulfate]

sodium azodisalicylate [now: olsalazine sodium]

sodium benzoate USAN, NF, JAN *antihyperammonemic; antifungal agent; preservative*

sodium benzoate & caffeine *analeptic for respiratory depression due to an overdose of CNS depressants* 250 mg/ mL injection

sodium benzoate & sodium phenylacetate *to prevent and treat hyperammonemia of urea cycle enzymopathy (orphan)*

sodium benzyl penicillin [see: penicillin G sodium]

sodium bicarbonate USP *electrolyte replenisher; systemic alkalizer; antacid* 325, 600, 650 mg oral; 0.5, 0.6, 0.9, 1 mEq/mL (4.2%, 5%, 7.5%, 8.4%) injection

sodium biphosphate *urinary acidifier; pH buffer*

sodium bisulfite NF *antioxidant*

sodium bitionolate INN *topical antiinfective* [also: bithionolate sodium]

sodium borate NF *alkalizing agent; antipruritic; bacteriostatic agent in cold creams, eye washes, and mouth rinses*

sodium borocaptate (^{10}B) INN *antineoplastic; radioactive agent* [also: borocaptate sodium B 10]

sodium cacodylate NF

sodium calcium edetate INN *heavy metal chelating agent* [also: edetate calcium disodium; sodium calciumedetate; calcium disodium edetate]

sodium calciumedetate BAN *heavy metal chelating agent* [also: edetate calcium disodium; sodium calcium edetate; calcium disodium edetate]

sodium caprylate *antifungal*

sodium carbonate NF *alkalizing agent*

sodium chloride (NaCl) USP *ophthalmic hypertonic; electrolyte replacement; abortifacient* [sterile isotonic solution] 650, 1000, 2250 mg oral; 0.45%, 0.9%, 3%, 5%, 14.6%, 23.4% injection/diluent

0.45% sodium chloride (½ normal saline; ½ NS) *electrolyte replacement*

0.9% sodium chloride (normal saline; NS) *electrolyte replacement* [also: saline solution]

sodium chloride, compound solution of INN *fluid and electrolyte replenisher* [also: Ringer's injection]

sodium chloride Na 22 USAN *radioactive agent*

sodium chondroitin sulfate [see: chondroitin sulfate sodium]

sodium chromate (^{51}Cr) INN *blood volume test; radioactive agent* [also: sodium chromate Cr 51]

sodium chromate Cr 51 USAN *blood volume test; radioactive agent* [also: sodium chromate (^{51}Cr)]

sodium citrate USP *systemic alkalizer; pH buffer; antacid; investigational (orphan) adjunct to leukapheresis procedures*

sodium colistin methanesulfonate [see: colistimethate sodium]

sodium cromoglycate [see: cromolyn sodium]

sodium cyclamate NF, INN

sodium cyclohexanesulfamate [see: sodium cyclamate]

sodium dehydroacetate NF *antimicrobial preservative*

sodium dehydrocholate INN [also: dehydrocholate sodium]

sodium denyl [see: phenytoin sodium]

sodium diatrizoate BAN *oral/rectal/parenteral radiopaque contrast medium (59.87% iodine)* [also: diatrizoate sodium; sodium amidotrizoate]

sodium dibunate INN, BAN

sodium dicloroacetate *investigational (orphan) for lactic acidosis and homozygous familial hypercholesterolemia*

sodium diethyldithiocarbamate [see: ditiocarb sodium]

sodium diiodomethanesulfonate [see: dimethiodal sodium]

sodium dioctyl sulfosuccinate INN *stool softener; surfactant* [also: docusate sodium]

sodium diphenylhydantoin [see: phenytoin sodium]

sodium diprotrizoate INN, BAN [also: diprotrizoate sodium]

Sodium Diuril powder for IV injection ℞ *diuretic* [chlorothiazide] 500 mg

sodium edetate [see: edetate sodium]

sodium estrone sulfate *estrogen replacement therapy for postmenopausal disorders* 0.625, 1.25, 2.5, 5 mg oral

sodium etasulfate INN *detergent* [also: sodium ethasulfate]

sodium ethasulfate USAN *detergent* [also: sodium etasulfate]

sodium feredetate INN [also: sodium ironedetate]

sodium ferric gluconate *hematinic for iron deficiency of chronic hemodialysis with erythropoietin therapy*

sodium fluoride USP *fluoride replacement therapy; dental caries preventative; investigational agent for treatment of postmenopausal osteoporosis* 1.1, 2.2 mg oral; 0.125 mg/drop oral

sodium fluoride F 18 USP

sodium fluoride & phosphoric acid USP *dental caries prophylactic*

sodium formaldehyde sulfoxylate NF *preservative*

sodium gammahydroxyburate [see: sodium oxybate]

sodium gentisate INN

sodium glucaspaldrate INN, BAN

sodium gluconate USP *electrolyte replenisher*

sodium glucosulfone USP

sodium glutamate

sodium glycerophosphate NF

sodium glycocholate [see: bile salts]

sodium gualenate INN [also: azulene sulfonate sodium]

sodium hyaluronate [see: hyaluronate sodium]

sodium hydroxide NF *alkalizing agent*

sodium hydroxybenzenesulfonate [see: phenolsulphonate sodium]

sodium 4-hydroxybutyrate [see: sodium oxybate]

sodium hypochlorite USP, JAN *disinfectant; bleach; used for utensils and equipment*

sodium hypochlorite, diluted NF [also: antiformin, dental]

sodium hypophosphite NF

sodium iodide USP *dietary iodine supplement*

sodium iodide (¹²³I) JAN *thyroid function test; radioactive agent* [also: sodium iodide I 123]

sodium iodide (¹²⁵I) INN *thyroid function test; radioactive agent* [also: sodium iodide I 125]

sodium iodide (¹³¹I) JAN *antineoplastic for thyroid carcinoma; radioactive agent for hyperthyroidism* [also: sodium iodide I 131]

sodium iodide I 123 USP *diagnostic aid for thyroid function; radioactive agent* [also: sodium iodide (¹²³I)] 3.7, 7.4 MBq oral

sodium iodide I 125 USAN, USP *thyroid function test; radioactive agent* [also: sodium iodide (¹²⁵I)]

sodium iodide I 131 USAN, USP, INN *antineoplastic for thyroid carcinoma; radioactive agent for hyperthyroidism* [also: sodium iodide (¹³¹I)] 0.75–100 mCi, 3.5–150 mCi oral

sodium iodohippurate (¹³¹I) INN, JAN *renal function test; radioactive agent* [also: iodohippurate sodium I 131]

sodium iodomethanesulfonate [see: methiodal sodium]

sodium iopodate JAN *oral radiopaque contrast medium for cholecystography (61.4% iodine)* [also: ipodate sodium; sodium ipodate]

sodium iotalamate (¹²⁵I) INN *radioactive agent* [also: iothalamate sodium I 125]

sodium iotalamate (¹³¹I) INN *radioactive agent* [also: iothalamate sodium I 131]

sodium iothalamate BAN *parenteral radiopaque contrast medium (59.9% iodine)* [also: iothalamate sodium]

sodium ioxaglate BAN *radiopaque contrast medium* [also: ioxaglate sodium]

sodium ipodate INN, BAN *oral radiopaque contrast medium for cholecystography (61.4% iodine)* [also: ipodate sodium; sodium iopodate]

sodium ironedetate BAN [also: sodium feredetate]

sodium lactate (SL) USP *electrolyte replenisher* 167 mEq/L (1/6 molar) injection

sodium lactate, compound solution of INN *electrolyte and fluid replenisher; systemic alkalizer* [also: Ringer's injection, lactated]

sodium lauryl sulfate NF *surfactant/wetting agent* [also: laurilsulfate]

sodium lignosulfonate [see: polignate sodium]

sodium metabisulfite NF *antioxidant*

sodium metrizoate INN *radiopaque contrast medium* [also: metrizoate sodium]

sodium monododecyl sulfate [see: sodium lauryl sulfate]

sodium monofluorophosphate USP *dental caries prophylactic*

sodium monomercaptoundecahydro-closo-dodecaborate *investigational (orphan) for boron neutron capture therapy (BNCT) for glioblastoma multiforme*

sodium morrhuate INN *sclerosing agent* [also: morrhuate sodium]

sodium nitrite USP *antidote to cyanide poisoning*

sodium nitroferricyanide [see: sodium nitroprusside]

sodium nitroferricyanide dihydrate [see: sodium nitroprusside]

sodium nitroprusside USP *emergency antihypertensive; vasodilator* 50 mg/dose injection

sodium noramidopyrine methanesulfonate [see: dipyrone]

sodium oxybate USAN *adjunct to anesthesia; investigational (orphan) for narcolepsy, cataplexy, sleep paralysis, and hypnagogic hallucinations*

sodium oxychlorosene [see: oxychlorosene sodium]

sodium paratoluenesulfan chloramide [see: chloramine-T]

Sodium P.A.S. tablets (discontinued 1996) ℞ *tuberculostatic* [aminosalicylate sodium] 500 mg

sodium penicillin G [see: penicillin G sodium]

sodium pentosan polysulfate [see: pentosan polysulfate sodium]

sodium perborate *topical antiseptic/ germicidal*

sodium perborate monohydrate USAN

sodium pertechnetate Tc 99m USAN, USP *radioactive agent*

sodium phenolate [see: phenolate sodium]

sodium phenylacetate USAN *antihyperammonemic*

sodium phenylacetate & sodium benzoate *to prevent and treat hyperammonemia of urea cycle enzymopathy (orphan)*

sodium phenylbutyrate USAN *antihyperammonemic for urea cycle disorders (orphan); investigational (orphan) for various sickling disorders*

sodium phosphate (^{32}P) INN *antineoplastic; antipolycythemic; neoplasm test* [also: sodium phosphate P 32]

sodium phosphate, dibasic USP *saline laxative; phosphorus replacement; pH buffer*

sodium phosphate, monobasic USP *saline laxative; phosphorus replacement; pH buffer*

sodium phosphate P 32 USAN, USP *antipolycythemic; radiopharmaceutical antineoplastic for various leukemias and skeletal metastases* [also: sodium phosphate (^{32}P)] *0.67 mCi/mL*

sodium picofosfate INN

sodium picosulfate INN

sodium polyphosphate USAN *pharmaceutic aid*

sodium polystyrene sulfonate USP *potassium-removing ion-exchange resin 15 g/60 mL oral*

sodium propionate NF *preservative; antifungal*

sodium propionate hydrate [see: sodium propionate]

sodium 2-propylvalerate [see: valproate sodium]

sodium psylliate NF

sodium pyrophosphate USAN *pharmaceutic aid*

sodium radiochromate [see: sodium chromate Cr 51]

sodium rhodanate [see: thiocyanate sodium]

sodium salicylate (SS) USP *analgesic; antipyretic; anti-inflammatory; antirheumatic 325, 650 mg oral*

sodium starch glycolate NF *tablet excipient*

sodium stearate NF *emulsifying and stiffening agent*

sodium stearyl fumarate NF *tablet and capsule lubricant*

sodium stibocaptate INN [also: stibocaptate]

sodium stibogluconate INN, BAN, DCF *investigational antiparasitic for leishmaniasis and trypanosomiasis*

Sodium Sulamyd eye drops, ophthalmic ointment ℞ *topical ophthalmic antibiotic* [sulfacetamide sodium] *10%, 30%; 10%*

sodium sulfacetamide [see: sulfacetamide sodium]

sodium sulfate USP *calcium regulator*

sodium sulfate S 35 USAN *radioactive agent*

sodium sulfocyanate [see: thiocyanate sodium]

sodium taurocholate [see: bile salts]

sodium tetradecyl (STD) sulfate INN *sclerosing agent; investigational (orphan) for bleeding esophageal varices*

sodium thiomalate, gold [see: gold sodium thiomalate]

sodium thiosalicylate *analgesic; antipyretic; anti-inflammatory; antirheumatic 50 mg/mL injection*

sodium thiosulfate USP *antidote to cyanide poisoning; antiseptic; antifungal 25% (250 mg/mL) IV injection*

sodium thiosulfate, gold [see: gold sodium thiosulfate]

sodium thiosulfate & hydroxocobalamin *investigational (orphan) for severe acute cyanide poisoning*

sodium timerfonate INN *topical anti-infective* [also: thimerfonate sodium]

sodium trimetaphosphate USAN *pharmaceutic aid*

sodium tyropanoate INN *oral radiopaque contrast medium for cholecystography (57.4% iodine)* [also: tyropanoate sodium]

sodium valproate [see: valproate sodium]

Sodol tablets ℞ *skeletal muscle relaxant* [carisoprodol]

Sodol Compound tablets ℞ *skeletal muscle relaxant; analgesic* [carisoprodol; aspirin] 200•325 mg

sofalcone INN

Sofarin tablets (discontinued 1995) ℞ *anticoagulant* [warfarin sodium] 2, 2.5, 5 mg

Sofenol 5 lotion OTC *moisturizer; emollient*

Sof/Pro-Clean; Sof/Pro-Clean (s.a.) solution (discontinued 1995) OTC *surfactant cleaning solution for soft contact lenses*

Soft Mate Comfort Drops for Sensitive Eyes OTC *rewetting solution for soft contact lenses*

Soft Mate Consept solution + aerosol spray OTC *two-step chemical disinfecting system for soft contact lenses* [hydrogen peroxide based] 3%

Soft Mate Daily Cleaning for Sensitive Eyes solution (discontinued 1995) OTC *surfactant cleaning solution for soft contact lenses*

Soft Mate Disinfecting for Sensitive Eyes solution OTC *chemical disinfecting solution for soft contact lenses*

Soft Mate Enzyme Plus Cleaner tablets (discontinued 1995) OTC *enzymatic cleaner for soft contact lenses*

Soft Mate Hands Off Daily Cleaner solution OTC *surfactant cleaning solution for soft contact lenses*

Soft Mate Saline for Sensitive Eyes solution (discontinued 1995) OTC *rinsing/storage solution for soft contact lenses* [sodium chloride (preserved saline solution)]

soft pine *medicinal herb* [see: white pine]

Soft Rinse 250 tablets (discontinued 1995) OTC *rinsing/storage solution for*

soft contact lenses [sodium chloride (normal saline solution)] 250 mg

Soft Sense lotion OTC *moisturizer; emollient*

Softabs (trademarked dosage form) *chewable tablets*

softgels (dosage form) *soft gelatin capsules*

Soft-Stress capsules (discontinued 1995) OTC *vitamin/mineral/calcium/iron supplement* [multiple vitamins & minerals; calcium; iron; folic acid; biotin] ±•50•4.5•0.05• ± mg

SoftWear solution OTC *rinsing/storage solution for soft contact lenses* [sodium chloride (preserved saline solution)]

sol particle immunoassay (SPIA) *detects hCG in urine for pregnancy testing*

Solanum dulcamara *medicinal herb* [see: bittersweet nightshade]

solapsone BAN [also: solasulfone]

Solaquin cream OTC *hyperpigmentation bleaching agent in a sunscreen base* [hydroquinone] 2%

Solaquin Forte cream, gel ℞ *hyperpigmentation bleaching agent; sunscreen* [hydroquinone; ethyl dihydroxypropyl PABA; dioxybenzone; oxybenzone] 4%•5%•3%•2%

Solarase (commercially available in Europe) ℞ *investigational (NDA filed) topical treatment for actinic keratosis* [hyaluronate sodium; diclofenac potassium]

Solarcaine aerosol spray, lotion OTC *topical local anesthetic; antiseptic* [benzocaine; triclosan] 20%•0.13%

Solarcaine cream (name changed to Solarcaine Aloe Extra Burn Relief in 1995)

Solarcaine Aloe Extra Burn Relief spray, gel, cream OTC *topical local anesthetic* [lidocaine] 0.5%

solasulfone INN [also: solapsone]

Solatene capsules (discontinued 1996) ℞ *vitamin A precursor* [beta carotene] 30 mg (50 000 IU)

soldier's woundwort *medicinal herb* [see: yarrow]

Solfoton tablets, capsules ℞ *long-acting barbiturate sedative, hypnotic and anticonvulsant* [phenobarbital] 16 mg

Solganal IM injection ℞ *antirheumatic* [aurothioglucose] 50 mg/mL

Solidago nemoralis; S. odora; S. virgaurea medicinal herb [see: goldenrod]

Solomon's seal *(Polygonatum multiflorum; P. odoratum)* root *medicinal herb used as an astringent, demulcent, emetic, and expectorant*

solpecainol INN

Soltice Quick-Rub OTC *topical analgesic; counterirritant* [methyl salicylate; camphor; menthol; eucalyptus oil]

soluble complement receptor [see: complement receptor type I, soluble recombinant human]

soluble ferric pyrophosphate [see: ferric pyrophosphate, soluble]

soluble gelatin (SG) [see: gelatin]

Soluble T4 ℞ *orphan status withdrawn 1996* [CD4, human truncated 369 AA polypeptide]

Solu-Cortef powder for IV or IM injection ℞ *corticosteroid; anti-inflammatory* [hydrocortisone sodium succinate] 100, 250, 500, 1000 mg/vial

Solu-Medrol powder for IV or IM injection ℞ *corticosteroid; anti-inflammatory; immunosuppressant* [methylprednisolone sodium succinate] 40, 125, 500, 1000, 2000 mg/vial

Solumol OTC *ointment base*

Solurex intra-articular, intralesional, soft tissue, or IM injection ℞ *corticosteroid; anti-inflammatory* [dexamethasone sodium phosphate] 4 mg/mL

Solurex LA intralesional, intra-articular, soft tissue, or IM injection ℞ *corticosteroid; anti-inflammatory* [dexamethasone acetate] 8 mg/mL

Soluspan (trademarked form) *injectable suspension*

Soluvite C.T. chewable tablets ℞ *pediatric vitamin supplement and dental caries preventative* [multiple vitamins; fluoride; folic acid] ± • 1 • 0.3 mg

Soluvite-f drops ℞ *pediatric vitamin supplement and dental caries preventa-*

tive [vitamins A, C, and D; fluoride] 1500 IU • 35 mg • 400 IU • 0.25 mg per 0.6 mL

Solvent-G OTC *liquid base*

Solvet (trademarked dosage form) *soluble tablet*

solypertine INN *antiadrenergic* [also: solypertine tartrate]

solypertine tartrate USAN *antiadrenergic* [also: solypertine]

Soma tablets ℞ *skeletal muscle relaxant* [carisoprodol] 350 mg

Soma Compound tablets ℞ *skeletal muscle relaxant; analgesic* [carisoprodol; aspirin] 200 • 325 mg

Soma Compound with Codeine tablets ℞ *skeletal muscle relaxant; analgesic* [carisoprodol; aspirin; codeine phosphate] 200 • 325 • 16 mg

Somagard ℞ *investigational (orphan) LHRH agonist for central precocious puberty* [deslorelin]

somagrebove USAN *veterinary galactopoietic agent*

somalapor USAN, INN, BAN *porcine growth hormone*

somantadine INN *antiviral* [also: somantadine HCl]

somantadine HCl USAN *antiviral* [also: somantadine]

SomatoKine ℞ *investigational (Phase II) treatment for muscle degradation following severe burns and hip fracture surgery* [IGF-BP3 complex]

somatomedin-C [see: mecasermin]

somatorelin INN *growth hormone-releasing factor (GH-RF)*

somatostatin (SS) INN, BAN *growth hormone-release inhibiting factor; investigational (orphan) for cutaneous gastrointestinal fistulas and bleeding esophageal varices*

somatotropin, human [see: somatropin]

Somatrel ℞ *investigational (orphan) diagnostic aid for pituitary release of growth hormone* [NG-29 (code name —generic name not yet assigned)]

somatrem USAN, INN, BAN *growth hormone for congenital growth failure* (orphan) or due to chronic renal insufficiency

somatropin USAN, INN, BAN, JAN growth hormone for adults or children with congenital or endogenous growth hormone deficiency, children with Turner syndrome or renal-induced growth failure, or AIDS-wasting syndrome (orphan); investigational (orphan) for severe burns [also: human growth hormone]

somatropin & glutamine investigational (orphan) for GI malabsorption due to short bowel syndrome

somavubove USAN, INN veterinary galactopoietic agent

somenopor USAN porcine growth hormone

sometribove USAN, INN, BAN veterinary growth stimulant

sometripor USAN, INN, BAN veterinary growth stimulant

somfasepor USAN veterinary growth stimulant

somidobove USAN, INN synthetic bovine growth hormone

Sominex tablets, caplets OTC antihistaminic sleep aid [diphenhydramine HCl] 25 mg; 50 mg

Sominex Pain Relief tablets OTC antihistaminic sleep aid; analgesic [diphenhydramine HCl; acetaminophen] 25•500 mg

Sonata ℞ investigational (NDA filed) nonbenzodiazepine sedative and hypnotic [zaleplon]

SonoRx oral suspension ℞ ultrasound imaging agent to reduce gas shadowing [simethicone-coated cellulose] 7.5 mg/mL

Soothaderm lotion OTC topical anesthetic; topical antihistamine; emollient [pyrilamine maleate; benzocaine; zinc oxide] 2.07•2.08•41.35 mg/mL

Soothe eye drops (discontinued 1995) OTC topical ophthalmic decongestant and vasoconstrictor [tetrahydrozoline HCl] 0.05%

Soothers Throat Drops lozenges (discontinued 1995) OTC topical analgesic; counterirritant; mild local anesthetic [menthol] 2 mg

sopecainol [see: solpecainol]

sopitazine INN

sopromidine INN

soquinolol INN

sorb apple medicinal herb [see: mountain ash]

sorbic acid NF antimicrobial agent; preservative

sorbide nitrate [see: isosorbide dinitrate]

sorbimacrogol laurate 300 [see: polysorbate 20]

sorbimacrogol oleate 300 [see: polysorbate 80]

sorbimacrogol palmitate 300 [see: polysorbate 40]

sorbimacrogol stearate [see: polysorbate 60]

sorbimacrogol tristearate 300 [see: polysorbate 65]

sorbinicate INN

sorbinil USAN, INN, BAN aldose reductase enzyme inhibitor

sorbitan laurate INN surfactant [also: sorbitan monolaurate]

sorbitan monolaurate USAN, NF surfactant [also: sorbitan laurate]

sorbitan monooleate USAN, NF surfactant [also: sorbitan oleate]

sorbitan monopalmitate USAN, NF surfactant [also: sorbitan palmitate]

sorbitan monostearate USAN, NF surfactant [also: sorbitan stearate]

sorbitan oleate INN surfactant [also: sorbitan monooleate]

sorbitan palmitate INN surfactant [also: sorbitan monopalmitate]

sorbitan sesquioleate USAN, INN surfactant

sorbitan stearate INN surfactant [also: sorbitan monostearate]

sorbitan trioleate USAN, INN surfactant

sorbitan tristearate USAN, INN surfactant

sorbitol NF flavoring agent; tablet excipient; urologic irrigant 3%, 3.3%

sorbitol (solution) USP flavoring agent; tablet excipient

Sorbitrate tablets, sublingual tablets, chewable tablets ℞ *antianginal; vasodilator* [isosorbide dinitrate] 5, 10, 20, 30, 40 mg; 2.5, 5 mg; 5, 10 mg

Sorbitrate SA sustained-action tablets (discontinued 1995) ℞ *antianginal; vasodilator* [isosorbide dinitrate]

Sorbsan pads, wound packing ℞ *topical local hemostatic* [calcium alginate fiber]

Sorbus americana; S. aucuparia *medicinal herb* [see: mountain ash]

Soriatane capsules ℞ *systemic antipsoriatic* [acitretin] 10, 25 mg

sorivudine USAN, INN, BAN *antiviral for varicella zoster and herpes zoster in immunocompromised patients; orphan status withdrawn 1997*

sornidipine INN

sorrel *(Rumex acetosa)* plant *medicinal herb used as an antiscorbutic, astringent, diuretic, laxative, refrigerant, and vermifuge*

sorrel, common; mountain sorrel; white sorrel *medicinal herb* [see: wood sorrel]

sorrel, Jamaica *medicinal herb* [see: hibiscus]

sotalol INN, BAN *antiarrhythmic; antiadrenergic (β-receptor)* [also: sotalol HCl]

sotalol HCl USAN *antiarrhythmic (β-blocker) for ventricular arrhythmias (orphan)* [also: sotalol]

soterenol INN *adrenergic; bronchodilator* [also: soterenol HCl]

soterenol HCl USAN *adrenergic; bronchodilator* [also: soterenol]

Sotradecol IV injection, Dosette (unit-of-use injection) ℞ *sclerosing agent; investigational (orphan) for bleeding esophageal varices* [sodium tetradecyl sulfate] 1%, 3%

sour dock *medicinal herb* [see: yellow dock]

sourberry; sowberry *medicinal herb* [see: barberry]

sourgrass *medicinal herb* [see: sorrel]

Southern ginseng *medicinal herb* [see: jiaogulan]

Soviet gramicidin [see: gramicidin S]

sowberry; sourberry *medicinal herb* [see: barberry]

soy; soya; soybean *(Glycine max) medicinal herb and food crop; isoflavone compounds provide phytoestrogens to alleviate menopausal symptoms, including osteoporosis, and provide antineoplastic, cardiovascular, and gastrointestinal benefits*

Soyalac; I-Soyalac liquid, powder OTC *hypoallergenic infant food* [soy protein formula]

soybean oil USP *pharmaceutic necessity*

SP-303 *investigational (Phase III) treatment for AIDS-related diarrhea*

spaglumic acid INN

Span C tablets OTC *dietary supplement* [vitamin C; citrus & rose hips bioflavonoids] 200•300 mg

Spancap No. 1 sustained-release capsules ℞ *CNS stimulant* [dextroamphetamine sulfate] 15 mg

Spancaps (dosage form) *timed-release capsules*

Span-FF controlled-release capsules (discontinued 1998) OTC *hematinic* [ferrous fumarate (source of iron)] 325 mg (106 mg)

Spanidin *investigational (orphan) immunosuppressant for acute renal graft rejection* [gusperimus]

Spanish chestnut *medicinal herb* [see: horse chestnut]

Spanish pepper *medicinal herb* [see: cayenne]

Spansule (trademarked dosage form) *sustained-release capsule*

sparfloxacin USAN, INN, BAN *fluoroquinolone antibacterial*

sparfosate sodium USAN *antineoplastic* [also: sparfosic acid]

sparfosic acid INN *antineoplastic* [also: sparfosate sodium]

Sparine tablets ℞ *conventional (typical) antipsychotic* [promazine HCl] 25, 50 mg

Sparine Tubex (cartridge-needle unit for IM injection) (discontinued 1998) ℞ *conventional (typical) antipsychotic* [promazine HCl] 50 mg/mL

Sparkles effervescent granules OTC *antacid; aid in endoscopic examination* [sodium bicarbonate; citric acid; simethicone] 2000•1500• ≟ mg/dose

sparsomycin USAN, INN *antineoplastic*

Spartaject ℞ *investigational (Phase II/III) intravenous delivery device*

sparteine INN *oxytocic* [also: sparteine sulfate]

sparteine sulfate USAN *oxytocic* [also: sparteine]

Spasmoject IM injection (discontinued 1996) ℞ *GI antispasmodic* [dicyclomine HCl] 10 mg/mL

Spasmolin capsules (discontinued 1995) ℞ *GI antispasmodic; anticholinergic; sedative* [atropine sulfate; scopolamine hydrobromide; hyoscyamine hydrobromide; phenobarbital] 0.0194•0.0065•0.1037•16.2 mg

Spasmolin tablets ℞ *GI antispasmodic; anticholinergic; sedative* [atropine sulfate; scopolamine hydrobromide; hyoscyamine hydrobromide; phenobarbital] 0.0194•0.0065•0.1037•16.2 mg

Spasmophen tablets, elixir (discontinued 1995) ℞ *GI antispasmodic; anticholinergic; sedative* [atropine sulfate; scopolamine hydrobromide; hyoscyamine hydrobromide; phenobarbital] 0.0194•0.0065•0.1037•15 mg; 0.0194•0.0065•0.1037•16.2 mg/5 mL

Spasquid elixir (discontinued 1995) ℞ *GI antispasmodic; anticholinergic; sedative* [atropine sulfate; scopolamine hydrobromide; hyoscyamine hydrobromide; phenobarbital] 0.0194•0.0065•0.1037•16.2 mg/5 mL

Spastosed chewable tablets OTC *antacid* [calcium carbonate; magnesium carbonate]

SPC3 *investigational (Phase I/II) treatment for HIV*

SPCA (serum prothrombin conversion accelerator) factor [see: factor VII]

spearmint NF

spearmint *(Mentha spicata)* leaves *medicinal herb for colds, colic, flu, gas, nausea, and vomiting*

spearmint oil NF

Spec-T lozenges OTC *topical oral anesthetic* [benzocaine] 10 mg

Spec-T Sore Throat/Cough Suppressant lozenges OTC *topical oral anesthetic; antitussive* [benzocaine; dextromethorphan hydrobromide] 10•10 mg

Spec-T Sore Throat/Decongestant lozenges OTC *decongestant; topical oral anesthetic* [phenylpropanolamine HCl; phenylephrine HCl; benzocaine] 10.5•5•10 mg

Spectazole cream ℞ *topical antifungal* [econazole nitrate] 1%

spectinomycin INN *antibiotic* [also: spectinomycin HCl]

spectinomycin HCl USAN, USP *antibiotic* [also: spectinomycin]

Spectrobid film-coated tablets ℞ *aminopenicillin antibiotic* [bacampicillin HCl] 400 mg

Spectrobid powder for oral suspension (discontinued 1997) ℞ *aminopenicillin antibiotic* [bacampicillin HCl] 125 mg/5 mL

Spectrocin Plus ointment OTC *topical antibiotic; local anesthetic* [neomycin sulfate; polymyxin B sulfate; bacitracin; lidocaine] 5000 U•3.5 mg•400 U•5 mg per g

Spectro-Jel liquid OTC *soap-free therapeutic skin cleanser*

speedwell *(Veronica officinalis)* flowering plant *medicinal herb used as a diuretic, expectorant, and stomachic*

speedwell, tall *medicinal herb* [see: Culver's root]

spenbolic [see: methandriol]

spermaceti, synthetic [see: cetyl esters wax]

spermicides *a class of topical contraceptive agents that kill the male sperm*

Spersadex ⓒ (U.S. product: Decadron Phosphate) eye drops ℞ *topical ophthalmic corticosteroidal anti-inflam-*

matory [dexamethasone sodium phosphate] 0.1%

Spexil ℞ *investigational (Phase III) broad-spectrum aminocyclitol antibiotic for respiratory, gynecologic, and abdominal infections* [trospectomycin]

Spherulin intradermal injection ℞ *diagnostic aid for coccidioidomycosis* [coccidioidin] 1:100, 1:10

SPIA (sol particle immunoassay) [q.v.]

spiceberry *medicinal herb* [see: wintergreen]

spiclamine INN

spiclomazine INN

spicy wintergreen *medicinal herb* [see: wintergreen]

spider bite antivenin [see: antivenin (Latrodectus mactans)]

spignet *medicinal herb* [see: spikenard]

spikenard *(Aralia racemosa)* root *medicinal herb for asthma, childbirth, cough, and rheumatism*

spindle tree *medicinal herb* [see: wahoo]

spiperone USAN, INN *antipsychotic*

spiradoline INN *analgesic* [also: spiradoline mesylate]

spiradoline mesylate USAN *analgesic* [also: spiradoline]

spiramide INN

spiramycin USAN, INN, BAN *macrolide antibiotic* [also: acetylspiramycin]

spirapril INN, BAN *angiotensin-converting enzyme (ACE) inhibitor* [also: spirapril HCl]

spirapril HCl USAN *angiotensin-converting enzyme (ACE) inhibitor* [also: spirapril]

spiraprilat USAN, INN *angiotensin-converting enzyme (ACE) inhibitor*

spirazine INN

spirazine HCl [see: spirazine]

spirendolol INN

spirgetine INN

spirilene INN, BAN

spirit of nitrous ether [see: ethyl nitrite]

spirobarbital sodium

spirofylline INN

spirogermanium INN, BAN *antineoplastic* [also: spirogermanium HCl]

spirogermanium HCl USAN *antineoplastic* [also: spirogermanium]

spirohydantoin mustard [now: spiromustine]

spiromustine USAN, INN *antineoplastic*

spironolactone USP, INN, BAN, JAN *antihypertensive; potassium-sparing diuretic; aldosterone antagonist* 25 mg oral

spiroplatin USAN, INN, BAN *antineoplastic*

spirorenone INN

spirotriazine HCl [see: spirazine]

spiroxamide [see: spiroxatrine]

spiroxasone USAN, INN *diuretic*

spiroxatrine INN

spiroxepin INN

spirulina *(Spirulina pratensis)* plant *medicinal herb for chronic disease, enhancing antibody production, lowering serum lipids and triglycerides, and reducing gastric secretory activity; also used as a blood builder and food supplement*

spizofurone INN

SPL (staphage lysate) [q.v.]

SPL-Serologic types I and III solution for subcu injection, nasal aerosol, nasal drop, oral, or topical irrigation ℞ *staphylococcal or polymicrobial vaccine* [staphage lysate (Staphylococcus aureus vaccine; Staphylococcus bacteriophage plaque-forming units)]

spoonwood *medicinal herb* [see: linden tree]

Sporanox capsules, PulsePak (one-week dose package), IV infusion ℞ *systemic triazole antifungal* [itraconazole] 100 mg; 28 × 100 mg; 10 mg/mL

Sporanox oral solution ("swish and swallow") ℞ *antifungal for esophageal and oropharyngeal candidiasis* [itraconazole] 10 mg/mL

Sporidin-G ℞ *investigational (orphan) for treatment of Cryptosporidium-induced diarrhea in immunocompromised patients* [Cryptosporidium parvum bovine colostrum IgG concentrate]

Sports Spray OTC *topical analgesic; counterirritant; antiseptic* [methyl sali-

cylate; menthol; camphor; alcohol
58%] 3.5% • 10% • 5%

Sportscreme OTC *topical analgesic* [tro-
lamine salicylate] 10%

Sportscreme Ice gel OTC *topical analgesic; counterirritant* [trolamine; men-
thol] 2 • 2%

spotted alder *medicinal herb* [see:
witch hazel]

spotted comfrey *medicinal herb* [see:
lungwort]

spotted cranesbill *medicinal herb* [see:
alum root]

spotted geranium *medicinal herb* [see:
alum root]

**spotted hemlock; spotted cowbane;
spotted parsley** *medicinal herb* [see:
poison hemlock]

spotted lungwort *medicinal herb* [see:
lungwort]

spotted thistle *medicinal herb* [see:
blessed thistle]

**SPPG (sulfated polysaccharide pep-
tidoglycan)** [see: tecogalan sodium]

Spray-U-Thin oral spray OTC *diet aid*
[phenylpropanolamine HCl] 6.58 mg

spring wintergreen *medicinal herb*
[see: wintergreen]

Sprinkle Caps (trademarked form)
powder

sprodiamide USAN *heart and CNS
imaging aid for MRI*

spruce (Picea excelsa; P. mariana)
young shoots *medicinal herb used as a
calmative, diaphoretic, expectorant,
and pectoral*

spruce, Norway *medicinal herb* [see:
spruce]

spruce, weeping *medicinal herb* [see:
hemlock]

SPS oral suspension ℞ *potassium-removing agent for hyperkalemia* [sodium
polystyrene sulfonate] 15 g/60 mL

S-P-T "liquid" capsules ℞ *thyroid
replacement therapy for hypothyroidism
or thyroid cancer* [thyroid, desiccated
porcine] 60, 120, 180, 300 mg

spurge laurel; spurge olive *medicinal
herb* [see: mezereon]

squalamine *natural remedy; investigational (Phase III) angiogenesis inhibitor
for the treatment of solid tumors* [also:
shark cartilage]

squalane NF *oleaginous vehicle*

square, carpenter's *medicinal herb*
[see: figwort]

squaw balm; squaw mint *medicinal
herb* [see: pennyroyal]

squaw root *medicinal herb* [see: black
cohosh; blue cohosh]

squaw tea *medicinal herb* [see: ephedra]

squaw vine (Mitchella repens) plant
*medicinal herb for easing childbirth,
lactation, and menstruation and for
uterine disorders*

squaw weed *medicinal herb* [see: life
root]

squawberry *medicinal herb* [see: squaw
vine]

**squill (Urginea indica; U. maritima;
U. scilla)** bulb *medicinal herb for
edema and inducing emesis and expectoration; also used as a rat poison*

squirrel pea, ground *medicinal herb*
[see: twin leaf]

85Sr [see: strontium chloride Sr 85]

85Sr [see: strontium nitrate Sr 85]

85Sr [see: strontium Sr 85]

SRC Expectorant liquid ℞ *narcotic
antitussive; decongestant; expectorant*
[hydrocodone bitartrate; pseudoephedrine HCl; guaifenesin; alcohol
12.5%] 5 • 60 • 200 mg/5 mL

SRF (skin respiratory factor) [q.v.]

SS (saline solution)

SS (sodium salicylate) [q.v.]

SS (somatostatin) [q.v.]

SSD (silver sulfadiazine) [q.v.]

SSD; SSD AF cream ℞ *broad-spectrum
bactericidal for adjunctive burn treatment* [silver sulfadiazine] 10 mg/g

SSKI oral solution ℞ *expectorant*
[potassium iodide] 1 g/mL

**SSRIs (selective serotonin reuptake
inhibitors)** [q.v.]

**S.S.S. High Potency Vitamin Tab-
lets** OTC *vitamin/mineral/iron supplement* [multiple vitamins & minerals;
iron; biotin] ± • 27 • 0.0225 mg

S.S.S. Vitamin and Mineral Complex oral liquid OTC *vitamin/mineral/iron supplement* [multiple vitamins & minerals; iron; biotin; alcohol 6.6%] ± •3•0.1 mg

S.T. 37 solution OTC *topical antiseptic* [hexylresorcinol] 0.1%

S-T Cort lotion ℞ *topical corticosteroidal anti-inflammatory* [hydrocortisone] 0.5%

S-T Forte 2 liquid ℞ *narcotic antitussive; antihistamine* [hydrocodone bitartrate; chlorpheniramine maleate] 2.5•2 mg/5 mL

ST1-RTA immunotoxin (SR 44163) *investigational for graft vs. host disease and B-chronic lymphocytic leukemia; orphan status withdrawn 1998*

Staarvisc intraocular injection ℞ *viscoelastic agent for ophthalmic surgery* [hyaluronate sodium] ?

stable factor [see: factor VII]

Stachys officinalis medicinal herb [see: betony]

Stadol IV or IM injection ℞ *narcotic agonist-antagonist analgesic* [butorphanol tartrate] 1, 2 mg/mL

Stadol NS nasal spray ℞ *narcotic agonist-antagonist analgesic; antimigraine agent* [butorphanol tartrate] 10 mg/mL

staff vine *medicinal herb* [see: bittersweet nightshade]

Stagesic capsules ℞ *narcotic analgesic* [hydrocodone bitartrate; acetaminophen] 5•500 mg

staggerweed *medicinal herb* [see: turkey corn]

staghorn *medicinal herb* [see: club moss]

Stahist sustained-release tablets ℞ *decongestant; antihistamine; anticholinergic* [phenylpropanolamine HCl; phenylephrine HCl; chlorpheniramine maleate; hyoscyamine sulfate; atropine sulfate; scopolamine hydrobromide] 50•25•8•0.19•0.04•0.01 mg

stallimycin INN *antibacterial* [also: stallimycin HCl]

stallimycin HCl USAN *antibacterial* [also: stallimycin]

Stamoist E sustained-release tablets ℞ *decongestant; expectorant* [pseudoephedrine HCl; guaifenesin] 120•500 mg

Stamoist LA sustained-release tablets ℞ *decongestant; expectorant* [phenylpropanolamine HCl; guaifenesin] 75•400 mg

standard VAC *chemotherapy protocol* [see: VAC standard (under VAC)]

Stanford V (mechlorethamine, doxorubicin, vinblastine, vincristine, bleomycin, VePesid, prednisone) *chemotherapy protocol*

stannous chloride USAN *pharmaceutic aid*

stannous fluoride USP *dental caries prophylactic*

stannous pyrophosphate USAN *skeletal imaging aid*

stannous sulfur colloid USAN *bone, liver and spleen imaging aid*

stanolone BAN *investigational (orphan) for AIDS-wasting syndrome* [also: androstanolone]

stanozolol USAN, USP, INN, BAN *androgen; anabolic steroid*

staphage lysate (SPL) *active bacterin for staphylococcal infections; investigational for renal dialysis*

Staphcillin powder for IV or IM injection (discontinued 1998) ℞ *penicillinase-resistant penicillin antibiotic* [methicillin sodium] 1, 4, 6, 10 g

StaphVAX ℞ *investigational (Phase III) vaccine against Staphylococcus aureus infection of end-stage renal disease*

Staphylococcus aureus vaccine [see: staphage lysate]

star anise (Illicium anisatum; I. verum) seeds *medicinal herb used as a carminative, stimulant, and stomachic; also added to other herbal medications to improve digestibility and taste*

star chickweed; starweed *medicinal herb* [see: chickweed]

star grass (Aletris farinosa) root and rhizome *medicinal herb for diarrhea, dysmenorrhea and menstrual discomfort, gas and colonic cramps, and rheumatism*

star root *medicinal herb* [see: star grass]
starch NF *dusting powder; pharmaceutic aid*
starch, pregelatinized NF *tablet excipient*
starch, topical USP *dusting powder*
starch carboxymethyl ether, sodium salt [see: sodium starch glycolate]
starch glycerite NF
starch 2-hydroxyethyl ether [see: hetastarch; pentastarch]
Star-Otic ear drops OTC *antibacterial; antifungal* [acetic acid; aluminum acetate; boric acid]
Starvisc [see: Staarvisc]
starwort; mealy starwort *medicinal herb* [see: chickweed; star grass]
Stat-Crit electrode device for professional use *in vitro diagnostic aid for hemoglobin/hematocrit measurement*
STATdose (trademarked device) *prefilled syringes for self-administration*
Staticin topical solution ℞ *topical antibiotic for acne* [erythromycin] 1.5%
"statins" *brief term for a class of antihyperlipidemics that include atorvastatin, cerivastatin, fluvastatin, lovastatin, pravastatin, and simvastatin* [see: HMG-CoA reductase inhibitors]
statolon USAN *antiviral* [also: vistatolon]
Stat-One gel OTC *topical antiseptic* [hydrogen peroxide] 3%
Stat-One gel OTC *topical antiseptic* [isopropyl alcohol] 70%
Stat-Pak (trademarked packaging form) *unit-dose package*
Statuss Expectorant liquid ℞ *narcotic antitussive; decongestant; expectorant* [codeine phosphate; phenylpropanolamine HCl; guaifenesin; alcohol 5%] 10•12.5•100 mg/5 mL
Statuss Green liquid ℞ *narcotic antitussive; decongestant; antihistamine* [hydrocodone bitartrate; phenylpropanolamine HCl; phenylephrine HCl; pyrilamine maleate; pheniramine maleate; alcohol 5%] 1.67•3.3•5•3.3•3.3 mg/5 mL
staunch, blood *medicinal herb* [see: fleabane; horseweed]
stavudine USAN, INN *antiviral for HIV*

Stay Trim gum, mints (discontinued 1995) OTC *diet aid* [phenylpropanolamine HCl] 8.33 mg; 12.5 mg
Stay-Wet solution (discontinued 1995) OTC *wetting/rewetting solution for hard contact lenses*
Stay-Wet 3; Stay-Wet 4 solution OTC *disinfecting/wetting/soaking solution for rigid gas permeable contact lenses*
STD (sodium tetradecyl sulfate) [q.v.]
steaglate INN *combining name for radicals or groups*
STEAM (streptonigrin, thioguanine, cyclophosphamide, actinomycin, mitomycin) *chemotherapy protocol*
stearethate 40 [see: polyoxyl 40 stearate]
stearic acid NF *emulsion adjunct; tablet and capsule lubricant*
stearyl alcohol NF *emulsion adjunct*
stearyl dimethyl benzyl ammonium chloride
stearylsulfamide INN
Stedicor *investigational antiarrhythmic* [azimilide dihydrochloride]
steffimycin USAN, INN *antibacterial; antiviral*
Stelazine film-coated tablets, oral concentrate, IM injection ℞ *conventional (typical) antipsychotic; anxiolytic* [trifluoperazine HCl] 1, 2, 5, 10 mg; 10 mg/mL; 2 mg/mL
Stellaria media *medicinal herb* [see: chickweed]
stem cell factor (SCF) *investigational (Phase III) agent for blood-related disorders and chemotherapy "rescue"*
stem cells, hematopoietic *investigational (Phase I/II) gene therapy for HIV*
Stemetil ⓒ (U.S. product: Compazine) film-coated tablets ℞ *conventional (typical) antipsychotic; antiemetic* [prochlorperazine bimaleate] 5, 10 mg
Stemetil ⓒ (U.S. product: Compazine) oral liquid, IV or IM injection ℞ *conventional (typical) antipsychotic; antiemetic* [prochlorperazine mesylate] 5 mg/5 mL; 5 mg/mL

Stemetil ⓒ (U.S. product: Compazine) suppositories ℞ *conventional (typical) antipsychotic; antiemetic* [prochlorperazine] 10 mg

Stemgen ℞ *investigational (NDA filed) hematopoietic growth factor; investigational (orphan) adjunct to myelosuppressive and myeloablative therapy* [ancestim]

stenbolone INN *anabolic steroid; also abused as a street drug* [also: stenbolone acetate]

stenbolone acetate USAN *anabolic steroid; also abused as a street drug* [also: stenbolone]

Step 2 creme rinse OTC *for use following a pediculicide shampoo to remove lice eggs from hair*

stepronin INN

Sterapred tablets, Unipak (dispensing pack) ℞ *corticosteroid; anti-inflammatory* [prednisone] 5 mg

Sterapred DS tablets, Unipak (dispensing pack) ℞ *corticosteroid; anti-inflammatory* [prednisone] 10 mg

Sterculia tragacantha; S. urens; S. villosa medicinal herb [see: karaya gum]

stercuronium iodide INN

Sterecyt ℞ *investigational antineoplastic for malignant non-Hodgkin's lymphomas; orphan status withdrawn 1998* [prednimustine]

Steri-Dose (trademarked delivery system) *prefilled disposable syringe*

SteriNail solution OTC *topical antifungal* [undecylenic acid; tolnaftate] 2 • 2

Steri-Vial (trademarked packaging form) *ampule*

Sterules (trademarked dosage form) *solution for nebulization*

stevaladil INN

stevia (*Stevia rebaudiana*) leaves *medicinal herb used as a non-caloric sugar substitute; also used for diabetes, food cravings, hypertension, obesity, and tobacco cravings*

stibamine glucoside INN, BAN

stibocaptate BAN [also: sodium stibocaptate]

stibophen NF

stibosamine INN

stickwort; sticklewort *medicinal herb* [see: agrimony]

stigmata maidis (corn silk) *medicinal herb* [see: Indian corn]

stilbamidine isethionate [see: stilbamidine isetionate]

stilbamidine isetionate INN

stilbazium iodide USAN, INN *anthelmintic*

stilbestroform [see: diethylstilbestrol]

stilbestrol [see: diethylstilbestrol] ⚠ Stilphostrol

stilbestronate [see: diethylstilbestrol dipropionate]

stilboestroform [see: diethylstilbestrol]

stilboestrol BAN *estrogen* [also: diethylstilbestrol]

stilboestrol DP [see: diethylstilbestrol dipropionate]

stillingia (*Stillingia ligustina*) root *medicinal herb for acne, eczema, and other skin disorders, blood cleansing, liver disorders, respiratory illnesses, and syphilis*

Stilnoct; Stilnox (European name for U.S. product Ambien)

stilonium iodide USAN, INN *antispasmodic*

Stilphostrol tablets, IV injection ℞ *hormonal antineoplastic for prostatic carcinoma* [diethylstilbestrol diphosphate] 50 mg; 250 mg ⚠ Disophrol; stilbestrol

stilronate [see: diethylstilbestrol dipropionate]

Stimate nasal spray ℞ *posterior pituitary hormone for hemophilia A and von Willebrand's disease (orphan)* [desmopressin acetate] 150 μg (600 IU)/dose

stimulants *a class of agents that excite the activity of physiological processes*

Stimulon ℞ *investigational (Phase I/II) immune system stimulant for AIDS vaccines* [QS-21 (code name—generic name not yet assigned)]

Sting-Eze concentrate OTC *topical antihistamine; antipruritic; anesthetic; bacteriostatic* [diphenhydramine HCl; camphor; phenol; benzocaine; eucalyptol]

stinging nettle *medicinal herb* [see: nettle]

Sting-Kill swabs OTC *topical local anesthetic* [benzocaine; menthol] 20% • 1%

stingless nettle *medicinal herb* [see: blind nettle]

stinking nightshade *medicinal herb* [see: henbane]

stirimazole INN, BAN

stiripentol USAN, INN *anticonvulsant*

stirocainide INN

stirofos USAN *veterinary insecticide*

stitchwort *medicinal herb* [see: chickweed]

Stoko Gard cream OTC *topical protection from the effects of poison ivy*

stomachics *a class of agents that promote the functional activity of the stomach*

stone root (Collinsonia canadensis) roots and leaves *medicinal herb used as a diuretic and vulnerary*

Stop gel ℞ *topical dental caries preventative* [stannous fluoride] 0.4%

storax USP

storax (Liquidambar orientalis; L. styraciflua) leaves and gum *medicinal herb for diarrhea, inducing expectoration, parasitic infections, promoting sweating and diuresis, skin sores and wounds, and sore throat*

Storzfen eye drops ℞ *topical ophthalmic decongestant and vasoconstrictor; mydriatic* [phenylephrine HCl] 2.5%

Storzine 2 eye drops ℞ *topical antiglaucoma agent; direct-acting miotic* [pilocarpine HCl] 2%

Storz-N-D eye drops ℞ *topical ophthalmic corticosteroidal anti-inflammatory; antibiotic* [dexamethasone sodium phosphate; neomycin sulfate] 0.1% • 0.35%

Storz-N-P-D eye drop suspension ℞ *topical ophthalmic corticosteroidal anti-inflammatory; antibiotic* [dexamethasone; neomycin sulfate; polymyxin B sulfate] 0.1% • 0.35% • 10 000 U/mL

Storz-Sulf eye drops ℞ *topical ophthalmic antibiotic* [sulfacetamide sodium] 10%

stramonium [see: jimsonweed]

strawberry (Fragaria vesca) leaves *medicinal herb for blood cleansing,* diarrhea, eczema, intestinal disorders, preventing miscarriage, and stomach cleansing

strawberry bush; strawberry tree *medicinal herb* [see: wahoo]

Strep Detect slide tests for professional use *in vitro diagnostic aid for streptococcal antigens in throat swabs*

Streptase powder for IV or intracoronary infusion ℞ *thrombolytic enzyme for lysis of thrombi and catheter clearance* [streptokinase] 250 000, 750 000, 1 500 000 IU ② Streptonase

streptococcus immune globulin, group B investigational for neonatal group B streptococcal infection; orphan status withdrawn 1998

streptodornase (SD) INN, BAN

streptoduocin USP

streptogramins *a class of antibiotics, isolated from Streptomyces pristinaespirales, used for gram-positive infections*

streptokinase (SK) INN *thrombolytic enzymes for myocardial infarction, thrombosis or embolism* ② Streptonase

streptomycin INN, BAN *aminoglycoside antibiotic; primary tuberculostatic* [also: streptomycin sulfate]

streptomycin sulfate USP *aminoglycoside antibiotic; primary tuberculostatic* [also: streptomycin]

Streptonase-B test kit for professional use *in vitro diagnostic test for DNAse-B streptococcal antigens in serum* ② Streptase; streptokinase

streptoniazid INN *antibacterial* [also: streptonicozid]

streptonicozid USAN *antibacterial* [also: streptoniazid]

streptonigrin (SN) USAN *antineoplastic* [also: rufocromomycin]

Strepto-Sec slide test for professional use (discontinued 1991) *in vitro diagnostic test for streptococcal antigens*

streptovarycin INN

streptozocin USAN, INN *nitrosourea-type alkylating antineoplastic for metastatic islet cell carcinoma of the pancreas*

streptozotocin [see: streptozocin]

Streptozyme slide tests for professional use *in vitro diagnostic test for streptococcal extracellular antigens in blood, plasma, and serum*

Stress 600 with Zinc tablets OTC *vitamin/mineral supplement* [multiple vitamins & minerals; folic acid; biotin] ± •400•45 μg

Stress B Complex tablets OTC *vitamin/mineral supplement* [multiple vitamins & minerals; folic acid; biotin] ± •400•45 μg

Stress B Complex with Vitamin C timed-release tablets OTC *vitamin/mineral supplement* [multiple B vitamins; vitamin C; zinc] ± •300•15 mg

Stress B with C tablets (discontinued 1995) OTC *vitamin supplement* [multiple B vitamins; vitamin C; folic acid; biotin] ± •250 mg•50 μg•12.5 μg

Stress Formula 600 tablets OTC *vitamin supplement* [multiple vitamins; folic acid; biotin] ± •400•45 μg

Stress Formula 600 plus Iron tablets OTC *antianemic* [ferrous fumarate, dried; vitamins C and E; multiple B vitamins; folic acid]

Stress Formula "605" tablets (discontinued 1995) OTC *vitamin supplement* [multiple vitamins; folic acid; biotin] ± •400•45 μg

Stress Formula "605" with Zinc tablets (discontinued 1995) OTC *vitamin/mineral supplement* [multiple vitamins & minerals; folic acid; biotin] ± •400•45 μg

Stress Formula Vitamins capsules, tablets OTC *vitamin supplement* [multiple vitamins; folic acid; biotin] ± •400•45 μg

Stress Formula with Iron film-coated tablets OTC *vitamin/iron supplement* [multiple B vitamins; vitamins C and E; ferrous fumarate; folic acid; biotin] ± •500 mg•30 IU•27 mg•0.4 mg•45 μg

Stress Formula with Zinc tablets OTC *vitamin/iron supplement* [multiple B vitamins; vitamins C and E; multiple minerals; folic acid; biotin] ± • 500 mg•30 IU• ± •0.4 mg•45 μg

Stresscaps capsules (discontinued 1995) OTC *vitamin supplement* [multiple B vitamins; vitamin C] ± •300 mg

StressForm "605" with Iron tablets OTC *vitamin/iron supplement* [multiple B vitamins; vitamins C and E; iron; folic acid; biotin] ± •605 mg•30 IU•27 mg•0.4 mg•45 μg

Stresstabs tablets OTC *vitamin supplement* [multiple vitamins; folic acid; biotin] ± •400•45 μg

Stresstabs 600 with Iron tablets OTC *antianemic* [ferrous fumarate, dried; vitamins E and C; multiple B vitamins; folic acid]

Stresstabs Advanced Formula tablets (name changed to Stresstabs in 1995)

Stresstabs + Iron film-coated tablets OTC *vitamin/iron supplement* [multiple B vitamins; vitamins C and E; ferrous fumarate; folic acid; biotin] ± •500 mg•30 IU•18 mg•0.4 mg•45 μg

Stresstabs + Zinc film-coated tablets OTC *vitamin/mineral supplement* [multiple vitamins & minerals; folic acid; biotin] ± •400•45 μg

Stresstein powder OTC *enteral nutritional therapy for moderate to severe stress or trauma* [multiple branched chain amino acids]

Stri-Dex pads OTC *topical keratolytic cleanser for acne* [salicylic acid; alcohol] 0.5%•28%, 2%•44%, 2%•54%

Stri-Dex Cleansing bar OTC *medicated cleanser for acne* [triclosan] 1%

Stri-Dex Clear gel OTC *topical acne treatment* [salicylic acid; alcohol] 2%•9.3%

Stri-Dex Face Wash solution OTC *medicated cleanser for acne* [triclosan] 1%

strinoline INN

striped alder *medicinal herb* [see: winterberry; witch hazel]

Stromectol tablets ℞ *anthelmintic for strongyloidiasis and onchocerciasis* [ivermectin] 6 mg

strong ammonia solution [see: ammonia solution, strong]

Strong Iodine solution, tincture ℞ *thyroid-blocking therapy; topical antimicrobial* [iodine; potassium iodide] 5%•10%; 7%•5%

stronger rose water [see: rose water, stronger]

strontium *element (Sr)*

strontium chloride Sr 85 USAN *radioactive agent*

strontium chloride Sr 89 USAN *radioactive agent; analgesic for metastatic bone pain*

strontium nitrate Sr 85 USAN *radioactive agent*

strontium salicylate NF

strontium Sr 85 USP

Strovite tablets ℞ *vitamin supplement* [multiple B vitamins; vitamin C; folic acid] ≛•500•0.5 mg

Strovite Plus; Strovite Forte caplets ℞ *geriatric vitamin/mineral therapy* [multiple vitamins & minerals; folic acid; biotin] ≛•800•150 μg; ≛• 1000•150 μg

structum *natural remedy* [see: chondroitin sulfate]

strychnine NF *an extremely poisonous CNS stimulant; occasionally abused as a street drug in combination with LSD*

strychnine glycerophosphate NF

strychnine nitrate NF

strychnine phosphate NF

strychnine sulfate NF

strychnine valerate NF

Stuart Formula tablets OTC *vitamin/mineral/iron supplement* [multiple vitamins & minerals; iron; folic acid] ≛•18•0.1 mg

Stuart Prenatal tablets OTC *vitamin/calcium/iron supplement* [multiple vitamins; calcium; iron; folic acid] ≛•200•60•0.8 mg

Stuartinic film-coated tablets (discontinued 1995) OTC *hematinic* [ferrous fumarate; multiple B vitamins; vitamin C] 100•≛•500 mg

Stuartnatal 1 + 1 tablets (name changed to Stuartnatal Plus in 1995)

Stuartnatal Plus tablets ℞ *vitamin/calcium/iron supplement* [multiple vitamins; calcium; iron; folic acid] ≛•200•65•1 mg

stugeron [see: cinnarizine]

stutgin [see: cinnarizine]

Stye ophthalmic ointment OTC *emollient* [white petrolatum; mineral oil; boric acid]

Stye ophthalmic ointment (discontinued 1995; replaced by Stye without yellow mercuric oxide) OTC *stye treatment (the FDA ruled yellow mercuric oxide "not safe and effective" in 1992)* [yellow mercuric oxide] 1%

styptics *a class of hemostatic agents that stop bleeding of the skin by astringent action* [see also: astringents; hemostatics]

Stypto-Caine solution OTC *to stop bleeding of minor cuts* [aluminum chloride; tetracaine HCl; oxyquinoline sulfate] 250•2.5•1 mg/g

styramate INN

styronate resins

SU-5416 *investigational (Phase III) angiogenesis inhibitor for lung and colorectal cancers; investigational (Phase II/III) for AIDS-related Kaposi sarcoma*

subathizone INN

subendazole INN

Sublimaze IV or IM injection ℞ *narcotic analgesic; anesthetic* [fentanyl citrate] 0.05 mg/mL

sublimed sulfur [see: sulfur, sublimed]

Sublingual B Total drops OTC *vitamin supplement* [multiple B vitamins; vitamin C] ≛•60 mg/mL

substance F [see: demecolcine]

substituted benzimidazoles *a class of gastric antisecretory agents that inhibit the ATPase "proton pump" within the gastric parietal cell* [also called: proton pump inhibitors; ATPase inhibitors]

Suby's G solution; Suby's solution G (citric acid, magnesium oxide, sodium carbonate) *urologic irrigant to dissolve phosphatic calculi*

succimer USAN, INN, BAN *heavy metal chelating agent for lead poisoning (orphan); investigational (orphan) for* *mercury poisoning and cysteine kidney stones*

succinchlorimide NF

succinimides *a class of anticonvulsants*

succinylcholine chloride USP *neuromuscular blocker; muscle relaxant; anesthesia adjunct* [also: suxamethonium chloride] 20 mg/mL injection

succinyldapsone [see: succisulfone]

succinylsulfathiazole USP

succisulfone INN

succory *medicinal herb* [see: chicory]

Succus Cineraria Maritima eye drops ℞ *treatment for optic opacity caused by cataract* [senecio compositae; hamamelis water; boric acid]

suclofenide INN, BAN

Sucostrin IV or IM injection (discontinued 1996) ℞ *muscle relaxant; anesthesia adjunct* [succinylcholine chloride] 20, 100 mg/mL

Sucraid oral solution ℞ *enzyme replacement therapy for congenital sucrase-isomaltase deficiency (orphan)* [sacrosidase] 8500 IU/mL

sucralfate USAN, INN, BAN *treatment of gastric ulcers; investigational (orphan) for oral mucositis and stomatitis following cancer radiation or chemotherapy* 1 g oral

sucralose BAN

sucralox INN, BAN

sucrase *orphan status withdrawn 1997* ☒ sucrose

Sucrets throat spray OTC *topical antipruritic/counterirritant; mild local anesthetic* [dyclonine HCl] 0.1%

Sucrets Children's Sore Throat; Vapor Lemon Sucrets; Sucrets Maximum Strength lozenges OTC *topical antipruritic/counterirritant; mild local anesthetic* [dyclonine HCl] 1.2 mg; 2 mg; 3 mg

Sucrets Cough Control; Sucrets 4-Hour Cough lozenges OTC *antitussive* [dextromethorphan hydrobromide] 5 mg; 15 mg

Sucrets Sore Throat lozenges OTC *oral antiseptic* [hexylresorcinol] 2.4 mg

sucrose NF *flavoring agent; tablet excipient* ☒ sucrase

sucrose octaacetate NF *alcohol denaturant*

sucrosofate potassium USAN *antiulcerative*

Sudafed tablets OTC *nasal decongestant* [pseudoephedrine HCl] 30, 60 mg

Sudafed, Children's chewable tablets OTC *nasal decongestant* [pseudoephedrine HCl] 15 mg

Sudafed, Children's liquid (discontinued 1996) OTC *nasal decongestant* [pseudoephedrine HCl] 30 mg/5 mL

Sudafed 12 Hour Caplets extended-release tablets OTC *nasal decongestant* [pseudoephedrine HCl] 120 mg

Sudafed Cold & Cough liquid caps OTC *antitussive; decongestant; expectorant; analgesic* [dextromethorphan hydrobromide; pseudoephedrine HCl; guaifenesin; acetaminophen] 10•30•100•250 mg

Sudafed Cough syrup (discontinued 1996) OTC *antitussive; decongestant; expectorant* [dextromethorphan hydrobromide; pseudoephedrine HCl; guaifenesin; alcohol 2.4%] 5•15•100 mg/5 mL

Sudafed Plus liquid (discontinued 1996) OTC *decongestant; antihistamine* [pseudoephedrine HCl; chlorpheniramine maleate] 30•2 mg/5 mL

Sudafed Plus tablets OTC *decongestant; antihistamine* [pseudoephedrine HCl; chlorpheniramine maleate] 60•4 mg

Sudafed Severe Cold caplets, tablets OTC *antitussive; decongestant; analgesic* [dextromethorphan hydrobromide; pseudoephedrine HCl; acetaminophen] 15•30•500 mg

Sudafed Sinus tablets, caplets OTC *decongestant; analgesic; antipyretic* [pseudoephedrine HCl; acetaminophen] 30•500 mg

Sudal 60/500 film-coated sustained-release tablets ℞ *decongestant; expectorant* [pseudoephedrine HCl; guaifenesin] 60•500 mg

Sudal 120/600 film-coated sustained-release tablets (discontinued 1998) ℞ *decongestant; expectorant* [pseudoephedrine HCl; guaifenesin] 120•600 mg

Sudex film-coated sustained-release tablets (discontinued 1996) ℞ *decongestant; expectorant* [pseudoephedrine HCl; guaifenesin] 120•600 mg

Sudex tablets (discontinued 1997) OTC *decongestant* [pseudoephedrine HCl] 30 mg

sudexanox INN

sudismase INN

sudorifics *a class of agents that promote profuse perspiration* [also called: diaphoretics]

sudoxicam USAN, INN *anti-inflammatory*

Sufenta IV injection ℞ *narcotic analgesic; anesthetic* [sufentanil citrate] 50 μg/mL

sufentanil USAN, INN, BAN *narcotic analgesic*

sufentanil citrate USAN *narcotic analgesic* 50 μg/mL injection

sufosfamide INN

sufotidine USAN, INN, BAN *antagonist to histamine H₂ receptors*

sugar, compressible NF *flavoring agent; tablet excipient*

sugar, confectioner's NF *flavoring agent; tablet excipient*

sugar, invert (50% dextrose & 50% fructose) USP *fluid and nutrient replenisher; caloric replacement*

sugar spheres NF *solid carrier vehicle*

Sulamyd [see: Sodium Sulamyd]

Sular extended-release tablets ℞ *calcium channel blocker for hypertension* [nisoldipine] 10, 20, 30, 40 mg

sulazepam USAN, INN *minor tranquilizer*

sulbactam INN, BAN *β-lactamase inhibitor; penicillin/cephalosporin synergist*

sulbactam benzathine USAN *β-lactamase inhibitor; penicillin/cephalosporin synergist*

sulbactam pivoxil USAN *β-lactamase inhibitor; penicillin/cephalosporin synergist* [also: pivsulbactam]

sulbactam sodium USAN, USP *β-lactamase inhibitor; penicillin/cephalosporin synergist*

sulbenicillin INN

sulbenox USAN, INN *veterinary growth stimulant*

sulbentine INN

sulbutiamine INN [also: bisibutiamine]

sulclamide INN

sulconazole INN, BAN *antifungal* [also: sulconazole nitrate]

sulconazole nitrate USAN, USP *topical antifungal* [also: sulconazole]

sulergine [see: disulergine]

sulesomab USAN *monoclonal antibody; diagnostic aid for infectious lesions* [also: technetium Tc 99m sulesomab]

Sulf-10 eye drops ℞ *topical ophthalmic antibiotic* [sulfacetamide sodium] 10% ⍰ Sulten-10

Sulf-15 eye drops (discontinued 1995) ℞ *topical ophthalmic antibiotic* [sulfacetamide sodium] 15%

sulfabenz USAN, INN *antibacterial; coccidiostat for poultry*

sulfabenzamide USAN, USP, INN *bacteriostatic antibiotic*

sulfabromomethazine sodium NF

sulfacarbamide INN [also: sulphaurea]

sulfacecole INN

sulfacetamide USP, INN *bacteriostatic antibiotic*

sulfacetamide sodium USP *bacteriostatic antibiotic* 10%, 30% eye drops

Sulfacet-R lotion ℞ *topical antibiotic for acne* [sulfacetamide sodium; sulfur] 10%•5%

sulfachlorpyridazine INN

sulfachrysoidine INN

sulfacitine INN *antibacterial* [also: sulfacytine]

sulfaclomide INN

sulfaclorazole INN

sulfaclozine INN

sulfacombin [see: sulfadiazine]

sulfacytine USAN *broad-spectrum bacteriostatic* [also: sulfacitine]

sulfadiasulfone sodium INN *antibacterial; leprostatic* [also: acetosulfone sodium]

sulfadiazine USP, INN, JAN *broad-spectrum sulfonamide bacteriostatic* [also: sulphadiazine] 500 mg oral

sulfadiazine & pyrimethamine *Toxoplasma gondii encephalitis treatment (orphan)*

sulfadiazine silver JAN *broad-spectrum bactericidal; adjunct to burn therapy* [also: silver sulfadiazine]

sulfadiazine sodium USP, INN *antibacterial* [also: sulphadiazine sodium]

sulfadicramide INN, DCF

sulfadicrolamide [see: sulfadicramide]

sulfadimethoxine NF [also: sulphadimethoxine]

sulfadimidine INN, BAN *antibacterial* [also: sulfamethazine]

sulfadoxine USAN, USP *bacteriostatic; antimalarial adjunct*

sulfaethidole NF, INN [also: sulphaethidole]

sulfafurazole INN *broad-spectrum sulfonamide bacteriostatic* [also: sulfisoxazole; sulphafurazole]

sulfaguanidine NF, INN

sulfaguanole INN

sulfaisodimidine [see: sulfisomidine]

Sulfalax Calcium capsules OTC *stool softener* [docusate calcium] 240 mg

sulfalene USAN, INN *antibacterial* [also: sulfametopyrazine]

sulfaloxic acid INN [also: sulphaloxic acid]

sulfamates *a class of broad-spectrum anticonvulsants*

sulfamazone INN

sulfamerazine USP, INN *broad-spectrum bacteriostatic*

sulfamerazine sodium NF, INN

sulfameter USAN *antibacterial* [also: sulfametoxydiazine; sulfamethoxydiazine]

sulfamethazine USP *broad-spectrum bacteriostatic* [also: sulfadimidine]

sulfamethizole USP, INN, JAN *broad-spectrum sulfonamide bacteriostatic* [also: sulphamethizole] ☒ sulfamethoxazole

sulfamethoxazole (SMX; SMZ) USAN, USP, INN, JAN *broad-spectrum sulfonamide antibiotic* [also: sulphamethoxazole; acetylsulfamethoxazole; sulfamethoxazole sodium] ☒ sulfamethizole

sulfamethoxazole sodium JAN *broad-spectrum sulfonamide antibiotic* [also: sulfamethoxazole; sulphamethoxazole; acetylsulfamethoxazole]

sulfamethoxydiazine BAN *antibacterial* [also: sulfameter; sulfametoxydiazine]

sulfamethoxypyridazine USP, INN [also: sulphamethoxypyridazine]

sulfamethoxypyridazine acetyl

sulfametin [see: sulfameter]

sulfametomidine INN

sulfametopyrazine BAN *antibacterial* [also: sulfalene]

sulfametoxydiazine INN *antibacterial* [also: sulfameter; sulfamethoxydiazine]

sulfametrole INN, BAN

sulfamidothiodiazol [see: glybuzole]

sulfamonomethoxine USAN, INN, BAN *antibacterial*

sulfamoxole USAN, INN *antibacterial* [also: sulphamoxole]

p-sulfamoylbenzoic acid [see: carzenide]

4'-sulfamoylsuccinanilic acid [see: sulfasuccinamide]

Sulfamylon cream ℞ *broad-spectrum bacteriostatic for second- and third-degree burns* [mafenide acetate] 85 mg/g

Sulfamylon topical solution ℞ *broad-spectrum bacteriostatic to prevent meshed autograft loss on second- and third-degree burns (orphan)* [mafenide acetate] 5%

sulfanilamide NF, INN *broad-spectrum sulfonamide antibiotic* 15% topical

sulfanilanilide [see: sulfabenz]

sulfanilate zinc USAN *antibacterial*

N-sulfanilylacetamide [see: sulfacetamide]

N-sulfanilylacetamide monosodium salt monohydrate [see: sulfacetamide sodium]

N-p-sulfanilylphenylglycine sodium [see: acediasulfone sodium]

N-sulfanilylstearamide [see: stearylsulfamide]

4'-sulfanilylsuccinanilic acid [see: succisulfone]

sulfanilylurea [see: sulfacarbamide]
sulfanitran USAN, INN, BAN *antibacterial; coccidiostat for poultry*
sulfaperin INN
sulfaphenazole INN [also: sulphaphenazole]
sulfaphtalythiazol [see: phthalysulfathiazole]
sulfaproxyline INN [also: sulphaproxyline]
sulfapyrazole INN, BAN *antibacterial* [also: sulfazamet]
sulfapyridine USP, INN *investigational (orphan) dermatitis herpetiformis suppressant* [also: sulphapyridine]
sulfapyridine sodium NF
sulfaquinoxaline INN, BAN
sulfarsphenamine NF, INN
sulfasalazine USAN, USP, INN *broad-spectrum bacteriostatic; antirheumatic; anti-inflammatory for ulcerative colitis* [also: sulphasalazine; salazosulfapyridine] 500 mg oral
Sulfasim ℞ *investigational (Phase I) immunomodulator for sulfamethoxazole allergy in AIDS patients*
sulfasomizole USAN, INN *antibacterial* [also: sulphasomizole]
sulfastearyl [see: stearylsulfamide]
sulfasuccinamide INN
sulfasymazine INN
sulfated polysaccharide peptidoglycan (SPPG) [see: tecogalan sodium]
sulfathiazole USP, INN *bacteriostatic antibiotic* [also: sulphathiazole] 🔲 sulfisoxazole
sulfathiazole sodium NF
sulfathiocarbamide [see: sulfathiourea]
sulfathiourea INN
sulfatolamide INN
Sulfatrim oral suspension ℞ *anti-infective; antibacterial* [trimethoprim; sulfamethoxazole] 40•200 mg/5 mL 🔲 Sulfa-Trip
sulfatroxazole INN
sulfatrozole INN
sulfazamet USAN *antibacterial* [also: sulfapyrazole]
sulfinalol INN *antihypertensive* [also: sulfinalol HCl]

sulfinalol HCl USAN *antihypertensive* [also: sulfinalol]
sulfinpyrazone USP, INN *uricosuric for gout* [also: sulphinpyrazone] 100, 200 mg oral
sulfiram INN [also: monosulfiram]
sulfisomidine [also: sulphasomidine]
sulfisoxazole USP, JAN *broad-spectrum sulfonamide antibiotic* [also: sulfafurazole; sulphafurazole] 500 mg oral 🔲 sulfathiazole
sulfisoxazole acetyl USP *broad-spectrum sulfonamide antibiotic*
sulfisoxazole diolamine USAN, USP *broad-spectrum sulfonamide antibiotic*
Sulfoam shampoo OTC *antiseborrheic; keratolytic* [salicylic acid] 2%
sulfobenzylpenicillin [see: sulbenicillin]
sulfobromophthalein sodium USP *hepatic function test*
sulfobromphthalein sodium [see: sulfobromophthalein sodium]
sulfogaiacol INN *expectorant* [also: potassium guaiacolsulfonate]
Sulfoil liquid OTC *soap-free therapeutic skin cleanser* [sulfonated castor oil]
sulfomyxin USAN, INN *antibacterial* [also: sulphomyxin sodium]
sulfonal [see: sulfonmethane]
sulfonamides *a class of broad-spectrum bacteriostatic antibiotics effective against both gram-positive and gram-negative organisms*
sulfonated hydrogenated castor oil [see: hydroxystearin sulfate]
sulfonethylmethane NF
sulfonmethane NF
sulfonterol INN *bronchodilator* [also: sulfonterol HCl]
sulfonterol HCl USAN *bronchodilator* [also: sulfonterol]
sulfonylureas *a class of antidiabetic agents that stimulate insulin production in the pancreas*
Sulforcin lotion OTC *topical acne treatment* [sulfur; resorcinol; alcohol] 5%•2%•11.65%
sulforidazine INN
sulfosalicylic acid

sulfoxone sodium USP *antibacterial; leprostatic* [also: aldesulfone sodium]

Sulfoxyl Regular; Sulfoxyl Strong lotion ℞ *topical keratolytic for acne* [benzoyl peroxide; sulfur] 5%•2%; 10%•5%

sulfur *element (S)* [see: sulfur, precipitated; sulfur, sublimed]

sulfur, precipitated USP *scabicide; topical antibacterial; topical exfoliant*

sulfur, sublimed USP *scabicide; topical antibacterial; topical exfoliant*

sulfur dioxide NF *antioxidant*

Sulfur Soap bar OTC *medicated cleanser for acne* [precipitated sulfur] 10%

sulfurated lime solution [see: lime, sulfurated]

sulfurated potash [see: potash, sulfurated]

sulfuric acid NF *acidifying agent*

sulfuric acid, aluminum ammonium salt, dodecahydrate [see: alum, ammonium]

sulfuric acid, aluminum potassium salt, dodecahydrate [see: alum, potassium]

sulfuric acid, aluminum salt, hydrate [see: aluminum sulfate]

sulfuric acid, barium salt [see: barium sulfate]

sulfuric acid, calcium salt [see: calcium sulfate]

sulfuric acid, copper salt pentahydrate [see: cupric sulfate]

sulfuric acid, disodium salt decahydrate [see: sodium sulfate]

sulfuric acid, magnesium salt [see: magnesium sulfate]

sulfuric acid, manganese salt [see: manganese sulfate]

sulfuric acid, zinc salt hydrate [see: zinc sulfate]

sulfurous acid, monosodium salt [see: sodium bisulfite]

sulglicotide INN [also: sulglycotide]

sulglycotide BAN [also: sulglicotide]

sulicrinat INN

sulindac USAN, USP, INN, BAN *antiarthritic; nonsteroidal anti-inflammatory drug (NSAID); analgesic* 150, 200 mg oral ⑨ Zoladex

sulisatin INN

sulisobenzone USAN, INN *ultraviolet screen*

sulmarin USAN, INN *hemostatic*

Sulmasque mask OTC *antibacterial and exfoliant for acne* [sulfur] 6.4%

sulmazole INN

sulmepride INN

sulnidazole USAN, INN *antiprotozoal (Trichomonas)*

sulocarbilate INN

suloctidil USAN, INN, BAN *peripheral vasodilator*

sulodexide INN

sulofenur USAN, INN *antineoplastic*

sulopenem USAN, INN *antibacterial*

sulosemide INN

sulotroban USAN, INN, BAN *treatment for glomerulonephritis*

suloxifen INN *bronchodilator* [also: suloxifen oxalate]

suloxifen oxalate USAN *bronchodilator* [also: suloxifen]

sulphabutin [see: busulfan]

sulphadiazine BAN *broad-spectrum bacteriostatic* [also: sulfadiazine]

sulphadiazine sodium BAN *antibacterial* [also: sulfadiazine sodium]

sulphadimethoxine BAN [also: sulfadimethoxine]

sulphaethidole BAN [also: sulfaethidole]

sulphafurazole BAN *broad-spectrum sulfonamide bacteriostatic* [also: sulfisoxazole; sulfafurazole]

sulphaloxic acid BAN [also: sulfaloxic acid]

sulphamethizole BAN *broad-spectrum sulfonamide bacteriostatic* [also: sulfamethizole]

sulphamethoxazole BAN *broad-spectrum sulfonamide bacteriostatic* [also: sulfamethoxazole; acetylsulfamethoxazole; sulfamethoxazole sodium]

sulphamethoxypyridazine BAN [also: sulfamethoxypyridazine]

sulphamoxole BAN *antibacterial* [also: sulfamoxole]

sulphan blue BAN *lymphangiography aid* [also: isosulfan blue]

sulphaphenazole BAN [also: sulfaphenazole]

sulphaproxyline BAN [also: sulfaproxyline]

sulphapyridine BAN *dermatitis herpetiformis suppressant* [also: sulfapyridine]

sulphasalazine BAN *broad-spectrum bacteriostatic; antirheumatic; anti-inflammatory for ulcerative colitis* [also: sulfasalazine; salazosulfapyridine]

sulphasomidine BAN [also: sulfisomidine]

sulphasomizole BAN *antibacterial* [also: sulfasomizole]

sulphathiazole BAN *antibacterial* [also: sulfathiazole]

sulphaurea BAN [also: sulfacarbamide]

sulphinpyrazone BAN *uricosuric for gout* [also: sulfinpyrazone]

sulphocarbolate sodium [see: phenolsulphonate sodium]

Sulpho-Lac cream, soap OTC *antibacterial and exfoliant for acne* [sulfur] 5%

Sulpho-Lac Acne Medication cream OTC *antibacterial; exfoliant* [sulfur; zinc sulfate] 5%•27%

sulphomyxin sodium BAN *antibacterial* [also: sulfomyxin]

sulphonal [see: sulfonmethane]

sulpiride USAN, INN *antidepressant*

Sulpred eye drop suspension Ɑ *topical ophthalmic corticosteroidal anti-inflammatory; antibiotic* [prednisolone acetate; sulfacetamide sodium]

sulprosal INN

sulprostone USAN, INN *prostaglandin*

Sulster eye drops (discontinued 1998) Ɑ *topical ophthalmic corticosteroidal anti-inflammatory; antibiotic* [prednisolone sodium phosphate; sulfacetamide sodium] 0.25%•1%

sultamicillin USAN, INN, BAN *antibacterial*

sulthiame USAN *anticonvulsant* [also: sultiame]

sultiame INN *anticonvulsant* [also: sulthiame]

sultopride INN

sultosilic acid INN

Sultrin Triple Sulfa vaginal tablets, vaginal cream Ɑ *broad-spectrum bacteriostatic* [sulfathiazole; sulfacetamide; sulfabenzamide] 172.5•143.75•184 mg; 3.42%•2.86%•3.7%

sultroponium INN

sulukast USAN, INN *antiasthmatic; leukotriene antagonist*

sulverapride INN

suma *(Pfaffia paniculata)* bark and root *medicinal herb for circulatory disorders, chronic disease, fatigue, hormone regulation, immune system stimulation, lowering cholesterol levels, and stress; also used as a tonic*

Sumacal powder OTC *carbohydrate caloric supplement* [glucose polymers]

sumacetamol INN, BAN

sumach *(Rhus glabra)* bark, leaves, and berries *medicinal herb used as an antiseptic, astringent, diaphoretic, diuretic, emmenagogue, febrifuge, and refrigerant*

sumarotene USAN, INN *keratolytic*

sumatriptan INN, BAN *vascular serotonin 5-HT$_1$ receptor agonist for migraine and cluster headaches* [also: sumatriptan succinate]

sumatriptan succinate USAN *vascular serotonin 5-HT$_1$ receptor agonist for migraine and cluster headaches* [also: sumatriptan]

sumetizide INN

summer savory *(Calamintha hortensis; Satureja hortensis)* leaves and stems *medicinal herb for diarrhea, nausea, promoting expectoration, relieving gas and flatulence, and stimulation of menstruation; also used as an aphrodisiac*

Summer's Eve Disposable Douche solution OTC *antifungal; vaginal cleanser and deodorizer; acidity modifier* [sodium benzoate; citric acid]

Summer's Eve Disposable Douche; Summer's Eve Disposable Douche Extra Cleansing solution OTC *vaginal cleanser and deodorizer; acidity modifier* [vinegar (acetic acid)]

Summer's Eve Feminine Bath liquid OTC *for external perivaginal cleansing*

Summer's Eve Feminine Powder OTC *absorbs vaginal moisture* [cornstarch; benzethonium chloride]

Summer's Eve Feminine Wash liquid, wipes OTC *for external perivaginal cleansing*

Summer's Eve Medicated Disposable Douche solution OTC *antiseptic/germicidal; vaginal cleanser and deodorizer* [povidone-iodine] 0.3%

Summer's Eve Post-Menstrual Disposable Douche solution OTC *vaginal cleanser and deodorizer; acidity modifier* [monosodium phosphate; disodium phosphate]

Sumycin syrup ℞ *broad-spectrum antibiotic* [tetracycline HCl] 125 mg/5 mL

Sumycin '250'; Sumycin '500' capsules, tablets ℞ *broad-spectrum antibiotic* [tetracycline HCl] 250 mg; 500 mg

sun rose *medicinal herb* [see: rock rose]

sunagrel INN

suncillin INN *antibacterial* [also: suncillin sodium]

suncillin sodium USAN *antibacterial* [also: suncillin]

sunepitron HCl USAN *anxiolytic; antidepressant*

SunKist Multivitamins Complete, Children's chewable tablets OTC *vitamin/mineral/iron supplement* [multiple vitamins & minerals; iron; folic acid; biotin] ± •18 mg•400 μg•40 μg

SunKist Multi-Vitamins + Extra C chewable tablets OTC *vitamin supplement* [multiple vitamins; folic acid] ± •0.3 mg

SunKist Multivitamins + Iron, Children's chewable tablets OTC *vitamin/iron supplement* [multiple vitamins; iron; folic acid] ± •15•0.3 mg

SunKist Vitamin C chewable tablets, caplets OTC *vitamin supplement* [ascorbic acid] 60, 250, 500 mg; 500 mg

Supac tablets OTC *analgesic; antipyretic; anti-inflammatory* [acetaminophen; aspirin; caffeine] 160•230•32 mg

Super CalciCaps tablets OTC *dietary supplement* [dibasic calcium phosphate; calcium gluconate; calcium carbonate; vitamin D] 400 mg (Ca)•42 mg (P)•133 IU

Super CalciCaps M-Z tablets OTC *dietary supplement* [vitamins A and D; multiple minerals] 1667 mg•133 IU

Super Calcium '1200' softgels OTC *dietary supplement* [calcium; vitamin D] 600 mg•200 IU

Super Citro Cee sustained-release tablets OTC *dietary supplement* [ascorbic acid; lemon & rose hips bioflavonoids; rutin] 500•1000•50 mg

Super Complex C-500 Caplets OTC *dietary supplement* [ascorbic acid; multiple bioflavonoids; citrus hesperidin; rutin] 500•200•25•50 mg

Super D Perles (capsules) OTC *vitamin supplement* [vitamins A and D] 10 000•400 IU

Super Hi Potency tablets OTC *vitamin/mineral supplement* [multiple vitamins & minerals; folic acid; biotin] ± •0.4 mg•0.075 mg

Super Quints-50 tablets OTC *vitamin supplement* [multiple B vitamins; folic acid; biotin] ± •400•50 μg

Superdophilus powder OTC *dietary supplement; fever blister treatment; not generally regarded as safe and effective as an antidiarrheal* [Lactobacillus acidophilus] 2 billion U/g

SuperEPA 1200; SuperEPA 2000 softgels OTC *dietary supplement* [omega-3 fatty acids] 1200 mg; 1000 mg

superoxide dismutase (SOD) [see: orgotein]

Superplex-T tablets OTC *vitamin supplement* [multiple B vitamins; vitamin C] ± •500 mg

supidimide INN

Suplena ready-to-use liquid OTC *enteral nutritional therapy for renal failure* [multiple essential amino acids]

Suppap-120; Suppap-650 suppositories (discontinued 1997) OTC *analgesic; antipyretic* [acetaminophen] 120 mg; 650 mg

Supprelin subcu injection ℞ *gonado-tropin-releasing hormone for central precocious puberty (orphan)* [histrelin acetate] 120, 300, 600 μg/0.6 mL

Suppress lozenges OTC *antitussive* [dextromethorphan hydrobromide] 7.5 mg

Supprette (trademarked dosage form) *suppository*

Suprane liquid for vaporization ℞ *inhalation general anesthetic* [desflurane]

Suprax film-coated tablets, powder for oral suspension ℞ *cephalosporin antibiotic* [cefixime] 200, 400 mg; 100 mg/5 mL

Suprefact ⓒ nasal solution ℞ *LHRH analog; hormonal antineoplastic for prostatic cancer and endometriosis* [buserelin acetate] 1 mg/mL

Suprefact; Suprefact Depot ⓒ subcu injection ℞ *LHRH analog; hormonal antineoplastic for prostatic cancer and endometriosis* [buserelin acetate] 1 mg/mL; 6.6 mg/dose

suproclone USAN, INN *sedative*

suprofen USAN, INN, BAN *ocular non-steroidal anti-inflammatory drug (NSAID); antimiotic*

Supule (trademarked dosage form) *suppository*

suramin hexasodium USAN *investigational (NDA filed, orphan) growth factor antagonist for prostate cancer*

suramin sodium USP, BAN *antiparasitic for African trypanosomiasis and onchocerciasis*

Surbex Filmtabs (film-coated tablets) OTC *vitamin supplement* [multiple B vitamins] ±

Surbex 750 with Iron Filmtabs (film-coated tablets) OTC *vitamin/iron supplement* [multiple B vitamins; vitamins C and E; ferrous sulfate, dried; folic acid] ±•750 mg•30 IU•27 mg•0.4 mg

Surbex 750 with Zinc Filmtabs (film-coated tablets) OTC *vitamin/zinc supplement* [multiple vitamins; zinc sulfate; folic acid] ±•22.5•0.4 mg

Surbex-T; Surbex with C Filmtabs (film-coated tablets) OTC *vitamin supplement* [multiple B vitamins; vitamin C] ±•500 mg; ±•250 mg

Surbu-Gen-T film-coated tablets OTC *vitamin supplement* [multiple B vitamins; vitamin C] ±•500 mg

Sure Cell Chlamydia Test reagent kit for professional use *in vitro diagnostic aid for Chlamydia trachomatis* [monoclonal antibody-based enzyme-linked immunosorbent assay]

Sure Cell hCG-Urine Test kit (name changed to Sure Cell Pregnancy in 1995)

Sure Cell Herpes (HSV) Test reagent kit for professional use *in vitro diagnostic aid for herpes simplex virus in genital, rectal, oral, or dermal swabs* [monoclonal antibody-based enzyme-linked immunosorbent assay (ELISA)]

Sure Cell Pregnancy test kit for professional use *in vitro diagnostic aid for urine pregnancy test* [monoclonal/polyclonal antibody ELISA test]

Sure Cell Strep A Test kit (name changed to Sure Cell Streptococci in 1995)

Sure Cell Streptococci test kit for professional use *in vitro diagnostic aid for Group A streptococcal antigens in blood and throat swabs* [enzyme-linked immunosorbent assay (ELISA)]

SureLac chewable tablets OTC *digestive aid for lactose intolerance* [lactase enzyme] 3000 U

surface active extract of saline lavage of bovine lungs [see: beractant]

surfactant TA [see: beractant]

surfactant TA, modified bovine lung surfactant extract [see: beractant]

Surfak Liquigels (capsules) OTC *stool softener* [docusate calcium] 50, 240 mg

Surfaxin ℞ *investigational (Phase II/III, orphan) pulmonary surfactant for acute respiratory distress syndrome (ARDS) and meconium aspiration syndrome (MAS)* [KL4 surfactant]

surfilcon A USAN *hydrophilic contact lens material*
Surfol Post-Immersion Bath Oil OTC *bath emollient*
surfomer USAN, INN *hypolipidemic*
Surgel vaginal gel OTC *lubricant* [propylene glycol; glycerin]
surgibone USAN *internal bone splint*
surgical catgut [see: suture, absorbable surgical]
surgical gut [see: suture, absorbable surgical]
Surgicel strips, Nu-knit pads ℞ *topical local hemostat for surgery* [cellulose, oxidized]
suricainide INN *antiarrhythmic* [also: suricainide maleate]
suricainide maleate USAN, INN *antiarrhythmic* [also: suricainide]
suriclone INN, BAN
Surinam wood *medicinal herb* [see: quassia]
suritozole USAN, INN *antidepressant*
Surmontil capsules ℞ *tricyclic antidepressant* [trimipramine maleate] 25, 50, 100 mg
Surodex intraocular injection ℞ *investigational (Phase II) corticosteroidal anti-inflammatory* [dexamethasone]
suronacrine INN *cholinesterase inhibitor* [also: suronacrine maleate]
suronacrine maleate USAN *cholinesterase inhibitor* [also: suronacrine]
Survanta suspension for intratracheal instillation ℞ *pulmonary surfactant for neonatal respiratory distress syndrome or respiratory failure (orphan)* [beractant] 25 mg/mL
Susano elixir ℞ *GI antispasmodic; anticholinergic; sedative* [atropine sulfate; scopolamine hydrobromide; hyoscyamine hydrobromide; phenobarbital] 0.0194•0.0065•0.1037•16.2 mg/5 mL
Susano tablets (discontinued 1995) ℞ *GI antispasmodic; anticholinergic; sedative* [phenobarbital; atropine sulfate; scopolamine hydrobromide; hyoscyamine hydrobromide] 0.0194•0.0065•0.1037•16.2 mg

Sus-Phrine subcu injection ℞ *sympathomimetic bronchodilator for bronchial asthma, bronchospasm and COPD; vasopressor for shock* [epinephrine] 1:200 (5 mg/mL)
Sustacal powder OTC *enteral nutritional therapy* [milk-based formula]
Sustacal pudding OTC *enteral nutritional therapy* [milk-based formula]
Sustacal ready-to-use liquid OTC *enteral nutritional therapy* [lactose-free formula]
Sustacal Basic; Sustacal Plus ready-to-use liquid OTC *enteral nutritional therapy* [lactose-free formula]
Sustagen powder OTC *enteral nutritional therapy* [milk-based formula]
Sustaire timed-release tablets ℞ *antiasthmatic; bronchodilator* [theophylline] 100, 300 mg
Sustiva capsules ℞ *antiviral non-nucleoside reverse transcriptase inhibitor (NNRTI) for HIV* [efavirenz] 50, 100, 200 mg
sutilains USAN, USP, INN, BAN *topical proteolytic enzymes for necrotic tissue debridement*
sutoprofen [see: suprofen]
suture, absorbable surgical USP *surgical aid*
suture, nonabsorbable surgical USP *surgical aid*
suxamethone [see: succinylcholine chloride]
suxamethonium chloride INN, BAN *neuromuscular blocking agent* [also: succinylcholine chloride]
suxemerid INN *antitussive* [also: suxemerid sulfate]
suxemerid sulfate USAN *antitussive* [also: suxemerid]
suxethonium chloride INN
suxibuzone INN
swallow wort, orange *medicinal herb* [see: pleurisy root]
swallow wort, silky *medicinal herb* [see: milkweed]
swamp cabbage *medicinal herb* [see: skunk cabbage]

swamp laurel; swamp sassafras *medicinal herb* [see: magnolia]

sweet, mountain *medicinal herb* [see: New Jersey tea]

sweet, winter *medicinal herb* [see: marjoram]

sweet anise; sweet chervil *medicinal herb* [see: sweet cicely]

sweet balm *medicinal herb* [see: lemon balm]

sweet basil *medicinal herb* [see: basil]

sweet bay *medicinal herb* [see: laurel]

sweet birch *medicinal herb* [see: birch]

sweet birch oil [see: methyl salicylate]

sweet cicely (Osmorhiza longistylis) root *medicinal herb used as a carminative, expectorant, and stomachic*

sweet clover *medicinal herb* [see: melilot]

sweet dock *medicinal herb* [see: bistort]

sweet elder *medicinal herb* [see: elderberry]

sweet elm *medicinal herb* [see: slippery elm]

sweet fennel *medicinal herb* [see: fennel]

sweet flag *medicinal herb* [see: calamus]

sweet grass *medicinal herb* [see: calamus]

sweet leaf *medicinal herb* [see: stevia]

sweet magnolia *medicinal herb* [see: magnolia]

sweet marjoram *medicinal herb* [see: marjoram]

sweet myrtle *medicinal herb* [see: calamus]

sweet orange peel tincture [see: orange peel tincture, sweet]

sweet potato vine, wild *medicinal herb* [see: wild jalap]

sweet root *medicinal herb* [see: calamus]

sweet rush *medicinal herb* [see: calamus]

sweet sedge *medicinal herb* [see: calamus]

sweet spirit of nitre [see: ethyl nitrite]

sweet vernal grass (Anthoxanthum odoratum) *natural flavoring banned by the FDA as it is not generally regarded as safe and effective*

sweet violet *medicinal herb* [see: violet]

sweet water lily; sweet-scented water lily *medicinal herb* [see: white pond lily]

sweet weed *medicinal herb* [see: marsh mallow]

sweet woodruff (Asperula odorata; Galium odoratum) plant *medicinal herb for diuresis, inducing expectoration, liver disorders, promoting wound healing, relieving gastrointestinal spasms, and sedation*

Sweet'n Fresh Clotrimazole-7 cream, vaginal suppositories OTC *antifungal* [clotrimazole] 1%; 100 mg

sweet-scented pond lily; sweet-scented water lily *medicinal herb* [see: white pond lily]

sweetwood *medicinal herb* [see: licorice]

Swim-Ear ear drops OTC *antiseptic* [isopropyl alcohol] 95%

swine snout *medicinal herb* [see: dandelion]

Syllact powder OTC *bulk laxative* [psyllium seed husks] 3.3 g/tsp.

Syllamalt powder OTC *bulk laxative* [malt soup extract; psyllium seed husks] 4•3 g/tsp.

Symadine capsules (discontinued 1996) ℞ *antiviral; dopaminergic antiparkinsonian agent* [amantadine HCl] 100 mg

symclosene USAN, INN *topical anti-infective*

symetine INN *antiamebic* [also: symetine HCl]

symetine HCl USAN *antiamebic* [also: symetine]

Symlin ℞ *investigational (Phase III) antidiabetic for type 1 and type 2 diabetes* [pramlintide acetate]

Symmetrel capsules, syrup ℞ *antiviral; dopaminergic antiparkinsonian agent* [amantadine HCl] 100 mg; 50 mg/5 mL

sympatholytics *a class of cardiovascular drugs that block the passage of impulses through the sympathetic nervous system* [also called: antiadrenergics]

sympathomimetics *a class of bronchodilators that relax the bronchial muscles, reducing bronchospasm; a class of cardiac agents that increase myocardial contractility, causing a vasopressor effect to counteract shock* *(inadequate tissue perfusion)* [also called: adrenergic agonists]

Symphytum officinale; S. tuberosum *medicinal herb* [see: comfrey]

Symplocarpus foetidus *medicinal herb* [see: skunk cabbage]

Synacol CF tablets OTC *antitussive; expectorant* [dextromethorphan hydrobromide; guaifenesin] 15•200 mg

Synacort cream Ṙ *topical corticosteroidal anti-inflammatory* [hydrocortisone] 1%, 2.5%

Synagis IM injection Ṙ *monoclonal antibody for prophylaxis of respiratory syncytial virus (RSV) in infants* [palivizumab] 100 mg

Synalar cream, ointment, topical solution Ṙ *topical corticosteroidal anti-inflammatory* [fluocinolone acetonide] 0.01, 0.25%; 0.025%; 0.01%

Synalar-HP cream Ṙ *topical corticosteroidal anti-inflammatory* [fluocinolone acetonide] 0.2%

Synalgos-DC capsules Ṙ *narcotic analgesic* [dihydrocodeine bitartrate; aspirin; caffeine] 16•356.4•30 mg

Synapton SR Ṙ *investigational (NDA filed) sustained-release acetylcholinesterase inhibitor for Alzheimer's disease* [physostigmine]

Synarel nasal spray Ṙ *gonadotropin-releasing hormone for central precocious puberty (orphan) and endometriosis* [nafarelin acetate] 2 mg/mL (200 μg/spray)

Synemol cream Ṙ *topical corticosteroidal anti-inflammatory* [fluocinolone acetonide] 0.025%

Synercid injection Ṙ *investigational (NDA filed) semi-synthetic streptogramin antibiotic for iatrogenic infections* [quinupristin; dalfopristin]

synestrin [see: diethylstilbestrol]

synnematin B [see: adicillin]

Synophylate-GG syrup Ṙ *antiasthmatic; bronchodilator; expectorant* [theophylline; guaifenesin; alcohol 10%] 150•100 mg/15 mL

Synovir (name changed to Thalomid upon marketing release in 1998)

Syn-Rx controlled-release tablets (14-day, 56-tablet treatment regimen) Ṙ *decongestant; expectorant* [pseudoephedrine HCl; guaifenesin] 60•600 mg

Synsorb-Pk Ṙ *investigational (Phase III, orphan) E. coli neutralizer for traveler's diarrhea and hemolytic uremic syndrome (HUS)* [8-methoxycarbonyloctyl oligosaccharides]

synthestrin [see: diethylstilbestrol]

synthetic lung surfactant [see: colfosceril palmitate]

synthetic paraffin [see: paraffin, synthetic]

synthetic spermaceti [now: cetyl esters wax]

synthoestrin [see: diethylstilbestrol]

Synthroid tablets, powder for injection Ṙ *thyroid hormone* [levothyroxine sodium] 25, 50, 75, 88, 100, 112, 125, 150, 175, 200, 300 μg; 200, 500 μg ② Euthroid

Syntocinon IV, IM injection (discontinued 1998) Ṙ *oxytocic for induction of labor, postpartum bleeding, and incomplete abortion* [oxytocin] 10 U/mL

Syntocinon nasal spray (discontinued 1998) Ṙ *oxytocic for initial milk letdown* [oxytocin] 40 U/mL

synvinolin [now: simvastatin]

Synvisc intra-articular injection Ṙ *viscoelastic lubricant and "shock absorber" for osteoarthritis* [hylan G-F 20] 16 mg/2 mL

Syprine capsules Ṙ *copper chelating agent for Wilson's disease (orphan)* [trientine HCl] 50 mg

Syracol CF tablets OTC *antitussive; expectorant* [dextromethorphan hydrobromide; guaifenesin] 15•200 mg

syrosingopine NF, INN, BAN

syrup NF *flavoring agent*

syrupus cerasi [see: cherry juice]

Syrvite liquid OTC *vitamin supplement* [multiple vitamins] ±

Syzygium aromaticum *medicinal herb* [see: cloves]

**T-2 protocol (dactinomycin, doxo-
rubicin, vincristine, cyclophosphamide, radiation)** *chemotherapy
protocol*

T₃ (liothyronine sodium) [q.v.]

T₄ (levothyroxine sodium) [q.v.]

T4, recombinant soluble human
*investigational (Phase I/II) antiviral for
HIV*

**T4 endonuclease V (T4N5), lipo-
some encapsulated** *investigational
(orphan) for prevent cutaneous neoplasms in xeroderma pigmentosum*

**T-10 protocol (methotrexate, doxo-
rubicin, cisplatin, bleomycin,
cyclophosphamide, dactinomycin)** *chemotherapy protocol*

T30177 *investigational (Phase I) antiviral oligonucleotide for AIDS*

T-61 ℞ *veterinary anesthesia; also for
veterinary euthanasia* [embutramide]

Tab-A-Vite tablets OTC *vitamin supplement* [multiple vitamins; folic acid]
± • 0.4 mg

Tab-A-Vite + Iron tablets OTC *vita-
min/iron supplement* [multiple vitamins; iron; folic acid] ± • 18 • 0.4 mg

***Tabebuia avellanedae; T. impetigi-
nosa*** *medicinal herb* [see: pau d'arco]

Tabernanthe iboga *street drug* [see:
iboga]

tabilautide INN

Tabloid (trademarked dosage form)
tablet with raised lettering

Tabron Filmseals (film-coated tablets)
(discontinued 1996) ℞ *hematinic*
[ferrous fumarate; multiple B vitamins; vitamins C and E; docusate
sodium; folic acid] 100 mg • ± • 500
mg • 30 IU • 50 mg • 1 mg

Tabules (dosage form) *tablets*

Tac-3 IM, intra-articular, intrabursal,
intradermal injection ℞ *corticosteroid; anti-inflammatory* [triamcinolone
acetonide] 3 mg/mL

Tac-40 suspension for injection ℞ *corticosteroid; anti-inflammatory* [triam-
cinolone acetonide] 40 mg/mL

Tacaryl syrup (discontinued 1997) ℞
antihistamine [methdilazine HCl] 4
mg/5 mL

Tace capsules (discontinued 1998) ℞
*hormone for estrogen replacement ther-
apy or inoperable prostatic carcinoma*
[chlorotrianisene] 12, 25 mg

TA-CIN *investigational cancer vaccine*

taclamine INN *minor tranquilizer* [also:
taclamine HCl]

taclamine HCl USAN *minor tranquilizer* [also: taclamine]

tacmahac *medicinal herb* [see: balm of
Gilead]

tacrine INN, BAN *reversible cholinesterase
inhibitor; cognition adjuvant for Alzheimer's dementia* [also: tacrine HCl]

tacrine HCl USAN *reversible cholinesterase inhibitor; cognition adjuvant for
Alzheimer's dementia* [also: tacrine]

tacrolimus USAN, INN *immunosuppressant*

**TAD (thioguanine, ara-C, dauno-
rubicin)** *chemotherapy protocol* [also:
DCT; DAT]

taeniacides *a class of agents that destroy
tapeworms* [see also: anthelmintics;
vermicides; vermifuges]

Tagamet film-coated tablets ℞ *histamine H₂ antagonist for gastric and duodenal ulcers and gastric hypersecretory
conditions* [cimetidine] 200, 300,
400, 800 mg ② Tegopen

Tagamet liquid, IV or IM injection,
premixed injection ℞ *histamine H₂
antagonist for gastric and duodenal
ulcers and gastric hypersecretory conditions* [cimetidine] 300 mg/5 mL;
300 mg/2 mL; 300 mg/vial

Tagamet 100 (British name for U.S.
product Tagamet HB [in 100 mg
strength])

Tagamet HB film-coated tablets, oral
suspension OTC *histamine H₂ antagonist
for episodic heartburn and acid indigestion* [cimetidine] 100, 200 mg; 200 mg

taglutimide INN

taheebo *medicinal herb* [see: pau d'arco]

TA-HPV ℞ *investigational (orphan) for cervical cancer* [vaccinia virus vaccine for human papillomavirus (HPV), recombinant]

tail, colt's; cow's tail; horse tail; mare's tail *medicinal herb* [see: fleabane; horseweed]

tail, lion's *medicinal herb* [see: motherwort]

tailed cubebs; tailed pepper *medicinal herb* [see: cubeb]

TAK-603 *investigational (orphan) for Crohn's disease*

Talacen caplets ℞ *narcotic agonist-antagonist analgesic; antipyretic* [pentazocine HCl; acetaminophen] 25•650 mg

talampicillin INN *antibacterial* [also: talampicillin HCl]

talampicillin HCl USAN *antibacterial* [also: talampicillin]

talastine INN

talbutal USP, INN *sedative; hypnotic*

talc USP, JAN *dusting powder; tablet and capsule lubricant*

talc, sterile aerosol *investigational (NDA filed, orphan) treatment for malignant pleural effusion and pneumothorax via intrapleural thoracoscopy administration*

taleranol USAN, INN *gonadotropin enzyme inhibitor*

talinolol INN

talipexole INN

talisomycin USAN, INN *antineoplastic*

tall speedwell *medicinal herb* [see: Culver's root]

tall veronica *medicinal herb* [see: Culver's root]

TALL-104 *investigational killer cell line derived from cells of a patient with a rare form of T-cell leukemia for metastatic cancer*

tallimustine INN *investigational antineoplastic for leukemia and solid tumors*

tallow shrub *medicinal herb* [see: bayberry]

tallysomycin A [now: talisomycin]

talmetacin USAN, INN *analgesic; antiinflammatory; antipyretic*

talmetoprim INN

talniflumate USAN, INN *anti-inflammatory; analgesic*

talopram INN *catecholamine potentiator* [also: talopram HCl]

talopram HCl USAN *catecholamine potentiator* [also: talopram]

talosalate USAN, INN *analgesic; antiinflammatory*

Taloxa (foreign name for U.S. product Felbatol)

taloximine INN, BAN

talsaclidine INN

talsaclidine fumarate USAN *muscarinic M_1 agonist for Alzheimer's disease*

talsupram INN

taltibride [see: metibride]

taltrimide INN

taludipine [see: teludipine]

taludipine HCl [see: teludipine HCl]

Talwin IV, subcu or IM injection ℞ *narcotic agonist-antagonist analgesic; also abused as a street drug* [pentazocine lactate] 30 mg/mL

Talwin Compound caplets ℞ *narcotic agonist-antagonist analgesic; antipyretic; also abused as a street drug* [pentazocine HCl; aspirin] 12.5•325 mg

Talwin NX tablets ℞ *narcotic agonist-antagonist analgesic; also abused as a street drug* [pentazocine HCl; naloxone HCl] 50•0.5 mg

tamarind (Tamarindus indica) fruit and leaves *medicinal herb used as an anthelmintic, laxative, and refrigerant*

Tambocor tablets ℞ *antiarrhythmic* [flecainide acetate] 50, 100, 150 mg

tameridone USAN, INN, BAN *veterinary sedative*

tameticillin INN

tametraline INN *antidepressant* [also: tametraline HCl]

tametraline HCl USAN *antidepressant* [also: tametraline]

Tamine S.R. sustained-release tablets ℞ *decongestant; antihistamine* [phenylpropanolamine HCl; phenylephrine HCl; brompheniramine maleate] 15•15•12 mg

tamitinol INN

tamoxifen INN, BAN *antiestrogen antineoplastic for breast cancer* [also: tamoxifen citrate]

tamoxifen citrate USAN, USP, JAN *antiestrogen antineoplastic for breast cancer; breast cancer prevention for high-risk patients* [also: tamoxifen] 10, 20 mg oral

tampramine INN *antidepressant* [also: tampramine fumarate]

tampramine fumarate USAN *antidepressant* [also: tampramine]

Tamp-R-Tel (trademarked packaging form) *tamper-evident cartridge-needle unit*

tamsulosin INN *alpha₁-adrenergic blocker for benign prostatic hypertrophy (BPH)* [also: tamsulosin HCl]

tamsulosin HCl USAN, JAN *alpha₁-adrenergic blocker for benign prostatic hypertrophy (BPH)* [also: tamsulosin]

Tanac gel OTC *topical oral anesthetic; vulnerary* [dyclonine HCl; allantoin] 1%•0.5%

Tanac liquid OTC *topical oral anesthetic; antiseptic* [benzocaine; benzalkonium chloride] 10%•0.12%

Tanac Dual Core stick OTC *topical oral anesthetic; antiseptic; astringent* [benzocaine; benzalkonium chloride; tannic acid] 7.5%•0.12%•6%

Tanacetum parthenium medicinal herb [see: feverfew]

Tanacetum vulgare medicinal herb [see: tansy]

Tanafed oral suspension ℞ *decongestant; antihistamine* [pseudoephedrine tannate; chlorpheniramine tannate] 75•4.5 mg/5 mL

tandamine INN *antidepressant* [also: tandamine HCl]

tandamine HCl USAN *antidepressant* [also: tandamine]

tandospirone INN, BAN *anxiolytic* [also: tandospirone citrate]

tandospirone citrate USAN *anxiolytic* [also: tandospirone]

taniplon INN

tannic acid USP, JAN *astringent; topical mucosal protectant*

tannic acid acetate [see: acetyltannic acid]

tannin [see: tannic acid]

tannyl acetate [see: acetyltannic acid]

Tanoral tablets ℞ *decongestant; antihistamine* [phenylephrine tannate; chlorpheniramine tannate; pyrilamine tannate] 25•8•25 mg

tansy (Chrysanthemum vulgare; Tanacetum vulgare) leaves and seeds *medicinal herb for inducing diaphoresis, promoting wound healing, relieving spasms, stimulating menstruation, and treating worm infections*

tantalum *element (Ta)*

Tantrum ℞ *investigational (orphan) radioprotectant for oral mucosa following radiation therapy for head and neck cancer* [benzydamine HCl]

Tao capsules ℞ *macrolide antibiotic* [troleandomycin] 250 mg

taoryi edisylate [see: caramiphen edisylate]

Tapanol tablets, caplets, gelcaps OTC *analgesic; antipyretic* [acetaminophen] 325, 500 mg; 500 mg; 500 mg

Tapazole tablets ℞ *antithyroid agent* [methimazole] 5, 10 mg

tape, adhesive USP *surgical aid*

taprostene INN

tar [see: coal tar]

tarweed *medicinal herb* [see: yerba santa]

Tarabine PFS subcu, intrathecal, or IV injection ℞ *antimetabolite antineoplastic for various leukemias* [cytarabine]

Taraphilic Ointment OTC *topical antipsoriatic; antiseborrheic* [coal tar] 1%

Taraxacum officinale medicinal herb [see: dandelion]

Targocid (commercially available in 13 foreign countries) ℞ *investigational (NDA filed) glycopeptide antibiotic* [teicoplanin]

Targretin capsules, topical ℞ *investigational (Phase II/III) synthetic retinoid analog antineoplastic for AIDS-related Kaposi sarcoma (clinical trials discontinued 1999); investigational for cutaneous T-cell lymphoma* [bexarotene] Ⓓ Tegopen; Tegrin

Tarka film-coated combination-release tablets ℞ *once-daily antihypertensive; angiotensin-converting enzyme (ACE) inhibitor; calcium channel blocker* [trandolapril (immediate release); verapamil HCl (extended release)] 2•180, 1•240, 2•240, 4•240 mg

Tarlene hair lotion OTC *antiseborrheic; antipsoriatic; keratolytic* [salicylic acid; coal tar] 2.5%•2%

tarragon (Artemisia dracunculus) flowering plant *medicinal herb used as a diuretic, emmenagogue, hypnotic, and stomachic*

Tarsum shampoo OTC *antipsoriatic; antiseborrheic; keratolytic* [coal tar; salicylic acid] 10%•5%

tartar emetic [see: antimony potassium tartrate]

tartaric acid NF *buffering agent*

Tasmar film-coated tablets ℞ *COMT inhibitor; adjunct to carbidopa and levodopa for Parkinson's disease* [tolcapone] 100, 200 mg

tasosartan USAN, INN *antihypertensive; angiotensin II antagonist (NDA withdrawn 1998)*

tasuldine INN

TAT antagonist *investigational (Phase I/II) antiviral for HIV*

taurine INN [also: aminoethylsulfonic acid]

taurocholate sodium [see: sodium taurocholate]

taurolidine INN, BAN *investigational antitoxin for the treatment of sepsis*

tauromustine INN *investigational treatment for renal cancer and multiple sclerosis*

tauroselcholic acid INN, BAN

taurultam INN, BAN

Tavist tablets, syrup ℞ *antihistamine* [clemastine fumarate] 2.68 mg; 0.67 mg/5 mL

Tavist-1 tablets (discontinued 1997) OTC *antihistamine* [clemastine fumarate] 1.34 mg

Tavist-D film-coated sustained-release tablets OTC *decongestant; antihista-*mine [phenylpropanolamine HCl; clemastine fumarate] 75•1.34 mg

taxanes; taxoids *a class of antineoplastics that inhibits cancer cell mitosis by disrupting the cells' microtubular network*

Taxol IV infusion ℞ *antineoplastic for AIDS-related Kaposi sarcoma (orphan), and breast and ovarian cancers* [paclitaxel] 30 mg/5 mL

Taxotere IV infusion ℞ *antineoplastic for advanced or metastatic breast cancer* [docetaxel] 20, 80 mg/vial

Taxus bacatta and other species *medicinal herb* [see: yew]

tazadolene INN *analgesic* [also: tazadolene succinate]

tazadolene succinate USAN *analgesic* [also: tazadolene]

tazanolast INN

tazarotene USAN, INN *retinoid prodrug; topical keratolytic for acne and psoriasis*

tazasubrate INN, BAN

tazeprofen INN

Tazicef powder or frozen premix for IV or IM injection ℞ *cephalosporin antibiotic* [ceftazidime] 1, 2, 6 g

Tazidime powder for IV or IM injection ℞ *cephalosporin antibiotic* [ceftazidime] 0.5, 1, 2, 6 g

tazifylline INN *antihistamine* [also: tazifylline HCl]

tazifylline HCl USAN *antihistamine* [also: tazifylline]

taziprinone INN

tazobactam USAN, INN, BAN *β-lactamase inhibitor; penicillin synergist*

tazobactam sodium USAN *β-lactamase inhibitor; penicillin synergist*

Tazocin (European name for U.S. product Zosyn)

tazofelone USAN *investigational (Phase II) treatment for ulcerative colitis and Crohn's disease*

tazolol INN *cardiotonic* [also: tazolol HCl]

tazolol HCl USAN *cardiotonic* [also: tazolol]

tazomeline citrate USAN *cholinergic agonist for Alzheimer's disease*

Tazorac gel ℞ *retinoid pro-drug; topical keratolytic for acne and psoriasis* [tazarotene] 0.05%, 0.1%

TBC-3B *investigational (Phase I) vaccine for AIDS*

TBC-11251 *investigational (Phase II) endothelin-A antagonist for congestive heart failure*

TBC-1269 *investigational (Phase II) selectin inhibitor for asthma*

TBZ (thiabendazole) [q.v.]

TC (thioguanine, cytarabine) *chemotherapy protocol*

99mTc [see: macrosalb (99mTc)]

99mTc [see: sodium pertechnetate Tc 99m]

99mTc [see: technetium Tc 99m albumin]

99mTc [see: technetium Tc 99m albumin aggregated]

99mTc [see: technetium Tc 99m albumin colloid]

99mTc [see: technetium Tc 99m albumin microaggregated]

99mTc [see: technetium Tc 99m antimony trisulfide colloid]

99mTc [see: technetium Tc 99m biciromab]

99mTc [see: technetium Tc 99m bicisate]

99mTc [see: technetium Tc 99m disofenin]

99mTc [see: technetium Tc 99m etidronate]

99mTc [see: technetium Tc 99m exametazine]

99mTc [see: technetium Tc 99m ferpentetate]

99mTc [see: technetium Tc 99m furifosmin]

99mTc [see: technetium Tc 99m gluceptate]

99mTc [see: technetium Tc 99m lidofenin]

99mTc [see: technetium Tc 99m mebrofenin]

99mTc [see: technetium Tc 99m medronate]

99mTc [see: technetium Tc 99m medronate disodium]

99mTc [see: technetium Tc 99m mertiatide]

99mTc [see: technetium Tc 99m oxidronate]

99mTc [see: technetium Tc 99m pentetate]

99mTc [see: technetium Tc 99m pentetate calcium trisodium]

99mTc [see: technetium Tc 99m (pyro- & trimeta-) phosphates]

99mTc [see: technetium Tc 99m pyrophosphate]

99mTc [see: technetium Tc 99m red blood cells]

99mTc [see: technetium Tc 99m sestamibi]

99mTc [see: technetium Tc 99m siboroxime]

99mTc [see: technetium Tc 99m succimer]

99mTc [see: technetium Tc 99m sulfur colloid]

99mTc [see: technetium Tc 99m teboroxime]

99mTc [see: technetium Tc 99m tetrofosmin]

99mTc [see: technetium Tc 99m tiatide]

TCC (trichlorocarbanilide) [see: triclocarban]

T-cell gene therapy *investigational (Phase III) treatment for HIV*

T-cell receptor (TCR) peptide *investigational (Phase II) theraccine for rheumatoid arthritis*

TCR (T-cell receptor) peptide [q.v.]

TD; Td (tetanus & diphtheria [toxoids]) *the designation TD (or DT) denotes the pediatric vaccine; Td denotes the adult vaccine* [see: diphtheria & tetanus toxoids, adsorbed]

T-Dry *sustained-release capsules (discontinued 1995)* OTC *decongestant; antihistamine* [pseudoephedrine HCl; chlorpheniramine maleate] 120•12 mg

tea, Canada; mountain tea; redberry tea *medicinal herb* [see: wintergreen]

tea tree oil (Melaleuca alternifolia) *medicinal herb for acne, boils, burns, Candida infections, cold sores, joint pain, skin disorders, staphylococcal and streptococcal infections, and sunburn;*

also used as a douche for trichomonal cervicitis and vaginal candidiasis

TEAB (tetraethylammonium bromide) [see: tetrylammonium bromide]

teaberry oil [see: methyl salicylate]

TEAC (tetraethylammonium chloride) [q.v.]

teamster's tea *medicinal herb* [see: ephedra]

Tear Drop eye drops (discontinued 1998) OTC *ophthalmic moisturizer/lubricant* [polyvinyl alcohol] 2

TearGard eye drops OTC *ocular moisturizer/lubricant* [hydroxyethylcellulose]

Teargen eye drops OTC *ophthalmic moisturizer/lubricant* [polyvinyl alcohol] 2

Tearisol eye drops OTC *ophthalmic moisturizer/lubricant* [hydroxypropyl methylcellulose] 0.5%

Tears Naturale; Tears Naturale II; Tears Naturale Free eye drops OTC *ophthalmic moisturizer/lubricant* [hydroxypropyl methylcellulose] 0.3%

Tears Plus eye drops OTC *ophthalmic moisturizer/lubricant* [polyvinyl alcohol] 1.4%

Tears Renewed eye drops OTC *ophthalmic moisturizer/lubricant* [hydroxypropyl methylcellulose] 0.3%

Tears Renewed ophthalmic ointment OTC *ocular moisturizer/lubricant* [white petrolatum; mineral oil]

Tebamide suppositories, pediatric suppositories R *anticholinergic; antiemetic* [trimethobenzamide HCl] 200 mg; 100 mg

tebatizole INN

tebethion [see: thioacetazone; thiacetazone]

tebufelone USAN, INN *analgesic; antiinflammatory*

tebuquine USAN, INN *antimalarial*

tebutate USAN, INN *combining name for radicals or groups*

TEC (thiotepa, etoposide, carboplatin) *chemotherapy protocol*

teceleukin USAN, INN, BAN *immunostimulant; investigational (orphan) for metastatic renal cell carcinoma and metastatic malignant melanoma*

teceleukin & interferon alfa-2a *investigational (orphan) for metastatic renal cell carcinoma and metastatic malignant melanoma*

technetium *element (Tc)*

technetium (^{99m}Tc) dimercaptosuccinic acid JAN *diagnostic aid for renal function testing* [also: technetium Tc 99m succimer]

technetium (^{99m}Tc) human serum albumin JAN *radioactive agent*

technetium (^{99m}Tc) labeled macroaggregated human albumin JAN [also: macrosalb (^{99m}Tc)]

technetium (^{99m}Tc) methylenediphosphonate JAN *radioactive diagnostic aid for skeletal imaging* [also: technetium Tc 99m medronate]

technetium (^{99m}Tc) phytate JAN *radioactive agent*

technetium Tc 99m albumin USP *radioactive agent*

technetium Tc 99m albumin aggregated USAN, USP *radioactive diagnostic aid for lung imaging*

technetium Tc 99m albumin colloid USAN, USP *radioactive agent*

technetium Tc 99m albumin microaggregated USAN *radioactive agent*

technetium Tc 99m antimelanoma murine MAb *investigational (orphan) for diagnostic imaging agent for metastases of malignant melanoma*

technetium Tc 99m antimony trisulfide colloid USAN *radioactive agent*

technetium Tc 99m apcitide *radiopharmaceutical diagnostic aid for acute venous thrombosis*

technetium Tc 99m arcitumomab USAN *radiopharmaceutical diagnostic aid for recurrent or metastatic thyroid and colorectal cancers*

technetium Tc 99m bectumomab *monoclonal antibody; investigational (Phase III, orphan) diagnostic aid for non-Hodgkin's B-cell lymphoma, AIDS-related lymphomas, and other acute and chronic B-cell leukemias* [also: bectumomab]

technetium Tc 99m biciromab *radioactive diagnostic aid for deep vein thrombosis*

technetium Tc 99m bicisate USAN, INN, BAN *radioactive diagnostic aid for brain imaging*

technetium Tc 99m depreotide [see: depreotide]

technetium Tc 99m disofenin USP *radioactive diagnostic aid for hepatobiliary function testing*

technetium Tc 99m DMSA (dimercaptosuccinic acid) [see: technetium Tc 99m succimer]

technetium Tc 99m DTPA (diethylenetriaminepentaacetic acid) [see: technetium Tc 99m pentetate]

technetium Tc 99m etidronate USP *radioactive agent*

technetium Tc 99m exametazine USAN *radioactive agent*

technetium Tc 99m ferpentetate USP *radioactive agent*

technetium Tc 99m furifosmin USAN, INN *radioactive agent; diagnostic aid for cardiac disease*

technetium Tc 99m gluceptate USP *radioactive agent*

technetium Tc 99m HSA (human serum albumin) [see: technetium Tc 99m albumin]

technetium Tc 99m iron ascorbate pentetic acid complex [now: technetium Tc 99m ferpentetate]

technetium Tc 99m lidofenin USAN, USP *radioactive agent*

technetium Tc 99m MAA (microaggregated albumin) [see: technetium Tc 99m albumin aggregated]

technetium Tc 99m MDP (methylenediphosphonate) [see: technetium Tc 99m medronate]

technetium Tc 99m mebrofenin USAN, USP *radioactive agent*

technetium Tc 99m medronate USP *radioactive diagnostic aid for skeletal imaging* [also: technetium (^{99m}Tc) methylenediphosphonate]

technetium Tc 99m medronate disodium USAN *radioactive agent*

technetium Tc 99m mertiatide USAN *radioactive diagnostic aid for renal function testing*

technetium Tc 99m murine MAb IgG$_2$a to B cell [now: technetium Tc 99m bectumomab]

technetium Tc 99m murine MAb to human alpha-fetoprotein (AFP) *investigational (orphan) for diagnostic aid for AFP-producing tumors, hepatoblastoma, and hepatocellular carcinoma*

technetium Tc 99m murine MAb to human chorionic gonadotropin (hCG) *investigational (orphan) for diagnostic aid for hCG-producing tumors*

technetium Tc 99m oxidronate USP *radioactive diagnostic aid for skeletal imaging*

technetium Tc 99m pentetate USP *radioactive agent* [also: human serum albumin diethylenetriaminepentaacetic acid technetium (^{99m}Tc)]

technetium Tc 99m pentetate calcium trisodium USAN *radioactive agent*

technetium Tc 99m pentetate sodium [now: technetium Tc 99m pentetate]

technetium Tc 99m (pyro- and trimeta-) phosphates USP *radioactive agent*

technetium Tc 99m pyrophosphate USP, JAN *radioactive agent*

technetium Tc 99m red blood cells USAN *radioactive agent*

technetium Tc 99m sestamibi USAN, INN, BAN *radioactive/radiopaque diagnostic aid for cardiac perfusion imaging and mammography*

technetium Tc 99m siboroxime USAN, INN *radioactive diagnostic aid for brain imaging*

technetium Tc 99m sodium gluceptate [now: technetium Tc 99m gluceptate]

technetium Tc 99m succimer USP *diagnostic aid for renal function testing* [also: technetium (^{99m}Tc) dimercaptosuccinic acid]

technetium Tc 99m sulesomab *monoclonal antibody; diagnostic aid for infectious lesions* [also: sulesomab]

technetium Tc 99m sulfur colloid (TSC) USAN, USP *radioactive agent*

technetium Tc 99m teboroxime USAN, INN, BAN *radioactive/radiopaque diagnostic aid for cardiac perfusion imaging*

technetium Tc 99m tetrofosmin *radioactive agent for cardiovascular imaging*

technetium Tc 99m tiatide BAN

technetium Tc 99m TSC (technetium sulfur colloid) [see: technetium Tc 99m sulfur colloid]

technetium Tc 99m-labeled CEA scan [see: arcitumomab]

Techtide [see: P829 Techtide]

teclothiazide INN, BAN

teclozan USAN, INN *antiamebic*

Tecnu Poison Oak-N-Ivy liquid OTC *topical poison ivy treatment* [deodorized mineral spirits] ≟

tecogalan sodium USAN *antiangiogenic antineoplastic*

Teczem film-coated extended-release tablets ℞ *antihypertensive; angiotensin-converting enzyme (ACE) inhibitor; calcium channel blocker* [diltiazem maleate; enalapril maleate] 180•5 mg

tedisamil INN *investigational calcium channel blocker for ischemic heart disease and arrhythmias*

Tedrigen tablets OTC *antiasthmatic; bronchodilator; decongestant; sedative* [theophylline; ephedrine HCl; phenobarbital] 120•22.5•7.5 mg

tefazoline INN

tefenperate INN

tefludazine INN

teflurane USAN, INN *inhalation anesthetic*

teflutixol INN

tegafur USAN, INN, BAN *antineoplastic; prodrug of fluorouracil*

Tegison capsules ℞ *systemic antipsoriatic* [etretinate] 10, 25 mg

Tegopen capsules, powder for oral solution (discontinued 1998) ℞ *penicillinase-resistant penicillin antibi-*otic [cloxacillin sodium] 250, 500 mg; 125 mg/5 mL ② Tagamet; Tegrin; Targretin

Tegretol chewable tablets, tablets, oral suspension ℞ *anticonvulsant; analgesic for trigeminal neuralgia; antipsychotic* [carbamazepine] 100 mg; 200 mg; 100 mg/5 mL ② Tegrin

Tegretol-XR extended-release tablets ℞ *twice-daily anticonvulsant; antipsychotic* [carbamazepine] 100, 200, 400 mg

Tegrin for Psoriasis cream, lotion, soap OTC *topical antipsoriatic; antiseborrheic; antiseptic* [coal tar solution] 5% ② Tegopen; Tegretol; Targretin

Tegrin Medicated gel shampoo, lotion shampoo OTC *antiseborrheic; antipsoriatic; antipruritic; antibacterial* [coal tar] 5%

Tegrin Medicated Extra Conditioning; Advanced Formula Tegrin shampoo OTC *antiseborrheic; antipsoriatic; antipruritic; antibacterial* [coal tar] 7%

Tegrin-HC ointment OTC *topical corticosteroidal anti-inflammatory* [hydrocortisone] 1%

Tegrin-LT shampoo/conditioner OTC *pediculicide for lice* [pyrethrins; piperonyl butoxide technical] 0.33%• 3.15%

teholamine [see: aminophylline]

TEIB (triethyleneiminobenzoquinone) [see: triaziquone]

teicoplanin USAN, INN, BAN *glycopeptide antibacterial antibiotic*

teicoplanin A_{2-1}, A_{2-2}, A_{2-3}, A_{2-4}, A_{2-5}, **and** A_{3-1} *components of teicoplanin*

Telachlor timed-release capsules (discontinued 1997) ℞ *antihistamine* [chlorpheniramine maleate] 8, 12 mg

Teladar cream ℞ *topical corticosteroidal anti-inflammatory* [betamethasone dipropionate] 0.05%

Teldrin timed-release capsules (discontinued 1997) OTC *antihistamine* [chlorpheniramine maleate] 12 mg ② Tedral

Teldrin 12-Hour Allergy Relief sustained-release capsules OTC *decongestant; antihistamine* [phenylpropanolamine HCl; chlorpheniramine maleate] 75•8 mg

Tel-E-Amp (trademarked packaging form) *unit dose ampule*

Tel-E-Dose (trademarked packaging form) *unit dose package*

Tel-E-Ject (trademarked delivery system) *prefilled disposable syringe*

telenzepine INN

Tel-E-Pack (trademarked packaging form) *packaging system*

Telepaque tablets ℞ *radiopaque contrast medium for cholecystography* [iopanoic acid (66.68% iodine)] 500 mg (333.4 mg)

Tel-E-Vial (trademarked packaging form) *unit dose vial*

telinavir USAN *antiviral; HIV protease inhibitor*

Teline; Teline-500 capsules (discontinued 1997) ℞ *broad-spectrum antibiotic* [tetracycline HCl] 250 mg; 500 mg

tellurium *element (Te)*

telmisartan USAN *antihypertensive; angiotensin II receptor antagonist*

teloxantrone INN *antineoplastic* [also: teloxantrone HCl]

teloxantrone HCl USAN *antineoplastic* [also: teloxantrone]

teludipine INN, BAN *antihypertensive; calcium channel antagonist* [also: teludipine HCl]

teludipine HCl USAN *antihypertensive; calcium channel antagonist* [also: teludipine]

temafloxacin INN, BAN *antibacterial; microbial DNA topoisomerase inhibitor* [also: temafloxacin HCl]

temafloxacin HCl USAN *antibacterial; microbial DNA topoisomerase inhibitor* [also: temafloxacin]

Temaril tablets, syrup, Spansules (sustained-release capsules) (discontinued 1996) ℞ *antihistamine* [trimeprazine tartrate] 2.5 mg; 2.5 mg/5 mL; 5 mg ⨂ Demerol; Tepanil

temarotene INN

tematropium methylsulfate USAN *anticholinergic* [also: tematropium metilsulfate]

tematropium metilsulfate INN *anticholinergic* [also: tematropium methylsulfate]

temazepam USAN, INN *benzodiazepine hypnotic; minor tranquilizer* 7.5, 15, 30 mg oral

Temazin Cold syrup OTC *decongestant; antihistamine* [phenylpropanolamine HCl; chlorpheniramine maleate] 12.5•2 mg/5 mL

Tembid (trademarked dosage form) *sustained-action capsule*

temefos USAN, INN *veterinary ectoparasiticide*

temelastine USAN, INN, BAN *antihistamine*

temocapril HCl USAN *antihypertensive*

temocillin USAN, INN, BAN *antibacterial*

Temodar capsules ℞ *alkylating antineoplastic for refractory anaplastic astrocytoma; investigational (NDA filed) for recurrent malignant glioma and metastatic malignant melanoma* [temozolomide]

temodox USAN, INN *veterinary growth stimulant*

temoporfin USAN, INN, BAN *photosensitizer for photodynamic cancer therapy*

Temovate ointment, gel, cream, scalp application ℞ *topical corticosteroidal anti-inflammatory* [clobetasol propionate] 0.05%

Temovate Emollient cream ℞ *topical corticosteroidal anti-inflammatory* [clobetasol propionate in an emollient base] 0.05%

temozolomide INN, BAN *investigational (NDA filed) alkylating antineoplastic for malignant glioma and metastatic malignant melanoma*

TEMP (tamoxifen, etoposide, mitoxantrone, Platinol) *chemotherapy protocol*

Tempo chewable tablets OTC *antacid; antiflatulent* [aluminum hydroxide; magnesium hydroxide; calcium car-

bonate; simethicone] 133•81•414•
20 mg

Tempra Quicklets (quickly dissolving tablets) OTC *analgesic; antipyretic* [acetaminophen] 80, 160 mg

Tempra, Children's ⊛ syrup OTC *analgesic; antipyretic* [acetaminophen] 16 mg/mL

Tempra 1 drops OTC *analgesic; antipyretic* [acetaminophen] 100 mg/mL

Tempra 2 syrup OTC *analgesic; antipyretic* [acetaminophen] 160 mg/5 mL

Tempra 3 chewable tablets OTC *analgesic; antipyretic* [acetaminophen] 80, 160 mg

Tempule (trademarked dosage form) *timed-release capsule or tablet*

temurtide USAN, INN, BAN *vaccine adjuvant*

10 Benzagel; 5 Benzagel gel ℞ *topical keratolytic for acne* [benzoyl peroxide] 10%; 5%

10% LMD IV injection ℞ *plasma volume expander for shock due to hemorrhage, burns, or surgery* [dextran 40] 10%

tenamfetamine INN

Tencet capsules ℞ *analgesic; antipyretic; sedative* [acetaminophen; caffeine; butalbital] 325•40•50 mg

Tencon capsules ℞ *analgesic* [acetaminophen; butalbital] 650•50 mg

tendamistat INN

Tenex tablets ℞ *antihypertensive; antiadrenergic* [guanfacine HCl] 1, 2 mg

tenidap USAN, INN *anti-inflammatory for osteoarthritis and rheumatoid arthritis; cytokine inhibitor*

tenidap sodium USAN *anti-inflammatory for osteoarthritis and rheumatoid arthritis*

tenilapine INN

teniloxazine INN

tenilsetam INN

teniposide USAN, INN, BAN *antineoplastic for refractory childhood acute lymphocytic leukemia (orphan)*

Ten-K controlled-release tablets ℞ *potassium supplement* [potassium chloride] 750 mg (10 mEq)

tenoate INN *combining name for radicals or groups*

tenocyclidine INN

Tenol-Plus tablets (discontinued 1995) OTC *analgesic; antipyretic; anti-inflammatory* [acetaminophen; aspirin; caffeine] 250•250•65 mg

tenonitrozole INN

Tenoretic 50; Tenoretic 100 tablets ℞ *antihypertensive; β-blocker; diuretic* [chlorthalidone; atenolol] 25•50 mg; 25•100 mg

Tenormin tablets, IV injection ℞ *antianginal; antihypertensive; β-blocker* [atenolol] 25, 50, 100 mg; 5 mg/10 mL

tenoxicam USAN, INN, BAN *anti-inflammatory*

Tensilon IV or IM injection ℞ *myasthenia gravis treatment; antidote to curare overdose* [edrophonium chloride] 10 mg/mL

Ten-Tab (trademarked dosage form) *controlled-release tablet*

Tenuate tablets, Dospan (controlled-release tablets) ℞ *anorexiant; CNS stimulant* [diethylpropion HCl] 25 mg; 75 mg

tenylidone INN

teoclate INN *combining name for radicals or groups* [also: theoclate]

teopranitol INN

teoprolol INN

T.E.P. tablets OTC *antiasthmatic; bronchodilator; decongestant; sedative* [theophylline; ephedrine HCl; phenobarbital]

Tepanil tablets, Ten-tab (sustained-release tablets) (discontinued 1995) ℞ *anorexiant; CNS stimulant* [diethylpropion HCl] 25 mg; 75 mg ⊠ Temaril; Tofranil

tepirindole INN

tepoxalin USAN, INN *antipsoriatic*

teprenone INN

teprosilate INN *combining name for radicals or groups*

teprotide USAN, INN *angiotensin-converting enzyme (ACE) inhibitor*

Tequin ℞ *investigational (NDA filed) broad-spectrum fluoroquinolone antibiotic* [gatifloxacin]

Terak ophthalmic ointment ℞ *topical ophthalmic antibiotic* [oxytetracycline HCl; polymyxin B sulfate] 5 mg• 10 000 U per g

Terazol 3 vaginal suppositories, vaginal cream ℞ *antifungal* [terconazole] 80 mg; 0.8%

Terazol 7 vaginal cream ℞ *antifungal* [terconazole] 0.4%

terazosin INN, BAN α_1-*adrenergic blocker for hypertension and benign prostatic hyperplasia* [also: terazosin HCl]

terazosin HCl USAN α_1-*adrenergic blocker for hypertension and benign prostatic hyperplasia* [also: terazosin]

terbinafine USAN, INN, BAN *allylamine antifungal* [also: terbinafine HCl]

terbinafine HCl JAN *allylamine antifungal* [also: terbinafine]

terbium *element (Tb)*

terbucromil INN

terbufibrol INN

terbuficin INN

terbuprol INN

terbutaline INN, BAN *sympathomimetic bronchodilator* [also: terbutaline sulfate]

terbutaline sulfate USAN, USP *sympathomimetic bronchodilator* [also: terbutaline]

terciprazine INN

terconazole USAN, INN, BAN *vaginal antifungal*

terfenadine USAN, USP, INN, JAN *piperidine antihistamine*

terflavoxate INN

terfluranol INN

terguride INN *investigational dopamine agonist for central nervous system disorders*

teriparatide USAN, INN *diagnostic aid for hypocalcemia; anabolic osteoporosis treatment for women*

teriparatide acetate USAN, JAN *diagnostic aid for parathyroid-induced hypocalcemia (orphan)*

terizidone INN

terlakiren USAN *antihypertensive; renin inhibitor*

terlipressin INN, BAN *investigational (orphan) for bleeding esophageal varices*

ternidazole INN

terodiline INN, BAN, JAN *coronary vasodilator* [also: terodiline HCl]

terodiline HCl USAN *coronary vasodilator; investigational agent for urinary incontinence* [also: terodiline]

terofenamate INN

teroxalene INN *antischistosomal* [also: teroxalene HCl]

teroxalene HCl USAN *antischistosomal* [also: teroxalene]

teroxirone USAN, INN *antineoplastic*

terpin hydrate USP *(disapproved for use as an expectorant in 1991)* 85 mg/5 mL oral

terpinol [see: terpin hydrate]

Terra-Cortril eye drop suspension ℞ *topical ophthalmic corticosteroidal anti-inflammatory; antibiotic* [hydrocortisone acetate; oxytetracycline HCl] 1.5%•0.5%

terrafungine [see: oxytetracycline]

Terramycin capsules ℞ *broad-spectrum tetracycline antibiotic* [oxytetracycline HCl] 250 mg ☑ Garamycin; Theramycin

Terramycin IM injection ℞ *broad-spectrum tetracycline antibiotic* [oxytetracycline; lidocaine] 50 mg•2%, 125 mg•2% per mL

Terramycin with Polymyxin B ophthalmic ointment ℞ *topical ophthalmic antibiotic* [oxytetracycline HCl; polymyxin B sulfate] 5 mg•10 000 U per g

Tersaseptic shampoo/cleanser OTC *soap-free therapeutic cleanser*

tertatolol INN, BAN

tertiary amyl alcohol [see: amylene hydrate]

tert-pentyl alcohol [see: amylene hydrate]

Tesamone IM injection ℞ *androgen replacement for delayed puberty or breast cancer* [testosterone] 100 mg/mL

tesicam USAN, INN *anti-inflammatory*

tesimide USAN, INN *anti-inflammatory*

Teslac tablets ℞ *adjunctive hormonal chemotherapy for advanced postmenopausal breast carcinoma* [testolactone] 50 mg

Teslascan IV injection ℞ *MRI contrast medium for liver imaging* [mangofodipir trisodium] 37.9 mg/mL (50 μmol/mL)

TESPA (triethylenethiophosphoramide) [see: thiotepa]

Tessalon Perles (capsules) ℞ *antitussive* [benzonatate] 100 mg

Test Pack kit for professional use *in vitro diagnostic aid for Group A streptococcal antigens in throat swabs* [enzyme immunoassay]

Testandro IM injection ℞ *androgen replacement for delayed puberty or breast cancer* [testosterone] 100 mg/mL

Tes-Tape reagent strips for home use (discontinued 1996) OTC *in vitro diagnostic aid for urine glucose*

Test-Estro Cypionates IM injection ℞ *estrogen/androgen for menopausal vasomotor symptoms* [estradiol cypionate; testosterone cypionate] 2•50 mg/mL

Testoderm; Testoderm with Adhesive transdermal patch (for scrotal area) ℞ *hormone replacement therapy for hypogonadism* [testosterone] 4, 6 mg/day (10, 15 mg)

Testoderm TTS transdermal patch (for nonscrotal skin) ℞ *hormone replacement therapy for hypogonadism* [testosterone] 5 mg/day

testolactone USAN, USP, INN *antineoplastic; androgen hormone* ☑ testosterone

Testopel pellets for subcu implantation ℞ *hormone replacement therapy for hypogonadism* [testosterone] 75 mg

testosterone USP, INN, BAN *androgen; investigational (orphan) for AIDS-wasting syndrome and delay of growth and puberty in boys; investigational (Phase III) for testosterone deficiency in men* ☑ testolactone

Testosterone Aqueous IM injection ℞ *androgen for hypogonadism, delayed puberty, and androgen-responsive metastatic cancers* [testosterone] 25, 50, 100 mg/mL

testosterone cyclopentanepropionate [see: testosterone cypionate]

testosterone cyclopentylpropionate [see: testosterone cypionate]

testosterone cypionate USP *parenteral androgen; sometimes abused as a street drug* 100, 200 mg/mL

testosterone enanthate USP *parenteral androgen; sometimes abused as a street drug* 100, 200 mg/mL injection

testosterone heptanoate [see: testosterone enanthate]

testosterone ketolaurate USAN, INN *androgen*

testosterone 3-oxododecanoate [see: testosterone ketolaurate]

testosterone phenylacetate USAN *androgen*

testosterone propionate USP *parenteral androgen; investigational (orphan) for vulvar dystrophies* 100 mg/mL injection

TestPack [see: Abbott TestPack]

Testred capsules ℞ *androgen for male hypogonadism, impotence and breast cancer* [methyltestosterone] 10 mg

tetanus antitoxin USP *passive immunizing agent*

tetanus & gas gangrene antitoxins NF

tetanus & gas gangrene polyvalent antitoxin [see: tetanus & gas gangrene antitoxins]

tetanus immune globulin USP *passive immunizing agent*

tetanus immune human globulin [now: tetanus immune globulin]

tetanus toxoid USP *active immunizing agent*

tetanus toxoid, adsorbed USP *active immunizing agent*

tetiothalein sodium [see: iodophthalein sodium]

tetnicoran [see: nicofurate]

tetrabarbital INN

tetrabenazine INN, BAN *investigational (orphan) for Huntington's disease and severe tardive dyskinesia*

TetraBriks (trademarked delivery form) *ready-to-use liquid containers*

tetracaine USP, INN *topical local anesthetic* [also: amethocaine]

tetracaine HCl USP, JAN *topical local anesthetic* [also: amethocaine HCl]

Tetracap capsules ℞ *broad-spectrum antibiotic* [tetracycline HCl] 250 mg

tetrachlorodecaoxide *investigational (Phase III) immunomodulator and growth factor for HIV and AIDS*

tetrachloroethylene USP

tetrachloromethane [see: carbon tetrachloride]

tetracosactide INN *adrenocorticotropic hormone* [also: cosyntropin; tetracosactrin]

tetracosactrin BAN *adrenocorticotropic hormone* [also: cosyntropin; tetracosactide]

tetracyclics *a class of antidepressants which enhance noradrenergic and serotonergic activity by blocking norepinephrine or serotonin uptake*

tetracycline USP, INN, BAN *bacteriostatic antibiotic; antirickettsial*

tetracycline HCl USP *bacteriostatic antibiotic; antirickettsial* 100, 250, 500 mg oral; 125 mg/5 mL oral

tetracycline phosphate complex USP, BAN *antibacterial*

tetracyclines *a class of bacteriostatic, antimicrobial antibiotics*

Tetracyn; Tetracyn 500 capsules ℞ *broad-spectrum antibiotic* [tetracycline HCl]

tetradecanoic acid, methylethyl ester [see: isopropyl myristate]

tetradonium bromide INN

tetraethylammonium bromide (TEAB) [see: tetrylammonium bromide]

tetraethylammonium chloride (TEAC)

tetraethylthiuram disulfide [see: disulfiram]

tetrafilcon A USAN *hydrophilic contact lens material*

tetraglycine hydroperiodide *source of iodine for disinfecting water*

tetrahydroacridinamine (THA) [see: tacrine HCl]

tetrahydroaminoacridine (THA) [see: tacrine HCl]

tetrahydrocannabinol (THC) [see: dronabinol]

tetrahydrolipstatin [see: orlistat]

tetrahydrozoline BAN *vasoconstrictor; nasal decongestant; topical ophthalmic decongestant* [also: tetrhydrozoline HCl; tetryzoline]

tetrahydrozoline HCl USP *vasoconstrictor; nasal decongestant; topical ophthalmic decongestant* [also: tetryzoline; tetrahydrozoline] 0.05% eye drops

tetraiodophenolphthalein sodium [see: iodophthalein sodium]

Tetralan syrup (discontinued 1997) ℞ *broad-spectrum antibiotic* [tetracycline HCl] 125 mg/5 mL

Tetralan "250"; Tetralan-500 capsules (discontinued 1997) ℞ *broad-spectrum antibiotic* [tetracycline HCl] 250 mg; 500 mg

tetrallobarbital [see: butalbital]

Tetram capsules (discontinued 1996) ℞ *broad-spectrum antibiotic* [tetracycline HCl] 250 mg

tetramal [see: tetrabarbital]

tetrameprozine [see: aminopromazine]

tetramethrin INN

tetramethylene dimethanesulfonate [see: busulfan]

tetramisole INN *anthelmintic* [also: tetramisole HCl]

tetramisole HCl USAN *anthelmintic* [also: tetramisole]

Tetramune IM injection ℞ *pediatric vaccine for diphtheria, pertussis, tetanus and Haemophilus influenzae type b* [diphtheria & tetanus toxoids & whole-cell pertussis (DTwP) vaccine; Hemophilus b conjugate vaccine] 0.5 mL

tetranitrol [see: erythrityl tetranitrate]

tetrantoin

TetraPaks (trademarked delivery form) *ready-to-use open system containers*

Tetrasine; Tetrasine Extra eye drops OTC *topical ophthalmic decongestant and vasoconstrictor* [tetrahydrozoline HCl] 0.05%

tetrasodium ethylenediaminete-traacetate [see: edetate sodium]

tetrasodium pyrophosphate [see: sodium pyrophosphate]

tetrazepam INN

tetrazolast INN *antiallergic; antiasthmatic* [also: tetrazolast meglumine]

tetrazolast meglumine USAN *antiallergic; antiasthmatic* [also: tetrazolast]

tetridamine INN *analgesic; anti-inflammatory* [also: tetrydamine]

tetriprofen INN

tetrofosmin USAN, INN, BAN *diagnostic aid*

tetronasin BAN [also: tetronasin 5930]

tetronasin 5930 INN [also: tetronasin]

tetroquinone USAN, INN *systemic keratolytic*

tetroxoprim USAN, INN *antibacterial*

tetrydamine USAN *analgesic; anti-inflammatory* [also: tetridamine]

tetrylammonium bromide INN

tetryzoline INN *vasoconstrictor; nasal decongestant; topical ocular decongestant* [also: tetrahydrozoline HCl; tetrahydrozoline]

tetryzoline HCl [see: tetrahydrozoline HCl]

tetterwort *medicinal herb* [see: bloodroot; celandine]

Teveten *investigational (NDA filed) agent for the treatment of hypertension* [eprosartan mesylate]

Texacort solution ℞ *topical corticosteroidal anti-inflammatory* [hydrocortisone] 1%

texacromil INN

6-TG (6-thioguanine) [see: thioguanine]

TG (thyroglobulin) [q.v.]

T-Gen suppositories, pediatric suppositories ℞ *anticholinergic; antiemetic* [trimethobenzamide HCl] 200 mg; 100 mg

T-Gesic capsules ℞ *narcotic analgesic* [hydrocodone bitartrate; acetaminophen] 5•500 mg

αTGI (α-triglycidyl isocyanurate) [see: teroxirone]

TH (theophylline) [q.v.]

TH (thyroid hormone) [see: levothyroxine sodium]

TH-9506 *investigational GRF 1-29 growth hormone-releasing factor analog*

THA (tetrahydroaminoacridine or tetrahydroacridinamine) [see: tacrine HCl]

thalidomide USAN, INN, BAN *sedative; hypnotic; immunomodulator for erythema nodosum leprosum (ENL) (orphan); investigational (Phase III, orphan) cytokine inhibitor for graft vs. host disease, AIDS-wasting syndrome, lupus, and mycobacterial infections; investigational (Phase II, orphan) for various cancers*

Thalitone tablets ℞ *antihypertensive; diuretic* [chlorthalidone] 15, 25 mg

thallium *element (Tl)* ⑨ Valium

thallous chloride Tl 201 USAN, USP *radiopaque contrast medium; radioactive agent*

Thalomid capsules ℞ *immunomodulator for erythema nodosum leprosum (ENL) (orphan); investigational (Phase III, orphan) for graft vs. host disease, AIDS-wasting syndrome, lupus, and mycobacterial infections; investigational (Phase II) for various cancers* [thalidomide] 50 mg

Tham IV infusion ℞ *corrects systemic acidosis associated with cardiac bypass surgery or cardiac arrest* [tromethamine] 18 g/500 mL (150 mEq/500 mL)

thaumatin BAN

THC (tetrahydrocannabinol) [see: dronabinol]

THC (thiocarbanidin)

thebacon INN, BAN

Theelin Aqueous IM injection (discontinued 1995) ℞ *estrogen replacement therapy; antineoplastic for prostatic and breast cancer* [estrone] 2 mg/mL

theine [see: caffeine]

thenalidine INN

thenium closilate INN *veterinary anthelmintic* [also: thenium closylate]

thenium closylate USAN *veterinary anthelmintic* [also: thenium closilate]

thenyldiamine INN

thenylpyramine HCl [see: methapyrilene HCl]

Theo-24 timed-release capsules ℞ *antiasthmatic; bronchodilator* [theophylline] 100, 200, 300 mg

Theobid Duracaps (sustained-release capsules) ℞ *antiasthmatic; bronchodilator* [theophylline] 260 mg

Theobid Jr. Duracaps (sustained-release capsules) (discontinued 1996) ℞ *antiasthmatic; bronchodilator* [theophylline] 130 mg

theobromine NF

theobromine calcium salicylate NF

theobromine sodium acetate NF

theobromine sodium salicylate NF

Theobromo cacao medicinal herb [see: cocoa]

Theochron extended-release tablets ℞ *antiasthmatic; bronchodilator* [theophylline] 100, 200, 300 mg

theoclate BAN *combining name for radicals or groups* [also: teoclate]

Theoclear L.A. extended-release capsules ℞ *antiasthmatic; bronchodilator* [theophylline] 130, 260 mg

Theoclear-80 oral solution ℞ *antiasthmatic; bronchodilator* [theophylline] 80 mg/15 mL ⧉ Theolair

theodrenaline INN, BAN

Theodrine tablets OTC *antiasthmatic; bronchodilator; decongestant* [theophylline; ephedrine HCl] 120•22.5 mg

Theo-Dur extended-release tablets ℞ *antiasthmatic; bronchodilator* [theophylline] 100, 200, 300, 450 mg

Theo-Dur Sprinkle sustained-release capsules (discontinued 1996) ℞ *antiasthmatic; bronchodilator* [theophylline] 50, 75, 125, 200 mg

theofibrate USAN *antihyperlipoproteinemic* [also: etofylline clofibrate]

Theolair tablets, liquid ℞ *antiasthmatic; bronchodilator* [theophylline] 125, 250 mg; 80 mg/15 mL ⧉ Theoclear; Thyrolar

Theolair-SR sustained-release tablets ℞ *antiasthmatic; bronchodilator* [theophylline] 200, 250, 300, 500 mg

Theolate liquid ℞ *antiasthmatic; bronchodilator; expectorant* [theophylline; guaifenesin] 150•90 mg/15 mL

Theomax DF pediatric syrup ℞ *antiasthmatic; bronchodilator; decongestant; antihistamine* [theophylline; ephedrine sulfate; hydroxyzine HCl; alcohol 5%] 97.5•18.75•7.5 mg/15 mL

Theo-Organidin elixir (discontinued 1995) ℞ *antiasthmatic; bronchodilator; expectorant* [theophylline; iodinated glycerol] 8•2 mg/mL

theophyldine [see: aminophylline]

theophyllamine [see: aminophylline]

Theophyllin KI elixir ℞ *antiasthmatic; bronchodilator; expectorant* [theophylline; potassium iodide] 80•130 mg/15 mL

theophylline (TH) USP, BAN *bronchodilator* 100, 125, 200, 300, 450 mg oral; 80 mg/15 mL oral

theophylline aminoisobutanol [see: ambuphylline]

theophylline calcium salicylate *bronchodilator*

theophylline ethylenediamine [now: aminophylline]

theophylline monohydrate [see: theophylline]

theophylline olamine USP

theophylline sodium acetate NF

theophylline sodium glycinate USP *smooth muscle relaxant*

Theo-Sav controlled-release tablets ℞ *antiasthmatic; bronchodilator* [theophylline] 100, 200, 300 mg

Theospan-SR timed-release capsules ℞ *antiasthmatic; bronchodilator* [theophylline] 130, 260 mg

Theostat 80 syrup ℞ *antiasthmatic; bronchodilator* [theophylline; alcohol 1%] 80 mg/15 mL

Theovent timed-release capsules ℞ *antiasthmatic; bronchodilator* [theophylline] 125, 250 mg

Theo-X controlled-release tablets ℞ *antiasthmatic; bronchodilator* [theophylline] 100, 200, 300 mg

Thera Hematinic tablets OTC *hematinic; vitamin supplement* [ferrous fumarate; multiple vitamins; folic acid] 66.7• ± •0.33 mg

Thera Multi-Vitamin liquid OTC *vitamin supplement* [multiple vitamins] ±

Therabid tablets OTC *vitamin supplement* [multiple vitamins] ±

Therac lotion OTC *topical acne treatment* [colloidal sulfur] 10%

theraccines *a class of vaccines with therapeutic action, usually used to help prevent the spread of cancer*

TheraCys powder for intravesical instillation ℞ *antineoplastic for urinary bladder cancer* [BCG vaccine, live] 81 mg

TheraDerm transdermal patch ℞ *investigational (orphan) for AIDS-wasting syndrome* [testosterone]

TheraDerm-MTX transdermal patch ℞ *investigational hormone replacement for female testosterone deficiency* [estradiol; testosterone]

Therafectin ℞ *investigational (NDA filed) anti-inflammatory for rheumatoid arthritis* [amiprilose HCl]

TheraFlu Flu, Cold & Cough; NightTime TheraFlu powder for oral solution OTC *antitussive; decongestant; antihistamine; analgesic* [dextromethorphan hydrobromide; pseudoephedrine HCl; chlorpheniramine maleate; acetaminophen] 20•60•4• 650 mg/packet; 30•60•4•1000 mg/packet ⑨ Thera-Flur

TheraFlu Flu & Cold Medicine powder for oral solution OTC *decongestant; antihistamine; analgesic* [pseudoephedrine HCl; chlorpheniramine maleate; acetaminophen] 60•4•650 mg/packet

TheraFlu Non-Drowsy powder for oral solution (name changed to TheraFlu Non-Drowsy Flu, Cold & Cough in 1995)

TheraFlu Non-Drowsy Flu, Cold & Cough powder for oral solution OTC *antitussive; decongestant; analgesic* [dextromethorphan hydrobromide; pseudoephedrine HCl; acetaminophen] 30•60•100 mg/packet

TheraFlu Non-Drowsy Formula caplets OTC *antitussive; decongestant; analgesic* [dextromethorphan hydrobromide; pseudoephedrine HCl; acetaminophen] 15•30•500 mg

Thera-Flur; Thera-Flur-N gel (for self-application) ℞ *topical dental caries preventative* [sodium fluoride] 1.1% ⑨ TheraFlu

Theragenerix tablets (name changed to Therapeutic in 1995)

Theragenerix-H tablets (name changed to Therapeutic-H in 1995)

Theragenerix-M tablets (name changed to Therapeutic-M in 1995)

Thera-Gesic cream OTC *topical analgesic; counterirritant* [methyl salicylate; menthol] 15%• ²

Theragran caplets OTC *vitamin supplement* [multiple vitamins; folic acid; biotin] ±•400•30 μg ⑨ Theragyn

Theragran liquid OTC *vitamin supplement* [multiple vitamins] ± ⑨ Phenergan

Theragran AntiOxidant softgels OTC *vitamin/mineral supplement* [vitamins A, C, and E; multiple minerals] 5000 IU•250 mg•200 IU• ±

Theragran Hematinic tablets ℞ *hematinic; vitamin/mineral supplement* [ferrous fumarate; multiple vitamins & minerals; folic acid] 66.7• ± •0.33 mg

Theragran Stress Formula tablets OTC *vitamin/iron supplement* [multiple B vitamins; vitamins C and E; ferrous fumarate; folic acid; biotin] ±•600 mg•30 IU•27 mg•0.4 mg•45 μg

Theragran-M caplets OTC *vitamin/mineral/calcium/iron supplement* [multiple vitamins & minerals; calcium; iron; folic acid; biotin] ±•40•27• 0.4•0.03 mg

Theragyn ℞ *investigational (Phase III, orphan) adjuvant treatment for ovarian cancer* ⑨ Theragran

Thera-Hist syrup OTC *decongestant; antihistamine* [phenylpropanolamine HCl; chlorpheniramine maleate] 12.5•2 mg/5 mL

Thera-Ject (trademarked delivery system) *prefilled disposable syringe*

Thera-M tablets OTC *vitamin/mineral/iron supplement* [multiple vitamins & minerals; iron; folic acid; biotin] ± • 27 mg•0.4 mg•35 μg

Theramine Expectorant liquid OTC *decongestant; expectorant* [phenylpropanolamine HCl; guaifenesin] 12.5• 100 mg/5 mL

Theramycin Z topical solution ℞ *topical antibiotic for acne* [erythromycin] 2% ⌦ Garamycin; Terramycin

TheraPatch transdermal patch OTC *external analgesic* [methyl salicylate; menthol; camphor]

Therapeutic tablets OTC *vitamin supplement* [multiple vitamins; folic acid; biotin] ± •400•30 μg

Therapeutic B with C capsules OTC *vitamin supplement* [multiple B vitamins; vitamin C] ± •300 mg

Therapeutic Bath lotion, oil OTC *moisturizer; emollient*

Therapeutic Mineral Ice; Therapeutic Mineral Ice Exercise Formula gel OTC *topical analgesic; counterirritant* [menthol] 2%; 4%

Therapeutic-H tablets OTC *hematinic; vitamin supplement* [ferrous fumarate; multiple vitamins; folic acid] 66.7• ± •0.33 mg

Therapeutic-M tablets OTC *vitamin/mineral/iron supplement* [multiple vitamins & minerals; iron; folic acid; biotin] ± •27 mg•0.4 mg•30 μg

Theraplex T shampoo OTC *antiseborrheic; antipsoriatic; antipruritic; antibacterial* [coal tar] 1%

Theraplex Z shampoo OTC *antiseborrheic; antibacterial; antifungal* [pyrithione zinc] 2%

Theratope-STn ℞ *investigational (Phase III) theraccine for recurrent or metastatic breast and colorectal cancer*

Theravee tablets OTC *vitamin supplement* [multiple vitamins; folic acid; biotin] ± •400•15 μg

Theravee Hematinic tablets OTC *hematinic; vitamin supplement* [ferrous fumarate; multiple vitamins; folic acid] 66.7• ± •0.33 mg

Theravee-M tablets OTC *vitamin/mineral/iron supplement* [multiple vitamins & minerals; iron; folic acid; biotin] ± •27 mg•0.4 mg•15 μg

Theravim tablets OTC *vitamin supplement* [multiple vitamins; folic acid; biotin] ± •400•35 μg

Theravim-M tablets OTC *vitamin/mineral/iron supplement* [multiple vitamins & minerals; iron; folic acid; biotin] ± •27 mg•0.4 mg•30 μg

Theravite liquid OTC *vitamin supplement* [multiple vitamins] ± ⌦ Therevac

Therems tablets OTC *vitamin supplement* [multiple vitamins; folic acid; biotin] ± •400•15 μg

Therems-M tablets OTC *vitamin/mineral/iron supplement* [multiple vitamins & minerals; iron; folic acid; biotin] ± •27 mg•0.4 mg•30 μg

Therevac-Plus suppository enema OTC *stool softener; local anesthetic* [docusate sodium; benzocaine] 283• 20 mg ⌦ Theravite

Therevac-SB suppository enema OTC *stool softener* [docusate sodium] 283 mg

Thermazene cream ℞ *broad-spectrum bactericidal for adjunctive burn treatment* [silver sulfadiazine] 10 mg/g

ThexForte caplets OTC *vitamin supplement* [multiple B vitamins; vitamin C] ± •500 mg

THF (thymic humoral factor) [q.v.]

thiabendazole (TBZ) USAN, USP *anthelmintic for strongyloidiasis (threadworm), larva migrans, and trichinosis* [also: tiabendazole]

thiabutazide [see: buthiazide]

thiacetarsamide sodium INN

thiacetazone BAN [also: thioacetazone]

thialbarbital INN [also: thialbarbitone]

thialbarbitone BAN [also: thialbarbital]

thialisobumal sodium [see: buthalital sodium]

thiamazole INN *thyroid inhibitor* [also: methimazole]

thiambutosine INN, BAN

Thiamilate enteric-coated tablets OTC *vitamin supplement* [thiamine HCl] 20 mg

thiamine INN *vitamin B₁; enzyme cofactor* [also: thiamine HCl]

thiamine HCl USP *vitamin B₁; enzyme cofactor* [also: thiamine] 50, 100, 250, 500 mg oral; 100 mg/mL injection

thiamine mononitrate USP *vitamin B₁; enzyme cofactor*

thiamine propyl disulfide [see: prosultiamine]

thiaminogen *medicinal herb* [see: rice bran oil]

thiamiprine USAN *antineoplastic* [also: tiamiprine]

thiamphenicol USAN, INN, BAN *antibacterial*

thiamylal USP *barbiturate general anesthetic*

thiamylal sodium USP, JAN *barbiturate general anesthetic*

thiazesim HCl USAN *antidepressant* [also: tiazesim]

thiazides *a class of diuretic agents that increase urinary excretion of sodium and chloride in approximately equal amounts*

thiazinamium chloride USAN *antiallergic*

thiazinamium metilsulfate INN

4-thiazolidinecarboxylic acid [see: timonacic]

thiazolidinediones *a class of antidiabetic agents that increase insulin sensitivity and reduce plasma insulin levels*

thiazolsulfone [see: thiazosulfone]

thiazosulfone INN

thiazothielite [see: antienite]

thiazothienol [see: antazonite]

thienamycins *a class of antibiotics*

thienobenzodiazepines *a class of novel (atypical) antipsychotic agents*

thiethylperazine USAN, INN *antiemetic; antidopaminergic*

thiethylperazine malate USP *antiemetic; antipsychotic*

thiethylperazine maleate USAN, USP *antiemetic*

thihexinol methylbromide NF, INN

thimbleberry *medicinal herb* [see: blackberry]

thimerfonate sodium USAN *topical anti-infective* [also: sodium timerfonate]

thimerosal USP *topical anti-infective; preservative (49% mercury)* [also: thiomersal] 1:1000 topical

thioacetazone INN, DCF [also: thiacetazone]

thiocarbanidin (THC)

thiocarlide BAN [also: tiocarlide]

thiocolchicine glycoside [see: thiocolchicoside]

thiocolchicoside INN

thioctan; thioctacid; thioctic acid *natural antioxidant* [see: alpha lipoic acid]

thiocyanate sodium NF

thiodiglycol INN

thiodiphenylamine [see: phenothiazine]

thiofuradene INN

thioguanine (6-TG) USAN, USP *antimetabolite antineoplastic* [also: tioguanine] 40 mg oral

thiohexallymal [see: thialbarbital]

thiohexamide INN

Thiola sugar-coated tablets ℞ *prevention of cystine nephrolithiasis in homozygous cystinuria (orphan)* [tiopronin] 100 mg

thiomebumal sodium [see: thiopental sodium]

thiomersal INN, BAN *topical anti-infective; preservative* [also: thimerosal]

thiomesterone BAN [also: tiomesterone]

thiomicid [see: thioacetazone; thiacetazone]

thioparamizone [see: thioacetazone; thiacetazone]

thiopental sodium USP, INN, JAN *barbiturate general anesthetic; anticonvulsant* [also: thiopentone sodium] 2%, 2.5% (20, 25 mg/mL) injection

thiopentone sodium BAN *general anesthetic; anticonvulsant* [also: thiopental sodium]

thiophanate BAN

thiophosphoramide [see: thiotepa]

Thioplex powder for IV, intracavitary, or intravesical injection ℞ *alkylating* antineoplastic for lymphomas and carcinoma of the breast, ovary, or bladder [thiotepa] 15 mg

thiopropazate INN [also: thiopropazate HCl]

thiopropazate HCl NF [also: thiopropazate]

thioproperazine INN, BAN *phenothiazine antipsychotic* [also: thioproperazine mesylate]

thioproperazine mesylate *phenothiazine antipsychotic* [also: thioproperazine]

thioproperazine methanesulfonate [see: thioproperazine mesylate]

thioridazine USAN, USP, INN *phenothiazine antipsychotic; sedative*

thioridazine HCl USP *phenothiazine antipsychotic; sedative* 10, 15, 25, 50, 100, 150, 200 mg oral; 30, 100 mg/mL oral

thiosalan USAN *disinfectant* [also: tiosalan]

Thiosulfil Forte tablets ℞ *broad-spectrum sulfonamide bacteriostatic* [sulfamethizole] 500 mg

thiosulfuric acid, disodium salt pentahydrate [see: sodium thiosulfate]

thiotepa USP, INN, BAN, JAN *alkylating antineoplastic for lymphomas and carcinoma of the breast, ovary, or bladder*

thiotetrabarbital INN

thiothixene USAN, USP, BAN *thioxanthene antipsychotic* [also: tiotixene] 1, 2, 5, 10, 20 mg oral

thiothixene HCl USAN, USP *thioxanthene antipsychotic* 5 mg/mL oral

thiouracil

thiourea *antioxidant*

thioxanthenes *a class of dopamine receptor antagonists with conventional (typical) antipsychotic activity*

thioxolone BAN [also: tioxolone]

thiphenamil HCl USAN *smooth muscle relaxant* [also: tifenamil]

thiphencillin potassium USAN *antibacterial* [also: tifencillin]

thiram USAN, INN *antifungal*

thistle, bitter; holy thistle; Saint Benedict thistle; spotted thistle *medicinal herb* [see: blessed thistle]

thistle, carline; ground thistle *medicinal herb* [see: carline thistle]

thonzonium bromide USAN, USP *detergent; surface-active agent* [also: tonzonium bromide]

thonzylamine HCl USAN, INN

Thorazine tablets, Spansules (capsules), IV or IM injection, syrup, suppositories, concentrate ℞ *conventional (typical) antipsychotic; antiemetic* [chlorpromazine] 10, 25, 50, 100, 200 mg; 30, 75, 150 mg; 25 mg/mL; 10 mg/5 mL; 25, 100 mg; 30, 100 mg/mL

thorium *element (Th)*

thorn, Egyptian *medicinal herb* [see: acacia]

thorn-apple *medicinal herb* [see: hawthorn; jimsonweed]

thousand-leaf; thousand seal *medicinal herb* [see: yarrow]

thozalinone USAN *antidepressant* [also: tozalinone]

THQ (tetrahydroxybenzoquinone) [see: tetroquinone]

THR (trishydroxyethyl rutin) [see: troxerutin]

Threamine DM syrup OTC *antitussive; decongestant; antihistamine* [dextromethorphan hydrobromide; phenylpropanolamine HCl; chlorpheniramine maleate] 10•12.5•2 mg/5 mL

Threamine Expectorant liquid OTC *decongestant; expectorant* [phenylpropanolamine HCl; guaifenesin; alcohol 5%] 12.5•100 mg/5 mL

3 in 1 Toothache Relief gum, liquid, lotion/gel OTC *topical oral anesthetic* [benzocaine]

three-leaved nightshade *medicinal herb* [see: birthroot]

3TC [now: lamivudine]

threonine (L-threonine) USAN, USP, INN *essential amino acid; symbols: Thr, T; investigational (orphan) for familial spastic paraparesis and amyotrophic lateral sclerosis* 500 mg oral

Threostat ℞ *investigational (orphan) for familial spastic paraparesis and amyo-*

trophic lateral sclerosis [L-threonine]
⑨ Triostat

Throat Discs lozenges OTC *analgesic; counterirritant* [capsicum; peppermint oil]

throatwort *medicinal herb* [see: figwort; foxglove]

Thrombate III powder for IV infusion ℞ *for thrombosis and pulmonary emboli of congenital AT-III deficiency (orphan)* [antithrombin III] 500, 1000 IU

thrombin USP, INN *topical local hemostatic*

Thrombinar powder ℞ *topical local hemostatic for surgery* [thrombin] 1000, 5000, 50 000 U

Thrombin-JMI powder ℞ *topical local hemostatic for surgery* [thrombin] 10 000, 20 000, 50 000 U

thrombinogen (prothrombin)

Thrombogen powder ℞ *topical local hemostatic for surgery* [thrombin] 1000, 5000, 10 000, 20 000 U

thrombolytics *a class of enzymes that dissolve blood clots, used emergently to treat stroke, pulmonary embolus, and myocardial infarct*

thromboplastin USP

thrombopoietin, recombinant human *investigational (orphan) adjunct to hematopoietic stem cell transplantation*

Thrombostat powder ℞ *topical local hemostatic for surgery* [thrombin] 5000, 10 000, 20 000 U

throw-wort *medicinal herb* [see: motherwort]

thulium *element (Tm)*

thunder god vine (*Tripterygium wilfordii*) *plant medicinal herb for abscesses, autoimmune diseases, boils, fever, inflammation, tumors, and viruses; also used as an insecticide to kill maggots or larvae and as a rat and bird poison*

Thylline-GG tablets (discontinued 1995) ℞ *antiasthmatic; bronchodilator; expectorant* [dyphylline; guaifenesin] 200•200 mg

thymalfasin USAN *vaccine enhancer for hepatitis C, cancer, and infectious dis-*

eases; investigational (Phase III, orphan) for chronic active hepatitis B; investigational (orphan) for DiGeorge syndrome with immune defects

thyme (*Thymus serpyllum; T. vulgaris*) *plant medicinal herb for acute bronchitis, colic, digestive disorders, gas, gout, headache, laryngitis, lung congestion, sciatica, and throat disorders*

thymic humoral factor, gamma 2 *investigational (Phase II) immunomodulator for HIV*

thymidylate synthase (TS) inhibitors *a class of folate-based antineoplastics*

thymocartin INN

thymoctonan INN *investigational antiviral for HIV infection, genital herpes, and chronic viral hepatitis*

Thymoglobulin ℞ *immunosuppressant for kidney transplants* [anti-human thymocyte immunoglobulin, rabbit]

thymol NF *stabilizer; topical antiseptic*

thymol iodide NF

Thymone ℞ *investigational (orphan) for infant respiratory distress syndrome of prematurity* [protirelin]

thymopentin USAN, INN, BAN *immunoregulator; investigational (Phase III) for asymptomatic HIV infection*

thymopoietin 32-36 [now: thymopentin]

thymosin alpha-1 [now: thymalfasin]

thymostimulin INN *investigational (Phase III) immunomodulator for AIDS*

thymotrinan INN

thymoxamine BAN [also: moxisylyte]

Thymus serpyllum; T. vulgaris *medicinal herb* [see: thyme]

Thypinone IV injection ℞ *diagnostic aid for thyroid function* [protirelin] 500 μg/mL

Thyrar tablets ℞ *thyroid replacement therapy for hypothyroidism or thyroid cancer* [thyroid, desiccated bovine] 30, 60, 120 mg ⑨ Thyrolar

Thyrel-TRH IV injection ℞ *diagnostic aid for thyroid function* [protirelin] 500 μg/mL

Thyro-Block tablets ℞ *thyroid-blocking therapy* [potassium iodide] 130 mg thyrocalcitonin [see: calcitonin]

Thyrogen injection ℞ *recombinant human thyroid-stimulating hormone (rhTSH); diagnostic aid for thyroid cancer (orphan); investigational (NDA filed, orphan) treatment for thyroid cancer* [thyrotropin alfa]

thyroglobulin (TG) USAN, USP, INN *thyroid hormone*

thyroid USP *thyroid hormone* 15, 30, 60, 90, 120, 180, 240, 300 mg oral ② euthroid

thyroid hormone (TH) [see: levo-thyroxine sodium]

Thyroid Strong tablets ℞ *thyroid replacement therapy for hypothyroidism or thyroid cancer* [thyroid, desiccated] 30, 60, 120, 180 mg

thyroid-stimulating hormone (TSH) [see: thyrotropin]

Thyrolar-0.25; -0.5; -1; -2; -3 tablets ℞ *thyroid hormone therapy* [liotrix] 15 mg; 30 mg; 60 mg; 120 mg; 180 mg ② Theolair; Thyrar

thyromedan HCl USAN *thyromimetic* [also: tyromedan]

thyropropic acid INN

thyrotrophic hormone [see: thyro-trophin]

thyrotrophin INN *thyroid-stimulating hormone* [also: thyrotropin]

thyrotropin *thyroid-stimulating hormone; in vivo diagnostic aid for thyroid function* [also: thyrotrophin]

thyrotropin alfa USAN *recombinant human thyroid-stimulating hormone (rhTSH); diagnostic aid for thyroid cancer (orphan); investigational (NDA filed, orphan) treatment for thyroid cancer*

thyrotropin-releasing hormone (TRH) [see: protirelin]

thyroxine BAN *thyroid hormone* [also: levothyroxine sodium]

D-**thyroxine** [see: dextrothyroxine sodium]

L-**thyroxine** [see: levothyroxine sodium]

thyroxine I 125 USAN *radioactive agent*

thyroxine I 131 USAN *radioactive agent*

Thytropar powder for IM or subcu injection ℞ *thyrotrophic hormone; in vivo diagnostic aid for thyroid function* [thyrotropin] 10 IU

TI-23 *investigational (Phase I) antiviral for cytomegalovirus retinitis*

tiabendazole INN *anthelmintic* [also: thiabendazole]

Tiabex (name changed to Gabitril upon marketing release in 1998)

tiacrilast USAN, INN *antiallergic*

tiacrilast sodium USAN *antiallergic*

tiadenol INN

tiafibrate INN

tiagabine INN *anticonvulsant*

tiagabine HCl USAN *anticonvulsant*

Tiamate extended-release film-coated tablets ℞ *antihypertensive; antianginal; antiarrhythmic; calcium channel blocker* [diltiazem maleate] 120, 180, 240 mg

tiamenidine USAN, INN *antihypertensive*

tiamenidine HCl USAN *antihypertensive*

tiametonium iodide INN

tiamiprine INN *antineoplastic* [also: thi-amiprine]

tiamizide INN *diuretic; antihypertensive* [also: diapamide]

tiamulin USAN, INN *veterinary antibacterial*

tiamulin fumarate USAN *veterinary antibacterial*

tianafac INN

tianeptine INN

tiapamil INN, BAN *antagonist to calcium* [also: tiapamil HCl]

tiapamil HCl USAN *antagonist to calcium* [also: tiapamil]

tiapirinol INN

tiapride INN

tiaprofenic acid INN *nonsteroidal anti-inflammatory drug (NSAID)*

tiaprost INN

tiaramide INN, BAN *antiasthmatic* [also: tiaramide HCl]

tiaramide HCl USAN *antiasthmatic* [also: tiaramide]

Tiazac extended-release capsules ℞ *antihypertensive; antianginal; antiar-rhythmic; calcium channel blocker* [diltiazem HCl] 120, 180, 240, 300, 360, 420 mg ② Dyazide; thiazides

tiazesim INN *antidepressant* [also: thiazesim HCl]

tiazesim HCl [see: thiazesim HCl]

tiazofurin USAN *antineoplastic* [also: tiazofurine]

tiazofurine INN *antineoplastic* [also: tiazofurin]

tiazuril USAN, INN *coccidiostat for poultry*

tibalosin INN

tibenelast sodium USAN *antiasthmatic; bronchodilator*

tibenzate INN

tibezonium iodide INN

tibolone USAN, INN, BAN *anabolic*

tibric acid USAN, INN *antihyperlipoproteinemic*

tibrofan USAN, INN *disinfectant*

ticabesone INN *corticosteroid; anti-inflammatory* [also: ticabesone propionate]

ticabesone propionate USAN *corticosteroid; anti-inflammatory* [also: ticabesone]

Ticar powder for IV or IM injection ℞ *extended-spectrum penicillin antibiotic* [ticarcillin disodium] 1, 3, 6, 20, 30 g ⍰ Tigan

ticarbodine USAN, INN *anthelmintic*

ticarcillin INN *extended-spectrum penicillin antibiotic* [also: ticarcillin disodium]

ticarcillin cresyl sodium USAN *extended-spectrum penicillin antibiotic*

ticarcillin disodium USAN, USP *extended-spectrum penicillin antibiotic* [also: ticarcillin]

Tice BCG dermal puncture injection for TB, intravesical instillation for cancer ℞ *tuberculosis immunizing agent; antineoplastic for urinary bladder cancer* [BCG vaccine, Tice strain] 50 mg

tickweed *medicinal herb* [see: pennyroyal]

ticlatone USAN, INN *antibacterial; antifungal*

Ticlid film-coated tablets ℞ *platelet aggregation inhibitor for stroke* [ticlopidine HCl] 250 mg

ticlopidine INN, BAN *platelet aggregation inhibitor* [also: ticlopidine HCl]

ticlopidine HCl USAN *platelet aggregation inhibitor for stroke* [also: ticlopidine] 250 mg oral

ticolubant USAN *leukotriene B_4 receptor antagonist for psoriasis*

Ticon IM injection ℞ *anticholinergic; antiemetic* [trimethobenzamide HCl] 100 mg/mL

ticrynafen USAN *diuretic; uricosuric; antihypertensive* [also: tienilic acid]

tidiacic INN

tiemonium iodide INN, BAN

tienilic acid INN *diuretic; uricosuric; antihypertensive* [also: ticrynafen]

tienocarbine INN

tienopramine INN

tienoxolol INN

tifemoxone INN

tifenamil INN *smooth muscle relaxant* [also: thiphenamil HCl]

tifenamil HCl [see: thiphenamil HCl]

tifencillin INN *antibacterial* [also: thiphencillin potassium]

tifencillin potassium [see: thiphencillin potassium]

tiflamizole INN

tiflorex INN

tifluadom INN

tiflucarbine INN

Tifolar ℞ *investigational antineoplastic* [pemetrexed disodium]

tiformin INN [also: tyformin]

tifurac INN *analgesic* [also: tifurac sodium]

tifurac sodium USAN *analgesic* [also: tifurac]

Tigan capsules, suppositories, pediatric suppositories, IM injection ℞ *antiemetic* [trimethobenzamide HCl] 100, 250 mg; 200 mg; 100 mg; 100 mg/mL/ ⍰ Ticar

tigemonam INN *antimicrobial* [also: tigemonam dicholine]

tigemonam dicholine USAN *antimicrobial* [also: tigemonam]

tigestol USAN, INN *progestin*

tigloidine INN, BAN

tiglylpseudotropine [see: tigloidine]

tiglyltropeine [see: tropigline]

tilactase INN *digestive enzyme*

Tilad (Spanish name for U.S. product Tilade)

Tilade oral inhalation aerosol ℞ *respiratory anti-inflammatory; antiasthmatic; bronchoconstriction inhibitor* [nedocromil sodium] 1.75 mg/dose

tilbroquinol INN

tiletamine INN *anesthetic; anticonvulsant* [also: tiletamine HCl]

tiletamine HCl USAN *anesthetic; anticonvulsant* [also: tiletamine]

Tilia americana; T. cordata; T. europaea; T. platyphyllos *medicinal herb* [see: linden tree]

tilidate HCl BAN *analgesic* [also: tilidine HCl; tilidine]

tilidine INN *analgesic* [also: tilidine HCl; tilidate HCl]

tilidine HCl USAN *analgesic* [also: tilidine; tilidate HCl]

tiliquinol INN

tilisolol INN

tilmicosin USAN, INN, BAN *veterinary antibacterial*

tilmicosin phosphate USAN *veterinary antibacterial*

tilomisole USAN, INN *immunoregulator*

tilorone INN *antiviral* [also: tilorone HCl]

tilorone HCl USAN *antiviral* [also: tilorone]

tilozepine INN

tilsuprost INN

Tiltab (trademarked dosage form) *film-coated tablets*

tiludronate disodium USAN *bisphosphonate bone resorption inhibitor for Paget's disease*

tiludronic acid INN

Timecap (trademarked dosage form) *sustained-release capsule*

Timecelle (trademarked dosage form) *timed-release capsule*

timefurone USAN, INN *antiatherosclerotic*

timegadine INN

Time-Hist sustained-release capsules ℞ *decongestant; antihistamine* [pseudoephedrine HCl; chlorpheniramine maleate] 120•8 mg

timelotem INN

Timentin powder or frozen premix for IV infusion ℞ *extended-spectrum penicillin antibiotic* [ticarcillin disodium; clavulanate potassium] 3•0.1 g

timepidium bromide INN

Timespan (trademarked dosage form) *timed-release tablets*

Timesules (dosage form) *sustained-release capsules*

timiperone INN

timobesone INN *topical adrenocortical steroid* [also: timobesone acetate]

timobesone acetate USAN *topical adrenocortical steroid* [also: timobesone]

Timodal ⒸⒶⓃ (U.S. product: Timoptic) eye drops ℞ *topical antiglaucoma agent (β-blocker)* [timolol maleate] 0.25%, 0.5%

timofibrate INN

Timolide 10-25 tablets ℞ *antihypertensive; β-blocker; diuretic* [timolol maleate; hydrochlorothiazide] 10•25 mg

timolol USAN, INN, BAN *antiadrenergic (β-receptor)* ② atenolol

timolol hemihydrate *topical antiglaucoma agent (β-blocker)*

timolol maleate USAN, USP *antianginal; antihypertensive; antiadrenergic (β-receptor); topical antiglaucoma agent; migraine preventative* 5, 10, 20 mg oral; 0.25%, 0.5% eye drops

timonacic INN

timoprazole INN

Timoptic Ocumeter (eye drops), Ocudose (single-use eye drop dispenser) ℞ *topical antiglaucoma agent (β-blocker)* [timolol maleate] 0.25%, 0.5%

Timoptic-XE ophthalmic gel ℞ *topical once-daily antiglaucoma agent (β-blocker)* [timolol maleate] 0.25%, 0.5%

Timunox ℞ *investigational (Phase III) immunomodulator for asymptomatic HIV infection* [thymopentin]

tin *element (Sn)*

tin chloride dihydrate [see: stannous chloride]

tin ethyl etiopurpurin *investigational (Phase III) treatment for various cancers by photodynamic therapy; investi-*

gational *(Phase III) for age-related macular degeneration (AMD)*

tin etiopurpurin dichloride *investigational (Phase I/II) photosensitizer for age-related macular degeneration (AMD)*

tin fluoride [see: stannous fluoride]

tinabinol USAN, INN *antihypertensive*

Tinactin cream, powder, spray powder, spray liquid, solution OTC *topical antifungal* [tolnaftate] 1% ② Taractan

Tinactin; Tinactin Plus ⓐ powder, aerosol powder OTC *topical antifungal* [tolnaftate] 1%

Tinactin for Jock Itch cream, spray powder OTC *topical antifungal* [tolnaftate] 1%

tinazoline INN

TinBen tincture OTC *skin protectant* [benzoin; alcohol 75–83%]

TinCoBen tincture OTC *skin protectant* [benzoin; aloe; alcohol 77%]

Tincture of Green Soap liquid OTC *antiseptic cleanser* [green soap; alcohol 28–32%]

Tindal sugar-coated tablets (discontinued 1995) ℞ *antipsychotic* [acetophenazine maleate] 20 mg

Tine Test OT [see: Tuberculin Tine Test, Old]

Tine Test PPD single-use intradermal puncture test device ℞ *tuberculosis skin test* [tuberculin purified protein derivative] 5 U

Ting cream, powder, spray powder, spray liquid (discontinued 1998) OTC *topical antifungal* [tolnaftate] 1%

tinidazole USAN, INN *antiprotozoal*

tinisulpride INN

tinofedrine INN

tinoridine INN

Tinver lotion ℞ *topical antifungal; keratolytic; antipruritic; anesthetic* [sodium thiosulfate; salicylic acid; alcohol 10%] 25%•1%

tinzaparin sodium USAN, INN, BAN *anticoagulant; antithrombotic*

tiocarlide INN [also: thiocarlide]

tioclomarol INN

tioconazole USAN, USP, INN, BAN, JAN *antifungal*

tioctilate INN

tiodazosin USAN, INN *antihypertensive*

tiodonium chloride USAN, INN *antibacterial*

tiofacic [see: stepronin]

tioguanine INN *antineoplastic* [also: thioguanine]

tiomergine INN

tiomesterone INN [also: thiomesterone]

tioperidone INN *antipsychotic* [also: tioperidone HCl]

tioperidone HCl USAN *antipsychotic* [also: tioperidone]

tiopinac USAN, INN *anti-inflammatory; analgesic; antipyretic*

tiopronin INN *prevention of cystine nephrolithiasis in homozygous cystinuria (orphan)*

tiopropamine INN

tiosalan INN *disinfectant* [also: thiosalan]

tiosinamine [see: allylthiourea]

tiospirone INN *antipsychotic* [also: tiospirone HCl]

tiospirone HCl USAN *antipsychotic* [also: tiospirone]

tiotidine USAN, INN *antagonist to histamine H_2 receptors*

tiotixene INN *thioxanthene antipsychotic* [also: thiothixene]

tioxacin INN

tioxamast INN

tioxaprofen INN

tioxidazole USAN, INN *anthelmintic*

tioxolone INN [also: thioxolone]

tipentosin INN, BAN *antihypertensive* [also: tipentosin HCl]

tipentosin HCl USAN *antihypertensive* [also: tipentosin]

tipepidine INN

tipetropium bromide INN

tipindole INN

tipranavir disodium USAN *antiviral protease inhibitor*

tipredane USAN, INN, BAN *topical adrenocortical steroid*

tiprenolol INN *antiadrenergic (β-receptor)* [also: tiprenolol HCl]

tiprenolol HCl USAN *antiadrenergic (β-receptor)* [also: tiprenolol]

tiprinast INN *antiallergic* [also: tiprinast meglumine]

tiprinast meglumine USAN *antiallergic* [also: tiprinast]

tipropidil INN *vasodilator* [also: tipropidil HCl]

tipropidil HCl USAN *vasodilator* [also: tipropidil]

tiprostanide INN, BAN

tiprotimod INN

tiqueside USAN, INN *antihyperlipidemic*

tiquinamide INN *gastric anticholinergic* [also: tiquinamide HCl]

tiquinamide HCl USAN *gastric anticholinergic* [also: tiquinamide]

tiquizium bromide INN

tirapazamine USAN, INN *antineoplastic*

tiratricol INN

tiratricol & levothyroxine sodium *investigational (orphan) to suppress thyroid-stimulating hormone (TSH) in thyroid cancer*

Tirend tablets (discontinued 1998) OTC *CNS stimulant; analeptic* [caffeine] 100 mg

tirilazad INN, BAN *lipid peroxidation inhibitor; 21-aminosteroid (lazaroid) antioxidant* [also: tirilazad mesylate]

tirilazad mesylate USAN *lipid peroxidation inhibitor; 21-aminosteroid (lazaroid) antioxidant; investigational (Phase I/II) protease inhibitor for HIV* [also: tirilazad]

tirofiban HCl USAN *glycoprotein (GP) IIb/IIIa receptor antagonist; platelet aggregation inhibitor for acute coronary syndrome, unstable angina, myocardial infarction, and cardiac surgery*

tiropramide INN

tisilfocon A USAN *hydrophobic contact lens material*

Tisit liquid, shampoo OTC *pediculicide for lice* [pyrethrins; piperonyl butoxide] 0.3%•2%; 0.3%•3%

Tisit Blue gel OTC *pediculicide for lice* [pyrethrins; piperonyl butoxide; petroleum distillate] 0.3%•3%•1.2%

tisocromide INN

TiSol solution OTC *anesthetic and antimicrobial throat irrigation* [benzyl alcohol; menthol] 1%•0.04%

tisopurine INN

tisoquone INN

tissue factor [see: thromboplastin]

tissue plasminogen activator (tPA; t-PA) [see: alteplase]

Tis-U-Sol solution ℞ *sterile irrigant* [physiological irrigating solution]

Titan solution OTC *cleaning solution for hard contact lenses*

titanium *element (Ti)*

titanium dioxide USP *topical protectant; astringent*

titanium oxide [see: titanium dioxide]

Titradose (trademarked dosage form) *scored tablet*

Titralac chewable tablets OTC *antacid* [calcium carbonate] 420, 750 mg

Titralac Plus chewable tablets, liquid OTC *antacid; antiflatulent* [calcium carbonate; simethicone] 420•21 mg; 500•20 mg/5 mL

tivanidazole INN

tivazine [see: piperazine citrate]

tixadil INN

tixanox USAN *antiallergic* [also: tixanoxum]

tixanoxum INN *antiallergic* [also: tixanox]

tixocortol INN *topical anti-inflammatory* [also: tixocortol pivalate]

tixocortol pivalate USAN *topical anti-inflammatory* [also: tixocortol]

Tixogel VP *investigational topical skin protectant for allergic contact dermatitis* [bentoquatam]

tizabrin INN

tizanidine INN, BAN *antispasmodic; central α₂ agonist* [also: tizanidine HCl]

tizanidine HCl USAN, JAN *antispasmodic for multiple sclerosis and spinal cord injury (orphan); central α₂ agonist* [also: tizanidine]

tizolemide INN

tizoprolic acid INN

TJ-9 *investigational herbal compound (Sho-Saiko-To) adjunct for HIV*

T-Koff liquid ℞ *narcotic antitussive; decongestant; antihistamine* [codeine phosphate; phenylpropanolamine HCl; phenylephrine HCl; chlorpheniramine maleate] 10•20•20•5 mg/5 mL

²⁰¹Tl [see: thallous chloride Tl 201]

TLC ABLC ℞ *investigational systemic antifungal for bone marrow transplants* [amphotericin B lipid complex (ABLC)]

TLC C-53 *investigational cell adhesion antagonist for adult respiratory distress syndrome*

TLC D-99 *investigational liposomal form of doxorubicin for Kaposi sarcoma*

T-lymphotrophic virus antigens [see: human T-lymphotropic virus type III (HTLV-III) gp-160 antigens]

TMB (trimedoxime bromide) [q.v.]

TMP (trimethoprim) [q.v.]

TMP-SMZ (trimethoprim & sulfamethoxazole) [q.v.]

TNF (tumor necrosis factor) [q.v.]

TNK-tPA ℞ *investigational (Phase II) second-generation tissue plasminogen activator for the treatment of acute myocardial infarction*

TNP-470 *investigational angiogenesis inhibitor for AIDS-related Kaposi sarcoma*

TNT (tumor necrosis therapy) [q.v.]

TOAP (thioguanine, Oncovin, [cytosine] arabinoside, prednisone) *chemotherapy protocol*

tobacco *dried leaves of the Nicotiana tabacum plant; sedative narcotic; emetic; diuretic; heart depressant; antispasmodic* [also see: nicotine]

tobacco, British *medicinal herb* [see: coltsfoot]

tobacco, Indian; wild tobacco *medicinal herb* [see: lobelia]

tobacco, sailor's *medicinal herb* [see: mugwort]

tobacco wood *medicinal herb* [see: witch hazel]

TOBI solution for inhalation ℞ *antibiotic for Pseudomonas aeruginosa lung infections in cystic fibrosis patients*

(orphan); investigational (Phase II) for bronchiectasis and pulmonary tuberculosis [tobramycin] 300 mg/5 mL

toborinone USAN *cardiotonic*

TobraDex eye drop suspension ℞ *topical ophthalmic corticosteroidal anti-inflammatory; antibiotic* [dexamethasone; tobramycin] 0.1%•0.3% ⑨ Tobrex

TobraDex ophthalmic ointment ℞ *topical ophthalmic corticosteroidal anti-inflammatory; antibiotic* [dexamethasone; tobramycin; chlorobutanol] 0.1%•0.3%•0.5%

tobramycin USAN, USP, INN, BAN *aminoglycoside antibiotic; inhalant for Pseudomonas aeruginosa lung infections in cystic fibrosis patients (orphan)* 0.3% eye drops ⑨ Trobicin

tobramycin sulfate USP *aminoglycoside antibiotic* 10, 40 mg/mL injection

Tobrex Drop-Tainers (eye drops), ophthalmic ointment ℞ *topical ophthalmic antibiotic* [tobramycin] 0.3%; 3 mg/g ⑨ TobraDex

tobuterol INN

tocainide USAN, INN, BAN *antiarrhythmic*

tocainide HCl USP *antiarrhythmic*

tocamphyl USAN, INN *choleretic*

Tocicodendron diversilobum *medicinal herb* [see: poison oak]

tocofenoxate INN

tocofersolan INN *vitamin E supplement* [also: tocophersolan]

tocofibrate INN

tocolytics *a class of drugs used to inhibit uterine contractions*

tocopherol, d-alpha [see: vitamin E]

tocopherol, dl-alpha [see: vitamin E]

tocopherols, mixed [see: vitamin E]

tocopherols excipient NF *antioxidant*

tocophersolan USAN *vitamin E supplement* [also: tocofersolan]

tocopheryl acetate, d-alpha [see: vitamin E]

tocopheryl acetate, dl-alpha [see: vitamin E]

tocopheryl acid succinate, d-alpha [see: vitamin E]

tocopheryl acid succinate, dl-alpha [see: vitamin E]

tocopheryl polyethylene glycol suc-cinate (TPGS) [see: tocophersolan]

Today vaginal sponge (discontinued 1995) OTC *spermicidal/barrier contra-ceptive* [nonoxynol 9] 1 g

todralazine INN, BAN

tofenacin INN *anticholinergic* [also: tofenacin HCl]

tofenacin HCl USAN *anticholinergic* [also: tofenacin]

tofesilate INN *combining name for radi-cals or groups*

tofetridine INN

tofisoline

tofisopam INN

Tofranil IM injection (discontinued 1999) ℞ *tricyclic antidepressant* [imip-ramine HCl] 25 mg/2 mL ☑ Tepanil

Tofranil sugar-coated tablets ℞ *tri-cyclic antidepressant; treatment for childhood enuresis* [imipramine HCl] 10, 25, 50 mg ☑ Tepanil

Tofranil-PM capsules ℞ *tricyclic anti-depressant* [imipramine pamoate] 75, 100, 125, 150 mg

tolamolol USAN, INN *vasodilator; anti-arrhythmic; antiadrenergic (β-receptor)*

tolazamide USAN, USP, INN, BAN *sulfo-nylurea antidiabetic* 100, 250, 500 mg oral

tolazoline INN *peripheral vasodilator* [also: tolazoline HCl]

tolazoline HCl USP *peripheral vasodila-tor for neonatal persistent pulmonary hypertension* [also: tolazoline]

tolboxane INN

tolbutamide USP, INN, BAN *sulfonyl-urea antidiabetic* 500 mg oral

tolbutamide sodium USP *diagnostic aid for diabetes*

tolcapone USAN, INN *antiparkinsonian; catechol-O-methyltransferase (COMT) inhibitor*

tolciclate USAN, INN *antifungal*

tolclotide [see: disulfamide]

toldimfos INN, BAN

Tolectin 200; Tolectin 600 tablets ℞ *nonsteroidal anti-inflammatory drug (NSAID); antiarthritic; analgesic* [tol-metin sodium] 200 mg; 600 mg

Tolectin DS capsules ℞ *nonsteroidal anti-inflammatory drug (NSAID); antiarthritic; analgesic* [tolmetin sodium] 400 mg

Tolerex powder OTC *enteral nutritional therapy* [lactose-free formula]

tolfamide USAN, INN *urease enzyme inhibitor*

tolfenamic acid INN, BAN

Tolfrinic film-coated tablets OTC *hema-tinic* [ferrous fumarate; cyanocobala-min; ascorbic acid] 200 mg•25 μg• 100 mg

tolgabide USAN, INN, BAN *anticonvulsant*

tolhexamide [see: glycyclamide]

tolimidone USAN, INN *antiulcerative*

Tolinase tablets ℞ *sulfonylurea antidia-betic* [tolazamide] 100, 250, 500 mg ☑ Orinase

tolindate USAN, INN *antifungal*

toliodium chloride USAN, INN *veteri-nary food additive*

toliprolol INN

tolmesoxide INN

tolmetin USAN, INN *nonsteroidal anti-inflammatory drug (NSAID); analgesic*

tolmetin sodium USAN, USP *antiar-thritic; nonsteroidal anti-inflammatory drug (NSAID); analgesic* 200, 400, 600 mg oral

tolnaftate USAN, USP, INN, BAN *anti-fungal* 1% topical

tolnapersine INN

tolnidamine INN

toloconium metilsulfate INN

tolofocon A USAN *hydrophobic contact lens material*

tolonidine INN

tolonium chloride INN *blue dye used in histology; diagnostic aid for oral cancer*

toloxatone INN

toloxichloral [see: toloxychlorinol]

toloxychlorinol INN

tolpadol INN

tolpentamide INN, BAN

tolperisone INN, BAN

tolpiprazole INN, BAN

tolpovidone I 131 USAN *hypoalbu-minemia test; radioactive agent* [also: radiotolpovidone I 131]

tolpronine INN, BAN
tolpropamine INN, BAN
tolpyrramide USAN, INN *antidiabetic*
tolquinzole INN
tolrestat USAN, INN, BAN *aldose reductase inhibitor for diabetic neuropathy*
tolterodine USAN *muscarinic receptor antagonist for urinary incontinence*
tolterodine tartrate *muscarinic receptor antagonist for urinary frequency, urgency, and incontinence*
toltrazuril USAN, INN, BAN *veterinary coccidiostat*
tolu balsam USP *pharmaceutic aid*
p-**toluenesulfone dichloramine** [see: dichloramine T]
tolufazepam INN
toluidine blue O [see: tolonium chloride]
toluidine blue O chloride [see: tolonium chloride]
Tolu-Sed DM syrup OTC *antitussive; expectorant* [dextromethorphan hydrobromide; guaifenesin; alcohol 10%] 10•100 mg/5 mL
tolycaine INN, BAN
tomelukast USAN, INN *antiasthmatic; leukotriene antagonist*
Tomocat concentrated oral suspension ℞ *radiopaque contrast medium for gastrointestinal imaging* [barium sulfate] 5%
tomoglumide INN
tomoxetine INN *antidepressant* [also: tomoxetine HCl]
tomoxetine HCl USAN *antidepressant* [also: tomoxetine]
tomoxiprole INN
Tomudex ℞ *antimetabolite antineoplastic; investigational (Phase III) thymidylate synthase inhibitor for colorectal cancer* [raltitrexed]
tonazocine INN *analgesic* [also: tonazocine mesylate]
tonazocine mesylate USAN *analgesic* [also: tonazocine]
tongue grass *medicinal herb* [see: chickweed]
tonics *a class of agents that restore normal tone to tissue and strengthen or*

invigorate organs (a term used in folk medicine)
tonka bean (*Dipteryx odorata; D. oppositifolia*) fruit and seed *medicinal herb for cramps, nausea, and schistosomiasis*
Tonocard film-coated tablets ℞ *antiarrhythmic* [tocainide HCl] 400, 600 mg
Tonopaque powder for oral suspension ℞ *radiopaque contrast medium for gastrointestinal imaging* [barium sulfate] 95%
tonzonium bromide INN *detergent; surface-active agent* [also: thonzonium bromide]
tooth, lion's *medicinal herb* [see: dandelion]
Toothache gel OTC *topical oral anesthetic* [benzocaine] 2
toothache bush; toothache tree *medicinal herb* [see: prickly ash]
Topamax coated tablets, sprinkle caps ℞ *broad-spectrum sulfamate anticonvulsant for partial-onset seizures; investigational (orphan) for Lennox-Gastaut syndrome* [topiramate] 25, 100, 200 mg; 15, 25 mg
Topic gel OTC *topical analgesic; counterirritant* [benzyl alcohol; camphor; menthol; alcohol 30%] 5%•2•2 �ⓑ Topicort
topical starch [see: starch, topical]
Topicort ointment, cream, gel ℞ *topical corticosteroidal anti-inflammatory* [desoximetasone] 0.25%; 0.25%; 0.05% ⓑ Topic
Topicort LP cream ℞ *topical corticosteroidal anti-inflammatory* [desoximetasone] 0.05%
Topicycline solution ℞ *topical antibiotic for acne* [tetracycline HCl] 2.2 mg/mL
Topiglan ℞ *investigational (Phase II/III) topical therapy for erectile dysfunction* [alprostadil]
topiramate USAN, INN, BAN *broad-spectrum sulfamate anticonvulsant for partial-onset seizures; investigational (orphan) for Lennox-Gastaut syndrome*
topoisomerase I inhibitors *a class of hormonal antineoplastics that prevent*

DNA *replication of tumors by inhibiting the re-ligation of naturally occurring single-strand breaks*

Toposar IV injection ℞ *antineoplastic for testicular and small cell lung cancers* [etoposide; alcohol 30.5%] 20 mg/mL

topotecan INN, BAN *antineoplastic/ topoisomerase I inhibitor for ovarian and small cell lung cancers* [also: topotecan HCl]

topotecan HCl USAN *antineoplastic/ topoisomerase I inhibitor for ovarian and small cell lung cancers* [also: topotecan]

toprilidine INN

Toprol XL film-coated extended-release tablets ℞ *antihypertensive; long-term antianginal; β-blocker* [metoprolol succinate] 50, 100, 200 mg

topterone USAN, INN *antiandrogen*

TOPV (trivalent oral poliovirus vaccine) [see: poliovirus vaccine, live oral]

toquizine USAN, INN *anticholinergic*

Toradol film-coated tablets, Tubex (cartridge-needle unit) for IM or IV injection ℞ *nonsteroidal anti-inflammatory drug (NSAID); analgesic for acute, moderately severe pain* [ketorolac tromethamine] 10 mg; 15, 30 mg/mL

torasemide INN, BAN *antihypertensive; loop diuretic* [also: torsemide]

torbafylline INN

Torecan suppositories (discontinued 1997) ℞ *antiemetic* [thiethylperazine maleate] 10 mg

Torecan tablets, IM injection ℞ *antiemetic* [thiethylperazine maleate] 10 mg; 5 mg/mL

toremifene INN, BAN *antiestrogen; antineoplastic* [also: toremifene citrate]

toremifene citrate USAN *antiestrogen antineoplastic for metastatic carcinoma of the breast (orphan); investigational (orphan) for desmoid tumors* [also: toremifene]

toripristone INN

tormentil *(Potentilla tormentilla; Tormentilla erecta)* root *medicinal herb used as an antiphlogistic, antiseptic, astringent, and hemostatic*

Tornalate oral inhalation aerosol, solution for inhalation ℞ *sympathomimetic bronchodilator* [bitolterol mesylate] 0.8%; 0.2%

torsemide USAN *antihypertensive; loop diuretic* [also: torasemide]

tosactide INN [also: octacosactrin]

tosifen USAN, INN *antianginal*

tosilate INN *combining name for radicals or groups* [also: tosylate]

tositumomab [see: iodine I 131 tositumomab]

tosufloxacin USAN, INN *antibacterial*

tosulur INN

tosylate USAN, BAN *combining name for radicals or groups* [also: tosilate]

tosylchloramide sodium INN [also: chloramine-T]

Totacillin capsules, powder for oral suspension ℞ *aminopenicillin antibiotic* [ampicillin] 250, 500 mg; 125, 250 mg/5 mL

Totacillin-N powder for IV or IM injection (discontinued 1998) ℞ *aminopenicillin antibiotic* [ampicillin sodium] 0.25, 0.5, 1, 2, 10 g

Total solution OTC *cleaning/soaking/wetting solution for hard contact lenses*

Total Formula; Total Formula-2 tablets OTC *vitamin/mineral/iron supplement* [multiple vitamins & minerals; iron; folic acid; biotin] ±•20• 0.4•0.3 mg

Total Formula-3 without Iron tablets OTC *vitamin/mineral supplement* [multiple vitamins & minerals; folic acid; biotin] ±•0.4•0.3 mg

touch-me-not; pale touch-me-not *medicinal herb* [see: celandine; jewelweed; Siberian ginseng]

toughened silver nitrate [see: silver nitrate, toughened]

Touro A & H timed-release capsules ℞ *decongestant; antihistamine* [pseudoephedrine HCl; brompheniramine maleate] 60•6 mg

Touro Ex sustained-release caplets ℞ *expectorant* [guaifenesin] 600 mg

Touro LA long-acting caplets ℞ *decongestant; expectorant* [pseudoephedrine HCl; guaifenesin] 120•500 mg

toxoids *a class of drugs used for active immunization that produce endogenous antibodies to toxins*

toywort *medicinal herb* [see: shepherd's purse]

tozalinone INN *antidepressant* [also: thozalinone]

TP-10 *investigational (Phase I/II) complement inhibitor for severe burns, adult respiratory distress syndrome, and reperfusion injury* [also: sCR1]

TP-20 *investigational complement/selectin inhibitor for vascular inflammation*

tPA; t-PA (tissue plasminogen activator) [see: alteplase]

TPCH (thioguanine, procarbazine, CCNU, hydroxyurea) *chemotherapy protocol*

TPDCV (thioguanine, procarbazine, DCD, CCNU, vincristine) *chemotherapy protocol*

TPGS (tocopheryl polyethylene glycol succinate) [see: tocophersolan]

T-Phyl timed-release tablets ℞ *antiasthmatic; bronchodilator* [theophylline] 200 mg

TPM Test kit for professional use *in vitro diagnostic aid for Toxoplasma gondii antibodies in serum* [indirect hemagglutination test]

TPN Electrolytes; TPN Electrolytes II; TPN Electrolytes III IV admixture ℞ *intravenous electrolyte therapy* [combined electrolyte solution]

traboxopine INN

Trac Tabs 2X tablets ℞ *urinary antibiotic; analgesic; antispasmodic; acidifier* [methenamine; phenyl salicylate; atropine sulfate; hyoscyamine sulfate; benzoic acid; methylene blue] 120•30•0.06•0.03•7.5•6 mg

tracazolate USAN, INN, BAN *sedative*

Trace Metals Additive in 0.9% NaCl IV injection ℞ *intravenous nutritional therapy* [multiple trace elements (metals)]

Tracelyte; Tracelyte II; Tracelyte with Double Electrolytes; Tracelyte II with Double Electrolytes IV admixture ℞ *intravenous nutritional therapy* [multiple trace elements (metals); electrolytes]

Tracer bG reagent strips for home use (discontinued 1995) OTC *in vitro diagnostic aid for blood glucose*

Tracrium IV infusion ℞ *nondepolarizing neuromuscular blocker; adjunct to anesthesia* [atracurium besylate] 10 mg/mL

trafermin USAN *investigational (Phase II/III) fibroblast growth factor for stroke and coronary artery disease*

tragacanth NF *suspending agent*

tralonide USAN, INN *corticosteroid; anti-inflammatory*

tramadol INN *central analgesic* [also: tramadol HCl]

tramadol HCl USAN *central analgesic* [also: tramadol]

tramazoline INN *adrenergic* [also: tramazoline HCl]

tramazoline HCl USAN *adrenergic* [also: tramazoline]

Trancopal caplets (discontinued 1998) ℞ *mild anxiolytic* [chlormezanone] 100, 200 mg

Trandate film-coated tablets, IV injection ℞ *antihypertensive; α- and β-blocker* [labetalol HCl] 100, 200, 300 mg; 5 mg/mL

trandolapril INN, BAN *antihypertensive; angiotensin converting enzyme (ACE) inhibitor*

trandolaprilat INN

tranexamic acid USAN, INN, BAN *systemic hemostatic; orphan status withdrawn 1996*

tranilast USAN, INN *antiasthmatic*

trans AMCHA (trans-aminomethyl cyclohexanecarboxylic acid) [see: tranexamic acid]

transcainide USAN, INN *antiarrhythmic*

transclomiphene [now: zuclomiphene]

Transderm Scōp transdermal patch ℞ *motion sickness preventative* [scopolamine hydrobromide] 1.5 mg

Transderm-Nitro transdermal patch
℞ *antianginal; vasodilator* [nitroglycerin] 12.5, 25, 50, 75, 100 mg
transforming growth factor beta 2 *investigational (orphan) growth stimulator for full-thickness macular holes*
Trans-Plantar transdermal patch (name changed to Trans-Ver-Sal Plantar-Patch in 1995)
Transplatin ℞ *investigational (orphan) alkylating antineoplastic for ovarian and colorectal cancers* [oxaliplatin]
trans-π-**oxocamphor** JAN *topical antipruritic; mild local anesthetic; counterirritant* [also: camphor]
trans-**retinoic acid** [see: tretinoin]
Trans-Ver-Sal Adult-Patch; Trans-Ver-Sal Pedia-Patch; Trans-Ver-Sal Plantar-Patch transdermal patch OTC *topical keratolytic* [salicylic acid] 15%
trantelinium bromide INN
Tranxene T-Tabs ("T"-imprinted tablets) ℞ *benzodiazepine anxiolytic; minor tranquilizer; anticonvulsant adjunct; alcohol withdrawal aid* [clorazepate dipotassium] 3.75, 7.5, 15 mg
Tranxene-SD single-dose tablets ℞ *benzodiazepine anxiolytic; minor tranquilizer; anticonvulsant adjunct; alcohol withdrawal aid* [clorazepate dipotassium] 11.25, 22.5 mg
tranylcypromine INN, BAN *antidepressant; MAO inhibitor* [also: tranylcypromine sulfate]
tranylcypromine sulfate USP *antidepressant; MAO inhibitor* [also: tranylcypromine]
trapencaine INN
trapidil INN
trapymin [see: trapidil]
trastuzumab *antineoplastic monoclonal antibody to HER2 (human epidermal growth factor receptor 2) protein for metastatic breast cancer*
Trasylol IV infusion ℞ *systemic hemostatic for coronary artery bypass graft (CABG) surgery (orphan)* [aprotinin] 10 000 KIU/mL (Kallikrein inhibitor units) ⊒ Travasol

TraumaCal ready-to-use liquid OTC *enteral nutritional therapy for moderate to severe stress or trauma* [multiple branched chain amino acids]
Travase ointment (discontinued 1996) ℞ *topical enzyme for biochemical debridement* [sutilains] 82 000 U/g
Travasol 2.75% in 5% (10%, 25%) Dextrose; Travasol 4.25% in 5% (10%, 25%) Dextrose IV infusion ℞ *total parenteral nutrition; peripheral parenteral nutrition* [multiple essential and nonessential amino acids; dextrose] ⊒ Trasylol
Travasol 3.5% (5.5%, 8.5%) with Electrolytes IV infusion ℞ *total parenteral nutrition (all except 3.5%); peripheral parenteral nutrition (all)* [multiple essential and nonessential amino acids; electrolytes] ±
Travasol 5.5% (8.5%, 10%) IV infusion ℞ *total parenteral nutrition; peripheral parenteral nutrition* [multiple essential and nonessential amino acids] ±
Travasorb Hepatic Diet powder (discontinued 1996) OTC *enteral nutritional therapy for hepatic failure* [multiple branched chain amino acids] ±
Travasorb HN; Travasorb MCT; Travasorb STD powder OTC *enteral nutritional therapy* [lactose-free formula]
Travasorb Renal Diet powder (discontinued 1998) OTC *enteral nutritional therapy for acute renal failure*
traveler's joy *medicinal herb* [see: blue vervain; woodbine]
Travert IV infusion ℞ *nonelectrolyte fluid and caloric replacement* [invert sugar (50% dextrose + 50% fructose)]
5% Travert and Electrolyte No. 2; 10% Travert and Electrolyte No. 2 IV infusion ℞ *intravenous nutritional/electrolyte therapy* [combined electrolyte solution; invert sugar (50% dextrose + 50% fructose)]
traxanox INN
Traypak (trademarked packaging form) *multivial carton*
trazitiline INN

trazium esilate INN

trazodone INN *antidepressant used for panic disorders, aggressive behavior, alcoholism, and cocaine withdrawal; serotonin uptake inhibitor* [also: trazodone HCl]

trazodone HCl USAN *antidepressant used for panic disorders, aggressive behavior, alcoholism, and cocaine withdrawal; serotonin uptake inhibitor* [also: trazodone] 50, 100, 150 mg oral

trazolopride INN

trebenzomine INN *antidepressant* [also: trebenzomine HCl]

trebenzomine HCl USAN *antidepressant* [also: trebenzomine]

trecadrine INN

Trecator-SC tablets ℞ *tuberculostatic* [ethionamide] 250 mg

trecovirsen sodium USAN *antisense antiviral for HIV and AIDS*

trefentanil HCl USAN *analgesic*

trefoil, bean; bitter trefoil; marsh trefoil *medicinal herb* [see: buckbean]

treloxinate USAN, INN *antihyperlipoproteinemic*

trembling poplar; trembling tree *medicinal herb* [see: poplar]

trenbolone INN, BAN *veterinary anabolic steroid, also abused as a street drug* [also: trenbolone acetate]

trenbolone acetate USAN *veterinary anabolic steroid, also abused as a street drug* [also: trenbolone]

trenbolone hexahydrobenzylcarbonate *veterinary anabolic steroid, also abused as a street drug*

Trendar tablets (discontinued 1996) OTC *nonsteroidal anti-inflammatory drug (NSAID); antiarthritic; analgesic* [ibuprofen] 200 mg

trengestone INN

trenizine INN

Trental film-coated controlled-release tablets ℞ *peripheral vasodilator to improve blood microcirculation in intermittent claudication* [pentoxifylline] 400 mg

treosulfan INN, BAN *investigational (orphan) for ovarian cancer*

trepibutone INN

trepipam INN *sedative* [also: trepipam maleate]

trepipam maleate USAN *sedative* [also: trepipam]

trepirium iodide INN

treptilamine INN

trequinsin INN

trestolone INN *antineoplastic; androgen* [also: trestolone acetate]

trestolone acetate USAN *antineoplastic; androgen* [also: trestolone]

tretamine INN, BAN [also: triethylenemelamine]

trethinium tosilate INN

trethocanic acid INN

trethocanoic acid [see: trethocanic acid]

tretinoin USAN, USP, INN, BAN *keratolytic; treatment for acute promyelocytic leukemia (orphan); investigational (orphan) for other leukemias and ophthalmic squamous metaplasia* 0.025%, 0.05%, 0.1% topical

Tretinoin LF ℞ *investigational (Phase III) antineoplastic for promyelocytic leukemia and Kaposi sarcoma*

tretoquinol INN

Trexan tablets (name changed to ReVia in 1995)

TRH (thyrotropin-releasing hormone) [see: protirelin]

Tri Vit with Fluoride drops ℞ *pediatric vitamin supplement and dental caries preventative* [vitamins A, C, and D; fluoride] 1500 IU•35 mg•400 IU•0.25 mg, 1500 IU•35 mg•400 IU•0.5 mg per mL

Triacana ℞ *investigational (orphan) for suppression of thyroid-stimulating hormone (TSH) in thyroid cancer* [tiratricol; levothyroxine sodium]

Triacet cream ℞ *topical corticosteroidal anti-inflammatory* [triamcinolone acetonide] 0.1%

triacetin USP, INN *antifungal*

triacetyloleandomycin BAN *macrolide antibiotic* [also: troleandomycin]

Triacin-C Cough syrup ℞ *narcotic antitussive; decongestant; antihistamine* [codeine phosphate; pseudoephedrine HCl; triprolidine HCl; alcohol] 10•30•1.25 mg/5 mL

triaconazole [now: terconazole]

Triactin syrup OTC *decongestant; antihistamine* [phenylpropanolamine HCl; chlorpheniramine maleate] 6.25•1 mg/5 mL

Triad capsules ℞ *sedative; analgesic* [acetaminophen; caffeine; butalbital] 325•40•50 mg

Triafed syrup (discontinued 1995) OTC *decongestant; antihistamine* [pseudo-ephedrine HCl; triprolidine HCl] 30•1.25 mg/5 mL ② Trifed

Triafed with Codeine syrup ℞ *narcotic antitussive; decongestant; antihistamine* [codeine phosphate; pseudo-ephedrine HCl; triprolidine HCl] 10•30•1.25 mg/5 mL

triafungin USAN, INN *antifungal*

Triam Forte IM injection ℞ *corticosteroid; anti-inflammatory* [triamcinolone diacetate] 40 mg/mL

Triam-A IM, intra-articular, intrabursal, intradermal injection ℞ *corticosteroid; anti-inflammatory* [triamcinolone acetonide] 40 mg/mL

triamcinolone USP, INN, BAN, JAN *corticosteroid* 4 mg oral ② Triaminicin

triamcinolone acetonide USP, JAN *corticosteroidal anti-inflammatory; treatment for chronic asthma and rhinitis* 0.025%, 0.1%, 0.5% topical; 40 mg/mL injection

triamcinolone acetonide sodium phosphate USAN *corticosteroid*

triamcinolone benetonide INN *corticosteroid*

triamcinolone diacetate USP, JAN *corticosteroid* 40 mg/mL injection

triamcinolone furetonide INN *corticosteroid*

triamcinolone hexacetonide USAN, USP, INN, BAN *corticosteroid*

Triaminic chewable tablets, syrup OTC *pediatric decongestant and antihistamine* [phenylpropanolamine HCl; chlorpheniramine maleate] 6.25•0.5

mg; 6.25•1 mg/5 mL ② Triaminicin; TriHemic

Triaminic oral infant drops ℞ *pediatric decongestant and antihistamine* [phenylpropanolamine HCl; pyrilamine maleate; pheniramine maleate] 20•10•10 mg/mL

Triaminic Allergy; Triaminic Cold tablets OTC *decongestant; antihistamine* [phenylpropanolamine HCl; chlorpheniramine maleate] 25•4 mg; 12.5•2 mg

Triaminic AM Cough & Decongestant Formula liquid OTC *pediatric antitussive and decongestant* [dextromethorphan hydrobromide; pseudoephedrine HCl] 7.5•15 mg/5 mL

Triaminic AM Decongestant Formula syrup OTC *decongestant* [pseudoephedrine HCl] 15 mg/5 mL

Triaminic Decongestant oral infant drops OTC *pediatric decongestant* [pseudoephedrine HCl] 7.5 mg/0.8 mL

Triaminic DM syrup OTC *antitussive; decongestant* [dextromethorphan hydrobromide; phenylpropanolamine HCl] 5•6.25 mg/5 mL

Triaminic DM Day time Ⓒᴬᴺ oral solution OTC *pediatric antitussive, decongestant, and expectorant* [dextromethorphan hydrobromide; phenylpropanolamine HCl; guaifenesin] 1.5•1.75•7.5 mg/mL

Triaminic DM Night time for Children Ⓒᴬᴺ (U.S. product: Triaminic Night Light) liquid OTC *pediatric antitussive, decongestant, and antihistamine* [dextromethorphan hydrobromide; pseudoephedrine HCl; chlorpheniramine maleate] 7.5•15•1 mg/5 mL

Triaminic Expectorant liquid OTC *decongestant; expectorant* [phenylpropanolamine HCl; guaifenesin] 6.25•50 mg/5 mL

Triaminic Expectorant DH liquid ℞ *narcotic antitussive; decongestant; antihistamine; expectorant* [hydrocodone bitartrate; phenylpropanolamine HCl; pyrilamine maleate; pheniramine

maleate; guaifenesin; alcohol 5%]
1.67•12.5•6.25•6.25•100 mg/5 mL

Triaminic Expectorant with Codeine liquid Ŗ *narcotic antitussive; decongestant; expectorant* [codeine phosphate; phenylpropanolamine HCl; guaifenesin; alcohol 5%] 10•12.5•100 mg/5 mL

Triaminic Nite Light liquid OTC *pediatric antitussive, decongestant, and antihistamine* [dextromethorphan hydrobromide; pseudoephedrine HCl; chlorpheniramine maleate] 7.5•15•1 mg/5 mL

Triaminic Sore Throat Formula liquid OTC *pediatric antitussive, decongestant, and analgesic* [dextromethorphan hydrobromide; pseudoephedrine HCl; acetaminophen] 7.5•15• 160 mg/5 mL

Triaminic-12 sustained-release tablets OTC *decongestant; antihistamine* [phenylpropanolamine HCl; chlorpheniramine maleate] 75•12 mg

Triaminicin Cold, Allergy, Sinus tablets OTC *decongestant; antihistamine; analgesic* [phenylpropanolamine HCl; chlorpheniramine maleate; acetaminophen] 25•4•650 mg ② triamcinolone; Triaminic

Triaminicol Multi-Symptom Cough and Cold tablets OTC *antitussive; decongestant; antihistamine* [dextromethorphan hydrobromide; phenylpropanolamine HCl; chlorpheniramine maleate] 10•12.5•2 mg

Triaminicol Multi-Symptom Relief liquid OTC *antitussive; decongestant; antihistamine* [dextromethorphan hydrobromide; phenylpropanolamine HCl; chlorpheniramine maleate] 10•12.5•2 mg/5 mL

Triaminicol Multi-Symptom Relief Colds with Cough liquid OTC *pediatric antitussive, decongestant, and antihistamine* [dextromethorphan hydrobromide; phenylpropanolamine HCl; chlorpheniramine maleate] 5•6.25•1 mg/5 mL

Triamolone 40 IM injection Ŗ *corticosteroid; anti-inflammatory* [triamcinolone diacetate] 40 mg/mL

Triamonide 40 IM, intra-articular, intrabursal, intradermal injection Ŗ *corticosteroid; anti-inflammatory* [triamcinolone acetonide] 40 mg/mL

triampyzine INN *anticholinergic* [also: triampyzine sulfate]

triampyzine sulfate USAN *anticholinergic* [also: triampyzine]

triamterene USAN, USP, INN, BAN, JAN *antihypertensive; potassium-sparing diuretic* ② trimipramine

trianisestrol [see: chlorotrianisene]

Triapine Ŗ *investigational (Phase I) anticancer agent* ② Triaprim

Triaprin capsules (discontinued 1998) Ŗ *analgesic; sedative* [acetaminophen; butalbital] 325•50 mg ② Triapine

Triavil 2-10; Triavil 2-25; Triavil 4-10; Triavil 4-25; Triavil 4-50 tablets Ŗ *conventional (typical) antipsychotic; antidepressant* [perphenazine; amitriptyline HCl] 2•10 mg; 2•25 mg; 4•10 mg; 4•25 mg; 4•50 mg

Tri-A-Vite F drops Ŗ *pediatric vitamin supplement and dental caries preventative* [vitamins A, C, and D; fluoride] 1500 IU•35 mg•400 IU•0.5 mg per mL

Triaz gel, skin cleanser (discontinued 1998) Ŗ *topical keratolytic for acne* [benzoyl peroxide] 6%, 10%; 10%

triaziquone INN, BAN

triazolam USAN, USP, INN *benzodiazepine sedative; hypnotic* 0.125, 0.25 mg oral

Triban; Pediatric Triban suppositories Ŗ *anticholinergic; antiemetic; anesthetic* [trimethobenzamide HCl; benzocaine] 200 mg•2%; 100 mg•2%

tribasic calcium phosphate [see: calcium phosphate, tribasic]

tribavirin BAN *antiviral for severe lower respiratory tract infections* [also: ribavirin]

tribendilol INN

tribenoside USAN, INN *sclerosing agent*

Tribiotic Plus ointment OTC *topical antibiotic; anesthetic* [polymyxin B sulfate; bacitracin; neomycin sulfate;

lidocaine] 5000 U•500 U•3.5 mg•
40 mg per g

tribromoethanol NF

tribromomethane [see: bromoform]

tribromsalan USAN, INN *disinfectant*

tribuzone INN

tricalcium phosphate [see: calcium phosphate, tribasic]

tricarbocyanine dye [see: indocyanine green]

tricetamide USAN *sedative*

Trichinella extract USP

Tri-Chlor liquid ℞ *cauterant; keratolytic* [trichloroacetic acid] 80%

trichlorethoxyphosphamide [see: defosfamide]

trichlorfon USAN, USP *veterinary anthelmintic; investigational (NDA filed) acetylcholinesterase inhibitor for Alzheimer's dementia* [also: metrifonate; metriphonate]

trichlorisobutylalcohol [see: chlorobutanol]

trichlormethiazide USP, INN *diuretic; antihypertensive* 4 mg oral

trichlormethine INN [also: trimustine]

trichloroacetic acid USP *strong keratolytic/cauterant*

trichlorocarbanilide (TCC) [see: triclocarban]

trichloroethylene NF, INN

trichlorofluoromethane [see: trichloromonofluoromethane]

trichlorofon [see: metrifonate]

trichloromonofluoromethane NF *aerosol propellant; topical anesthetic*

trichlorphon [see: metrifonate]

Tricholomopsis edodes medicinal herb [see: shiitake mushrooms]

Trichophyton extract *diagnosis and treatment of Trichophyton-induced skin infections*

trichorad [see: acinitrazole]

Trichosanthes kirilowii medicinal herb [see: Chinese cucumber]

trichosanthin *investigational (Phase II) antiviral for AIDS and ARC*

Trichotine Douche powder OTC *antiseptic/germicidal; vaginal cleanser and*

deodorizer; acidity modifier [sodium perborate]

Trichotine Douche solution OTC *antiseptic/germicidal; vaginal cleanser and deodorizer; acidity modifier* [sodium borate]

triciribine INN *antineoplastic* [also: triciribine phosphate]

triciribine phosphate USAN *antineoplastic* [also: triciribine]

tricitrates (sodium citrate, potassium citrate, and citric acid) USP *systemic alkalizer; urinary alkalizer; antiurolithic*

triclabendazole INN

triclacetamol INN

triclazate INN

triclobisonium chloride NF, INN

triclocarban USAN, INN *disinfectant*

triclodazol INN

triclofenate INN *combining name for radicals or groups*

triclofenol piperazine USAN, INN *anthelmintic*

triclofos INN *hypnotic; sedative* [also: triclofos sodium]

triclofos sodium USAN *hypnotic; sedative* [also: triclofos]

triclofylline INN

triclonide USAN, INN *anti-inflammatory*

triclosan USAN, INN, BAN *disinfectant/antiseptic*

Tricodene Cough and Cold liquid ℞ *narcotic antitussive; antihistamine* [codeine phosphate; pyrilamine maleate] 8.2•12.5 mg/5 mL

Tricodene Forte; Tricodene NN liquid OTC *antitussive; decongestant; antihistamine* [dextromethorphan hydrobromide; phenylpropanolamine HCl; chlorpheniramine maleate] 10•12.5•2 mg/5 mL

Tricodene Pediatric Cough & Cold liquid OTC *pediatric antitussive and decongestant* [dextromethorphan hydrobromide; phenylpropanolamine HCl] 10•12.5 mg/5 mL

Tricodene Sugar Free liquid OTC *antitussive; antihistamine* [dextromethorphan hydrobromide; chlorpheniramine maleate] 10•2 mg/5 mL

Tricom tablets (discontinued 1995) oTC *decongestant; antihistamine; analgesic* [pseudoephedrine HCl; chlorpheniramine maleate; acetaminophen] 60•4•650 mg

Tricor capsules ℞ *antihyperlipidemic for hypertriglyceridemia* [fenofibrate] 67 mg

tricosactide INN

Tricosal film-coated tablets ℞ *analgesic; antipyretic; antirheumatic* [choline magnesium trisalicylate] 500, 750, 1000 mg

tricyclamol chloride INN

Tri-Cyclen [see: Ortho Tri-Cyclen]

tricyclics *a class of antidepressants which inhibit reuptake of amines, norepinephrine, and serotonin*

Triderm cream ℞ *topical corticosteroidal anti-inflammatory* [triamcinolone acetonide] 0.1%

Tridesilon cream, ointment ℞ *topical corticosteroidal anti-inflammatory* [desonide] 0.05%

Tridesilon Otic [see: Otic Tridesilon]

Tri-Desogen (name changed to Mircette upon marketing release in 1998)

tridihexethyl chloride USP *peptic ulcer adjunct*

tridihexethyl iodide INN

Tridil IV infusion ℞ *antianginal; vasodilator; perioperative antihypertensive; for congestive heart failure with myocardial infarction* [nitroglycerin] 0.5, 5 mg/mL

Tridione capsules, Dulcets (chewable tablets) ℞ *anticonvulsant* [trimethadione] 300 mg; 150 mg

Tridione oral solution (discontinued 1995) ℞ *anticonvulsant* [trimethadione] 40 mg/mL

Tridrate Bowel Evacuant Kit oral solution + 3 tablets + 1 suppository oTC *pre-procedure bowel evacuant* [magnesium citrate (solution); bisacodyl (tablets and suppository)] 300 mL; 5 mg; 10 mg

trientine INN *chelating agent* [also: trientine HCl; trientine dihydrochloride]

trientine dihydrochloride BAN *chelating agent* [also: trientine HCl; trientine]

trientine HCl USAN, USP *copper chelating agent for Wilson's disease (orphan)* [also: trientine; trientine dihydrochloride]

triethanolamine [now: trolamine]

triethyl citrate NF *plasticizer*

triethyleneiminobenzoquinone (TEIB) [see: triaziquone]

triethylenemelamine NF [also: tretamine]

triethylenethiophosphoramide (TSPA; TESPA) [see: thiotepa]

Trifed tablets (discontinued 1995) ℞ *decongestant; antihistamine* [pseudoephedrine HCl; triprolidine HCl] 60•2.5 mg ② Triafed

Trifed-C Cough syrup ℞ *narcotic antitussive; decongestant; antihistamine* [codeine phosphate; pseudoephedrine HCl; triprolidine HCl; alcohol 4.4%] 10•30•1.25 mg/5 mL

trifenagrel USAN, INN *antithrombotic*

trifezolac INN

triflocin USAN, INN *diuretic*

Tri-Flor-Vite with Fluoride drops ℞ *pediatric vitamin supplement and dental caries preventative* [vitamins A, C, and D; fluoride] 1500 IU•35 mg•400 IU•0.25 mg per mL

triflubazam USAN, INN *minor tranquilizer*

triflumidate USAN, INN *anti-inflammatory*

trifluomeprazine INN, BAN

trifluoperazine INN *phenothiazine antipsychotic; sedative* [also: trifluoperazine HCl]

trifluoperazine HCl USP *phenothiazine antipsychotic; sedative; anxiolytic* [also: trifluoperazine] 1, 2, 5, 10 mg oral; 10 mg/mL oral; 2 mg/mL injection

N-trifluoroacetyl adriamycin-14-valerate *investigational for carcinoma in situ of the urinary bladder; orphan status withdrawn 1998*

trifluorothymidine [see: trifluridine]

trifluperidol USAN, INN *antipsychotic*

triflupromazine USP, INN *phenothiazine antipsychotic; antiemetic*

triflupromazine HCl USP *phenothiazine antipsychotic; antiemetic*

trifluridine USAN, INN *ophthalmic antiviral*

Triflusal ℞ *investigational agent for the prevention of stroke and dementia*

triflusal INN *investigational treatment for stroke and vascular dementia*

triflutate USAN, INN *combining name for radicals or groups*

Trifolium pratense medicinal herb [see: red clover]

Trigesic tablets (discontinued 1995) OTC *analgesic; antipyretic; anti-inflammatory* [acetaminophen; aspirin; caffeine] 125•230•30 mg

trigevolol INN

α-triglycidyl isocyanurate (αTGI) [see: teroxirone]

Trigonella foenum-graecum medicinal herb [see: fenugreek]

TriHemic 600 film-coated tablets ℞ *hematinic* [ferrous fumarate; cyanocobalamin; ascorbic acid; vitamin E; intrinsic factor concentrate; docusate sodium; folic acid] 115 mg•25 μg•600 mg•30 IU•75 mg•50 mg• 1 mg ② Triaminic

Trihexy-2; Trihexy-5 tablets ℞ *anticholinergic; antiparkinsonian* [trihexyphenidyl HCl] 2 mg; 5 mg

trihexyphenidyl INN *anticholinergic; antiparkinsonian* [also: trihexyphenidyl HCl; benzhexol]

trihexyphenidyl HCl USP *anticholinergic; antiparkinsonian* [also: trihexyphenidyl; benzhexol] 2, 5 mg oral

TriHIBit IM injection ℞ *immunization against diphtheria, tetanus, and pertussis* [diphtheria & tetanus toxoids & acellular pertussis (DTaP) vaccine]

Tri-Hydroserpine tablets ℞ *antihypertensive; vasodilator; diuretic* [hydrochlorothiazide; reserpine; hydralazine HCl] 15•0.1•25 mg

Tri-Immunol IM injection ℞ *immunization against diphtheria, tetanus and pertussis* [diphtheria & tetanus toxoids & whole-cell pertussis (DTwP) vaccine, adsorbed] 0.5 mL

triiodothyronine sodium, levo [see: liothyronine sodium]

Tri-K liquid ℞ *potassium supplement* [potassium acetate; potassium bicarbonate; potassium citrate] 45 mEq/15 mL (K)

trikates USP *electrolyte replenisher*

Tri-Kort IM, intra-articular, intrabursal, intradermal injection ℞ *corticosteroid; anti-inflammatory* [triamcinolone acetonide] 40 mg/mL

Trilafon coated tablets, oral concentrate, IV or IM injection ℞ *conventional (typical) antipsychotic; antiemetic* [perphenazine] 2, 4, 8, 16 mg; 16 mg/5 mL; 5 mg/mL

Trileptal (commercially available in Argentina, Finland, and the Netherlands) ℞ *investigational (NDA filed) antiepileptic* [oxcarbazepine]

triletide INN

Tri-Levlen tablets ℞ *triphasic oral contraceptive; emergency "morning after" contraceptive* [levonorgestrel; ethinyl estradiol] Phase 1: 0.05 mg•30 μg; Phase 2: 0.075 mg•40 μg; Phase 3: 0.125 mg•30 μg

Trilisate tablets, liquid ℞ *analgesic; antipyretic; anti-inflammatory; antirheumatic* [choline salicylate; magnesium salicylate] 750, 1000 mg; 500 mg/5 mL

trilithium citrate tetrahydrate [see: lithium citrate]

Trillium erectum; T. grandiflorum; T. pendulum medicinal herb [see: birthroot]

Trilog IM, intra-articular, intrabursal, intradermal injection ℞ *corticosteroid; anti-inflammatory* [triamcinolone acetonide] 40 mg/mL

Trilone IM injection ℞ *corticosteroid; anti-inflammatory* [triamcinolone diacetate] 40 mg/mL

trilostane USAN, INN, BAN *adrenocortical suppressant; antisteroidal antineoplastic*

Trimazide capsules, suppositories, pediatric suppositories ℞ *anticholinergic; antiemetic* [trimethobenzamide HCl] 100 mg; 200 mg; 100 mg

trimazosin INN, BAN *antihypertensive* [also: trimazosin HCl]

trimazosin HCl USAN *antihypertensive* [also: trimazosin]

trimebutine INN GI *antispasmodic*

trimecaine INN

trimedoxime bromide INN

trimegestone USAN *progestin for postmenopausal hormone deficiency*

trimeperidine INN, BAN

trimeprazine BAN *phenothiazine antihistamine; antipruritic* [also: trimeprazine tartrate; alimemazine; alimemazine tartrate] ⊡ trimipramine

trimeprazine tartrate USP *phenothiazine antihistamine; antipruritic* [also: alimemazine; trimeprazine; alimemazine tartrate]

trimeproprimine [see: trimipramine]

trimetamide INN

trimetaphan camsilate INN *antihypertensive* [also: trimethaphan camsylate; trimetaphan camsylate]

trimetaphan camsylate BAN *antihypertensive* [also: trimethaphan camsylate; trimetaphan camsilate]

trimetazidine INN, BAN

trimethadione USP, INN *anticonvulsant* [also: troxidone]

trimethamide [see: trimetamide]

trimethaphan camphorsulfonate [see: trimethaphan camsylate] ⊡ trimethoprim

trimethaphan camsylate USP *emergency antihypertensive* [also: trimetaphan camsilate; trimetaphan camsylate]

trimethidinium methosulfate NF, INN

trimethobenzamide INN *antiemetic; anticholinergic* [also: trimethobenzamide HCl]

trimethobenzamide HCl USP *antiemetic; anticholinergic* [also: trimethobenzamide] 250 mg oral; 100, 200 mg suppositories; 100 mg/mL injection

trimethoprim (TMP) USAN, USP, INN, BAN *antibacterial antibiotic* 100, 200 mg oral ⊡ trimethaphan

trimethoprim & dapsone *investigational for Pneumocystis carinii pneumonia; orphan status withdrawn 1998*

trimethoprim sulfate USAN *antibacterial*

trimethoquinol [see: tretoquinol]

trimethylammonium chloride carbamate [see: bethanechol chloride]

trimethylene [see: cyclopropane]

trimethyltetradecylammonium bromide [see: tetradonium bromide]

trimetozine USAN, INN *sedative*

trimetrexate USAN, INN, BAN *antimetabolic antineoplastic; systemic antiprotozoal*

trimetrexate glucuronate USAN *antimetabolic antineoplastic; antiprotozoal for Pneumocystis carinii pneumonia of AIDS (orphan); investigational (orphan) for multiple cancers*

trimexiline INN

Triminol Cough syrup OTC *antitussive; decongestant; antihistamine* [dextromethorphan hydrobromide; phenylpropanolamine HCl; chlorpheniramine maleate] 10•12.5•2 mg/5 mL

trimipramine USAN, INN *tricyclic antidepressant* ⊡ imipramine; triamterene; trimeprazine

trimipramine maleate USAN *tricyclic antidepressant*

trimolide [see: trimetozine]

trimopam maleate [now: trepipam maleate]

trimoprostil USAN, INN *gastric antisecretory*

Trimo-San vaginal jelly OTC *antibacterial; astringent; antipruritic* [oxyquinoline sulfate; boric acid; sodium borate] 0.025%•1%•0.7%

Trimox capsules, powder for oral suspension, pediatric drops ℞ *aminopenicillin antibiotic* [amoxicillin] 250, 500 mg; 125, 250 mg/5 mL; 50 mg/mL

trimoxamine INN *antihypertensive* [also: trimoxamine HCl]

trimoxamine HCl USAN *antihypertensive* [also: trimoxamine]

Trimpex tablets ℞ *anti-infective; antibacterial* [trimethoprim] 100 mg

Trimstat tablets (discontinued 1996) ℞ *anorexiant; CNS stimulant* [phendimetrazine tartrate] 35 mg

trimustine BAN [also: trichlormethine]

Trinalin Repetabs (repeat-action tablets) ℞ *decongestant; antihistamine* [pseudoephedrine sulfate; azatadine maleate] 120•1 mg

Trind liquid (discontinued 1995) OTC *decongestant; antihistamine* [phenylpropanolamine HCl; chlorpheniramine maleate; alcohol 5%] 12.5•2 mg/5 mL

Tri-Nefrin tablets OTC *decongestant; antihistamine* [phenylpropanolamine HCl; chlorpheniramine maleate] 25•4 mg

Trinipatch Ⓒᴬᴺ transdermal patch ℞ *antianginal; vasodilator* [nitroglycerin] 22.4, 44.8, 67.2 mg (0.2, 0.4, 0.6 mg/hr.)

trinitrin [see: nitroglycerin]

trinitrophenol NF

Tri-Norinyl tablets ℞ *triphasic oral contraceptive* [norethindrone; ethinyl estradiol] Phase 1: 0.5 mg•35 μg; Phase 2: 1 mg•35 μg; Phase 3: 0.5 mg•35 μg

Trinsicon capsules ℞ *hematinic* [ferrous fumarate; cyanocobalamin; ascorbic acid; intrinsic factor concentrate; folic acid] 110 mg•15 μg•75 mg•240 mg•0.5 mg

Triofed syrup OTC *decongestant; antihistamine* [pseudoephedrine HCl; triprolidine HCl] 30•1.25 mg/5 mL

triolein I 125 USAN *radioactive agent*

triolein I 131 USAN *radioactive agent*

trional [see: sulfonethylmethane]

Triostat IV injection ℞ *thyroid hormone; treatment of myxedema coma or precoma (orphan)* [liothyronine sodium] 10 μg/mL ② Threostat

Triotann pediatric oral suspension (discontinued 1995) ℞ *decongestant; antihistamine* [phenylephrine tannate; chlorpheniramine tannate; pyrilamine tannate] 5•2•12.5 mg/5 mL

Triotann tablets ℞ *decongestant; antihistamine* [phenylephrine tannate; chlorpheniramine tannate; pyrilamine tannate] 25•8•25 mg

Tri-Otic ear drops ℞ *topical corticosteroidal anti-inflammatory; topical local anesthetic; antiseptic* [hydrocortisone; pramoxine HCl; chloroxylenol] 10•10•1 mg/mL

trioxifene INN *antiestrogen* [also: trioxifene mesylate]

trioxifene mesylate USAN *antiestrogen* [also: trioxifene]

trioxsalen USAN, USP *systemic psoralens for repigmentation of idiopathic vitiligo; also used to enhance pigmentation and increase tolerance to sunlight* [also: trioxysalen]

trioxyethylrutin [see: troxerutin]

trioxymethylene [see: paraformaldehyde]

trioxysalen INN *systemic psoralens for repigmentation of idiopathic vitiligo; also used to enhance pigmentation and increase tolerance to sunlight* [also: trioxsalen]

Tri-P oral infant drops ℞ *decongestant; antihistamine* [phenylpropanolamine HCl; pyrilamine maleate; pheniramine maleate] 20•10•10 mg/mL

Tri-Pain tablets (discontinued 1995) OTC *analgesic; antipyretic; anti-inflammatory* [acetaminophen; aspirin; salicylamide; caffeine] 162•162•162•16.2 mg

Tripalgen Cold syrup (discontinued 1995) OTC *decongestant; antihistamine* [phenylpropanolamine HCl; chlorpheniramine maleate] 12.5•2 mg/5 mL

tripamide USAN, INN *antihypertensive; diuretic*

triparanol INN *(withdrawn from market)*

Tripedia IM injection ℞ *immunization against diphtheria, tetanus and pertussis* [diphtheria & tetanus toxoids & acellular pertussis (DTaP) vaccine] 6.7 LfU•5 LfU• 46.8 μg per 0.5 mL

tripelennamine INN *ethylenediamine antihistamine* [also: tripelennamine citrate]

tripelennamine citrate USP *ethylenediamine antihistamine* [also: tripelennamine]

tripelennamine HCl USP *ethylenediamine antihistamine*

Triphasil tablets ℞ *triphasic oral contraceptive; emergency "morning after" contraceptive* [levonorgestrel; ethinyl estradiol] Phase 1: 0.05 mg•30 μg; Phase 2: 0.075 mg•40 μg; Phase 3: 0.125 mg•30 μg

Tri-Phen-Chlor syrup, pediatric syrup, pediatric drops ℞ *decongestant; antihistamine* [phenylpropanolamine HCl; phenylephrine HCl; chlorpheniramine maleate; phenyltoloxamine citrate] 20•5•2.5•7.5 mg/5 mL; 5•1.25•0.5•2 mg/5 mL; 5•1.25•0.5•2 mg/mL

Tri-Phen-Chlor T.R. timed-release tablets ℞ *decongestant; antihistamine* [phenylpropanolamine HCl; phenylephrine HCl; chlorpheniramine maleate; phenyltoloxamine citrate] 40•10•5•15 mg

Tri-Phen-Mine syrup, drops ℞ *pediatric decongestant and antihistamine* [phenylpropanolamine HCl; phenylephrine HCl; chlorpheniramine maleate; phenyltoloxamine citrate] 5•1.25•0.5•2 mg/5 mL; 5•1.25•0.5•2 mg/mL

Tri-Phen-Mine S.R. timed-release tablets ℞ *decongestant; antihistamine* [phenylpropanolamine HCl; phenylephrine HCl; chlorpheniramine maleate; phenyltoloxamine citrate] 40•10•5•15 mg

Triphenyl syrup OTC *decongestant; antihistamine* [phenylpropanolamine HCl; chlorpheniramine maleate] 6.25•1 mg/5 mL

Triphenyl Expectorant liquid OTC *decongestant; expectorant* [phenylpropanolamine HCl; guaifenesin; alcohol 5%] 12.5•100 mg/5 mL

Triple Antibiotic ointment OTC *topical antibiotic* [polymyxin B sulfate; neomycin sulfate; bacitracin] 5000 U•3.5 mg•400 U per g

Triple Antibiotic ophthalmic ointment ℞ *topical ophthalmic antibiotic* [polymyxin B sulfate; neomycin sulfate; bacitracin zinc] 5000 U•3.5 mg•400 U per g

Triple Sulfa vaginal cream ℞ *broad-spectrum bacteriostatic* [sulfathiazole; sulfacetamide; sulfabenzamide] 3.42%•2.86%•3.7%

triple sulfa (sulfathiazole, sulfacetamide, and sulfabenzamide) [q.v.]

Triple Sulfa No. 2 tablets (discontinued 1995) ℞ *broad-spectrum bacteriostatic* [trisulfapyrimidines] 500 mg

Triple Vitamin ADC with Fluoride drops ℞ *pediatric vitamin supplement and dental caries preventative* [vitamins A, C, and D; fluoride] 1500 IU•35 mg•400 IU•0.5 mg per mL

Triple Vitamins with Fluoride chewable tablets ℞ *vitamin supplement; dental caries preventative* [vitamins A, C, and D; fluoride]

Triple X Kit liquid + shampoo OTC *pediculicide for lice* [pyrethrins; piperonyl butoxide; petroleum distillate] 0.3%•3%• ?

Triposed tablets, syrup OTC *decongestant; antihistamine* [pseudoephedrine HCl; triprolidine HCl] 60•2.5 mg; 30•1.25 mg/5 mL

tripotassium citrate monohydrate [see: potassium citrate]

triproamylin [see: pramlintide]

triprolidine INN *antihistamine* [also: triprolidine HCl]

triprolidine HCl USP *antihistamine* [also: triprolidine]

Tripterygium wilfordii *medicinal herb* [see: thunder god vine]

Triptone long-acting caplets OTC *antinauseant; antiemetic; antivertigo; motion sickness preventative* [dimenhydrinate] 50 mg

triptorelin USAN, INN *antineoplastic*

triptorelin pamoate *antineoplastic; orphan status withdrawn 1996*

trisaccharides A & B *investigational (orphan) for newborn hemolytic disease and ABO blood incompatibility of organ or bone marrow transplants*

trisodium citrate [see: sodium citrate]

trisodium citrate dihydrate [see: sodium citrate]

trisodium hydrogen ethylenediaminetetraacetate [see: edetate trisodium]

Trisoralen tablets ℞ *systemic psoralens for repigmentation of idiopathic vitiligo; also used to enhance pigmentation and increase tolerance to sunlight* [trioxsalen] 5 mg

Tri-Statin II cream ℞ *topical corticosteroidal anti-inflammatory; antifungal* [triamcinolone acetonide; nystatin] 0.1%•100 000 U per g

Tristoject IM injection ℞ *corticosteroid; anti-inflammatory* [triamcinolone diacetate] 40 mg/mL

trisulfapyrimidines USP (a mixture of sulfadiazine, sulfamerazine, and sulfamethazine) *broad-spectrum bacteriostatic*

Tritan tablets ℞ *decongestant; antihistamine* [phenylephrine tannate; chlorpheniramine tannate; pyrilamine tannate] 25•8•25 mg

Tritann Pediatric oral suspension (discontinued 1995) ℞ *pediatric antihistamine and decongestant* [phenylephrine tannate; chlorpheniramine tannate; pyrilamine tannate] 5•2•12.5 mg/5 mL

Tri-Tannate tablets, pediatric oral suspension ℞ *decongestant; antihistamine* [phenylephrine tannate; chlorpheniramine tannate; pyrilamine tannate] 25•8•25 mg; 5•2•12.5 mg/5 mL

Tri-Tannate Plus Pediatric oral suspension ℞ *pediatric antitussive, decongestant, and antihistamine* [carbetapentane tannate; phenylephrine tannate; ephedrine tannate; chlorpheniramine tannate] 30•5•5•4 mg/5 mL

Tritec film-coated tablets ℞ *histamine H₂ antagonist for duodenal ulcers with H. pylori infection* [ranitidine bismuth citrate] 400 mg

tritheon [see: acinitrazole]

tritiated water USAN *radioactive agent*

Triticum repens *medicinal herb* [see: couch grass]

Tri-Tinic capsules ℞ *antianemic* [ferrous fumarate; intrinsic factor concentrate; vitamins B₁₂ and C; folic acid]

tritiozine INN

tritoqualine INN

Triva Douche powder OTC *antiseptic/germicidal; vaginal cleanser and deodorizer* [oxyquinoline sulfate] 2%

trivalent oral poliovirus vaccine (TOPV) [see: poliovirus vaccine, live oral]

Tri-Vi-Flor chewable tablets, drops ℞ *pediatric vitamin supplement and dental caries preventative* [vitamins A, C, and D; sodium fluoride] 2500 IU•60 mg•400 IU•1 mg; 1500 IU•35 mg•400 IU•0.25 mg, 1500 IU•35 mg•400 IU•0.5 mg per mL

Tri-Vi-Flor with Iron drops ℞ *pediatric vitamin/iron supplement and dental caries preventative* [vitamins A, C, and D; iron; sodium fluoride] 1500 IU•35 mg•400 IU•0.25 mg per mL

Tri-Vi-Sol drops OTC *pediatric vitamin supplement* [vitamins A, C, and D] 1500 IU•35 mg•400 IU per mL

Tri-Vi-Sol with Iron drops OTC *vitamin/iron supplement* [vitamins A, C, and D; ferrous sulfate] 1500 IU•35 mg•400 IU•10 mg per mL

Trivitamin Fluoride chewable tablets, drops ℞ *pediatric vitamin supplement and dental caries preventative* [vitamins A, C, and D; fluoride] 2500 IU•60 mg•400 IU•1 mg; 1500 IU•35 mg•400 IU•0.25 mg, 1500 IU•35 mg•400 IU•0.5 mg per mL

Tri-Vitamin Infants' Drops OTC *vitamin supplement* [vitamins A, C, and D] 1500 IU•35 mg•400 IU per mL

Tri-Vitamin with Fluoride drops ℞ *pediatric vitamin supplement and dental caries preventative* [vitamins A, C, and D; fluoride] 1500 IU•35 mg•400 IU•0.5 mg per mL

Trivora-28 tablets ℞ *triphasic oral contraceptive* [levonorgestrel; ethinyl estradiol] Phase 1: 0.05 mg•30 µg; Phase 2: 0.075 mg•40 µg; Phase 3: 0.125 mg•30 µg

trixolane INN

trizoxime INN

Trizyme (ingredient) OTC *digestive enzymes* [amylolytic, proteolytic and cellulolytic enzymes (amylase; protease; cellulase)]

Trobicin powder for IM injection ℞ *antibiotic* [spectinomycin HCl] 400 mg/mL ☑ tobramycin

Trocaine lozenges OTC *topical oral anesthetic* [benzocaine] 10 mg

Trocal lozenges OTC *antitussive* [dextromethorphan hydrobromide] 7.5 mg

trocimine INN

troclosene potassium USAN, INN *topical anti-infective*

trofosfamide INN

troglitazone USAN, INN *thiazolidinedione antidiabetic; increases cellular response to insulin without increasing insulin secretion*

trolamine USAN, NF *alkalizing agent; analgesic*

trolamine polypeptide oleate-condensate *cerumenolytic to emulsify and disperse ear wax*

troleandomycin USAN, USP *macrolide antibiotic; investigational (orphan) for severe asthma* [also: triacetyloleandomycin]

trolnitrate INN

trolnitrate phosphate [see: trolnitrate]

tromantadine INN

trometamol INN, BAN *alkalizer for cardiac bypass surgery* [also: tromethamine]

tromethamine USAN, USP *alkalizer for cardiac bypass surgery* [also: trometamol]

Tronolane anorectal cream OTC *topical local anesthetic* [pramoxine HCl] 1% ☑ Tronothane

Tronolane rectal suppositories OTC *astringent; emollient* [zinc oxide] 11%

Tronothane HCl cream OTC *topical local anesthetic* [pramoxine HCl] 1% ☑ Tronolane

tropabazate INN

Tropaeolum majus medicinal herb [see: Indian cress]

tropanserin INN, BAN *migraine-specific serotonin receptor antagonist* [also: tropanserin HCl]

tropanserin HCl USAN *migraine-specific serotonin receptor antagonist* [also: tropanserin]

tropapride INN

tropatepine INN

tropenziline bromide INN

TrophAmine 6%; TrophAmine 10% IV infusion ℞ *total parenteral nutrition; peripheral parenteral nutrition* [multiple essential and nonessential amino acids]

Troph-Iron liquid (name changed to Trophite + Iron in 1995)

Trophite liquid (discontinued 1995) OTC *vitamin supplement* [vitamins B_1 and B_{12}] 10 mg•25 μg per 5 mL

Trophite + Iron liquid OTC *hematinic* [ferric pyrophosphate; vitamins B_1 and B_{12}] 60 mg•30 mg•75 μg per 15 mL

trophosphamide [see: trofosfamide]

Tropicacyl eye drops ℞ *cycloplegic; mydriatic* [tropicamide] 0.5%, 1%

tropicamide USAN, USP, INN *ophthalmic anticholinergic; cycloplegic; short-acting mydriatic*

tropigline INN, BAN

tropirine INN

tropisetron INN, BAN *investigational treatment for nausea and vomiting related to chemotherapy*

Tropi-Storz eye drops ℞ *cycloplegic; mydriatic* [tropicamide] 0.5%, 1%

tropodifene INN

troquidazole INN

trospectomycin INN, BAN *broad-spectrum aminocyclitol antibiotic* [also: trospectomycin sulfate]

trospectomycin sulfate USAN *broad-spectrum aminocyclitol antibiotic* [also: trospectomycin]

trospium chloride INN

trovafloxacin mesylate USAN *broad-spectrum fluoroquinolone antibacterial*

Trovan IV infusion ℞ *broad-spectrum fluoroquinolone antibiotic* [alatrofloxacin mesylate] 5 mg/mL ☑ Atrovent

Trovan tablets ℞ *broad-spectrum fluoroquinolone antibiotic* [trovafloxacin mesylate] 100, 200 mg

Trovan/Zithromax Compliance Pak ℞ *single-dose antibiotic treatment for sexually transmitted diseases* [Trovan (trovafloxacin mesylate); Zithromax (azithromycin)] 100 mg tablet; 1 g packet for oral suspension

Trovert ℞ *investigational (Phase II, orphan) growth hormone antagonist for acromegaly* [B2036-PEG (code name —generic name not yet assigned)] ⑨ Provir; Provera

troxerutin INN, BAN *vitamin P₄* *vitamin P_4*

troxidone BAN *anticonvulsant* [also: trimethadione]

troxipide INN

troxolamide INN

troxonium tosilate INN [also: troxonium tosylate]

troxonium tosylate BAN [also: troxonium tosilate]

troxundate INN *combining name for radicals or groups*

troxypyrrolium tosilate INN [also: troxypyrrolium tosylate]

troxypyrrolium tosylate BAN [also: troxypyrrolium tosilate]

true ivy *medicinal herb* [see: English ivy]

T.R.U.E. Test patch ℞ *diagnostic aid for contact dermatitis* [skin test antigens (23 different) plus 1 negative control]

Truphylline suppositories ℞ *antiasthmatic; bronchodilator* [aminophylline] 250, 500 mg

Truquant BR RIA test for professional use *in vitro diagnostic aid for breast cancer recurrence* [radioimmunoassay (RIA) test for CA27.29 antigen]

Trusopt eye drops ℞ *topical carbonic anhydrase inhibitor for glaucoma* [dorzolamide HCl] 2%

truxicurium iodide INN

truxipicurium iodide INN

trypaflavine [see: acriflavine HCl]

tryparsamide USP, INN

trypsin, crystallized USP *topical proteolytic enzyme; necrotic tissue debridement*

tryptizol [see: amitriptyline]

tryptizol HCl [see: amitriptyline HCl]

tryptophan (L-tryptophan) USAN, USP, INN *essential amino acid; serotonin precursor (The FDA has recalled all OTC tryptophan supplements.)*

Trysul vaginal cream ℞ *broad-spectrum bacteriostatic* [sulfathiazole; sulfacetamide; sulfabenzamide] 3.42%• 2.86%•3.7%

TSC (technetium sulfur colloid) [see: technetium Tc 99m sulfur colloid]

T/Scalp liquid OTC *topical corticosteroidal anti-inflammatory* [hydrocortisone] 1%

TSH (thyroid-stimulating hormone) [see: thyrotropin]

TSPA (triethylenethiophosphoramide) [see: thiotepa]

TST (tuberculin skin test) [see: tuberculin]

T-Stat topical solution, medicated pads ℞ *topical antibiotic for acne* [erythromycin] 2%

Tsuga canadensis medicinal herb [see: hemlock]

T-Tabs (trademarked form) *"T"-imprinted tablets*

tuaminoheptane USP, INN *adrenergic; vasoconstrictor*

tuaminoheptane sulfate USP

tuberculin USP *dermal tuberculosis test*

tuberculin, crude [see: tuberculin]

tuberculin, old (OT) [see: tuberculin]

tuberculin purified protein derivative (PPD) [see: tuberculin]

Tuberculin Tine Test, Old single-use intradermal puncture test device ℞ *tuberculosis skin test* [old tuberculin] 5 U

tuberculosis vaccine [see: BCG vaccine]

Tubersol intradermal injection ℞ *tuberculosis skin test* [tuberculin purified protein derivative] 1, 5, 250 U/0.1 mL

Tubex (trademarked delivery system) *cartridge-needle unit*

tubocurarine chloride USP, INN, BAN *neuromuscular blocker; muscle relaxant* 3 mg (20 U)/mL injection

tubocurarine chloride HCl pentahydrate [see: tubocurarine chloride]

tubulozole INN *antineoplastic; microtubule inhibitor* [also: tubulozole HCl]

tubulozole HCl USAN, INN *antineoplastic; microtubule inhibitor* [also: tubulozole]

tucaresol INN, BAN *investigational (Phase I/II) immunopotentiator for HIV*

Tucks; Tucks Take-Alongs cleansing pads OTC *moisturizer and cleanser for the perineal area; astringent* [witch hazel; glycerin] 50% • 10%

Tucks Clear gel OTC *astringent* [hamamelis water; glycerin] 50% • 10%

Tucks Hemorrhoidal cream (discontinued 1995) OTC *astringent* [hamamelis water] 50%

tuclazepam INN

Tuinal Pulvules (capsules) ℞ *sedative; hypnotic; also abused as a street drug* [amobarbital sodium; secobarbital sodium] 50 • 50, 100 • 100 mg ⧉ Luminal; Tylenol

tulobuterol INN, BAN, JAN [also: tulobuterol HCl]

tulobuterol HCl JAN [also: tulobuterol]

tulopafant INN

tumeric root *medicinal herb* [see: goldenseal]

tumor necrosis factor (TNF) *investigational (Phase I) antiviral for HIV; investigational treatment for septic shock* [also see: anti-TNF]

tumor necrosis factor-binding protein I and II *investigational (orphan) for symptomatic AIDS patients*

tumor necrosis therapy (TNT) *investigational (orphan) radioactive chimeric monoclonal antibody for malignant glioma and astrocytoma*

Tums; Tums E-X chewable tablets OTC *antacid* [calcium carbonate] 500 mg; 750 mg

Tums 500; Tums Ultra chewable tablets OTC *antacid* [calcium carbonate] 1.25 g; 1 g

tung seed *(Aleurites cordata; A. moluccana)* seed and oil *medicinal herb for asthma, bowel evacuation, and tumors; not generally regarded as safe and effective as it is highly toxic*

tungsten *element (W)*

Turbinaire (trademarked delivery system) *nasal inhalation aerosol*

Turbuhaler (trademarked delivery system) *dry powder in a metered-dose inhaler*

turkey corn *(Corydalis formosa)* root *medicinal herb used as an antisyphilitic, bitter tonic, and diuretic*

turkey pea; wild turkey pea *medicinal herb* [see: turkey corn]

turmeric *(Curcuma domestica; C. longa)* rhizomes *medicinal herb for flatulence, hemorrhage, hepatitis and jaundice, topical analgesia, and ringworm*

Turnera aphrodisiaca; T. diffusa; T. microphylla *medicinal herb* [see: damiana]

turosteride INN

turpentine *(Pinus palustris)* gum *natural treatment for colds, cough, and toothache; also used topically as a counterirritant for muscle pain and rheumatic disorders*

turtlebloom *(Chelone glabra)* leaves *medicinal herb used as an anthelmintic, aperient, cholagogue, and detergent*

Tusibron syrup OTC *expectorant* [guaifenesin; alcohol 3.5%] 100 mg/5 mL ⧉ Tussigon

Tusibron-DM syrup OTC *antitussive; expectorant* [dextromethorphan hydrobromide; guaifenesin] 15 • 100 mg/5 mL

Tusquelin syrup ℞ *antitussive; decongestant; antihistamine; analgesic* [dextromethorphan hydrobromide; phenylpropanolamine HCl; phenylephrine HCl; chlorpheniramine maleate; alcohol 5%] 15 • 5 • 5 • 2 mg/5 mL

Tussafed syrup, pediatric drops ℞ *antitussive; decongestant; antihistamine* [dextromethorphan hydrobromide; pseudoephedrine HCl; carbinoxamine maleate; menthol] 15•60•4 mg/5 mL; 4•25•2 mg/mL ℞ Tussafin

Tussafed HC syrup ℞ *narcotic antitussive; decongestant; expectorant* [hydrocodone bitartrate; phenylephrine HCl; guaifenesin] 2.5•7.5•50 mg/5 mL

Tussafin Expectorant liquid ℞ *narcotic antitussive; decongestant; expectorant* [hydrocodone bitartrate; pseudoephedrine HCl; guaifenesin; alcohol 12.5%] 5•60•200 mg/5 mL ℞ Tussafed

Tuss-Allergine Modified T.D. capsules ℞ *antitussive; decongestant* [caramiphen edisylate; phenylpropanolamine HCl] 40•75 mg

Tussanil DH syrup ℞ *narcotic antitussive; decongestant; antihistamine* [hydrocodone bitartrate; phenylephrine HCl; chlorpheniramine maleate; alcohol 5%] 2.5•10•4 mg/5 mL

Tussanil DH tablets ℞ *narcotic antitussive; decongestant; expectorant; analgesic* [hydrocodone bitartrate; phenylpropanolamine HCl; guaifenesin; salicylamide] 1.66•25•100•300 mg

Tussanil Plain syrup (discontinued 1995) ℞ *decongestant; antihistamine* [phenylephrine HCl; chlorpheniramine maleate; alcohol 5%] 10•4 mg/5 mL

Tussar DM syrup OTC *antitussive; decongestant; antihistamine* [dextromethorphan hydrobromide; pseudoephedrine HCl; chlorpheniramine maleate] 15•30•2 mg/5 mL

Tussar SF; Tussar-2 liquid ℞ *narcotic antitussive; antihistamine; expectorant* [codeine phosphate; pseudoephedrine HCl; guaifenesin; alcohol 2.5%] 10•30•100 mg/5 mL

Tuss-DM tablets OTC *antitussive; expectorant* [dextromethorphan hydrobromide; guaifenesin] 10•200 mg

Tussend syrup ℞ *narcotic antitussive; decongestant; antihistamine* [hydrocodone bitartrate; pseudoephedrine HCl; chlorpheniramine maleate; alcohol 5%] 2.5•30•2 mg/5 mL

Tussex Cough syrup OTC *antitussive; decongestant; expectorant* [dextromethorphan hydrobromide; phenylephrine HCl; guaifenesin] 10•5• 100 mg/5 mL ℞ Tussionex; Tussirex

Tussgen liquid (discontinued 1995) ℞ *narcotic antitussive; decongestant* [hydrocodone bitartrate; pseudoephedrine HCl; alcohol 5%] 5•60 mg/5 mL

Tuss-Genade Modified sustained-release capsules (discontinued 1995) ℞ *antitussive; decongestant* [caramiphen edisylate; phenylpropanolamine HCl] 40•75 mg

Tussi-12 oral suspension ℞ *pediatric antitussive, decongestant, and antihistamine* [carbetapentane tannate; phenylephrine tannate; chlorpheniramine tannate] 30•5•4 mg/5 mL

Tussigon tablets ℞ *narcotic antitussive; anticholinergic* [hydrocodone bitartrate; homatropine methylbromide] 5•1.5 mg ℞ Tusibron

Tussilago farfara medicinal herb [see: coltsfoot]

Tussionex Pennkinetic extended-release suspension ℞ *narcotic antitussive; antihistamine* [hydrocodone polistirex; chlorpheniramine polistirex] 10•8 mg/5 mL ℞ Tussex; Tussirex

Tussi-Organidin DM NR; Tussi-Organidin DM-S NR liquid (S includes a 10 mL oral syringe) ℞ *antitussive; expectorant* [dextromethorphan hydrobromide; guaifenesin] 10•100 mg/5 mL

Tussi-Organidin NR; Tussi-Organidin-S NR liquid (S includes a 10 mL oral syringe) ℞ *narcotic antitussive; expectorant* [codeine phosphate; guaifenesin] 10•100 mg/5 mL

Tussirex syrup, sugar-free liquid ℞ *narcotic antitussive; decongestant; antihistamine; expectorant; analgesic* [codeine phosphate; phenylephrine HCl; pheniramine maleate; sodium citrate; sodium salicylate; caffeine citrate] 10•4.17•13.33•83.3•83.33•25 mg/5 mL ℞ Tussex; Tussionex

Tuss-LA sustained-release tablets ℞ *decongestant; expectorant* [pseudo-ephedrine HCl; guaifenesin] 120•500 mg

Tusso-DM liquid ℞ *antitussive; expectorant* [dextromethorphan hydrobromide; iodinated glycerol] 10•30 mg/5 mL

Tussogest extended-release capsules ℞ *antitussive; decongestant* [caramiphen edisylate; phenylpropanolamine HCl] 40•75 mg

Tuss-Ornade Spansules (sustained-release capsules), liquid (discontinued 1997) ℞ *antitussive; decongestant* [caramiphen edisylate; phenylpropanolamine HCl] 40•75 mg; 6.7•12.5 mg/5 mL

Tusstat syrup ℞ *antihistamine; antitussive* [diphenhydramine HCl; alcohol 5%] 12.5 mg/5 mL

tuvatidine INN

tuvirumab USAN, INN *investigational (Phase II) antiviral monoclonal antibody for hepatitis B*

TVC-2 Dandruff Shampoo (discontinued 1998) OTC *antiseborrheic; antibacterial; antifungal* [pyrithione zinc] 2%

T-Vites tablets OTC *vitamin/mineral supplement* [multiple vitamins & minerals; biotin] ±•30 μg

12 Hour nasal spray OTC *nasal decongestant* [oxymetazoline HCl] 0.05%

12 Hour Antihistamine Nasal Decongestant sustained-release tablets (discontinued 1995) OTC *decongestant; antihistamine* [pseudo-ephedrine sulfate; dexbrompheniramine maleate] 120•6 mg

12 Hour Cold sustained-release capsules (discontinued 1995) OTC *decongestant; antihistamine* [phenylpropanolamine HCl; chlorpheniramine maleate] 75•4 mg

12 Hour Cold sustained-release tablets OTC *decongestant; antihistamine* [pseudoephedrine sulfate; dexbrompheniramine maleate] 120•6 mg

Twice-A-Day nasal spray OTC *nasal decongestant* [oxymetazoline HCl] 0.05%

Twilite caplets OTC *antihistaminic sleep aid* [diphenhydramine HCl] 50 mg

twin leaf *(Jeffersonia diphylla)* root *medicinal herb used as an antirheumatic, antispasmodic, antisyphilitic, diuretic, emetic, and expectorant*

Twin-K liquid ℞ *potassium supplement* [potassium gluconate; potassium citrate] 20 mEq/15 mL (K)

TwoCal HN ready-to-use liquid OTC *enteral nutritional therapy* [lactose-free formula]

Two-Dyne capsules (discontinued 1998) ℞ *analgesic; sedative* [acetaminophen; caffeine; butalbital] 325•40•50 mg

tybamate USAN, NF, INN, BAN *minor tranquilizer*

Ty-Cold tablets (discontinued 1995) OTC *antitussive; decongestant; antihistamine; analgesic* [dextromethorphan hydrobromide; pseudoephedrine HCl; chlorpheniramine maleate; acetaminophen] 15•30•2•325 mg

tyformin BAN [also: tiformin]

tylcalsin [see: calcium acetylsalicylate]

tylemalum [see: carbubarb]

Tylenol tablets, caplets, gelcaps, liquid OTC *analgesic; antipyretic* [acetaminophen] 325, 500 mg; 325, 650 mg; 500 mg; 500 mg/15 mL ② Tuinal

Tylenol, Children's chewable tablets, liquid OTC *analgesic; antipyretic* [acetaminophen] 80 mg; 160 mg/5 mL

Tylenol, Children's ⓐ suspension OTC *analgesic; antipyretic* [acetaminophen] 32 mg/mL

Tylenol Allergy Sinus caplets, gelcaps OTC *decongestant; antihistamine; analgesic* [pseudoephedrine HCl; chlorpheniramine maleate; acetaminophen] 30•2•500 mg

Tylenol Allergy Sinus NightTime caplets OTC *decongestant; antihistamine; analgesic* [pseudoephedrine HCl; diphenhydramine HCl; acetaminophen] 30•25•500 mg

Tylenol Arthritis Extended Relief
extended-release caplets OTC *analgesic;
antipyretic* [acetaminophen] 650 mg

Tylenol Cold effervescent tablets (discontinued 1995) OTC *decongestant;
antihistamine; analgesic* [phenylpropanolamine HCl; chlorpheniramine
maleate; acetaminophen] 12.5•2•
325 mg

Tylenol Cold, Children's chewable
tablets, liquid OTC *pediatric decongestant, antihistamine and analgesic*
[pseudoephedrine HCl; chlorpheniramine maleate; acetaminophen]
7.5•0.5•80 mg; 15•1•160 mg/5 mL

Tylenol Cold, Multi-Symptom caplets, tablets OTC *antitussive; decongestant; antihistamine; analgesic* [dextromethorphan hydrobromide;
pseudoephedrine HCl; chlorpheniramine maleate; acetaminophen] 10•
30•2•325 mg

Tylenol Cold & Flu powder for oral
solution (name changed to Tylenol
Multi-Symptom Hot Medication in
1995)

Tylenol Cold & Flu No Drowsiness
powder for oral solution (discontinued 1995) OTC *antitussive; decongestant; analgesic* [dextromethorphan
hydrobromide; pseudoephedrine
HCl; acetaminophen] 30•60•650
mg/packet

**Tylenol Cold Multi Symptom Plus
Cough, Children's** liquid OTC
*pediatric antitussive, decongestant,
antihistamine, and analgesic* [dextromethorphan hydrobromide; pseudoephedrine HCl; chlorpheniramine
maleate; acetaminophen] 5•15•1•
160 mg/5 mL

Tylenol Cold Night Time liquid (discontinued 1995) OTC *decongestant;
antihistamine; analgesic* [pseudoephedrine HCl; diphenhydramine
HCl; acetaminophen; alcohol 10%]
2•1.66•21.66 mg

Tylenol Cold No Drowsiness caplets,
gelcaps OTC *antitussive; decongestant;
analgesic* [dextromethorphan hydro-

bromide; pseudoephedrine HCl;
acetaminophen] 15•30•325 mg

Tylenol Cold Plus Cough, Children's chewable tablets OTC *antitussive; decongestant; antihistamine;
analgesic* [dextromethorphan hydrobromide; pseudoephedrine HCl;
chlorpheniramine maleate; acetaminophen] 2.5•7.5•0.5•80 mg

Tylenol Cough liquid (name changed
to Multi-Sympton Tylenol Cough in
1995)

Tylenol Cough, Multi-Symptom
liquid OTC *antitussive; analgesic* [dextromethorphan hydrobromide; acetaminophen; alcohol 5%] 10•216.7
mg/5 mL

Tylenol Cough with Decongestant
liquid (name changed to Multi-
Symptom Tylenol Cough with
Decongestant in 1995)

**Tylenol Cough with Decongestant,
Multi-Symptom** liquid OTC *antitussive; decongestant; analgesic* [dextromethorphan hydrobromide; pseudoephedrine HCl; acetaminophen;
alcohol 5%] 10•20•200 mg/5 mL

Tylenol Extended Relief (name
changed to Tylenol Arthritis
Extended Relief in 1998)

Tylenol Flu gelcaps OTC *antitussive;
decongestant; analgesic* [dextromethorphan hydrobromide; pseudoephedrine
HCl; acetaminophen] 15•30•500 mg

Tylenol Flu NightTime gelcaps, powder OTC *decongestant; antihistamine;
analgesic* [pseudoephedrine HCl;
diphenhydramine HCl; acetaminophen] 30•25•500 mg; 60•50•1000
mg/packet

Tylenol Fruit; Tylenol Junior Fruit
⊛ chewable tablets OTC *analgesic;
antipyretic* [acetaminophen] 80 mg;
160 mg

Tylenol Headache Plus caplets OTC
analgesic; antipyretic; antacid [acetaminophen; calcium carbonate] 500•
250 mg

Tylenol Infants' Drops solution OTC *analgesic; antipyretic* [acetaminophen] 100 mg/mL

Tylenol Infants' Drops ⒸⒶⓃ suspension OTC *analgesic; antipyretic* [acetaminophen] 80 mg/mL

Tylenol Junior Strength chewable tablets OTC *analgesic; antipyretic* [acetaminophen] 160 mg

Tylenol Multi-Symptom Hot Medication powder for oral solution OTC *antitussive; decongestant; antihistamine; analgesic* [dextromethorphan hydrobromide; pseudoephedrine HCl; chlorpheniramine maleate; acetaminophen] 30•60•4•650 mg/packet

Tylenol No. 2, No. 3, and No. 4 [see: Tylenol with Codeine]

Tylenol PM tablets, caplets, gelcaps OTC *antihistaminic sleep aid; analgesic* [diphenhydramine HCl; acetaminophen] 25•500 mg

Tylenol Severe Allergy caplets OTC *antihistamine; analgesic* [diphenhydramine HCl; acetaminophen] 12.5•500 mg

Tylenol Sinus tablets, caplets, geltabs, gelcaps OTC *decongestant; analgesic; antipyretic* [pseudoephedrine HCl; acetaminophen] 30•500 mg

Tylenol with Codeine elixir ℞ *narcotic analgesic* [codeine phosphate; acetaminophen] 12•120 mg/5 mL

Tylenol with Codeine No. 2, No. 3, and No. 4 tablets ℞ *narcotic analgesic; sometimes abused as a street drug* [codeine phosphate; acetaminophen] 15•300 mg; 30•300 mg; 60•300 mg

tylosin INN, BAN

Tylox capsules ℞ *narcotic analgesic* [oxycodone HCl; acetaminophen] 5•500 mg

tyloxapol USAN, USP, INN, BAN *detergent; wetting agent; cleaner/lubricant for artificial eyes; investigational (orphan) for cystic fibrosis*

Tympagesic ear drops ℞ *topical local anesthetic; analgesic; decongestant* [benzocaine; antipyrine; phenylephrine HCl] 5%•5%•0.25%

Typherex (commercially available in England) ℞ *investigational vaccine for typhoid fever*

Typhim Vi IM injection ℞ *typhoid vaccine for adults and children over 2 years* [typhoid vaccine, Vi polysaccharide] 25μg/0.5 mL

typhoid vaccine USP *active bacterin for typhoid fever (Salmonella typhi Ty21a, attenuated)*

Typhoid Vaccine (AKD) subcu injection by jet injectors only ℞ *typhoid vaccine for military use only* [typhoid vaccine, acetone-killed and dried] 8 U/mL

Typhoid Vaccine (H-P) subcu injection (incompatible with jet injectors) ℞ *typhoid vaccine for adults and children* [typhoid vaccine, heat- and phenol-inactivated] 8 U/mL

typhoid Vi capsular polysaccharide vaccine *active bacterin for typhoid fever (Salmonella typhi Ty2, inactivated)*

typhus vaccine USP

"typical" antipsychotics [see: conventional antipsychotics]

Tyrex-2 powder OTC *enteral nutritional therapy for tyrosinemia type II*

Tyrodone liquid ℞ *antitussive; decongestant* [hydrodocone bitartrate; pseudoephedrine HCl; alcohol 5%] 5•60 mg/5 mL

tyromedan INN *thyromimetic* [also: thyromedan HCl]

tyromedan HCl [see: thyromedan HCl]

Tyromex-1 powder OTC *formula for infants with tyrosinemia type I*

tyropanoate sodium USAN, USP *oral radiopaque contrast medium for cholecystography (57.4% iodine)* [also: sodium tyropanoate]

tyrosine (L-tyrosine) USAN, USP, INN *nonessential amino acid; symbols: Tyr, Y*

Tyrosum Cleanser liquid, packets OTC *topical cleanser for acne* [isopropanol; acetone] 50%•10%

tyrothricin USP, INN *antibacterial*

Tyzine nasal spray, nose drops, pediatric drops ℞ *nasal decongestant* [tetra-hydrozoline HCl] 0.1%; 0.1%; 0.05%

U89 *investigational (Phase I/II) reverse transcriptase inhibitor for AIDS*

UAA sugar-coated tablets ℞ *urinary antibiotic; analgesic; antispasmodic; acidifier* [methenamine; phenyl salicylate; atropine sulfate; methylene blue; hyoscyamine sulfate; benzoic acid] 40.8•18.1•0.03•5.4•0.03•4.5 mg

UAD cream, lotion ℞ *topical anti-infective; corticosteroidal anti-inflammatory* [clioquinol; hydrocortisone]

UAD Otic ear drop suspension ℞ *topical corticosteroidal anti-inflammatory; antibiotic* [hydrocortisone; neomycin sulfate; polymyxin B sulfate] 1%•5 mg•10 000 U per mL

ubenimex INN

ubidecarenone INN

ubiquinone [see: coenzyme Q10]

ubisindine INN

UBT Breath Test for H. pylori test for professional use *diagnostic aid for the detection of ulcers*

Ucephan oral solution ℞ *to prevent and treat hyperammonemia of urea cycle enzymopathy (orphan)* [sodium benzoate; sodium phenylacetate] 10•10 g/100 mL

UCG Beta Slide Monoclonal II slide tests for professional use *in vitro diagnostic aid for urine pregnancy test*

UCG Slide tests for professional use *in vitro diagnostic aid for urine pregnancy test* [latex agglutination test]

U·Cort cream (discontinued 1997) ℞ *topical corticosteroidal anti-inflammatory* [hydrocortisone acetate] 1%

UDIP (trademarked packaging form) *unit-dose identification package*

Uendex ℞ *investigational (Phase II) antiviral for HIV and AIDS; investiga-tional (orphan) for cystic fibrosis* [dextran sulfate]

ufenamate INN

ufiprazole INN

UFT ℞ *investigational antimetabolite antineoplastic* [tegafur; uracil] 4:1

U·Ject (trademarked delivery system) *prefilled disposable syringe*

UK-109,496 *investigational (Phase II) antifungal for HIV-related candidiasis and aspergillosis*

Ulcerease mouth rinse OTC *topical antipruritic/counterirritant; mild local anesthetic* [phenol] 0.6%

uldazepam USAN, INN *sedative*

ulinastatin INN

Ulmus fulva; U. rubra medicinal herb [see: slippery elm]

ulobetasol INN *topical corticosteroidal anti-inflammatory* [also: halobetasol propionate]

ULR-LA long-acting tablets ℞ *decongestant; expectorant* [phenylpropanolamine HCl; guaifenesin] 75•400 mg

Ultane liquid for vaporization ℞ *inhalation general anesthetic* [sevoflurane]

Ultiva powder for IV infusion ℞ *short-acting narcotic analgesic for general anesthesia* [remifentanil HCl] 1 mg/mL

Ultra Derm lotion, bath oil OTC *moisturizer; emollient*

Ultra KLB6 tablets OTC *dietary supplement* [vitamin B_6; multiple food supplements] 16.7•≜ mg

Ultra Mide 25 lotion OTC *moisturizer; emollient; keratolytic* [urea] 25%

Ultra Tears eye drops OTC *ophthalmic moisturizer/lubricant* [hydroxypropyl methylcellulose] 1%

Ultra Vent (trademarked delivery system) *jet nebulizer*

Ultra Vita Time tablets OTC *dietary supplement* [multiple vitamins & minerals; multiple food products; iron; folic acid; biotin] ± •6•0.4•1 mg

UltraBrom sustained-release capsules ℞ *decongestant; antihistamine* [pseudoephedrine HCl; brompheniramine maleate] 120•12 mg

UltraBrom PD timed-release capsules ℞ *pediatric decongestant and antihistamine* [pseudoephedrine HCl; brompheniramine maleate] 60•6 mg

Ultracal liquid OTC *enteral nutritional therapy* [lactose-free formula]

Ultra-Care solution + tablets OTC *two-step chemical disinfecting system for soft contact lenses* [hydrogen peroxide-based] 3%

Ultracef capsules, tablets, oral suspension (discontinued 1995) ℞ *cephalosporin antibiotic* [cefadroxil] 500 mg; 1 g; 125, 250 mg/5 mL

Ultra-Freeda; Ultra Freeda, Iron Free tablets OTC *geriatric vitamin/mineral supplement* [multiple vitamins & minerals; folic acid; biotin] ± •270•100 μg

UltraJect prefilled syringe ℞ *narcotic analgesic* [morphine sulfate]

Ultralan liquid OTC *enteral nutritional therapy* [lactose-free formula]

Ultram film-coated tablets ℞ *central analgesic* [tramadol HCl] 50 mg

Ultrase MT 12; Ultrase MT 20 capsules ℞ *digestive enzymes* [lipase; protease; amylase] 12 000•39 000•39 000 U; 20 000•65 000•65 000 U

Ultravate ointment, cream ℞ *topical corticosteroidal anti-inflammatory* [halobetasol propionate] 0.05%

Ultravist IV injection ℞ *radiopaque contrast medium for imaging of the head, heart, peripheral vascular system, and genitourinary tract* [iopromide (39% iodine)] 311.7, 498.72, 623.4, 768.86 mg/mL (150, 240, 300, 370 mg/mL)

Ultrazyme Enzymatic Cleaner effervescent tablets OTC *enzymatic cleaner for soft contact lenses* [subtilisin A]

umespirone INN

uña de gato *medicinal herb* [see: cat's claw]

Unasyn powder for IV or IM injection ℞ *aminopenicillin antibiotic plus synergist* [ampicillin sodium; sulbactam sodium] 1•0.5, 2•1, 10•5 g ☒ Anacin; Unisom

Uncaria guianensis; U. tomentosa *medicinal herb* [see: cat's claw]

10-undecenoic acid [see: undecylenic acid]

10-undecenoic acid, calcium salt [see: calcium undecylenate]

undecoylium chloride-iodine

undecylenic acid USP *antifungal*

Unguentine aerosol spray (discontinued 1995) OTC *topical local anesthetic* [benzocaine] 0.99 g/oz.

Unguentine ointment OTC *minor burn treatment* [phenol; zinc oxide; eucalyptus oil] 1% • ? • ?

Unguentine Plus cream OTC *topical local anesthetic* [lidocaine HCl; phenol] 2%•0.5%

Unguentum Bossi cream ℞ *topical antipsoriatic; anti-infective; bactericidal* [ammoniated mercury; methenamine sulfosalicylate; coal tar] 5%•2%•2%

Uni-Ace drops OTC *analgesic; antipyretic* [acetaminophen] 100 mg/mL

Uni-Amp (trademarked packaging form) *single-dose ampule*

Unibase OTC *ointment base*

Uni-Bent Cough syrup OTC *antihistamine; antitussive* [diphenhydramine HCl; alcohol 5%] 12.5 mg/5 mL

Unicap capsules, tablets OTC *vitamin supplement* [multiple vitamins; folic acid] ± •0.4 mg

Unicap Jr. chewable tablets OTC *vitamin supplement* [multiple vitamins; folic acid] ± •0.4 mg

Unicap M; Unicap T tablets OTC *vitamin/mineral/iron supplement* [multiple vitamins & minerals; iron; folic acid] ± •18•0.4 mg

Unicap Plus Iron tablets OTC *vitamin/iron supplement* [multiple vitamins; iron; folic acid] ± •22.5•0.4 mg

Unicap Sr. tablets OTC *vitamin/mineral/iron supplement* [multiple vitamins & minerals; iron; folic acid] ≛ •10•0.4 mg

Unicomplex T & M tablets OTC *vitamin/mineral/iron supplement* [multiple vitamins & minerals; iron; folic acid] ≛•18•0.4 mg

Uni-Decon sustained-release tablets ℞ *decongestant; antihistamine* [phenylpropanolamine HCl; phenylephrine HCl; chlorpheniramine maleate; phenyltoloxamine citrate] 40•10•5•15 mg

Uni-Dur extended-release tablets ℞ *once-daily antiasthmatic/bronchodilator* [theophylline] 400, 600 mg

Unifiber powder OTC *bulk laxative* [powdered cellulose]

unifocon A USAN *hydrophobic contact lens material*

Unilax capsules OTC *stimulant laxative; stool softener* [phenolphthalein; docusate sodium] 130•230 mg

Unimatic (trademarked delivery system) *prefilled disposable syringe*

Uni-nest (trademarked packaging form) *ampule*

Unipak (packaging form) *dispensing pack*

Unipen capsules ℞ *penicillinase-resistant penicillin antibiotic* [nafcillin sodium] 250 mg ⍰ Omnipen

Unipen film-coated tablets, powder for IV or IM injection (discontinued 1998) ℞ *penicillinase-resistant penicillin antibiotic* [nafcillin sodium] 500 mg; 0.5, 1, 2, 10 g ⍰ Omnipen

Uniphyl timed-release tablets ℞ *antiasthmatic; bronchodilator* [theophylline] 400, 600 mg

Unipres tablets (discontinued 1996) ℞ *antihypertensive; vasodilator; diuretic* [hydrochlorothiazide; reserpine; hydralazine HCl] 15•0.1•25 mg

Uniquin (foreign name for U.S. product Maxaquin)

Uniretic tablets ℞ *antihypertensive; angiotensin-converting enzyme (ACE) inhibitor; diuretic* [moexipril HCl;

hydrochlorothiazide] 7.5•12.5, 15•25 mg

Uni-Rx (trademarked packaging form) *unit-dose containers and packages*

Unisert (trademarked dosage form) *suppository*

Unisol; Unisol 4 solution OTC *rinsing/storage solution for soft contact lenses* [sodium chloride (saline solution)]

Unisol Plus aerosol solution OTC *rinsing/storage solution for soft contact lenses* [sodium chloride (saline solution)]

Unisom Nighttime Sleep-Aid tablets OTC *antihistaminic sleep aid* [doxylamine succinate] 25 mg ⍰ Anacin; Unasyn

Unisom SleepGels (capsules) OTC *antihistaminic sleep aid* [diphenhydramine HCl] 50 mg ⍰ Anacin; Unasyn

Unisom with Pain Relief tablets OTC *antihistaminic sleep aid; analgesic* [diphenhydramine citrate; acetaminophen] 50•650 mg ⍰ Anacin; Unasyn

Unistep hCG test kit for professional use *in vitro diagnostic aid for urine pregnancy test*

Unitrol timed-release capsules OTC *diet aid* [phenylpropanolamine HCl] 75 mg

Unituss HC syrup ℞ *narcotic antitussive; decongestant; antihistamine* [hydrocodone bitartrate; phenylephrine HCl; chlorpheniramine maleate] 2.5•5•2 mg/5 mL

Uni-Tussin syrup OTC *expectorant* [guaifenesin; alcohol 3.5%] 100 mg/5 mL

Uni-Tussin DM syrup OTC *antitussive; expectorant* [dextromethorphan hydrobromide; guaifenesin] 10•100 mg/5 mL

Univasc tablets ℞ *antihypertensive; angiotensin-converting enzyme (ACE) inhibitor* [moexipril HCl] 7.5, 15 mg

Universal Antidote (discontinued 1996) *general-purpose gastric adsorbent/detoxicant* [activated charcoal; magnesium hydroxide; tannic acid] ≛

Univial (trademarked form) *single-dose vials*

Unna's boot [see: Dome-Paste bandage]

Uracid capsules ℞ *urinary acidifier to control ammonia production* [raceme-

thionine] 200 mg ⑫ uracil; Urised;
Urocit

uracil USAN *antineoplastic potentiator
for tegafur (not available separately;
combined with tegafur in a 1:4 ratio)*

uracil mustard USAN, USP *nitrogen
mustard-type alkylating antineoplastic*
[also: uramustine] ⑫ Uracel; Uracid

uradal [see: carbromal]

uralenic acid [see: enoxolone]

uramustine INN, BAN *nitrogen mustard-type alkylating antineoplastic*
[also: uracil mustard]

uranin [see: fluorescein sodium]

uranium *element (U)*

urapidil INN, BAN

urea USP *osmotic diuretic; keratolytic;
emollient*

urea peroxide [see: carbamide peroxide]

Ureacin-10 lotion OTC *moisturizer;
emollient; keratolytic* [urea] 10%

Ureacin-20 cream OTC *moisturizer;
emollient; keratolytic* [urea] 20%

Ureacin-40 cream (discontinued
1995) ℞ *for removal of dystrophic
nails* [urea] 40%

Ureaphil IV infusion ℞ *osmotic diuretic*
[urea] 40 g/150 mL

Urecholine tablets, subcu injection ℞
*cholinergic urinary stimulant for post-
surgical and postpartum urinary retention* [bethanechol chloride] 5, 10,
25, 50 mg; 5 mg/mL

uredepa USAN, INN *antineoplastic*

uredofos USAN, INN *veterinary anthelmintic*

urefibrate INN

***p*-ureidobenzenearsonic acid** [see:
carbarsone]

urethan NF [also: urethane]

urethane INN, BAN [also: urethan]

urethane polymers [see: polyurethane
foam]

Urex tablets ℞ *urinary antibiotic* [meth-
enamine hippurate] 1 g ⑫ Eurax;
Serax

***Urginea indica; U. maritima; U.
scilla*** *medicinal herb* [see: squill]

Uricult culture paddles *for professional
use in vitro diagnostic aid for nitrate,
uropathogens, or bacteria in the urine*

uridine 5'-triphosphate *investigational
(Phase I/II, orphan) for cystic fibrosis
and primary ciliary dyskinesia*

Uridon Modified sugar-coated tablets
℞ *urinary antibiotic; analgesic; antispasmodic; acidifier* [methenamine;
phenyl salicylate; atropine sulfate;
methylene blue; hyoscyamine sulfate; benzoic acid] 40.8•18.1•0.03•
5.4•0.03•4.5 mg

Urimar-T tablets ℞ *urinary antibiotic;
antiseptic; analgesic; antispasmodic*
[methenamine; sodium biphosphate;
phenyl salicylate; methylene blue;
hyoscyamine sulfate] 81.6•40.8•
36.2•10.8•0.12 mg

Urinary Antiseptic No. 2 tablets ℞
*urinary antibiotic; analgesic; antispas-
modic; acidifier* [methenamine;
phenyl salicylate; atropine sulfate;
methylene blue; hyoscyamine sulfate; benzoic acid] 40.8•18.1•0.03•
5.4•0.03•4.5 mg

Urised sugar-coated tablets ℞ *urinary
antibiotic; analgesic; antispasmodic;
acidifier* [methenamine; phenyl salicylate; atropine sulfate; methylene
blue; hyoscyamine sulfate; benzoic
acid] 40.8•18.1•0.03•5.4•0.03•4.5
mg ⑫ Uracel; Uracid; Urispas

Urisedamine tablets ℞ *urinary antibiotic; antispasmodic* [methenamine mandelate; hyoscyamine] 500•0.15 mg

Urispas film-coated tablets ℞ *urinary
antispasmodic* [flavoxate HCl] 100
mg (200 mg available in Canada) ⑫
Urised

Uristat tablets ℞ *urinary analgesic*
[phenazopyridine HCl] 95 mg

Uristix; Uristix 4 reagent strips *in
vitro diagnostic aid for multiple urine
products*

Uri-Tet capsules (discontinued 1997)
℞ *broad-spectrum tetracycline antibiotic* [oxytetracycline HCl] 250 mg

Uritin tablets ℞ *urinary antibiotic;
analgesic; antispasmodic; acidifier*

[methenamine; phenyl salicylate; atropine sulfate; methylene blue; hyoscyamine sulfate; benzoic acid] 40.8•18.1•0.03•5.4•0.03•4.5 mg

Urobak tablets ℞ *broad-spectrum bacteriostatic* [sulfamethoxazole] 500 mg

Urobiotic-250 capsules (discontinued 1997) ℞ *urinary anti-infective; urinary analgesic* [oxytetracycline HCl; sulfamethizole; phenazopyridine HCl] 250•250•50 mg ⚕ Otobiotic

Urocit-K tablets ℞ *urinary alkalizer for nephrolithiasis and hypocitruria prevention (orphan)* [potassium citrate] 5, 10 mEq ⚕ Uracid

Urodine tablets (discontinued 1997) ℞ *urinary analgesic* [phenazopyridine HCl] 100, 200 mg

urofollitrophin BAN *follicle-stimulating hormone (FSH)* [also: urofollitropin]

urofollitropin USAN, INN *follicle-stimulating hormone (FSH); ovulation stimulant for polycystic ovarian disease (orphan) and assisted reproductive techniques (ARTs); investigational (orphan) for spermatogenesis in hormone-deficient males* [also: urofollitrophin]

urogastrone *investigational (orphan) for recovery from corneal transplant surgery*

Urogesic tablets ℞ *urinary analgesic* [phenazopyridine HCl] 100 mg

Urogesic Blue sugar-coated tablets ℞ *urinary antibiotic; antiseptic; analgesic; antispasmodic* [methenamine; sodium biphosphate; phenyl salicylate; methylene blue; hyoscyamine sulfate] 81.6•40.8•36.2•10.8•0.12 mg

urokinase USAN, INN, BAN, JAN *plasminogen activator; thrombolytic enzyme*

urokinase alfa USAN *plasminogen activator; thrombolytic enzyme*

Uro-KP-Neutral film-coated tablets ℞ *urinary acidifier; phosphorus supplement* [sodium phosphate; potassium phosphate; monobasic sodium phosphate] 250 mg (P)

Urolene Blue tablets ℞ *urinary anti-infective and antiseptic; antidote to cyanide poisoning* [methylene blue] 65 mg

Uro-Mag capsules OTC *antacid; magnesium supplement* [magnesium oxide] 140 mg

uronal [see: barbital]

Uro-Phosphate film-coated tablets ℞ *urinary antibiotic; acidifier* [methenamine; sodium biphosphate] 300•434.78 mg

Uroqid-Acid No. 2 film-coated tablets ℞ *urinary antibiotic; acidifier* [methenamine mandelate; sodium acid phosphate] 500•500 mg

Urovist Cysto intracavitary instillation (discontinued 1999) ℞ *radiopaque contrast medium for cystourethrography* [diatrizoate meglumine (46.67% iodine)] 30% (14.1%)

Urovist Meglumine DIU/CT injection (discontinued 1999) ℞ *radiopaque contrast medium* [diatrizoate meglumine (46.67% iodine)] 30%

Urovist Sodium 300 injection (discontinued 1999) ℞ *radiopaque contrast medium* [diatrizoate sodium (59.87% iodine)] 50%

Ursinus Inlay-Tabs (tablets) OTC *decongestant; analgesic; antipyretic* [pseudoephedrine HCl; aspirin] 30•325 mg

Urso tablets ℞ *bile acid for primary biliary cirrhosis (orphan); investigational for hypercholesterolemia, type IIa and IIb* [ursodiol] 250 mg

ursodeoxycholic acid INN, BAN *naturally occurring bile acid; anticholelithogenic* [also: ursodiol]

ursodiol USAN *naturally occurring bile acid for primary biliary cirrhosis (orphan); investigational for hypercholesterolemia, type IIa and IIb* [also: ursodeoxycholic acid]

ursulcholic acid INN

Urtica dioica; U. urens medicinal herb [see: nettle]

Uticort cream, lotion, gel (discontinued 1996) ℞ *topical corticosteroidal anti-inflammatory* [betamethasone benzoate] 0.025%

uva ursi *(Arbutus uva ursi; Arctostaphylos uva ursi)* leaves *medicinal herb for bladder and kidney infections,*

Bright's disease, constipation, diabetes, gonorrhea, nephritis, spleen disorders, urethritis, and uterine ulcerations

Uvadex extracorporeal solution (leukocytes are collected, photoactivated with the UVAR Photopheresis System, then reinfused) ℞ *palliative treatment for cutaneous T-cell lymphoma (CTCL); investigational (orphan) treatment of diffuse systemic sclerosis and to prevent rejection of cardiac allografts* [methoxsalen] 20 μg/mL

VA (vincristine, actinomycin D) *chemotherapy protocol*

VA-10367 *investigational neurophilic compound that accelerates functional recovery and nerve regeneration in spinal cord and peripheral nerve injury*

VAAP (vincristine, asparaginase, Adriamycin, prednisone) *chemotherapy protocol*

VAB; VAB-I (vinblastine, actinomycin D, bleomycin) *chemotherapy protocol*

VAB-II (vinblastine, actinomycin D, bleomycin, cisplatin) *chemotherapy protocol*

VAB-III (vinblastine, actinomycin D, bleomycin, cisplatin, chlorambucil, cyclophosphamide) *chemotherapy protocol*

VAB-V (vinblastine, actinomycin D, bleomycin, cyclophosphamide, cisplatin) *chemotherapy protocol*

VAB-6 (vinblastine, actinomycin D, bleomycin, cyclophosphamide, cisplatin) *chemotherapy protocol*

VABCD (vinblastine, Adriamycin, bleomycin, CCNU, DTIC) *chemotherapy protocol*

VAC (vincristine, Adriamycin, cisplatin) *chemotherapy protocol*

VAC; VAC pulse; VAC standard (vincristine, actinomycin D, cyclophosphamide) *chemotherapy protocol*

VAC; VAC pulse; VAC standard (vincristine, Adriamycin, cyclophosphamide) *chemotherapy protocol* [also: CAV]

VACA (vincristine, actinomycin D, cyclophosphamide, Adriamycin) *chemotherapy protocol*

VACAD (vincristine, actinomycin D, cyclophosphamide, Adriamycin, dacarbazine) *chemotherapy protocol*

VACAdr-IfoVP (vincristine, actinomycin D, cyclophosphamide, Adriamycin, ifosfamide, VePesid) *chemotherapy protocol*

vaccines *a class of drugs used for active immunization that consist of antigens which induce endogenous production of antibodies*

vaccinia immune globulin (VIG) USP *passive immunizing agent*

vaccinia immune human globulin [now: vaccinia immune globulin]

vaccinia virus vaccine for human papillomavirus (HPV), recombinant *investigational (orphan) for cervical cancer*

Vaccinium edule; V. erythrocarpum; V. macrocarpon; V. oxycoccos; V. vitis medicinal herb [see: cranberry]

Vaccinium myrtillus medicinal herb [see: bilberry]

VACP (VePesid, Adriamycin, cyclophosphamide, Platinol) *chemotherapy protocol*

VAD (vincristine, Adriamycin, dactinomycin) *chemotherapy protocol*

VAD (vincristine, Adriamycin, dexamethasone) *chemotherapy protocol*

Vademin-Z capsules OTC *vitamin/mineral supplement* [multiple vitamins & minerals] ±

vadocaine INN
VAdrC (vincristine, Adriamycin, cyclophosphamide) chemotherapy protocol
VAD/V (vincristine, Adriamycin, dexamethasone, verapamil) chemotherapy protocol
VAFAC (vincristine, amethopterin, fluorouracil, Adriamycin, cyclophosphamide) chemotherapy protocol
Vagifem film-coated vaginal tablets ℞ estrogen replacement for postmenopausal atrophic vaginitis [estradiol hemihydrate] 25 μg
Vagi-Gard; Vagi-Gard Advanced Sensitive Formula vaginal cream OTC topical local anesthetic; keratolytic; antifungal [benzocaine; resorcinol] 20%•3%; 5%•2%
Vaginex vaginal cream OTC topical antihistamine [tripelennamine HCl]
Vagisec Douche solution ℞ vaginal cleanser and deodorizer
Vagisec Plus vaginal suppositories ℞ antibacterial [aminacrine HCl] 6 mg
Vagisil cream OTC topical local anesthetic; antipruritic; antifungal [benzocaine; resorcinol] 5%•2%
Vagisil powder OTC absorbs vaginal moisture [cornstarch; aloe]
Vagistat-1 vaginal ointment in prefilled applicator OTC antifungal [tioconazole] 6.5%
VAI (vincristine, actinomycin D, ifosfamide) chemotherapy protocol
valaciclovir INN antiviral for herpes zoster and herpes simplex [also: valacyclovir HCl]
valacyclovir HCl USAN antiviral for herpes zoster and herpes simplex [also: valaciclovir]
valconazole INN
valdetamide INN
valdipromide INN
valepotriate [see: valtrate]
Valergen 10 IM injection (discontinued 1995) ℞ estrogen replacement therapy for postmenopausal disorders; antineoplastic for prostatic cancer [estradiol valerate in oil] 10 mg/mL

Valergen 20; Valergen 40 IM injection ℞ estrogen replacement therapy for postmenopausal disorders; antineoplastic for prostatic cancer [estradiol valerate in oil] 20 mg/mL; 40 mg/mL
valerian (Valeriana officinalis) root medicinal herb for convulsions, hypertension, hysteria, hypochondria, nervousness, pain, and sedation
valerian, false medicinal herb [see: life root]
Valertest No. 1 IM injection ℞ estrogen/androgen for menopausal vasomotor symptoms [estradiol valerate; testosterone enanthate] 4•90 mg/mL
valethamate bromide NF
valganciclovir HCl USAN antiviral
valine (L-valine) USAN, USP, INN, JAN essential amino acid; symbols: Val, V
valine & isoleucine & leucine investigational (orphan) for hyperphenylalaninemia
Valisone ointment, cream, lotion ℞ topical corticosteroidal anti-inflammatory [betamethasone valerate] 0.1%
Valisone Reduced Strength cream ℞ topical corticosteroidal anti-inflammatory [betamethasone valerate] 0.01%
Valium tablets, IV or IM injection, Tel-E-Ject syringes ℞ benzodiazepine sedative; anxiolytic; anticonvulsant; skeletal muscle relaxant; also abused as a street drug [diazepam] 2, 5, 10 mg; 5 mg/mL; 10 mg ⊡ thallium; Valpin
Valium Roche Oral ⓒⒶⓃ tablets ℞ benzodiazepine sedative; anxiolytic; anticonvulsant; skeletal muscle relaxant; also abused as a street drug [diazepam] 5, 10 mg
valnoctamide USAN, INN tranquilizer
valofane INN
valperinol INN
valproate pivoxil INN
valproate semisodium INN anticonvulsant; antipsychotic for manic episodes; migraine prophylaxis [also: divalproex sodium; semisodium valproate]
valproate sodium USAN anticonvulsant 250 mg/5 mL oral

valproic acid USAN, USP, INN, BAN *anticonvulsant* 250 mg oral

valpromide INN

Valrelease sustained-release capsules (discontinued 1996) ℞ *benzodiazepine sedative; anxiolytic; skeletal muscle relaxant; anticonvulsant adjunct* [diazepam] 15 mg

valrubicin *anthracycline antibiotic antineoplastic for bladder cancer (orphan)*

valsartan USAN, INN *antihypertensive; angiotensin II receptor antagonist*

Valstar intravesical solution ℞ *anthracycline antibiotic antineoplastic for bladder cancer (orphan)* [valrubicin] 40 mg/mL

valtrate INN

Valtrex film-coated caplets ℞ *antiviral for herpes zoster, herpes simplex, and genital herpes* [valacyclovir HCl] 500 mg

VAM (vinblastine, Adriamycin, mitomycin) *chemotherapy protocol*

VAM (VP-16-213, Adriamycin, methotrexate) *chemotherapy protocol*

VAMP (vincristine, actinomycin, methotrexate, prednisone) *chemotherapy protocol*

VAMP (vincristine, Adriamycin, methylprednisolone) *chemotherapy protocol*

VAMP (vincristine, amethopterin, mercaptopurine, prednisone) *chemotherapy protocol*

vanadium *element (V)*

Vancenase Pockethaler (nasal inhalation aerosol) ℞ *corticosteroidal anti-inflammatory for seasonal or perennial rhinitis* [beclomethasone dipropionate] 42 μg/dose

Vancenase AQ nasal spray ℞ *corticosteroidal anti-inflammatory for seasonal or perennial rhinitis* [beclomethasone dipropionate] 0.084%

Vanceril; Vanceril Double Strength oral inhalation aerosol ℞ *corticosteroidal anti-inflammatory for chronic asthma* [beclomethasone dipropionate] 42 μg/dose; 84 μg/dose

Vancocin Pulvules (capsules), powder for oral solution, powder for IV or IM injection ℞ *tricyclic glycopeptide antibiotic* [vancomycin HCl] 125, 250 mg; 1, 10 g; 0.5, 1, 10 g

Vancoled powder for IV or IM injection ℞ *tricyclic glycopeptide antibiotic* [vancomycin HCl] 0.5, 1, 5 g

vancomycin INN, BAN *tricyclic glycopeptide antibiotic* [also: vancomycin HCl]

vancomycin HCl USP *tricyclic glycopeptide antibiotic* [also: vancomycin] 1 g oral; 0.5, 1, 5, 10 g/vial injection

vaneprim INN

Vanex Expectorant liquid ℞ *narcotic antitussive; decongestant; expectorant* [hydrocodone bitartrate; pseudoephedrine HCl; guaifenesin; alcohol 5%] 2.5•30•100 mg/5 mL

Vanex Forte sustained-release caplets ℞ *decongestant; antihistamine* [phenylpropanolamine HCl; phenylephrine HCl; chlorpheniramine maleate; pyrilamine maleate] 50•10•4•25 mg

Vanex Forte-R sustained-release capsules ℞ *decongestant; antihistamine* [phenylpropanolamine HCl; chlorpheniramine maleate] 75•12 mg

Vanex-HD liquid ℞ *narcotic antitussive; decongestant; antihistamine* [hydrocodone bitartrate; phenylephrine HCl; chlorpheniramine maleate] 1.67•5•2 mg/5 mL

Vanex-LA long-acting tablets (discontinued 1996) ℞ *decongestant; expectorant* [phenylpropanolamine HCl; guaifenesin] 75•400 mg

Vanicream OTC *cream base*

vanilla NF *flavoring agent*

vanilla (Vanilla fragrans; V. planifolia; V. tahitensis) bean *medicinal herb for CNS stimulation, fever, and flatulence; also used as an aphrodisiac*

vanillin NF *flavoring agent*

N-vanillylnonamide [see: nonivamide]

N-vanillyloleamide [see: olvanil]

vanitiolide INN

Vanoxide lotion OTC *topical keratolytic for acne* [benzoyl peroxide] 5%

Vanoxide-HC lotion ℞ *topical corticosteroidal anti-inflammatory and keratolytic for acne* [benzoyl peroxide; hydrocortisone] 5%•0.5%

Vanquish caplets OTC *analgesic; antipyretic; anti-inflammatory* [acetaminophen; aspirin; caffeine] 194•227•33 mg

Vanseb cream, lotion OTC *antiseborrheic; keratolytic* [sulfur; salicylic acid]

Vansil capsules ℞ *anthelmintic for schistosomiasis (flukes)* [oxamniquine] 250 mg

Vanticon (German name for U.S. product Accolate)

Vantin film-coated tablets, granules for suspension ℞ *broad-spectrum cephalosporin antibiotic* [cefpodoxime proxetil] 100, 200 mg; 50, 100 mg/5 mL ☑ Banthine; Bantron

vanyldisulfamide INN

VAP (vinblastine, actinomycin D, Platinol) *chemotherapy protocol*

VAP (vincristine, Adriamycin, prednisone) *chemotherapy protocol*

VAP (vincristine, Adriamycin, procarbazine) *chemotherapy protocol*

VAP (vincristine, asparaginase, prednisone) *chemotherapy protocol*

vapiprost INN, BAN *antagonist to thromboxane* A_2 [also: vapiprost HCl]

vapiprost HCl USAN *antagonist to thromboxane* A_2 [also: vapiprost]

Vaponefrin solution for inhalation (discontinued 1999) OTC *sympathomimetic bronchodilator* [racepinephrine] 2%

Vaporole (trademarked dosage form) *crushable ampule for inhalation*

vapreotide USAN *antineoplastic*

Vaqta IM injection ℞ *immunization against hepatitis A virus (HAV)* [hepatitis A vaccine, inactivated] 25 U/0.5 mL (pediatric), 50 U/mL (adult)

varicella virus vaccine *live, attenuated vaccine for chickenpox*

varicella-zoster immune globulin (VZIG) USP *passive immunizing agent* 10%–18% (125 U/2.5 mL)

Varivax powder for subcu injection ℞ *vaccine for chickenpox* [varicella virus vaccine, live attenuated] 1350 PFU/0.5 mL

Varoniscastrum virgincum medicinal herb [see: Culver's root]

Vascor film-coated tablets ℞ *antianginal* [bepridil HCl] 200, 300, 400 mg

Vascoray injection ℞ *radiopaque contrast medium* [iothalamate meglumine; iothalamate sodium (51.3% total iodine)] 520•260 mg/mL (400 mg/mL)

vascular endothelial growth factor (VEGF) *investigational (Phase II) gene therapy for peripheral vascular disease and coronary artery disease*

vascular serotonin 5-HT_1 receptor agonists *a class of antimigraine agents that constrict cranial blood vessels and inhibit the release of inflammatory neuropeptides*

Vaseretic 5-12.5; Vaseretic 10-25 tablets ℞ *antihypertensive; angiotensin-converting enzyme (ACE) inhibitor; diuretic* [enalapril maleate; hydrochlorothiazide] 5•12.5 mg; 10•25 mg

vasoactive intestinal polypeptide (VIP) *investigational (NDA filed) treatment for male sexual dysfunction; investigational (orphan) for acute esophageal food impaction*

VasoCare ℞ *investigational agent that reduces stress* ☑ VasoClear

Vasocidin eye drops ℞ *topical ophthalmic corticosteroidal anti-inflammatory; antibiotic* [prednisolone sodium phosphate; sulfacetamide sodium] 0.25%•10% ☑ Vasodilan

Vasocidin ophthalmic ointment ℞ *topical ophthalmic corticosteroidal anti-inflammatory; antibiotic* [prednisolone acetate; sulfacetamide sodium] 0.5%•10%

Vasocine ophthalmic ointment ℞ *topical ophthalmic corticosteroidal anti-inflammatory; antibiotic* [prednisolone acetate; sulfacetamide sodium] 0.5%•10% ☑ Vaseline

VasoClear eye drops OTC *topical ophthalmic decongestant and lubricant*

[naphazoline HCl; polyvinyl alcohol; polyethylene glycol 400] 0.02%•0.25%•1% ⊠ VasoCare

VasoClear A eye drops OTC *topical ophthalmic decongestant and astringent* [naphazoline HCl; zinc sulfate] 0.02%•0.25%

Vasocon Regular eye drops ℞ *topical ophthalmic decongestant and vasoconstrictor* [naphazoline HCl] 0.1%

Vasocon-A eye drops ℞ *topical ophthalmic decongestant and antihistamine* [naphazoline HCl; antazoline phosphate] 0.05%•0.5%

vasoconstrictors *a class of cardiovascular drugs that narrow the blood vessels*

Vasoderm; Vasoderm-E cream ℞ *topical corticosteroidal anti-inflammatory* [fluocinonide]

Vasodilan tablets ℞ *peripheral vasodilator* [isoxsuprine HCl] 10, 20 mg ⊠ Vasocidin

vasodilators *a class of cardiovascular drugs that dilate the blood vessels*

Vasoflux ℞ *investigational (Phase II) anticoagulant for use in acute myocardial infarction patients* ⊠ Vasoprost; Vasosulf

Vasomax ℞ *investigational (NDA filed) oral treatment for erectile dysfunction* [phentolamine mesylate]

vasopressin (VP) USP, INN *posterior pituitary hormone; antidiuretic* 20 U/mL injection

vasopressin tannate USP *posterior pituitary hormone; antidiuretic*

vasopressors *a class of posterior pituitary hormones that raise blood pressure by causing contraction of capillaries and arterioles; a class of sympathomimetic agents that raise blood pressure by increasing myocardial contractility* [also called: vasopressins]

Vasoprost ℞ *investigational (orphan) prostaglandin for severe peripheral arterial occlusive disease* [alprostadil] ⊠ Vasoflux

Vasosulf eye drops ℞ *topical ophthalmic antibiotic and decongestant* [sulfacetamide sodium; phenylephrine HCl] 15%•0.125% ⊠ Velosef; Vasoflux

Vasotate HC ear drops ℞ *topical corticosteroidal anti-inflammatory; antibacterial; antifungal* [hydrocortisone; acetic acid] 1%•2%

Vasotec tablets ℞ *antihypertensive; angiotensin-converting enzyme (ACE) inhibitor* [enalapril maleate] 2.5, 5, 10, 20 mg

Vasotec I.V. injection ℞ *antihypertensive; angiotensin-converting enzyme (ACE) inhibitor* [enalaprilat] 1.25 mg/mL

Vasoxyl IV or IM injection ℞ *vasopressor for hypotensive shock during surgery* [methoxamine HCl] 20 mg/mL

VAT (vinblastine, Adriamycin, thiotepa) *chemotherapy protocol*

VATD; VAT-D (vincristine, ara-C, thioguanine, daunorubicin) *chemotherapy protocol*

VATH (vinblastine, Adriamycin, thiotepa, Halotestin) *chemotherapy protocol*

Vatronol [see: Vicks Vatronol]

VAV (VP-16-213, Adriamycin, vincristine) *chemotherapy protocol*

Vaxigrip ⓐ (U.S. product: Fluogen) IM injection ℞ *flu vaccine* [influenza split-virus vaccine] 0.5 mL/dose

VaxSyn HIV-1 ℞ *investigational (orphan) antiviral (therapeutic, Phase II) and vaccine (preventative, Phase I) for HIV and AIDS* [gp160 antigens]

VB (vinblastine, bleomycin) *chemotherapy protocol*

VBA (vincristine, BCNU, Adriamycin) *chemotherapy protocol*

VBAP (vincristine, BCNU, Adriamycin, prednisone) *chemotherapy protocol*

VBC (VePesid, BCNU, cyclophosphamide) *chemotherapy protocol*

VBC (vinblastine, bleomycin, cisplatin) *chemotherapy protocol*

VBD (vinblastine, bleomycin, DDP) *chemotherapy protocol*

VBM (vincristine, bleomycin, methotrexate) *chemotherapy protocol*

VBMCP (vincristine, BCNU, melphalan, cyclophosphamide, prednisone) *chemotherapy protocol*

VBMF (vincristine, bleomycin, methotrexate, fluorouracil) *chemotherapy protocol*

VBP (vinblastine, bleomycin, Platinol) *chemotherapy protocol*

VC (VePesid, carboplatin) *chemotherapy protocol*

VC (vincristine) [q.v.]

VC (vinorelbine, cisplatin) *chemotherapy protocol*

VCAP (vincristine, cyclophosphamide, Adriamycin, prednisone) *chemotherapy protocol* [see also: V-CAP III]

V-CAP III (VP-16-213, cyclophosphamide, Adriamycin, Platinol) *chemotherapy protocol* [see also: VCAP]

VCF (vaginal contraceptive film) OTC *spermicidal contraceptive* [nonoxynol 9] 28%

VCF (vincristine, cyclophosphamide, fluorouracil) *chemotherapy protocol*

V-Cillin K powder for oral solution (discontinued 1997) ℞ *natural penicillin antibiotic* [penicillin V potassium] 125, 250 mg/5 mL ⊘ Bicillin; Wycillin

V-Cillin K tablets (discontinued 1998) ℞ *natural penicillin antibiotic* [penicillin V potassium] 125, 250, 500 mg ⊘ Bicillin; Wycillin

VCMP (vincristine, cyclophosphamide, melphalan, prednisone) *chemotherapy protocol*

VCP (vincristine, cyclophosphamide, prednisone) *chemotherapy protocol*

VCP 205 *investigational (Phase I) vaccine for HIV*

VCR (vincristine) [q.v.]

VDA (vincristine, daunorubicin, asparaginase) *chemotherapy protocol*

V-Dec-M sustained-release tablets ℞ *decongestant; expectorant* [pseudoephedrine HCl; guaifenesin] 120•500 mg

VDP (vinblastine, dacarbazine, Platinol) *chemotherapy protocol*

VDP (vincristine, daunorubicin, prednisone) *chemotherapy protocol*

Vectrin capsules ℞ *tetracycline antibiotic* [minocycline HCl] 50, 100 mg

vecuronium bromide USAN, INN, BAN *nondepolarizing neuromuscular blocker; muscle relaxant; adjunct to anesthesia* 10, 20 mg injection

Veetids film-coated tablets ℞ *natural penicillin antibiotic* [penicillin V potassium] 250, 500 mg

Veetids '125'; Veetids '250' powder for oral solution ℞ *natural penicillin antibiotic* [penicillin V potassium] 125 mg/5 mL; 250 mg/5 mL

vegetable oil, hydrogenated NF *tablet and capsule lubricant*

vegetable tallow; vegetable wax *medicinal herb* [see: bayberry]

VEGF (vascular endothelial growth factor) [q.v.]

Vehicle/N; Vehicle/N Mild OTC *lotion base*

VeIP (Velban, ifosfamide, Platinol) *chemotherapy protocol*

Velban powder for IV injection ℞ *antineoplastic for lung, breast and testicular cancers, lymphomas, sarcomas, and neuroblastoma* [vinblastine sulfate] 10 mg ⊘ Valpin

Veldona low-dose oral ℞ *investigational (Phase I) cytokine for AIDS and hepatitis B* [interferon alfa]

velnacrine INN, BAN *cholinesterase inhibitor* [also: velnacrine maleate]

velnacrine maleate USAN *cholinesterase inhibitor for Alzheimer's disease* [also: velnacrine]

Velosef capsules, oral suspension, powder for IV or IM injection ℞ *cephalosporin antibiotic* [cephradine] 250, 500 mg; 125, 250 mg/5 mL; 250, 500, 1000, 2000 mg ⊘ Vasosulf

Velosulin Human BR subcu injection OTC *antidiabetic* [human insulin (the rDNA version is replacing the semisynthetic version)] 100 U/mL

Veltane tablets (discontinued 1997) ℞ *antihistamine* [brompheniramine maleate] 4 mg

Velvachol OTC *cream base*

Vendona ℞ *investigational cytokine for AIDS*

Venice turpentine *medicinal herb* [see: larch]

venlafaxine INN, BAN *antidepressant; anxiolytic; serotonin and norepineph-rine reuptake inhibitor* [also: venlafax-ine HCl]

venlafaxine HCl USAN *antidepressant; anxiolytic; serotonin and norepinephrine reuptake inhibitor* [also: venlafaxine]

Venoglobulin-I powder for IV infusion ℞ *passive immunizing agent for HIV and idiopathic thrombocytopenic purpura (ITP)* [immune globulin] 50 mg/mL

Venoglobulin-S IV infusion ℞ *passive immunizing agent for HIV and idio-pathic thrombocytopenic purpura (ITP)* [immune globulin, solvent/detergent treated] 5%, 10%

Venomil subcu or IM injection ℞ *venom sensitivity testing (subcu); venom desensitization therapy (IM)* [extracts of honeybee, yellow jacket, yellow hornet, white-faced hornet, mixed vespid, and wasp venom]

Ventolin inhalation aerosol ℞ *sympa-thomimetic bronchodilator* [albuterol] 90 μg/dose ☑ phentolamine

Ventolin Rotacaps (encapsulated pow-der for inhalation), tablets, solution for inhalation, Nebules (unit-dose solution for inhalation), syrup ℞ *sympathomimetic bronchodilator* [albu-terol sulfate] 200 μg; 2, 4 mg; 0.05%; 0.083%; 2 mg/5 mL

VePesid IV injection, capsules ℞ *anti-neoplastic for testicular and small cell lung cancers* [etoposide] 20 mg/mL; 50 mg

Veracolate tablets OTC *stimulant laxa-tive* [phenolphthalein; cascara sagrada extract; capsicum oleoresin] 32.4•75•0.05 mg

veradoline INN *analgesic* [also: verado-line HCl]

veradoline HCl USAN *analgesic* [also: veradoline]

veralipride INN

verapamil USAN, INN, BAN *coronary vasodilator; calcium channel blocker*

verapamil HCl USAN, USP *antianginal; antiarrhythmic; antihypertensive; cal-cium channel blocker* 40, 80, 120, 180, 240 mg oral; 5 mg/2 mL injection

Veratrum species *medicinal herb* [see: hellebore]

veratrylidene-isoniazid [see: verazide]

verazide INN, BAN

Verazinc capsules OTC *zinc supplement* [zinc sulfate] 220 mg

Verbascum nigrum; V. phlomoides; V. thapsiforme; V. thapsus *medicinal herb* [see: mullein]

Verbena hastata *medicinal herb* [see: blue vervain]

Verdia ℞ *investigational angiotensin II receptor antagonist for hypertension (NDA withdrawn 1998)* [tasosartan]

Verelan sustained-release capsules ℞ *antihypertensive; antianginal; antiar-rhythmic; calcium channel blocker* [ver-apamil HCl] 120, 180, 240, 360 mg

Verelan PM delayed-onset, extended-release capsules ℞ *antihypertensive; calcium channel blocker* [verapamil HCl] 100, 200, 300 mg

Vergon capsules OTC *anticholinergic; antihistamine; antivertigo agent; motion sickness preventative* [mecli-zine HCl] 30 mg

verilopam INN *analgesic* [also: verilo-pam HCl]

verilopam HCl USAN *analgesic* [also: verilopam]

verlukast USAN, INN *bronchodilator; antiasthmatic*

Verluma technetium Tc 99 prep kit ℞ *monoclonal antibody imaging agent for small cell lung cancer* [nofetumomab merpentan]

vermicides; vermifuges *a class of drugs effective against parasitic infec-tions* [also called: anthelmintics]

Vermox chewable tablets ℞ *anthel-mintic for trichuriasis, enterobiasis,* *ascariasis, and uncinariasis* [mebenda-zole] 100 mg

verofylline USAN, INN *bronchodilator; antiasthmatic*

veronal [see: barbital]

veronal sodium [see: barbital sodium]

veronica, tall *medicinal herb* [see: Culver's root]

Veronica beccabunga medicinal herb [see: brooklime]

Veronica officinalis medicinal herb [see: speedwell]

Verr-Canth liquid (discontinued 1997) ℞ *topical keratolytic* [cantharidin] 0.7%

Verrex liquid (discontinued 1997) ℞ *topical keratolytic* [salicylic acid; podophyllum] 30% • 10%

Verrusol liquid (discontinued 1996) ℞ *topical keratolytic* [salicylic acid; podophyllum; cantharidin] 30% • 5% • 1%

Versacaps prolonged-action capsules ℞ *decongestant; expectorant* [pseudoephedrine HCl; guaifenesin] 60 • 300 mg

Versed IV or IM injection, Tel-E-Ject syringes, pediatric syrup ℞ *short-acting benzodiazepine general anesthetic adjunct for preoperative sedation* [midazolam HCl] 1, 5 mg/mL; 2 mg/mL

versetamide USAN *stabilizer; carrier agent for gadoversetamide*

Versiclear lotion ℞ *topical antifungal; keratolytic; antipruritic; anesthetic* [sodium thiosulfate; salicylic acid; alcohol 10%] 25% • 1%

Vertab capsules (discontinued 1995) OTC *antinauseant; antiemetic; antivertigo; motion sickness preventative* [dimenhydrinate] 50 mg

verteporfin USAN *antineoplastic (used with phototherapy); investigational (Phase III) treatment for age-related macular degeneration (AMD)*

vervain *medicinal herb* [see: blue vervain]

Vesanoid capsules ℞ *antineoplastic for acute promyelocytic leukemia (orphan); investigational (orphan) for other leukemias and ophthalmic squamous metaplasia* [tretinoin] 10 mg

vesicants *a class of agents that cause blisters*

vesnarinone USAN, INN *cardiotonic; investigational inotropic for congestive heart failure (clinical trials discontinued 1996)*

vesperal [see: barbital]

Vesprin IV or IM injection ℞ *conventional (typical) antipsychotic; antiemetic* [triflupromazine HCl] 10, 20 mg/mL

vetrabutine INN, BAN

Vetuss HC syrup ℞ *narcotic antitussive; decongestant; antihistamine* [hydrocodone bitartrate; phenylpropanolamine HCl; phenylephrine HCl; pyrilamine maleate; pheniramine maleate; alcohol 5%] 1.7 • 3.3 • 5 • 3.3 • 3.3 mg/5 mL

Vexol eye drop suspension ℞ *topical ophthalmic corticosteroidal anti-inflammatory* [rimexolone] 1%

V-Gan 25; V-Gan 50 injection (discontinued 1996) ℞ *antihistamine; sedative; antiemetic; motion sickness relief* [promethazine HCl] 25 mg/mL; 50 mg/mL

Viactiv chewable tablets OTC *calcium supplement* [calcium carbonate; vitamin D; vitamin K] 1.25 g • 100 IU • 40 μg

Viaflex (trademarked form) *ready-to-use IV*

ViaFoam ℞ *investigational (Phase III) corticosteroid foam for psoriasis of the scalp* [clobetasol propionate]

Viagra film-coated tablets ℞ *selective vasodilator for erectile dysfunction* [sildenafil citrate] 25, 50, 100 mg

Vianain ℞ *investigational (orphan) proteolytic enzymes for debridement of severe burns* [ananain; comosain; bromelains]

vibesate

Vibramycin capsules, powder for IV injection ℞ *tetracycline antibiotic* [doxycycline hyclate] 50, 100 mg; 100, 200 mg

Vibramycin powder for oral suspension ℞ *tetracycline antibiotic* [doxycycline] 25 mg/5 mL

Vibramycin syrup ℞ *tetracycline antibiotic* [doxycycline calcium] 50 mg/5 mL

Vibra-Tabs tablets ℞ *tetracycline antibiotic* [doxycycline hyclate] 100 mg

Viburnum opulus *medicinal herb* [see: cramp bark]

VIC (VePesid, ifosfamide [with mesna rescue], carboplatin) *chemotherapy protocol* [also: CVI]

VIC (vinblastine, ifosfamide, CCNU) *chemotherapy protocol*

Vicam injection ℞ *parenteral vitamin therapy* [multiple B vitamins; vitamin C] ± • 50 mg/mL

Vicef capsules OTC *vitamin/iron supplement* [multiple vitamins; iron; folic acid]

Vicks 44 Non-Drowsy Cold & Cough LiquiCaps (capsules) OTC *antitussive; decongestant* [dextromethorphan hydrobromide; pseudoephedrine HCl] 30 • 60 mg

Vicks 44 Pediatric syrup (name changed to Vicks Pediatric 44d Dry Hacking Cough and Head Congestion in 1994)

Vicks 44D Cough & Head Congestion; Vicks Formula 44D Cough & Decongestant; Vicks Pediatric Formula 44d Cough & Decongestant liquid OTC *antitussive; decongestant* [dextromethorphan hydrobromide; pseudoephedrine HCl] 10 • 20 mg/5 mL; 10 • 20 mg/5 mL; 5 • 10 mg/5 mL

Vicks 44E liquid OTC *antitussive; expectorant* [dextromethorphan hydrobromide; guaifenesin] 6.7 • 66.7 mg/5 mL

Vicks 44M Cold, Flu & Cough LiquiCaps (capsules) OTC *antitussive; decongestant; antihistamine; analgesic* [dextromethorphan hydrobromide; pseudoephedrine HCl; chlorpheniramine maleate; acetaminophen] 10 • 30 • 2 • 250 mg

Vicks Cough Drops; Vicks Menthol Cough Drops OTC *topical analgesic; counterirritant; mild local anesthetic* [menthol] 10 mg; 8.4 mg

Vicks Cough Silencers lozenges OTC *antitussive; topical oral anesthetic* [dextromethorphan hydrobromide; benzocaine] 2.5 • 1 mg

Vicks Dry Hacking Cough syrup OTC *antitussive* [dextromethorphan hydrobromide; alcohol 10%] 15 mg/5 mL

Vicks Inhaler OTC *nasal decongestant* [l-desoxyephedrine] 50 mg

Vicks NyQuil products [see: NyQuil]

Vicks Pediatric 44d Dry Hacking Cough and Head Congestion syrup OTC *antitussive* [dextromethorphan hydrobromide] 15 mg/15 mL

Vicks Pediatric Formula 44e liquid OTC *antitussive; expectorant* [dextromethorphan hydrobromide; guaifenesin] 3.3 • 33.3 mg/5 mL

Vicks Pediatric Formula 44m Multi-Symptom Cough & Cold liquid OTC *pediatric antitussive, decongestant, and antihistamine* [dextromethorphan hydrobromide; pseudoephedrine HCl; chlorpheniramine maleate] 5 • 10 • 0.67 mg/5 mL

Vicks Sinex products [see: Sinex]

Vicks VapoRub vaporizing ointment, cream OTC *counterirritant* [camphor; menthol; eucalyptus oil] 4.7% • 2.6% • 1.2%

Vicks Vitamin C Drops (lozenges) OTC *vitamin supplement* [sodium ascorbate & ascorbic acid] 60 mg

Vicodin; Vicodin ES; Vicodin HP tablets ℞ *narcotic analgesic* [hydrocodone bitartrate; acetaminophen] 5 • 500 mg; 7.5 • 750 mg; 10 • 660 mg

Vicodin Tuss syrup ℞ *narcotic antitussive; expectorant* [hydrocodone bitartrate; guaifenesin] 5 • 100 mg/5 mL ② Hycodan; Hycomine

Vicon Forte capsules ℞ *vitamin/mineral supplement* [multiple vitamins & minerals; folic acid] ± • 1 mg

Vicon Plus capsules OTC *vitamin/mineral supplement* [multiple vitamins & minerals] ±

Vicon-C capsules OTC *vitamin/mineral supplement* [multiple B vitamins & minerals; vitamin C] ± • 300 mg

Vicoprofen film-coated tablets ℞ *narcotic analgesic* [hydrocodone bitartrate; ibuprofen] 7.5•200 mg

vicotrope [see: cosyntropin]

vidarabine USAN, USP, INN, BAN *antiviral* ⑨ cytarabine

vidarabine monohydrate [see: vidarabine]

vidarabine phosphate USAN *antiviral*

vidarabine sodium phosphate USAN *antiviral*

Vi-Daylin chewable tablets OTC *vitamin supplement* [multiple vitamins; folic acid] ± •0.3 mg

Vi-Daylin ADC drops OTC *vitamin supplement* [vitamins A, C, and D] 1500 IU•35 mg•400 IU per mL

Vi-Daylin ADC Vitamins + Iron drops OTC *vitamin/iron supplement* [vitamins A, C, and D; ferrous gluconate] 1500 IU•35 mg•400 IU•10 mg per mL

Vi-Daylin Multivitamin liquid, drops OTC *vitamin supplement* [multiple vitamins] ±

Vi-Daylin Multivitamin + Iron chewable tablets OTC *vitamin/iron supplement* [multiple vitamins; iron; folic acid] ± •12•0.3 mg

Vi-Daylin Multivitamin + Iron liquid, drops OTC *vitamin/iron supplement* [multiple vitamins; ferrous gluconate] ± •10 mg/5 mL; ± •10 mg/mL

Vi-Daylin/F ADC drops ℞ *pediatric vitamin supplement and dental caries preventative* [vitamins A, C, and D; sodium fluoride] 1500 IU•35 mg• 400 IU•0.25 mg per mL

Vi-Daylin/F ADC + Iron drops ℞ *pediatric vitamin/iron supplement and dental caries preventative* [vitamins A, C, and D; sodium fluoride; ferrous sulfate] 1500 IU•35 mg•400 IU• 0.25 mg•10 mg per mL

Vi-Daylin/F Multivitamin chewable tablets ℞ *pediatric vitamin supplement and dental caries preventative* [multiple vitamins; sodium fluoride; folic acid] ± •1•0.3 mg

Vi-Daylin/F Multivitamin drops ℞ *pediatric vitamin supplement and dental caries preventative* [multiple vitamins; sodium fluoride] ± •0.25 mg/mL

Vi-Daylin/F Multivitamin + Iron chewable tablets ℞ *pediatric vitamin/ iron supplement and dental caries preventative* [multiple vitamins; sodium fluoride; ferrous sulfate; folic acid] ± •1•12•0.3 mg

Vi-Daylin/F Multivitamin + Iron drops ℞ *pediatric vitamin/iron supplement and dental caries preventative* [multiple vitamins; sodium fluoride; ferrous sulfate] ± •0.25•10 mg/mL

Videx chewable/dispersible tablets, powder for oral solution, powder for pediatric oral solution ℞ *antiviral for advanced HIV infection and AIDS* [didanosine] 25, 50, 100, 150 mg; 100, 167, 250, 375 mg/packet; 2, 4 g

VIE (vincristine, ifosfamide, etoposide) *chemotherapy protocol*

vifilcon A USAN *hydrophilic contact lens material*

vifilcon B USAN *hydrophilic contact lens material*

Vi-Flor [see: Poly-Vi-Flor; Tri-Vi-Flor]

VIG (vaccinia immune globulin) [q.v.]

vigabatrin USAN, INN, BAN *anticonvulsant for tardive dyskinesia*

Vigomar Forte tablets OTC *vitamin/ mineral/iron supplement* [multiple vitamins & minerals; iron] ± •12 mg

Vigortol liquid OTC *geriatric vitamin/ mineral supplement* [multiple B vitamins & minerals; alcohol 18%] ±

VIL ℞ *investigational (orphan) for hyperphenylalaninemia* [valine; isoleucine; leucine]

viloxazine INN, BAN *bicyclic antidepressant* [also: viloxazine HCl]

viloxazine HCl USAN *bicyclic antidepressant* [also: viloxazine]

Viminate liquid OTC *geriatric vitamin/ mineral supplement* [multiple B vitamins & minerals] ±

viminol INN

VIMRxyn ℞ *investigational (Phase I) antiviral for HIV and AIDS* [hypericin (synthetic)]

vinafocon A USAN *hydrophobic contact lens material*

vinbarbital NF, INN [also: vinbarbitone]

vinbarbital sodium NF

vinbarbitone BAN [also: vinbarbital]

vinblastine INN *antineoplastic* [also: vinblastine sulfate]

vinblastine sulfate USAN, USP *antineoplastic* [also: vinblastine] 10 mg/vial, 1 mg/mL injection

vinburnine INN

vinca alkaloids *a class of natural antineoplastics*

Vinca major; V. minor medicinal herb [see: periwinkle]

vincaleukoblastine sulfate [see: vinblastine sulfate]

vincamine INN, BAN

vincanol INN

vincantenate [see: vinconate]

vincantril INN

Vincasar PFS IV injection ℞ *antineoplastic* [vincristine sulfate] 1 mg/mL

vincofos USAN, INN *anthelmintic*

vinconate INN

vincristine (VC; VCR) INN *antineoplastic* [also: vincristine sulfate]

vincristine sulfate USAN, USP *antineoplastic* [also: vincristine] 1 mg/mL injection

vindeburnol INN

vindesine USAN, INN, BAN *antineoplastic*

vindesine sulfate USAN, JAN *antineoplastic*

vinegar [see: acetic acid]

vinepidine INN *antineoplastic* [also: vinepidine sulfate]

vinepidine sulfate USAN *antineoplastic* [also: vinepidine]

vinformide INN

vinglycinate INN *antineoplastic* [also: vinglycinate sulfate]

vinglycinate sulfate USAN *antineoplastic* [also: vinglycinate]

vinleurosine INN *antineoplastic* [also: vinleurosine sulfate]

vinleurosine sulfate USAN *antineoplastic* [also: vinleurosine]

vinmegallate INN

vinorelbine INN *antineoplastic* [also: vinorelbine tartrate]

vinorelbine tartrate USAN *antineoplastic* [also: vinorelbine]

vinpocetine USAN, INN

vinpoline INN

vinrosidine INN *antineoplastic* [also: vinrosidine sulfate]

vinrosidine sulfate USAN *antineoplastic* [also: vinrosidine]

vintiamol INN

vintoperol INN

vintriptol INN

vinyl alcohol polymer [see: polyvinyl alcohol]

vinyl ether USP

vinyl gamma-aminobutyric acid [see: vigabatrin]

vinylbital INN [also: vinylbitone]

vinylbitone BAN [also: vinylbital]

vinylestrenolone [see: norgesterone]

vinymal [see: vinylbital]

vinyzene [see: bromchlorenone]

vinzolidine INN *antineoplastic* [also: vinzolidine sulfate]

vinzolidine sulfate USAN *antineoplastic* [also: vinzolidine]

Vioform cream, ointment OTC *topical antifungal; antibacterial* [clioquinol] 3%

Viogen-C capsules OTC *vitamin/mineral supplement* [multiple B vitamins & minerals; vitamin C] ±•300 mg

Viokase tablets, powder ℞ *digestive enzymes* [lipase; protease; amylase] 8000•30 000•30 000 U; 16 800•70 000•70 000 U/0.7 g

Viola odorata medicinal herb [see: violet]

Viola tricolor medicinal herb [see: pansy]

violet (Viola odorata) flowers and leaves *medicinal herb for asthma, bronchitis, cancer, colds, cough, sinus congestion, tumors, and ulcers*

violet, garden medicinal herb [see: pansy]

violetbloom medicinal herb [see: bittersweet nightshade]

viomycin INN [also: viomycin sulfate]

viomycin sulfate USP [also: viomycin]

viosterol in oil [see: ergocalciferol]

Vioxx tablets, oral suspension ℞ *COX-2 inhibitor anti-inflammatory and analgesic for osteoarthritis, acute pain, and primary dysmenorrhea* [rofecoxib] 12.5, 25 mg; 12.5, 25 mg/5 mL

VIP (vasoactive intestinal polypeptide) [q.v.]

VIP; VIP-1; VIP-2 (VePesid, ifosfamide [with mesna rescue], Platinol) *chemotherapy protocol*

VIP (vinblastine, ifosfamide [with mesna rescue], Platinol) *chemotherapy protocol*

VIP-B (VP-16, ifosfamide, Platinol, bleomycin) *chemotherapy protocol*

Viprinex Ⓒ subcu injection, IV infusion ℞ *anticoagulant for deep vein thrombosis (DVT) and severe chronic peripheral circulatory disorders* [ancrod] 70 IU/mL

viprostol USAN, INN, BAN *hypotensive; vasodilator*

viprynium embonate BAN *anthelmintic* [also: pyrvinium pamoate]

viqualine INN

viquidil INN

Viquin Forte cream ℞ *hyperpigmentation bleaching agent; sunscreen* [hydroquinone; padimate O; dioxybenzone; oxybenzone] 4%•8%•3%•2%

Vira-A IV infusion (discontinued 1995) ℞ *antiviral for herpes simplex and herpes zoster* [vidarabine] 200 mg/mL

Vira-A ophthalmic ointment ℞ *topical antiviral for acute keratoconjunctivitis and recurrent epithelial keratitis due to herpes simplex virus infection* [vidarabine] 3%

Viracept tablets, powder for oral solution ℞ *antiretroviral HIV-1 protease inhibitor* [nelfinavir mesylate] 250 mg; 50 mg/g

Viractin cream, gel OTC *topical anesthetic for cold sores and fever blisters* [tetracaine HCl] 2%

Viramune tablets, oral suspension ℞ *antiviral non-nucleoside reverse transcriptase inhibitor (NNRTI) for HIV-1* [nevirapine] 200 mg; 50 mg/5 mL

Virazole powder for inhalation aerosol ℞ *antiviral for severe lower respiratory tract infections; investigational (Phase II/III) for HIV; investigational (orphan) for hemorrhagic fever with renal syndrome* [ribavirin] 6 g/100 mL vial (20 mg/mL reconstituted)

Virend ℞ *investigational (Phase II) antiviral for AIDS-related genital herpes* [SP-303 (code name—generic name not yet assigned)]

Virginia mountain mint; Virginia thyme *medicinal herb* [see: wild hyssop]

Virginia silk *medicinal herb* [see: milkweed]

virginiamycin USAN, INN *antibacterial; veterinary food additive*

virginiamycin factor M₁ [see: virginiamycin]

virginiamycin factor S [see: virginiamycin]

virgin's bower *medicinal herb* [see: woodbine]

viridofulvin USAN, INN *antifungal*

Virilon capsules ℞ *androgen for male hypogonadism, impotence and breast cancer* [methyltestosterone] 10 mg

Virogen Herpes slide test for professional use *in vitro diagnostic aid for herpes simplex virus antigen in lesions or cell cultures* [latex agglutination test]

Virogen Rotatest slide test for professional use *in vitro diagnostic aid for fecal rotavirus* [latex agglutination test]

Virogen Rubella; Virogen Rubella Microlatex slide test for professional use (discontinued 1995) *in vitro diagnostic aid for rubella virus antibodies in serum* [latex agglutination test]

Viro-Med tablets (discontinued 1995) OTC *antitussive; decongestant; antihistamine; analgesic* [dextromethorphan hydrobromide; pseudoephedrine HCl; chlorpheniramine maleate; acetaminophen] 15•30•2•500 mg

Viroptic Drop-Dose (eye drops) ℞ *ophthalmic antiviral for keratoconjunctivitis*

and epithelial keratitis due to herpes simplex virus infection [trifluridine] 1%

viroxime USAN, INN antiviral

viroxime component A [see: zinviroxime]

viroxime component B [see: enviroxime]

Virulizin investigational agent for malignant melanoma; investigational (Phase I/II) agent for HIV-related Kaposi sarcoma; investigational (Phase I/II) immunostimulant for pancreatic cancer

Viscoat prefilled syringes ℞ viscoelastic agent for ophthalmic surgery [hyaluronate sodium; chondroitin sulfate sodium] 30•40 mg/mL

Viscum album medicinal herb [see: mistletoe]

Visine eye drops (discontinued 1996) OTC topical ophthalmic decongestant and vasoconstrictor [tetrahydrozoline HCl] 0.05%

Visine A.C. eye drops (name changed to Visine Allergy Relief in 1995)

Visine Allergy Relief eye drops OTC topical ophthalmic decongestant and astringent [tetrahydrozoline HCl; zinc sulfate] 0.05%•0.25%

Visine Extra eye drops (name changed to Visine Moisturizing in 1995)

Visine L.R. eye drops OTC topical ophthalmic decongestant and vasoconstrictor [oxymetazoline HCl] 0.025%

Visine Moisturizing eye drops OTC topical ophthalmic decongestant, vasoconstrictor, and lubricant [tetrahydrozoline HCl; polyethylene glycol 400] 0.05%•1%

Vision Care Enzymatic Cleaner tablets OTC enzymatic cleaner for soft contact lenses [pork pancreatin]

Visipak (trademarked packaging form) reverse-numbered package

Visipaque intra-arterial or IV injection ℞ radiopaque contrast medium for CT, x-ray and visceral digital subtraction angiography [iodixanol (49.1% iodine)] 550, 653 mg/mL (270, 320 mg/mL)

Visken tablets ℞ antihypertensive; antianginal; β-blocker [pindolol] 5, 10 mg

visnadine INN, BAN

visnafylline INN

Vi-Sol [see: Ce-Vi-Sol; Poly-Vi-Sol; Tri-Vi-Sol]

Vistacon IM injection (discontinued 1998) ℞ anxiolytic; antiemetic [hydroxyzine HCl] 50 mg/mL

Vistaject-25; Vistaject-50 IM injection (discontinued 1996) ℞ anxiolytic; antiemetic [hydroxyzine HCl] 25 mg/mL; 50 mg/mL

Vistaquel 50 IM injection (discontinued 1997) ℞ anxiolytic [hydroxyzine HCl] 50 mg/mL

Vistaril capsules, oral suspension ℞ anxiolytic; minor tranquilizer; antihistamine for allergic pruritus [hydroxyzine pamoate] 25, 50, 100 mg; 25 mg/5 mL ⑨ Restoril

Vistaril IM injection ℞ anxiolytic; antiemetic; antihistamine for allergic pruritus [hydroxyzine HCl] 25, 50 mg/mL ⑨ Restoril; Zestril

vistatolon INN antiviral [also: statolon]

Vistazine 50 IM injection ℞ anxiolytic; antiemetic; antihistamine for allergic pruritus [hydroxyzine HCl] 50 mg/mL

Vistide IV infusion ℞ nucleoside antiviral for AIDS-related cytomegalovirus retinitis [cidofovir] 75 mg/mL

Visual-Eyes ophthalmic solution OTC extraocular irrigating solution [sterile isotonic solution]

Visudyne ℞ investigational (Phase III) treatment for age-related macular degeneration (AMD) [verteporfin]

Vita Bee C-800 tablets (discontinued 1995) OTC vitamin supplement [multiple B vitamins; vitamins C and E] ≛ •800•45 mg

Vita-bee with C Captabs (capsule-shaped tablets) OTC vitamin supplement [multiple B vitamins; vitamin C] ≛ •300 mg

Vita-Bob softgel capsules OTC vitamin supplement [multiple vitamins; folic acid] ≛ •0.4 mg

Vita-C crystals OTC *vitamin supplement* [ascorbic acid] 4 g/tsp.

VitaCarn oral solution ℞ *dietary amino acid for primary and secondary genetic carnitine deficiency (orphan); investigational (orphan) for end-stage renal disease and pediatric cardiomyopathy* [levocarnitine]

Vit-A-Drops eye drops (discontinued 1995) OTC *ocular moisturizer/lubricant* [vitamin A]

Vita-Feron tablets (discontinued 1998) OTC *hematinic* [iron; folic acid; vitamin B₁₂] 150•0.8•0.006 mg

Vitafōl syrup ℞ *hematinic* [ferric pyrophosphate; multiple B vitamins; folic acid] 90• ± •0.75 mg/15 mL

Vitafōl; Vitafōl-PN film-coated caplets ℞ *hematinic; vitamin supplement* [ferrous fumarate; multiple vitamins; folic acid] 65 mg• ± •1 mg

Vita-Kid chewable wafers OTC *vitamin supplement* [multiple vitamins; folic acid] ± •0.3 mg

Vital B-50 timed-release tablets OTC *vitamin supplement* [multiple B vitamins; folic acid; biotin] ± •100•50 μg

Vital High Nitrogen powder OTC *enteral nutritional therapy* [lactose-free formula] 79 g

Vitalets chewable tablets OTC *vitamin/mineral/iron supplement* [multiple vitamins & minerals; iron; biotin] ± •10 mg•25 μg

VitalEyes capsules (discontinued 1995) OTC *vitamin/mineral supplement* [vitamins A, C, and E; multiple minerals] 10 000 IU•200 mg•100 IU• ±

Vitalize SF liquid OTC *hematinic* [ferric pyrophosphate; multiple B vitamins; lysine] 66• ± •300 mg/15 mL

vitamin A USP *vitamin; antixerophthalmic; topical emollient* 10 000, 25 000, 50 000 IU oral

vitamin A acid [see: tretinoin]

vitamin A palmitate

vitamin A₁ [see: retinol]

Vitamin B Complex 100 injection ℞ *parenteral vitamin therapy* [multiple B vitamins] ±

vitamin B₁ [see: thiamine HCl]

vitamin B₁ mononitrate [see: thiamine mononitrate]

vitamin B₂ [see: riboflavin]

vitamin B₃ [see: niacin; niacinamide]

vitamin B₅ [see: calcium pantothenate]

vitamin B₆ [see: pyridoxine HCl]

vitamin B₈ [see: adenosine phosphate]

vitamin B₁₂ [now: cyanocobalamin; hydroxocobalamin]

vitamin B_c [see: folic acid]

vitamin B_t [see: carnitine]

vitamin C [see: ascorbic acid]

vitamin D [see: ergocalciferol (D₂); cholecalciferol (D₃)]

Vitamin D Oral Drops OTC *vitamin supplement* [ergocalciferol (vitamin D₂)] 8000 IU/mL

vitamin D₁ [see: dihydrotachysterol]

vitamin D₂ [see: ergocalciferol]

vitamin D₃ [see: cholecalciferol]

vitamin E USP *vitamin E supplement; topical emollient* 100, 200, 400, 500, 600, 1000 IU oral

vitamin E-TPGS (tocopheryl polyethylene glycol succinate) [see: tocophersolan]

vitamin G [see: riboflavin]

vitamin H [see: biotin]

vitamin K₁ [see: phytonadione]

vitamin K₂ [see: menaquinone]

vitamin K₃ [see: menadione]

vitamin K₄ [see: menadiol sodium diphosphate]

vitamin M [see: folic acid]

vitamin P [see: bioflavonoids]

vitamin P₄ [see: troxerutin]

Vitamin-Mineral Supplement liquid OTC *vitamin/mineral supplement* [multiple B vitamins & minerals; alcohol 18%]

vitamins A & D (topical) *emollient*

Vitaneed liquid OTC *enteral nutritional therapy* [lactose-free formula]

Vita-Plus E softgels OTC *vitamin supplement* [vitamin E] 400 IU

Vita-Plus G softgel capsules OTC *geriatric vitamin/mineral supplement* [multiple vitamins & minerals]

Vita-Plus H softgel capsules OTC *vitamin/mineral/iron supplement* [multiple vitamins & minerals; iron] ± • 13.4 mg

Vita-PMS; Vita-PMS Plus tablets OTC *vitamin/mineral supplement; digestive enzymes* [multiple vitamins & minerals; folic acid; biotin; amylase; protease; lipase; betaine acid HCl] ± • 0.33 mg • 10.4 μg • 2500 U • 2500 U • 200 U • 16.7 mg

Vitarex tablets OTC *vitamin/mineral/iron supplement* [multiple vitamins & minerals; iron] ± • 15 mg

Vitaxin ℞ *investigational (Phase II) angiogenesis inhibitor for leiomyosarcoma*

Vite E cream OTC *emollient* [vitamin E] 50 mg/g

Vitec cream OTC *emollient* [vitamin E]

vitellin *natural remedy* [see: lecithin]

Vitex agnus-castus *medicinal herb* [see: chaste tree]

Vitinoin ⓒⒶⓝ (U.S. product: Retin-A) cream, gel ℞ *topical keratolytic for acne* [tretinoin] 0.025%, 0.05%, 0.1%; 0.025%

Vitis coigetiae; V. vinifera *medicinal herb* [see: grape seed]

Vitrase ℞ *investigational (Phase III) agent to clear vitreous hemorrhage*

Vitrasert intraocular implant (5–8 months' duration) ℞ *antiviral for AIDS-related CMV retinitis (orphan)* [ganciclovir] 4.5 mg

Vitravene intravitreal injection ℞ *ophthalmic antiviral for AIDS-related CMV retinitis* [fomivirsen sodium] 6.6 mg/mL

Vitron-C chewable tablets OTC *hematinic* [iron (from ferrous fumarate); ascorbic acid] 66 • 125 mg ② Vytone

Vitron-C-Plus tablets (discontinued 1998) OTC *hematinic* [iron (from ferrous fumarate); ascorbic acid] 132 • 250 mg

Vivactil film-coated tablets ℞ *tricyclic antidepressant* [protriptyline HCl] 5, 10 mg

Viva-Drops eye drops OTC *ocular moisturizer/lubricant*

Vivarin tablets OTC *CNS stimulant; analeptic* [caffeine] 200 mg

Vivelle; Vivelle-Dot transdermal patch ℞ *estrogen replacement therapy for postmenopausal disorders* [estradiol] 37.5, 50, 75, 100 μg/day

Vivonex T.E.N. powder OTC *enteral nutritional therapy* [lactose-free formula]

Vivotif Berna enteric-coated capsules ℞ *typhoid fever vaccine* [typhoid vaccine, live attenuated] $2–6 \times 10^9$ viable CFU + $5–50 \times 10^9$ nonviable cells

Vi-Zac capsules OTC *vitamin/zinc supplement* [vitamins A, C, and E; zinc] 5000 IU • 500 mg • 50 mg • 18 mg

V-Lax powder OTC *bulk laxative* [psyllium hydrophilic mucilloid] 50%

VLP (vincristine, L-asparaginase, prednisone) *chemotherapy protocol*

VM (vinblastine, mitomycin) *chemotherapy protocol*

VM-26 [see: teniposide]

VM-26PP (teniposide, procarbazine, prednisone) *chemotherapy protocol*

VMAD (vincristine, methotrexate, Adriamycin, actinomycin D) *chemotherapy protocol*

VMCP (vincristine, melphalan, cyclophosphamide, prednisone) *chemotherapy protocol*

VML-262 *investigational (Phase II) topical treatment for psoriasis*

VMP (VePesid, mitoxantrone, prednimustine) *chemotherapy protocol*

VOCAP (VP-16-213, Oncovin, cyclophosphamide, Adriamycin, Platinol) *chemotherapy protocol*

volatile nitrites *amyl nitrite, butyl nitrite, and isobutyl nitrite vapors that produce coronary stimulant effects, abused as street drugs* [see also: nitrous oxide; petroleum distillate inhalants]

volazocine USAN, INN *analgesic*

Volmax extended-release tablets ℞ *sympathomimetic bronchodilator* [albuterol sulfate] 4, 8 mg

Voltaren delayed-release enteric-coated tablets ℞ *nonsteroidal anti-inflammatory drug (NSAID); antiarthritic; analgesic* [diclofenac sodium] 25, 50, 75 mg

Voltaren eye drops ℞ *ocular nonsteroidal anti-inflammatory drug (NSAID) for postoperative treatment following cataract extraction* [diclofenac sodium] 0.1%

Voltaren ⓒᴬᴺ tablets, suppositories ℞ *nonsteroidal anti-inflammatory drug (NSAID); antiarthritic; analgesic* [diclofenac sodium] 25, 50 mg; 50, 100 mg

Voltaren Rapide ⓒᴬᴺ (U.S. product: Cataflam) tablets ℞ *nonsteroidal anti-inflammatory drug (NSAID); antiarthritic; analgesic for primary dysmenorrhea* [diclofenac potassium] 50 mg

Voltaren SR ⓒᴬᴺ (U.S. product: Voltaren XR) slow-release tablets ℞ *once-daily antiarthritic for osteoarthritis and rheumatoid arthritis* [diclofenac sodium] 75, 100 mg

Voltaren XR extended-release tablets ℞ *once-daily antiarthritic for osteoarthritis and rheumatoid arthritis* [diclofenac sodium] 100 mg

von Willebrand's factor [see: antihemophilic factor]

Vontrol tablets (discontinued 1998) ℞ *antiemetic; antivertigo agent* [diphenidol HCl] 25 mg ▣ Bontril

vorozole USAN, INN, BAN *antineoplastic; aromatase inhibitor*

vortel [see: clorprenaline HCl]

VōSol HC Otic ear drops ℞ *topical corticosteroidal anti-inflammatory; antibacterial; antifungal* [hydrocortisone; acetic acid] 1%•2%

VōSol Otic ear drops ℞ *antibacterial; antifungal* [acetic acid] 2%

votumumab USAN *monoclonal antibody for cancer imaging and therapy*

voxergolide INN

Voxsuprine tablets ℞ *peripheral vasodilator* [isoxsuprine HCl] 10, 20 mg

VP (vasopressin) [q.v.]

VP (vincristine, prednisone) *chemotherapy protocol*

VP + A (vincristine, prednisone, asparaginase) *chemotherapy protocol*

VP-16 (VePesid; etoposide) [q.v.]

VPB (vinblastine, Platinol, bleomycin) *chemotherapy protocol*

VPBCPr (vincristine, prednisone, vinblastine, chlorambucil, procarbazine) *chemotherapy protocol*

VPCA (vincristine, prednisone, cyclophosphamide, ara-C) *chemotherapy protocol*

VPCMF (vincristine, prednisone, cyclophosphamide, methotrexate, fluorouracil) *chemotherapy protocol*

VP-L-asparaginase (vincristine, prednisone, L-asparaginase) *chemotherapy protocol*

VPP (VePesid, Platinol) *chemotherapy protocol*

V-TAD (VePesid, thioguanine, ara-C, daunorubicin) *chemotherapy protocol*

vulneraries *a class of agents that promote wound healing*

Vumon IV infusion ℞ *antineoplastic for acute lymphocytic leukemia (orphan) and bladder cancer* [teniposide] 50 mg (10 mg/mL)

V.V.S. vaginal cream ℞ *broad-spectrum bacteriostatic* [sulfathiazole; sulfacetamide; sulfabenzamide] 3.42%•2.86%•3.7%

VX-497 *investigational (Phase II) inosine monophosphate dehydrogenase (IMPDH) inhibitor for the oral treatment of hepatitis C and autoimmune diseases*

VX-740 *investigational anti-inflammatory agent*

Vytone cream ℞ *topical corticosteroidal anti-inflammatory; antifungal; antibacterial* [hydrocortisone; iodoquinol] 1%•1% ▣ Hytone; Vitron

VZIG (varicella-zoster immune globulin) [q.v.]

wahoo *(Euonymus atropurpureus)* bark *medicinal herb used as a diuretic, expectorant, and laxative*

wakerobin *medicinal herb* [see: birthroot]

wallflower; western wallflower *medicinal herb* [see: dogbane]

walnut *(Juglans* **spp.)** *medicinal herb* [see: black walnut; butternut; English walnut]

walnut, lemon; white walnut *medicinal herb* [see: butternut]

Walpole tea *medicinal herb* [see: New Jersey tea]

Wampole One-Step hCG test kit for professional use (discontinued 1995) *in vitro diagnostic aid for urine/serum pregnancy test*

wandering milkweed *medicinal herb* [see: dogbane]

warfarin INN, BAN *coumarin-derivative anticoagulant* [also: warfarin potassium]

warfarin potassium USP *coumarin-derivative anticoagulant* [also: warfarin]

warfarin sodium USP *coumarin-derivative anticoagulant* 1, 2, 2.5, 4, 5, 7.5, 10 mg oral

Wart Remover liquid OTC *topical keratolytic* [salicylic acid in flexible collodion] 17%

Wartec ⒶⒷ (U.S. product: Condylox) solution ℞ *topical antimitotic for external genital warts* [podofilox] 0.5%

Wart-Off liquid OTC *topical keratolytic* [salicylic acid in flexible collodion] 17%

water, purified USP *solvent*

water, tritiated [see: tritiated water]

water cabbage *medicinal herb* [see: white pond lily]

water dock *(Rumex aquaticus) medicinal herb* [see: yellow dock]

water eryngo *(Eryngium aquaticum)* root *medicinal herb used as a diaphoretic, diuretic, emetic, expectorant, and stimulant*

water fern *medicinal herb* [see: buckhorn brake]

water flag *medicinal herb* [see: blue flag]

water hemlock; water parsley *medicinal herb* [see: poison hemlock]

water lily *medicinal herb* [see: blue flag; white pond lily]

water lily, sweet; sweet-scented water lily; white water lily *medicinal herb* [see: white pond lily]

water moccasin snake antivenin [see: antivenin (Crotalidae) polyvalent]

water O 15 USAN *radioactive diagnostic aid for vascular disorders*

water pepper *medicinal herb* [see: knotweed]

water pimpernel; water purslain *medicinal herb* [see: brooklime]

water shamrock *medicinal herb* [see: buckbean]

water smartweed *medicinal herb* [see: knotweed]

[^{15}O]water [see: water O 15]

watercress *(Nasturtium officinale)* plant *medicinal herb for anemia, cramps, kidney and liver disorders, nervousness, and rheumatism*

water-d$_2$ [see: deuterium oxide]

wax, carnauba NF *tablet-coating agent*

wax, emulsifying NF *emulsifying and stiffening agent*

wax, microcrystalline NF *stiffening and tablet-coating agent*

wax, white NF *stiffening agent* [also: beeswax, white]

wax, yellow NF *stiffening agent* [also: beeswax, yellow]

wax cluster *medicinal herb* [see: wintergreen]

wax myrtle *medicinal herb* [see: bayberry]

weeping spruce *medicinal herb* [see: hemlock]

Wehdryl injection (discontinued 1996) ℞ *antihistamine; motion sickness preventative; sleep aid; antiparkinsonian* [diphenhydramine HCl] 50 mg/mL

Wehgen IM injection (discontinued 1996) ℞ *estrogen replacement therapy; antineoplastic for prostatic and breast cancer* [estrone] 2 mg/mL

Wehless capsules, Timecelles (sustained-release capsules) (discontinued 1996) ℞ *anorexiant; CNS stimulant* [phendimetrazine tartrate] 35 mg; 105 mg

Weightrol tablets (discontinued 1996) ℞ *anorexiant; CNS stimulant* [phendimetrazine tartrate] 35 mg

Wellbutrin tablets ℞ *aminoketone antidepressant* [bupropion HCl] 75, 100 mg

Wellbutrin SR sustained-release film-coated tablets ℞ *aminoketone antidepressant* [bupropion HCl] 100, 150 mg

Wellcovorin powder for IV infusion ℞ *chemotherapy "rescue" agent (orphan)* [leucovorin calcium] 100 mg/vial

Wellcovorin tablets ℞ *chemotherapy "rescue" agent (orphan); antidote to folic acid antagonist overdose* [leucovorin calcium] 5, 25 mg

Wellferon subcu or IM injection ℞ *biological response modifier for chronic hepatitis C (orphan); investigational (Phase III) for HIV* [interferon alfa-n1] 3 MU/mL (a MU or "megaunit" is 10^6 IU)

Wellferon ⒶⓃ subcu or IM injection ℞ *biological response modifier for hairy cell leukemia, laryngeal papillomatosis, condyloma acuminata, and chronic hepatitis B and C* [interferon alfa-n1] 3, 5, 10 MU/mL (a MU or "megaunit" is 10^6 IU)

Westcort ointment, cream ℞ *topical corticosteroidal anti-inflammatory* [hydrocortisone valerate] 0.2%

western wallflower *medicinal herb* [see: dogbane]

Wet-N-Soak solution OTC *rewetting solution for rigid gas permeable contact lenses*

Wet-N-Soak Plus solution OTC *disinfecting/wetting/soaking solution for rigid gas permeable contact lenses* [note: RGP contact indication different from hard contact indication for same product]

Wet-N-Soak Plus solution OTC *wetting/soaking solution for hard contact lenses* [note: hard contact indication

different from RGP contact indication for same product]

Wetting solution OTC *wetting solution for hard contact lenses*

Wetting & Soaking solution OTC *disinfecting/wetting/soaking solution for rigid gas permeable contact lenses* [note: one of two different products with the same name]

Wetting & Soaking solution OTC *wetting/soaking solution for hard contact lenses* [note: one of two different products with the same name]

wheat germ oil (octacosanol) *natural supplement for increasing muscle endurance*

WHF Lubricating Gel OTC *vaginal antimicrobial and lubricant* [chlorhexidine gluconate; glycerin]

white bay *medicinal herb* [see: magnolia]

white beeswax [see: beeswax, white]

White Cloverine Salve ointment OTC *skin protectant* [white petrolatum] 97%

White Cod Liver Oil Concentrate capsules, chewable tablets OTC *vitamin supplement* [vitamins A, D, and E] 10 000•400• ̱ ̱ IU; 4000•200• ̱ ̱ IU

White Cod Liver Oil Concentrate with Vitamin C chewable tablets OTC *vitamin supplement* [vitamins A, C, and D] 4000 IU•50 mg•200 IU

white cohosh (Actaea alba; A. pachypoda; A. rubra) plant and root *medicinal herb for arthritis, bowel evacuation, colds, cough, itching, promoting labor, reviving those near death, rheumatism, stimulating menses, stomach disorders, and urogenital disorders*

white endive *medicinal herb* [see: dandelion]

white fringe *medicinal herb* [see: fringe tree]

white hellebore (Veratrum album) [see: hellebore]

white horehound *medicinal herb* [see: horehound]

white lotion USP *astringent; topical protectant*

white mineral oil [see: petrolatum, white]

white mustard; white mustard seed *medicinal herb* [see: mustard]

white nettle *medicinal herb* [see: blind nettle]

white oak (Quercus alba) bark *medicinal herb for internal and external bleeding, menstrual disorders, mouth sores, skin irritation, toothache, strep throat, ulcers, and urinary bleeding*

white ointment [see: ointment, white]

white petrolatum [see: petrolatum, white]

white phenolphthalein [see: phenolphthalein]

white pine (Pinus strobus) bark *medicinal herb for bronchitis, dysentery, laryngitis, and mucous build-up*

white pond lily (Nymphaea odorata) root *medicinal herb used as an antiseptic, astringent, demulcent, discutient, and vulnerary*

white root *medicinal herb* [see: pleurisy root]

white sorrel *medicinal herb* [see: wood sorrel]

white walnut *medicinal herb* [see: butternut]

white water lily *medicinal herb* [see: white pond lily]

white wax [see: wax, white]

white willow (Salix alba) *medicinal herb* [see: willow]

whitethorn *medicinal herb* [see: hawthorn]

Whitfield's ointment OTC *topical antifungal; keratolytic* [benzoic acid; salicylic acid] 6%•3%

Whitfield's ointment [see: benzoic & salicylic acids]

whole blood [see: blood, whole]

whole root rauwolfia [see: rauwolfia serpentina]

whorlywort *medicinal herb* [see: Culver's root]

Wibi lotion OTC *moisturizer; emollient*

widow spider species antivenin [now: antivenin (Latrodectus mactans)]

Wigraine suppositories ℞ *migraine-specific vasoconstrictor* [ergotamine tartrate; caffeine; tartaric acid] 2•100•21.5 mg

Wigraine tablets ℞ *migraine-specific vasoconstrictor* [ergotamine tartrate; caffeine] 1•100 mg

wild bergamot (Monarda fistulosa) leaves *medicinal herb used as a carminative and stimulant*

wild black cherry (Prunus serotina) bark *medicinal herb used as an astringent, pectoral, sedative, and stimulant*

wild carrot *medicinal herb* [see: carrot]

wild cherry (Prunus virginiana) bark *medicinal herb for asthma, bronchitis, cough, fever, hypertension, and mucosal inflammation with discharge; also used as an expectorant*

wild cherry syrup USP

wild chicory *medicinal herb* [see: chicory]

wild clover *medicinal herb* [see: red clover]

wild cranesbill *medicinal herb* [see: alum root]

wild daisy (Bellis perennis) flowers and leaves *medicinal herb used as an analgesic, antispasmodic, demulcent, digestive, expectorant, laxative, and purgative*

wild endive *medicinal herb* [see: dandelion]

wild fennel *medicinal herb* [see: fennel]

wild geranium *medicinal herb* [see: alum root]

wild ginger (Asarum canadense) root *medicinal herb used as a carminative, diaphoretic, expectorant, and irritant; sometimes used as a substitute for ginger (Zingiber)*

wild hydrangea *medicinal herb* [see: hydrangea]

wild hyssop *medicinal herb* [see: blue vervain]

wild hyssop (Pycnanthemum virginianum) plant *medicinal herb used as an antispasmodic, carminative, diaphoretic, and stimulant*

wild indigo (Baptisia tinctoria) plant *medicinal herb used as an antiseptic,* astringent, emetic, purgative, and stimulant

wild jalap (Ipomoea pandurata) root medicinal herb used as a strong cathartic

wild lemon medicinal herb [see: mandrake]

wild lettuce (Lactuca virosa) leaves, flowers, and seeds medicinal herb for asthma, bronchitis, chronic pain, circulatory disorders, cramps, laryngitis, nervous disorders, stimulating lactation, swollen genitals, and urinary tract infections

wild marjoram medicinal herb [see: marjoram]

wild Oregon grape medicinal herb [see: Oregon grape]

wild pepper medicinal herb [see: mezereon; Siberian ginseng]

wild potato; wild scammony; wild sweet potato vine medicinal herb [see: wild jalap]

wild red raspberry medicinal herb [see: red raspberry]

wild senna medicinal herb [see: senna]

wild snowball medicinal herb [see: New Jersey tea]

wild strawberry medicinal herb [see: strawberry]

wild tobacco medicinal herb [see: lobelia]

wild turkey pea medicinal herb [see: turkey corn]

wild valerian, great medicinal herb [see: valerian]

wild woodbine medicinal herb [see: American ivy]

wild yam (Dioscorea villosa) root medicinal herb for arthritis, bilious colic, bowel spasms, gas, menstrual cramps, morning sickness, and spasmodic asthma

Willard water natural remedy for acne, alopecia, anxiety, arthritis, hypertension, and stomach ulcers

willow (Salix alba; S. caprea; S. nigra; S. purpurea) bark and buds medicinal herb for analgesia, diuresis, eczema, fever, inducing diaphoresis, headache, nervousness, rheumatism, and ulcerations; also used as an anaphrodisiac, antiseptic, and astringent

wind root medicinal herb [see: pleurisy root]

wineberry medicinal herb [see: currant]

winged elm medicinal herb [see: slippery elm]

WinRho SD; WinRho SDF IV or IM injection ℞ obstetric Rh factor immunity suppressant; treatment for immune thrombocytopenic purpura (orphan) [Rh_0(D) immune globulin] 600, 1500 IU (120, 300 µg)

Winstrol tablets ℞ anabolic steroid for hereditary angioedema [stanozolol] 2 mg

winter bloom medicinal herb [see: witch hazel]

winter clover medicinal herb [see: squaw vine]

winter marjoram; winter sweet medicinal herb [see: marjoram]

winter savory (Calamintha montana; Satureja montana; S. obovata) leaves and stems medicinal herb for diarrhea, nausea, promoting expectoration, relieving gas and flatulence, and stimulation of menstruation; also used as an aphrodisiac

winterberry (Ilex verticillata) bark and fruit medicinal herb used as an astringent, bitter tonic, and febrifuge

wintergreen (Gaultheria procumbens) leaves and oil medicinal herb for aches and pains, colds, gout, lumbago, and migraine headache; also used topically as an astringent and rubefacient

wintergreen, bitter; false wintergreen medicinal herb [see: pipsissewa]

wintergreen oil [see: methyl salicylate]

winterlein medicinal herb [see: flaxseed]

Wintersteiner's compound F [see: hydrocortisone]

winterweed medicinal herb [see: chickweed]

witch hazel (Hamamelis virginiana) bark medicinal herb for bruises, burns, colds, colitis, diarrhea, dysentery, eye irritations, hemorrhoids, internal and external bleeding, mucous membrane *inflammation of mouth, gums, and throat, tuberculosis, and varicose veins*

withania (Withania somnifera) fruit and roots *medicinal herb for diuresis, inducing emesis, liver disorders, inflammation, sedation, tuberculosis, and tumors*

withe; withy *medicinal herb* [see: willow]

wolf claw *medicinal herb* [see: club moss]

Women's Daily Formula capsules OTC *vitamin/calcium/iron supplement* [multiple vitamins; calcium; iron; folic acid] ±•450•25•0.4 mg

Wonder Ice gel OTC *topical analgesic; counterirritant* [menthol] 5.25%

Wonderful Dream salve (discontinued 1998) OTC *topical antiseptic and antimicrobial* [phenylmercuric nitrate] 1:5000

Wondra lotion OTC *moisturizer; emollient* [lanolin]

wood betony *medicinal herb* [see: betony]

wood creosote [see: creosote carbonate]

wood sanicle *medicinal herb* [see: sanicle]

wood sorrel (Oxalis acetosella) plant *medicinal herb used as an anodyne, diuretic, emmenagogue, irritant, and stomachic*

wood strawberry *medicinal herb* [see: strawberry]

woodbine (Clematis virginiana) leaves *medicinal herb for bowel evacuation, cancer, edema, fever, hypertension, inflammation, insomnia, itching, kidney disorders, skin cuts and sores, tuberculous cervical lymphadenitis, tumors, and venereal eruptions; not generally regarded as safe and effective*

woodbine; American woodbine; wild woodbine *medicinal herb* [see: American ivy]

woodruff *medicinal herb* [see: sweet woodruff]

woody nightshade *medicinal herb* [see: bittersweet nightshade]

Woolley's antiserotonin [see: benanserin HCl]

wooly parsnip *medicinal herb* [see: masterwort]

wormwood (Artemisia absinthium) plant and leaves *medicinal herb for aiding digestion, constipation, debility, fever, intestinal worms, jaundice, labor pains, menstrual cramps, and stomach and liver disorders; not generally regarded as safe and effective*

wound weed *medicinal herb* [see: goldenrod]

woundwort (Prunella vulgaris) plant *medicinal herb used as an antispasmodic, astringent, bitter tonic, diuretic, hemostatic, vermifuge, and vulnerary*

woundwort, soldier's *medicinal herb* [see: yarrow]

WOWtabs (trademarked dosage form) *quickly dissolving "without water" tablets*

Wyamine Sulfate IV or IM injection ℞ *vasopressor for hypotensive shock* [mephentermine sulfate] 15, 30 mg/mL

Wyanoids Relief Factor rectal suppositories OTC *emollient* [cocoa butter; shark liver oil] 79%•3%

Wycillin IM injection, Tubex (cartridge-needle units) ℞ *natural penicillin antibiotic* [penicillin G procaine] 600 000, 1 200 000, 2 400 000 U ⊠ Bicillin; V-Cillin

Wydase IV or subcu injection, powder for injection ℞ *adjuvant to increase absorption and dispersion of injected drugs* [hyaluronidase] 150 U/mL; 150, 1500 U/vial ⊠ Lidex

Wygesic tablets ℞ *narcotic analgesic* [propoxyphene HCl; acetaminophen] 65•650 mg

wymote *medicinal herb* [see: marsh mallow]

Wymox capsules, powder for oral suspension ℞ *aminopenicillin antibiotic* [amoxicillin] 250, 500 mg; 125, 250 mg/5 mL

Wyseal (trademarked dosage form) *film-coated tablet*

Wytensin tablets ℞ *antihypertensive* [guanabenz acetate] 4, 8 mg

Xalatan eye drops ℞ *prostaglandin agonist for glaucoma and ocular hypertension* [latanoprost] 0.005% (50 μg/mL) ⊇ Dilantin

xamoterol USAN, INN, BAN *cardiac stimulant*

xamoterol fumarate USAN *cardiac stimulant*

Xanax tablets ℞ *benzodiazepine anxiolytic* [alprazolam] 0.25, 0.5, 1, 2 mg ⊇ Zantac

xanomeline USAN *cholinergic agonist for Alzheimer's disease*

xanomeline tartrate USAN *cholinergic agonist for Alzheimer's disease*

xanoxate sodium USAN *bronchodilator*

xanoxic acid INN

xanthan gum NF *suspending agent*

xanthines, xanthine derivatives *a class of bronchodilators*

xanthinol niacinate USAN *peripheral vasodilator* [also: xantinol nicotinate]

xanthiol INN

xanthiol HCl [see: xanthiol]

xanthocillin BAN [also: xantocillin]

Xanthorhiza simplicissima medicinal herb [see: yellow root]

xanthotoxin [see: methoxsalen]

Xanthoxylum americanum; X. fraxineum medicinal herb [see: prickly ash]

xantifibrate INN

xantinol nicotinate INN *peripheral vasodilator* [also: xanthinol niacinate]

xantocillin INN [also: xanthocillin]

xantofyl palmitate INN

^{127}**Xe** [see: xenon Xe 127]

^{133}**Xe** [see: xenon Xe 133]

Xeloda film-coated tablets ℞ *antineoplastic for metastatic breast cancer; investigational (NDA filed) for colorectal cancer* [capecitabine] 150, 500 mg

xemilofiban HCl USAN *antianginal; investigational (Phase II) antithrombotic to prevent reocclusion of coronary arteries after PTCA (clinical trials discontinued 1999)*

xenalamine [see: xenazoic acid]

xenaldial [see: xenygloxal]

xenalipin USAN, INN *hypolipidemic*

xenazoic acid INN

xenbucin USAN, INN *antihypercholesterolemic*

xenbuficin [see: xenbucin]

Xenical capsules ℞ *lipase inhibitor for weight loss* [orlistat] 120 mg

xenipentone INN

xenon *element (Xe)*

xenon (^{133}Xe) INN *radioactive agent* [also: xenon Xe 133]

xenon Xe 127 USP *diagnostic aid; medicinal gas; radioactive agent*

xenon Xe 133 USAN, USP *radioactive agent* [also: xenon (^{133}Xe)]

xenthiorate INN

xenygloxal INN

xenyhexenic acid INN

xenysalate INN, BAN *topical anesthetic; antibacterial; antifungal* [also: biphenamine HCl]

xenysalate HCl [see: biphenamine HCl]

xenytropium bromide INN

Xerac AC liquid ℞ *topical cleanser for acne* [aluminum chloride; alcohol] 6.25%•96%

Xerecept *investigational (Phase I/II, orphan) agent for peritumoral brain edema* [corticotropin-releasing factor]

Xeroderm lotion (discontinued 1998) OTC *moisturizer; emollient*

xibenolol INN

xibornol INN, BAN

xilobam USAN, INN *muscle relaxant*

ximoprofen INN

xinafoate USAN, INN, BAN *combining name for radicals or groups*

xinidamine INN

xinomiline INN

xipamide USAN, INN *antihypertensive; diuretic*

xipranolol INN

XomaZyme-791 *orphan status withdrawn 1996* [anti-TAP-72 immunotoxin]

XomaZyme-H65 *orphan status withdrawn 1997* [CD5-T lymphocyte immunotoxin]

Xopenex inhalation solution ℞ *sympathomimetic bronchodilator* [levalbuterol HCl] 0.63, 1.25 mg/3 mL dose

xorphanol INN *analgesic* [also: xorphanol mesylate]

xorphanol mesylate USAN *analgesic* [also: xorphanol]

X-Prep liquid OTC *pre-procedure bowel evacuant* [senna extract; alcohol 7%] 74 mL

X-Prep Bowel Evacuant Kit-1 liquid, tablet & suppository in a kit OTC *pre-procedure bowel evacuant* [X-Prep liquid (q.v.); Senokot-S tablets (q.v.); Rectolax suppository (q.v.)]

X-Prep Bowel Evacuant Kit-2 liquid, granules & suppository in a kit OTC *pre-procedure bowel evacuant* [X-Prep liquid (q.v.); Citralax granules (q.v.); Rectolax suppository (q.v.)]

XRT (x-ray therapy) *adjunct to chemotherapy* [not a pharmaceutical agent]

X-Seb shampoo OTC *antiseborrheic; keratolytic* [salicylic acid] 4%

X-Seb Plus shampoo OTC *antiseborrheic; keratolytic; antibacterial; antifungal* [salicylic acid; pyrithione zinc] 2%•1%

X-Seb T shampoo OTC *antiseborrheic; antipsoriatic; keratolytic* [coal tar; salicylic acid] 10%•4%

X-Seb T Plus shampoo OTC *antiseborrheic; antipsoriatic; keratolytic* [coal tar; salicylic acid; menthol] 10%•3%•1%

xylamidine tosilate INN *serotonin inhibitor* [also: xylamidine tosylate]

xylamidine tosylate USAN *serotonin inhibitor* [also: xylamidine tosilate]

xylazine INN *analgesic; veterinary muscle relaxant* [also: xylazine HCl]

xylazine HCl USAN *analgesic; veterinary muscle relaxant* [also: xylazine]

xylitol NF *sweetened vehicle*

Xylocaine injection ℞ *injectable local anesthetic* [lidocaine HCl] 0.5%, 1%, 2%

Xylocaine liquid, solution, ointment, jelly ℞ *mucous membrane anesthetic* [lidocaine HCl] 5%; 4%; 5%; 2%

Xylocaine ointment OTC *topical local anesthetic* [lidocaine] 2.5%

Xylocaine 10% Oral spray ℞ *mucous membrane anesthetic* [lidocaine HCl] 10%

Xylocaine HCl injection ℞ *injectable local anesthetic* [lidocaine HCl; dextrose] 1.5%•7.5%

Xylocaine HCl injection ℞ *injectable local anesthetic* [lidocaine HCl; epinephrine] 0.5%•1:200 000, 1%•1:100 000, 1%•1:200 000, 2%•1:50 000, 2%•1:100 000, 2%•1:200 000

Xylocaine HCl IV for Cardiac Arrhythmias IV injection, IV admixture ℞ *antiarrhythmic* [lidocaine HCl] 1%, 2%, 4%, 20%

Xylocaine MPF injection ℞ *injectable local anesthetic* [lidocaine HCl] 0.5%, 1%, 1.5%, 2%, 4%

Xylocaine MPF injection ℞ *injectable local anesthetic* [lidocaine HCl; epinephrine] 1%•1:200 000, 1.5%•1:200 000, 2%•1:200 000

Xylocaine MPF injection ℞ *injectable local anesthetic* [lidocaine HCl; glucose] 5%•7.5%

Xylocaine Viscous solution ℞ *mucous membrane anesthetic* [lidocaine HCl] 2%

xylocoumarol INN

xylofilcon A USAN *hydrophilic contact lens material*

xylometazoline INN, BAN *vasoconstrictor; nasal decongestant* [also: xylometazoline HCl]

xylometazoline HCl USP *vasoconstrictor; nasal decongestant* [also: xylometazoline]

Xylo-Pfan tablets OTC *diagnostic aid for intestinal function* [xylose] 25 g

xylose (D-xylose) USP *diagnostic aid for intestinal function*

xyloxemine INN

Xyrem ℞ *investigational (orphan) treatment for cataplexy* [sodium oxybate]

Y

yam *medicinal herb* [see: wild yam]

yarrow (Achillea millefolium) flower *medicinal herb for bowel hemorrhage, colds, fever, flu, hypertension, inducing sweating, measles, mucosal inflammation with discharge, nosebleed, reducing heavy menstrual bleeding and pain, thrombosis, and topical hemostasis*

yatren [see: chiniofon]

169Yb [see: pentetate calcium trisodium Yb 169]

169Yb [see: ytterbium Yb 169 pentetate]

yeast, dried NF

yeast cell derivative *claimed to promote wound healing*

Yeast-Gard vaginal suppositories OTC *for vaginal irritations, itching, and burning* [pulsatilla 28x; Candida albicans 28x]

Yeast-Gard; Yeast-Gard Sensitive Formula vaginal cream (name changed to Vagi-Gard in 1998)

Yeast-Gard Medicated Disposable Douche Premix solution OTC *antifungal; vaginal cleanser and deodorizer; acidity modifier* [sodium benzoate; lactic acid]

Yeast-Gard Medicated Douche; Yeast-Gard Medicated Disposable Douche solution OTC *antiseptic/germicidal; vaginal cleanser and deodorizer* [povidone-iodine] 10%; 0.3%

Yeast-X powder (discontinued 1998) OTC *absorbs vaginal moisture; astringent* [cornstarch; zinc oxide]

Yeast-X vaginal suppositories OTC *for vaginal irritations, itching, and burning* [pulsatilla 28x]

Yelets tablets OTC *vitamin/mineral/iron supplement* [multiple vitamins & minerals; ferrous fumarate; folic acid] ±•20•0.1 mg

yellow bedstraw; yellow cleavers *medicinal herb* [see: bedstraw]

yellow beeswax [see: beeswax, yellow]

yellow dock (Rumex crispus) root *medicinal herb for anemia, blood cleansing, constipation, itching, liver congestion, rheumatism, skin problems, and eyelid ulcerations; also used as a dentifrice*

yellow ferric oxide [see: ferric oxide, yellow]

yellow fever vaccine USP *active immunizing agent for yellow fever*

yellow gentian *medicinal herb* [see: gentian]

yellow ginseng *medicinal herb* [see: blue cohosh]

yellow Indian paint *medicinal herb* [see: goldenseal]

yellow jessamine *medicinal herb* [see: gelsemium]

yellow mercuric oxide [see: mercuric oxide, yellow]

yellow ointment [see: ointment, yellow]

yellow paint root; yellow root *medicinal herb* [see: goldenseal]

yellow petrolatum JAN *ointment base; emollient/protectant* [also: petrolatum]

yellow phenolphthalein [see: phenolphthalein, yellow]

yellow precipitate [see: mercuric oxide, yellow]

yellow puccoon *medicinal herb* [see: goldenseal]

yellow root (Xanthorhiza simplicissima) *medicinal herb used for diabetes and hypertension*

yellow root; yellow paint root *medicinal herb* [see: goldenseal]

yellow wax [see: wax, yellow]

yellow wood; yellow wood berries *medicinal herb* [see: prickly ash]

yerba maté (Ilex paraguariensis) leaves *medicinal herb used as a CNS stimulant, diuretic, and purifier*

yerba santa (Eriodictyon californicum) leaves *medicinal herb for asthma, bronchial congestion, colds, hay fever, inducing expectoration, inflammation, rheumatic pain, and tuberculosis*

yew (Taxus bacatta and other species) leaves *medicinal herb for* *liver disorders, rheumatism, and urinary tract disorders*

YF-Vax subcu injection ℞ *yellow fever vaccine* [yellow fever vaccine] 0.5 mL

YKP-10A *investigational (Phase II) antidepressant*

Yocon tablets ℞ *no FDA-approved uses; sympatholytic; mydriatic; aphrodisiac* [yohimbine HCl] 5.4 mg

Yodoxin tablets, powder ℞ *amebicide* [iodoquinol] 210, 650 mg; 25 g

yohimbe (*Corynanthe johimbe; Pausinystalia johimbe*) bark *medicinal herb for angina, hypertension, and impotence and other sexual dysfunction; also used as an aphrodisiac*

yohimbic acid INN

yohimbine HCl *alpha$_2$-adrenergic blocker; claimed to be an aphrodisiac; no FDA-sanctioned uses* 5.4 mg oral

Yohimex tablets ℞ *no FDA-approved uses; sympatholytic; mydriatic; aphrodisiac* [yohimbine HCl] 5.4 mg

Your Choice Non-Preserved Saline solution OTC *rinsing/storage solution for soft contact lenses* [sodium chloride (saline solution)]

Your Choice Sterile Preserved Saline solution OTC *rinsing/storage solution for soft contact lenses* [sodium chloride (preserved saline solution)]

youthwort *medicinal herb* [see: masterwort]

ytterbium *element (Yb)*

ytterbium Yb 169 pentetate USP *radioactive agent*

yttrium *element (Y)*

yttrium Y 90 murine MAb (2B8-MXDTPA) & indium In 111 murine MAb (2B8-MXDTPA) *investigational (orphan) for non-Hodgkin's B-cell lymphoma*

yucca (*Yucca glauca*) root *medicinal herb for arthritis, colitis, hypertension, migraine headache, and rheumatism*

yuma *medicinal herb* [see: wild yam]

Yurelax (Spanish name for U.S. product Flexeril)

Yutopar IV infusion ℞ *uterine relaxant to arrest preterm labor* [ritodrine HCl] 10, 15 mg/mL

Yutopar tablets (discontinued 1995) ℞ *uterine relaxant to arrest preterm labor* [ritodrine HCl] 10 mg

zabicipril INN

zacopride INN *antiemetic; peristaltic stimulant* [also: zacopride HCl]

zacopride HCl USAN, INN *antiemetic; peristaltic stimulant* [also: zacopride]

Zacutex IV injection ℞ *investigational (Phase III) platelet activating factor (PAF) antagonist for acute pancreatitis* [lexipafant]

Zadaxin (commercially available in several countries) ℞ *investigational (Phase III) influenza vaccine and vaccine enhancer for lung cancer; investigational (Phase III, orphan) for chronic hepatitis B; investigational (orphan) for DiGeorge syndrome with immune defects* [thymalfasin]

Zaditen ℞ *investigational (NDA filed) antiasthmatic* [ketotifen fumarate]

Zaditor eye drops ℞ *topical ophthalmic antihistamine and mast cell stabilizer for allergic conjunctivitis* [ketotifen fumarate] 0.025%

zafirlukast USAN, INN, BAN *antiasthmatic; leukotriene receptor antagonist (LTRA)*

zafuleptine INN

Zagam film-coated tablets ℞ *once-daily broad-spectrum fluoroquinolone antibiotic* [sparfloxacin] 200 mg

zalcitabine USAN *antiviral for AIDS (orphan)*

zaleplon USAN *investigational (NDA filed) sedative and hypnotic*

zalospirone INN *anxiolytic* [also: zalospirone HCl]

zalospirone HCl USAN *anxiolytic* [also: zalospirone]

zaltidine INN, BAN *antagonist to histamine H₂ receptors* [also: zaltidine HCl]

zaltidine HCl USAN *antagonist to histamine H₂ receptors* [also: zaltidine]

zamifenacin INN, BAN *investigational treatment for irritable bowel syndrome*

Zanaflex tablets ℞ *antispasmodic for multiple sclerosis and spinal cord injury (orphan)* [tizanidine HCl] 4 mg

zanamivir USAN *influenza neuraminidase inhibitor for the treatment of acute influenza types A and B*

zankiren HCl USAN *antihypertensive*

Zanosar powder for IV injection ℞ *nitrosourea-type alkylating antineoplastic for metastatic islet cell carcinoma of pancreas* [streptozocin] 1 g (100 mg/mL)

zanoterone USAN *antiandrogen*

Zantac film-coated tablets, syrup, IV or IM injection ℞ *histamine H₂ antagonist for gastric and duodenal ulcers* [ranitidine HCl] 150, 300 mg; 15 mg/mL; 0.5, 25 mg/mL ② Xanax

Zantac 75 tablets OTC *histamine H₂ antagonist for episodic heartburn* [ranitidine HCl] 75 mg

Zantac EFFERdose effervescent tablets, effervescent granules ℞ *histamine H₂ antagonist for gastric and duodenal ulcers* [ranitidine HCl] 150 mg; 150 mg/packet

Zantac GELdose capsules ℞ *histamine H₂ antagonist for gastric and duodenal ulcers* [ranitidine HCl] 150, 300 mg

Zanthorhiza apiifolia medicinal herb [see: yellow root]

Zantryl capsules ℞ *anorexiant; CNS stimulant* [phentermine HCl] 30 mg

Zanzibar aloe medicinal herb [see: aloe]

zapizolam INN

zaprinast INN, BAN

zardaverine INN

Zarontin capsules, syrup ℞ *anticonvulsant* [ethosuximide] 250 mg; 250 mg/5 mL ② Zaroxolyn

Zaroxolyn tablets ℞ *antihypertensive; diuretic* [metolazone] 2.5, 5, 10 mg ② Zarontin; Zeroxin

Zartan capsules (discontinued 1995) ℞ *cephalosporin antibiotic* [cephalexin] 500 mg

zatosetron INN, BAN *antimigraine* [also: zatosetron maleate]

zatosetron maleate USAN *antimigraine* [also: zatosetron]

Zavedos (European name for U.S. product Idamycin)

Z-Bec tablets OTC *vitamin/zinc supplement* [multiple vitamins; zinc sulfate] ±•22.5 mg

ZBT Baby powder OTC *topical diaper rash treatment* [talc]

ZD 4522 *investigational (Phase III) HMG-CoA reductase inhibitor for hyperlipidemia*

ZE Caps soft capsules OTC *dietary supplement* [vitamin E; zinc gluconate] 200•9.6 mg

Zea mays medicinal herb [see: Indian corn]

Zeasorb AF ⓒ (U.S. product: Tinactin) topical solution OTC *topical antifungal* [tolnaftate] 10 mg/mL

Zeasorb-AF powder OTC *topical antifungal* [miconazole nitrate] 2%

Zebeta film-coated tablets ℞ *antihypertensive; β-blocker* [bisoprolol fumarate] 5, 10 mg

Zecnil (discontinued 1997) ℞ *investigational (orphan) for secreting cutaneous gastrointestinal fistulas and bleeding esophageal varices* [somatostatin]

Zefazone powder or frozen premix for IV injection ℞ *cephalosporin antibiotic* [cefmetazole sodium] 1, 2 g ② cefazolin

Zeffix ℞ *investigational oral treatment for hepatitis B* [lamivudine]

zein NF *coating agent*

Zeldox ℞ *investigational (NDA filed) antipsychotic for schizophrenia (NDA disapproved in 1998)* [ziprasidone HCl]

Zemaphyte ℞ *investigational (Phase III) treatment for eczema*

Zemplar IV injection ℞ *synthetic vitamin D analog for hyperparathyroidism secondary to chronic renal failure* [paricalcitol] 5 μg/mL

Zemuron IV injection ℞ *neuromuscular blocking agent for anesthesia* [rocuronium bromide] 10 mg/mL

Zenapax injection ℞ *preventative for acute renal allograft rejection and acute graft vs. host disease following organ or bone marrow transplant* (orphan) [dacliximab] 25 mg/5 mL

Zenate, Advanced Formula film-coated tablets ℞ *vitamin/iron supplement* [multiple vitamins; iron; folic acid] ± • 65 • 1 mg

zenazocine mesylate USAN *analgesic*

zepastine INN

Zephiran Chloride tincture, tincture spray, aqueous solution, towelettes, disinfectant concentrate OTC *topical antiseptic* [benzalkonium chloride] 1:750; 1:750; 1:750; 1:750; 17%

zephirol [see: benzalkonium chloride]

Zephrex film-coated tablets ℞ *decongestant; expectorant* [pseudoephedrine HCl; guaifenesin] 60 • 400 mg

Zephrex LA timed-release tablets ℞ *decongestant; expectorant* [pseudoephedrine HCl; guaifenesin] 120 • 600 mg

zeranol USAN, INN *anabolic*

Zerit capsules, oral solution, powder for oral solution ℞ *antiviral for HIV infection* [stavudine] 15, 20, 30, 40 mg; 1 mg/mL; 1 mg/mL

Zestoretic tablets ℞ *antihypertensive; angiotensin-converting enzyme (ACE) inhibitor; diuretic* [hydrochlorothiazide; lisinopril] 12.5 • 10, 25 • 20 mg

Zestril tablets ℞ *antihypertensive; angiotensin-converting enzyme (ACE) inhibitor* [lisinopril] 2.5, 5, 10, 20, 40 mg ② Restoril; Vistaril

Zetar shampoo OTC *antiseborrheic; antipsoriatic; antipruritic; antibacterial* [coal tar] 1%

Zetar Emulsion bath oil ℞ *antipsoriatic; antiseborrheic; antipruritic; emollient* [coal tar] 30%

zetidoline INN, BAN

Zetran IV or IM injection (discontinued 1996) ℞ *benzodiazepine sedative; anxiolytic; skeletal muscle relaxant; anticonvulsant adjunct* [diazepam] 5 mg/mL

Z-gen tablets OTC *vitamin/zinc supplement* [multiple vitamins; zinc] ± • 22.5 mg

Zhuzishen (Panax pseudoginseng) medicinal herb [see: ginseng]

Ziac tablets ℞ *antihypertensive; β-blocker; diuretic* [hydrochlorothiazide; bisoprolol fumarate] 6.25 • 2.5, 6.25 • 5, 6.25 • 10 mg

Ziagen film-coated tablets, oral solution ℞ *antiviral nucleoside reverse transcriptase inhibitor for HIV* [abacavir sulfate] 300 mg; 20 mg/mL

ziconotide *investigational (Phase III) calcium channel blocker for chronic malignant pain of cancer or AIDS; investigational (Phase II) for acute postsurgical pain*

zidapamide INN

zidometacin USAN, INN *anti-inflammatory*

zidovudine USAN, INN, BAN *nucleoside antiviral for AIDS and AIDS-related complex* (orphan)

zifrosilone USAN *acetylcholinesterase inhibitor for Alzheimer's disease*

Ziks cream OTC *topical analgesic; counterirritant* [methyl salicylate; menthol; capsaicin] 12% • 1% • 0.025% ② Vicks

Zilactin Medicated gel OTC *astringent for oral canker and herpes lesions* [tannic acid; alcohol 80%] 7%

Zilactin-B Medicated gel OTC *topical oral anesthetic* [benzocaine; alcohol 76%] 10%

Zilactin-L liquid OTC *topical local anesthetic* [lidocaine] 2.5%

ZilaDent gel (discontinued 1995) OTC *topical oral anesthetic* [benzocaine; alcohol 74.9%] 6%

zilantel USAN, INN *anthelmintic*

zileuton USAN, INN, BAN *5-lipoxygenase inhibitor; leukotriene receptor inhibitor; for prophylaxis and chronic treatment of asthma*

zilpaterol INN

zimeldine INN, BAN *antidepressant* [also: zimeldine HCl]

zimeldine HCl USAN *antidepressant* [also: zimeldine]

zimelidine HCl [now: zimeldine HCl]

zimidoben INN

Zinacef powder or frozen premix for IV or IM injection Ṟ *cephalosporin antibiotic* [cefuroxime sodium] 0.75, 1.5, 7.5 g

zinc *element (Zn)*

Zinc 15 tablets OTC *zinc supplement* [zinc sulfate] 66 mg

zinc acetate USP *copper blocking/complexing agent for Wilson's disease (orphan)*

zinc acetate, basic INN

zinc acetate dihydrate [see: zinc acetate]

zinc bacitracin [see: bacitracin zinc]

zinc caprylate *antifungal*

zinc carbonate USAN *zinc supplement*

zinc chloride USP *astringent; dentin desensitizer; dietary zinc supplement*

zinc chloride Zn 65 USAN *radioactive agent*

zinc complex bacitracins [see: bacitracin zinc]

zinc gelatin USP

zinc gluconate USP *dietary zinc supplement* 10, 15, 50, 78 mg oral

Zinc Lozenges OTC *topical anti-infective to relieve sore throat* [zinc citrate and zinc gluconate] 23 mg

zinc mesoporphyrin & hemin *investigational (orphan) for acute porphyric syndromes*

zinc oleate NF

zinc oxide USP, JAN *astringent; topical protectant; emollient; antiseptic* 20% topical

zinc peroxide, medicinal USP

zinc phenolsulfonate NF *not generally regarded as safe and effective as an antidiarrheal*

zinc propionate *antifungal*

zinc pyrithione [see: pyrithione zinc]

zinc stearate USP *dusting powder; tablet and capsule lubricant; antifungal*

zinc sulfate USP, JAN *ophthalmic astringent; dietary zinc supplement* 200, 220, 250 mg oral; 1, 5 mg/mL injection

zinc sulfate heptahydrate [see: zinc sulfate]

zinc sulfate monohydrate [see: zinc sulfate]

zinc sulfocarbolate [see: zinc phenolsulfonate]

zinc undecylenate USP *antifungal*

zinc valerate USP

Zinc-220 capsules OTC *zinc supplement* [zinc sulfate] 220 mg

Zinca-Pak IV injection Ṟ *intravenous nutritional therapy* [zinc sulfate] 1, 5 mg/mL

Zincate capsules Ṟ *zinc supplement* [zinc sulfate] 220 mg

zinc-eugenol USP

Zincfrin Drop-Tainers (eye drops) OTC *topical ocular decongestant and astringent* [phenylephrine HCl; zinc sulfate] 0.12%•0.25%

Zincon shampoo OTC *antiseborrheic; antibacterial; antifungal* [pyrithione zinc] 1%

Zincvit capsules Ṟ *vitamin/mineral supplement* [multiple vitamins & minerals; folic acid] ≚•1 mg

zindotrine USAN, INN *bronchodilator*

zindoxifene INN

Zinecard powder for IV drip or push Ṟ *cardioprotectant for doxorubicin-induced cardiomyopathy (orphan)* [dexrazoxane] 250, 500 mg/vial

Zingiber officinale *medicinal herb* [see: ginger]

zinoconazole INN *antifungal* [also: zinoconazole HCl]

zinoconazole HCl USAN *antifungal* [also: zinoconazole]

zinostatin USAN, INN *antineoplastic* � Sandostatin; simvastatin

zinterol INN *bronchodilator* [also: zinterol HCl]

zinterol HCl USAN *bronchodilator* [also: zinterol]

Zintevir Ṟ *investigational (Phase II) integrase inhibitor for HIV* [AR-177 (code name—generic name not yet assigned)]

zinviroxime USAN, INN *antiviral*

zipeprol INN

ziprasidone *investigational (NDA filed) antipsychotic for schizophrenia*

ziprasidone HCl *investigational (NDA filed) antipsychotic for schizophrenia (NDA disapproved in 1998)*

Ziradryl lotion OTC *topical antihistamine; astringent; antiseptic* [diphenhydramine HCl; zinc oxide; alcohol 2%] 1%•2%

zirconium *element (Zr)*

zirconium oxide *astringent*

Zithromax tablets, powder for oral suspension, powder for IV or IM injection ℞ *macrolide antibiotic* [azithromycin] 250, 600 mg; 100, 200 mg/5 mL, 1 g packet; 500 mg

Zithromax Ⓒᴬᴺ capsules, tablets, powder for oral suspension ℞ *macrolide antibiotic* [azithromycin] 250 mg; 250 mg; 300, 600 mg/15 mL, 900 mg/22.5 mL

Zixoryn ℞ *investigational (orphan) for neonatal hyperbilirubinemia* [flumecinol]

Z-Max (Mexican name for U.S. product Vasomax)

⁶⁵Zn [see: zinc chloride Zn 65]

ZNP cleansing bar OTC *antiseborrheic; antibacterial; antifungal* [pyrithione zinc] 2%

zocainone INN

Zocor film-coated tablets ℞ *HMG-CoA reductase inhibitor for hyperlipidemia and coronary heart disease* [simvastatin] 5, 10, 20, 40, 80 mg

Zodeac-100 tablets ℞ *hematinic; vitamin/mineral supplement* [ferrous fumarate; multiple vitamins & minerals; folic acid; biotin] 60 mg•±•1 mg•300 μg

zofenopril INN, BAN *angiotensin-converting enzyme (ACE) inhibitor* [also: zofenopril calcium]

zofenopril calcium USAN *angiotensin-converting enzyme (ACE) inhibitor* [also: zofenopril]

zofenoprilat INN *antihypertensive* [also: zofenoprilat arginine]

zofenoprilat arginine USAN *antihypertensive* [also: zofenoprilat]

zoficonazole INN

Zofran film-coated tablets, oral solution, IV infusion, IM injection ℞ *5-HT₃ antagonist; antiemetic for chemotherapy and radiotherapy* [ondansetron HCl] 4, 8 mg; 4 mg/5 mL; 32 mg/50 mL; 2 mg/mL

Zofran ODT (orally disintegrating tablets) ℞ *5-HT₃ antagonist; antiemetic for chemotherapy and radiotherapy* [ondansetron HCl] 4, 8 mg

Zoladex subcu implant in preloaded syringe ℞ *hormonal antineoplastic for palliative treatment of prostatic carcinoma, breast cancer, and endometriosis* [goserelin acetate] 3.6 mg (1-month implant), 10.8 mg (3-month implant) ⊉ sulindac

zolamine INN *antihistamine; topical anesthetic* [also: zolamine HCl]

zolamine HCl USAN *antihistamine; topical anesthetic* [also: zolamine]

zolazepam INN, BAN *sedative* [also: zolazepam HCl]

zolazepam HCl USAN *sedative* [also: zolazepam]

zoledronate disodium USAN *bone resorption inhibitor for osteoporosis*

zoledronate trisodium USAN *bone resorption inhibitor for osteoporosis*

zoledronic acid USAN *bone resorption inhibitor for osteoporosis*

zolenzepine INN

zolertine INN *antiadrenergic; vasodilator* [also: zolertine HCl]

zolertine HCl USAN *antiadrenergic; vasodilator* [also: zolertine]

Zolicef powder for IV or IM injection ℞ *cephalosporin antibiotic* [cefazolin sodium] 0.5, 1 g

zolimidine INN

zolimomab aritox USAN *anti-T lymphocyte monoclonal antibody*

zoliprofen INN

zoliridine [see: zolimidine]

zolmitriptan USAN *vascular serotonin 5-HT₁ receptor agonist for migraine headache*

Zoloft film-coated tablets ℞ *selective serotonin reuptake inhibitor (SSRI) for depression, obsessive-compulsive disorder (OCD), and panic disorder* [sertraline HCl] 25, 50, 100 mg

Zoloft ⊛ capsules ℞ *selective serotonin reuptake inhibitor (SSRI) for depression, obsessive-compulsive disorder (OCD), and panic disorder* [sertraline HCl] 25, 50, 100 mg

zoloperone INN

zolpidem INN, BAN *imidazopyridine sedative/hypnotic* [also: zolpidem tartrate]

zolpidem tartrate USAN *imidazopyridine sedative/hypnotic* [also: zolpidem]

Zomaril ℞ *investigational (Phase III) treatment for schizophrenia* [iloperidone]

zomebazam INN

zomepirac INN, BAN *analgesic; anti-inflammatory* [also: zomepirac sodium]

zomepirac sodium USAN, USP *analgesic; anti-inflammatory* [also: zomepirac]

zometapine USAN *antidepressant*

Zomig film-coated tablets ℞ *vascular serotonin 5-HT$_1$ receptor agonist for migraine headache* [zolmitriptan] 2.5, 5 mg ▣ Flomax; Slow-Mag

Zonalon cream ℞ *topical antihistamine and antipruritic* [doxepin HCl] 5%

Zone-A Forte lotion ℞ *topical corticosteroidal anti-inflammatory; local anesthetic* [hydrocortisone acetate; pramoxine] 2.5%•1%

Zonegran capsules ℞ *investigational (NDA filed) benzisoxazole anticonvulsant* [zonisamide]

zoniclezole INN *anticonvulsant* [also: zoniclezole HCl]

zoniclezole HCl USAN *anticonvulsant* [also: zoniclezole]

zonisamide USAN, INN, BAN *investigational (NDA filed) benzisoxazole anticonvulsant*

Zonite Douche solution concentrate OTC *antiseptic; antipruritic/counterirritant; vaginal cleanser and deodorizer* [benzalkonium chloride; menthol; thymol]

Zophren (European name for U.S. product Zofran)

zopiclone INN, BAN, JAN *sedative; hypnotic*

zopolrestat USAN *antidiabetic; aldose reductase inhibitor*

zorbamycin USAN *antibacterial*

ZORprin Zero Order Release tablets ℞ *analgesic; antipyretic; anti-inflammatory; antirheumatic* [aspirin] 800 mg

zorubicin INN *antineoplastic* [also: zorubicin HCl]

zorubicin HCl USAN *antineoplastic* [also: zorubicin]

Zostrix; Zostrix-HP cream OTC *topical analgesic* [capsaicin] 0.025%; 0.075%

Zosyn powder or frozen premix for IV injection ℞ *extended-spectrum penicillin antibiotic* [piperacillin sodium; tazobactam sodium] 2•0.25, 3•0.375, 4•0.5, 36•4.5 g

zotepine INN, JAN *investigational antipsychotic*

Zoto-HC ear drops ℞ *topical corticosteroidal anti-inflammatory; antibacterial; local anesthetic* [hydrocortisone; chloroxylenol; pramoxine HCl] 10%•1%•10%

Zovia tablets ℞ *monophasic oral contraceptive* [ethynodiol diacetate; ethinyl estradiol] 1 mg•35 µg; 1 mg•50 µg

Zovirax powder for IV infusion ℞ *antiviral for herpes infections* [acyclovir sodium] 500, 1000 mg

Zovirax tablets, capsules, oral suspension, ointment ℞ *antiviral for herpes simplex, herpes zoster, and adult-onset chickenpox* [acyclovir] 400, 800 mg; 200 mg; 200 mg/5 mL; 5%

zoxazolamine NF, INN

zucapsaicin USAN *topical analgesic*

zuclomifene INN

zuclomiphene USAN

zuclopenthixol INN, BAN *thioxanthene antipsychotic*

Zurinol tablets ℞ *xanthine oxidase inhibitor for gout* [allopurinol]

Zyban film-coated sustained-release tablets ℞ *non-nicotine aid to smoking cessation* [bupropion HCl] 150 mg

Zydis ℞ *investigational (orphan) treatment for late-stage Parkinson's disease* [apomorphine HCl]

Zydone tablets, capsules ℞ *narcotic analgesic* [hydrocodone bitartrate; acetaminophen] 5•400, 7.5•400, 10•400 mg; 5•500 mg

Zyflo film-coated tablets ℞ *5-lipoxygenase inhibitor; leukotriene receptor inhibitor; prophylaxis and treatment for chronic asthma* [zileuton] 600 mg

zylofuramine INN

Zyloprim injection ℞ *antineoplastic for leukemia, lymphoma, and solid tumor malignancies (orphan)* [allopurinol sodium]

Zyloprim tablets ℞ *xanthine oxidase inhibitor for gout and hyperuricemia* [allopurinol] 100, 300 mg

Zymacap capsules OTC *vitamin supplement* [multiple vitamins; folic acid] ±•0.4 mg

Zymase capsules containing enteric-coated spheres ℞ *digestive enzymes* [lipase; protease; amylase] 12 000•24 000•24 000 U

Zyprexa film-coated tablets ℞ *novel (atypical) antipsychotic* [olanzapine] 2.5, 5, 7.5, 10 mg

Zyrkamine *investigational (orphan) for non-Hodgkin's lymphoma* [mitoguazone]

Zyrtec film-coated tablets, syrup ℞ *nonsedating antihistamine* [cetirizine HCl] 5, 10 mg; 5 mg/5 mL

Zyvox ℞ *investigational (Phase II) antibiotic against gram-positive bacteria* [linezolid]

APPENDIX **A**
Sound-Alikes

Listed below are 716 drug names that may be confused in transcription, followed by one or more possible "sound-alike" names. The list is not all-inclusive, and we would appreciate hearing of any additions the reader might suggest. These sound-alikes have also been included in the main section of the book. Look for the "ear" icon (🔊).

Accurbron	Accutane
Accutane	Accurbron
Achromycin	actinomycin; Aureomycin
Actidil	Actifed
Actifed	Actidil
actinomycin	Achromycin; Aureomycin
Adapin	Atabrine; Ativan; Betapen
adrenaline	adrenalone
adrenalone	adrenaline
Advil	Avail
Afrin	aspirin
Agoral	Argyrol
AK-Mycin	Akne-Mycin
Akne-mycin	Ak-Mycin
Alamag	Alma-Mag
Alco-Gel	aloe gel
Aldactazide	Aldactone
Aldactone	Aldactazide
Aldoril	Elavil; Eldepryl; Enovil; Equanil; Mellaril
Allergan	allergen; Auralgan
aloe	Alco-Gel
ALOMAD	Alomide
Alomide	ALOMAD
Ambenyl	Aventyl
Amicar	Amikin
Amikin	Amicar
amitriptyline	nortriptyline
amoxapine	amoxicillin; Amoxil
amoxicillin	amoxapine
Amoxil	amoxapine
Amphojel	Amphocil
Anacin	Unisom; Unasyn
Anafranil	enalapril
Analpram	Analbalm
Ancobon	Oncovin
Anturane	Artane

Anusol	Aplisol
Aplisol	Anusol; Apresoline
Appedrine	aprindine; ephedrine
aprindine	Appedrine; ephedrine
ara-C	ERYC
Aralen	Arlidin
Aricept	Erycette
Artane	Anturane
aspirin	Afrin
Atarax	Marax
atenolol	timolol
Ativan	Adapin; Avitene
Atrovent	Trovan
Auralgan	Allergan; allergen
Aureomycin	Achromycin; actinomycin
Avail	Advil
Aventyl	Ambenyl; Bentyl
Avita	Evista
Avitene	Ativan
Axid	Biaxin
azolimine	Azulfidine
Azulfidine	azolimine; Silvadene
Bacid	Banacid
bacitracin	Bacitrin; Bactrim
Bactocill	Pathocil
Bactrim	bacitracin
Banophen	Barophen
Banthīˉne	Brethine; Vantin
Bantron	Vantin
Barophen	Banophen
Beminal	Benemid
Benadryl	Bentyl; Benylin; Caladryl
Benemid h	Beminal
Benoxyl	PanOxyl
Bentyl	Aventyl; Benadryl; Bontril
Benylin	Benadryl
Betagan	Betagen
Betagen	Betagan
Betapen	Adapin; Phenaphen
Biaxin	Axid
Bichloracetic Acid	dichloroacetic acid
Bicillin	V-Cillin; Wycillin
bleomycin	Cleocin
Bontril	Bentyl; Vontrol
Boyol	boil
Brethine	Banthine
Bretylol	Brevital
Brevital	Bretylol
Bromfed	Bromphen
Bromophen	Bromphen

Bromphen	Bromfed; Bromophen
Broncholate	Brondelate
Brondelate	Broncholate
butabarbital	butalbital
butalbital	butabarbital; Butibel
Butibel	butalbital
Butisol Sodium	Butazolidin
Byclomine	Hycomine
Bydramine	Hydramine
Caladryl	Benadryl
Calamox	Camalox
Calan	kaolin; Kaon
calcitonin	calcitriol
calcitriol	calcitonin
Capastat	Cepastat
Capitrol	captopril
captopril	Capitrol
Cardene	Cardizem
Cardizem	Cardene
Catapres	Catarase; Combipres; Ser-Ap-Es
Catarase	Catapres
Cefadyl	Cefzil
cefazolin	cephalothin; Zefazone
cefotaxime	cefoxitin
cefoxitin	cefotaxime
ceftizoxime	cefuroxime
cefuroxime	ceftizoxime
Cefzil	Cefadyl; Kefzol
Celebrex	Cerebyx
Ce⁻pastat	Capastat
cephalexin	cefazolin; cephalothin
cephalothin	cefazolin
cephapirin	cephradine
cephradine	cephapirin
Cerebyx	Celebrex
chlorpheniramine	chlorphentermine
chlorphentermine	chlorpheniramine
cimetidine	dimethicone
Cipro	Septa; Septra
Citracal	Citrucel
Citrucel	Citracal
clara cell	Clearasil
claretin	Claritin; Clarityne
Claritin	claretin; Clarityne
Clarityne	claretin; Claritin
Clearasil	clara cell
Cleocin	bleomycin; Lincocin
Clinoxide	clioxanide; Clipoxide
clioxanide	Clinoxide
Clipoxide	Clinoxide

clomiphene	clonidine
clonidine	clomiphene; Klonopin; quinidine
clotrimazole	co-trimoxazole
Codegest	Codehist
Codehist	Codegest
codeine	Kaodene
Colestid	colistin
colestipol	colistin
colistin	Colestid; colestipol
Combipres	Catapres
Cort-Dome	Cortone
Cortenema	quart enema
Cortin	Cotrim
cortisone	Cortizone
Cortizone	cortisone
Cortone	Cort-Dome
Cotrim	Cortin
co-trimoxazole	clotrimazole
Coumadin	Kemadrin
Covera	Provera
cytarabine	vidarabine
dacarbazine	Dicarbosil; procarbazine
Dalmane	Dialume
danthron	Dantrium
Dantrium	danthron
Daranide	Daraprim
Daraprim	Daranide
Daricon	Darvon
Darvocet-N	Darvon-N
Darvon	Daricon
daunorubicin	doxorubicin
Decadron	Decaderm; Percodan
Deconsal	Deconal
Delcort	Dilacor
Demolin	Demulen
Demulen	Demerol; Demolin
Dermacort	DermiCort
DermiCort	Dermacort
deserpidine	desipramine
Desferal	Disophrol
desipramine	deserpidine
desoximetasone	dexamethasone
Desoxyn	digitoxin; digoxin
dexamethasone	desoximetasone
Dexedrine	dextran
dextran	Dexedrine; dextrin
dextrin	dextran
Dialume	Dalmane
Dicarbosil	dacarbazine
dichloroacetic acid	Bichloracetic acid

dicumarol	Demerol
digitoxin	Desoxyn; digoxin
digoxin	Desoxyn; digitoxin
Dilacor	Delcort
Dilantin	Milontin; Mylanta; Xalatan
Dimacol	dimercaprol
dimenhydrinate	diphenhydramine
dimercaprol	Dimacol
Dimetabs	Dimetane; Dimetapp
Dimetane	Dimetabs
Dimetapp	Dimetabs
dimethicone	cimetidine
diphenhydramine	dimenhydrinate
Diphenylan	Diphenylin
Disophrol	Desferal; disoprofol; Stilphostrol
disoprofol	Disophrol
Ditropan	Intropin
Diutensen	Salutensin
dobutamine	dopamine
Donnagel	Donnatal
Donnatal	Donnagel
Donnazyme	Entozyme
dopamine	dobutamine; Dopram
Dopar	Dopram
Dopram	dopamine; Dopar
doxepin	Doxidan; Loxitane
Doxidan	doxepin
doxorubicin	daunorubicin
Dramanate	Dommanate
Dyazide	thiazides; Tiazac
Dymelor	Demerol; Pamelor
Dyrenium	Pyridium
Ecotrin	Edecrin
Edecrin	Ecotrin; Ethaquin
Elavil	Aldoril; Eldepryl; Enovil; Equanil; Mellaril
Eldepryl	Aldoril; Elavil; Enovil; Equanil; Mellaril
emetine	Emetrol
Emetrol	emetine
Enbrel	Incel
Endal	Intal
Enduron	Imuran; Inderal
Enduronyl	Inderal
Enovil	Aldoril; Elavil; Eldepryl; Equanil; Mellaril
ephedrine	Appedrine; aprindine
Epifrin	epinephrine; EpiPen
Epinal	Epitol
epinephrine	Epifrin
EpiPen	Epifrin
Epitol	Epinal
Epogen	"amp and gent" (ampicillin & gentamicin)

Equanil	Aldoril; Elavil; Eldepryl; Enovil; Mellaril
ERYC	ara-C
Erycette	Aricept
erythromycin	clarithromycin
Esidrix	Lasix
Esimil	Estinyl; Isomil
Estinyl	Esimil
Estraderm	Estradurin
Estratab	Ethatab
ethacridine	ethacrynic
ethacrynic acid	ethacridine
Ethaquin	Edecrin
Ethatab	Estratab
ethinamate	ethionamide
Ethiodol	ethynodiol
ethionamide	ethinamate
ethynodiol	Ethiodol
Eurax	Serax; Urex
Evac-Q-Kit	Evac-Q-Kwik
Evac-Q-Kwik	Evac-Q-Kit
Evista	Avita
Femiron	Remeron
fentanyl	Sentinel
Feosol	Feostat; Fer-In-Sol; Festal
Feostat	Feosol
Fer-In-Sol	Feosol
Feverall	Fiberall
Fiberall	Feverall
Fioricet	Lorcet
Fiorinal	Florinef
Flaxedil	Flexeril
Flexeril	Flaxedil
Flomax	Slow-Mag; Zomig
Florinef	Fiorinal
folacin	Fulvicin
Fostex	pHisoHex
Fulvicin	folacin; Furacin
Furacin	Fulvicin
Gabitril	Carbatrol
Gamastan	Garamycin
Gantrisin	Gantanol
Garamycin	Gamastan; kanamycin; Terramycin; Theramycin
Gelfoam	Ger-O-Foam
Genatap	Genapap
Generet	Gentap
gentamicin	Jenamicin; kanamycin
glucose	Glutose
Glutose	glucose
Glycotuss	Glytuss
Glytuss	Glycotuss

Gonak	Gonic
Gonic	Gonak
guaifenesin	guanfacine
guanethidine	guanidine
guanfacine	guaifenesin
guanidine	guanethidine
Guiatuss	Guiatussin
Guiatussin	Guiatuss
Haldol	Halenol; Halog
Halog	Haldol
Halotestin	Halotex; Halotussin
Halotex	Halotestin
Halotussin	Halotestin
Hespan	Histatan
Hexadrol	Hexalol
Hexalen	Hexalol
Hycodan	Hycomine; Vicodin
Hycomine	Byclomine; Hycodan; Vicodin
Hydergine	Hydramine
Hydramyn	Hydramine; Hytramyn
Hygroton	Regroton
HyperHep	Hyper-Tet; Hyperstat
Hyperstat	Hyper-Tet; HyperHep; Nitrostat
Hyper-Tet	HyperHep; Hyperstat
Hytone	Vytone
Ilosone	inosine
imipramine	Imferon; Norpramin; trimipramine
Imuran	Enduron; Imferon
Incel	Enbrel
Inderal	Enduron; Enduronyl; Inderide
Inderide	Inderal
Indocin	Lincocin; Minocin
inosine	Ilosone
insulin	inulin
Intal	Endal
Intropin	Ditropan; Isoptin
inulin	insulin
Ismelin	Ritalin
Isomil	Esimil
Isoptin	Intropin
Isopto Carpine	Isopto Eserine
Isordil	Isuprel
Isuprel	Isordil
kanamycin	Garamycin; gentamicin
Kaochlor	K-Lor
Kaodene	codeine
kaolin	Calan; Kaon
Kaon	Calan; kaolin
Kaopectate	Kapectalin
Kapectolin	Kaopectate

Kay Ciel	KCl
KCl (potassium chloride)	Kay Ciel
Keflex	Keflet; Keflin
Keflin	Keflet; Keflex
Kefzol	Cefzil
Kemadrin	Coumadin
Kenalog	Ketalar
Ketalar	Kenalog
Klonopin	clonidine
K-Lor	Kaochlor
Klotrix	Liotrix
Koromex	Komex
lanolin	Lanoline
Lasix	Esidrix; Lidex
levallorphan	levorphanol
levodopa	methyldopa
levorphanol	levallorphan
levothyroxine	liothyronine
Lidex	Lasix; Lidox; Wydase
Lidox	Lidex
Lincocin	Cleocin; Indocin
liothyronine	levothyroxine
liotrix	Klotrix
Loniten	clonidine
Lonox	Lovenox
Lorcet	Fioricet
Lotrimin	Otrivin
Lovenox	Lonox
Loxitane	doxepin
Luminal	Tuinal
Lupron	Mepron; Napron
Maalox	Marax
Mandol	nadolol
Marax	Atarax; Maalox
Marcaine	Narcan
Maxzide	Microzide
mazindol	mebendazole
Mebaral	Medrol
mebendazole	mazindol
Meclan	Meclomen; Mezlin
meclizine	mescaline
Meclomen	Meclan
meclozine	mescaline
Medrol	Mebaral
Mellaril	Aldoril; Elavil; Eldepryl; Enovil; Equanil; Moderil
meperidine	meprobamate
mephenytoin	Mephyton; Mesantoin
Mephyton	mephenytoin; methadone
meprobamate	meperidine
Mepron	Lupron; Napron

Meprospan	Naprosyn
Mesantoin	mephenytoin; Mestinon; Metatensin
mescaline	meclizine
Mestinon	Mesantoin; Metatensin
Metahydrin	Metandren
metaproterenol	metoprolol
Metatensin	Mesantoin; Mestinon
metaxalone	metolazone
metesind	medicine
methadone	Mephyton
methenamine	methionine
methionine	methenamine
methixene	methoxsalen
methoxsalen	methixene
methyldopa	levodopa
metolazone	metaxalone
Metopirone	metyrapone
metoprolol	metaproterenol
metyrapone	Metopirone; metyrosine
metyrosine	metyrapone
Mezlin	Meclan
MICRhoGAM	microgram
Microzide	Maxzide
Midrin	Mydfrin
Milontin	Dilantin; Miltown; Mylanta
Miltown	Milontin
Minocin	Indocin; Mithracin; niacin
Mithracin	Minocin
mithramycin	mitomycin
mitomycin	mithramycin; Mutamycin
Moban	Mobidin; Modane
Mobidin	Moban
Modane	Moban; Mudrane
Moderil	Mellaril
Modicon	Mylicon
Moi-Stir	moisture
Monocaps	Monoclate; Monoket
Monocete	Monocid
Monocid	Monocete
Monoclate	Monocaps; Monoket
Monoket	Monocete
Mudrane	Modane
Mutamycin	mitomycin
Myambutol	Nembutal
Mydfrin	Midrin; Myfedrine
Mylanta	Dilantin; Milontin
Myleran	Mylicon
Mylicon	Modicon; Myleran
nadolol	Nandol
Naldecon	Nalfon

Nalfon	Naldecon
Napron	Lupron; Mepron
Naprosyn	Meprospan; Natacyn
Narcan	Marcaine
Nardil	Norinyl
Natacyn	Naprosyn
Nembutal	Myambutal
Neomixin	neomycin
neomycin	Neomixin
Neovastat	Novastan
niacin	Minocin
Nicobid	Nitro-Bid
Nilstat	Nitrostat; nystatin
Nitro-Bid	Nicobid
nitroglycerin	Nitroglyn
Nitroglyn	nitroglycerin
Norinyl	Nardil
Norlutate	Norlutin
Norlutin	Norlutate
Norpramin	imipramine
nortriptyline	amitriptyline
Novastan	Neovastat; Ovastat
nystatin	Nilstat; Nitrostat
Omnipen	Unipen
Oncovin	Ancobon
Ophthocort	Ophthochlor
Orabase	Orinase
orarsan	Oracin; Orasone
Orasone	Oracin; orarsan
Oretic	Oreton
Oreton	Oretic
Orinase	Orabase; Ornade; Ornex; Tolinase
Ornade	Orinase; Ornex
Ornex	Orex; Orinase; Ornade
Orthoclone	Ortho-Creme
Otobiotic	Urobiotic
Otrivin	Lotrimin
OvaRex	O-Vax
Ovastat	Novastan
O-Vax	Ovarex
oxymetazoline	oxymetholone
oxymetholone	oxymetazoline; oxymorphone
oxymorphone	oxymetholone
Pamelor	Dymelor
Panasol	Panscol
Panorex	Panarex
Panoxyl	Benoxyl
Panscol	Panasol
Parafon	Pantopon
paramethadione	paramethasone

paramethasone	paramethadione
Pathilon	Pathocil
Pathocil	Bactocill; Pathilon; Placidyl
Pavabid	Pavased
Pavatine	Pavatym
Paverolan	Pavulon
Pavulon	Paverolan
penicillamine	penicillin
penicillin	penicillamine; Polycillin
Pentazine	Phenazine
pentobarbital	phenobarbital
Pentothal	pentrinitrol
Pentothal	pentrinitrol;
pentrinitrol	Pentothal
Percodan	Decadron
Perdiem	Pyridium
Periactin	Taractan
Persantine	Pertofrane
Pertofrane	Persantine
Phazyme	Pherazine
phenacetin	phenazocine
Phenazine	Pentazine; phenelzine; Phenoxine; Pherazine
phenazocine	phenacetin
phenelzine	Phenazine; Phenylzin
Phenergan	Phenaphen; Theragran
phenobarbital	pentobarbital
Phenoxine	Phenazine
phentermine	phentolamine
phentolamine	phentermine; Ventolin
pHisoHex	Fostex
physostigmine	pyridostigmine; Prostigmin
piperacetazine	piperazine
piperazine	piperacetazine
piracetam	piroxicam
piroxicam	piracetam
Pitocin	Pitressin
Pitressin	Pitocin
Placidyl	Pathocil
Podofin	podophyllin
podophyllin	Podofin
Polycillin	penicillin
Ponstel	Pronestyl
Posicor	Proscar
pralidoxime	pyridoxine; pramoxine
Pramosone	pramoxine
pramoxine	pralidoxime; Pramosone
Pravachol	Primacor
prazepam	prazepine; prazosin
prazepine	prazepam
prazosin	prazepam

prednisolone	prednisone
prednisone	prednisolone
Preven	Preveon
Preveon	Preven
Prilosec	Prozac
Primacor	Pravachol
Priscoline	Apresoline
procaine	Procan
Procan	procaine
procarbazine	dacarbazine
proline	Prolene
promazine	Promethazine
Pronestyl	Ponstel
Proscar	Posicor
Prostigmin	physostigmine
Protopam	Protamine
Provera	Covera; Provir; Trovert
Provir	Provera; Trovert
Prozac	Prilosec
Pyridium	Dyrenium; pyridoxine; pyrithione; pyritidium
pyridostigmine	physostigmine
pyridoxine	pralidoxime; Pyridium
pyrithione sodium	Pyridium
pyritidium bromide	Pyridium
Quarzan	Questran
quinacrine HCl	quinidine
quinidine	clonidine; quinacrine; Quinatime; quinine
quinine	quinidine
Re⁻gain	Rogaine
Reglan	Regonol
Regonol	Reglan
Regroton	Hygroton
Remeron	Femiron
Repan	Riopan
Restoril	Risperdal; Vistaril; Zestril
Rheumatex	Rheumatrex
Rheumatrex	Rheumatex
Rifadin	Ritalin
Risperdal	Restoril
Ritalin	Ismelin; Rifadin
Robaxisal	Robaxacet
Rogaine	Re⁻gain
Salutensin	Diutensen
Sandostatin	simvastatin; zinostatin
Sentinel	fentanyl
Septa	Cipro; Septra
Septra	Cipro; Septa
Ser-Ap-Es	Catapres
Serax	Eurax; Urex; Xerac
Serentil	Surital

Silvadene	Azulfidine
Simplet	Singlet
simvastatin	Sandostatin; zinostatin
Singlet	Simplet
Slow-Mag	Flomax; Zomig
stilbestrol	Stilphostrol
Stilphostrol	Disophrol; stilbestrol
Streptase	Streptonase
streptokinase	Streptonase
Streptonase	Streptase; streptokinase
sucrase	sucrose
sucrose	sucrase
Sulf-10	Sulten-10
sulfamethizole	sulfamethoxazole
sulfamethoxazole	sulfamethizole
sulfathiazole	sulfisoxazole
Sulfatrim	Sulfa-Trip
sulfisoxazole	sulfathiazole
sulindac	Zoladex
Synthroid	Euthroid
Tagamet	Tegopen
Targretin	Tegopen; Tegrin
Tegopen	Tagamet; Tegrin; Targretin
Tegretol	Tegrin
Tegrin	Tegopen; Tegretol; Targretin
Teldrin	Tedral
Temaril	Demerol; Tepanil
Tepanil	Temaril; Tofranil
Terramycin	Garamycin; Theramycin
testolactone	testosterone
testosterone	testolactone
thallium	Valium
Theoclear	Theolair
Theolair	Theoclear; Thyrolar
TheraFlu	Thera-Flur
Thera-Flur	TheraFlu
Theragran	Theragyn; Phenergan
Theragyn	Theragran
Theramycin	Garamycin; Terramycin
Theravite	Therevac
Therevac	Theravite
Threostat	Triostat
Thyrar	Thyrolar
thyroid	euthroid
Thyrolar	Theolair; Thyrar
Tiazac	Dyazide; thiazides
Ticar	Tigan
Tigan	Ticar
timolol	atenolol
Tinactin	Taractan

TobraDex	Tobrex
tobramycin	Trobicin
Tobrex	TobraDex
Tofranil	Tepanil
Tolinase	Orinase
Topic	Topicort
Topicort	Topic
Trasylol	Travasol
Travasol	Trasylol
Triafed	Trifed
triamcinolone	Triaminicin
Triaminic	Triaminicin; TriHemic
Triaminicin	triamcinolone; Triaminic
triamterene	trimipramine
Triapine	Triaprim
Triaprin	Triapine
Trifed	Triafed
TriHemic	Triaminic
trimeprazine	trimipramine
trimethaphan	trimethoprim
trimethoprim	trimethaphan
trimipramine	imipramine; triamterene; trimeprazine
Triostat	Threostat
Trobicin	tobramycin
Tronolane	Tronothane
Tronothane	Tronolane
Trovan	Atrovent
Trovert	Provir; Provera
Tuinal	Luminal; Tylenol
Tusibron	Tussigon
Tussafed	Tussafin
Tussafin	Tussafed
Tussex	Tussionex; Tussirex
Tussigon	Tusibron
Tussionex	Tussex; Tussirex
Tussirex	Tussex; Tussionex
Tylenol	Tuinal
Unasyn	Anacin; Unisom
Unipen	Omnipen
Unisom	Anacin; Unasyn
Uracid	uracil; Urised; Urocit
uracil	Uracel; Uracid
Urex	Eurax; Serax
Urised	Uracel; Uracid; Urispas
Urispas	Urised
Urobiotic	Otobiotic
Urocit	Uracid
Valium	thallium; Valpin
Vantin	Banthine; Bantron
VasoCare	VasoClear

Vasocidin	Vasodilan
Vasocine	Vaseline
VasoClear	VasoCare
Vasodilan	Vasocidin
Vasoflux	Vasoprost; Vasosulf
Vasoprost	Vasoflux
Vasosulf	Velosef; Vasoflux
V-Cillin K	Bicillin; Wycillin
Velban	Valpin
Velosef	Vasosulf
Ventolin	phentolamine
Vicodin	Hycodan; Hycomine
vidarabine	cytarabine
Vistaril	Restoril; Zestril
Vitron	Vytone
Vontrol	Bontril
Vytone	Hytone; Vitron
Wycillin	Bicillin; V-Cillin
Wydase	Lidex
Xalatan	Dilantin
Xanax	Zantac
Zantac	Xanax
Zarontin	Zaroxolyn
Zaroxolyn	Zarontin; Zeroxin
Zefazone	cefazolin
Zestril	Restoril; Vistaril
Ziks	Vicks
zinostatin	Sandostatin; simvastatin
Zoladex	sulindac
Zomig	Flomax; Slow-Mag

Abbreviations Used with Medications and Dosages

Abbreviation	Literally	Meaning
a.c.	ante cibum	before meals or food
ad	ad	to, up to
A.D., AD	auris dextra	right ear
ad lib.	ad libitum	at pleasure
A.L.	auris laeva	left ear
a.m., A.M.	ante meridiem	morning
Aq.	aqua	water
A.S., AS	auris sinistra	left ear
A.U., AU*	auris uterque	each ear
b.i.d.	bis in die	twice daily
b.m.	bowel movement	
cc, cm^3	cubic centimeter	
d.	die	day
et	et	and
g	gram(s)	
gt. (plural gtt.)	gutta (plural guttae)	a drop (drops)
h.	hora	hour
h.s.	hora somni	at bedtime
IM†	intramuscular	
IV†	intravenous	
mcg, μg	microgram(s)	
mg	milligram(s)	
mEq	milliequivalent(s)	
mL, ml	milliliter(s)	
O.D.	oculus dexter	right eye
O.L.	oculus laevus	left eye
O.S.	oculus sinister	left eye
O.U.§	oculus uterque	each eye
p.c.	post cibum	after meals
p.m., P.M.	post meridiem	afternoon or evening
p.o.	per os	by mouth
p.r.n.	pro re nata	as needed
q.a.d.	quaque alterni die	every other day
q.d.	quaque die	every day
q.h.	quaque hora	every hour
q.i.d.	quater in die	four times a day
q.o.d.		every other day
q.s.	quantum satis	sufficient quantity

Abbreviation	Literally	Meaning
q.s. ad	quantum satis ad	a sufficient quantity to make
℞, Rx	recipe	take; a recipe
Sig.	signetur	label
s.o.s.	si opus sit	if there is need
stat	statim	at once, immediately
t.i.d.	ter in die	three times a day
tsp.	teaspoonful	
μg, mcg	microgram(s)	

---

[*] Although some references have aures unitas (Latin, both ears), this cannot be justified by classical Latin.

[†] Some references suggest that IM and IV be typed with periods to distinguish from Roman numerals, but we believe context is sufficient to make this distinction.

[§] Although some references have oculi unitas (Latin, both eyes), this cannot be justified by classical Latin.

Therapeutic Drug Levels

Drug	Class	Serum Levels metric units (SI units)
amantadine	antiviral	300 ng/mL
amikacin	aminoglycoside	16-32 μg/mL
amiodarone	antiarrhythmic	0.5-2.5 μg/mL
amitriptyline	antidepressant	110-250 ng/mL
amoxapine	antidepressant	200-500 ng/mL
amrinone	cardiotonic	3.7 μg/mL
bretylium	antiarrhythmic	0.5-1.5 μg/mL
bupropion	antidepressant	25-100 ng/mL
carbamazepine	anticonvulsant	4-12 μg/mL (17-51 μmol/L)
chloramphenicol	antibiotic	10-20 μg/mL (31-62 μmol/L)
chlorpromazine	antipsychotic	30-500 ng/mL
clomipramine	antidepressant	80-100 ng/mL
cyclosporine	immunosuppressive	250-800 ng/mL (whole blood, RIA*)
trough values:		50-300 ng/mL (plasma, RIA*)
desipramine	antidepressant	125-300 ng/mL
digitoxin	antiarrhythmic	9-25 μg/L (11.8-32.8 nmol/L)
digoxin	antiarrhythmic	0.5-2.2 ng/mL (0.6-2.8 nmol/L)
disopyramide	antiarrhythmic	2-8 μg/mL (6-18 μmol/L)
doxepin	antidepressant	100-200 ng/mL
flecainide	antiarrhythmic	0.2-1 μg/mL
fluphenazine	antipsychotic	0.13-2.8 ng/mL
gentamicin	aminoglycoside	4-8 μg/mL
haloperidol	antipsychotic	5-20 ng/mL
hydralazine	antihypertensive	100 ng/mL
imipramine	antidepressant	200-350 ng/mL
kanamycin	aminoglycoside	15-40 μg/mL
lidocaine	antiarrhythmic	1.5-6 μg/mL (4.5-21.5 μmol/L)
lithium	antipsychotic	0.5-1.5 mEq/L (0.5-1.5 mmol/L)
maprotiline	antidepressant	200-300 ng/mL
mexiletine	antiarrhythmic	0.5-2 μg/mL
netilmicin	aminoglycoside	6-10 μg/mL

Drug	Class	*Serum Levels* *metric units (SI units)*
nortriptyline	antidepressant	50-150 ng/mL
perphenazine	antipsychotic	0.8-1.2 ng/mL
phenobarbital	anticonvulsant	15-40 μg/mL (65-172 μmol/L)
phenytoin	anticonvulsant	10-20 μg/mL (40-80 μmol/L)
primidone	anticonvulsant	5-12 μg/mL (25-46 μmol/L)
procainamide	antiarrhythmic	4-8 μg/mL (17-34 μmol/L)
propranolol	antiarrhythmic	50-200 ng/mL (190-770 nmol/L)
protriptyline	antidepressant	100-200 ng/mL
quinidine	antiarrhythmic	2-6 μg/mL (4.6-9.2 μmol/L)
salicylate	analgesic	100-200 mg/L (725 1448 μmol/L)
streptomycin	aminoglycoside	20-30 μg/mL
sulfonamide	antibiotic	5-15 mg/dL
terbutaline	bronchodilator	0.5-4.1 ng/mL
theophylline	bronchodilator	10-20 μg/mL (55-110 μmol/L)
thiothixene	antipsychotic	2-57 ng/mL
tobramycin	aminoglycoside	4-8 μg/mL
tocainide	antiarrhythmic	4-10 μg/mL
trazodone	antidepressant	800-1600 ng/mL
valproic acid	anticonvulsant	50-100 μg/mL (350-700 μmol/L)
vancomycin	antibiotic	30-40 ng/mL (peak)
verapamil	antiarrhythmic	0.08-0.3 μg/mL

---

* radioimmunoassay

The Most Prescribed Drugs

Drug	Class/Indications
Accolate (zafirlukast)	antiasthmatic
Accupril (quinapril HCl)	antihypertensive, ACE inhibitor
acetaminophen with codeine	analgesic, anti-inflammatory
Adalat CC (nifedipine)	antianginal, antihypertensive
Adderall (mixed amphetamines)	CNS stimulant for ADHD
albuterol sulfate	bronchodilator
Alesse (levonorgestrel, ethinyl estadiol)	monophasic oral contraceptive
Allegra (fexofenadine HCl)	nonsedating antihistamine
allopurinol	treatment for gout and hyperuricemia
alprazolam	anxiolytic, sedative
Altace (ramipril)	antihypertensive, ACE inhibitor
Amaryl (glimepiride)	oral sulfonylurea antidiabetic
Ambien (zolpidem tartrate)	sedative, hypnotic
amitriptyline HCl	tricyclic antidepressant
amoxicillin trihydrate	antibiotic
Amoxil (amoxicillin trihydrate)	antibiotic
atenolol	antiadrenergic
Atrovent (ipratropium bromide)	bronchodilator
Augmentin (amoxicillin trihydrate, clavulanate potassium)	antibiotic
Axid (nizatidine)	histamine antagonist for gastric ulcers
Azmacort (triamcinolone acetonide)	corticosteroid for asthma
Bactroban (mupirocin)	topical antibiotic
Biaxin (clarithromycin)	antibiotic
BuSpar (buspirone HCl)	anxiolytic
Cardizem CD (diltiazem HCl)	antihypertensive, antianginal
Cardura (doxazosin mesylate)	antihypertensive, antiadrenergic
carisoprodol	skeletal muscle relaxant
Ceftin (cefuroxime axetil)	antibiotic
Cefzil (cefprozil)	antibiotic
cephalexin	antibiotic
cimetidine	antiulcer
Cipro (ciprofloxacin)	antibiotic
Claritin (loratadine)	antihistamine
Claritin-D (loratadine, pseudoephedrine sulfate)	antihistamine, decongestant
Climara (estradiol)	transdermal estrogen for menopause
clonazepam	anticonvulsant
clonidine	antihypertensive
Coumadin (warfarin sodium)	anticoagulant
Cozaar (losartan potassium)	antihypertensive

cyclobenzaprine HCl	skeletal muscle relaxant
Cycrin (medroxyprogesterone acetate)	progestin
Daypro (oxaprozin)	NSAID
Deltasone (prednisone)	glucocorticoid
Depakote (divalproex sodium)	anticonvulsant
Desogen (ethinyl estradiol, desogestrel)	monophasic oral contraceptive
diazepam	anxiolytic, skeletal muscle relaxant
Diflucan (fluconazole)	systemic antifungal
Dilantin (phenytoin sodium)	anticonvulsant
Diovan (valsartan)	antihypertensive; angiotensin II blocker
Dyazide (hydrochlorothiazide, triamterene)	diuretic, antihypertensive
Effexor (venlafaxine)	antidepressant
Elocon (mometasone furoate)	topical corticosteroid
Ery-Tab (erythromycin)	antibiotic
Estrace (estradiol)	topical estrogen
Estraderm (estradiol)	estrogen replacement
estradiol	estrogen replacement
Flonase (fluticasone propionate)	steroidal anti-inflammatory
Flovent (fluticasone propionate)	steroidal anti-inflammatory
Fosamax (alendronate sodium)	postmenopausal osteoporosis treatment
furosemide	diuretic, antihypertensive
gemfibrozil	antihyperlipidemic
glipizide	antidiabetic
Glucophage (metformin HCl)	antidiabetic
Glucotrol XL (glipizide)	antidiabetic
glyburide	antidiabetic
guaifenesin with phenylpropanolamine	expectorant, decongestant
Humulin 70/30, N, R (human insulin)	antidiabetic
hydrochlorothiazide	diuretic, antihypertensive
hydrocodone with acetaminophen	antitussive, analgesic
Hytrin (terazosin HCl)	antihypertensive
Hyzaar (losartin potassium; hydro-chlorothiazide)	antihypertensive; angiotensin II receptor antagonist; diuretic
ibuprofen	NSAID
Imdur (isosorbide mononitrate)	antianginal
Imitrex (sumatriptan succinate)	antimigraine
K-Dur (potassium chloride)	potassium supplement
Klor-Con (potassium chloride)	potassium supplement
Lanoxin (digoxin)	antiarrhythmic
Lasix (furosemide)	diuretic
Lescol (fluvastatin sodium)	antihyperlipidemic
Levaquin (levofloxacin)	fluoroquinolone antibiotic
Levoxyl (levothyroxine sodium)	thyroid hormone
Lipitor (atorvastatin calcium)	antihyperlipidemic
Lodine (etodolac)	NSAID, analgesic, antiarthritic
Loestrin Fe (norethindrone acetate, ethinyl estradiol, ferrous fumarate)	monophasic oral contraceptive with iron
Lo/Ovral (ethinyl estradiol, norgestrel)	monophasic oral contraceptive
Lorabid (loracarbef)	antibiotic

lorazepam	anxiolytic, tranquilizer
Lotensin (benazepril HCl)	antihypertensive, ACE inhibitor
Lotrel (amlodipine besylate, benazepril HCl)	antihypertensive, ACE inhibitor, calcium channel blocker
Lotrisone (betamethasone dipropionate, clotrimazole)	topical corticosteroid, antifungal
Macrobid (nitrofurantoin macrocrystals, nitrofurantoin monohydrate)	urinary antibacterial
medroxyprogesterone	progestin
methylprednisolone	corticosteroidal anti-inflammatory
metoprolol tartrate	antiadrenergic
Mevacor (lovastatin)	antihyperlipidemic
Miacalcin (calcitonin salmon)	calcium regulator for osteoporosis
Monopril (fosinopril sodium)	antihypertensive, ACE inhibitor
naproxen sodium	NSAID, antiarthritic, analgesic
Necon (norethindrone, ethinyl estradiol)	monophasic oral contraceptive
neomycin/polymyxin/hydrocortisone	antibiotic, steroidal anti-inflammatory
Neurontin (gabapentin)	anticonvulsant
Nitrostat (nitroglycerin)	antianginal
Norvasc (amlodipine)	antianginal, antihypertensive
Ortho-Cept (ethinyl estradiol, desogestrel)	monophasic oral contraceptive
Ortho-Cyclen (norgestimate, ethinyl estradiol)	monophasic oral contraceptive
Ortho-Novum 7/7/7 (norethindrone, ethinyl estradiol)	triphasic oral contraceptive
Ortho Tri-Cyclen (norgestimate, ethinyl estradiol)	triphasic oral contraceptive
Paxil (paroxetinc HCl)	antidepressant
penicillin VK (penicillin V potassium)	natural antibiotic
Pepcid (famotidine)	antiulcer
Phenergan (promethazine HCl)	antihistamine, antiemetic, sedative
Plendil (felodipine)	antihypertensive
potassium chloride	potassium supplement
Pravachol (pravastatin sodium)	antihyperlipidemic
prednisone	corticosteroidal anti-inflammatory
Premarin (conjugated estrogens)	estrogen replacement
Prempro (conjugated estrogens, medroxyprogesterone acetate)	hormone replacement therapy
Prevacid (lansoprazole)	antisecretory, antiulcer
Prilosec (omeprazole)	antiulcer
Prinivil (lisinopril)	antihypertensive, ACE inhibitor
Procardia XL (nifedipine)	antianginal, antihypertensive
promethazine HCl	antihistamine, antiemetic
Propacet 100 (propoxyphene napsylate, acetaminophen)	narcotic analgesic
propoxyphene napsylate with acetaminophen	narcotic analgesic
propranolol HCl	antihypertensive, antiarrhythmic
Propulsid (cisapride)	gastroesophageal reflux

Provera (medroxyprogesterone acetate)	progestin replacement
Prozac (fluoxetine HCl)	antidepressant
ranitidine	histamine antagonist for gastric ulcers
Relafen (namubetone)	NSAID, antiarthritic
Retin-A (tretinoin)	topical keratolytic
Rezulin (troglitazone)	oral antidiabetic agent
Rhinocort (budesonide)	intranasal steroidal anti-inflammatory
Risperdal (risperidone)	antipsychotic
Roxicet (oxycodone HCl, acetaminophen)	narcotic analgesic
Serevent (salmeterol xinafoate)	antiasthmatic, bronchodilator
Serzone (nefazodone HCl)	antidepressant
Sumycin (tetracycline HCl)	broad-spectrum antibiotic
Synthroid (levothyroxine sodium)	thyroid replacement
tamoxifen citrate	antineoplastic for breast cancer
temazepam	tranquilizer, hypnotic
Timoptic-XE (timolol maleate)	antiglaucoma beta-blocker
Tobradex (tobramycin, dexamethasone)	ophthalmic antibiotic and steroid
Toprol XL (metoprolol succinate)	antihypertensive, antianginal
trazodone HCl	tetracyclic antidepressant
triamterene with hydrochlorothiazide	diuretic, antihypertensive
Tri-Levlen (levonorgestrel, ethinyl estradiol)	triphasic oral contraceptive
trimethoprim with sulfamethoxazole	anti-infective, antibacterial
Trimox (amoxicillin trihydrate)	antibiotic
Triphasil (levonorgestrel, ethinyl estradiol)	triphasic oral contraceptive
Ultram (tramadol HCl)	analgesic
Vancenase AQ, DS (beclomethasone dipropionate)	steroidal anti-inflammatory
Vasotec (enalaprilat maleate)	antihypertensive, ACE inhibitor
Veetids (penicillin V potassium)	antibiotic
verapamil HCl	antianginal, antiarrhythmic, calcium channel blocker
Viagra (sildenafil citrate)	vasodilator for erectile dysfunction
warfarin	anticoagulant
Wellbutrin SR (bupropion HCl)	antidepressant
Xalatan (latanoprost)	antiglaucoma
Xanax (alprazolam)	anxiolytic
Zantac (ranitidine HCl)	histamine antagonist for gastric ulcers
Zestoretic (hydrochlorothiazide, lisinopril)	antihypertensive, ACE inhibitor, diuretic
Zestril (lisinopril)	antihypertensive
Ziac (hydrochlorothiazide, bisoprolol fumarate)	antihypertensive
Zithromax (azithromycin dihydrate)	antibiotic
Zocor (simvastatin)	antihyperlipidemic
Zoloft (sertraline)	antidepressant
Zyban (bupropion HCl)	smoking cessation aid
Zyrtec (cetirizine HCl)	antihistamine

Dropped from the previous list:

Calan SR (verapamil HCl)	antianginal, antiarrhythmic, antihypertensive
cefaclor	antibiotic
Darvocet-N 100 (propoxyphene napsylate, acetaminophen)	narcotic analgesic
Demulen 1/35 (ethynodiol diacetate, ethinyl estradiol)	monophasic oral contraceptive
dicyclomine HCl	antispasmodic, anticholinergic
doxycycline hyclate	antibacterial
Floxin (ofloxacin)	antibiotic
Genora 1/35 (norethindrone, ethinyl estradiol)	monophasic oral contraceptive
Glynase (glyburide)	antidiabetic
Klonopin (clonazepam)	anticonvulsant
methylphenidate HCl	CNS stimulant for ADHD
Nitro-Dur (nitroglycerin)	antianginal
Ortho-Novum 1/35 (norethindrone, ethinyl estradiol)	monophasic oral contraceptive
oxycodone HCl with acetaminophen	narcotic analgesic
phentermine	anorexiant, CNS stimulant
Pondimin (fenfluramine HCl)	anorexiant, CNS depressant
promethazine with codeine	narcotic antitussive, antihistamine
Proventil aerosol (albuterol)	bronchodilator
Redux (dexfenfluramine HCl)	anorexiant, CNS depressant
Suprax (cefixime)	antibiotic
Trusopt (dorzolamide HCl)	glaucoma treatment
Vanceril (beclomethasone dipropionate)	corticosteroid for bronchial asthma
Ventolin (albuterol)	bronchodilator
Zovirax (acyclovir)	antiviral